OSKI'S PEDIATRIC CERTIFICATION AND RECERTIFICATION BOARD REVIEW

OSKI'S PEDIATRIC CERTIFICATION AND RECERTIFICATION BOARD REVIEW

Editors

Carmen M. Coombs, MD, MPH

Pediatric Emergency Medicine Fellow
Children's Hospital of Pittsburgh
Pittsburgh, Pennsylvania

Arethusa Stevens Kirk, MD, FAAP

Associate Medical Director, Pediatrics
Total Health Care, Inc.
Clinical Instructor
Johns Hopkins University School of Medicine
Baltimore, Maryland

Advisor

Julia A. McMillan, MD

Professor of Pediatrics
Vice Chair for Education
Department of Pediatrics
Director, Residency Training Program
Associate Dean for Graduate Medical Education
Johns Hopkins University School of Medicine
Johns Hopkins Hospital
Baltimore, Maryland

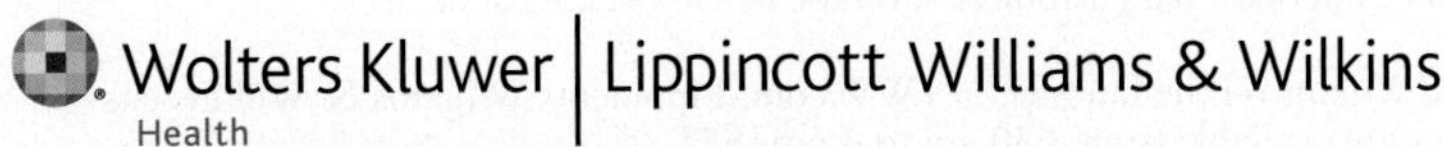

Philadelphia • Baltimore • New York • London
Buenos Aires • Hong Kong • Sydney • Tokyo

Acquisitions Editor: Sonya Seigafuse
Product Manager: Nicole Walz
Vendor Manager: Bridgett Dougherty
Senior Manufacturing Manager: Benjamin Rivera
Marketing Manager: Lisa Lawrence
Design Coordinator: Holly Reid McLaughlin
Production Service: Aptara, Inc.

Two Commerce Square
2001 Market Street
Philadelphia, PA 19103 USA
LWW.com

Printed in China

Library of Congress Cataloging-in-Publication Data

Coombs, Carmen M.
Oski's pediatric certification and recertification board review / Carmen M. Coombs, Arethusa Stevens Kirk, Julia A. McMillan.
p. ; cm.
Other title: Pediatric certification and recertification board review
Includes bibliographical references and index.
Summary: "Oski's Pediatric Certification and Recertification Board Review provides comprehensive coverage of all of the areas focused on in the board exam. Features include more than 300 board-style review questions, a full-color design and illustrations, and numerous Points to Remember"—Provided by publisher.
ISBN 978-1-60547-134-1 (pbk. : alk. paper)
1. Pediatrics—Outlines, syllabi, etc. 2. Pediatrics—Examinations, questions, etc. I. Kirk, Arethusa Stevens. II. McMillan, Julia A. III. Oski, Frank A. IV. Title. V. Title: Pediatric certification and recertification board review.
[DNLM: 1. Pediatrics—Examination Questions. 2. Pediatrics—Outlines. 3. Certification—Examination Questions. 4. Certification—Outlines. WS 18.2]
RJ48.3.C66 2012
618.92—dc22

2010033883

To purchase additional copies of this book, call our customer service department at (800) 638-3030 or fax orders to (301) 223-2320. International customers should call (301) 223-2300.

Visit Lippincott Williams & Wilkins on the Internet: at LWW.com. Lippincott Williams & Wilkins customer service representatives are available from 8:30 am to 6 pm, EST.

10 9 8 7 6 5 4 3

DEDICATION

This book is dedicated to our patients and their families who continually inspire us to better ourselves.

CONTRIBUTORS

Kristin W. Baranano, MD, PhD
Fellow
Department of Neurogenetics
Kennedy Krieger Institute;
Department of Neurology
Johns Hopkins University School of Medicine
Baltimore, Maryland

Shazia Bhombal, MD
Neonatal Fellow
USC Division of Neonatal Medicine
LAC+USC Medical Center and Children's
Hospital of Los Angeles
Keck School of Medicine, University of Southern California
Los Angeles, California

Margaret Brewinski, MD, MPH, FAAP, FACPM
Senior Advisor
Bureau of Global Health, Office of HIV/AIDS
United States Agency for International Development
Washington, District of Colombia

Joseph B. Cantey, MD
Fellow
Department of Pediatric Infectious Diseases
University of Texas, Southwestern
Dallas, Texas

Carmen M. Coombs, MD, MPH
Pediatric Emergency Medicine Fellow
Children's Hospital of Pittsburgh
Pittsburgh, Pennsylvania

Katherine S. Dahab, MD
Fellow
Pediatric Sports Medicine
University of Wisconsin Hospitals and Clinics
Madison, Wisconsin

Hema Dave, MD, MPH
Clinical Fellow
Pediatric Hematology/Oncology
Johns Hopkins Hospital
Baltimore, Maryland;
Clinical Fellow
Pediatric Oncology Branch
National Institutes of health/
National Cancer Institute
Bethesda, Maryland

Joan H. Dunlop, MD, FAAP
Assistant Clinical Professor
Department of Pediatrics
George Washington University School of Medicine;
Clinical Associate
Department of Emergency Medicine
Children's National Medical Center
Washington, District of Colombia

Michelle B. Dunn, MD
Attending Physician
General Pediatrics
Children's Hospital of Philadelphia
Philadelphia, Pennsylvania

Eva Granzow, MD
USC Division of Neonatal Medicine of the LAC+USC Medical
Center and Children's
Hospital of Los Angeles
Keck School of Medicine
University of Southern California
Los Angeles, California

Raegan D. Hunt, MD, PhD
Resident Physician
Department of Pediatrics
Johns Hopkins University School of Medicine
Baltimore, Maryland

Calvin K. Lee, MD
Clinical Fellow
Pediatric Hematology/Oncology
Johns Hopkins University School of Medicine/
National Cancer Institute
Baltimore, Maryland

Jessica Hebert Mouledoux, MD
Fellow
Department of Pediatrics, Division of Cardiology
Vanderbilt University
Nashville, Tennessee

Rachel E. Rau, MD
Clinical Fellow
Department of Pediatric Oncology
Johns Hopkins University School of Medicine
Baltimore, Maryland

Ashley Hall Shoemaker, MD
Clinical Fellow
Department of Pediatric Endocrinology
Monroe Carell Jr. Children's Hospital at Vanderbilt
Nashville, Tennessee

Joelle N. Simpson, MD, MPH
Fellow
Emergency Medicine
Children's National Medical Center
Washington, District of Colombia

Daniel J. Sklansky, MD
Hospitalist Fellow
Department of Pediatrics
Hospital for Sick Children
Toronto, Ontario, Canada

Arvind Iyengar Srinath, MD
Clinical Fellow
Department of Pediatric Gastroenterology
Children's Hospital of Pittsburgh
Pittsburgh, Pennsylvania

Arethusa Stevens Kirk, MD, FAAP
Associate Medical Director, Pediatrics
Total Health Care, Inc.
Clinical Instructor
Johns Hopkins University School of Medicine
Baltimore, Maryland

Laura L. Steinberg, MD
General Pediatrician
Capitol Pediatrics
Raleigh, North Carolina

Pranita D. Tamma, MD
Pediatric Infectious Diseases Fellow
Department of Pediatric Infectious Diseases
The Johns Hopkins University School of Medicine
Baltimore, Maryland

Jade Marie Tan, MD
Pediatrician
Department of Pediatrics
Total Health Care, Inc.
Baltimore, Maryland

Megan Marie Tschudy, MD
Fellow
Division of General Pediatrics and Adolescent Medicine
Johns Hopkins University School of Medicine
Baltimore, Maryland

Amy E. Valasek, MD
Towson Orthopaedic Associates
Sports Medicine Pediatrician
Baltimore, Maryland

Hilary Tinkel Vernon, MD, PhD
Resident
McKusick-Nathans Institute of Genetic Medicine
Johns Hopkins University School of Medicine
Baltimore, Maryland

Sabrina R. Vineberg, MD
Instructor in Pediatrics
Harvard Medical School;
Assistant in Medicine
Children's Hospital Boston
Boston, Massachusetts

Michael F. Walsh, MD
Resident
Department of Pediatrics
Johns Hopkins Hospital;
Resident
McKusick-Nathans Institute of Genetic Medicine
Baltimore, Maryland

Dakara Rucker Wright, MD
Pediatric Dermatology Fellow/Clinical Instructor
Department of Dermatology
Johns Hopkins University School of Medicine
Baltimore, Maryland

PREFACE

As Pediatricians, the pediatric board examination represents the culmination of years of hard work dedicated to mastering the knowledge, skills, and qualities required to care for children. We have all successfully prepared for many standardized examinations in the past but none more important than the pediatric boards. *Oski's Pediatric Certification and Recertification Board Review* was written for both the first-time pediatric board examinee and the recertifying practitioner. We trust that you will not be disappointed.

The purpose of this text is to provide a concise yet comprehensive review book. The content contained in these chapters was formulated on the basis of the American Board of Pediatrics examination content outline. The format of the pages was designed with efficiency and readability in mind: uniform organization of content, images woven within the text, wide margins on each page in which to write notes, and "Points to Remember" throughout each chapter to highlight key points. Each chapter ends with a series of practice questions for review of chapter content and refinement of test-taking skills.

Enjoy and good luck!

Carmen M. Coombs, MD, MPH
Pediatric Emergency Medicine Fellow
Children's Hospital of Pittsburgh
Pittsburgh, Pennsylvania

Arethusa Stevens Kirk, MD, FAAP
Associate Medical Director, Pediatrics
Total Health Care, Inc.
Baltimore, Maryland

ACKNOWLEDGMENTS

This book would not have been possible without the encouragement and dedicated intellect of our mentor and friend Dr. Julia A. McMillan. This review is as much a product of her editorial eye as ours, and we are forever grateful to her. We owe a special thanks to the individual chapter authors who voluntarily committed endless time and energy to this project. We are incredibly appreciative of the time they took out of their busy schedules and the sacrifices they made to ensure a quality product. We thank Sarah Granlund for her expertise in shaping the content into its finalized form and Nicole Walz and Lippincott Williams & Wilkins for the opportunity to produce this book. It has been an unforgettable experience for us, and we are honored to bring the finished product to the market. Finally, a special thanks to our families and friends who sacrificed time away from us on nights and weekends while we intently plunked away on our computers—we celebrate our successful conclusion of this challenge with you!

FOREWORD

The vision for this book began when we were senior residents in the pediatric residency program at Johns Hopkins University School of Medicine preparing for our pediatric board examination. We both successfully passed the boards and then committed ourselves to creating a focused board review book that would be useful for our rising colleagues as we were not satisfied with the current products on the market during our preparation.

As a National Health Service Corps Scholar, Arethusa is realizing her dream of caring for underserved inner city children and fullfilling her commitment at a Federally Qualified Health Center in Baltimore, Maryland where she is the Associate Medical Director for Pediatrics and a General Pediatrician.

After finishing residency, Carmen completed her Masters of Public Health at the Johns Hopkins Bloomberg School of Public Health and then served for an additional year as the Chief Resident of Pediatrics. She is currently a pediatric emergency medicine fellow at Children's Hospital of Pittsburgh.

Carmen and Arethusa

CONTENTS

CHAPTER 1 ■ PREPARING FOR THE EXAMINATION

ARETHUSA STEVENS KIRK AND CARMEN M. COOMBS

ABMS	American Board of Medical Specialties
ABP	American Board of Pediatrics
AAP	American Academy of Pediatrics
CME	Continued Medical Education
MOC	Maintenance of Certification

CHAPTER OBJECTIVES

1. Understand how to register for the Initial and Recertification Pediatric Board Examinations
2. Learn where to find a current outline of the examination content
3. Understand the requirements for MOC
4. Provide a guide to study for the examination along with test taking strategies
5. Understand what constitutes a passing score.

INTRODUCTION

Whether you are a first-time test taker of the ABP Certifying examination, just completing your residency, or a returning examinee maintaining your certification, it is our hope that this review book will provide you the necessary tools to prepare for the examination with efficiency. To ensure the comprehensive review of all possible examination topics, the outline and content of this book were developed to mirror the content examination outline available by the ABP. With a consistent, steady approach to study of these chapters, their questions, and suggested readings we are certain that you will arrive at examination day with a sense of confidence in your mastery of the material.

About the American Board of Pediatrics

The ABP, founded in 1933, is one of 24 certifying boards of the ABMS: http://www.abms.org. It is an independent, nonprofit organization whose certificate is a credential signifying a high level of physician competence, which is recognized throughout the world. The ABP is led by a board of directors who are distinguished and recognized pediatricians in research, education, and clinical practice. Included within the Board are also one or more persons, nonphysicians in profession, with notable interest in the health and welfare of children. It is the mission of the ABP to improve training of pediatricians, to set the rules and regulations for its examinations, and to establish the requirements for certification. Certification, though voluntary, is sought by nearly all qualified pediatricians as it represents dedication to the highest level of professionalism in patient care.

General Pediatrics Initial Certification

The following requirements must be met to sit for the ABP certifying examination:

- **Graduation** from an accredited medical school in the United States, Canada, or from a foreign medical school recognized by the World Health Organization.
- **Completion** of 3 years of postgraduation training in Pediatrics at an accredited residency program involving the care of children and adolescents both in the outpatient and hospital setting.

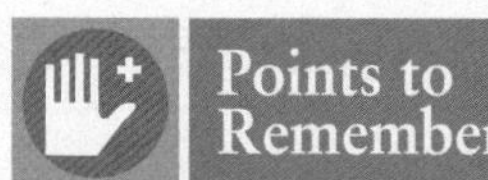

Points to Remember

- **The initial examination is offered once a year, usually in October. The recertification examination is offered 6 days a week excluding holidays and the months of July and August.**

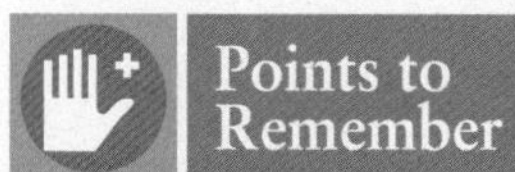

Points to Remember

- **Keep your ABP Personal Physician Portfolio username and password secure.**

- **Verification** of the completion of a pediatric residency training program, which includes the proof of achievements in clinical competence as well as the demonstration of ethical behavior befitting the profession.
- **Attainment** of a valid, unrestricted state license to practice medicine.

The general pediatrics initial certifying examination is administered once a year, traditionally in the fall. Applications to register are not available all year round therefore planning is necessary. All applications and current information about the examination and registration dates are available only from the ABP Web site—please refer there for updates.

Steps to Register for the Examination

You will need to create a "Personal Physician Portfolio" on the ABP Web site. To create your portfolio, you must be able to provide a valid e-mail address as well as your social security number, full name, date of birth, and the name of the school where your final year of training was completed. Your username and password must remain secure as you will need these unique codes to access your online portfolio. This portfolio will be your repository for necessary registration documents needed by the ABP as well as your source of information, validation of acceptance of your application, and eventual posting of your examination scores and status.

Examination Fee Schedule

These fees are paid by credit card (Visa or MasterCard) during the online application process (Table 1.1).

Examination Content Outline

This book was designed with close attention to the 2009 ABP examination content outline. Although we are confident that the contents of this book cover the outline specifications as well as additional content the outline does very slightly from year to year. Annual updates are posted on the ABP Web site and we encourage you to print out the most recent update for your reference while studying for both the initial and recertification examinations.

Maintenance of Certification

Since 1988 certificates issued from the ABP have been time limited. As of 2000, the ABP, along with 23 other Member Boards of the ABMS, redesigned their recertification program to a continuous professional development curriculum otherwise referred to as MOC. Although, in the past, certificates expired after 7 years, now the Board is transitioning to a 10-year renewal schedule for the secure examination component (cognitive expertise) and 5-year renewal schedule for the remaining three MOC components. MOC requirements are designed to demonstrate a commitment to competency in the ever-evolving field of Pediatrics and to assure the public of each diplomate's ability to deliver safe, quality care.

There are four core components to the MOC:

1. Evidence of professional standing—possession of a valid medical license.
2. Evidence of life-long learning—CME and other such activities as approved by the ABP.
3. Proof of cognitive expertise—passing a secure Board recertification examination.
4. Evidence of satisfactory performance in practice—ABP approved quality improvement projects.

TABLE 1.1

EXAMINATION REGISTRATION FEES

Initial Examination		MOC Examination	
Registration type	2010 Calendar year fees	Enrollment fee	2010 Calendar year fees
Regular registration	$2,030.00	Initial	$1,030.00
Late registration	$2,335.00	Lapsed	$1,530.00
Late fee	$305.00	Retake fee	$240

To demonstrate competency in these four areas the MOC requires that the same six competencies by pediatric residency training continue to be met. The six MOC competencies are the following:

1. Patient care
2. Medical knowledge
3. Practice-based learning and improvement
4. Interpersonal and communication skills
5. Professionalism
6. Systems-based practice

Preparation for the Certifying or Recertification Examination

It is vital that you not wait until the day before, the week before, or even the month before the examination to start studying. This is particularly true for first-time test takers who would do well to begin a study schedule 2 to 3 months prior to the examination date. A sample study guide organized by the chapters is included in Appendix 1.1. It is suggested that you review each chapter at least twice, along with the questions. For test takers who also benefit from review of a

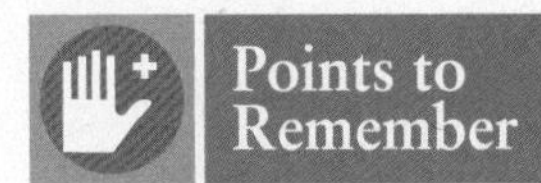

Organizing the Material

- Key Point: Do not wait until 2 weeks before the examination to start studying.

APPENDIX 1.1

OSKI BOARD REVIEW STUDY GUIDE

No.	Chapter	First Review	Chapter Review Questions	Second Review	Relevant PREP Questions	Select Review Articles
2	Adolescent Health					
3	Allergy & Immunology					
4	Cardiology					
5	Connective Tissue Diseases					
6	Critical Care and Emergency Medicine					
7	Pediatric Dermatology					
8	Dysmorphology					
9	Ear, Nose, and Throat					
10	Endocrinology					
11	Fluids & Electrolytes					
12	Gastroenterology					
13	Metabolism					
14	Growth and Development					
15	Hematology					
16	Infectious Diseases					
17	Neonatology					
18	Neurology					
19	Nutrition					
20	Oncology					
21	Pediatric Ophthalmology					
22	Orthopedics					
23	Preventive Pediatrics, Biostatistics, & Ethics					
24	Pulmonary					
25	Renal and Genitourinary Disorders					

Suggestion: Plot out this study guide over a 6- to 8-week time period; this will likely mean you will need to carve out study time approximately 5 days a week. Attention to selected review articles and extra question review is recommended for those subject areas that you know you need additional time. For first-time test takers, refer to the analysis of your in-service examination to identify the areas in which your performance was weakest and focus the most concentrated study there.

TABLE 1.2

EXAMINATION PASS RATES FOR FIRST-TIME TEST TAKERS

	2004	2005	2006	2007	2008
Number	2,993	2,850	2,892	3,009	2,916
%	79.1	76.6	75.8	76.5	77.7

Data from the American Board of Pediatrics (https://www.abp.org/abpwebsite/stats/abp_esic.pdf).

multitude of questions prior to the examination, the AAP produces an excellent series each year titled PREP, which can be another helpful additional study resource. Be cautioned, it is important to read and review, not simply complete practice questions, to prepare for this examination.

Examination Format

Question Format: The examination consists of single best-answer multiple-choice questions similar to the sample review questions in this book. The majority of the questions will use patient-based formats used to evaluate the cognitive abilities needed for clinical decision making. Graphical illustrations (photographs and radiographic images) are used to complement approximately 5% to 10% of the ABP questions.

Examination Length

- Initial certification: One day with AM and PM sessions each lasting 3.5 hs (200 questions a session).
- Recertification: Half day 3.5-h session consisting of 200 questions.

Scoring

The score is determined by the number of questions answered correctly with no penalty for guessing.

Test Results

Examination pass requirements differ between the initial general practice examination and the MOC examination. A higher score is required for those initiating certification than for those returning for maintenance of their board license.

1. Initial examination: Although this is not published by the ABP, a passing score has traditionally been approximately 420 and above.
2. MOC examination: No score is published although a minimum passing score is traditionally lower that for the initial certification examination.

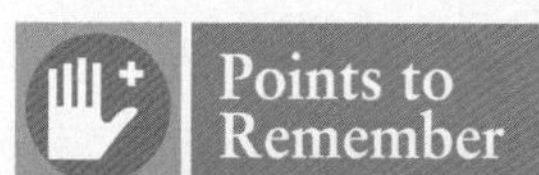

- **There is no penalty for guessing, make sure you answer all the questions.**

Notification of results traditionally has occurred 60 days after completion of the examination but with the advent of computerized test taking, an electronic scoring process may allow for a more expedient scoring and notification. Examination pass rates for first-time test takers are presented in Table 1.2.

Final Words

Anyone who is eligible to take the Pediatric Board Examination has taken over hundreds of tests during their medical career. Keep in mind that the study and test taking skills you have honed from years of practice will continue to serve you well as you prepare for and take this examination. We truly hope this book provides you a concise yet comprehensive review to help you to successfully pass the examination. Enjoy the journey and good luck!

SUGGESTED READINGS

Althouse LA, Du Y, Ham HP. Confirming the validity of the general pediatrics certification examinations: a practice analysis. *J Pediatr.* 2009;155(2):155–156.e1

Althouse LA, McGuinness GA. The in-training examination: an analysis of its predictive value on performance on the general pediatrics certification examination. *J Pediatr.* 2008;153(3):425–428.

CHAPTER 2 ■ ADOLESCENT HEALTH

JOELLE N. SIMPSON

CAH	Congenital adrenal hyperplasia	OCP	Oral contraceptive pill
BMI	Body mass index	PCOS	Polycystic ovarian syndrome
DFA	Direct fluorescent antibody	PCR	Polymerase chain reaction
DGI	Disseminated gonococcal infection	PMN	Polymorphonuclear leucocyte
		PID	Pelvic inflammatory disease
DMPA	Depot form of medroxyprogesterone acetate	RPR	Rapid plasma regain
		SIL	Squamous intraepithelial lesion
DUB	Dysfunctional uterine bleeding		
ECG	Electrocardiogram	STI	Sexually transmitted infection
FSH	Follicle-stimulating hormone	PT	Prothrombin time
FTA-ABS	Fluorescent treponemal antibody absorbed	PTT	Partial thromboplastin time
		DHEAS	Dehydroepiandrosterone sulfate
HPV	Human papilloma virus		
HSV	Herpes simplex virus	TMA	Transcription-mediated amplification
LE	Leucocyte esterase		
LH	Luteinizing hormone	TOA	Tuboovarian abscess
MRI	Magnetic resonance imaging	TSH	Thyroid-stimulating hormone
MMR	Measles, mumps, and rubella vaccine	VDRL	Venereal disease research laboratory
NAA	Nucleic acid amplification	MHA-TP	Treponema pallidum hemagglutination assays
NSAID	Nonsteroidal anti-inflammatory drug		

This chapter reviews normal adolescent development as well as failures and variations in achieving adult physiology. It highlights key preventive health guidelines as well as common infections and mental health conditions seen in the adolescent population.

CHAPTER OBJECTIVES

1. To identify normal adolescent development, physiology, and key preventive health guidelines
2. To highlight variations and abnormalities in achieving adult physiology
3. To present common STIs including diagnostic criteria and treatment plans
4. To identify mental health conditions including eating disorders and behavioral disorders commonly seen in the adolescent population.

ADOLESCENT DEVELOPMENT

Physiologic Development in Males and Females

Tanner stages of pubic hair development in females (Fig. 2.1) are the following:

Stage 1: Preadolescent, no pubic hair.

Stage 2: Sparse growth of hair appearing chiefly along the labia. Mean age 11.7 years (9.3 to 14.1) (Pubarche).

Stage 3: Hair is considerably darker, coarser, and curlier. The hair spreads sparsely over the junction of the pubes. Mean age 12.4 years (10.2 to 14.6).

Stage 4: Hair has adult texture but with sparser distribution than adults. There is no spread to the medial surface of the thighs. Mean age 13.0 years (10.8 to 15.1).

Stage 5: Hair is adult in quantity and type, distributed as an inverse triangle and spreads to the medial surface of the thighs. Mean age 14.4 years (12.2 to 16.7).

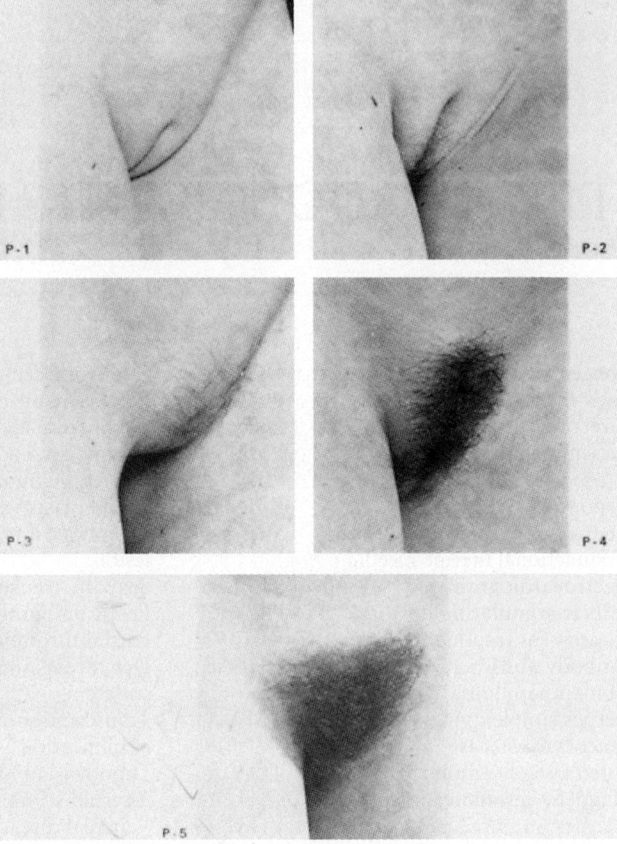

FIGURE 2.1. Tanner stages of pubic hair development in girls. (Reprinted with permission from McMillan JA, Feigin RD, DeAngelis C, et al. *Oski's Pediatrics: Principles and Practice*. 4th ed. Philadelphia, PA: Lippincott Williams & Wilkins, 2006.)

Points to Remember

- *Fast facts*: The size of the ovaries and uterus of an adolescent increases five to sevenfold during puberty. The penis doubles in size, and the volume of the testicles increases from approximately 2 to 18 mL.

Tanner stages of breast development in females are the following:

Stage 1: Preadolescent, no palpable breast tissue.
Stage 2: Breast tissue palpable only under the areola. Mean age 11.2 years (9 to 13.4) (Thelarche).
Stage 3: The breast tissue extends beyond the areola to form a distinct mound. Mean age 12.2 (10 to 14.3).
Stage 4: The areola and papilla form a secondary mound distinct from the underlying breast tissue. Mean age 13.1 years (10.8 to 15.4).
Stage 5: The areola and breast tissue form a smooth contour (no separation of areola and breast tissue). Mean age 15.3 years (11.9 to 18.8).

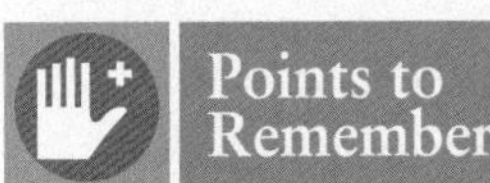

- Menarche occurs, on average, 2 years after the start of thelarche.

Tanner stages of pubic hair and genital development in males are given below (Fig. 2.2).

Stage 1: Preadolescent; testes, scrotum, and penis are approximately the same size and proportion as in early childhood, there is no pubic hair. Normal testicular volume is less than 3 mL or a maximum length of 2 cm.
Stage 2: The scrotum and testes have enlarged; change in the texture and some reddening of the scrotal skin. Sparse growth of long, slightly pigmented hair at the base of the penis. Mean age 11.4 years (9.5 to 13.8).
Stage 3: Elongation of the penis with some growth of testes and scrotum. Darker, coarser, and curlier hair, which spreads sparsely over the junction of the pubes. Mean age 12.9 years (10.8 to 14.9).
Stage 4: Enlargement of the penis in length and breadth with development of the glans. Testes and scrotum are also further enlarged. Scrotal skin darkens and hair is adult texture but less distribution than an adult usually sparing the medial surface of the thighs. Mean age 13.8 years (11.7 to 15.8).
Stage 5: Genitalia are adult in size and shape. Testicular volume may be between 12 and 30 mL or a length of 4 to 5 cm. Hair is adult in quantity and type, distributed as an inverse triangle and spreads to the medial surface of the thighs. Mean age 14.9 years (13 to 17.3) (Table 2.1).

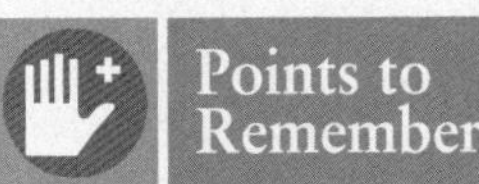

- *Fast facts*: The peak growth spurt in girls occurs approximately 1 year after onset of puberty, between Tanner stages 2 and 3, and growth is largely completed by the time girls begin to menstruate. In boys, the growth spurt occurs 2 years after the onset of genital enlargement.

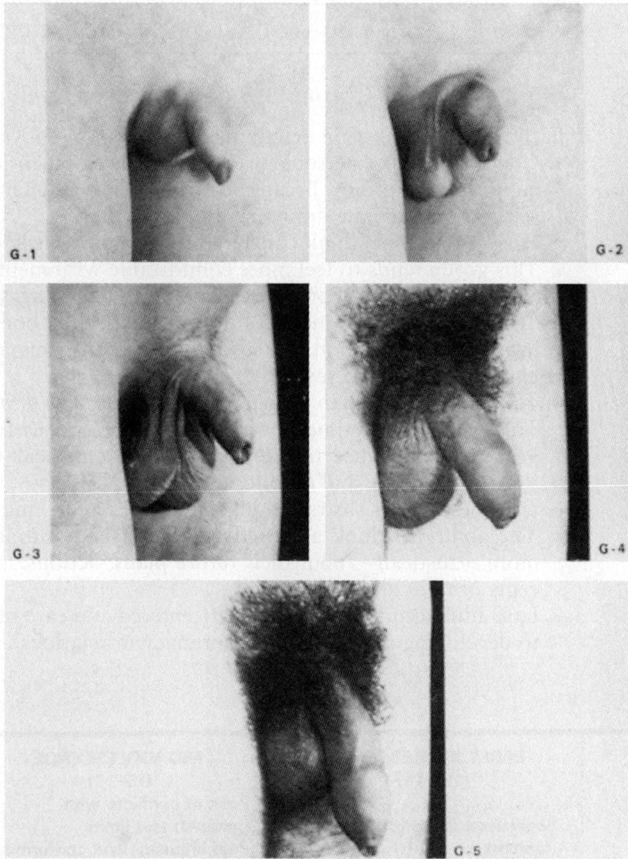

FIGURE 2.2. Tanner stages of pubic hair and genital development in males. (Reprinted with permission from McMillan JA, Feigin RD, DeAngelis C, et al. *Oski's Pediatrics: Principles and Practice*. 4th ed. Philadelphia, PA: Lippincott Williams & Wilkins, 2006.)

TABLE 2.1

PRIMARY ACTION OF MAJOR HORMONES OF PUBERTY

Hormone	Gender	Action
Follicle-stimulating hormone (FSH)	Male	Stimulates gametogenesis
	Female	Stimulates development of primary ovarian follicles; stimulates activation of enzymes in ovarian granulosa cells to increase estrogen production
Luteinizing hormone (LH)	Male	Stimulates testicular Leydig cells to produce testosterone
	Female	Stimulates ovarian theca cells to produce androgens and the corpus luteum to synthesize progesterone; mid-cycle surge includes ovulation
Estradiol	Male	Increases rate of epiphyseal fusion; advances bone age; increases bone mineral density
	Female	Stimulates breast development. Low level enhances linear growth; high level increases the rate of epiphyseal-fusion. Triggers mid-cycle surge of luteinizing hormone; stimulates development of labia, vagina, uterus, and ducts of the breasts; stimulates development of a proliferative endometrium in the uterus; increases fat mass of the body
Testosterone	Male	Accelerates linear growth; increases rate of epiphyseal fusion; stimulates development of the penis, scrotum, prostate, and seminal vesicles; stimulates growth of pubic, facial, and axillary hair; increases larynx size and thus deepens the voice; stimulates sebaceous gland secretion of oil; increases libido; increases muscles mass; increases red blood cell mass
	Female	Accelerates linear growth; stimulates growth of pubic and axillary hair
Progesterone	Female	Converts a proliferative uterine endometrium to a secretory endometrium; stimulates lobuloalveolar breast development
Adrenal	Male and female	Stimulates pubic hair and linear growth androgens

Reprinted with permission from McMillan JA, Feigin RD, DeAngelis C, et al. *Oski's Pediatrics: Principles and Practice*. 4th ed. Philadelphia, PA: Lippincott Williams & Wilkins, 2006.

Psychologic Growth and Development

Chronology of Cognitive Development

- Early adolescence—Concrete thinkers (ages 10 to 13 years) (Fig. 2.3)
  - Concerns of how personal growth and development deviate from that of peers preoccupy this age group. Because of rapid physical changes, concept of body image and self-esteem fluctuate dramatically.
  - **Early adolescents think concretely** and cannot easily conceptualize the future.
  - This group tends to feel more comfortable with members of the same sex.
- Middle adolescence—Formal operational thinkers (ages 14 to 16 years)
  - This group becomes more comfortable with their bodies, but intense emotional swings in mood are common. As sexuality develops, this age group may begin dating and experimenting with sex.
  - Thinking progresses to formal operations and **they develop the ability to think abstractly.** This age group is primarily narcissistic with a sense of personal invulnerability.
  - Peer group influence and conflicts with parents peak at this age group as they struggle for independence and autonomy.
- Late adolescence—Abstract thinkers (ages 17 years and older)
  - **The ability to think abstractly is established** and allows older adolescents to think more realistically about their future plans, actions, and careers. They have solid concepts of right and wrong.
  - Late adolescents become less self-centered and care more about others and focus shifts to developing the capacity for intimacy in relationships.

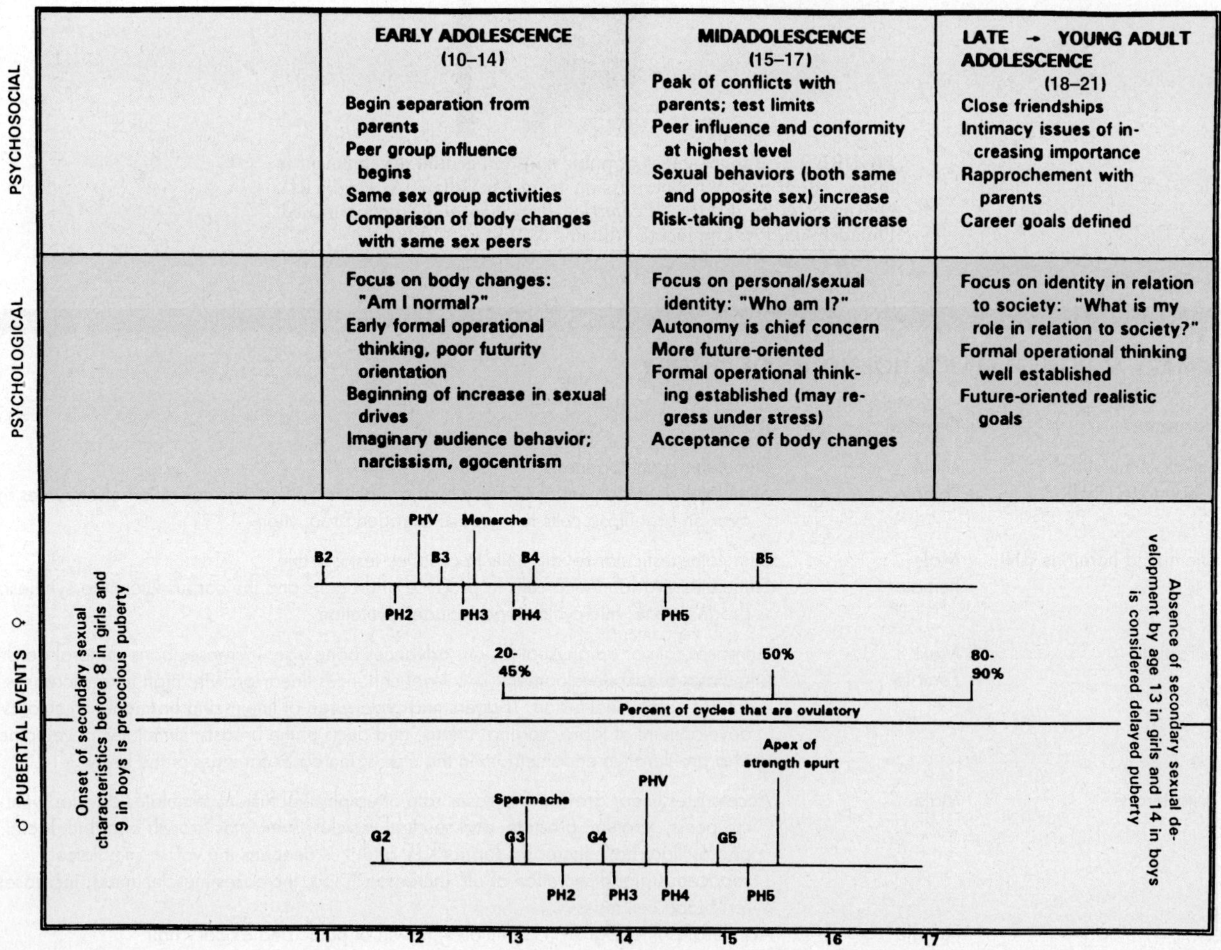

FIGURE 2.3. This figure shows the temporal relation between the biological, psychologic, and psychosocial events of adolescence. Key: B2, B3, B4, B5, breast stage 2, 3, and so forth; G2, G3, G4, G5, genital stage 2, 3, and so forth; PH2, PH3, PH4, PH5, pubic hair stage 2, 3, and so forth; PHV, peak height velocity. (Reprinted with permission from McMillan JA, Feigin RD, DeAngelis C, et al. *Oski's Pediatrics: Principles and Practice*. 4th ed. Philadelphia, PA: Lippincott Williams & Wilkins, 2006.)

Failures and Variations in Achievement of Adult Physiology

Constitutional Delay of Growth and Puberty. A nonpathologic condition characteristically seen in healthy patients who have short stature in comparison to familial height and have a significant delay in pubertal development. They may be below the third percentile for age and usually have a family history of constitutional delay or "late bloomers." Their target height is calculated as mid-parental stature ± 4 inches. They have bone age x-rays that are delayed compared with their chronological age by 2 to 4 years, but their predicted height falls within their genetic target range. (See further discussion in the chapter on Endocrinology.)

Points to Remember

- *Fast facts*: This equation can be used to help predict adult height in boys (paternal height + maternal height + 5 inches)/2 and also in girls (paternal height + maternal height − 5 inches)/2.

Delayed Puberty. Puberty, on average, is completed in 4 years for girls and in 3 years for boys.

An evaluation for pubertal delay is indicated if no signs of puberty are observed in a girl by the time she reaches 13 years of age or in a boy by 14 years of age or if there is an arrest in pubertal maturation.

For further discussion of this topic refer to the chapter on Endocrinology.

Points to Remember

- *Fast facts*: Children with constitutional growth delay will grow at a low normal growth rate but have a decreased growth velocity as puberty approaches.

HEALTH ISSUES OF ADOLESCENCE

Health Maintenance—General Preventive Health

Medical Screening

All adolescents should have a complete physical examination done, including genitalia inspection annually. Their weight, height, BMI, and blood pressure should be recorded and percentiles for age noted.

Points to Remember

- Pubertal delay is indicated if no signs of puberty observed in a girl by the age of 13 years or in a boy by the age of 14 years.

Psychosocial Screening

Psychosocial screening should be performed at every adolescent visit using the pneumonic HEADSS and the CAGE questions.

- Home: Home environment: Safety, stability, support, responsibilities, privileges.
- Education: Educational achievement, skills, strengths, plans, employment.
- Activities: Pastimes, sports; religious; civic and community involvement.
- Drugs: Tobacco, alcohol, and other drug use by friends, family, personal use
  - C: Have you ever felt the need to Cut down?
  - A: Have others Annoyed you by commenting on your use?
  - G: Have you ever felt Guilty about your use or about something you said or did while using?
  - E: Have you ever needed and Eye-opener?
- Sexuality: Satisfaction with body and self, involvement and concerns about sexuality, sexual activity and sexual identity.
- Suicidality: Symptoms of depression, anxiety, mood disorder, thinking problems.

Laboratory Screening Tests

1. Hemoglobin and hematocrit levels: Obtain once during puberty for males and at least once after menarche for females to screen for anemia.
2. Urinalysis and microscopic evaluation: Obtain once during puberty to screen for renal disease.
3. Sexually transmitted diseases annual screening for sexually active adolescents:
   a. Males: First-part voided urine screen for gonorrhea and chlamydia. For homosexual males, depending on sexual behaviors, consider testing throat for gonorrhea and rectum for gonorrhea and chlamydia; hepatitis B screening if not immunized.
   b. Females: Detection tests for gonorrhea and chlamydia, wet prep, cervical Gram stain if microscope available, Papanicolaou test, and mid-vaginal pH.
   c. Both sexes: Syphilis and HPV.
   d. HIV screening should be discussed with all adolescents and encouraged for those who are sexually active. Although parental involvement in an adolescent's health care is usually desirable, it typically is not required when the adolescent consents to HIV testing.
4. Cholesterol screening performed once during puberty and earlier if family history is positive for early cardiovascular disease or hyperlipidemia.
5. Purified protein derivative placement if positive history for exposure to active TB or live/works in a high-risk situation, for example, homeless shelter, jail, or health care facility.

CBC
Lipid panel
TSH
UA
PPD

Vaccinations

Ideally, all vaccinations should be administered at the 11- to 12-year-old well child visit.

1. Hepatitis B: Vaccinate any adolescent who are not previously vaccinated.
2. Hepatitis A: Vaccinate if at risk for hepatitis A infection.

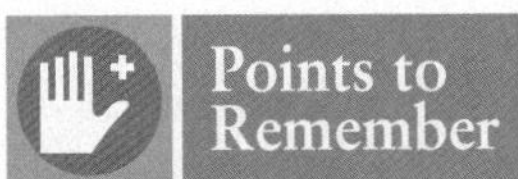

- See Preventive Medicine chapter for full review of cholesterol screening, tuberculosis screening, vaccines, and recommended vaccine schedules.

3. Varicella: Offer vaccine if no reliable history of chicken pox or prior vaccination. Varicella should not be administered to pregnant adolescents.
4. Tetanus-diphtheria-pertussis booster (Tdap) more than 5 years after fourth DTaP (usually at 11- to 12-year visit); Routine Td boosters should be administered every 10 years.
5. HPV vaccine available for 9 to 26 years of age and routinely recommended for girls aged 11 to 12 years; now FDA approved for males as well.
6. Adolescents should receive a second dose of MMR at the age of 11 to 12 years, unless there is documentation of two vaccinations earlier during childhood. MMR should not be administered to pregnant adolescents.
7. Conjugated *Neisseria meningitidis* vaccine for ages above 11 years.
8. Pneumococcal polysaccharide (23 valent) vaccine for immunocompromised patients.
9. Influenza vaccine annually for all adolescents.

Gynecology

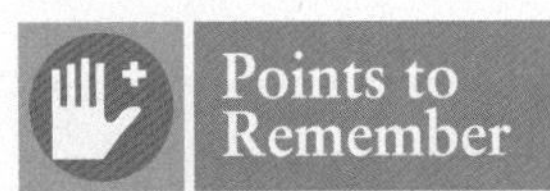

- Chlamydia and gonorrhea can cause vaginal discharge. These topics will be covered later in the chapter.

Vaginal Discharge

See Table 2.2 for the clinical and laboratory features of disorders causing vaginal discharge in adolescents.

Menstrual Abnormalities

Definitions of uterine bleeding

Oligomenorrhea: cycle length greater than 35 days.

Polymenorrhea: cycle length less than 21 days.

Amenorrhea: may be primary (absence of menarche by 16 years of age) or secondary (absence of menses for more than three cycle intervals or 6 months if previously menstruating).

Menorrhagia: prolonged (more than 7 days) or heavy bleeding occurring at regular intervals.

TABLE 2.2

CLINICAL AND LABORATORY FEATURES OF DISORDERS CAUSING VAGINAL DISCHARGE IN ADOLESCENTS

Vaginal Discharge	Color, Consistency pH	Pelvic Examination Findings	Microscopy	Treatment	Management of Sex Partners
Physiologic leukorrhea	Clear or white discharge, pH <4.5	Normal, no odor	Epithelial cells with some lactobacilli	Proper hygiene. Douching not recommended	None
Yeast vaginitis (*Candida albicans* or other yeast)	Increased white discharge with clumpy appearance, pH <4.5	Vulvar itching and irritation; notable inflammation of the vulva	Leukocytes, epithelial cells, yeast, mycelia, or pseudomycelia	Oral fluconazole, miconazole, or clotrimazole vaginal suppository	None; topical if symptomatic
Trichomoniasis (*Trichomonas vaginalis*)	Malodorous, yellow-green purulent discharge, sometimes frothy, pH >5.0	Vulvar itching; notable inflammation of the vulva and vaginal epithelium	Leukocytes and motile trichomonads in saline prep	Metronidazole single dose or 7-day course	Treatment
Bacterial vaginosis (BV) (*Gardnerella vaginalis*, anaerobic bacteria and mycoplasma)	Malodorous, white/gray discharge, pH >4.5	Three out of four criteria to diagnose BV clinically: ■ Thin, homogenous discharge that smoothly coats the vaginal walls; ■ Positive whiff-amine test[1]; ■ Vaginal pH >4.5; ■ >20% clue cells in saline wet mount per high-power microscopic field (most reliable of the four criteria).	Clue cells and few leukocytes in saline prep, anaerobic species on gram stain	Oral or topical metronidazole or oral clindamycin	Examine for STI; routine treatment not recommended

[1]Whiff amine test—a "fishy" odor produced when a drop of 10% KOH is added to vaginal discharge.
STI, sexually transmitted infection.

Box 2.1 Differential Diagnoses of Dysfunctional Uterine Bleeding

Hormonal causes
- Polycystic ovary syndrome
- Thyroid dysfunction
- Hyperprolactinemia
- Adrenal gland abnormalities
- Use of hormonal contraception

Pregnancy-related bleeding
- Threatened, spontaneous, and elective abortion
- Molar or ectopic pregnancy
- Postabortion endometritis
- Placenta previa or abruption

Local pathologic features
- Sexually transmitted disease (e.g., gonorrhea and infection with *Chlamydia* or *Trichomonas*), retained foreign body in the vagina (e.g., retained tampon) or uterus (e.g., intrauterine device)
- Laceration
- Polyp
- Uterine arteriovenous malformation
- Uterine dysplasia or malignancy

Bleeding diatheses
- Idiopathic thrombocytopenic purpura
- von Willebrand disease
- Abnormal platelet function resulting from drugs (e.g., aspirin) or systemic illness (e.g., renal failure)
- Bone marrow suppression (e.g., chemotherapy) or infiltration (e.g., leukemia)
- Coagulopathy resulting from inherited clotting factor deficiency, systemic illness (e.g., liver failure), or anticoagulant therapy (e.g., warfarin)

Adapted from Sergio R. Russon Buzzini, Melanie A. Gold. Menstrual disorders. In: Julia A. McMillan, Ralph D. Feigin, Catherine DeAngelis, M. Douglas Jones, Jr., eds. *Oski's Pediatrics: Principles & Practice,* 4th ed. Philadelphia, PA: Lippincott Williams & Wilkins, 2006.

Metrorrhagia: irregular and frequent episodes of vaginal bleeding.
Menometrorrhagia: prolonged uterine bleeding occurring at unpredictable intervals.
Abnormal uterine bleeding: any change in the frequency of menses, duration of flow, or volume of blood loss.

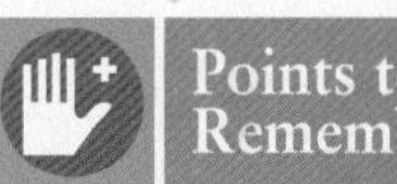

- *Fast facts*: Menstrual bleeding lasting longer than 8 days and occurring at a frequency less than 20 days or greater than 40 days is considered abnormal.

Dysfunctional Uterine Bleeding

Definition: Painless, excessive, prolonged, and unpatterned endometrial bleeding in the absence of structural pathologic features or medical illness. The differential diagnosis of DUB falls into four general categories: hormonal, pregnancy-related, local pathologic, and related to bleeding diatheses.

Physical Examination
- Weight and BMI.
- Evaluate for abnormal bruising, acanthosis nigricans, and hirsutism.
- Perform a pelvic examination to evaluate for estrogenization of vaginal mucosa as well as foreign bodies, condylomata acuminata, cervicitis, and uterine/adnexal tenderness.

Laboratory Evaluation
- Pregnancy test.
- Gonorrhea and chlamydia and a wet preparation to rule out trichomoniasis.
- Complete blood cell count with platelet count.
- TSH level.
- Coagulation studies (e.g., PT/PTT, bleeding time, and von Willebrand disease) are indicated in patients who have a family history of bleeding disorders, have significant blood loss at menarche, or heavy cyclic menses.
- FSH and LH, prolactin, and serum androgens (total and free testosterone, androstenedione, 17-hydroxyprogesterone, and DHEA-S).
- Pelvic ultrasonography or MRI can be helpful when a pelvic mass is felt or a structural disorder is suspected.

Treatment. Focus is on reassurance, prevention of anemia, and follow up.

Mild DUB:
- Hemoglobin level above 12 g/dL without active bleeding.
- Reassurance and prophylactic iron should be given with re-evaluation in 3 months.

Points to Remember

- *Fast facts*: In the rare cases when hemostasis cannot be achieved medically, dilation and curettage are indicated both for diagnosis and treatment.

Moderate DUB:
- Hemoglobin level between 10 and 12 g/dL with moderate to heavy blood flow.
- Hormonal management with oral contraceptives and therapeutic iron supplementation.

Severe DUB:
- Hemoglobin level below 10 g/dL with heavy bleeding or initial hemoglobin level below 7 g/dL, or if orthostatic signs are present—inpatient monitoring is recommended.
- Transfusion should be considered if there are clinical signs of acute blood loss or the hemoglobin level is extremely low.
- IV conjugated estrogens may be given initially until the bleeding slows.
- A combined OCP should be taken until the bleeding stops, and the dose should be tapered until the hemoglobin level is above 12 g/dL.
- A progestin must be added as soon as possible to the IV conjugated estrogen regimen to stabilize the endometrium and to prevent heavy estrogen withdrawal bleeding.

Amenorrhea

Points to Remember

- *Fast facts*: Girls who have not menstruated by the age of 15 years or who have failed to menstruate within 4 years of the onset of breast budding should be evaluated for primary amenorrhea.

Definition:
- Primary amenorrhea is the absence of menses by the age of 16 years in the presence of breast development or by the age of 14 years in the absence of breast development.
- Secondary amenorrhea is the cessation of regular menses for more than three cycles or more than 6 months any time after menarche.
- Amenorrhea may be caused by disorders of hypothalamus, pituitary, ovaries, and outflow tract, or by androgen excess (Table 2.3).

Evaluation of Primary Amenorrhea. For the adolescent with primary amenorrhea and an unremarkable history, review of systems, general physical examination, and no evidence of vaginal outlet obstruction, the physician needs to determine if a uterus is present.

TABLE 2.3

CAUSES OF PRIMARY AND SECONDARY AMENORRHEA

- Pregnancy
- Hypothyroidism and hyperthyroidism
- Disorders of the hypothalamus
  - Hypothalamic suppression caused by constitutional delay of puberty; stress; intense exercise; chronic or systemic illnesses (e.g., inflammatory bowel disease, cystic fibrosis, chronic renal failure)
  - Drug use (e.g., opiate, phenothiazine, marijuana)
  - Obesity
  - Eating disorders
  - Space-occupying lesions (e.g., craniopharyngioma, meningioma, glioma)
  - Syndromes associated with hypothalamic dysfunction and pubertal delay (e.g., Kallmann, Prader-Willi, and Laurence-Moon-Biedl syndromes)
- Disorders of pituitary
  - Idiopathic hypopituitarism
  - Hyperprolactinemia (caused by tumors, psychoactive drugs [e.g., haloperidol, phenothiazines, opiates, cocaine], breast stimulation, renal failure, infiltrative processes, or infarction)
- Disorders of the ovary
  - Congenital causes: Turner syndrome, Turner mosaic or chromosomal incompetence, pure gonadal dysgenesis, gonadotropin resistant ovary syndrome, inborn deficiency of 17alpha-hydroxylase, and galactosemia
  - Acquired causes: premature ovarian failure (e.g., autoimmune oophoritis, radiation and/or chemotherapy), trauma, and other disorders (e.g., tuberculosis, sarcoidosis, gonococcal salpingitis, mumps oophoritis)
- Disorders of outflow tract
  - Müllerian agenesis
  - Androgen insensitivity
  - Vaginal septum
  - Imperforate hymen
  - Spontaneous testicular regression and specific gonadal enzyme deficiencies
  - Uterine synechiae
- Androgen excess
  - Functional ovarian hyperandrogenism or polycystic ovary syndrome (PCOS)
  - Late-onset 21-hydroxylase deficiency
  - Androgen-producing ovarian or adrenal tumors
  - Ovarian stromal hypertrophy (hyperthecosis)
  - Cushing syndrome
  - Use of extraneous androgens

Box 2.2 Causes of Primary and Secondary Amenorrhea

Pregnancy
Hypothyroidism and hyperthyroidism
Disorders of the hypothalamus
- Hypothalamic suppression caused by constitutional delay of puberty; stress; intense exercise; chronic or systemic illnesses (e.g., inflammatory bowel disease, cystic fibrosis, chronic renal failure)
- Drug use (e.g., opiate, phenothiazine, marijuana)
- Obesity
- Eating disorders
- Space-occupying lesions (e.g., craniopharyngioma, meningioma, glioma)
- Syndromes associated with hypothalamic dysfunction and pubertal delay (e.g., Kallmann, Prader-Willi, and Laurence-Moon-Biedl syndromes)

Disorders of pituitary
- Idiopathic hypopituitarism
- Hyperprolactinemia (caused by tumors, psychoactive drugs [e.g., haloperidol, phenothiazines, opiates cocaine], breast stimulation, renal failure, infiltrative processes, or infarction)

Disorders of the ovary
- Congenital causes: Turner syndrome, Turner mosaic or chromosomal incompetence, pure gonadal dysgenesis, gonadotropin resistant ovary syndrome, inborn deficiency of 17alpha-hydroxylase, and galactosemia
- Acquired causes: premature ovarian failure (e.g., autoimmune oophoritis, radiation and/or chemotherapy), trauma, and other disorders (e.g., tuberculosis, sarcoidosis, gonococcal salpingitis, mumps oophoritis)

Disorders of outflow tract
- Müllerian agenesis
- Androgen insensitivity
- Vaginal septum
- Imperforate hymen
- Spontaneous testicular regression and specific gonadal enzyme deficiencies
- Uterine synechiae

Androgen excess
- Functional ovarian hyperandrogenism or polycystic ovary syndrome
- Late-onset 21-hydroxylase deficiency
- Androgen-producing ovarian or adrenal tumors
- Ovarian stromal hypertrophy (hyperthecosis)
- Cushing syndrome
- Use of extraneous androgens

Adapted from Sergio R. Russon Buzzini, Melanie A. Gold. Menstrual disorders. In: Julia A. McMillan, Ralph D. Feigin, Catherine DeAngelis, M. Douglas Jones, Jr., eds. *Oski's Pediatrics: Principles & Practice,* 4th ed. Philadelphia, PA: Lippincott Williams & Wilkins, 2006.

- If no uterus is present, karyotyping and serum testosterone levels should be determined to screen for müllerian agenesis, androgen insensitivity, gonadal enzyme deficiency, or testicular regression.
- If the uterus is present, serum FSH and LH levels will help to distinguish between ovarian failure and problems at the pituitary or hypothalamic levels.

Evaluation of Secondary Amenorrhea

- Secondary amenorrhea occurs when estrogen is unopposed and the endometrium is maintained in the proliferative phase. It is most commonly caused by pregnancy, stress, and PCOS.
- A thorough history should be obtained with a focus on stressors, illness, weight change, contraceptive use, drugs, or evidence of the female athlete triad (amenorrhea, disordered eating, and osteoporosis).
- Physical examination: Tanner staging, ophthalmoscopic and visual field examination, thyroid palpation, blood pressure, compression of areola to check for galactorrhea, signs of hyperandrogenism (hirsutism, clitoromegaly, severe acne, ovarian enlargement).
- If virilization is present on examination, obtain levels of free testosterone, 17-hydroxyprogesterone, and DHEAS to distinguish PCOS from adrenal causes of virilization and amenorrhea.

Points to Remember

- *Fast facts*: Disorders at the level of the hypothalamus or the pituitary gland present with low or normal levels of gonadotropins (FSH and LH) (hypogonadotropic hypogonadism), whereas high levels of gonadotropins suggest ovarian failure (hypergonadotropic hypogonadism).

Points to Remember

- *Fast facts*: The female athlete triad refers to a combination of three conditions: amenorrhea, disordered eating, and osteoporosis. Treatment focuses on nutritional counseling, calcium supplementation, oral contraceptives and at times psychiatric counseling.

Points to Remember

- *Fast facts*: A progesterone challenge test is used to determine whether the uterus is primed with estrogen. If any amount of bleeding occurs within 7 days after progesterone, a diagnosis of anovulation is made. If no bleeding occurs after progesterone, either the uterus outflow tract is abnormal or endogenous estrogen production is inadequate or absent. To distinguish between these conditions, the estrogen-progesterone challenge should be performed, which involves priming the uterus with exogenous estrogen and repeating the progesterone challenge (Fig. 2.4).

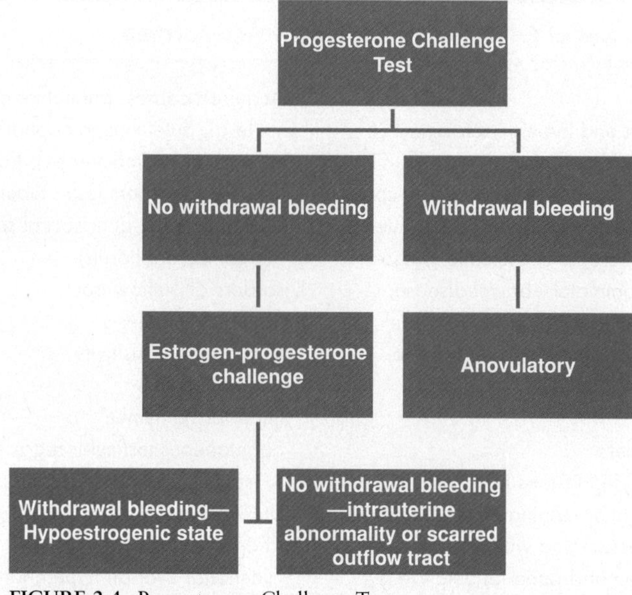

FIGURE 2.4. Progesterone Challenge Test.

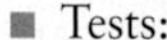

- Tests:
  - Urine pregnancy test.
    - If not pregnant: Check TSH, free thyroxine (T4), and prolactin to rule out primary or central hypothyroidism, hyperthyroidism, or hyperprolactinemia, respectively.
      - If TSH, free T4, and prolactin levels are normal proceed to a progesterone challenge test. This assesses endogenous estrogen production, endometrial response, and outflow tract competency.
- If withdrawal flow occurs, obtain FSH and LH levels
  - ✓ High FSH/LH → Premature ovarian failure. Send karyotype and antiovarian antibodies.
  - ✓ Low FSH/LH → Likely central nervous system etiology such as prolactinoma, craniopharyngioma, pituitary infarction or another chronic disease.
  - ✓ High LH:FSH ratio → Evaluate for PCOS.
- If no withdrawal bleeding, obtain a pelvic ultrasound to identify outflow tract obstruction such as Asherman syndrome.

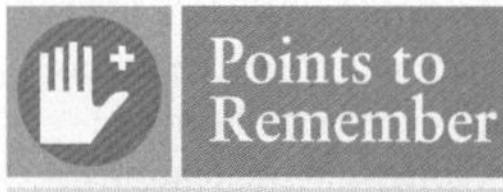

Points to Remember

- **Asherman syndrome is an acquired condition characterized by intrauterine adhesions secondary to scarring usually seen in patients who have had uterine instrumentation such as a D&C (dilatation & curettage).**

Treatment of Primary or Secondary Amenorrhea. Treatment is focused on the underlying etiology. Patients often require referral to a gynecologist or endocrinologist. See management for PCOS in the following section.

Polycystic Ovarian Syndrome

Diagnosis is clinical based on two of the following three findings:

1. Evidence of hyperandrogenism on examination (hirsutism, clitoromegaly, severe acne) or measured elevated androgen levels.
2. Irregular menses or amenorrhea.
3. Presence of polycystic ovaries on ultrasonography in the absence of other causes such as CAH or other androgenic disorders. Polycystic ovaries are defined as 12 or more follicles in at least 1 ovary measuring 2 to 9 mm in diameter or a total ovarian volume of more than 10 cm^3.

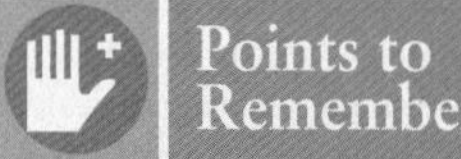

Points to Remember

- **Hyperandrogenism physical examination findings: acne vulgaris, hirsutism, weight gain, menstrual irregularities.**

Generally, girls who have PCOS also have hyperinsulinism, obesity, hirsutism, severe acne, male-pattern alopecia, voice deepening, and acanthosis nigricans.

Treatment is aimed at the management of metabolic derangements, anovulation, hirsutism, and menstrual irregularity.

- Oral contraceptives: to inhibit androgen production and re-establish cycles.
- Diet and exercise: to promote weight loss and improve insulin resistance. Metformin therapy may also be added to treat hyperinsulinism.
- Antiandrogen medication such as spironolactone is effective for hirsutism but should be taken with oral contraceptives because of its potential teratogenic effects.

Dysmenorrhea

Definition: Dysmenorrhea is pain with menstruation, usually cramping in nature and centered in the lower abdomen. Dysmenorrhea is the most common menstrual problem in adolescents, occurring in approximately 60% of 12- to 17-year-old postmenarchal girls.

Etiology. *Primary dysmenorrhea* results from myometrial contractions because of the increased production of prostaglandins. It is often associated with headaches, nausea and vomiting, bloating, backache, and diarrhea, which can all be explained by the increased secretion of prostaglandins. The symptoms tend to be most severe during the first few days of the menstrual cycle when prostaglandin levels are highest. There is often a positive family history of menstrual pain.

Secondary dysmenorrhea is associated with organic disease. Common causes include endometriosis, PID, uterine fibroids, and polyps, presence of an intrauterine device, pelvic adhesions, and ovarian cyst, or mass. Secondary dysmenorrhea should be suspected if the pain is unusually severe, if it began at menarche, if it is increasing in severity, or if it is isolated and related to only one painful period.

Physical Examination. A complete pelvic examination may not be necessary in a virginal patient with a history suggestive of primary dysmenorrhea. If the pain is mild and the patient has a normal physical examination including the hymen, a speculum examination is not necessary.

A complete pelvic examination is indicated at the initial evaluation if the patient is sexually active or the pain is severe. The examination helps to detect a genital tract obstruction, adnexal and/or uterosacral pain suggestive of endometriosis, evidence of sexually transmitted disease or PID, and an adnexal or uterine mass.

Laboratory Evaluation

- No diagnostic tests are needed for the assessment and treatment of primary dysmenorrhea. A PID workup should be initiated if the patient is sexually active and meets clinical criteria. All sexually active adolescents should have testing for STIs and pregnancy.
- A pelvic ultrasound or MRI studies may help with the diagnosis of a congenital anomaly.
- If pain is severe and unresponsive to medical management, diagnostic laparoscopy to rule out endometriosis may be indicated.

Treatment. The two most effective treatments for primary dysmenorrhea are NSAIDs and combined oral contraceptives.

- NSAIDs inhibit the synthesis and/or action of prostaglandins. Adolescents should be advised to begin taking the medication the day before the menses or at the first sign of menses and then continue taking the medication around the clock for the first 2 or 3 days of menses.
- Combined oral contraceptives may also be used and work directly by limiting endometrial growth and indirectly by inhibiting ovulation and progesterone secretion.

Treatment of secondary dysmenorrhea is specific to the etiology discovered.

Pregnancy

- Female adolescents often present with delayed or missed menses and may request a pregnancy test. For some there may be an element of denial resulting in a variety of somatic complaints. Certain complaints should trigger the physician to obtain a urine pregnancy test such as: abdominal pain, urinary frequency, dizziness, and other nonspecific symptoms.
- Pregnant adolescents are at greater risk than adult women for pre-eclampsia, eclampsia, iron deficiency anemia, cephalopelvic disproportion, prolonged labor, premature labor, and maternal death.
- Adolescents have the highest mortality rate from ectopic pregnancy. Risk factors include history of PID or chlamydial infection. There should be a high level of suspicion for ectopic pregnancy in an adolescent presenting with vaginal bleeding and abdominal pain.

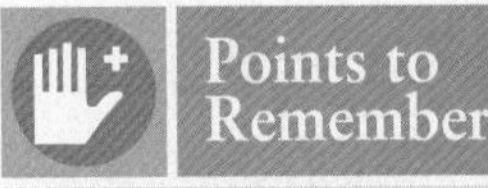

- There should be a high level of suspicion for ectopic pregnancy in an adolescent presenting with vaginal bleeding and abdominal pain.

Prevention—Contraceptive Technologies

1. Physical barriers
   a. Condoms—The only contraceptive device that protects against STIs.
   b. Diaphragm—Inserted by females to cover the cervix. May confer an increased risk for urinary tract infections and toxic shock syndrome.
2. OCPs
   a. OCPs have three mechanisms of action: (1) suppression of ovulation; (2) thickening of cervical mucus; (3) endometrial atrophy.
   b. Combination OCPs contain both estrogen and progestin and are available in pill form, patch, or insertable vaginal ring.
   c. OCPs may be used to treat dysmenorrhea, menorrhagia, DUB, and acne.
   d. Contraindications to OCPs include pregnancy, lactation (recommended to wait 6 weeks postpartum), history of thromboembolic or cerebrovascular disease, breast cancer, structural heart disease, severe migraines, liver disease, severe hypertension, and major surgery with prolonged immobilization.
   e. Progestin-only pills are used in women who have a contraindication to estrogen-containing pills or significant side effects from estrogen. Progestin-only pills have less predictable menstrual patterns and are thus not routinely used in adolescents.

3. Contraceptive patch—Delivers the same medication as oral contraceptives but protection extends for 1 week.
4. Injectable hormonal contraceptives
   a. DMPA or Depo-Provera is a long-acting injectable progestational contraceptive given as a single injection every 12 weeks.
   b. DMPA works by blocking the LH surge and suppressing ovulation while thickening the cervical mucus and inhibiting endometrial implantation.
5. Intrauterine device: This is a long-acting, reversible contraceptive method. It requires insertion or removal by a practitioner intrauterine devices change the lining of the uterus and fallopian tubes such that fertilization is inhibited. There is no STI protection.
6. Emergency contraception
   a. Combination of estrogen and progestin OCP or a progestin-only pill taken within 72 hours of unprotected intercourse, with a second dose 12 hours later.
   b. Mechanism of action includes delaying ovulation or altering the endometrial lining to prevent implantation.
   c. Emergency contraception does not interfere with an already existing pregnancy and is not considered an abortifacient drug.

Social and Emotional Aspects of Adolescent Pregnancy

A pregnant adolescent should have options discussed with her (abortion, adoption, raising the baby) and assistance telling her parents.

Significant psychosocial consequences for an adolescent mother and her infant exist. These include decreased educational attainment, lower occupational attainment and prestige, less stable marital relationships, higher rates of single parenthood, and higher rate of unintended repeat pregnancies.

Sexually Transmitted Diseases

Chlamydia trachomatis

The most common reportable STI is in the United States. Complications from *Chlamydia* include urethritis, cervicitis, vaginitis, salpingitis, PID, perihepatitis (Fitzhugh-Curtis syndrome), conjunctivitis, and Reiter syndrome (reactive arthritis) for both men and women. Men may also develop epididymitis.

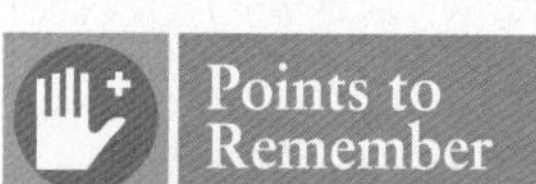

Points to Remember

- Discussion of neonatal chlamydial conjunctivitis covered in the Infectious Diseases chapter.

Clinical Manifestations are multiple with several reviewed below. Urethritis and cervicitis are the most common manifestations. When present, symptoms generally appear about 2 weeks after

Box 2.3 Etiology of Common Sexually Transmitted Infections

Discharge Syndromes (Urethritis, Cervicitis, Vaginitis)
- *Chlamydia trachomatis*
- *Neisseria gonorrhoeae*
- *Trichomonas vaginalis*
- *Mycoplasma genitalium*
- *Ureaplasma urealyticum*
- Herpes simplex virus
- *Candida* species

Ulcer Syndromes
- *Treponema pallidum*
- Herpes simplex virus
- *Haemophilus ducreyi*
- *Calymmatobacterium granulomatis* (granuloma inguinale, rare in the United States)
- *Chlamydia trachomatis serovars* Ll, L2, or L3 (lymphogranuloma venereum, rare in the United States)

Pelvic Inflammatory Disease
- *Neisseria gonorrhoeae*
- *Chlamydia trachomatis*
- "Normal vaginal flora, e.g., anaerobes, *Gardnerella vaginalis, Haemophilus influenzae*, enteric gram-negative rods, and *Streptococcus agalactiae*
- Uncommon: *Mycoplasma genitalium*, cytomegalovirus, *Mycoplasma hominis, Ureaplasma urealyticum*

Epididymitis
- *Chlamydia trachomatis*
- *Neisseria gonnorrhoeae*
- Enteric organisms, e.g., *Escherichia coli*

Dermatologic
- *Treponema pallidum*
- *Neisseria gonorrhoeae* (disseminated gonococcal infection)
- Acute human immunodeficiency virus (See Chapter 139)

Adapted from Richard B. Heyman. Adolescent substance abuse and other high-risk behaviors. In: Julia A. McMillan, Ralph D. Feigin, Catherine DeAngelis, M. Douglas Jones, Jr., eds. *Oski's Pediatrics: Principles & Practice*, 4th ed. Philadelphia, PA: Lippincott Williams & Wilkins, 2006.

TABLE 2.4

CLINICAL FINDINGS IN EPIDIDYMITIS AND TESTICULAR TORSION

Epididymitis	Testicular Torsion
Acute scrotal pain and swelling. May have pain relief with scrotal elevation (Prehn sign)	Acute scrotal pain and swelling. No pain relief with scrotal elevation.
Urinalysis often abnormal with pyuria	Normal urinalysis
Cremasteric reflex present	Cremasteric reflex absent

sexual contact, although this is quite variable. Urethritis symptoms are usually mild and include frequency and dysuria. Urethral discharge tends to be mucoid and scant; however, it may mimic the typical purulent discharge of gonorrhea.

Diagnosis: For females, symptoms include odorless vaginal discharge and at times intermenstrual or postcoital spotting. The examination may be normal or may demonstrate cervical friability (bleeding when lightly swabbed with a cotton-tipped applicator) and mucopurulent exudate in the endocervical canal.

Evidence of inflammation includes more than five PMNs/oil-immersion field on Gram stain or positive LE on the first 10 to 20 mL of urine specimen. Diagnostic tests are based on tissue culture, antigen detection, and amplification of nucleic acid sequences of *C. trachomatis*.

Epididymitis: Male adolescents with epididymitis usually present with unilateral testicular pain; swelling and tenderness along with a hydrocele are present on examination. Almost all have an asymptomatic urethritis as demonstrated by more than five PMNs on Gram stain of urethral swab or LE in a first-specimen urine sample. May have bacterial etiology (*Gonococcus*, *Chlamydia*) but often the organism remains undetermined (Table 2.4).

Lymphogranuloma venereum (LGV): LGV occurs in three stages

a. Primary stage—Painless herpetiform ulceration at the site of inoculation.
b. Secondary stage—Painful supperative lymphatic infection of the femoral and/or inguinal nodes. Patients may experience constitutional symptoms, which can include fever, headache, malaise, chills, nausea, vomiting, and arthralgias.
c. Tertiary stage—This stage occurs years after the initial infection and manifests as rectal stricture or elephantiasis of the genitalia.

Points to Remember

- *Fast facts*: Reiter syndrome: "Can't see, Can't pee, Can't climb a tree" is a common mnemonic for this syndrome characterized by urethritis, bilateral conjunctivitis, and arthritis.

Treatment

- For uncomplicated genital infection, doxycycline × 7 days (preferred treatment in patients older than 8 years), azithromycin × 1 dose, ofloxacin × 7 days, or erythromycin × 7 days.
- For males with epididymitis, bed rest, scrotal elevation, and analgesics are also recommended until symptoms have subsided.
- Patients with Reiter syndrome may require analgesics and physical therapy.

Points to Remember

- Neonatal gonococcal disease is discussed in the chapter on Infectious Diseases.

Neisseria gonorrhoeae

Clinical Manifestations. *N. gonorrhoeae* is associated with the clinical syndromes or symptoms of urethritis, cervicitis, pharyngitis, proctitis, and conjunctivitis. Complications include epididymitis in males, PID and TOA in females and DGI in both. Coinfection with *C. trachomatis* is common.

DGI results from gonococcal bacteremia causing petechial or pustular acral skin lesions, asymmetric arthralgia/arthritis, tenosynovitis, or septic arthritis. Mucosal surface(s) provide the entry point; DGI may be complicated by perihepatitis and rarely meningitis or endocarditis.

Points to Remember

- Rectal and pharyngeal gonorrhea infections are often asymptomatic. It is imperative to ask about oral and anal sex.

Gonococcal urethritis may be mild (scant mucoid discharge, dysuria, frequency) or more severe, with intense pain on urination and penile edema. Approximately 50% of girls and women with gonococcal genitourinary infection remain asymptomatic. Presentation and findings of uncomplicated infection in girls and women are similar to those caused by *C. trachomatis*.

Points to Remember

- *Fast facts:* Adolescents infected with either gonorrhea or chlamydia are often coinfected and should be evaluated for all common STIs when either is diagnosed.

Diagnosis. Gonococcal urethritis is reliably diagnosed in boys and men by observation of intracellular Gram-positive diplococci on Gram stain of the urethral exudate. NAA tests are highly sensitive and specific and may be used on urethral, endocervical, and urine specimens. These may include PCR, TMA, and strand displacement assays. The TMA assay is the only NAA test approved for testing vaginal swabs in postmenarcheal females. NAA tests are not recommended for pharyngeal or rectal swabs.

Treatment. Ceftriaxone × 1 dose or cefixime × 1 dose. Note: As of 2007, the Centers for Disease Control no longer recommends fluoroquinolones for the treatment of gonorrhea.

Pelvic Inflammatory Disease

Definition: PID refers to a group of infections of the upper genital tract: endometritis, salpingitis, TOA, and pelvic peritonitis. PID is associated with significant morbidity, including tubal adhesions and increased risk for ectopic pregnancy, infertility, and chronic pelvic pain.

Epidemiology: *C. trachomatis* or *N. gonorrhoeae* is identified from cervical or tubal specimens in about 30% of cases of acute PID from ambulatory settings and up to two-thirds of women hospitalized for acute PID. Other vaginal flora (anaerobes and bacteroides species, enteric Gram-negative rods, coliforms, *Haemophilus influenzae*, *Gardnerella vaginalis*, and *Streptococcus agalactiae*) have been identified in the endocervix and upper genital tract. Infection with anaerobes and multiple organisms appears to be common among those with more severe disease and TOA.

Diagnosis. Minimum diagnostic criteria for PID are the following:

- Sexually active women with pelvic or lower abdominal pain unexplained by other etiology.
- Cervical motion tenderness or uterine tenderness or adnexal tenderness.

The following additional criteria can be used to enhance the specificity of the minimum criteria and support a diagnosis of PID:

- Oral temperature >101°F (>38.3°C).
- Abnormal cervical or vaginal mucopurulent discharge.
- Presence of abundant numbers of WBC on saline microscopy of vaginal secretions.
- Elevated erythrocyte sedimentation rate.
- Elevated C-reactive protein.
- Laboratory documentation of cervical infection with *N. gonorrhoeae* or *C. trachomatis*.

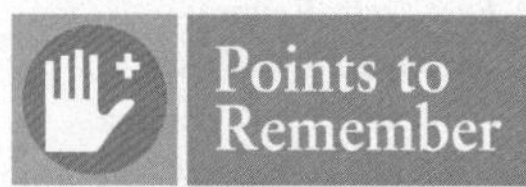

Points to Remember

- If cervical discharge appears normal and no WBCs are observed on the wet preparation of vaginal fluid, the diagnosis of PID is unlikely, and alternative causes of pain should be investigated.

Treatment

- Outpatient: Ceftriaxone 250 mg IM in a single dose and doxycycline 100 mg orally twice a day × 14 days ± metronidazole 500 mg orally twice a day for 14 days.
- Inpatient: Cefotetan 2 g IV every 12 hours or cefoxitin 2 g IV every 6 hours and doxycycline 100 mg orally or IV every 12 hours.

Criteria for hospitalization include the following:

- Surgical emergency (e.g., appendicitis) cannot be excluded.
- Pregnancy.
- Lack of clinical response to oral antimicrobial therapy.
- Inability to follow or tolerate an outpatient oral regimen.
- Severe illness, nausea and vomiting, or high fever.
- TOA.

Points to Remember

- Refer to http://www.cdc.gov/STD/treatment/2006/updated-regimens.htm for additional alternative enteral and parenteral PID treatment regimens.

Treponema pallidum (Syphilis)

Primary Syphilis. The first clinical sign of infection is a local lesion that appears approximately 14 to 21 days after sexual contact at the site of inoculation, which is usually a moist mucous membrane. This progresses to a shallow, **painless, indurated ulcer (chancre).** Rubbery, painless regional lymphadenopathy develops approximately 1 week later. Untreated, the lesion heals in 3 to 6 weeks and progresses to secondary syphilis.

Secondary Syphilis. Without treatment of primary syphilis, there is widespread dissemination of *T. pallidum* about 3 to 6 weeks after the appearance of the chancre. An evanescent macular rash is often the initial clinical manifestation of systemic spread. This is followed by several other eruption types:

- Symmetric papular eruptions involving the trunk and extremities including the palms and soles.
- Small aphthous ulcers.
- "Moth-eaten" alopecia.
- Condylomata lata (large, raised, verrucous whitish-gray lesions) adjacent to the primary site of infection.

Points to Remember

- Congenital syphilis will be discussed the chapter Neonatology.

Other common constitutional symptoms include malaise, sore throat, headaches, weight loss, fever, and myalgia. More than 75% of individuals develop a rash, and 50% to 86% have widespread lymphadenopathy.

Points to Remember

- All adolescents diagnosed with syphilis should be tested for HIV.

Latent or Tertiary Syphilis. Without treatment, symptoms resolve spontaneously in 3 to 12 weeks, and the patient does not demonstrate clinical manifestations of the disease but remains seroreactive. There are two stages to late syphilis—early latent and late latent. The tertiary stage can be marked by aortitis, gumma formation affecting multiple organs and neurosyphilis.

Diagnosis. Diagnosis is based on clinical suspicion and a confirmatory laboratory test. Patients at risk should have a nontreponemal serum screen—RPR or VDRL test—and if positive then a specific treponemal test should be performed—FTA-ABS or MHA-TP to confirm the diagnosis.

Dark field examinations and DFA tests of exudates or tissue can help diagnose early syphilis.

Treatment

- Primary, secondary, and early latent syphilis
  - Benzathine penicillin G 50,000 units/kg IM, up to the adult dose of 2.4 million units in a single dose.
- Late latent syphilis or latent syphilis of unknown duration.
- Benzathine penicillin G 50,000 units/kg IM, up to the adult dose of 2.4 million units, administered as three doses at 1-week intervals (total 150,000 units/kg up to the adult total dose of 7.2 million units).
- Tertiary syphilis
  - Benzathine penicillin G 7.2 million units total, administered as three doses of 2.4 million units IM each at 1-week intervals.
- Neurosyphilis
  - Aqueous crystalline penicillin G 18 to 24 million units per day, administered as 3 to 4 million units IV every 4 hours or continuous infusion, for 10 to 14 days.

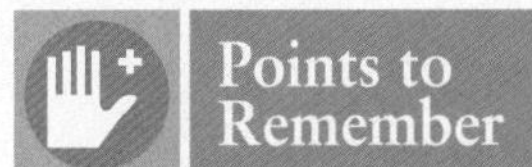

- FTA-ABS is a treponemal blood serum screening that detects specific antibodies directed against *T. pallidum.* The FTA-ABS test is often used as a confirmatory test after first screening a patient with a VDRL or RPR test. The VDRL is a nontreponemal serological screening test for syphilis that is also used to assess response to therapy.

Herpes Simplex Virus

Infection with HSV types 1 and 2 is common. HSV-2 is most commonly associated with genital infection and HSV-1 with oral infection; however, both organisms may infect either site (Fig. 2.5).

Clinical Manifestations. Initial (primary) infections tend to be associated with systemic symptoms such as malaise, myalgia, headache, and fever. Local genital and rectal symptoms include dysuria, urethral and cervical discharge, and pain on defecation, tenesmus, or mucoid discharge (proctitis).

Sequence of events:

- Incubation period of 1 week (2 to 12 days).
- Virus is shed for at least 10 to 12 days following an initial infection.
- Eruption of painful, discrete groups of vesicles at the site(s) of inoculation.
- Lesions resolve 15 to 20 days after the appearance of the vesicles.

More than 90% of those with genital HSV-2 have a recurrence of symptoms within 1 year, during which there is active viral shedding. Most patients develop multiple recurrences, which may be asymptomatic. Genital herpes during pregnancy may lead to congenital or intrapartum transmission resulting in neonatal herpes. Please see the Neonatology chapter for details on neonatal HSV.

Diagnosis. Material should be obtained from unroofed vesicles. Cell culture techniques require about 3 days and can differentiate HSV-1 and HSV-2, but they are dependent on live virus; antigen tests include detection using DFA and PCR.

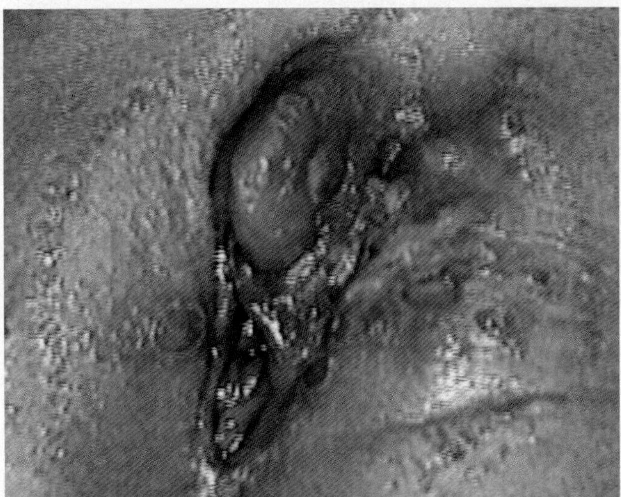

FIGURE 2.5. Herpes simplex virus. Multiple, painful, erythematous ulcerations on the labia of a 4-year-old girl who reported penile genital contact with an adult relative. Culture was positive for herpes simplex virus type II. (Courtesy of Allan R. De Jong, MD.)

Treatment. Patients with primary disease should be treated with a 7- to 10-day course of acyclovir. Other antiviral agents include famciclovir and valacyclovir. Patients with recurrent disease should be treated with acyclovir as early as the onset of prodromal symptoms such as itching skin, burning, pain, or abnormal tingling sensation. Topical preparations are not considered effective and are thus not recommended.

Daily suppressive therapy is useful for individuals with frequent recurrent episodes (four or more annually).

Genital Human Papillomavirus

HPVs are small, nonenveloped DNA viruses that infect basal epithelial cells. Most infections are subclinical and asymptomatic. HPV types are divided into low-risk and high-risk on the basis of their association with clinical sequelae (Table 2.5). More than 90% of women with cervical cancer have been infected with HPV.

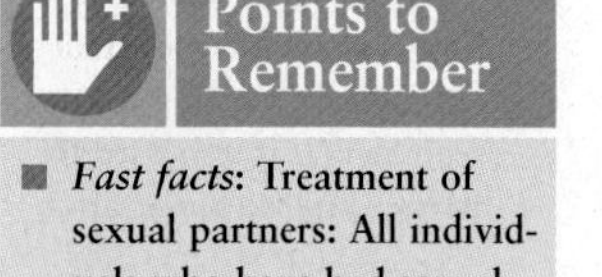

- *Fast facts*: Treatment of sexual partners: All individuals who have had sexual contact within 60 days with a patient treated for an STI (except HPV or HSV) should be evaluated and empirically treated. Syphilis, gonorrhea, chlamydia, and HIV are reportable diseases in every state; HIV infection and chancroid are reportable in many states.

TABLE 2.5

LOW-RISK AND HIGH-RISK HPV SUBTYPES

Low-risk HPV Subtypes	High-risk HPV Subtypes
6, 11	16, 18, 31, 33, and 45
Associated with exophytic warts	Associated with 95% of cervical cancers

Clinical Manifestations. Exophytic warts of the genitals and anus are common. In most immunocompetent people with anogenital warts, spontaneous regression eventually occurs. As with cervical infections, some progress to malignancy.

Diagnosis. Most anogenital HPV infections are subclinical and are recognized only if cellular abnormalities are identified on a Papanicolaou test. Cervical infection can be visualized with the application of 5% acetic acid solution, which whitens affected tissue.

Reasons to refer for colposcopy after Papanicolaou test are the following:

- Identification of high-risk HPV types with atypical squamous cells of undetermined signified (ASCUS).
- Any diagnosis of high-grade SILs or persistent low-grade SILs.

Treatment. Podophyllin, 25% benzoin tincture applied directly to warts (not used in intravaginal or urethral lesions). Trichloroacetic acid applied directly to external warts, cryotherapy, or electrocautery.

Breast Disorders

Pubertal Male Gynecomastia

Definition: Breast development commonly seen in teenage boys between Tanner stages 2 or 3 which may last for approximately 2 years. Physical exam reveals a palpable disk of rubbery, freely mobile, occasionally tender, breast tissue directly under the areola. It can be distinguished from adipose tissue by the absence of discrete mass of breast tissue. Masses not consisting of breast tissue are usually not centered directly beneath the areola (Fig. 2.6).

- Pathologic causes of gynecomastia include the following:
  - *Endocrine*: Hypogonadism (e.g., Klinefelter syndrome [47XXY]), partial androgen insensitivity, partial blocks in testosterone biosynthesis, hyperthyroidism.
  - *Oncologic*: Adrenal, testicular, or LH and hCG-producing tumors; liver tumors or disease.
  - *Nutrition:* Chronic debilitating illness causing malnutrition.
  - *Pharmacologic*: Side effect of a variety of drugs including androgens, estrogens, psychoactive drugs (e.g., phenothiazines), *marijuana and other street drugs* and alcohol, testosterone antagonists (e.g., ketoconazole, cimetidine, spironolactone), and antituberculosis and cytotoxic agents.

Treatment

- Patients with pubertal gynecomastia should be reassured and carefully re-examined at routine physicals. Breast tissue usually regresses in less than 2 years. Medication or drug use/abuse implicated in gynecomastia should be discontinued, and the patient should be re-examined in 2 to 3 months for improvement in symptoms.

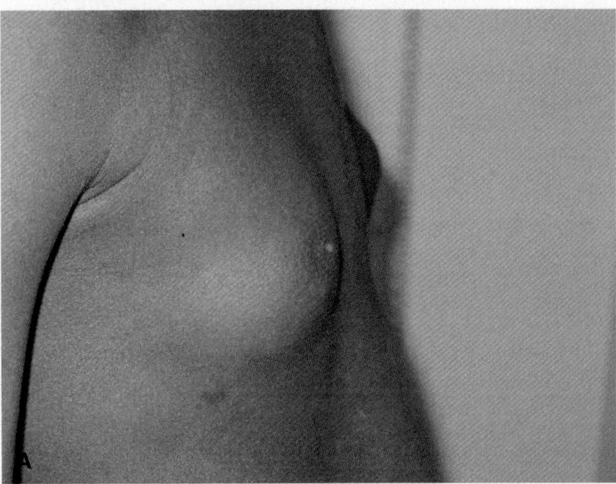

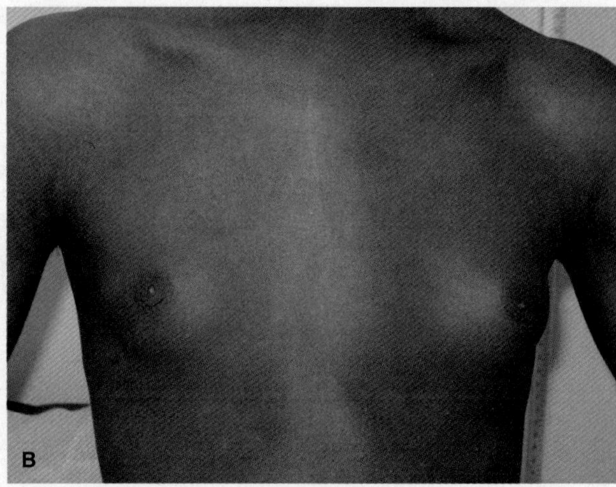

FIGURE 2.6. Gynecomastia. (**A**) Adolescent male with Tanner III–IV genital staging and bilateral breast development with palpable breast buds, side view. (**B**) Adolescent male with Tanner 111–IV genital staging and bilateral breast development with palpable breast buds, front view. (Images courtesy of Christine Finck, MD.)

- If gynecomastia persists for more than 2 years, or if features of the history or physical examination suggest systemic disease referral to an endocrinologist or adolescent medicine specialist may be warranted.

Breast Masses

A thorough history and examination should highlight potential infectious or oncologic etiologies. In the absence of signs suggestive of infection or malignancy, the patient can be observed through at least one complete menstrual cycle. If the mass disappears, it was probably a cyst or fibrocystic breast change.

Although many benign breast masses persist for more than 8 weeks, persistent masses should be evaluated with a combination of physical examination, ultrasound (to assess the dimensions and to distinguish cystic from solid masses), and referral to a gynecologist or breast specialist for fine needle aspiration or core biopsy.

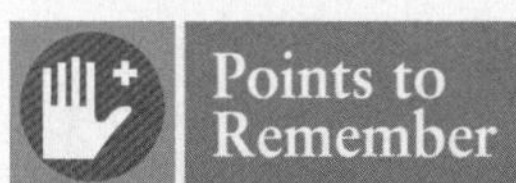

- *Fast facts*: Mammography is not useful because of the density of adolescent breasts and because of the low risk for malignancy. However, a breast ultrasound may be helpful to distinguish cystic versus solid masses.

Types of Common Breast Masses (Table 2.6)

Breast Abscess

- Tender, cystic, erythematous, and warm fluctuant mass.
- Treatment includes incision and drainage and antibiotics. Warm compresses and analgesics ease discomfort. If the patient is febrile, blood cultures should also be obtained.

Clinical findings suggestive of breast cancer include a hard, fixed, irregular mass with overlying skin changes and nipple retraction.

Breast Pain

Mastalgia (breast pain) can be noncyclic but is more commonly cyclic, with premenstrual worsening. It usually presents as bilateral heaviness or soreness that resolves during menses. The history should document the duration and location of the pain, its relation to menses, and the possibility of pregnancy.

With a normal physical examination and a negative pregnancy test, patients can be reassured that mastalgia is common and usually self-limited. Potential treatments include heat, a well-fitting supportive bra, and over-the-counter analgesics.

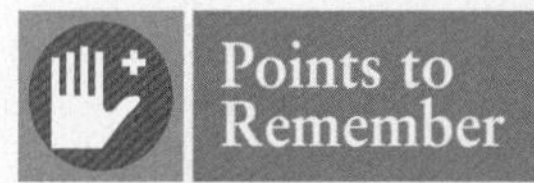

- *Fast fact*: Many young women are concerned about breast cancer when a mass is detected. However, breast cancer is rare in women younger than 20 years.

Nipple Discharge—Galactorrhea

Definition: Nipple discharge in an adolescent is most commonly galactorrhea (inappropriate lactation). Galactorrhea usually arises from multiple ducts of both breasts.

Physical examination should include breast examination, palpation of the thyroid gland, and neurologic assessment including visual fields. To elicit nipple discharge, either the examiner or the patient may massage the breast from the outside in toward the nipple.

- Purulent discharge indicates infection.
- Yellow, brown, or green sticky discharge may indicate duct ectasia (dilated ducts with stagnant secretions).
- Serous or serosanguinous discharge can be seen with intraductal papilloma, fibrocystic changes, duct ectasia, or cancer.

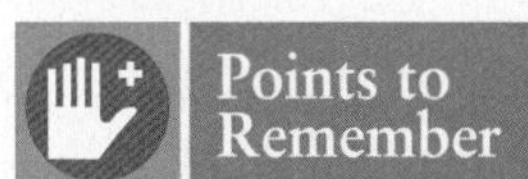

- *Fast fact*: Most complaints of breast lumps in adolescents are diagnosed as physiologic breast tissue or benign fibrocystic changes.

TABLE 2.6

TYPES OF COMMON BREAST MASSES AND ASSOCIATED CLINICAL FINDINGS

Benign Fibrocystic Changes	Fibroadenomas
■ Found in more than 50% of reproductive-age women as a painless breast mass or at times may be associated with cyclic tenderness ■ On exam notable nodularity and diffuse cordlike thickening.	■ Most common surgically excised breast lesion in adolescents representing 70% to 90% of benign breast lesions ■ Firm, rubbery, mobile, 2 to 3 cm well circumscribed lesions, typically nontender and most commonly found in the upper outer quadrant of the breast ■ Giant (or juvenile) fibroadenomas are >5 cm in size and often grow much more rapidly. These may require excisional biopsy.
Cystosarcoma Phyllodes	**Intraductal Papilloma**
■ A rare primary tumor with firm, mobile lesions that can grow quickly to >13 cm. ± association with bloody nipple discharge and skin discoloration. ■ Diagnose by ultrasound. If malignant, these may metastasize to the chest so a chest CT would be indicated. ■ May require a wide-margin excisional biopsy or if malignant, chemotherapy, radiation and hormonal treatment.	■ A small benign tumor arising from the ductal epithelium usually associated with nipple discharge ■ Most are benign but may require excision for cytologic diagnosis

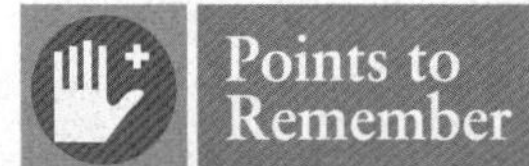

■ *Note*: Consultation with a gynecologist should be considered for the evaluation of nonmilky discharge.

Laboratory evaluation includes the following:

- Urine pregnancy test.
- Prolactin level: prolactin level of more than 100 ng/mL suggests a prolactin-secreting tumor. For the most accurate result, the prolactin level should be obtained between 8 and 10 o'clock in the morning with the patient fasting and several hours after any breast manipulation, including breast examination.
- TSH—used to rule out primary hypothyroidism. Patients with primary hypothyroidism have increased production of thyrotropin-releasing hormone, which may stimulate prolactin release.
- Blood urea nitrogen and creatinine—some patients with chronic renal failure have increased levels of prolactin possibly due to decreased renal clearance.

Galactorrhea associated with unexplained hyperprolactinemia, amenorrhea or oligomenorrhea, or symptoms suggestive of an intracranial mass requires neuroimaging (MRI) to detect a pituitary adenoma.

Galactorrhea with normal prolactin levels, normal neuroimaging, and history of regular menses do not require treatment unless the patient finds the discharge bothersome, in which case a dopamine agonist can be used.

Male Genitourinary Disorders

Hydrocele

Definition: A collection of fluid between the parietal and visceral layers if the tunica vaginalis.
Diagnosis: Hydroceles are usually soft, painless, and fluctuant fluid filled masses that transilluminate when a light is shone behind the testicle. These occur in 0.5% to 1% of males and may appear at any age.

Treatment: If the hydrocele is tense, painful or associated with a hernia it is called a communicating hydrocele and surgical intervention is advised. Otherwise, no treatment is necessary as the hydrocele may resolve spontaneously.

Spermatocele

Definition: This mass is a retention cyst of the epididymis that contains spermatozoa. The incidence of spermatoceles is less than 1%.
Diagnosis: They are usually located above the head if the epididymis and behind the testes. Spermatoceles usually separate from and are above the testicle. Most are less than 1 cm in diameter

and are freely movable, painless, and will transilluminate. Microscopic examination of aspirated fluid shows dead spermatozoa and the fluid is typically, thin, white, and cloudy.

Treatment: Usually require no therapy unless large enough to annoy the patient in which cause they can be (electively) excised.

Hernia

Definition: A sac-like protrusion through the inguinal ring into the scrotum.
Diagnosis: May resemble a hydrocele but can usually be reduced when the patient is in a supine position and will not descend with traction on the testicle. It may be associated with bowel sounds in the scrotum.

Treatment: Surgical correction is usually warranted.

Varicocele

Definition: These are elongated, dilated, tortuous veins of the pampiniform plexus within the spermatic cord formed from incompetent and dilated internal and external spermatic veins. This is the most common scrotal mass among adolescents; Most are asymptomatic but occasionally can be associated with an ache or "dragging" sensation or like a "bag of worms" along the spermatic cord.

Diagnosis: Usually the varicocele is most prominent when the patient is standing and less obvious when he is lying down. They occur more often on the left side possibly as a consequence of retrograde blood flow from the left renal vein. Testicular hypotrophy or growth arrest of affected side is the hallmark of testicular damage.

Treatment: In the adolescent, indications for ligation of the internal spermatic vein, which corrects the varicocele, are pain, ipsilateral testicular atrophy, or size.

Testis Tumor

Regular testicular examinations should be encouraged for all male adolescents. On examination, a testicular tumor will be well circumscribed, nontender, and will not transilluminate. Refer to the Oncology chapter for further discussion of testicular tumors.

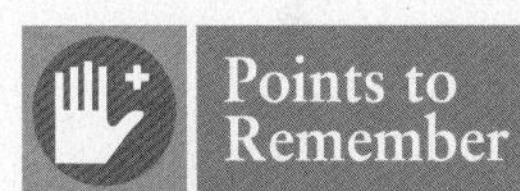

- *Fast facts*: **If an undescended testis is diagnosed after puberty, an orchiectomy is recommended because of the risk for malignant changes.**

Eating Disorders

Factors predisposing an individual to develop an eating disorder include (1) being female; (2) possessing traits such as perfectionism, obsessive/compulsiveness, or moodiness; (3) having low self-esteem; (4) engaging in activities that place a high value on thinness, such as classic ballet or modeling, or in which the body is exposed during competition, such as gymnastics, track, or swimming; and (5) being in a weight-conscious environment. Eating disorders may be managed on an outpatient basis; however, please refer to Table 2.9 on admission criteria for inpatient management.

Anorexia Nervosa

Diagnostic criteria for anorexia nervosa include the following:

- Refusal to maintain body weight at or above a minimally normal weight for age and height (Usually 15% below the norm).
- Intense fear of gaining weight or becoming fat, even though underweight.
- Disturbance in the perception of one's body weight or shape.

TABLE 2.7

KEY CLINICAL FINDINGS ASSOCIATED WITH WEIGHT LOSS

History	Physical Examination
Cold intolerance	Hypothermia, acrocyanosis, cold extremities
Fatigue, weakness	Decreased muscle mass
Dizziness, lightheadedness	Bradycardia with orthostasis
Difficulty concentrating	Normal neurologic examination
Early satiety	Scaphoid abdomen with no organomegaly
Amenorrhea	Dry skin, lanugo hair on body, loss of scalp hair

Reprinted with permission from McMillan JA, Feigin RD, DeAngelis C, et al. *Oski's Pediatrics: Principles and Practice.* 4th ed. Philadelphia, PA: Lippincott Williams & Wilkins, 2006.

TABLE 2.8

KEY CLINICAL FINDINGS ASSOCIATED WITH BINGE EATING AND VOMITING

History	Physical Examination
Bloating and fullness	Normal to overweight
Facial swelling	Salivary gland enlargement Dental enamel erosion Subconjunctival hemorrhage Knuckle calluses
Rapid weight changes	Evidence of hypokalemia
Heart palpitations	Dysrhythmias

Reprinted with permission from McMillan JA, Feigin RD, DeAngelis C, et al. *Oski's Pediatrics: Principles and Practice*. 4th ed. Philadelphia, PA: Lippincott Williams & Wilkins, 2006.

- Amenorrhea in postmenarchal females (three consecutive missed periods in absence of pregnancy).

Bulimia Nervosa

Diagnostic criteria for bulimia nervosa include the following:

- Recurrent episodes of binge eating (i.e., eating an amount of food that is definitely larger than most people would eat in a given time frame and a sense of lack of control over eating during the episodes).
- Recurrent inappropriate or compensatory behavior to prevent weight gain such as self-induced vomiting, use of laxatives, diuretics or enemas, fasting, or excessive exercise.
- Binge eating and inappropriate compensatory behavior both occur at least twice per week for 3 months.
- Poor insight into disorder secondary to disturbance in perception of body shape and weight.

Clinical Manifestations of Anorexia and Bulimia

Common laboratory abnormalities include the following:

- Low WBC count with normal differential and hemoglobin level.
- Hypokalemic, hypochloremic metabolic alkalosis with severe vomiting.
- Elevated liver enzymes, cholesterol, and cortisol levels.
- Low gonadotropins.
- Low blood glucose level.
- Usually normal total protein, albumin, and renal function.
- An ECG may reveal profound bradycardia or arrhythmia; the ECG usually has low voltage, with nonspecific ST- or T-wave changes.

Criteria for hospital admission for eating disorders are given in Table 2.9.

TABLE 2.9

CRITERIA FOR HOSPITAL ADMISSION FOR EATING DISORDERS

Anorexia Nervosa	Bulimia Nervosa
<75% ideal body weight or ongoing weight loss despite intensive management	Syncope
Refusal to eat	Serum potassium concentration: 3.2 mEq/L (3.2 mmol/L)
Body fat <10%	Serum chloride concentration: 88 mEq/L (88 mmol/L)
Heart rate <50 beats/min daytime or <45 beats/min nighttime	Esophageal tears
Systolic pressure <90 mmHg	Cardiac arrhythmias, including prolonged QTc
Temperature <96°F (35.6°C)	Hypothermia
Arrhythmia	Suicide risk
	Intractable vomiting
	Hematemesis
	Failure to respond to outpatient treatment

Box 2.4 Key Clinical Findings Associated with Weight Loss

History	Physical Examination
Cold intolerance	Hypothermia, acrocyanosis, cold extremities
Fatigue, weakness	Decreased muscle mass
Dizziness, lightheadedness	Bradycardia with orthostasis
Difficulty concentrating	Normal neurologic examination
Early satiety	Scaphoid abdomen with no organomegaly
Amenorrhea	Dry skin, lanugo hair on body, loss of scalp hair

Treatment. The assessment of an eating disorder should focus on health and the exploration of underlying factors. The first step in assessment is to determine if weight loss is intentional and to detect any unrecognized medical disorders.

Various levels of care are usually required for patients with eating disorders including intensive outpatient, partial hospitalization, or residential treatment centers. Behavioral therapy, nutritional support/monitoring, psychotherapy, and antidepressants are often necessary.

The other "eating disorder" affecting the adolescent population in epidemic proportions is obesity. The prevalence of being overweight has nearly tripled in the last three decades in the United States. For a full discussion on this topic see the chapters on Prevention and Nutrition.

Mental Health

Substance Abuse

Early signs of substance abuse are the following:

- Mood changes, secretive and erratic behavior, distancing from the family or friends, or frequently in conflict with others.

Box 2.5 Signs of Substance Abuse

Early Signs of Substance Abuse

- Mood changes, secretive and erratic behavior, distancing from the family and family activities
- Being away from the home more, spending more time locked away in own room
- Abandoning old friends, associating with new friends, having strangers call and visit
- Change in appearance, dress, hygiene, taste in music, sleep behavior
- Things (perhaps alcohol, prescribed medications, jewelry, electronics) and money missing
- Physical signs, including cough (may request cough medicine), red eyes (may use ocular vasoconstrictor), dermatitis (may use lotions), sniffles and congestion (may use nose spray), bruises, changes in mental/neurologic status (including slurred speech, abnormal pupils)
- Odor of petrochemicals or alcohol on clothes or in room
- Conflicts with teachers, coaches, other young people

Later Signs of Substance Abuse

- Decline in school performance, truancy, loss of interest in extracurricular activities
- No association with old friends, who may, in fact, express concern
- Refusal to participate in family events or even leave own room
- Large blocks of unaccounted-for time, breaking curfews
- Finding drug paraphernalia in the home, including alcohol containers, pipes, rolling papers, empty containers of volatile substances
- Encounters with the police for theft, shoplifting, vagrancy

Adapted from Donald P. Orr, Margaret J. Blythe. Sexually transmitted diseases. In: Julia A. McMillan, Ralph D. Feigin, Catherine DeAngelis, M. Douglas Jones, Jr., eds. *Oski's Pediatrics: Principles & Practice*, 4th ed. Philadelphia, PA: Lippincott Williams & Wilkins, 2006.

- Being away from the home more or spending more time locked away in own room.
- Change in appearance, dress, hygiene, taste in music, sleep behavior.
- Physical signs, including cough (may request cough medicine), red eyes (may use ocular vasoconstrictor), dermatitis (may use lotions), sniffles and congestion (may use nose spray), bruises, changes in mental/neurologic status (including slurred speech, abnormal pupils).

Later signs of substance abuse are the following:

- Decline in school performance, truancy, loss of interest in extracurricular activities, breaking curfews.
- No association with old friends, who may, in fact, express concern.
- Refusal to participate in family events or even leave own room.
- Finding drug paraphernalia in the home, including alcohol containers, pipes, rolling papers, empty containers of volatile substances.
- Encounters with the police for theft, shoplifting, vagrancy.

Between 50% and 80% of drug-using teens suffer concurrently with a coexisting psychiatric disorder.

Treatment. Substance abuse counseling, self-help groups, and close clinical follow up are used to treat adolescents with substance abuse problems.

Depression

Definition: Depression is a pervasive emotional disorder manifested by negative mood. Irritability, deterioration in school performance, difficulty in peer relationships, and problems in conduct may be the presenting symptoms.

Diagnostic Criteria for Major Depressive Episode (Box 2.6):

Five (or more) of the following symptoms have been present during the same 2-week period and represent a change from previous functioning; at least one of the symptoms is either (1) depressed mood or (2) loss of interest or pleasure.

- Depressed mood most of the day, sadness or in children and adolescents can be irritable mood.
- Markedly diminished interest or pleasure in activities most of the day.
- Weight loss when not dieting or weight gain.
- Insomnia or hypersomnia nearly every day.
- Psychomotor agitation or retardation nearly every day.
- Fatigue or loss of energy nearly every day.
- Feelings of worthlessness or excessive or inappropriate guilt.
- Diminished ability to think or concentrate, or indecisiveness.
- Recurrent thoughts of death (not just fear of dying), recurrent suicidal ideation without a specific plan, or a suicide attempt or a specific plan for committing suicide.

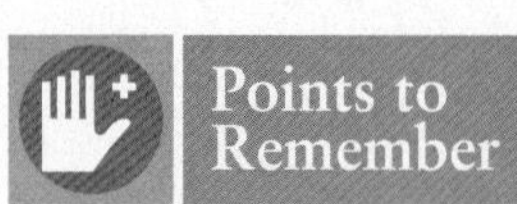

- Fluoxetine is the only antidepressant approved by the United States Food and Drug Administration for the treatment of children and adolescents.

Treatment

- Patients with mild depressive symptoms may respond to counseling, problem-solving discussions, and education of family members.
- For more severe depressive symptoms, referral to a child psychiatrist/psychologist is necessary.
- Other treatment approaches include pharmacotherapy with antidepressants such as selective-serotonin reuptake inhibitors either alone or in combination with psychotherapy, cognitive behavioral therapy, and interpersonal therapy.

Psychotic Disorders

Schizophrenia. Schizophrenia is a chronic deterioration from a previous level of functioning for at least 6 months with psychotic features and without organic etiology or drug abuse. Typical age of onset is late adolescence and earlier onset is associated with worse prognosis.

The characteristic features include the following:

- Disorders in thinking—Thoughts are often incoherent, and the train of thought is lost.
- Delusional beliefs, which may take on a paranoid form in older children.
- Hallucinatory experience—A false perception that occurs without external sensory stimulation. Hallucinations are primarily auditory and are described as voices outside the child or adolescent's head that may speak with him or her directly or make reference to him or her in the third person.
- Disturbance of mobility—Purposeless agitation, catatonia, extreme negativism, abnormal posturing, mutism, echolalia, or echopraxia.

Treatment. Referral to child psychiatrist with parental education and counseling.

Atypical antipsychotics are most commonly used to treat schizophrenia.

Bipolar Disorder. Bipolar disorder is characterized by episodes of depression with manic or hypomanic episodes. During a manic or hypomanic episode, mood is elevated, and rapid and

Box 2.6 Diagnostic Criteria for Major Depressive Episode

A. Five (or more) of the following symptoms have been present during the same 2-week period and represent a change from previous functioning; at least one of the symptoms is either (1) depressed mood or (2) loss of interest or pleasure. Note: Symptoms that are clearly due to a general medical condition or mood-incongruent delusions or hallucinations should not be included.
   1. Depressed mood most of the day, nearly every day, as indicated by either subjective report (e.g., feels sad or empty) or observation made by others (e.g., appears tearful). Note: In children and adolescents, can be irritable mood.
   2. Markedly diminished interest or pleasure in all, or almost all, activities most of the day, nearly every day (as indicated by either subjective account or observation made by others).
   3. Significant weight loss when not dieting or weight gain (e.g., a change of more than 5% of body weight in a month), or decrease or increase in appetite nearly every day. Note: In children, consider failure to make expected weight gains.
   4. Insomnia or hypersomnia nearly every day.
   5. Psychomotor agitation or retardation nearly every day (observable by others, not merely subjective feelings of restlessness or being slowed down).
   6. Fatigue or loss of energy nearly every day.
   7. Feelings of worthlessness or excessive or inappropriate guilt (which may be delusional) nearly every day (not merely self-reproach or guilt about being sick).
   8. Diminished ability to think or concentrate, or indeci-siveness, nearly every day (either by subjective account or as observed by others).
   9. Recurrent thoughts of death (not just fear of dying) recurrent suicidal ideation, without a specific plan, or a suicide attempt or a specific plan for committing suicide.

B. The symptoms do not meet criteria for a mixed episode (manic episode and depressive episode).

C. The symptoms cause clinically significant distress or impairment in social, occupational, or other important areas of functioning.

D. The symptoms are not due to the direct physiologic effects of a substance (e.g., a drug; of abuse, a medication) or a general medical condition (e.g., hypothyroidism).

E. The symptoms are not better accounted for by bereave ment (i.e., after the loss of a loved one); the symptoms persist for longer than 2 months or are characterized by marked functional impairment, morbid preoccupation with worthlessness, suicidal ideation, psychotic symptoms, or psychomotor retardation.

Reprinted with permission from American Psychiatric Association. *Diagnostic and statistical manual of mental disorders,* 4th ed. Text revision. Washington, DC: American Psychiatric Association, 2000.

pressured speech and irritability are observed. The patient may be overly energetic, disinhibited in their behavior, and sleep less than usual. For example, an affected adolescent may wear flamboyant clothing, drive a car recklessly, distribute gifts, and show inappropriate sexual behavior.

Treatment. *Pharmacologic*: Neuroleptic medications are used to deal with acute symptoms, and initiation of a mood stabilizer (lithium carbonate or sodium valproate) may be added for long-term treatment.

Psychotherapy: Supportive psychotherapy for the child and family is needed to deal with the consequences of the irrational behavior and its effects on family and friends.

Somatoform Disorders

The somatoform disorders are a group of psychological disorders in which a patient experiences physical symptoms despite the absence of an underlying medical condition that can fully explain their presence.

Conversion Disorder. The most common somatoform disorders of adolescence are conversion disorders or conversion reaction. This is a psychophysiologic process in which unpleasant feelings such as anxiety, depression, and/or guilt are expressed as a physical symptom. This may be an unconscious manifestation.

Common symptoms include seizures, paralysis, dizziness, syncope, hyperventilation, abdominal pain, nausea and vomiting, or mimicking a close relative's symptoms (e.g., chest pain in a girl whose father died of a heart attack).

Somatization Disorder

- Four different pain sites (e.g., head, abdomen, back, joints, extremities, chest, rectum) or functions (e.g., menstruation, sexual intercourse, urination).
- Two gastrointestinal symptoms other than pain (e.g., nausea, bloating, vomiting not caused by diarrhea, or intolerance of several different foods).
- One sexual or reproductive symptom other than pain (e.g., erectile or ejaculatory dysfunction, irregular menses, excessive menstrual bleeding).
- One pseudoneurological symptom (e.g., impaired balance, paralysis, aphonia, urinary retention).

Pain Disorder. A pain disorder is a variant of conversion disorder if the symptoms are dominated by pain dysfunction.

Body Dysmorphic Disorder. Body dysmorphic disorder is the preoccupation with an imagined defect in appearance or excessive concern over a slight physical anomaly. The distressing preoccupation may involve any part of the body.

Hypochondriasis. Hypochondriasis is defined as a preoccupation with fears of having or the idea that one has a serious disease based on misinterpretation of bodily symptoms. This preoccupation persists despite appropriate medical evaluation and reassurance.

Laboratory Evaluation. If indicated, specific studies used to rule out somatization due to general medical conditions including the following:

- Thyroid function studies.
- Pheochromocytoma screen.
- Drug screen (urine and serum) for agents including cannabis, amphetamine, hallucinogens, cocaine, opioids, benzodiazepines.
- Referral for psychological testing.

Treatment. Medication is rarely helpful. Referral for psychotherapy is recommended and regular appointments should be scheduled with the patient and family to encourage compliance with psychotherapy. The goals are to maintain or improve overall functioning, care for the patient, and rule out concurrent physical disorders.

Behavioral Health Issues

Disruptive Behavior Disorders

Oppositional Defiant Disorder. An ongoing pattern of uncooperative, defiant, and hostile behavior toward authority figures that seriously interferes with the individual's daily functioning and persists for at least 6 months.

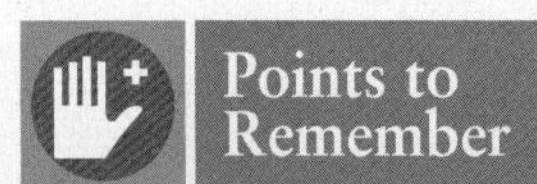

- Consent and Confidentiality: Covered in Preventive Pediatrics, Biostatistics, & Ethics Chapter

Conduct Disorder. This disorder refers to a group of behavioral and emotional problems that are viewed by others to be "bad" or delinquent, rather than mentally ill. Some behaviors of patients with conduct disorder include aggression to people and animals, destruction of property, deceitfulness, lying, stealing, truancy, or criminal offenses.

Treatment. Behavior therapy and psychotherapy are usually necessary to help the patient appropriately express and control anger. Treatment is more successful when initiated early and must include medical, mental health, and educational components as well as family support.

Important Concepts in the Care of Adolescents

Consent is a function of the adolescent's capacity to understand treatment choices presented to him or her, including the risks and benefits, and to choose among them. A minor who is not emancipated is capable of consenting to and refusing medical care in most circumstances, as long as he or she is of reasonable intelligence and is able to understand the implications of what is being said or recommended.

Confidentiality refers to the control and protection of health information shared between the adolescent and the physician. To gain the trust and confidence of a young person, some statement of confidentiality should be made. Confidentiality must have limits, however, and children or adolescents who are severely ill or in danger of hurting themselves or others must receive help even if confidentiality is breached.

SAMPLE BOARD REVIEW QUESTIONS

1. An 11-year-old girl presents for routine health maintenance examination. She is concerned about frequent vaginal discharge seen on her underwear. She is otherwise asymptomatic and denies vaginal itching, dysuria, or abdominal pain. She is premenarcheal. On your examination you note sticky, whitish vaginal discharge on her underwear. On physical examination, she has sparse pubic hair growth and breast tissue only palpable below the areola. Microscopic examination of a saline preparation of the discharge reveals many epithelial cells. The vaginal pH is less than 4.5. Of the following, the most appropriate next step in the management of this patient is
   a. Culture of the discharge for bacteria
   b. Explanation and reassurance
   c. Pelvic ultrasound
   d. Treatment with ceftriaxone and doxycycline
   e. Sitz baths

   Answer: B. Physiologic leukorrhea—discharge caused by the desquamation of vaginal epithelial cells in response to the effect of estrogen on the vaginal mucosa at the onset of puberty.

2. You are evaluating a 17-year-old girl who has anorexia nervosa for possible hospital admission. Of the following physical findings, the most appropriate indication for hospitalization includes
   a. Bradycardia
   b. Hypertension
   c. Pedal edema
   d. Fever
   e. Tachypnea

   Answer: A. Refer to Table 2.9 for criteria for hospital admission for a patient with anorexia.

3. A 15-year-old boy presents to your office with complaints of breast development over the past 2 months. Physical examination reveals a palpable disk of rubbery, freely mobile, breast tissue directly under the areola. He is otherwise well appearing and has a Sexual Maturity Rating of 3 by genital examination. Which of the following screening health maintenance questions would be MOST pertinent given his examination findings?
   a. Marijuana use/abuse
   b. History of sexually transmitted diseases
   c. Educational level attained
   d. Home environment
   e. History of depression

   Answer: A. One of the pathologic causes of gynecomastia includes marijuana use/abuse.

4. A 16-year-old girl presents with a history of dysmenorrhea that has caused her to miss multiple days of school during her menses. She has tried naproxen with some improvement but is interested in treatment with oral contraceptives. Of the following, an absolute contraindication for the use of oral contraceptives in this patient is a history of
   a. Smoking
   b. Breast fibroadenoma
   c. Atrial septal defect
   d. STIs
   e. Migraine with aura

   Answer: E. Contraindications to using OCPs include pregnancy, lactation (recommended to wait 6 weeks postpartum), history of thromboembolic or cerebrovascular disease, breast cancer, structural heart disease, severe migraines, liver disease, severe hypertension, major surgery with prolonged immobilization.

5. A 14-year-old girl complains of lower abdominal cramps during the first few days of her menstrual cycle. These cramps are often associated with feeling "bloated" and loose bowel movements. Sometimes the cramps are so severe she has had to miss school. She has tried acetaminophen in the past but says that it "does nothing." Her menstrual cycle occurs regularly, lasts 6 days and began when she was 11 years of age. Which of the following is the most appropriate management for these symptoms?

a. Peppermint tea
b. Acetaminophen with codeine
c. Naproxen sodium
d. Fluoxetine
e. Montelukast

Answer: C. Primary dysmenorrhea is caused by prostaglandin release; Naproxen sodium is a long acting NSAID, which has been shown to effectively inhibit prostaglandin release.

6. A 16-year-old girl presents to your office with a 6-month history of amenorrhea. Eight months ago she joined the swimming team at school and has subsequently gotten very involved in dance. Prior to her athletic participation her menstrual cycle occurred every 28 days. Before her periods stopped altogether she noticed her menstrual flow was decreased. She has lost 3 to 4 pounds since your last visit but her BMI remains 50%. She denies a desire to lose weight or purging. You suspect exercise as the cause for her amenorrhea. Of the following, what is most likely to be associated with stress fractures and low bone density in this patient?
a. Early onset puberty
b. Use of antidepressant medication
c. Average BMI
d. Use of oral contraceptives
e. Cigarette smoking

Answer: E. Cigarette smoking increases the risk for stress fractures. This patient should also be advised to reduce the intensity of her athletic training and to increase her calorie and calcium intake. To prevent further bone mineralization, it is important to restore the natural rhythm of her menstrual cycle.

7. A 17-year-old girl presents to the emergency department complaining of right upper quadrant pain, nausea, and occasional right shoulder pain. She is sexually active and has been using OCPs for the past year. An ultrasound of her gallbladder is normal and a urine pregnancy test result is negative. What is the next most important step in evaluation of this patient's symptoms?
a. Hydrogen breath test
b. Ultrasound of the abdomen
c. CT scan of the liver
d. Hepatobiliary scintography
e. Pelvic examination

Answer: E. The next most appropriate step is a pelvic examination to assess for signs of salpingitis or PID. This patient's symptoms raise suspicion for Fitz-Hugh-Curtis or perihepatitis, which is a complication of PID. Treatment of PID often results in significant improvement of the right upper quadrant pain within 48 hours.

8. A 15-year-old boy presents with complaints of missing her menses for the past 8 months. She is a star gymnast and has been successful in numerous national competitions. She has been competing regularly over the past year and has lost 25 lb in the process. Her height plots in the 50th percentile and her weight in the 5th percentile. You make a diagnosis of secondary amenorrhea. Which of the following tests may be the most likely to be abnormal given her history?
a. Prolactin level
b. Head MRI
c. Bone density
d. TSH level
e. Pelvic ultrasound

Answer: C. The patient's presentation is highly consistent with the female athlete triad of amenorrhea, disordered eating, and osteoporosis.

9. The mother of your 15-year-old patient with depression recently obtained a mental health referral for further testing and treatment of her son. She calls you with concerns about the safety and efficacy of psychiatric medications in adolescents. You explain to her that the antidepressant approved by the Food and Drug Administration and often recommended for adolescents is
a. Fluoxetine
b. Amitriptyline
c. Citalopram
d. Bupropion
e. Sertraline

Answer: A.

10. You are asked by a local high school principle to give a presentation on adolescent substance abuse to the Parent Teacher Association. Of the following statements about adolescents, which is most true?

a. Homosexual youth have the lowest rates of alcohol and marijuana use
b. Since 1980 marijuana use among 12th graders has decreased
c. Daily use of cigarettes has decreased among 8th graders over the last 10 years
d. Athletes who use drugs to enhance their athletic performance are less likely to use other illicit drugs
e. Inhalant use is more prevalent among 8th grade students than 12th grade students

Answer: E. Inhalant use is more common among the younger adolescents although across all age groups alcohol continues to be the most widely used drug of use and abuse.

SUGGESTED READINGS

Brigham KS, Goldstein MA. Adolescent immunizations. *Pediatr Rev*. 2009;30:47–56.

Centers for Disease Control and Prevention. 2006. Guidelines for treatment of sexually transmitted diseases. *MMWR Morb Mortal Wkly Rep*. 2006;55(No. RR-11):1–100.

Centers for Disease Control and Prevention. Updated recommended treatment regimens for gonococcal infections and associated conditions—United States, April 2007. Available online only at http://www.cdc.gov/STD/treatment/2006/updated-regimens.htm. Accessed July 11, 2010.

Emans SJ. Amenorrhea in the adolescent. In: Emans SJ, Laufer MR, Goldstein DP, eds. *Pediatric and Adolescent Gynecology*. 5th ed. Philadelphia, PA: Lippincott Williams & Wilkins; 2005:214–269.

Jellinek M. Depression. In: Parker S, Zuckerman B, Augustyn M, eds. *Developmental and Behavioral Pediatrics: A Handbook for Primary Care*. 2nd ed. Philadelphia, PA: Lippincott Williams & Wilkins; 2005:163–166.

Neinstein LS. Breast disease in adolescents and young women. *Pediatr Clin North Am*. 1999;46:607–629.

Prager LM. Depression and suicide in children and adolescents. *Pediatr Rev*. 2009;30:199–206.

CHAPTER 3 ■ ALLERGY & IMMUNOLOGY

RAEGAN D. HUNT

ADA	Adenosine deaminase	MMR	Measles, mumps, and rubella vaccine
AFP	Alpha fetoprotein		
ANC	Absolute neutrophil count	NADPH	Nicotinamide adenine dinucleotide phosphate (reduced form)
ATM	Ataxia telangiectasia-mutated		
CGD	Chronic granulomatous disease		
CH50	Total hemolytic complement	NBT	Nitroblue tetrazolium
CVID	Common variable immunodeficiency	NK cells	Natural killer cells
		PCP	*Pneumocystis jiroveci*
CXR	Chest x-ray	PFTs	Pulmonary function tests
FISH	Fluorescent in situ hybridization	RAST	Radioallergosorbent testing
GI	Gastrointestinal	SCID	Severe combined immunodeficiency
GVHD	Graft versus host disease		
IgG	Immunoglobulin G	SBDS	Shwachman-Bodian-Diamond syndrome
IVIG	Intravenous immunoglobulin		
LAD	Leukocyte adhesion deficiency	TMP-SMX	Trimethoprim-sulfamethoxazole
MAC	Membrane attack complex		

CHAPTER OBJECTIVES

1. To recognize signs and symptoms that should prompt an evaluation for an immunodeficiency
2. To differentiate between the major categories of immunodeficiencies
3. To understand the classic features, diagnosis, and treatment of the most common immunodeficiency syndromes in children
4. To understand the pathophysiology of allergic diseases in children
5. To understand the clinical manifestations, diagnosis, and treatment of common allergic diseases in children.

PRIMARY IMMUNODEFICIENCY

Children with normal immune systems may have an average of one routine, self-resolving illness per month. **Immunodeficiency syndromes should be considered in children with recurrent infections, infections with unusual organisms, severe infections, and/or failure to thrive.**

Immunodeficiencies manifest differently based on which component of the immune system is affected. The four major categories are (1) defective antibody-mediated immunity, (2) defective cell-mediated immunity, (3) defective complement function, and (4) defects in phagocytosis. Specific laboratory tests are available for each of the major limbs of the immune system. Susceptibility to certain types of infections guides clinical suspicion to the defective area of the immune system and informs efficient laboratory testing. Table 3.1 summarizes typical patterns of illness and screening tests for different categories of immunodeficiencies.

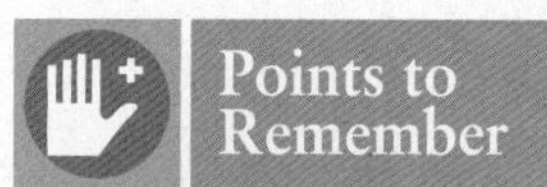

- **Many immunodeficiency syndromes are X-linked—be especially suspicious in boys.**
- **Many immunodeficiency syndromes are associated with increased risk of malignancy and autoimmune disorders.**

ANTIBODY-MEDIATED (B-CELL) IMMUNODEFICIENCY

Defects in antibody-mediated immunity result from **inability to produce normal levels of immunoglobulins** and represent **the most common primary immunodeficiencies.** Patients who suffer from these disorders experience frequent infections with *Streptococcus pneumoniae*, *Haemophilus influenzae*, *Staphylococcus aureus*, and *Pseudomonas* species, as well as giardia. They often fail to improve with standard antibiotic treatment courses. Diagnosis is confirmed by

TABLE 3.1

PATTERNS OF ILLNESS AND LABORATORY TESTING FOR PRIMARY IMMUNODEFICIENCIES

Disorder	Infection Susceptibility	Laboratory Test
Antibody mediated (Humoral)	Illness beginning after 6 months when maternal antibodies wane Infections with encapsulated bacteria *Haemophilus influenzae, pneumococcus, staphylococcus, giardia*	Quantitative immunoglobulin levels (IgM, IgG, IgA) Antibody response to vaccines (titers)
Cell mediated	Fungal infections (especially aspergillus and candida) Unusually severe viral infections Pneumocystis, mycobacteria	Lymphocyte count T-cell subsets (CD4, CD8) Delayed type hypersensitivity reaction (*candida* skin test)
Complement	*Neisseria meningitidis and Neisseria gonorrhea* Sepsis with encapsulated bacteria	Total hemolytic complement (CH50)
Phagocytes	Abscesses, skin infections Poor wound healing *Mycobacteria, fungal infections* Catalase-positive organisms *(Staphylococcus, Escherichia coli, serratia, klebsiella, pseudomonas, aspergillus)*	White blood cell count with differential Nitroblue tetrazolium test Chemotaxis assay

quantifying specific total immunoglobulin levels or by evaluating antibody response to vaccines. Treatment of these disorders generally consists of prophylactic antibiotics and/or IVIG infusions.

Points to Remember

- Defects in humoral immunity account for almost 50% of primary immunodeficiencies in kids.
- Antibody-mediated immunodeficiency syndromes often manifest around 6 months of age as maternal IgG antibody levels in the infant decline.
- Risks of long-term IVIG treatment include exposure to bloodborne pathogens and insidious-onset chronic lung disease (check PFTs every 1 to 2 years).
- Some important encapsulated bacteria are S. pneumoniae, group B streptococcus, H. influenzae type b, and Neisseria meningitidis.

Bruton's Agammaglobulinemia

Bruton's agammaglobulinemia is an **X-linked** disorder and therefore affects only **males**. Development of the B-lymphocyte lineage is disrupted in these patients because of a deficiency of Bruton's tyrosine kinase enzyme. Because of the lack of B cells, antibodies cannot be produced. This illness typically manifests at about 6 months of life, when protection from maternal antibodies subsides.

Clinical Manifestations

- **Small or absent tonsils,** no palpable lymph nodes.
- Susceptibility to **pyogenic bacterial infections of the respiratory tract, skin, and joints.**
- Risk of life-threatening ***pseudomonal*** **infections.**
- **Enterovirus infections** (e.g., Coxsackie, polio) are severe and can be fatal.

Diagnosis

- Suggested by absent or very low levels of all immunoglobulin classes.
- Confirmation: demonstrate absence of B cells on flow cytometry (<1% of normal values).

Treatment

- Targeted treatment of associated infections.
- IVIG replacement every 3 to 4 weeks.
- Avoidance of live virus vaccines.

Points to Remember

- Live vaccines (e.g., MMR, varicella) in children with primary or acquired immunodeficiency can lead to life-threatening infection with vaccine viruses.

Common Variable Immunodeficiency

CVID describes a heterogeneous group of disorders characterized by hypogammaglobulinemia with phenotypically normal B cells that fail to mature appropriately into antibody-producing plasma cells. No recognizable pattern of inheritance exists for most patients, although there is clearly a genetic component. The infection susceptibility pattern is similar to that for X-linked agammaglobulinemia, although most patients do not manifest symptoms until after the first decade of life.

Points to Remember

- In contrast to Bruton's X-linked agammaglobulinemia, CVID occurs equally in both sexes, and lymphoid tissue and B-cell numbers are normal.

Clinical Manifestations

- Susceptibility to infections of the upper and lower respiratory tract (e.g., pneumonia, sinusitis, etc.).
- Chronic diarrhea due to infectious agents (e.g., giardia, etc.), bacterial overgrowth, and/or inflammatory bowel diseases.
- Increased risk of lymphoma, amyloidosis, rheumatologic disorders, and noncaseating granulomas of the spleen, liver, lungs, and skin.

Diagnosis

- Hypogammaglobulinemia with normal B-cell numbers.

Treatment

- Targeted treatment of associated infections.
- IVIG replacement.
- Many patients with CVID require immunosuppressive treatment for their rheumatologic disorders.

Selective IgA Deficiency

IgA deficiency is the most common immunodeficiency syndrome, occurring in approximately 1 out of 600 people. Incidence is increased in families with CVID. IgA-deficient patients do not have IgA to protect their **mucosal surfaces** and, as a result, are more susceptible to bacterial and viral infections involving mucosal surfaces.

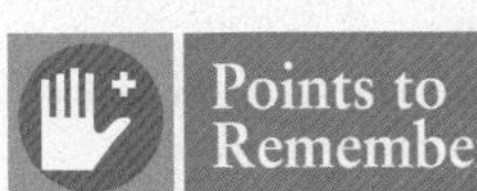

- **Patients with IgA deficiency should receive blood products only from other individuals with IgA deficiency because trace amounts of IgA may trigger anaphylaxis. Think about undiagnosed IgA deficiency in a patient with anaphylaxis to a blood product.**

Clinical Manifestations

- Typically asymptomatic or mild.
- Increased susceptibility to bacterial and viral respiratory infections, urinary tract infections, and GI tract infections.
- **Anaphylaxis from blood transfusions** and IVIG-containing IgA.
- Can be associated with a sprue-like syndrome.

Diagnosis

- Serum IgA <5 mg/dL.

Treatment

- Targeted treatment of associated infections.
- IVIG is not indicated as these patients make IgG normally.
- If present, sprue-like syndrome may respond to a gluten-free diet.

IgG Subclass Deficiency

IgG is made up of four subclasses (IgG1, IgG2, IgG3, IgG4) that differ in biological activity. The IgG immune response to protein antigens versus polysaccharide antigens differs by subclass.

Clinical Manifestations

- Recurrent upper respiratory tract infections caused by the polysaccharide-encapsulated pathogens (similar to those that affect patients with B-cell deficiency).

Diagnosis

- Total IgG levels are normal to borderline low.
- Specific IgG subclasses (IgG1, IgG2, IgG3, IgG4) are low.
- Antibody response to T-cell–dependent vaccines (e.g., diphtheria and tetanus toxoid) and T-cell–independent vaccines (e.g., unconjugated pneumococcal polysaccharide) may be inappropriate.

Treatment

- Targeted treatment of associated infections.
- IVIG therapy is indicated only if patient lacks response to a wide variety of antigens.
- May benefit from antibiotic prophylaxis.

Hyper IgM Syndrome

IgM is the first antibody generated in response to an antigen, and class switch recombination allows for the subsequent production of antigen-specific IgA, IgG, and IgE. Patients with hyper

IgM syndrome have a defect in the class switch recombination mechanism. Several genetic variants of this syndrome exist. One variant is X-liked recessive and associated with ectodermal dysplasia.

Clinical Manifestations

- Susceptible to the infection pattern typical of humoral immunodeficiencies.
- Many patients also have abnormal T-cell function and are susceptible to infections caused by opportunistic organisms such as PCP, *Cryptococcus neoformans*, cryptosporidium, and mycobacteria.

Diagnosis

- Normal or increased levels of IgM with reduced levels of IgA, IgG, and IgE.

Treatment

- Targeted treatment of associated infections.
- Monthly IVIG replacement.

Transient Hypogammaglobulinemia of Infancy

Transient hypogammaglobulinemia of infancy describes a transient delay of antibody production. While a few of these patients progress to develop a true primary immunodeficiency, **most regain normal immune function by 3 to 6 years of age.**

Clinical Manifestations

- Increased susceptibility to recurrent infection of the respiratory and GI tracts.
- Sepsis and meningitis are rare but can occur.

Diagnosis

- Low immunoglobulin levels with normal B lymphocyte numbers.
- Predicted antibody rise in response to vaccinations may be delayed.

Treatment

- Targeted treatment of associated infections.
- Most can be managed expectantly and do not require IVIG.

T-CELL IMMUNITY DISORDERS

T-cell immunity is critical for protection against viral, fungal, and intracellular infections. Because of decreased immune surveillance, patients with defective T-cell function also have increased susceptibility to certain malignancies and autoimmune disorders. Furthermore, disorders of T-cell function often result in compromised B-cell antibody production because B-cells require support from T cells to function properly. These combination immunodeficiency states are severe with great morbidity and decreased survival and are discussed in the following section. DiGeorge syndrome is the only recognized, isolated congenital T-cell immunodeficiency. HIV infection results in acquired isolated T-cell immunodeficiency.

Diagnosis of T-cell disorders may be difficult and often requires specialized laboratory services. Lymphopenia is often present, as the majority of circulating lymphocytes in normal children are T cells. Abnormal T cells will fail to proliferate in vitro with mitogen stimulation tests. Patients with T-cell immunodeficiency are anergic (do not respond to skin antigen testing for delayed type hypersensitivity).

DiGeorge Syndrome

DiGeorge syndrome, also known as 22q deletion syndrome, results from abnormal development of the third and fourth branchial pouches. This leads to a characteristic pattern of abnormalities which includes thymic hypoplasia. Because thymus tissue is required for normal T-cell maturation, defective T-cell immunity results. The severity of immunodeficiency in DiGeorge syndrome depends on the degree of thymic hypoplasia.

Points to Remember

- DiGeorge syndrome typically presents in infancy with facial dysmorphism, cardiac disease, and/or hypocalcemic tetany.

Points to Remember

- The pneumonic "CATCH 22" can be used to remember the features of DiGeorge syndrome: Cardiac defects, Abnormal facies, Thymic hypoplasia, Cleft palate, Hypocalcemia, and 22q deletion.

Clinical Manifestations ("CATCH-22")

- C—Cardiac defects (conotruncal congenital heart defects including tetralogy of Fallot, truncus arteriosus, interrupted aortic arch, and/or ventricular septal defects; can also see vascular rings).
- A—Abnormal facies (e.g., micrognathia, low set ears, short philtrum, small mouth) (see Fig. 3.1).
- T—Thymic hypoplasia and T-cell immunodeficiency.
- C—Cleft palate.
- H—Hypoparathyroidism (10% to 30% of patients have hypocalcemic tetany from hypoparathyroidism during the first week of life).

Diagnosis

- Suggested by characteristic facies, hypocalcemia, and/or **absence of thymic shadow on CXR.**
- Confirmation via FISH for 22q11 deletion.
- May have lymphopenia and poor response to mitogen proliferation tests.

Treatment

- Repair of any associated cardiac defects and/or cleft palate.
- Calcium supplementation.
- Patients with severe T-cell immunodeficiency may require thymic tissue or bone marrow transplantation.

Chronic Mucocutaneous Candidiasis

Chronic mucocutaneous candidiasis is a syndrome of chronic candidal infections of **mucosa, skin, and nails** that generally manifests before the age of 3 years. The susceptibility to candidal infection may be the result of defects in general T-cell immunity or may be due to the lack of specific anticandidal response. Chronic mucocutaneous candidiasis has a good prognosis as infections are not generally invasive. There is a rare, but serious risk of mycotic aneurysms. The syndrome may occur in the context of DiGeorge syndrome, AIDS, thymoma,

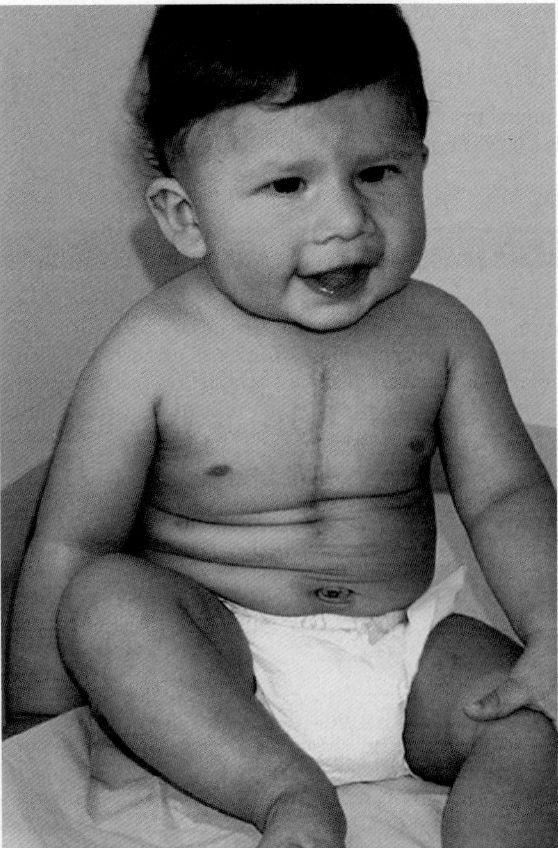

FIGURE 3.1. An infant with DiGeorge syndrome. The surgical scar on the chest indicates repair of heart disease caused by truncus arteriosus or interrupted aortic arch, which is common in this syndrome. The infant also has the facial features of a child with DiGeorge syndrome, as illustrated by hypertelorism, low-set ears, hypoplastic mandible, and bowing upward of the upper lip. (Reprinted with permission from Roberts R. *Atlas of Infectious Diseases*. In: Wilfert CM, ed. Mandell G, series ed. Philadelphia, PA: Current Medicine, Inc. Copyright 1998.)

or other T-cell deficiency syndromes. There is an inherited form of chronic mucocutaneous candidiasis that is associated with multiple endocrinological abnormalities and ectodermal dystrophy.

COMBINED IMMUNODEFICIENCY DISORDERS

Because B cells depend on T cells to present antigens for antibody production, most congenital T-cell disorders result in both B-cell and T-cell immunodeficiency. Patients with combined B-cell and T-cell immunodeficiency exhibit low immunoglobulin levels, abnormal response to delayed type hypersensitivity testing, and low circulating lymphocyte counts. Most combined B-cell and T-cell immunodeficiencies manifest within the first year of life and are quite severe.

Severe Combined Immunodeficiency

SCID is a group of genetic disorders that result in severe T-cell dysfunction and resultant humoral immunodeficiency. Autosomal recessive and X-linked forms of SCID exist. Approximately 40% of autosomal recessive SCID is due to **ADA deficiency**. The incidence of SCID is high within the Navajo population, and because some forms are X-linked, there is a slight predominance in males. SCID **presents in infancy**; the mean age of diagnosis is 6 months. The immune deficiency is severe, and most children die of infection during the first 2 years of life without immune reconstitution or strict isolation.

Clinical Manifestations

- Failure to thrive.
- Increased susceptibility to pneumonia, diarrhea, sepsis, skin infections, recurrent thrush, and opportunistic infections such as PCP pneumonia.
- Patients with SCID may suffer from **GVHD** from engrafted maternal T cells or cells within nonirradiated blood transfusions. GVHD manifestations include morbilliform erythroderma, lymphadenopathy, hepatosplenomegaly, and GI disease.
- ADA-deficient patients with SCID may have bony abnormalities, and a CXR with a radiographic appearance similar to the rachitic rosary may suggest the diagnosis.

Diagnosis

- Lymphopenia, decreased T-cell subpopulations, and hypogammaglobulinemia.
- Genetic testing for known mutations.

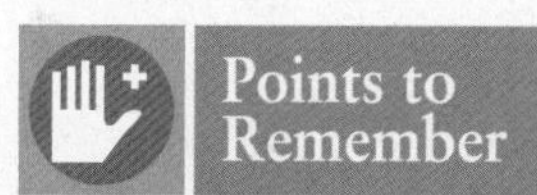

- **"Severe" is the key word in SCID—without treatment, most patients with SCID will die of infection within the first year or two of life.**

Treatment

- Bone marrow transplant is curative.
- IVIG replacement and PCP prophylaxis until bone marrow transplantation can be performed.
- Enzyme replacement therapy has some efficacy in ADA-deficient patients with SCID but the immunocompetence achieved is less than with bone marrow transplant.

Ataxia Telangiectasia

Ataxia telangiectasia is an **autosomal recessive** disorder due to a genetic defect in ATM, a **DNA repair enzyme**. It is characterized by **oculocutaneous telangiectasias, progressive ataxia**, and **combined B- and T-cell immunodeficiency**. The immunodeficiency component is variable and progressive and results from accumulation of unrepaired mutations in immunoglobulin and T-cell receptor genes.

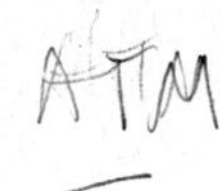

Clinical Manifestations

- Truncal ataxia (onset during first few years of life; progressive with patients becoming wheelchair bound in adolescence).
- Telangiectasias (usually absent at birth, develop in early childhood).
- Combined immunodeficiency (usually does not present within the first year of life).
- Increased risk of leukemia and lymphoma due to impaired immune surveillance.
- Cognitive deficits are common.

Diagnosis

- Normal IgM and IgG levels; specific deficiencies of IgA and IgG2.
- Elevated serum AFP.
- Definitive diagnosis via sequencing the ATM gene and measuring the ATM protein level.

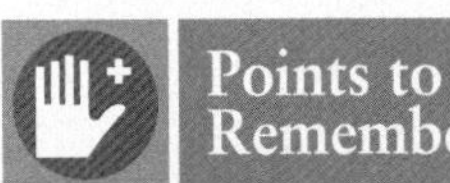

■ The most common causes of death in patients with ataxia telangiectasia (often in the second or third decades of life) are lymphoreticular malignancies and progressive neurologic disease.
■ Ocular telangiectasias in patients with ataxia telangiectasia can be mistaken for conjunctivitis.

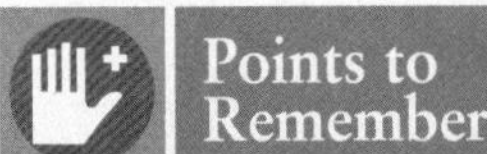

■ Abnormally small platelets are strongly suggestive of Wiskott-Aldrich syndrome.
■ Splenectomy may be required to manage the thrombocytopenia in Wiskott-Aldrich syndrome, further increasing the risk of infection from encapsulated bacteria.

Treatment

- Primarily supportive.
- Immunodeficiency is treated with IVIG, targeted therapy of associated infections, and avoidance of live vaccines.

Wiskott-Aldrich Syndrome

Wiskott-Aldrich syndrome is an X-linked recessive combined immunodeficiency disorder characterized by small platelet size, thormboctopenia, and eczema. The average age of diagnosis is 8 months, and the average age of death is 8 years.

Clinical Manifestations

- Severe flexural eczematous rash.
- Easy bleeding/bruising and petechiae.
- Combined immunodeficiency.
- Recurrent otitis media, sinusitis, and pneumonia.
- Early in life, most infections are due to encapsulated bacteria, especially *S. pneumoniae.*
- Opportunistic infections become a problem later in life.
- Increased risk of autoimmune disease and malignancy.
- EBV-induced lymphoreticular infection is an important cause of death.

Diagnosis

- T-cell lymphopenia.
- Normal IgG, decreased IgM, and increased IgA and IgE.
- Peripheral smear reveals thrombocytopenia and small platelets.

Treatment

- Targeted therapy of associated infections.
- IVIG.
- Splenectomy for severe thrombocytopenia.
- Bone marrow transplant.

DISORDERS OF PHAGOCYTOSIS, CHEMOTAXIS, AND/OR CELL ADHERENCE

Disorders of phagocytosis, chemotaxis, and/or cell adherence are described in Table 3.2.

DISORDERS OF COMPLEMENT

Depending on which component is defective, disorders of complement result in susceptibility to **infection, angioedema,** and **autoimmune-like illnesses. The CH50 assay effectively screens for all disorders of the complement system.** After screening, specific testing can be done for individual proteins in the classical and alternative complement pathway. Disorders of both early and late complement components have **autosomal recessive** inheritance.

Early Complement Deficiency (C1-C4)

Early complement deficiencies predispose patients to **rheumatologic disorders,** including glomerulonephritis, as well as **pyogenic bacterial infections.** Defects in early complement impair opsonization of encapsulated bacteria such that bacteria recognized by specific IgG antibodies cannot be cleared. Thus, susceptibility to encapsulated bacteria such as pneumococcus and *H. influenzae* is characteristic of disorders of early complement and of the humoral (B-cell–mediated) immune system.

Late Complement Deficiency (C5-C9)

Deficiency in late (terminal) complement proteins results in defective MAC formation, leaving patients susceptible to recurrent infections with ***Neisseria meningitidis*** and ***Neisseria gonorrhea.*** Patients may develop disseminated gonococcal infections, meningococcal sepsis, and meningitis.

TABLE 3.2

DISORDERS OF PHAGOCYTOSIS, CHEMOTAXIS, AND CELL ADHERENCE

	Etiology	Genetics	Clinical Manifestations	Diagnosis	Treatment
Chronic granulomatous disease	Neutrophils lack NADPH-mediated "oxidative burst" that is critical for destruction of catalase-positive bacteria and some fungi	2/3 are X-linked 1/3 are autosomal recessive Autosomal dominant form has also been described	Recurrent abscesses in lymph nodes, skin, liver, spleen, and lungs Failure to thrive Granulomas in respiratory, GI, and urogenital tracts	Nitroblue tetrazolium test	Life-long prophylaxis with TMP-SMX Gamma interferon in severe cases
Hyper IgE recurrent infection syndrome (Job's syndrome)	Abnormal neutrophil migration	Autosomal dominant	Course facial features Delayed exfoliation of primary teeth Eczema Recurrent abscess and respiratory infections Recurrent fractures and increased risk of osteomyelitis	IgE >2,000 Eosinophilia Neutrophil chemotaxis assay	Antistaphylococcal antimicrobial prophylaxis
Chediak-Higashi syndrome	Impaired natural killer cell function, neutrophil chemotaxis, and phagocytosis	Autosomal recessive	Oculocutaneous albinism Easy bruising Recurrent skin and respiratory tract infections Severe gingivitis and periodontal disease Almost all develop a proliferative lymphoma-like illness prior to age 10 years; typically fatal	Giant granules in neutrophils, eosinophils, and granulocytes Variable amount of neutropenia and thrombocytopenia	Bone marrow transplantation
Leukocyte adhesion deficiency (LAD)	Impaired ability of leukocytes to attach to vessels and migrate to sites of infection		Recurrent nonpurulent local infections LAD-1 is associated with delayed separation of umbilical stump LAD-2 is associated with mental retardation and severe growth impairment	Flow cytometry to detect CD11/CD18 antigens on white blood cells	Bone marrow transplantation
Shwachman-Bodian-Diamond syndrome (SBDS)	Severe neutropenia and neutrophil chemotaxis abnormalities	Autosomal recessive	Growth retardation Pancreatic exocrine dysfunction Steatorrhea Chondrodysplasia Bone marrow hypoplasia Severe and recurrent infections Increased risk of leukemias	Neutropenia Genetic testing for the SBDS gene (7q11)	Pancreatic enzyme replacement Targeted antibiotic therapy
Kostmann syndrome	Severe congenital neutropenia	Autosomal recessive	Severe infections beginning in infancy Mortality in the first year of life is 70% without treatment	Severe neutropenia (ANC <200)	G-CSF Bone marrow or stem cell transplantation

ANC, absolute neutrophil count; IgE, immunoglobulin E; NADPH, nicotinamide adenine dinucleotide phosphate (reduced form); TMP-SMX, trimethoprim-sulfamethoxazole.

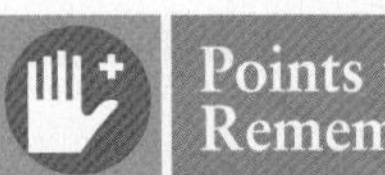

Points to Remember

- The X-linked form of CGD is often diagnosed in toddler age children; the autosomal recessive form is more often detected during the teenage years.
- Common microorganisms that cause infection in patients with CGD are as follows:
  - Gram positive, catalase-positive organisms—*S. aureus*
  - Gram negative, catalase-positive organisms—*Escherichia coli, Klebsiella, Enterobacter* species, *Serratia marcescens, Salmonellae* species, *Pseudomonas* species
  - Fungi—*Aspergillus* species, *Candida albicans*
- Shwachman-Bodian-Diamond syndrome should be considered in any infant or child with steatorrhea, depressed cell counts, poor growth, and recurrent infections.
- Despite severe neutropenia, patients with Kostmann syndrome often have normal total leukocyte counts because of an increased number of monocytes.
- LAD-1 is due to a defect in the CD18 adhesion molecule. LAD-2 is due to lack of proper expression of the Sialyl-Lewis-X protein that binds selectins.

ALLERGY

Allergic reactions are nonadaptive immune system responses to environmental stimuli due to overproduction of allergen-specific IgE. Chronic and acute exposures in sensitized individuals by contact, ingestion, or inhalation trigger symptoms varying from mild rhinitis to overwhelming anaphylaxis. Although the genetics are not completely understood, children of parents with allergic disease are at significantly increased risk of developing allergic disease. Other significant epidemiologic risk factors for allergic disease include early sensitization to allergens, exposure to tobacco smoke, and early introduction of cow milk and/or solid foods during infancy. Breastfeeding does not decrease the risk of allergic disease but may delay the onset.

Children with chronic allergic disease may be recognizable by characteristic physical findings:

- **Allergic crease**—horizontal line just proximal to the fleshy tip of the nose formed by repeatedly rubbing an itchy nose upwards.
- **Allergic shiners**—purplish discoloration beneath the lower eyelids due to venous stasis; present in 60% of allergic patients (Fig. 3.2).
- Dennie-Morgan folds—symmetric arced skin folds extending from inner canthus beneath the lower eyelid.

Certain laboratory studies and skin testing are also helpful in patients with suspected allergic disease:

- Peripheral blood eosinophilia.
- Elevated IgE levels.
- Presence of eosinophils in nasal and/or bronchial secretions.
- **RAST**: a serum test that quantifies the IgE level for a given antigen; less sensitive than skin testing but safer and not influenced by skin disease or medications.
- Skin testing: allergen is introduced intradermally into skin and causes IgE mediated local mast cell degranulation leading to a wheal and flare reaction; more sensitive than RAST testing but caries risk of anaphylaxis and is influenced by skin disease and medications.

Urticaria/Angioedema

Urticaria describes the formation of hives (pruritic, wheal-like skin lesions that come and go over several hours) caused by release of inflammatory contents of mast cells in response to a stimulus such as food, drug, virus, or physical exposure. Angioedema describes the same reaction in deeper subcutaneous or submucosal tissue layers. Degranulation of the mast cells may be triggered by **allergy-mediated IgE reactions** and **nonallergic stimuli** such as sunlight, cold, heat, or pressure.

Acute urticaria is defined as symptoms **less than 6 weeks;** a trigger is identified at least half of the time. **Chronic urticaria** is defined as symptoms **more than 6 weeks;** a trigger is almost never identified. Chronic urticaria usually resolve spontaneously, but the course often lasts 1 to

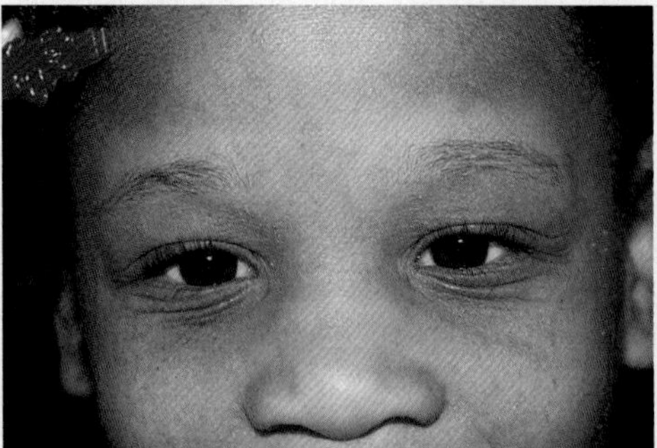

FIGURE 3.2. Eyelid atopic dermatitis. Note lichenification and the characteristic double-fold (Dennie-Morgan line) that extends from the inner to the outer canthus of the lower eyelid and the "allergic shiners," the darkening color of the periorbital areas. (From Goodheart HP. *Goodheart's Photoguide of Common Skin Disorders*. 2nd ed. Philadelphia, PA: Lippincott Williams & Wilkins, 2003.)

3 years before resolution. Antihistamines (H1 ± H2 blockers) are the mainstay of treatment for both acute and chronic urticaria and angioedema.

Cold urticaria deserves special consideration, as a total body exposure to cold water may result in extensive vasodilation, hypotension, and death. To test for cold urticaria, an ice cube is applied to the patient's body for 10 to 15 minutes. The result is positive if the patient develops hives with rewarming of the chilled area. Patients with cold urticaria should be counseled not to swim or submerge themselves in cold water due to the risk of hypotension and death with rewarming.

Anaphylaxis

Anaphylaxis is a sudden IgE-mediated reaction that involves **three or more organ systems.** Symptoms occur within minutes of the exposure and can include tongue swelling, tongue itching, tightness of the throat, nausea, abdominal pain, emesis, wheezing, chest pain, and dyspnea. Hypotensive shock may occur in severe cases. **The most common allergens responsible for anaphylactic reactions are food allergens.** Peanuts, tree nuts (e.g., almonds, Brazil nuts, cashews, chestnuts, filbert/hazelnuts, macadamia nuts, pecans, pine nuts, pistachios, walnuts), and seafood are the most common food triggers. Patients with spina bifida and genitourinary disorders are at risk for anaphylaxis with exposure to latex. Emergency management of anaphylaxis is reviewed in Chapter 6. Desensitization therapy is not effective for food allergies but is recommended for anaphylaxis in response to insect stings (reviewed later). All patients with a history of anaphylaxis should be instructed in the use of an epinephrine pen and carry it with them at all times.

Anaphylactoid Reactions

Anaphylactoid reactions are similar to anaphylaxis but are not IgE mediated. Instead, they are the result of direct degranulation of mast cells. Common triggers include **IV contrast material** for radiology and **opiates.** Anaphylactoid reactions are managed similarly to anaphylaxis. The severity of an anaphylactoid reaction can be reduced by pretreatment with antihistamines and corticosteroids.

Drug Allergy

Drug allergies can be IgE mediated or non-IgE mediated and can manifest in various ways including rash, anaphylaxis, fixed drug eruptions, and serum sickness. The most common allergy to medication is penicillin allergy. There is approximately **20% cross reactivity of allergy between penicillins and cephalosporins,** so cephalosporins should be used cautiously in patients with penicillin allergies. If necessary, a patient can be desensitized to penicillin in an intensive care unit setting.

A **fixed drug eruption** refers to development of one or more annular erythematous lesions after exposure to a medication. These lesions frequently **resolve with residual hyperpigmentation.** On re-exposure to the offending drug, this lesion will often reappear in the same location and other erythematous lesions may also develop.

Serum Sickness

Serum sickness is an **immune complex–**mediated disease that begins **1 to 3 weeks after an allergic exposure.** A foreign antigen in the blood, most often a **medication,** triggers the development of circulating **antigen-antibody immune complexes** that deposit in small vessels and cause vasculitis. Common medications responsible for serum sickness include anti-venom prepared in another animal host, animal hormones, and antibiotics.

Clinical Manifestations

- Patients are usually **ill-appearing** with **fever, rash, arthralgias,** myalgias, abdominal cramping, and diarrhea.
- Rarely, glomerulonephritis, carditis, or peripheral neuritis may develop.

Diagnosis

- Lab abnormalities include thrombocytopenia, elevated ESR, and depressed C3 and C4 levels; WBC may be normal, decreased, or elevated.
- Peripheral blood smear demonstrates increased numbers of plasma cells.
- In some cases, serum antibodies to an offending allergen can be measured.
- Skin biopsy of a lesion reveals immune complex formation.

Points to Remember

- Immunotherapy for allergy involves the gradual introduction of increasing amounts of allergen to decrease sensitization. It should be considered in patients with insect venom sensitivity and for refractory rhinoconjunctivitis that creates significant disability. It is not effective for food allergies. Treatments must be performed in a facility equipped to handle emergencies.

Treatment

- Mild cases can be managed with nonsteroidal anti-inflammatory drugs and antihistamines.
- Moderate and severe cases require corticosteroids for 7 to 10 days followed by a slow taper and/or plasmapheresis.

Insect Sting Allergy

The majority of insect venom reactions originate from members of the order of **Hymenoptera** (e.g., honeybees, bumble bees, hornets, yellow jackets, and fire ants). Yellow jackets are the most aggressive insects in this group. The insect venom contains enzymes that break down tissue and cause local edema. Swelling 2 inches or less lasting for 1 day or less is considered a normal reaction. **Large local reactions** occur in 10% of children and are characterized by tender swelling greater than 2 inches that persists between 1 and 7 days. **Generalized systemic reactions** may be confined to the skin with rash and angioedema or may be life-threatening anaphylactic reactions, which develop within 5 to 10 minutes and are rare in children. **Patients who have experienced a life-threatening systemic reaction and have positive venom RAST testing must be referred for desensitization immunotherapy and should be prescribed an emergency epinephrine pen.**

Points to Remember

- Food intolerance (such as lactose intolerance) differs from food allergy in that it results from lack of an enzyme required to process the food rather than a true immunological response to the food.

Allergic/Atopic March

The "allergic march" refers to the typical sequence of IgE antibody development and disease evolution in allergic patients (Fig. 3.3). Not all patients have all components of allergic disease. Typically, food allergies (milk protein, egg, etc.) manifest early in infancy and are followed by the development of eczema in late infancy. In early childhood years, patients develop IgE-mediated wheezing and asthma symptoms. Allergic rhinitis tends to develop later during childhood or adolescence.

Food Allergies	→	Eczema	→	Asthma	→	Allergic Rhinitis
(early infancy)		(late infancy)		(early childhood)		(late childhood/early adolescence)

FIGURE 3.3. Allergic March.

Points to Remember

- "Oral allergy syndrome" is a type of local food allergy primarily seen with the ingestion of fresh fruits and vegetables that consists of swelling, irritation, and pruritus of the oral cavity (lips, tongue, throat).
- Heiner's syndrome manifests as pulmonary hemosiderosis, GI bleeding, iron-deficiency anemia, and failure to thrive; it has been reported in association with allergy to cow's milk and egg.

Food Allergy

Food allergies can be IgE mediated or non-IgE mediated. The most common offending foods include cow's milk protein, egg, peanuts, tree nuts, fish, shellfish, wheat, soy, and seeds. Symptoms occur shortly after ingestion of the offending food.

Clinical Manifestations

- Dermatologic: rash, pruritus, urticaria, angioedema.
- GI: nausea, vomiting, diarrhea, abdominal pain, GI bleeding.
- Respiratory: rhinorrhea, wheezing, shortness of breath.
- Cardiovascular: hypotension.

Diagnosis

- For non–life-threatening allergic reactions, diagnosis can be made clinically if symptoms improve with elimination of the suspected food from the diet during a 2-week trial (if removal of the food does not impact nutrition).
- Skin and RAST testing are useful if the diagnosis is unclear and/or for more severe allergies.
- The gold standard test is the double blind placebo controlled oral food challenge (must be done in a controlled setting with emergency equipment available).

Points to Remember

- The vast majority of children are allergic only to one or two foods. If a parent reports multiple food allergies, further testing is warranted to avoid overrestricting the child's diet and compromising nutrition.

Treatment

- Food allergy to cow's milk, egg, and soy are usually outgrown, whereas allergy to peanuts, tree nuts, shellfish, and fish tend to be life-long allergies.
- **The only proven therapy for food allergy is strict avoidance.** Desensitization therapy is not effective for food allergy.
- Formula-fed infants with milk protein allergy should be fed hydrolysate formulas such as Nutramigen, Pregestimil, and Alimentum. Soy formula is not a good alternative due to a high level of cross reactivity with milk protein antigens.
- Mothers of breast-feeding infants with milk protein allergy should eliminate all milk and soy products from their diet.

- Infants almost universally outgrow milk protein allergy and can transition successfully to cow's milk at 12 months of age.

Eczema (Atopic Dermatitis)

Eczema, or atopic dermatitis, is an inflammatory allergic skin disease. Skin is **pruritic** and **dry,** and over time, becomes **lichenified.** The diagnosis of eczema is clinical. Patients may improve with **elimination of allergen exposure, good skin hydration,** and **topical corticosteroids** to control inflammation. Atopic dermatitis is associated with increased risk for the development of asthma and allergic rhinitis as well as other allergic diseases. Please refer to Chapter 7 for a more thorough discussion of eczema.

Asthma

Acute asthma attacks are triggered by both allergic and nonallergic irritant exposures. Common allergens include **dust mites, pet dander,** and **cockroaches.** Activation of IgE bound to mast cells triggers the release of inflammatory cellular contents and results in bronchoconstriction, airway edema, and mucous plug formation. Patients experience wheezing, coughing, chest tightness, and respiratory distress. Please refer to Chapter 24 for a more thorough discussion of asthma.

Allergic Rhinitis

Allergic rhinitis is IgE-mediated inflammation of the nasal passages that manifests as profuse rhinorrhea, nasal congestion, and itching. The **nasal mucosa appears boggy and pale.** Patients may have noisy breathing, dental malocclusion from mouth breathing, cough from postnasal drip, and/or an allergic crease. **Perennial symptoms are generally due to indoor allergens, whereas seasonal symptoms are usually due to outdoor airborne exposures.** Tree pollens are the predominant allergen in early spring, grass pollens in late spring, and ragweed in the fall. Diagnosis is primarily clinical but, if obtained, a smear of nasal secretions will reveal eosinophils and peripheral blood eosinophilia may also be present. Education is centered on avoidance of allergens. If avoidance is not feasible, treatment is initiated with **oral antihistamine** medications and **topical nasal corticosteroids.** Poorly controlled allergic rhinitis is a risk factor for recurrent sinusitis.

Allergic Conjunctivitis

Allergic conjunctivitis describes inflammation of the eye due to an IgE-mediated response to airborne pathogens. Allergic conjunctivitis symptoms are generally seasonal and include intense itching, bilateral conjunctival injection, watery eye discharge, chemosis (conjunctival swelling), cobblestoning of palpebral conjunctiva, and eyelid edema. Diagnosis is primarily clinical. Testing for severe cases or when the diagnosis is uncertain may include conjunctival scrapings to look for eosinophils and RAST and/or skin testing for airborne antigens. Treatment includes avoidance of allergens, **oral H1-antihistamines,** and **topical ophthalmic antihistamines.**

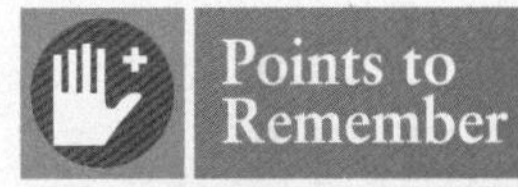

- **Seasonal allergic rhinitis and allergic conjunctivitis require sensitization to the allergen, making them very unlikely to occur before 2 or 3 years of age.**

Hereditary Angioedema (C1 Esterase Inhibitor Deficiency)

C1 esterase inhibitor protein is a regulator of the classical complement pathway. C1 esterase inhibitor deficiency (hereditary angioedema) is an **autosomal dominant** disorder characterized by **noninflammatory edema** of the skin and mucous membranes that is **provoked by trauma or stress** and may be life-threatening. Patients are typically treated prophylactically with antifibrinolytic agents (e.g., aminocaproic acid) or modified androgens (e.g., danzol). They **require prophylaxis prior to surgical procedures.** C1 esterase inhibitor deficiency is not associated with immunodeficiency.

SAMPLE BOARD REVIEW QUESTIONS

1. A 5-month-old boy with failure to thrive, recurrent thrush, and two prior hospital admissions for diarrhea is found to have leukopenia with a decreased absolute lymphocyte count. After immunologic testing, he is diagnosed with SCID due to ADA deficiency. Which of the following abnormalities are you most likely to find in this child?
   a. Preauricular pits
   b. Coarctation of the aorta
   c. Bony abnormalities
   d. Horseshoe kidney
   e. Hypoplastic thymus

Answer: c. SCID is an inherited immunodeficiency syndrome characterized by lymphopenia and poor T-cell function, which results in hypogammaglobulinemia from impaired signaling between T and B lymphocytes. Inheritance may be X-linked or autosomal recessive. Without treatment, most children with SCID would die before the age of 2 years. In general, SCID is treated with IVIG infusions and TMP/SMX prophylaxis until bone marrow transplant can be done to reconstitute the immune system. It is important to distinguish the subpopulation of autosomal recessive SCID due to ADA enzyme deficiency. This subpopulation accounts for approximately 40% of cases of autosomal recessive SCID and may respond well to ADA enzyme replacement therapy. In ADA deficient SCID, 50% of children have bony abnormalities. Bony abnormalities are not seen in other forms of SCID.

2. A 9-month-old boy has suffered from two episodes of acute otitis media and two radiographically proven pneumonias. He is the youngest of six children. His family history is significant for a brother who died at age 10 months from enteroviral meningitis. On examination, he is febrile to 102° F with mild tachycardia. He has bulging, erythematous tympanic membranes bilaterally and an erythematous posterior oropharynx. No cervical lymph nodes are palpable and you cannot visualize palatal tonsils. From your examination findings, which of the following immunodeficiencies is most likely in this patient?
   a. Bruton's X-linked agammaglobulinemia
   b. Chediak-Higashi syndrome
   c. Complement deficiency
   d. CVID
   e. Job's syndrome

Answer: a. Bruton's agammaglobulinemia is an X-linked disorder characterized by abnormal B-cell development. Affected males have hypogammaglobulinemia, no circulating B cells, small or absent tonsils, and no palpable lymph nodes. They frequently suffer from pyogenic upper respiratory tract infections, joint infections, and skin infections. They are particularly susceptible to life-threatening enteroviral infections (e.g., coxsackie, polio). They are treated with lifelong IVIG infusions and should not receive live virus vaccines.

3. A 6-year-old girl with a history of recurrent pneumonias and sinus infections over the past 2 years is brought to your office with a chief complaint of pink eye. On examination, she is noted to have bilateral conjunctival injection without eye discharge. She has been followed by neurology for poor coordination since she was 2 years old. What laboratory test result is expected to be abnormal?
   a. IgE
   b. C3 and C4
   c. Absolute neutrophil count
   d. AFP
   e. Platelet count

Answer: d. This patient has features of ataxia telangiectasia, an autosomal recessive disorder characterized by progressive truncal ataxia, telangiectasias, and immunodeficiency. Ataxia usually appears by 2 years of age and telangiectasias generally develop between 3 and 5 years of age and become increasingly extensive over time. Conjunctival telangiectasias can be mistaken for viral or bacterial conjunctivitis. Death usually occurs during the second decade of life as the result of infection or malignancy. Serum AFP is elevated in patients with ataxia telangiectasia.

4. What immunological screening test should be ordered first in a patient who develops overwhelming sepsis from a gonorrheal infection?
   a. IgG
   b. CH50
   c. Absolute neutrophil count
   d. C3, C4
   e. NBT test

Answer: b. Late complement deficiencies (C5-C9) predispose patients to severe disseminated gonococcal infections, meningococcal sepsis, and meningitis. CH50 is a screening test for all deficiencies in the complement system and the result will be abnormal in patients with late complement deficiencies.

5. A previously healthy 17-year-old girl experiences an anaphylactic reaction during an emergent blood transfusion after a motor vehicle accident. What underlying condition should you suspect?
   a. CVID
   b. IgA deficiency
   c. Hyper IgM syndrome

d. Job's syndrome
e. C4, C4 deficiency

Answer: b. Selective IgA deficiency is the most common immunodeficiency syndrome. Patients with IgA deficiency are susceptible to upper respiratory tract, GI, and urinary tract infections as they do not have IgA to protect their mucosal surfaces. These patients can receive only IgA-depleted blood products, because exposure to trace amounts of IgA can trigger an anaphylactic reaction.

6. A 28-month-old boy has had five episodes of *S. aureus* skin abscesses in the past year and has a history of *Klebsiella* bacteremia after a severe diarrheal illness. Which of the following tests result is most likely to be abnormal in this patient?
   a. Immunoglobulin levels
   b. CH50
   c. Neutrophil chemotaxis studies
   d. NBT test
   e. T-cell subsets

Answer: d. CGD is an immunodeficiency that results from defective oxidative burst function in neutrophils. In two-thirds of cases, its inheritance is x-linked. Patients with CGD are susceptible to infection with catalase-positive organisms (e.g., *S. aureus, E. coli, Klebsiella, Enterobacter* species, *Serratia marcescens, Salmonellae* species, *Pseudomonas*) and fungal infections. They frequently develop recurrent abscesses in skin, lymph nodes, liver, and spleen. The NBT test assesses the oxidative burst function of neutrophils and the result is abnormal in patients with CGD.

7. A 10-month-old boy with severe eczema has recurrent draining ear infections. Which of the following laboratory abnormalities is the patient most likely to have?
   a. Neutropenia
   b. Thrombocytopenia
   c. Hypogammaglobulinemia
   d. Eosinophilia
   e. Elevated IgE levels

Answer: b. Wiskott-Aldrich syndrome is characterized by eczematous dermatitis, small platelet size, and thrombocytopenia. Patients develop recurrent otitis media, sinusitis, and pneumonia. Because of the thrombocytopenia, they may experience easy bleeding and bruising. Patients with Wiskott-Aldrich syndrome are at increased risk of autoimmune disease and malignancy.

8. A 6-year-old girl presents to your office 2 days after being stung by a yellow jacket on her right forearm. Physical examination is significant for a 4-inch well-demarcated oval lesion on her right forearm at the site of the injury that is edematous, erythematous, and tender to palpation. Her physical examination is otherwise normal, and her mother denies any respiratory distress at the time of the yellow jacket sting. What is the correct diagnosis in this patient?
   a. Retained foreign body reaction
   b. Generalized systemic reaction
   c. Anaphylactoid reaction
   d. Normal insect sting reaction
   e. Large local reaction to insect sting

Answer: e. Large local reactions to insect bites are characterized by areas of tenderness, swelling, and erythema that are greater than 2 inches in diameter and persist for 1 to 7 days after the initial incident. A normal insect bite reaction consists of less than 2 inches of swelling, tenderness, and/or erythema and resolves within 1 day.

9. A 5-month-old girl presents with a respiratory rate of 86 breaths per minute and subcostal retractions. Her CXR reveals bilateral patchy infiltrates. Her weight is 3% for age. Complete blood cell count reveals a hemoglobin level of 6.4 g/dL. Stool hemoccult studies are positive. Bronchoscopic lavage detects hemosiderin- laden macrophages. What is the diagnosis?
   a. Histiocytosis
   b. Chediak-Higashi syndrome
   c. Heiner's syndrome
   d. Wiskott-Aldrich syndrome
   e. Shwachman-Bodian-Diamond syndrome

Answer: c. Severe cow's milk allergy may result in Heiner's syndrome, which consists of pulmonary hemosiderosis (due to recurrent bleeding into the lungs), GI bleeding, iron-deficiency anemia, and failure to thrive. Treatment is restriction of lactose from the diet. Soy products should also be avoided because of the risk of cross-reactivity.

10. Desensitization to allergens through tolerance-inducing immunotherapy is appropriate for which of the following allergens?
   a. Milk
   b. Peanuts
   c. Soy
   d. IV contrast
   e. Hymenoptera venom

Answer: e. Immunological tolerance therapy is appropriate and effective for the treatment of insect venom hypersensitivity. It should also be considered to treat severe rhinoconjunctivitis (seasonal or perennial) that creates significant disability and is refractory to medication. It is not effective for food allergies.

11. A 12-year-old boy suffers from rhinorrhea and nasal congestion on a daily basis most months of the year. He and his mother are not aware of any seasons when his symptoms remit. A nasal discharge smear reveals eosinophils. What is most likely to be the allergen responsible for his symptoms?
   a. Tree pollens
   b. Ragweed
   c. Grasses
   d. Dust mites
   e. Weed pollens

Answer: d. The patient described suffers from a year-round allergic rhinitis, supported by evidence of eosinophils on nasal smear. Perennial allergic rhinitis most often represents an allergy to a trigger present within the home, such as dust mites. Tree pollens cause allergy symptoms in early spring. Grass pollens are responsible for most allergy symptoms in late spring. The predominant fall allergen is ragweed.

12. Patients with spina bifida are at increased risk for anaphylaxis on exposure to which of the following agents?
   a. Peanuts
   b. Wasp sting
   c. Milk protein
   d. Latex
   e. IV contrast

Answer: d. Patients with spina bifida and congenital genitourinary abnormalities are at risk for anaphylaxis upon exposure to latex.

13. A previously healthy 11-year-old boy suddenly collapses upon climbing out of the pool during an early evening swim. Emergency responders arrive and find the boy confused, lethargic, hypotensive, and in shock. What underlying condition is he likely to have?
   a. Cholinergic urticaria
   b. Cold urticaria
   c. Chlorine allergy
   d. Dermatographism
   e. Hereditary angioedema

Answer: b. Patients with cold urticaria may experience massive vasodilation, hypotension, and death upon rewarming after whole body exposure to cold temperatures. The test to detect cold urticaria involves placing an ice cube on the patient's body for 10 to 15 minutes. The test result is positive if the patient develops hives as the skin rewarms after the ice cube is removed.

14. A 17-year-old girl develops a 6-cm annular reddish-purple colored lesion on her chest. She reports that she had a similar patch of discoloration in the exact location of this lesion about 4 months ago. The last time this occurred, the affected skin area gradually improved but remained slightly darker than her normal skin color. Her medications include a daily multivitamin, oral contraceptive tablets, and over-the-counter Excedrin as needed for headaches. What is the most likely explanation?
   a. Fixed drug eruption
   b. Hormone-induced hyperpigmentation
   c. Generalized drug eruption
   d. Erythema multiforme
   e. Pseudoporphyria

Answer: a. A fixed drug eruption is characterized by one or more round erythematous patches of skin that develop after exposure to a medication. These lesions usually occur within 8 hours of taking the drug and frequently resolve with residual dark discoloration. On re-exposure to the offending drug, this lesion will often reappear in the same location. Medications that have been implicated in fixed drug reactions include acetaminophen, ibuprofen, and tetracycline antibiotics.

15. Which of the following food allergies is a child least likely to outgrow?
   a. Milk protein
   b. Egg
   c. Soy
   d. Peanut
   e. Wheat

Answer: d. Allergies to peanuts and shellfish tend to be life-long, whereas allergies to soy, milk, wheat, and egg commonly resolve with age.

SUGGESTED READINGS

Braganza S, Adam H. Food allergy. *Pediatr Rev.* 2003;24:393–394.
Iseki M, Heiner DC. Immunodeficiency disorders. *Pediatr Rev.* 1993;14;226–236.
Nimmagadda S, Evans R. Allergy: etiology and epidemiology. *Pediatr Rev.* 1999;20:110–116.
Stehim ER. Clinical and laboratory evaluation of the child with immunodeficiency. *Pediatr Rev.* 1985;7:53–61.
Tatachar P, Kumar S. Food-induced anaphylaxis and oral allergy syndrome. *Pediatr Rev.* 2008; 29:e23–e27.
Waibel K. Anaphylaxis. *Pediatr Rev.* 2008;29:255–263.

CHAPTER 4 ■ CARDIOLOGY

JESSICA HEBERT MOULEDOUX

ABG	Arterial blood gas
ACE-I	Angiotension converting enzyme inhibitor
ARB	Angiotensin-receptor blocker
AD	Autosomal dominant
AS	Aortic stenosis
ASO	Antistreptolysin O
ASD	Atrial septal defect
AV	Atrioventricular
BP	Blood pressure
bpm	Beats per minute
BT	Blalock-Taussig
BUN	Blood urea nitrogen
BVH	Biventricular hypertrophy
CCB	Calcium channel blocker
CHD	Congenital heart disease
CHF	Congestive heart failure
CK-MB	Creatine kinase, MB type
COA	Coarctation of the aorta
CNS	Central nervous system
CXR	Chest x-ray
DCM	Dilated cardiomyopathy
ECD	Endocardial cushion defect
GAS	Group A streptococcus
GER	Gastroesophageal reflux
GI	Gastrointestinal
GU	Genitourinary
HCM	Hypertrophic cardiomyopathy
HLHS	Hypoplastic left heart syndrome
HSV	Herpes simplex virus
HTN	Hypertension
ICD	Implantable cardioverter-defibrillator
IE	Infective endocarditis
IM	Intramuscular
IV	Intravenous
IVIG	Intravenous immunoglobulin
JVD	Jugular venous distention
JVP	Jugular venous pressure
LAE	Left atrial enlargement
LLSB	Left lower sternal border
Lt	Left
LQTS	Long QT syndrome
LUSB	Left upper sternal border
LV	Left ventricle
LVH	Left ventricular hypertrophy
LVOT	Left ventricular outflow tract
MI	Myocardial infarction
MLSB	Mid-left sternal border
MR	Mitral regurgitation
MRSA	Methicillin-resistant *S. aureus*
MVP	Mitral valve prolapse
NHBPEP	National High Blood Pressure Education Program
OCP	Oral contraceptive pills
PA	Pulmonary artery
PAC	Premature atrial contraction
PALS	Pediatric Advanced Life Support
PBF	Pulmonary blood flow
PCO_2	Partial pressure of carbon dioxide
PDA	Patent ductus arteriosus
PGE_1	Prostaglandin E_1
PO_2	Partial pressure of oxygen
PPHN	Persistent pulmonary hypertension of the newborn
PS	Pulmonary stenosis
PVC	Premature ventricular contraction
PVM	Pulmonary vascular marking
PVR	Pulmonary vascular resistance
RA	Right atrium
RAD	Right axis deviation
RAE	Right atrial enlargement
RAH	Right atrial hypertrophy
RBBB	Right bundle branch block
RPA	Right pulmonary artery
Rt	Right
RV	Right ventricle
RVH	Right ventricular hypertrophy
RVOT	Right ventricular outflow tract
SCD	Sudden cardiac death
SEM	Systolic ejection murmur
SVC	Superior vena cava
SVR	Systemic vascular resistance
SVT	Supraventricular tachycardia
TAPVR	Total anomalous pulmonary venous return
TGA	Transposition of the great arteries
TOF	Tetralogy of Fallot
URI	Upper respiratory tract infection
VSD	Ventricular septal defect
VT	Ventricular tachycardia
WPW	Wolff-Parkinson-White

CHAPTER OBJECTIVES

1. To recognize the varied presentations of CHD and to use appropriate diagnostic tools in formulating a differential diagnosis
2. To be familiar with the diagnosis and management of acquired heart disease
3. To recognize, determine pathology of, and direct management of classic arrhythmias
4. To evaluate complaints of chest pain and syncope for cardiac pathology and to recognize signs and symptoms that are associated with sudden cardiac death
5. To properly diagnose HTN and recognize underlying disease in patients with secondary HTN.

INNOCENT MURMURS

Physiologic (functional, innocent) murmurs are very common and are noted on examination in 80% of patients sometime during childhood. Distinguishing between innocent and pathologic murmurs is essential in diagnosis and management. Innocent murmurs are usually **systolic ejection** type, begin early in systole, are of **short duration** and **low intensity** (grade 1 or 2), and have a **vibratory** or **musical quality**. Common innocent murmurs are described in **Table 4.1**.

Features of murmurs and associated findings indicating possible pathology and need for cardiac consultation include the following:

- Long duration or high intensity (≥ grade 3).
- Diastolic murmur.
- Abnormal heart sounds (gallop, rub, etc.).
- Symptoms of heart disease (chest pain, dyspnea, exercise intolerance, syncope, etc.)
- Cyanosis.
- Unequal or abnormally strong or weak pulses.
- High BP or differential BPs in upper and lower extremities.
- Cardiomegaly or increased pulmonary vascularity on CXR.
- Abnormal EKG.

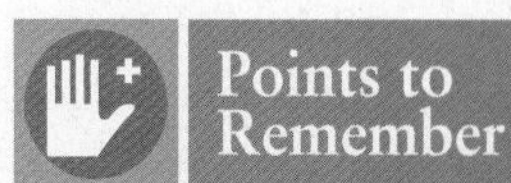

- **If the history and physical examination are reassuring for a benign murmur, no further evaluation (CXR, EKG, etc) is needed.**

TABLE 4.1

COMMON INNOCENT HEART MURMURS

Type (Timing)	Description of Murmur	Age Group
Classic vibratory murmur (Still's murmur) (systolic)	Maximal at MLSB or between LLSB and apex Grades 2 to 3/6 Low-frequency vibratory, "twanging string," groaning, squeaking, or musical	3–6 y Occasionally in infancy
Pulmonary ejection murmur (systolic)	Maximal at ULSB Early to midsystolic Grades 1 to 3/6 in intensity Blowing in quality	8–14 y
Pulmonary flow murmur of newborn (systolic)	Maximal at ULSB Transmits well to the left and right chest, axilla, and back Grades 1 to 2/6 in intensity	Premature and full-term newborns Usually disappears by 3–6 mo of age
Venous hum (continuous)	Maximal at right (or left) supraclavicular and infraclavicular areas Grades 1 to 3/6 in intensity Inaudible in the supine position Intensity changes with rotation of the head and compression of the jugular vein	3–6 y
Carotid brunt (systolic)	Right supraclavicular area and over the carotids Grades 2 to 3/6 in intensity Occasional thrill over a carotid	Any age

LLSB, lower left sternal border: MLSB, midleft sternal border: ULSB, upper left sternal border.
Reprinted with permission from Park MK. Pediatric Cardiology for Practitioners. 5th ed. Philadelphia, PA: Elsevier Health Sciences, 2008.

CONGENITAL HEART DISEASE

Presentation of Congenital Heart Disease in Neonates

The presentation of CHD in infancy can vary significantly. Some infants present in severe distress due to cardiogenic shock or CHF. Other infants may be solely cyanotic or may be well-appearing and present with subtle signs of CHD (presence of a murmur, HTN, abnormal pulses, or failure to thrive). Understanding the pathophysiology of specific defects can assist in formulating and narrowing a differential diagnosis of suspected CHD.

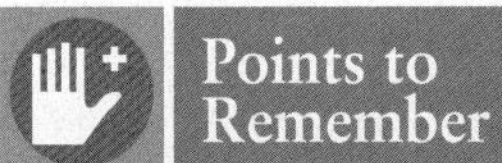

- Normally, the ductus arteriosus functionally closes by 12 to 24 hours of life, but anatomic closure is not typically complete until 2 to 3 weeks of age.

Cardiogenic Shock

Poor myocardial function or an obstruction to blood flow decreases cardiac output and leads to inadequate tissue perfusion. Shock in the neonate with CHD is typically secondary to **left heart obstruction** (HLHS, severe COA or interrupted aortic arch, critical AS, obstructive TAPVR). Systemic perfusion in these lesions is often **dependant on a patent ductus arteriosus** and symptoms worsen with ductus closure.

Clinical Manifestations

- Hypotension and tachypnea.
- Poor perfusion with diminished pulses, mottled skin, and lactic acidosis.
- Tachycardia progressing to bradycardia in advanced shock.
- Signs of congestion—hepatomegaly, pulmonary crackles.
- Cyanosis.

Treatment

- **PGE_1** is used to maintain patency of the ductus arteriosus, thus **preserving systemic blood flow.**
- Beware of excess O_2 administration (O_2 is a pulmonary vasodilator; thus, O_2 administration decreases PVR and can result in increased blood flow toward pulmonary circulation and away from systemic circulation, further decreasing systemic perfusion).
- Gentle fluid resuscitation (use smaller volumes of 10 cc/kg and continually reassess the patient for signs of fluid overload as excess fluid can worsen CHF).
- Inotropic agents to improve function and cardiac output (e.g., dobutamine, dopamine, epinephrine).

Congestive Heart Failure

Infants with CHD can present with CHF due to pressure and/or volume overload. CHF is discussed extensively later in this chapter.

Cyanosis

An increased concentration of reduced hemoglobin ($\geq$5 g/dL) results in bluish discoloration of skin and mucous membranes. Cyanosis is defined as **central** (desaturation of arterial blood) or **peripheral** (normal arterial blood saturation). Types of peripheral cyanosis include **acrocyanosis** (bluish hue of fingers and toes) and **circumoral cyanosis** (bluish skin color surrounding the mouth) and reflect sluggish capillary blood flow.

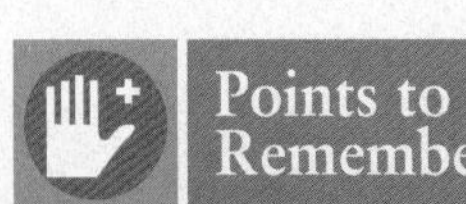

- Hemoglobin levels influence the perception of cyanosis. Approximately 5 g/dL of reduced hemoglobin is necessary before most people can appreciate cyanosis. In infants with normal hemoglobin levels, cyanosis becomes apparent at a saturation of 75% to 80%. Polycythemic infants will have apparent cyanosis at higher oxygen saturations, and anemic infants will not appear cyanotic until more significant desaturation occurs.

Diagnosis and Evaluation

Central cyanosis always warrants evaluation. The most common causes of central cyanosis are CHD, pulmonary disease, and CNS depression.

- CXR—may uncover pulmonary pathology or demonstrate cardiomegaly ± changes in PVMs consistent with CHD.
- EKG—assists in differentiating among CHD lesions.
- ABG (done with patient on room air)—low PO_2 confirms central cyanosis; elevated PCO_2 may be present in pulmonary or CNS disease.
- Hyperoxia test (response to 100% oxygen via oxyhood or endotracheal tube)—assists in differentiating cardiac verses pulmonary etiology.
  - PO_2 >100 mmHg, or a rise in PO_2 >30 mmHg above that on room air—suggests pulmonary etiology.
  - PO_2 <100 mmHg, or a rise in PO_2 <10 to 30 mmHg—suggestive of intracardiac right-to-left shunt (usually due to CHD or PPHN) or a mixing lesion.
- Pre- and postductal saturations—evaluate for the presence of right-to-left shunt across a PDA with pulmonary pressure > systemic pressure.
  - Preductal > postductal—present in **PPHN** and cardiac conditions with decreased systemic pressures (**obstructive lesions of the LV**—AS, interrupted arch, COA).
  - Postductal > preductal—**TGA with associated obstruction** (interrupted arch or COA).

TABLE 4.2

ACYANOTIC LESIONS

Lesion	Presentation and Clinical Manifestations	Physical Examination	CXR	EKG	Management	Comment
Ventricular septal defect (VSD)	Small defects can be asymptomatic. Large defects can present with CHF at 6–8 weeks of life	**Loud, harsh, holosystolic murmur** at LLSB; ± thrill; Murmur may not be present in a newborn	Cardiomegaly; ↑PVM	**LVH** ± LAE	Small defects, especially muscular VSDs, close spontaneously Larger defects require surgery Medical treatment of CHF	Most common congenital heart defect requiring follow-up or intervention
Patent ductus arteriosus (PDA)	Can be asymptomatic; Premature infants can present with hemodynamic instability	**Continuous machinery-like** murmur at LUSB **Bounding pulses** with **wide pulse pressure**	Cardiomegaly; ↑PVM	LVH, BVH with large lesion	Medical treatment (premature infants): **indomethacin, ibuprofen** Some require closure via cardiac catheterization or surgery	Common in premature infants PDA normally closes by 72 h of life
Atrial septal defect (ASD)	Rarely become symptomatic until third or fourth decade of life then may present with CHF and pulmonary hypertension	**Wide, fixed split S2** ± SEM at the LUSB (PS murmur)	Cardiomegaly ± RA and RV enlargement	RAD, RVH, RBBB (rsR′ in V1)	Small or moderate ASDs may resolve spontaneously	Atrial arrhythmias may occur in adults
Complete endocardial cushion defect (AV canal)	Similar to VSD, CHF at 4–6 weeks	Holosystolic murmur of VSD	Cardiomegaly with four-chamber enlargement, ↑PVM	**Superior QRS axis,** RVH or RBBB	Surgical repair	Very common in patients with **Down syndrome**

BVH, biventricular hypertrophy; CHF, congestive heart failure; LAE, left atrial enlargement; LLSB, left lower sternal border; LUSB, left upper sternal border; LVH, left ventricular hypertrophy; PS, pulmonary stenosis; PVM, pulmonary vascular marking; RA, right atrium; RAD, right axis deviation; RBBB, right bundle branch block; RV, right ventricle; RVH, right ventricular hypertrophy; SEM, systolic ejection murmur.

Treatment
Cyanosis in CHD results from right-to-left shunting lesions and mixing lesions, which allow deoxygenated blood to enter the systemic circulation and also result in decreased PBF. PGE_1 can be helpful in these situations by maintaining the patency of the PDA and preserving PBF.

Specific Congenital Heart Defects

Specific CHDs can be categorized as acyanotic lesions, obstructive lesions, and cyanotic lesions.

Acyanotic Lesions

- Defects causing left-to-right shunts, typically resulting in increased PBF.
- Specific defects are described in **Table 4.2.**

Obstructive Lesions

- Defects obstructing blood flow from the ventricles to the pulmonary or systemic circulation.
- Specific defects are described in **Table 4.3.**

Cyanotic Lesions

- Defects producing central cyanosis via right-to-left shunting or complete mixing of pulmonary and systemic blood flow.
- Specific defects are described in **Table 4.4.**

TABLE 4.3

OBSTRUCTIVE LESIONS

Lesion	Presentation and Clinical Manifestations	Physical Examination	CXR	EKG	Management	Miscellaneous
Pulmonary stenosis (PS)	Mild lesions: asymptomatic Critical lesions: **cyanosis,** tachypnea, exertional dyspnea, fatigue, CHF	**Loud SEM** at ULSB radiating to **back and lung fields**	Prominent PA segment, normal to decreased PVM	RAD, RVH	PGE_1 for pulmonary perfusion Balloon valvuloplasty or surgical correction	
Aortic stenosis (AS)	Neonates: hypoperfusion, respiratory distress, **cyanosis** with Rt to Lt ductal flow Children: chest pain, syncope, dyspnea	**Ejection click, harsh midsystolic murmur** **Systolic thrill** at **suprasternal notch**	Critical AS: cardiomegaly, ↑PVM	LVH ± strain	PGE_1 to maintain systemic perfusion Balloon valvuloplasty or surgical correction	Supravalvular AS is common in **Williams syndrome**
Coarctation of the aorta (COA)	Symptomatic infants: CHF, respiratory distress, **shock,** diminished pulses and cyanosis of lower extremities, BP differential (Rt arm > leg)	No murmur in 50%	Cardiomegaly, ↑PVM	RVH or RBBB	PGE_1 for systemic perfusion and treatment of CHF Surgical correction	Present in 30% of **Turner's syndrome** patients 70% of patients with coarctation have an associated aortic valve abnormality
	Asymptomatic infants and children: **hypertension in right arm,** diminished femoral pulses	Ejection click, SEM	**Three sign** of descending aorta (**E-shaped esophagus** on barium esophagram), **rib notching** (Fig. 4.1)	LAD, LVH	Primary surgical correction in infants Balloon angioplasty for recoarctation post surgical repair or as primary intervention in older child	

CHF, congestive heart failure; Lt, left; LVH, left ventricular hypertrophy; PA, pulmonary artery; PGE_1, prostaglandin E_1; PVM, pulmonary vascular marking; RAD, right axis deviation; RBBB, right bundle branch block; Rt, right; RVH, right ventricular hypertrophy; SEM, systolic ejection murmur; ULSB, upper left sternal border.

Staged Surgical Repair of HLHS

Surgical repair of HLHS is accomplished via a staged approach that includes three operations: the Norwood operation, the Bidirectional Glenn operation, and the Fontan operation. Similar repair technique is used in other congenital heart defects with single ventricle physiology (tricuspid atresia, pulmonary atresia with intact ventricular septum, etc.)

Norwood

- A neoaorta is created to supply systemic blood flow by connecting the proximal PA to the hypoplastic aorta with an allograft.
- An atrial septectomy improves intra-atrial mixing.
- Pulmonary blood flow is provided by a systemic-to-PA shunt (BT shunt) or **Sano modification** (a central RV-to-PA shunt).
- RV supplies both pulmonary and systematic blood flow.

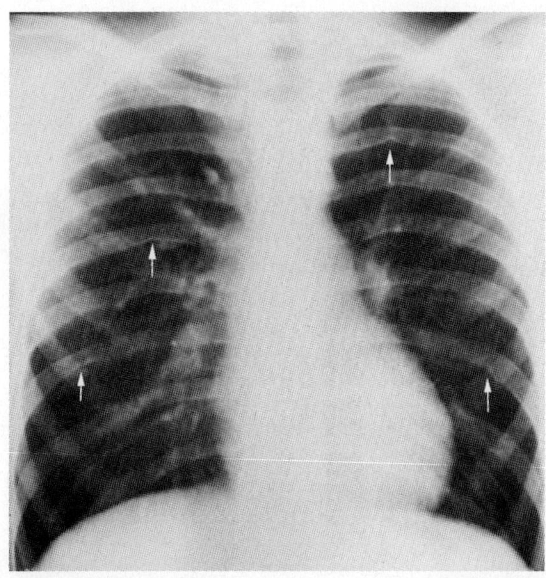

FIGURE 4.1. Posteroanterior chest film with rib notching (*arrows*) and a three-sign identified in a 7-year-old child. (Reprinted with permission from McMillan JA, Feigin RD, DeAngelis C, et al. *Oski's Pediatrics: Principles and Practice*. 4th ed. Philadelphia, PA: Lippincott Williams & Wilkins, 2006.)

Bidirectional Glenn

- An SVC-to-RPA shunt is constructed and the prior BT shunt or Sano is removed.
- Pulmonary blood flow is provided by systemic venous return via the SVC.
- The IVC returns systemic venous blood to the RA.

Fontan

- The IVC is directed to the RPA via an intra-atrial tubular pathway.
- All systemic venous blood is then routed directly to the lungs, bypassing a pumping chamber, and thus separating pulmonary and systemic blood flow.

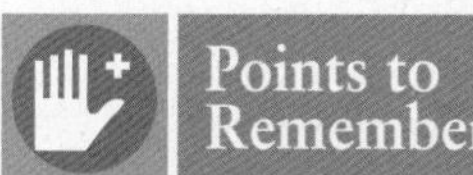

Points to Remember

- Tet spells, also called hypoxic or hypercyanotic spells, consist of paroxysms of hyperpnea, worsening cyanosis, and diminished murmur.
- Caused by decreased SVR or increased PVR with subsequent increase in right-to-left flow across VSD.

Treatment

- Knee-chest position to ↑SVR and calm infant
- Supplemental oxygen
- Morphine ↓ respiratory drive → ↓ hyperpnea
- Sodium bicarbonate to treat metabolic acidosis
- Vasoconstrictors (phenylephrine) ↑ SVR
- Propranolol (acute and prophylactic) ↓ heart rate
- Ketamine ↑SVR and sedates patient

CONGESTIVE HEART FAILURE

Heart failure occurs when the heart is incapable of supplying enough blood to the body to meet its needs. The syndrome of CHF is caused by volume overload, pressure overload, or both.

Clinical Manifestations

Symptoms vary depending on the age of the patient.

- Infants commonly exhibit **difficulty feeding** (prolonged duration of feeds or sweating with feeds), tiring, shortness of breath, **poor weight gain**, **tachypnea**, and excessive perspiration.
- Older children exhibit **shortness of breath**, exercise intolerance, orthopnea, **easy fatigue**, and dependant edema.
- Physical examination is notable for **tachycardia**, **gallop rhythm**, signs of pulmonary congestion (tachypnea, wheezing, **basilar crackles**), and signs of systemic venous congestion (**hepatomegaly**, **edema**).

Etiologies of CHF

The most likely etiologies of CHF in children can be broken down by age and include CHD, acquired heart disease, and myocardial disease. See Table 4.5 for age-specific etiologies of CHF.

Diagnosis and Evaluation

- CXR—**cardiomegaly, ± increased PVMs.**
- EKG— ± chamber enlargement; evaluates for **arrhythmia** as underlying etiology.

TABLE 4.4

CYANOTIC LESIONS

	Lesion	Presentation and Clinical Manifestations	Physical Examination	CXR	EKG	Management	Miscellaneous
Right-to-left shunting lesions (decreased pulmonary blood flow)	Tetralogy of Fallot (TOF), [Large VSD, RVOT obstruction (PS), RVH, overriding aorta]	Initially **cyanosis,** dyspnea on exertion; later **hypoxic (Tet) spells** Occasionally acyanotic and asymptomatic	Single S2; long, loud **SEM at mid-upper LSB**	↓PVM, **"boot-shaped" heart,** right aortic arch in 25%	RAD, **RVH**	PGE_1 if cyanotic Primary surgical repair preferred, occasionally palliative **Blalock-Taussig (BT) shunt** (subclavian artery to ipsilateral PA) is performed	Degree of cyanosis and symptoms related to severity of PS. **Most common cyanotic CHD**
	Tricuspid Atresia	Severe cyanosis and tachypnea in patients with normally related great vessels	Murmur from associated lesions (VSD, PDA)	↓PVM	Leftward or **superior QRS axis, RAE,** minimal positive forces in V_1 and V_2	PGE_1, rarely balloon atrial septostomy. Typically a BT shunt is the first stage of surgical repair to ↑PBF, definitive repair is a single ventricle Fontan-type repair	Associated mixing defects (ASD, VSD, PDA) needed for survival 30% with TGA
	Pulmonary atresia with intact ventricular septum	Severe cyanosis and tachypnea in the neonatal period. Intra-atrial communication necessary for survival	**Single S_2,** murmur usually **absent,** occasionally **PDA** murmur	↓PVM, dark lung fields	LVH, RAH	PGE_1 for pulmonary blood flow. Surgery or interventional cath for perforation of PV. Repair depends on size of RV (small = single ventricle repair)	Commonly associated with **coronary artery anomalies**
	Ebstein's anomaly (downward displacement of TV, resulting functional RV hypoplasia)	Cyanosis, arrhythmias (SVT) ASD or PFO always present	**Triple** or **quadruple rhythm** (wide split S_2, ± split S_1, S_3, or S_4)	↓PVM, massive cardiomegaly with **"balloon-shaped" heart**	RBBB, RAH, **first-degree AV block, delta wave**	PGE_1 for pulmonary blood flow. If needed, type of surgical repair depends on size of RV	**WPW** is frequently associated

Total mixing lesions	Transposition of the great arteries (TGA)	Severe cyanosis, signs of **CHF** (dyspnea, feeding difficulty) **in the first week of life**	Single S_2, often **no murmur**	↑PVM, **"egg-shaped" heart,** or "egg on a string"	RAD, RVH	PGE_1 and oxygen, CHF therapy, **balloon atrial septostomy** if severe cyanosis. Arterial switch operation	VSD present in 30%–40%
	Truncus arteriosus	Mild cyanosis immediately after birth, **CHF in days to weeks** Large VSD located beneath truncal valve	**Single S_2, systolic ejection click** at the apex, murmur of VSD **Bounding pulses,** wide pulse pressure	↑PVM, cardiomegaly, **right aortic arch** in 30%	BVH	Surgical repair directing LV flow to truncus with a homograft/conduit connecting RV and PA	**Coronary artery anomalies** are common, **DiGeorge syndrome** is present in one-third of patients
	Total anomalous pulmonary venous return (TAPVR)	Respiratory distress, CHF Types vary with vessel insertion: supracardiac—SVC **(most common);** cardiac—RA or coronary sinus; infracardiac—portal veins, IVC	**Quadruple rhythm** (S_1, widely split S_2, and S_3 or S_4), hepatomegaly	Cardiomegaly, **significantly ↑PVM, "snowman" sign"** or **"figure-of-8"** configuration (Fig. 4.2)	RVH, **rsR′ in V_1**	PGE_1, rarely balloon atrial septostomy; surgical correction redirects pulmonary blood flow to LA	**Obstruction** to venous return commonly occurs in infracardiac type PGE_1 may worsen condition in obstructed TAPVR
	Hypoplastic left heart syndrome (HLHS)	Respiratory distress, **shock,** and **CHF** within **first week of life**	Loud, single S_2, commonly **no murmur,** hepatomegaly	↑PVM, pulmonary venous congestion, edema ± cardiomegaly	**RVH, RAE,** minimal positive forces in V_5 and V_6	PGE_1 to maintain systemic perfusion; staged operative single ventricle repair or transplant	

BVH, biventricular hypertrophy; CHD, congenital heart disease; CHF, congestive heart failure; LV, left ventricle; LVH, left ventricular hypertrophy; PA, pulmonary artery; PBF, pulmonary blood flow; PDA, patent ductus arteriosus; PGE_1, prostaglandin E_1; PS, pulmonary stenosis; PVM, pulmonary vascular marking; RA, right atrium; RAD, right axis deviation; RAE, right atrial enlargement; RAH, right atrial hypertrophy; RBBB, right bundle branch block; RV, right ventricle; RVH, right ventricular hypertrophy; RVOT, right ventricular outflow tract; SEM, systolic ejection murmur; SVC, superior vena cava; SVT, supraventricular tachycardia; TGA, transposition of the great arteries; VSD, ventricular septal defect; WPW, Wolff-Parkinson-White.

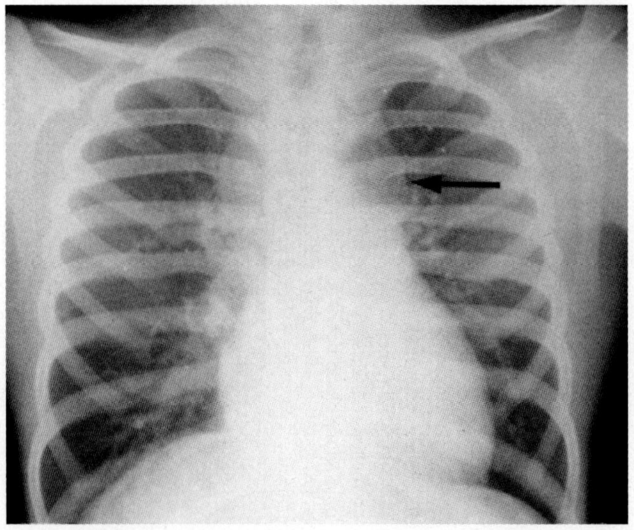

FIGURE 4.2. Supracardiac total anomalous pulmonary venous return (TAPVR). Chest radiograph in a child with connection to the left innominate vein demonstrating figure-of-eight or "snowman" appearance. The arrow points to an anomalous vertical vein. (Reprinted with permission from McMillan JA, Feigin RD, DeAngelis C, et al. *Oski's Pediatrics: Principles and Practice.* 4th ed. Philadelphia, PA: Lippincott Williams & Wilkins, 2006.)

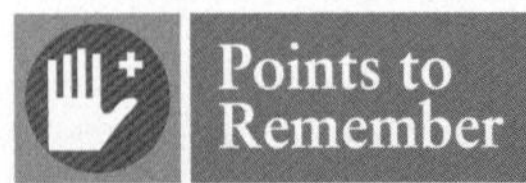

Points to Remember

- **Large left-to-right shunts (VSD, PDA) do not typically cause CHF before 4 to 8 weeks of age because pulmonary resistance does not decrease enough to cause significant shunting until this age.**

- Laboratories—B-type natriuretic peptide is commonly elevated in CHF and can help distinguish pulmonary edema secondary to heart failure from that associated with pulmonary disease.
- Echocardiogram—evaluates heart structure and function and can be used to quantify shortening fraction.
- Cardiac catheterization—endomyocardial biopsy to investigate underlying etiology.

Treatment

- Management of underlying etiology is critical.
- Drug therapy includes the following:
  - **Diuretics** decrease **pulmonary and systemic venous congestion**; furosemide is the drug of choice.

TABLE 4.5

ETIOLOGIES OF CONGESTIVE HEART FAILURE

Birth and First Week of Life	1–4 Weeks	Infants >1 Month of Age	Children
Severe obstructive CHD ■ HLHS ■ Critical AS or PS ■ Obstructive TAPVR ■ Interrupted aortic arch TGA Volume overload ■ Severe tricuspid or pulmonary insufficiency ■ Systemic arterio-venous fistula Genetic or metabolic cardiomyopathy	More favorable obstructive lesions ■ Coarctation of the aorta ■ AS or PS ■ TAPVR Truncus arteriosus Genetic or metabolic cardiomyopathy	Large left-to-right shunts ■ ECD at 4–6 weeks ■ Large VSD or PDA at 6–8 weeks Arrhythmias (SVT) Myocarditis Genetic or metabolic cardiomyopathy	Inflammatory processes—Kawasaki, myocarditis, rheumatic fever Acute hypertension (hemolytic-uremic syndrome) Genetic or metabolic cardiomyopathy

CHD, congenital heart disease; ECD, endocardial cushion defect ; HLHS, hypoplastic left heart syndrome; PDA, patent ductus arteriosus; PS, pulmonary stenosis; SVT, supraventricular tachycardia; TAPVR, total anomalous pulmonary venous return; TGA, transposition of the great arteries; VSD, ventricular septal defect.

- **Afterload reduction** agents include ACE-Is, milrinone, nitroprusside, and hydralazine.
- **Inotropes** increase contractility; dopamine and dobutamine are fast-acting agents used in critically ill children; digoxin can be used in more stable patients.
- **β-Blockers** are an essential component in the treatment of **chronic CHF.**
- Infants with poor weight gain and/or difficulty feeding often require fortification of breast milk or formula and use of nasogastric feeds to increase caloric intake.

Points to Remember

- Surgical correction of CHD leading to CHF should be performed as soon as possible if patient fails medical management.

ACQUIRED HEART DISEASE

Rheumatic Fever

Rheumatic fever is an inflammatory disease of connective tissue, which develops as a delayed complication of an untreated or inadequately treated **group A β-hemolytic streptococcal pharyngitis.** It is most common in patients aged 5 to 15 years and is **rare in children younger than 4 years.** Onset is usually 1 to 5 weeks postpharyngitis. Rheumatic fever is rare in the United States but is still common in developing countries.

Points to Remember

- Noncardioselective β-blockers like propranolol are contraindicated in asthmatics because of bronchoconstrictive effects.

Clinical Manifestations and Diagnosis

The diagnosis of rheumatic fever rests on a combination of clinical and laboratory findings. Diagnosis according to the **JONES criteria** requires the following:

- Laboratory evidence of a prior streptococcal infection (e.g., positive throat culture, elevated ASO titer) **PLUS.**
- Two major criteria or one major criterion and two minor criteria (see Table 4.6).

Points to Remember

- Rheumatic fever does occur after GAS pharyngitis but does not occur after GAS skin infections.

Treatment

- Antimicrobial
  - Acute—benzathine penicillin IM or oral penicillin G.
  - Prophylaxis—long-term prophylaxis with monthly benzathine penicillin IM or daily oral penicillin G is required and dramatically reduces risk of recurrence.

Points to Remember

- Rheumatic fever cannot be diagnosed in the absence of laboratory evidence of a prior strep infection.

TABLE 4.6

JONES CRITERIA FOR DIAGNOSIS OF ACUTE RHEUMATIC FEVER

Major Criteria	
J = Joints (Arthritis)	Migratory polyarthritis of large joints
O = Carditis	1) Endocarditis—new murmur; mitral valve most commonly affected followed by aortic value; can lead to valvular insufficiency and/or stenosis 2) Myocarditis—tachycardia; myocardial strain on EKG 3) Pericarditis—pericardial friction rub, effusion, ST changes on EKG
N = Nodules, subcutaneous	Located on the extensor surfaces of extremities; histologically composed of Aschoff bodies (Fig. 4.3), the pathognomic histologic lesion of rheumatic fever
E = Erythema marginatum	Expanding erythema with central clearing mainly on trunk and extremities (Fig. 4.4)
S = Sydenham chorea	Neuropsychiatric disorder characterized by emotional lability, personality changes, and involuntary uncoordinated movements; late manifestation with up to a 6-month latent period; female > male
Minor Criteria	
Arthralgia	
Prolonged PR interval (first-degree AV block)	
Fever	
Elevated ESR and/or CRP	
Elevated WBC count	
Previous rheumatic fever	

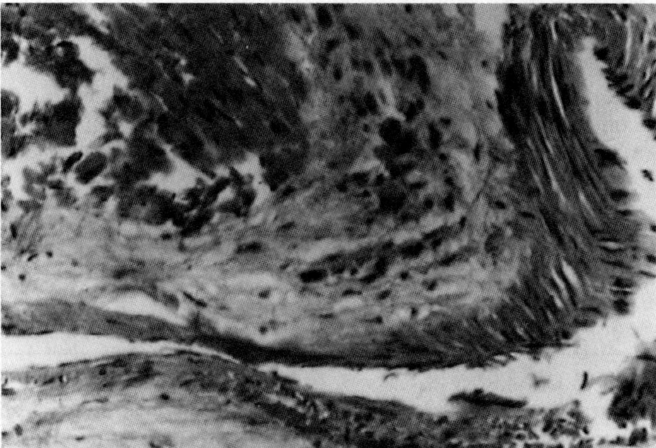

FIGURE 4.3. A paravascular Aschoff body, which consists of granulomatous inflammation of connective tissue with fibrinoid changes. Aschoff bodies can be found subcutaneously (in nodules) and also in the myocardium of those with rheumatic fever. (Reprinted with permission from McMillan JA, Feigin RD, DeAngelis C, et al. *Oski's Pediatrics: Principles and Practice.* 4th ed. Philadelphia, PA: Lippincott Williams & Wilkins, 2006.)

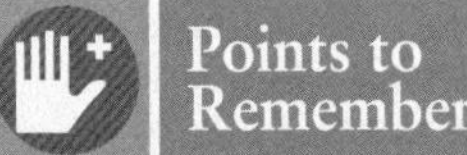

Points to Remember

- The most common murmur noted in patients with rheumatic fever is that of mitral regurgitation (a regurgitant systolic murmur at the apex with radiation to the axilla).
- The arthritis associated with rheumatic fever is remarkably responsive to salicylates.

- Symptomatic
  - Arthritis—salicylate therapy.
  - Carditis—corticosteroids and/or aspirin; medical management of CHF; surgical valve replacement may be necessary.
  - Chorea—quiet atmosphere with minimal environmental stimuli; pharmacologic options include haloperidol, phenobarbital, and chlorpromazine.

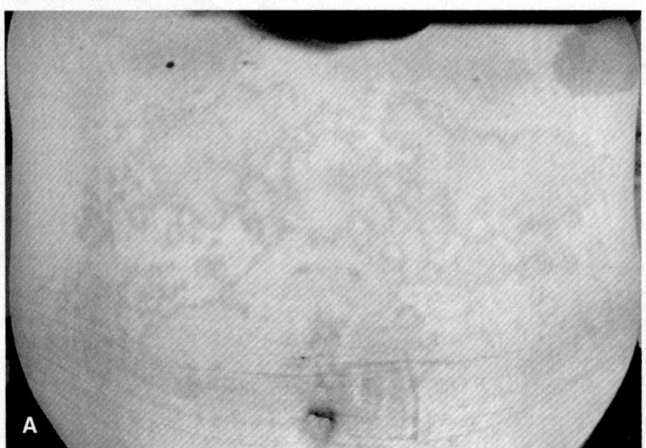

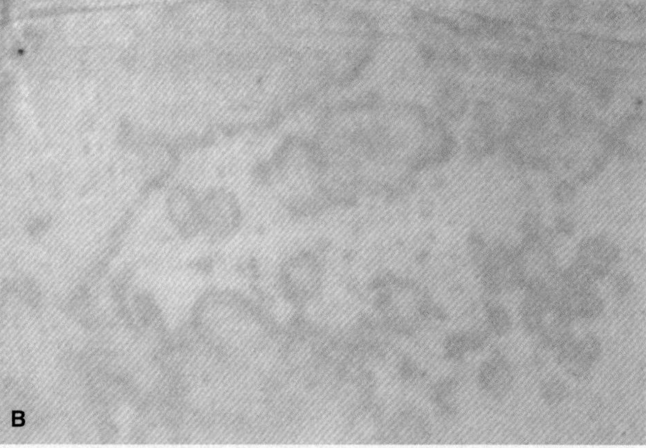

FIGURE 4.4. The rash of erythema marginatum begins as a serpiginous area of erythema and the margins of the rash progress as the center clears. Primarily occurs over the trunk and proximal extremities. (A) Erythema marginatum in an adult with rheumatic fever. (B) Closer view of rash. (Courtesy P. Witman, Mayo Clinic. Reprinted with permission from Koopman WJ, Moreland LW. *Arthritis and Allied Conditions. A Textbook of Rheumatology*. 15th ed. Philadelphia, PA: Lippincott Williams & Wilkins, 2005.)

Points to Remember

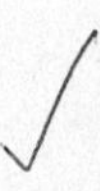

- Kawasaki disease is the most common cause of acquired heart disease in children in the United States. Rheumatic heart disease remains the most common cause of acquired heart disease in children worldwide.

Kawasaki Disease

Kawasaki disease is an acute febrile syndrome of **vasculitis** that occurs in children and has predilection for medium-sized arteries including the **coronary arteries.** It is a self-limited illness but is associated with significant morbidity and mortality due to its cardiac sequelae. This section will focus on the cardiac manifestations of Kawasaki disease. A more comprehensive discussion of the disease is included in the Chapter 5.

Cardiovascular Manifestations of Kawasaki Disease

- Acute phase (first 10 days): Pancarditis may occur but is usually mild and self-limited; signs and symptoms can include those of myocarditis, pericarditis, and/or endocarditis.

- Subacute phase (11 to 25 days after onset): **Coronary artery aneurysms.**
  - **Without treatment, 20% of patients will develop coronary artery aneurysms. With IVIG treatment, this risk is reduced to 5%.**
  - Aneurysms typically develop between days 7 and 28 of the illness.
  - Risk factors for the development of aneurysms include male gender, age below 1 year, prolonged fever (>14 days), and high fevers.
  - More than 50% of non-giant aneurysms resolve within 1 to 2 years of illness. Giant aneurysms (>8 mm) usually persist and are associated with increased risk of future stenosis and/or occlusion.

Points to Remember

- All patients with Kawasaki disease need a baseline echocardiogram at the time of diagnosis and at least one or two follow-up echocardiograms; patients with aneurysms require serial echocardiograms to monitor disease evolution.

Treatment

Goals of the treatment include decreasing coronary artery and myocardial inflammation and inhibiting platelet aggregation.

- **IVIG** reduces the risk of developing aneurysms and should be given within 10 days of disease onset (earlier is better). It is usually given as a single dose, although subsequent doses may be needed for patients with refractory disease.
- **High-dose aspirin** is given initially and continued until 48 to 72 hours after resolution of fevers. Aspirin is then continued at lower doses for a minimum of 6 to 8 weeks to reduce the risk of thrombus formation (longer course is needed with persistent coronary manifestations).

Points to Remember

- Beware of the risk of Reye syndrome in patients receiving aspirin who develop concurrent viral illnesses.

Prognosis

Kawasaki disease is largely self-limited, but cardiovascular complications can result in long-term sequelae and death.

- Deaths in the acute phase of illness are rare but can result from pancarditis.
- Patients with coronary artery aneurysms are at increased risk of MI related to thrombosis of aneurysms or stenosis of coronary arteries. **Most infarctions occur within 1 year of illness** without preceding signs or symptoms.

Points to Remember

- An MI in an apparently healthy child should make you think of previously unrecognized Kawasaki disease.

Lyme Carditis

Lyme disease is a tick borne illness caused by the spirochete *Borrelia burgdorferi*. Lyme disease has multisystem effects and causes cardiac manifestations in up to 10% of those with disseminated infection. This section will focus on the cardiac manifestations of Lyme disease—a more comprehensive discussion is included in the Chapter 16.

Points to Remember

- All patients who present with new heart block should have Lyme titers as part of their diagnostic evaluation.
- All patients with disseminated Lyme disease should have an EKG as part of their evaluation.

Cardiovascular Manifestations of Lyme Disease

- Cardiac involvement typically occurs several weeks post tick bite.
- The most common cardiac complication is AV block and can be first-, second-, or third-degree.
- Myocarditis, pericarditis, and LV dysfunction can also occur.

Treatment

Antimicrobial therapy for Lyme disease is dependant on disease stage and degree of systemic involvement. Recommendations for Lyme carditis are as follows:

- IV ceftriaxone or penicillin G for 14 days.
- Oral therapy (amoxicillin for young children; doxycycline for those older than 8 years) may be considered with mild cardiac involvement.
- Temporary pacing may be indicated for third-degree AV block.

Prognosis

AV block is antibiotic responsive and typically has a good prognosis, especially if treated early. However, a few patients may develop permanent heart block requiring pacemaker placement.

Myocarditis

Myocarditis is the inflammation of the walls of the heart characterized by inflammatory infiltrate and myocyte necrosis. Myocardial damage is considered secondary to a cell-mediated immunologic reaction. Myocarditis is almost always caused by viruses, particularly **enteroviruses (coxsackievirus)** and **adenovirus**. Other viral pathogens include rubella, HSV, varicella, and influenza. Less common causes of myocarditis include rheumatic fever, Kawasaki disease, collagen vascular diseases, and toxins.

Points to Remember

- Coxsackievirus is the most common cause of viral myocarditis.

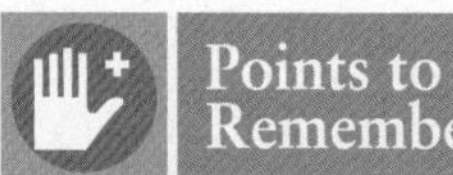

Points to Remember

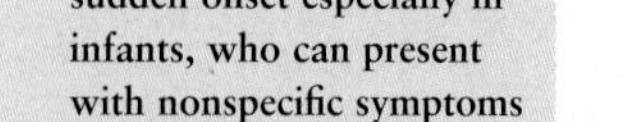

- Myocarditis can have a sudden onset especially in infants, who can present with nonspecific symptoms of poor feeding, emesis, and lethargy.

Clinical Manifestations

Wide spectrum of disease severity. Presentation ranges from vague URI symptoms and low-grade fevers to signs and symptoms of CHF. Chest pain may or may not be present. In subtle cases, look for **tachycardia out of proportion to fever** or the presence of a gallop on examination.

Diagnosis and Evaluation

- CXR—**cardiomegaly,** pulmonary edema.
- EKG—low QRS voltages, ST-T changes, PR and QT prolongation, and arrhythmias (PACs, PVCs, tachyarrhythmias, etc.).
- Laboratories—troponin level and CK-MB may be elevated.
- Echocardiogram—decreased ventricular function and chamber enlargement.
- Endomyocardial biopsy early in disease process can confirm diagnosis and may help elucidate the specific etiology.

Treatment

Supportive therapy to maintain cardiac output and limit further myocardial damage includes the following:

- Bed rest.
- Treat CHF—digoxin, diuretics, afterload reduction (ACE-I).
- Treat arrhythmias aggressively.
- Use inotropes (dopamine, dobutamine) if needed.
- IVIG has been shown to be beneficial in some studies, but its use remains controversial. If used, it must be given early in the course.
- Some patients go on to require a cardiac transplant.

Points to Remember

- Signs of cardiac tamponade include the Beck triad (↑ JVP, hypotension, and ↓ heart sounds due to acute compression of the heart), pulsus paradoxus, and tachycardia.
- Pulsus paradoxus is a decrease in systolic BP by 10 mmHg or more with inspiration (i.e., an exaggeration of the normal decrease in BP that occurs with inspiration).

Pericarditis

Pericarditis is the inflammation of the visceral and parietal surfaces of the pericardium and often leads to an associated pericardial effusion. Causes of pericarditis are similar to those of myocarditis with viral infections being the most common etiology. In addition, pericarditis can occur as a complication of an oncologic disease or its treatment (e.g., chemotherapy agents, radiation), in association with autoimmune disorders, or secondary to uremia.

Clinical Manifestations

- Typically presents with URI symptoms and fever followed by **precordial chest pain** that radiates to the shoulder and neck, is **relieved by leaning forward,** and is worsened when in supine position or with deep inspiration.
- Classic examination finding is the presence of a **pericardial friction rub.** Physical examination may also reveal diminished heart sounds if effusion is present. In severe cases, signs of **cardiac tamponade** from acute compression of the myocardium may be present.

Diagnosis

- EKG—**diffuse ST segment elevation,** T wave inversion, **low-voltage QRS.**
- CXR—cardiomegaly, pear-shaped or water-bottle shaped heart if a large effusion is present.
- Echocardiogram—diagnostic of effusion with or without tamponade.

Treatment

- Pericardiocentesis is both diagnostic and therapeutic and will aid in evaluating the underlying etiology. Pericardiocentesis is indicated immediately for tamponade physiology.
- Treat underlying etiology.
- Salicylates or corticosteroids for symptomatic relief.

Endocarditis

Endocarditis is an infection of the endocardium, valves, or related structures resulting from a combination of bacteremia and endothelial damage. Most children with endocarditis have a **history of congenital or acquired heart disease** and often have prosthetic materials in place. There is also an increased risk of endocarditis with IV drug use. Common pathogens include ***Staphylococcus aureus, S. viridans,*** **and enterococci** with increased prevalence of **HACEK** organisms (*Haemophilus, Actinobacillus, Cardiobacterium, Eikenella, Kingella*) and fungi in neonates and immunocompromised patients.

Clinical Manifestations

Endocarditis may present acutely with overwhelming sepsis but can also have a more indolent course with prolonged low-grade **fevers** and nonspecific symptoms including malaise, anorexia, weight loss, and fatigue.

Physical examination findings include the following:

- New or changing **heart murmur.**
- Splenomegaly occurs in more than 40% of patients.
- Dental caries or gingivitis is often present.
- Petechiae are the most common skin finding. More disease-specific skin lesions include **Janeway lesions** (hemorrhagic plaques on the palms and soles), **Osler nodes** (tender nodules on the pads of fingers and toes), and **splinter hemorrhages** (subungual linear hemorrhagic lesions) but are rare in children.
- Distant organ involvement due to emboli is common. The lungs, kidneys, and brain are most commonly affected. Retinal hemorrhages (**Roth spots**) are rare but can occur.

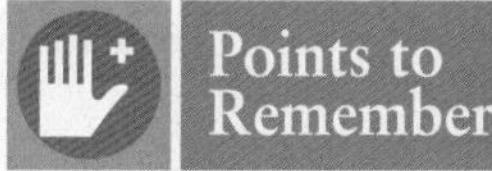

- **Large volume blood cultures and an echocardiogram should be obtained in any patient suspected to have endocarditis.**
- **An echocardiogram may show vegetations consistent with endocarditis, but a negative echo does not rule out endocarditis!**
- **EKG will be normal in most patients with endocarditis but may reveal associated arrhythmias or conduction abnormalities (AV or bundle branch block) depending on the location and extent of disease.**

Diagnosis

Modified **Duke criteria** are used for the diagnosis of IE. A definite diagnosis is made with the presence of two major criteria, one major and two minor criteria, or five minor criteria.

Major Duke criteria:

1. **Positive blood culture**: typical organism with two positive cultures more than 12 hours apart.
2. **Echocardiographic evidence** of endocardial involvement: vegetative mass, abscess, dehiscence of a prosthetic valve, or new valvular regurgitation.

Minor Duke criteria:

1. Predisposition: congenital or acquired heart disease, IV drug use.
2. Fever.
3. Embolic events: pulmonary infarct, intracranial abscess or focal infarct, conjunctival hemorrhage, Janeway lesions.
4. Immunologic events: + rheumatoid factor, glomerulonephritis, or Osler nodes.
5. Positive blood culture without meeting major criterion.

Treatment

- Initial empiric IV antibiotic therapy typically includes an antistaphylococcal penicillin (oxacillin, nafcillin) and an aminoglycoside (gentamicin). Vancomycin is added if MRSA is a concern (e.g., recent cardiac surgery).
- Patients should receive a total of 4 to 6 weeks of IV antibiotics, with selection of specific regimen ultimately guided by identification and sensitivity of infectious organism.
- Operative intervention is warranted for severe CHF, malfunction of prosthetic valves, persistently positive blood cultures with more than 2 weeks of treatment, fungal endocarditis, and relapse.

Prognosis

Overall case fatality is approximately 20%. Staphylococcal infection, fungal infection, and prosthetic valve infection worsen prognosis.

Prevention

Infective endocarditis is much more likely to occur as a result of bacteremia due to daily activities rather than bacteremia associated with dental or medical procedures. Proper **oral health and hygiene** is critical in the prevention of IE. The American Heart Association revised prophylaxis guidelines for prevention of procedure associated IE in 2007. Prophylaxis is indicated for high-risk patients (see Table 4.7) undergoing dental procedures or procedures on the respiratory tract, infected skin, or infected musculoskeletal tissue. Prophylaxis is no longer indicated for moderate-risk patients or for patients undergoing GU or GI tract procedures. See Table 4.8 for the recommended antibiotic regimens.

TABLE 4.7

CARDIAC CONDITIONS ASSOCIATED WITH THE HIGHEST RISK OF ADVERSE OUTCOME FROM INFECTIVE ENDOCARDITIS

- Prosthetic valve or prosthetic material used for valve repair
- Previous IE
- CHD:
  - Unrepaired or partially repaired cyanotic CHD disease (including palliative shunts and conduits)
  - Completely repaired CHD with prosthetic material for 6 months after procedure
  - Repaired CHD disease with residual defect near prosthetic material
- Cardiac transplant patients with valvulopathy

CHD, congenital heart disease; IE, infective endocarditis.

TABLE 4.8

RECOMMENDED ENDOCARDITIS PROPHYLAXIS FOR HIGH RISK PATIENTS

	Procedure Type	
Regimen Type and Route of Drug Administration	Dental and Respiratory Procedure	Procedures Involving Skin and Musculoskeletal Tissue
Standard oral regimens	**Amoxicillin**	Antistaphylococcal penicillin (**dicloxacillin**) **OR** oral cephalosporin
Standard IV regimens	**Ampicillin** or cefazolin or ceftriaxone	Antistaphylococcal penicillin (**nafcillin or oxacillin**) **or** parenteral cephalosporin
Oral regimens for penicillin allergy	Cephalexin or clindamycin or azithromycin or clarithromycin	Clindamycin
IV regimens for penicillin allergy	Cefazolin or ceftriaxone or clindamycin	Vancomycin or clindamycin

Adapted from Wilson W, Taubert KA, Gewitz M, et al. Prevention of infective endocarditis. *Circulation*. 2007;116:1736–1754.

TABLE 4.9

CARDIOMYOPATHY

	Dilated	Hypertrophic	Restrictive
Overview	↑ Ventricular size, ↓contractility (systolic dysfunction), MR is common	Hypertrophied LV and/or RV, commonly asymmetric septal hypertrophy and LVOT obstruction, stiff LV (diastolic dysfunction)	Myocardial fibrosis with stiff ventricular walls and impaired diastolic filling (diastolic dysfunction), atrial enlargement
Prevalence	55%	35%	5%
Etiology	Primarily idiopathic, 30% familial, can occur post myocarditis, secondary to toxins/meds (**doxorubicin**) or metabolic disturbances	AD inheritance in 50% due to sarcomere mutations, others with sporadic mutations	Myocardial fibrosis, hypertrophy or infiltration (amyloidosis, sarcoidosis, mucopolysaccharidosis)
Clinical manifestations	Signs and symptoms of CHF, S3 gallop, murmur of MR	Varies—can be asymptomatic, dizziness, palpitations, syncope, chest pain, sudden death, S_4 gallop, SEM due to LVOT obstruction	Exercise intolerance, chest pain, dyspnea, JVD, gallop
Diagnosis	**CXR**—cardiomegaly, pulmonary congestion **EKG**—tachycardia, LVH, ST-T waves changes **Echocardiogram**—biventricular dilatation, atrial enlargement, poor ventricular function, apical thrombus	**CXR**—LV enlargement, globular-shaped heart **EKG**—LVH, deep Q waves, ST-T wave changes **Echocardiogram**—thickened LV (± RV) wall, small LV chamber size, ↑ LV contractility	**CXR**—cardiomegaly, pulmonary congestion **EKG**—atrial hypertrophy, atrial arrhythmias **Echocardiogram**—biatrial enlargement, normal ventricular volume and function, atrial thrombus
Treatment	■ CHF treatment—diuretics, ACE-I, β-blockers ■ Anticoagulation ■ Antiarrhythmic ■ ± ICD ■ Cardiac transplant	■ Activity restriction ■ β-Blockers and CCB to improve ventricular filling ■ Antiarrhythmic ■ ICD placement ■ Myomectomy **Digoxin and diuretics are contraindicated**	■ Diuretics (congestive symptoms) ■ CCB (increase diastolic compliance) ■ Anticoagulants ■ Cardiac transplant
Prognosis	Progressive; 50% of patients die within 5 years of diagnosis	Variable from asymptomatic to progressive symptoms. **Sudden death in 5%** of patients per year (secondary to arrhythmias), 10%–20% develop DCM	Poor; 5-year survival rate is <30%

ACE-I, angiotensin converting enzyme inhibitors; CCB, calcium channel blocker; CHF, congestive heart failure; DCM, dilated cardiomyopathy; ICD, implantable cardioverter-defibrillator; JVD, jugular venous distention; LV, left ventricle; LVH, left ventricular hypertrophy; LVOT, left ventricular outflow tract; MR, mitral regurgitation; RV, right ventricle; SEM, systolic ejection murmur.

CARDIOMYOPATHY

Cardiomyopathy is a disease of the heart muscle. It can be classified into three major categories on the basis of clinical manifestations and functional features: dilated, hypertrophic, and restrictive. See Table 4.9 for complete discussion of cardiomyopathy.

ARRHYTHMIAS

Arrhythmias in children can be idiopathic but are often secondary to underlying pathology including CHD, myocardial disease (e.g., myocarditis, cardiomyopathy), or post surgical correction of heart defects. The risks of an arrhythmia are development of a rate too fast or too slow to supply adequate cardiac output or degeneration to a critical arrhythmia. Significant arrhythmia can result in syncope, heart failure, or sudden death.

Atrial Arrhythmias

Premature Atrial Contraction

A premature P wave (P′) usually but not always followed by a premature QRS. PACs commonly appear in normal children and have no hemodynamic significance (Fig. 4.5A).

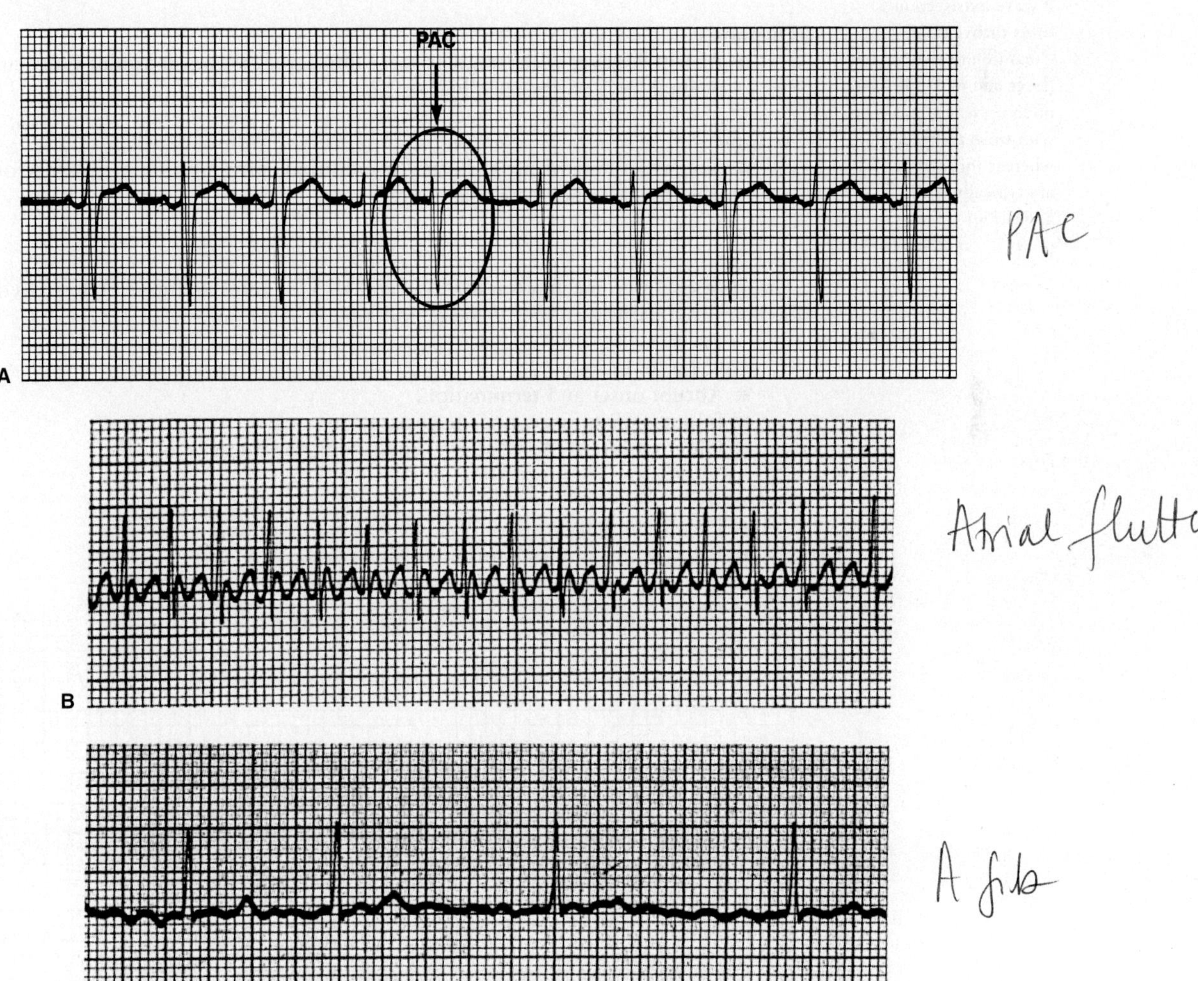

FIGURE 4.5. Atrial arrhythmias. (**A**) Premature atrial contraction (PAC). A premature P wave is followed by a premature QRS complex; there is a compensatory pause after the premature beat. (**B**) Atrial flutter. Note the normal appearing QRS complexes with a baseline "saw-tooth" patter of flutter waves. (**C**) Atrial fibrillation demonstrates the absence of P waves and a baseline of rapid fibrillatory waves with irregular QRS complexes. (**A:** Reprinted with permission from Nettina SM. *The Lippincott Manual of Nursing Practice*. 7th ed. Philadelphia, PA: Lippincott Williams & Wilkins, 2001. **B, C:** Reprinted with permission from Fleisher GR, Ludwig S, Henretig FM, et al. *Textbook of Pediatric Emergency Medicine*. 5th ed. Philadelphia, PA: Lippincott Williams & Wilkins, 2005.)

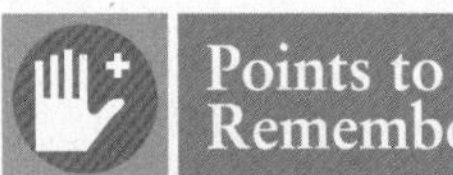

- SVT associated with WPW syndrome most commonly occurs though an AV reentrant tachycardia.

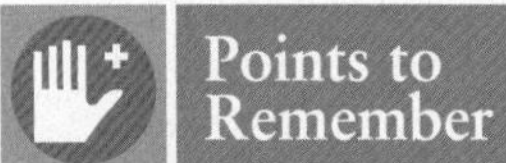

- Sinus tachycardia can be differentiated from SVT by the following:
  - Rate (>230 bpm is almost always SVT)
  - Variability (heart rate in SVT does not vary)
  - P wave axis (upright P waves in leads I and aVF indicate a normal P wave axis seen in sinus tachycardia)
  - Condition of the patient (fever and irritability are often present in patients with sinus tachycardia, whereas those with SVT are typically well appearing)

Atrial Flutter

Atrial flutter originates from an ectopic atrial focus and results in an intra-atrial "circus movement." Atrial rate is 250 to 400 bpm, but because there is almost always some degree of AV block, a ventricular response typically occurs every second to fourth atrial beat (note: fetuses and newborns can conduct a slow flutter 1:1). Atrial flutter usually suggests **significant cardiac pathology** but can occur in infants with structurally normal hearts. It can also be secondary to digitalis toxicity. Long-standing arrhythmia can lead to intra-atrial **thrombus** with risk of **embolic complications.**

Diagnosis

- Rapid, regular **"saw-toothed" flutter waves** with normal QRS complexes (Fig. 4.5B).

Treatment

- Acutely, synchronized **cardioversion** is the treatment of choice; amiodarone, ibutilide, and procainamide can also be effective.
- With arrhythmia lasting 24 to 48 hours or more, patients are at risk of cerebral embolic events because of thrombi and require **anticoagulation** prior to cardioversion.
- **Ablation** may be considered for refractory cases.

Atrial Fibrillation

Less common than atrial flutter in children. Atrial excitation is chaotic with a very rapid rate (350 to 600 bpm) and **irregularly irregular** ventricular response. Atrial fibrillation is usually associated with **atrial dilation** secondary to structural heart disease.

Diagnosis

- **Absent P waves** with **irregular rapid fibrillatory waves, irregular ventricular response,** and normal QRS complexes (Fig. 4.5C).

Treatment

- Similar to that of atrial flutter. In addition, propranolol, verapamil, or digoxin can be used to slow the ventricular rate.

Re-entrant Tachycardia

The **most common mechanism for SVT** and also the **most common tachyarrhythmia in children;** involves two pathways: the AV node and an accessory pathway.

Clinical Manifestations

- **Abrupt onset and termination.**
- Infants—irritability, poor feeding, tachypnea.
- Older children—palpitations, chest pain, shortness of breath.

Diagnosis

- **Unvarying heart rate of 240 ± 40 bpm or more.**
- **P waves** are either **abnormal** or **not visible** (Fig. 4.6).

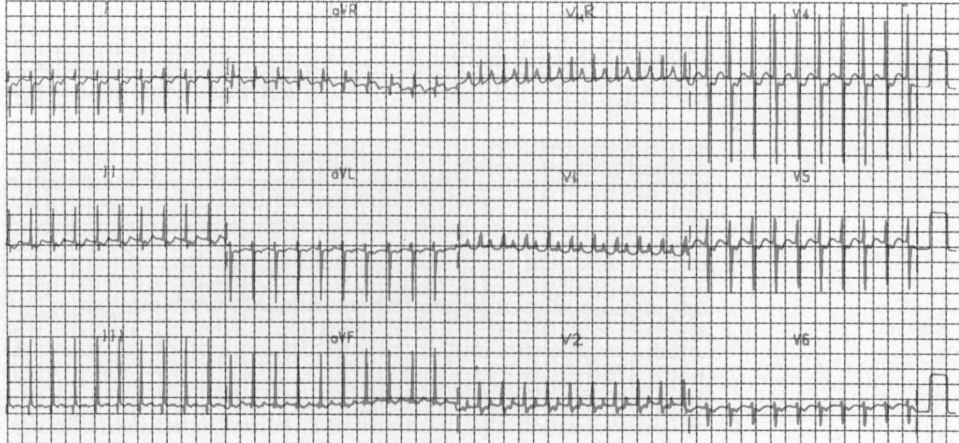

FIGURE 4.6. Supraventricular tachycardia. Narrow complex tachycardia with an unvarying rate and either abnormal or nonvisible P waves. In this EKG, the heart rate is 250 bpm and the P waves occur after the QRS complexes (best seen in lead V_2). (Reprinted with permission from McMillan JA, Feigin RD, DeAngelis C, et al. *Oski's Pediatrics: Principles and Practice.* 4th ed. Philadelphia, PA: Lippincott Williams & Wilkins, 2006.)

Treatment

- Acute management:
  - Vagal stimulation—ice-water bag on the face of infants; valsalva maneuvers in older children.
  - **Adenosine**—drug of choice; very effective.
  - Cardioversion—may be indicated with concomitant CHF or if patient fails adenosine treatment.
- Long-term management:
  - β-Blockers.
  - Ablation—may be indicated for recurrent arrhythmias or failure of medical management.

Ectopic Atrial Tachycardia

Increased automaticity of an **ectopic atrial focus** causes this uncommon arrhythmia. On EKG, P waves are visible with an abnormal P wave axis and a **variable** heart rate of 110 to 160 bpm. There can be multiple atrial foci and ectopic atrial tachycardia is very difficult to treat.

Supraventricular Tachycardia

This group of arrhythmias includes narrow QRS complex tachycardias that originate above the bifurcation of the bundle of His and can be divided into two main groups: **re-entrant** (reciprocating) tachycardias and **ectopic** (non-reciprocating) tachycardias.

Ventricular Arrhythmias

Premature Ventricular Contraction

Occasional PVCs often occur in healthy children, but PVCs can also be pathologic and result from myocardial and structural heart disease, LQTS, and secondary to drugs (caffeine, amphetamines, digoxin).

Diagnosis

- **Premature wide QRS complex** not preceded by a P wave, typically followed by a compensatory pause (Fig. 4.7).

Treatment

- **Occasional PVCs are benign** in children and require reassurance only.
- Rarely, PVCs can degenerate into severe arrhythmias. Patients with associated underlying heart disease or syncope, runs of PVCs, increased frequency of PVCs with activity, and multiform PVCs are at increased risk and may require **suppressive therapy.**

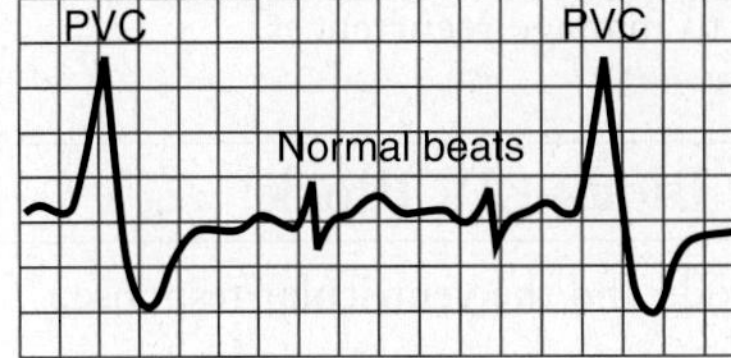

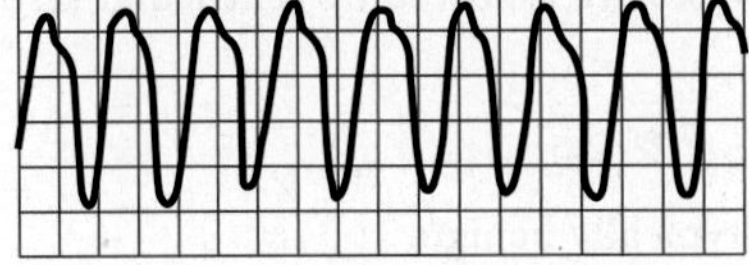

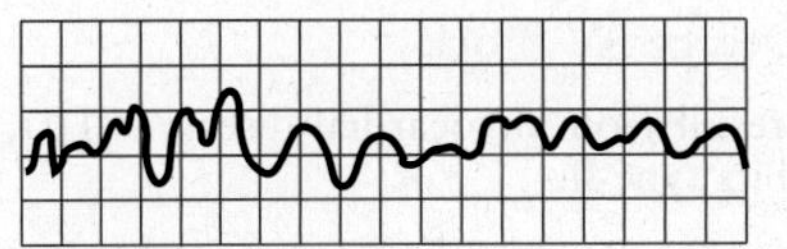

FIGURE 4.7. Ventricular arrhythmias. Electrocardiographic (ECG) tracings of ventricular arrhythmias. Premature ventricular contractions (PVCs) (top tracing) originate from an ectopic focus in the ventricles, causing a distortion of the QRS complex. Because the ventricle usually cannot repolarize sufficiently to respond to the next impulse that arises in the sinoatrial node, a PVC frequently is followed by a compensatory pause. Ventricular tachycardia (middle tracing) is characterized by a rapid ventricular rate of 70 to 250 bpm and the absence of P waves. In ventricular fibrillation (bottom tracing), there are no regular or effective ventricular contractions, and the ECG tracing is totally disorganized. (Reprinted with permission from Porth CM, *Pathophysiology Concepts of Altered Health States*. 7th ed. Philadelphia, PA: Lippincott Williams & Wilkins, 2005.

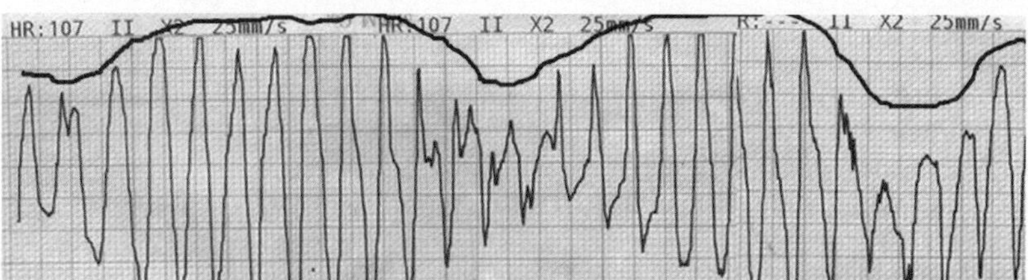

FIGURE 4.8. This rhythm strip of Torsades de pointes shows the characteristic change of the QRS amplitude delineated by the *blue line.* (http://en.wikipedia.org/wiki/File:Tosadesdepointes.jpg.)

Ventricular Tachycardia

Defined by three or more PVCs with a heart rate of 120 to 200 bpm. Children may tolerate rapid ventricular rates for hours; however, VT must be treated quickly as hypotension and degeneration to ventricular fibrillation may result. VT can occur in otherwise healthy children but is more common in children with underlying heart disease, long QT, and metabolic disturbances (electrolyte abnormalities, hypoxia).

Points to Remember

- Torsades de pointes—"Twisting of the points"—A type of polymorphic VT characterized by QRS amplitude that gradually increases then decreases. (Fig. 4.8).

Diagnosis

- Wide QRS complex tachycardia with AV dissociation (no relationship between P waves and the VT) (Fig. 4.7).

Treatment

Management guided by PALS algorithm.

- Immediate synchronized **cardioversion** in symptomatic patients.
- Pharmacologic conversion can be attempted with amiodarone, procainamide, or lidocaine but should not delay cardioversion.
- Prevention may require β-blockers or other antiarrhythmic medication and/or ICD placement.

Ventricular Fibrillation (VF)

Rapid, irregular arrhythmia with odd and varied QRS complexes. Rare in children. Usually results from degeneration of VT and is **rapidly fatal** unless effective ventricular contraction is quickly re-established (Fig. 4.7).

Treatment

Management guided by PALS algorithm

- Immediate defibrillation and IV epinephrine.
- Survivors often require ICD placement to manage recurrences.

Points to Remember

- Think of VT secondary to hyperkalemia with degeneration to VF in a renal patient with a sudden cardiac arrest.

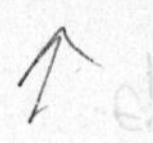

Atrioventricular Block (AV Block)

A conduction disturbance between the sinus node and the ventricular response.

First-Degree AV Block

Prolongation of the PR interval. All atrial impulses are followed by ventricular response (see Fig. 4.9A).

Treatment/Prognosis

- No treatment required as condition is **typically benign.**
- Occasionally can progress to more significant AV block.

Second-Degree AV Block

Often appears in healthy children but can result from myocardial disease, CHD, and digitalis toxicity. Two forms: Mobitz type I and Mobitz type II.

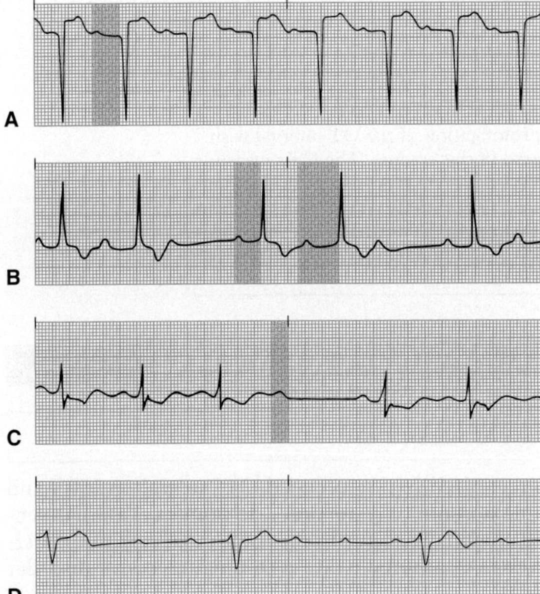

FIGURE 4.9. Atrioventricular block. (A) First-degree AV block. The shaded area demonstrates prolongation of the PR interval. (B) Type I second-degree AV block. The shaded areas show progressive lengthening of the PR interval followed by a P wave with a dropped QRS complex. (C) Type II second-degree AV block. The shaded area highlights a P wave with no corresponding QRS, note there is no change of the PR interval. (D) Third-degree AV block with complete disassociation of atrial and ventricular contractions. (Reprinted with permission from Springhouse. *ECG Facts Made Incredibly Easy*. 2nd ed. Ambler, PA: Wolters Kluwer Health, 2010.)

Mobitz Type I (Wenckebach Phenomenon)

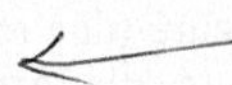

Progressive lengthening of the PR interval until a QRS complex is dropped (see Fig. 4.9B).

Treatment/Prognosis

- Underlying causes should be treated if present.
- Does not usually progress to complete AV block.

Mobitz Type II

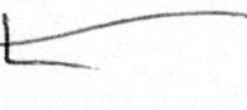

No change in the PR interval, but occasional atrial contractions do not conduct to the ventricle and a QRS complex is dropped (see Fig. 4.9C).

Treatment/Prognosis

- Underlying causes should be treated if present.
- **May progress to complete heart block.**

Third-Degree AV Block

Complete dissociation of atrial and ventricular contraction. Etiology can be congenital or acquired. Some forms of congenital disease result from maternal connective tissue disease (**systemic lupus erythematosus**, Sjögren's syndrome). Other etiologies include CHD, cardiac surgery, myocarditis, and **Lyme carditis.**

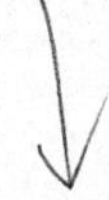

Clinical Manifestations

- CHF can develop in infancy.
- **Low heart rate** can result in syncope or sudden death.
- Some children may be asymptomatic.

Diagnosis

- P waves are regular with a rate similar to a normal heart rate.
- QRS complexes are also regular, but the rate is significantly slower than the P rate.
- P waves and QRS complexes are not associated (see Fig. 4.9D).

Treatment

- Symptomatic patients require pacemaker therapy.
- Atropine or isoproterenol can be given until pacing is established.

Points to Remember

- **Maternal SLE can result in complete heart block in the newborn (some previously undiagnosed cases of maternal SLE may even be picked up because of heart block in the newborn).**

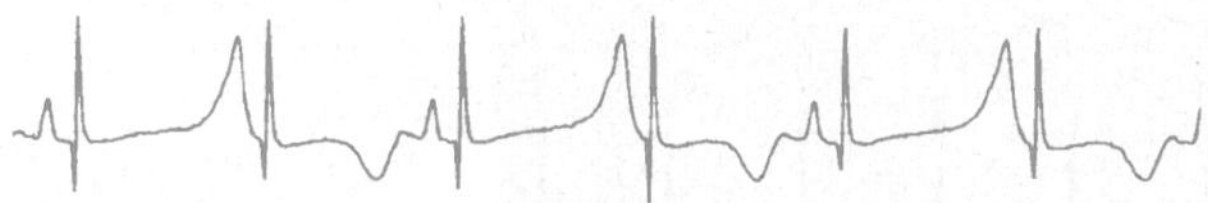

FIGURE 4.10. Congenital prolongation of the QT interval with T wave alternans is demonstrated in this tracing. The QTc measures 0.68 seconds. The T waves have a bizarre morphology and at times may be mistaken for P waves. (Reprinted with permission from McMillan JA, Feigin RD, DeAngelis C, et al. *Oski's Pediatrics: Principles and Practice*. 4th ed. Philadelphia, PA: Lippincott Williams & Wilkins, 2006.)

Points to Remember

- Prolongation of the QT interval can occur with anorexia nervosa and improves with caloric rehabilitation.
- Many medications can cause QT prolongation and should be avoided in patients with LQTS. Examples: antimicrobials (macrolides, fluoroquinolones, trimethoprim-sulfamethoxazole) stimulants (methylphenidate), antidepressants (tricyclics, selective serotonin reuptake inhibitors), antipsychotics (chlorpromazine, thioridazine, risperidone, haloperidol), antiarrhythmics: (amiodarone, procainamide, quinidine, sotalol), decongestants (pseudoephedrine).

ABNORMALITIES IN SINUS RHYTHM

Long QT syndrome

A disorder of ventricular repolarization characterized by a prolonged QT interval on EKG and association with ventricular arrhythmias, most commonly **torsades de pointes.** Familial syndromes cause approximately 50% of cases. **Romano-Ward syndrome** is the most common inherited form and is AD. **Jervell and Lange-Nielsen syndrome** is an autosomal recessive disorder characterized by LQTS and **congenital deafness.**

Clinical Manifestations

- Can be asymptomatic but can also present with syncope and/or palpitations with exertion, intense emotion, sudden noise, swimming.
- Seizure (due to hypoperfusion with associated ventricular arrhythmias).
- Ventricular arrhythmias (torsades de pointes).
- Cardiac arrest with or without sudden death.

Diagnosis

The normal length of the QT interval varies slightly with age, but in general a QTc >0.46 seconds is considered long. (QTc = QT/square root of the R-R interval) (Fig. 4.10).

Treatment

- Acute treatment of associated arrhythmias.
- β-Blockers reduce incidence of syncope and SCD.
- ICD placement.

Points to Remember

- Digoxin and verapamil can increase impulse conduction through the accessory pathway in WPW and should be avoided.

Wolff-Parkinson-White Syndrome

Pre-excitation due to an anomalous conduction pathway between the atria and ventricles with an associated episode of tachycardia (pre-excitation alone is not diagnostic of WPW).

Diagnosis

- EKG findings: short PR interval, **delta wave,** wide QRS complex (Fig. 4.11).
- Episode of tachycardia (SVT).

Treatment

- Acute management: management of SVT and/or resulting CHF.
- Long-term management: propranolol and atenolol for arrhythmia prevention.

Points to Remember

- Less than 5% of children with chest pain have underlying cardiac disease.

CHEST PAIN

Chest pain is a common complaint in children that usually has a benign etiology and is only rarely associated with underlying cardiac disease. **The most common causes of chest pain in children are costochondritis, musculoskeletal, respiratory, psychogenic, and idiopathic.** Noncardiac and cardiac etiologies of chest pain as well as associated clinical manifestations are reviewed in **Tables 4.10, 4.11, and 4.12.**

Diagnosis

- History—important elements include duration, quality, location, radiation, severity, precipitating factors, and associated symptoms.

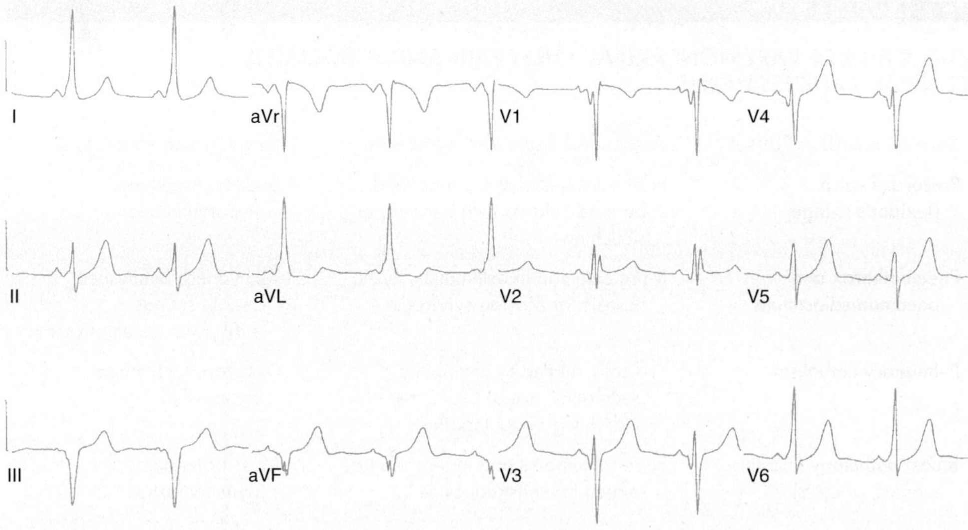

FIGURE 4.11. EKG evidence of Wolff-Parkinson-White (WPW) is seen on this strip with notable short PR interval, widened QRS complex, and delta wave. (Reprinted with permission from McMillan JA, Feigin RD, DeAngelis C, et al. *Oski's Pediatrics: Principles and Practice*. 4th ed. Philadelphia, PA: Lippincott Williams & Wilkins, 2006.)

- Red flags that should heighten suspicion for a cardiac etiology
  - Chest pain that occurs **with exercise.**
  - **Anginal type pain** (precordial or substernal pain described as a heavy pressure, choking or crushing with radiation to the neck, jaw, back, arms, or abdomen).
  - **Recurrent pain.**
  - Pain associated with **syncope, dizziness, palpitations,** or **dyspnea.**
- Examination—pertinent findings for specific etiologies are noted in **Tables 4.10, 4.11, and 4.12.** Patients with abnormal physical exam findings or symptoms suggestive of organic disease should undergo further evaluation.

TABLE 4.10

ETIOLOGIES OF COMMON NONCARDIAC CHEST PAIN AND ASSOCIATED CLINICAL MANIFESTATIONS, AND TREATMENT

Common Noncardiac Causes	Associated Signs and Symptoms	Examination Findings	Treatment
Costochondritis	Anterior chest pain, usually unilateral with tenderness at the costochondral joint. May follow respiratory illnesses or physical activity.	**Reproducible pain with palpation**	Rest, NSAIDs or acetaminophen
Musculoskeletal	Secondary to stain of chest wall muscles (related to exercise or coughing) or trauma.	Tenderness of the chest wall, signs of trauma (bruises)	Rest, NSAIDs or acetaminophen
Respiratory (Exercise-induced asthma, pneumonia, bronchitis)	**Chest tightness** or pain may occur with exercise induced bronchospasm. Other complaints include shortness of breath, decreased exercise tolerance, or cough.	Tachypnea, crackles, wheezing, or increased work of breathing. Fever with pneumonia.	Asthma—inhaled β-agonists; pneumonia and bronchitis—appropriate antimicrobial therapy
Psychogenic	More common in children older than 12 years and girls. Often related to anxiety or stressful events. Vague associated somatic complaints include headache and abdominal pain.	Normal or nonspecific	Reassurance, address life stressors
Gastrointestinal (GER, esophageal spasm, foreign body, or ingestion)	Burning substernal pain, relief or exacerbation with eating, worse when in supine position	Epigastric tenderness	Antacids, hydrogen ion inhibitors, or proton pump inhibitors. Referral to a gastroenterologist

GER, gastroesophageal reflux; NSAID, nonsteroidal anti-inflammatory drugs.

TABLE 4.11

ETIOLOGIES OF RARE NONCARDIAC CHEST PAIN AND ASSOCIATED CLINICAL MANIFESTATIONS

Rare Noncardiac Causes	Associated Signs and Symptoms	Examination Findings
Precordial catch (Texidor's twinge)	Brief episodes of sharp localized pain associated with bending or slouching	Shallow breathing, hyperventilation
Pneumothorax and pneumomediastinum	More common in asthmatics, cystic fibrosis, or Marfan syndrome	Tachypnea, diminished breath sounds, subcutaneous emphysema
Pulmonary embolism	Typically related to immobility, pregnancy, use of OCPs, or underlying coagulopathy	Dyspnea, tachypnea, hypoxemia
Breast pathology (mastitis, masses, or cysts)	Pubertal females and males, may be related to menstrual cycle	Mass or tenderness, gynecomastia

OCP, oral contraceptive pill.

- Initial studies:
  - CXR—may show evidence of pneumonia, asthma, foreign body, or other pulmonary disorder; in cardiac disease, **cardiomegaly** or vascular abnormalities may be apparent.
  - EKG— **LVH** may indicate obstructive disease or cardiomyopathy; **ischemic changes** are concerning for coronary anomalies; **diffuse ST segment elevation** is characteristic of pericarditis; **ST-T wave anomalies** are seen in myocarditis; **arrhythmias** may be evident.
  - Laboratory studies—cardiac enzymes are indicated if concern for MI.
- Further workup by a cardiologist for suspected cardiac disease may include Holter monitor, exercise stress test, echocardiogram, and/or cardiac catheterization.

Treatment

- Depends on underlying etiology; treatment options for common noncardiac causes are listed in Table 4.10.

TABLE 4.12

ETIOLOGIES OF CARDIAC CHEST PAIN AND ASSOCIATED CLINICAL MANIFESTATIONS

Cardiac Causes	Associated Signs and Symptoms	Examination Findings
Severe obstructive lesions (aortic or pulmonary stenosis)	Pain associated **with exercise,** and is often **recurrent. Anginal pain** may be present	Loud harsh systolic murmur
Cardiomyopathy	Pain may be **ischemic** or **arrhythmic** in origin. Syncope or palpitations may also be present.	Normal or SEM
Coronary artery disease (anomalous origin, vasospasm)	History of **Kawasaki disease**, pain with intense physical activity, anginal pain, diaphoresis, nausea, dyspnea, syncope	Normal, possible gallop, or SEM of mitral insufficiency
Aortic dissection or aneurysm	**Severe tearing pain** with radiation to the **back.** Patients with Marfan syndrome, Turner syndrome, and Noonan's syndromes are at risk.	Stigmata of associated syndrome
Inflammatory (pericarditis, myocarditis)	Sharp, stabbing precordial pain, improved with upright position or leaning forward, signs of tamponade, evidence of fever, or recent illness	Pericardial friction rub, tachycardia, muffled heart sounds
Arrhythmias	Sensation of "heart pounding," palpitations, syncope, abrupt onset, and termination	Tachycardia, irregular rhythm
Toxins (cocaine, methamphetamines, sympathomimetic decongestants)	Social history of use or abuse, anginal pain, possible palpitations related to arrhythmia, may present similar to coronary artery disease	Tachycardia, hypertension

SEM, systolic ejection murmur.

SYNCOPE

Syncope is defined as a temporary loss of consciousness and muscle tone secondary to decreased cerebral perfusion. In most cases, the duration of unconsciousness is less than 1 minute. Approximately 15% of children experience a syncopal event prior to 18 years of age. Although syncope is often benign, the possibility of underlying pathology must be investigated. Etiologies of syncope with corresponding manifestations are listed in **Table 4.13**.

Points to Remember

- 75% of patients with syncope have autonomic causes.

Diagnosis

- History—a detailed history is the key to diagnosis in most cases of syncope; historical elements including the time of day, position of patient, relationship to exercise or stress, duration of episode, and associated symptoms can guide diagnosis of etiology and further workup.
- EKG—necessary in all patients with syncope; can identify arrhythmias, long QT syndrome, and WPW syndrome; can be suggestive of obstructive lesions or myocardial dysfunction.
- Holter monitor—can be used to correlate heart rhythm and symptoms for a 24-hour period if arrhythmia is suspected but not detected on EKG.
- Exercise stress test—used in cases of syncope associated with exercise.
- Echocardiogram—can identify structural abnormalities (AS, cardiomyopathy, etc.)
- Tilt-table test—useful in the diagnosis of orthostatic intolerance (vasovagal, orthostatic hypotension). Neither specific nor sensitive.
- EEG—if seizure is suspected.

TABLE 4.13

ETIOLOGIES OF SYNCOPE AND ASSOCIATED CLINICAL MANIFESTATIONS

Differential Diagnosis			Clinical Manifestations
Autonomic	Orthostatic Intolerance	Vasovagal syncope	Prodrome of dizziness, lightheadedness, nausea, pallor, palpitations, visual changes, headache, and shortness of breath. May be precipitated by acute illness or noxious stimuli (pain, fear). Heart rate and blood pressure drop acutely with symptoms.
Autonomic	Orthostatic Intolerance	Orthostatic hypotension	≥20/10 mmHg drop in blood pressure after assuming an upright position Lightheadedness without extensive prodrome Exacerbated by dehydration and prolonged bed rest.
Autonomic	Orthostatic Intolerance	Postural orthostatic tachycardia syndrome (POTS)	Orthostatic symptoms (fatigue, lightheadedness, recurrent near syncope) associated with 30 bpm increase in heart rate with upright positioning. Associated with chronic fatigue syndrome.
Autonomic	Situational syncope		Related to breathholding spells, cough, micturition, defecation.
Cardiac	Arrhythmias (SVT, VT)		Suggested by occurrence of events in a supine or sitting position, can be provoked by exercise.
Cardiac	Obstructive lesions (AS, PS, HCM)		May be accompanied by chest pain or palpitations.
Cardiac	Myocardial dysfunction (Coronary artery anomalies, Kawasaki disease)		
Neuropsychiatric	Hyperventilation		Unnoticed apprehension and deep sighing respirations Associated with emotional disturbances Reproducible with intentional hyperventilation
Neuropsychiatric	Seizure		Unusual eye or limb movements Postictal confusion Prolonged duration of unconsciousness (>1 minute)
Neuropsychiatric	Migraine		Headache, nausea, vomiting, photophobia, relief by sleep
Neuropsychiatric	Hysteria		Prolonged episode occurring only in the presence of others; rare before age 10 years
Metabolic	Hypoglycemia		Symptoms may include pallor, perspiration, lightheadedness; duration of onset and recovery are gradual
Metabolic	Electrolyte disturbances Drugs/Toxins		Varied dependant on the underlying etiology

HCM, hypertrophic cardiomyopathy; PS, pulmonary stenosis; SVT, supraventricular tachycardia; VT, ventricular tachycardia.

Treatment

- Orthostatic intolerance, the most common cause of syncope, can be treated with nonpharmacologic therapy (e.g., **increased water** and **sodium intake**, elastic support hose). Pharmacologic management consists of **fludrocortisone**, β-blockers, or α-agonists.
- Treatment of other etiologies of syncope depends on the underlying disorder.

SUDDEN CARDIAC DEATH

The incidence of SCD in children and adolescents in the United States ranges from 0.8 to 6.2 per 100,000 per year resulting in approximately 500 deaths.

Clinical Manifestations

Patients are often **asymptomatic** before the event. If preceding symptoms do occur, they may include chest pain, syncope, palpitations or dyspnea. **Exercise** often **precipitates death.**

Differential Diagnosis/Etiology

Myocardial Disease

- Cardiomyopathy— **HCM is the most common cause of SCD in adolescents**; among those with HCM, risk factors for SCD include family history of sudden death, symptomatic disease, ventricular arrhythmias, and young age. Dilated cardiomyopathy is also associated with SCD.
- Myocarditis—SCD can result from overt heart failure, heart block, or arrhythmias.

Coronary Artery Disease

- **Anomalous origin** or anomalous tract of the coronary arteries (most commonly, anomalous origin of the left main coronary artery), leading to ischemia and predisposing patients to arrhythmias and SCD.
- Acquired coronary artery disease—coronary artery aneurysm related to **Kawasaki disease** and atherosclerosis related to **familial hyperbetalipoproteinemia.**

Conduction Anomalies

- **LQTS**—leads to ventricular arrhythmias (most commonly torsades de pointes) and SCD
- **WPW syndrome**—predisposes to SVTs.
- Complete heart block—SCD is caused by bradycardia and ventricular arrhythmias.
- Sick sinus syndrome—arrhythmia-related death.

Congenital Heart Disease

- **Valvular AS**—congenital defect most commonly associated with sudden death in children.
- Following CHD repair—increased incidence of ventricular arrhythmias following **TOF** repair; increased incidence of atrial arrhythmias post **Fontan.**
- **Mitral valve prolapse**—typically benign, but those with associated ventricular arrhythmias, regurgitation, prolonged QT, and/or history of syncope are at high risk of SCD.

Others

- Commotio cordis—fatal development of ventricular fibrillation classically unresponsive to resuscitation after blunt nonpenetrating chest trauma.
- Marfan syndrome—most common cause of SCD is rupture of a dilated aortic root.
- Pulmonary HTN—significant risk factor for SCD in patients with heart disease and concurrent pulmonary HTN and also in primary pulmonary HTN.

Diagnosis/Treatment

Evaluation for and management of potentially treatable causes of SCD is imperative in patients presenting with syncope, chest pain, and palpitations. However, many patients are asymptomatic until the event causing death. Family members of those who suffer SCD should be evaluated for genetic causes (e.g., LQTS, HCM).

TABLE 4.14

NATIONAL HIGH BLOOD PRESSURE EDUCATION PROGRAM (NHBPEP) CLASSIFICATION OF BLOOD PRESSURE LEVELS

BP Classification	Systolic or Diastolic BP
Normotensive	<90th percentile
Prehypertension	90th–95th percentile
Stage 1 hypertension	95th–99th percentile + 5 mmHg on ≥3 **occasions**
Stage 2 hypertension	>99th percentile + 5 mmHg on ≥3 **occasions**

HYPERTENSION

In children, normal BP varies with age, gender, and height; therefore, elevated BP is statistically defined on the basis of normative BP standards. Elevated BP is defined by the Fourth Report of the NHBPEP in Table 4.14.

The most likely etiology of HTN is age dependant. In infants and younger children, HTN is usually secondary to another disease process (**secondary HTN**). In adolescents, **primary** or **essential HTN** in which there is no specific cause is more common and is often contributed to by obesity, genetics, diet, and stress.

Points to Remember

- **To ensure correct BP determination, the cuff must be the correct size. The bladder width of the cuff should be at least 40% of the arm circumference, and the length should be 125% to 155% of the arm diameter.**

Clinical Manifestations

- Essential HTN—**usually asymptomatic; mild elevations** in BP; patients are often **overweight.**
- Secondary HTN—**BP elevation varies** from **mild to severe**; most patients remain **asymptomatic** unless BP quickly changes or maintains substantial elevation; clinical manifestations of the underlying disease may be present.
- Significant or acute HTN can cause headache, epistaxis, visual changes, dizziness, nausea, and vomiting. Hypertensive encephalopathy can develop and manifest as seizure.

Points to Remember

- **10% to 30% of overweight children have elevated BP.**
- **Both primary and secondary HTN are most often asymptomatic. If a patient is symptomatic, however, secondary HTN is more likely than primary HTN.**

Etiologies of Secondary HTN

Many disease entities can cause secondary HTN, but it is most commonly attributed to renal parenchymal disease, renovascular disease, and COA.

- **Renal parenchymal disease** (e.g., glomerulonephritis, pyelonephritis, congenital anomalies, obstructive uropathies) and **renovascular disease** (e.g., renal artery stenosis, renal vein thrombosis).
- Cardiovascular disease (**COA**).
- Endocrinopathies (e.g., hyperthyroidism, pheochromocytoma, neuroblastoma, congenital adrenal hyperplasia, Cushing's syndrome, hyperaldosteronism).
- Drugs (e.g., steroids, caffeine, cocaine, tobacco, oral contraceptives, nasal decongestants, stimulants, immunosuppressive agents).

Diagnosis and Evaluation

Once diagnosis is established, the NHBPEP has suggested a management algorithm shown in Figure 4.12.

- Recommended diagnostic workup evaluates for causes of secondary HTN and includes a complete history and physical examination to evaluate for signs and symptoms of underlying disease processes, specifically related to the renal and cardiovascular systems.
- Initial laboratory evaluation and imaging should include the following:
  - BUN, creatinine, and electrolytes.
  - Urinalysis and urine culture.
  - Renal ultrasound.
- Evaluation for target-organ damage in selected patients should include the following:
  - Echocardiogram—LVH suggests sustained HTN and risk for future heart disease.
  - Retinal examination.

Treatment

The goal of therapy is to reduce BP to below the 95th percentile. Initial treatment for essential HTN in overweight patients includes **therapeutic lifestyle changes** (weight reduction, increased physical activity, reduction of sodium intake).

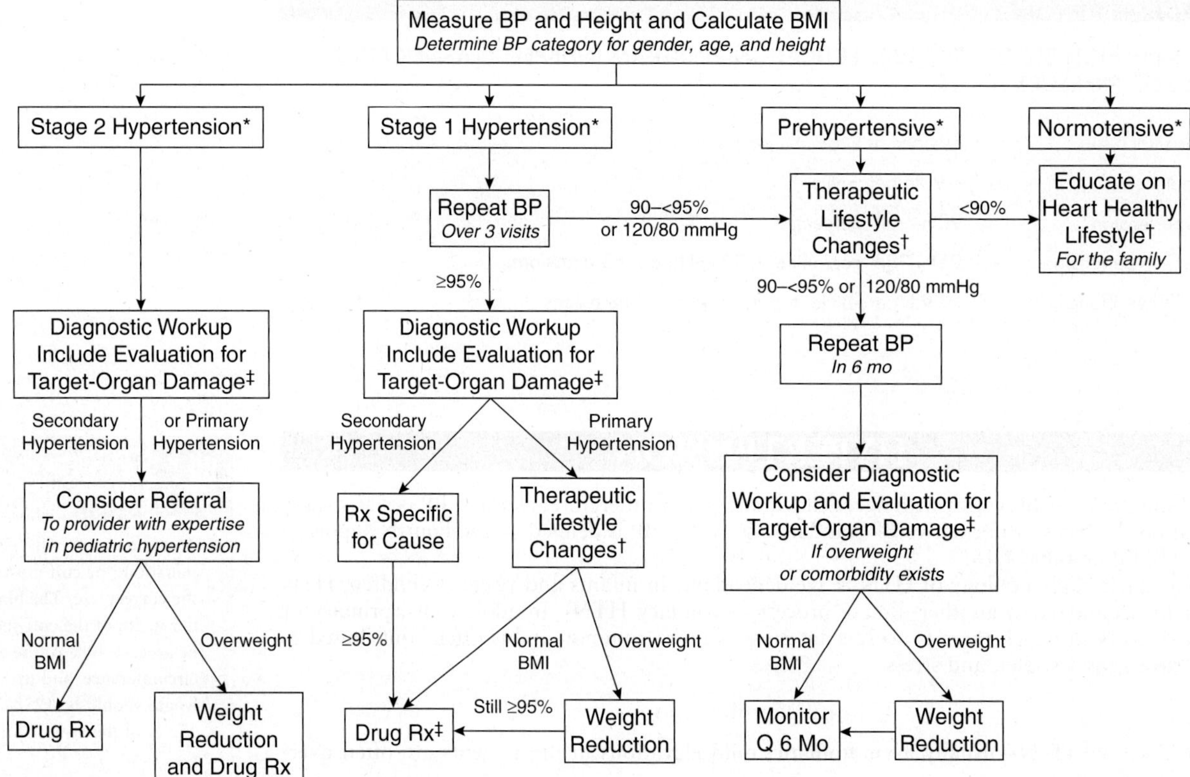

FIGURE 4.12. Algorithm for the management of high blood pressure. Rx indicates prescription; Q, every; *, See Table 4.14 for definitions; †, diet modification and physical activity; ‡, especially is younger, very high BP, little or no family history, diabetic, or other risk factors. (Reprinted with permission from The fourth report on the diagnosis, evaluation, and treatment of high blood pressure in children and adolescents. *Pediatrics*. 2004;114(2 Suppl):555–576.)

TABLE 4.15

SYNDROMES COMMONLY ASSOCIATED WITH CARDIAC LESIONS

Syndrome	Frequency of Cardiac Disease (%)	Associated Lesions	Genetic Anomaly
Alagille (arteriohepatic dysplasia)	85	Peripheral PS	AD, mutations of 20p12
CHARGE	65	TOF, truncus arteriosus, aortic arch anomalies	Sporadic
DiGeorge (Velocardiofacial)	85	TOF, truncus arteriosus, IAA, VSD, PDA	Microdeletion of 22q11.2
Down	40–50	ECD, VSD, ASD	Trisomy 21
Marfan	80–100	Aortic root dilation → aortic aneurysm/ dissection, MVP	AD, mutations of fibrillin gene
Noonan	85	PS (dystrophic pulmonary valve), HCM	Sporadic, AD; mutation of 12q24.1
Smith-Lemli-Opitz	45	VSD, PDA	AR, defect in cholesterol synthesis
Turner	35	COA, bicuspid aortic valve, AS, hypertension	45, XO
VATER/VACTERAL	>50	VSD, TOF, ASD, PDA	Sporadic
Williams	60	Supravalvular AS, valvular, and peripheral PS	Sporadic, AD; deletion of 7q11.23

AD, autosomal dominant; AR, autosomal recessive; ASD, atrial septal defect; AS, aortic stenosis; CHARGE, coloboma, heart defects, atresia choanae, retardation of growth and mentation, genitourinary anomalies, and ear anomalies; COA, coarctation of the aorta; ECD, endocardial cushion defect; HCM, hypertrophic cardiomyopathy; IAA, interrupted aortic arch; MVP, mitral valve prolapse; PDA, patent ductus arteriosus; PS, pulmonary stenosis; TOF, tetralogy of Fallot; VACTERL, vertebral defects, anal atresia, cardiac defects, tracheoesophageal fistula, renal dysplasia, limb anomalies; VSD, ventricular septal defect.

Indications for drug therapy are as follows:

- Symptomatic HTN
- Secondary HTN
- Target-organ damage
- Diabetes
- Persistent primary HTN despite nonpharmacologic treatment

Commonly used antihypertensive agents for chronic management include ACE-Is, ARBs, β-blockers, CCBs, and diuretics. Because of side effect profile, first-line agents are generally ACE-Is, ARBs, and CCBs.

Note: Acute management of hypertensive urgency and emergency are discussed in the Chapter 6.

Syndromes Associated with Cardiac Lesions

Many syndromes are commonly associated with cardiovascular anomalies. Syndromes commonly associated with cardiac lesions are listed in Table 4.15.

SAMPLE BOARD REVIEW QUESTIONS

1. A 10-year-old girl presents to your clinic for well-child care. She is growing and developing well. Your examination is notable for a grade 2, soft, SEM heard best at the LUSB. The remainder of the examination, including heart rate, BP, and pulses, is normal. The patient is asymptomatic. What is the next step in management of this patient?
   a. Order a CXR and EKG
   b. Refer patient to a cardiologist for evaluation
   c. No intervention, offer reassurance to patient and parent
   d. Order echocardiogram
   e. Refer patient to the local emergency department

   Answer: c. The description of the murmur is consistent with a benign pulmonary ejection murmur and is a common finding in the 8- to 14-year age group. Given that the murmur does not demonstrate characteristics of a pathologic murmur, the patient is asymptomatic, and the remainder of the examination (including vital signs) is normal, no further evaluation is needed.

2. You are an emergency department physician evaluating a 1-week-old full-term infant presenting with complaints of poor feeding and fast breathing. The patient's heart rate is 180 bpm, respiratory rate is 70, oxygen saturation in the right arm is 92%, and BP is 50/25. On examination, you note that the patient is in respiratory distress with cyanosis of the lower extremities; there is no murmur on examination. What is the most likely cause of the patient's condition?
   a. Ventricular septal defect
   b. Coarctation of the aorta
   c. Tetralogy of Fallot
   d. Aortic stenosis
   e. Transposition of the great arteries

   Answer: b. The patient is in cardiogenic shock, likely related to the closing of the patient's PDA. Left-sided obstructive lesions (e.g., HLHS, AS, COA, or interrupted aortic arch) are the most common cardiac etiology of shock in a neonate. In addition, this patient does not have central cyanosis, decreasing the likelihood of cyanotic lesions (e.g., TOF, TGA). Of the obstructed lesions listed, COA is the most likely diagnosis given that the examination was without a murmur and that the patient exhibited differential cyanosis.

3. Regarding the patient described in Question 2, what is the most important intervention in treating the patient's cardiogenic shock?
   a. A normal saline fluid bolus of 20 cc/kg
   b. Administration of 100% oxygen via endotracheal tube
   c. Transfer to the nearest tertiary care pediatric hospital
   d. Administration of PGE_1
   e. Administration of antibiotics

   Answer: d. The patient has COA, and maintaining patency of the PDA via the administration of PGE_1 is essential in providing the patient with systemic perfusion. Fluid administration may also be necessary, but it is not as important as PGE_1 and should be accomplished gently with smaller 10 cc/kg normal saline boluses and close monitoring for signs of congestion (e.g., rales, hepatomegaly) as fluid may worsen CHF. Oxygen may also be needed in a resuscitative effort; however, it should be used judiciously as excess oxygen administration can worsen systemic perfusion by diverting blood flow to the lungs.

4. You are called to the nursery to see a newborn infant. The prenatal course was notable for poor prenatal care. Syndromes commonly associated with cardiac lesions are listed in Table 4.15. The nurse informs you that the patient was tachypneic upon arrival to the nursery and the patient's oxygen saturation is currently 72% on RA. On examination, you note significant cyanosis and a single S2 but no murmur. CXR is notable for dark lung fields and EKG is remarkable for LVH. What lesion is most likely responsible for the patient's condition?
   a. Pulmonary atresia with intact ventricular septum
   b. Tetralogy of Fallot
   c. Transposition of the great arteries
   d. Pulmonary stenosis
   e. Complete endocardial cushion defect

   Answer: a. The combination of cyanosis, CXR, EKG, and examination findings makes pulmonary atresia with intact ventricular septum the most likely diagnosis. Patients with ECD are generally not cyanotic. TGA is a total mixing lesion and typically results in increased PVMs. Single S2 can be seen in TOF; however, patients with both TOF and PS typically exhibit an SEM at the ULSB. In addition, both TOF and PS demonstrate RVH (as opposed to LVH) on EKG.

5. A 6-week-old infant presents for well-child care. The patient's mother is concerned because the infant has been feeding poorly. At triage, the patient's heart rate is 185 bpm, respiratory rate is 65, and oxygen saturation is 93% on RA. On examination, there is a grade 3 harsh, holosystolic murmur at the LLSB, bilateral wheezes are present, and the patient's liver is palpable 3 cm below the right costal margin. CXR is notable for cardiomegaly and pulmonary vascular congestion. EKG demonstrates LVH. You review the patient's chart and note that no murmur was appreciated in the newborn nursery. What is most likely responsible for the patient's clinical presentation?
   a. Complete endocardial cushion defect
   b. Pulmonary stenosis
   c. Myocarditis
   d. Supraventricular tachycardia
   e. Ventricular septal defect

   Answer: e. The patient is in CHF secondary to a large VSD. The murmur described is a classic VSD murmur; however, like the patient in question, some infants do not have a murmur in the neonatal period. Patients with large VSDs can develop heart failure with increased left-to-right shunting as PVR falls with age. A VSD murmur is also seen in ECDs, but an EKG is likely to demonstrate a superior axis and RVH or RBBB. Myocarditis and SVT can both cause CHF in this age group but these diagnoses are not consistent with the cardiac examination and EKG findings in this infant.

6. A 10-year-old boy presents to your clinic with a complaint of knee pain. The patient reports his right knee is swollen and tender to touch. Several days ago, his left ankle was also swollen and tender but is now improved. Review of systems reveals that the patient had a sore throat and fever approximately 1 month ago but did not go to the doctor and improved after a few days. On examination, you note arthritis of the right knee and a new grade 3, regurgitant systolic murmur at the apex, radiating to the left axilla. You are concerned that the patient has acute rheumatic fever. What other piece of information is needed to confirm your suspicion?
   a. Subcutaneous nodules on the anterior surface of the patient's knee
   b. Fever
   c. Current group A streptococcal infection
   d. ASO titer consistent with prior GAS infection
   e. Improvement of arthritis with use of salicylates

   Answer: d. A diagnosis of acute rheumatic fever requires evidence of a prior GAS infection (either a positive throat culture or a positive streptococcal antibody test, i.e., ASO) plus the presence of two major criteria or one major and two minor criteria. The patient has evidence of carditis (a new mitral regurgitation murmur) and arthritis, both major criteria. With proof of a prior GAS infection, the patient meets diagnostic criteria for acute rheumatic fever.

7. A previously healthy 15-year-old girl presents to your clinic with a chief complaint of shortness of breath. She mentions that a few weeks ago, she had a cold, which subsequently resolved. Now she reports difficulty breathing when walking up the steps in her

high school. On examination, the patient's BP is 85/50 and heart rate is 150 bpm. A gallop rhythm is present as well as lower extremity edema. CXR is notable for cardiomegaly and pulmonary congestion. EKG demonstrates low QRS voltages and ST-T segment changes. Echocardiogram demonstrates depressed left ventricular function. What is the most likely etiology of the patient's clinical presentation?

a. Myocarditis
b. Acute hypertension
c. Pericarditis
d. Rheumatic heart disease
e. Coarctation of the aorta

Answer: a. The patient is in CHF secondary to myocarditis. The diagnosis of myocarditis is suggested by the patient's tachycardia, EKG, CXR, and echocardiographic findings. Patients with myocarditis can present solely with vague URI symptoms, but may also present in fulminant CHF. Acute HTN and rheumatic valvular heart disease are other potential causes of CHF in the patient's age group but have different clinical manifestations.

8. What is the most common cause of myocarditis in infants and children?

a. Influenza
b. Rheumatic heart disease
c. Coxsackievirus
d. Herpes simplex virus
e. Kawasaki disease

Answer: c. Viral pathogens are responsible for most cases of myocarditis (and pericarditis as well) in infants and children. Enteroviruses, particularly coxsackieviruses, are the most common etiology. Although all of the above choice can cause myocarditis, they are not as common as coxsackievirus.

9. According to the American Heart Association 2007 guidelines, which of the following patients should receive antibiotic prophylaxis before a dental procedure?

a. An 8-year-old who is 1 year post cardiac transplant
b. A 2-year-old with a history of a spontaneously closed VSD
c. A 4-year-old who underwent full repair of an ECD with use of prosthetic material at 8 months of age
d. A 17-year-old with Marfan's disease and mitral valve prolapse
e. A 9-year-old status post TOF repair with a small residual VSD near prosthetic material

Answer: e. The patient has a residual defect near prosthetic material, which places the patient at highest risk of adverse outcome from IE. The 2007 American Heart Association guidelines significantly altered the practice of procedural antibiotic prophylaxis related to heart disease. Only those at highest risk of adverse outcome are recommended to receive prophylaxis. In addition, prophylaxis is no longer recommended for GI and GU procedures.

10. A 15-year-old male basketball player has been experiencing palpitations and occasional chest pain with activity. His family history is notable for an aunt who died suddenly while running track in college and a mother who has an ICD and history of arrhythmias. The patient's CXR shows a globular-shaped heart and his EKG demonstrates LVH and LV strain. What would you expect to find on his cardiac examination?

a. A harsh midsystolic murmur at second left intercostal space
b. A pericardial friction rub
c. An SEM at the LLSB
d. A harsh holosystolic murmur at the LLSB
e. A continuous machinery like murmur at the LUSB

Answer: c. The patient has HCM. If a murmur is present, it commonly is a SEM due to the LVOT obstruction created by LV hypertrophy. In addition, a gallop rhythm or a murmur of mitral regurgitation (a soft regurgitant murmur at the apex) could also be present in patients with HCM. An AS murmur is described in A, a VSD murmur is described in D, and a PDA murmur is described in E.

11. SVT can be difficult to distinguish from sinus tachycardia. Which of the descriptions below is most consistent with SVT as opposed to sinus tachycardia?

a. A heart rate of 170 bpm in a 1-year-old
b. Tachycardia that is without variability
c. Tachycardia in a child who is febrile and ill-appearing
d. An EKG with upright P waves in leads I and aVF
e. A irregularly irregular ventricular response

Answer: b. SVT is diagnosed by the presence of an unvarying heart rate (usually greater than 240 ± 40 bpm) and abnormal or absent P waves. A, B, and D describe sinus tachycardia, and E is a classic description of atrial fibrillation.

12. A 6-year-old with a history of LQTS presents to the emergency department with a chief complaint of palpitations and shortness of breath. The patient's heart rate is 160 bpm and her EKG demonstrates a wide QRS complex tachycardia. On examination, the patient's perfusion is poor, but pulses are present. What is the next step in management of this patient?

a. Synchronized cardioversion
b. Immediate placement of an ICD
c. Defibrillation
d. Delay cardioversion by administering adenosine
e. Administration of propranolol

Answer: a. The patient has symptomatic VT with pulses and poor perfusion; therefore, immediate synchronized cardioversion is indicated. If the patient was experiencing a pulseless arrest in VT, CPR, and immediate defibrillation would be indicated. SVT with aberrancy can be difficult to distinguish from VT; however, the administration of adenosine should never delay cardioversion. Both ICD placement and use of β-blockers may be indicated for prevention of VT.

13. A 15-year-old girl presents to your clinic with a complaint of chest pain. She reports the pain began 1 month ago, occurs in the center of her chest, and is a stabbing pain, which does not radiate. The pain typically lasts 10 to 15 minutes, occurs multiple times per day, and is not dependant on activity. There are no aggravating or alleviating factors. The patient denies associated shortness of breath, palpitations, and dizziness. She has never fainted. The patient's mother confides in you that she and the patient's father are currently undergoing a messy divorce. Your examination of the patient is unrevealing. What is the most likely etiology of the patient's symptoms?

a. Myocardial infarction
b. Asthma
c. Pericarditis
d. Psychogenic
e. Gastroesophageal reflux

Answer: d. The patient's age, gender, and recent life stressor increase the likelihood of a psychogenic cause of chest pain. There is no association of the pain with exercise and no associated symptoms or physical examination findings suggestive of an underlying organic etiology.

14. A 12-year-old girl presents to your clinic in the afternoon after fainting at school. The patient remembers sitting in her desk after completing an extensive standardized test. She arose from her desk to exit the classroom, felt faint, and then remembers waking up on the floor of the room surrounded by her teacher and classmates. She has never passed out before. She does occasionally feel lightheaded upon getting out of bed in the morning. What would you expect to find upon examination and investigation of this patient's syncopal episode?

a. An unvarying heart rate of 220 bpm with absent P waves on EKG
b. A 20 mmHg drop in the patient's systolic BP with assuming an upright position
c. A blood glucose level of 50 mg/dL
d. A loud SEM at the ULSB
e. Reproduction of the event with hyperventilation

Answer: b. The patient has orthostatic hypotension, which manifests clinically as a 20/10 mmHg are more drop in BP after assuming an upright position. In addition, feeling faint or lightheaded when standing up after prolonged sitting or bed rest is also consistent with a diagnosis of orthostatic hypotension. The description in A is consistent with SVT, and the murmur in D can be present in patient with PS, both of which are unlikely causes of syncope in this patient. Syncope secondary to hyperventilation can be reproduced by intentional hyperventilation.

15. During a preparticipation sports physical for a 12-year-old obese male, you discover that his BP is between the 90th and 95th percentile for his age and height. The patient's review of systems is unremarkable and physical examination is significant only for obesity. What is the next step in evaluation and treatment of this patient?

a. Begin a calcium channel blocker
b. Order an echocardiogram
c. Refer the patient to an ophthalmologist for retinal examination
d. Order laboratory testing including BUN, creatinine, and electrolyte levels
e. Recommend therapeutic lifestyle changes

Answer: e. A BP between the 90th and 95th percentile for age, sex, and height is classified as prehypertensive. The initial treatment of this patient with likely obesity-related essential HTN would be to institute therapeutic lifestyle changes (weight reduction, increased physical activity, and reduction of sodium intake). The patient's BP should be repeated in 6 months. The laboratory testing in D is recommended as part of a diagnostic workup for those with stage 1 or stage 2 HTN. In addition, evaluation for end-organ damage (B and C) should also occur in those with stage 1 or stage 2 HTN. Pharmacologic treatment is not indicated for prehypertension.

SUGGESTED READINGS

Feld LG, Corey H. Hypertension in childhood. *Pediatr Rev*. 2007;28(8):283–298.
Menashe V. Heart murmurs. *Pediatr Rev*. 2007;28(4):e19–e22.
Park MK. *Pediatric Cardiology for Practitioners*. 5th ed. Philadelphia, PA: Mosby Elsevier, 2008.
Silberbach M, Hannon D. Presentation of congenital heart disease in the neonate and young infant. *Pediatr Rev*. 2007;28(4):123–131.

CHAPTER 5 ■ CONNECTIVE TISSUE DISEASES

MICHAEL F. WALSH

ANA	Antinuclear antibody	EDS	Ehlers-Danlos syndrome
AST	Aspartate aminotransferase	ESR	Erythrocyte sedimentation rate
c-ANCA	Cytoplasmic staining antineutrophil cytoplasmic antibody	GERD	Gastroesophageal reflux disease
BS	Behcet syndrome	GI	Gastrointestinal
BUN	Blood urea nitrogen	HLA	Human leukocyte antigen
CHF	Congestive heart failure	HSP	Henoch-Schonlein purpura
CK	Creatine kinase	JRA	Juvenile rheumatoid arthritis
CNS	Central nervous system	NSAID	Nonsteroidal anti-inflammatory drug
CRP	C reactive protein	PAN	Polyarteritis nodosa
CS	Churg-Strauss syndrome	SLE	Systemic lupus erythematosus
CT	Computerized tomography	WBC	White blood cell
		WG	Wegener's granulomatosis

CHAPTER OBJECTIVES

1. To understand the epidemiology, inheritance patterns, clinical manifestations, diagnosis, and treatment of the heritable connective tissue diseases including Marfan syndrome and Ehrlos-Danlos syndrome
2. To understand the epidemiology, clinical manifestations, diagnosis, and treatment of the rheumatic connective tissues diseases including SLE, JRA, scleroderma, and dermatomyositis
3. To understand the epidemiology, clinical manifestations, diagnosis, and treatment of the vasculitic connective tissue diseases including HSP, Kawasaki disease, PAN, WG, CS, BS, and Takayasu arteritis.

HERITABLE CONNECTIVE TISSUE DISEASES

Marfan Syndrome

Marfan syndrome is an autosomal dominant connective tissue disease that affects the skeleton, cardiovascular system, eyes, lungs, and integument. It results from a mutation in the fibrillin gene on chromosome 15 and has an incidence of approximately 1/5,000. Disease severity is variable, even amongst individuals in the same family. The increased mortality associated with Marfan syndrome is primarily related to cardiovascular events.

Clinical Manifestations

Skeletal (Fig. 5.1)

- Increased arm span to height ratio >1.05.
- Arachnodactyly.
- Pectus excavatum or pectus carinatum.
- Scoliosis ± kyphosis.
- Spondylolisthesis.
- Dolichocephaly.
- Malar hypoplasia.
- High arched palate giving rise to dental crowding or occlusion.
- Dural ectasia.
- Decreased flexibility at the elbow.

Points to Remember

- Acute onset of severe chest pain in a patient with Marfan syndrome should be assumed to be aortic dissection until proven otherwise. The differential diagnosis also includes spontaneous pneumothorax.

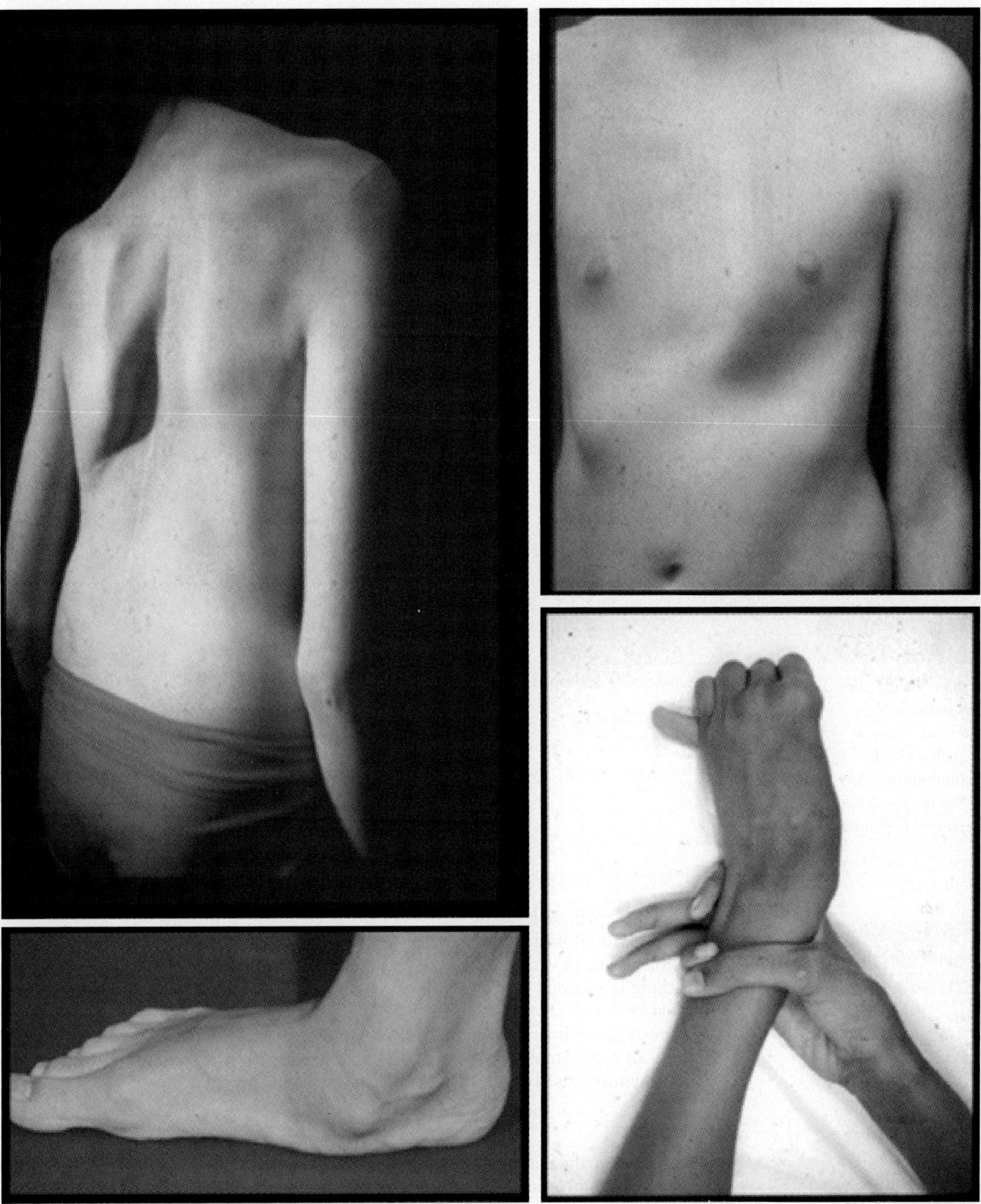

FIGURE 5.1. Major skeletal manifestations of Marfan syndrome such as scoliosis, pectus carinatum, pes planum, and positive wrist and thumb signs. (Reprinted with permission from McMillan JA, Feigin RD, DeAngelis C, et al. *Oski's Pediatrics: Principles and Practice*. 4th ed. Philadelphia, PA: Lippincott Williams & Wilkins, 2006.)

Cardiovascular

- Mitral valve prolapse (can lead to mitral regurgitation with risk of CHF and dysrhythmia).
- Aortic root dilation with predisposition to aortic root dissection and rupture.

Ophthalmology

- Subluxation or complete dislocation of the lens.
- Myopia.
- Retinal detachment.

Pulmonary

- Blebs.
- Pneumothorax.

TABLE 5.1

DIAGNOSTIC CRITERIA FOR MARFAN SYNDROME

	Major Criteria	Minor Criteria	Involvement
Skeletal	Any four of the following: - Pectus carinatum - Pectus excavatum - Arm span/height >1.05 - Wrist and thumb signs - Scoliosis, spondylolisthesis - Hyperextension at elbow - Pes planus	Pectus excavatum Joint hypermobility High arched palate Facial appearance	Two components of major criteria OR One component of major criteria and two minor criteria
Ocular	Ectopia lentis	Flat cornea Myopia Hypoplastic iris	Two minor criteria
Cardiovascular	Dilated ascending aorta Dissection of ascending aorta	Mitral valve prolapse Dilated pulmonary artery Calcification of mitral annulus Dilation/dissection of descending aorta	One major criteria OR One minor criteria
Pulmonary	None	Spontaneous pneumothorax Apical blebs	One minor criteria
Skin/Integument	Lumbosacral dural ectasia	Stria atrophicae Recurrent or incisional herniae	One major criteria OR One minor criteria

Adapted from McMillan JA, Feigin RD, DeAngelis C, et al. *Oski's Pediatrics: Principles and Practice.* 4th ed. Philadelphia, PA: Lippincott Williams & Wilkins, 2006.

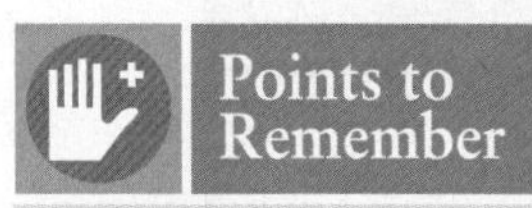

Points to Remember

- Because many of the clinical manifestations of Marfan disease occur as isolated findings in the general community, many cases of Marfan syndrome go undiagnosed until later in life.

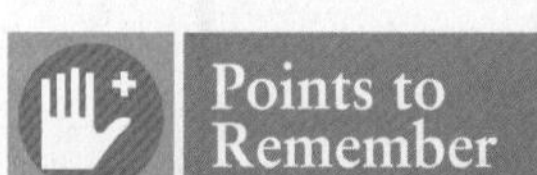

Points to Remember

- Loeys-Dietz syndrome is a connective tissue disorder that shares many of the features of Marfan syndrome. It follows an autosomal dominant inheritance pattern and is characterized by hypertelorism, cleft palate, bifid uvula, and aortic aneurysm with arterial tortuosity.

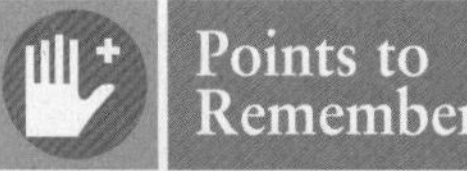

Points to Remember

- Patients with vascular type EDS are at risk for organ rupture. There is a 15% mortality associated with pregnancy in women with vascular type EDS because of the risk of uterine rupture.

Diagnosis

- Diagnosis is primarily clinical and is also affected by family history (see Table 5.1)
  - An individual with no family history requires major criteria in two organ systems and involvement of a third.
  - If there is a family history, major criteria must be met in one organ system and another must be involved.
- Gene testing for fibrillin 1 is helpful in some cases but is problematic as there are a large number of separate causative mutations and related but distinct conditions (e.g., Ehrlos-Danlos syndromes) can be caused by mutations in the same gene.

Management

- Yearly echocardiograms to detect cardiovascular abnormalities and allow for appropriate medical and/or surgical intervention.
- Propranolol to slow the rate of aortic root dilatation and reduce the risk of aortic dissection; there is also evidence that losartan prevents aneurysm formation in mice.
- Regular moderate aerobic activity with restriction of contact sports, weight lifting, and activities which require closure of the airway and bearing down.
- Clinical and radiographic monitoring for scoliosis which may require bracing and or surgical intervention.
- Physical therapy and occupational therapy as needed for management of hypermobile joints.
- Yearly ophthalmology examinations and intervention for specific conditions as needed.
- Regular dental visits and intervention as needed for overcrowding.

Ehlers-Danlos Syndromes

EDSs are a heterogeneous group of disorders in which abnormalities of collagen production affect the skin, joints, and blood vessels. EDS maybe inherited in an autosomal dominant or autosomal recessive manner. The six main types include classic (I/II), hypermobile (III), vascular (IV), ocular-scoliotic (VI), arthrochalasia (VII), dermatosparaxis (VII), and periodontal (VIII).

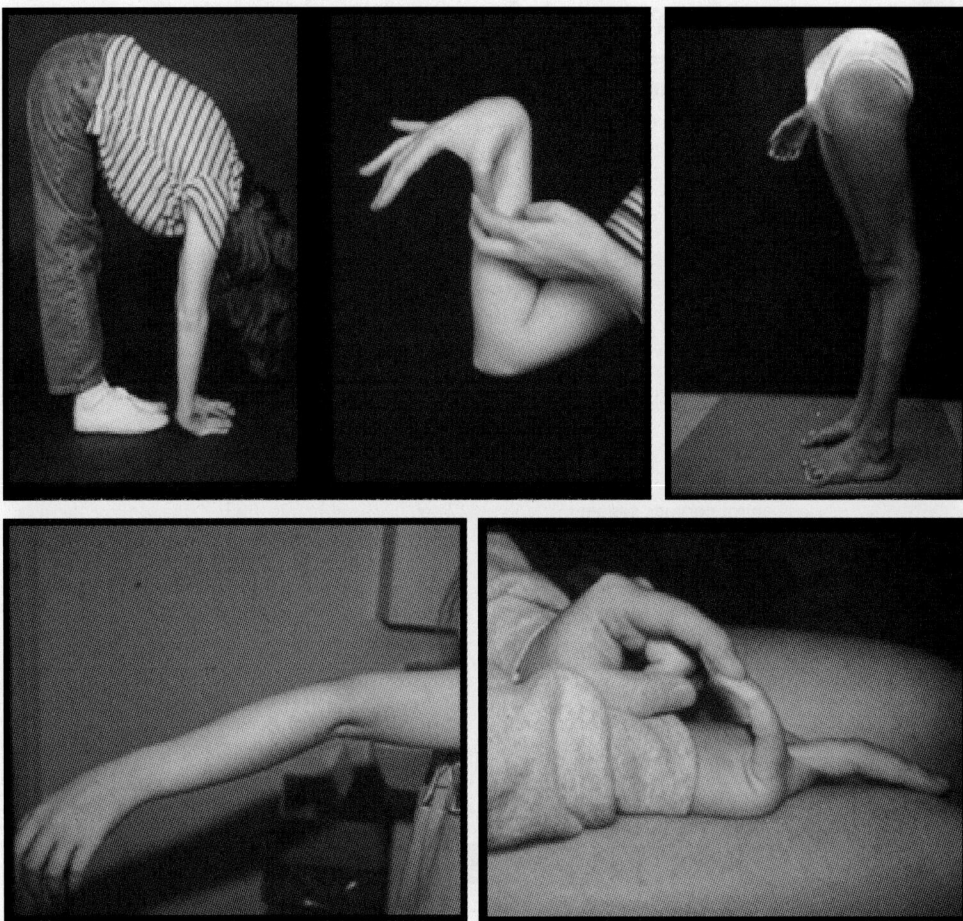

FIGURE 5.2. Joint hypermobility as seen in Ehlers-Danlos syndromes: ability to put hands flat on the ground, thumb abduction sign, and hyperextension of fingers, elbows, and knees. (Reprinted with permission from McMillan JA, Feigin RD, DeAngelis C, et al. *Oski's Pediatrics: Principles and Practice*. 4th ed. Philadelphia, PA: Lippincott Williams & Wilkins, 2006.)

Clinical Manifestations

- Hyperextensible skin with a velvety texture that is loose and fragile.
- Dystrophic scarring.
- Easy bruising.
- Joint hypermobility and frequent dislocations with or without chronic joint pain (see Fig. 5.2).
- Connective tissue fragility (e.g., poor wound healing, vascular tearing/rupture).
- Muscle weakness, developmental motor delay.

Diagnosis

- Genetic testing is available for vascular, classical, kyphoscoliosis, and arthrochalasis types.
- Diagnosis for the other types is clinical.

Management

Medical intervention is focused on prophylaxis, symptomatic treatment, and psychosocial support.

- Avoidance of injury via use of protective pads and gear.
- Regular participation in non—weight-bearing exercises (e.g., swimming) to stabilize joints, diminish pain, and improve psychosocial status.
- Avoidance of contact sports.
- Bracing, splinting, and pain management as needed.
- Avoidance of elective surgery given wound healing problems.
- Serial echocardiograms to assess for valvular and aortic disease.
- Genetic counseling and psychosocial support.

TABLE 5.2

CLINICAL PRESENTATION AND COURSE OF SYSTEMIC LUPUS ERYTHEMATOSUS IN CHILDREN

Presentation	At Onset (%)	During Course (%)
Nephritis	84	86
Hypertension	10	28
Arthritis	72	76
Dermatitis	69	76
Malar erythema	51	56
Photosensitivity	16	16
Alopecia	16	20
Oral or nasopharyngeal ulcerations	12	16
Pericarditis	40	47
Pleuritis	31	36
Central nervous system disease	9	31
Raynaud phenomenon	16	24
Hepatomegaly	43	47
Splenomegaly	20	20
Anemia	43	47
Leukopenia	60	71
Thrombocytopenia	22	24

Reprinted with permission from McMillan JA, Feigin RD, DeAngelis C, et al. *Oski's Pediatrics: Principles and Practice.* 4th ed. Philadelphia, PA: Lippincott Williams & Wilkins, 2006.

RHEUMATIC CONNECTIVE TISSUE DISEASE

Systemic Lupus Erythematosus

SLE is the most common connective tissue disease. Clinical manifestations are highly variable and can range from a benign isolated rash to multisystem organ failure. The pathologic findings resulting in SLE arise from excessive autoantibody production, immune complex formation, and immunologically mediated tissue injury. Onset in children usually occurs after 5 years of age and is increasingly common during the adolescent years. The female to male ratio is 8:1. Ten to fifteen percentage of affected individuals have a first-degree family member with SLE.

Clinical Manifestations

Table 5.2 shows the clinical presentation and course of SLE in children. Figure 5.3 shows the malar erythematous rash characteristic of SLE.

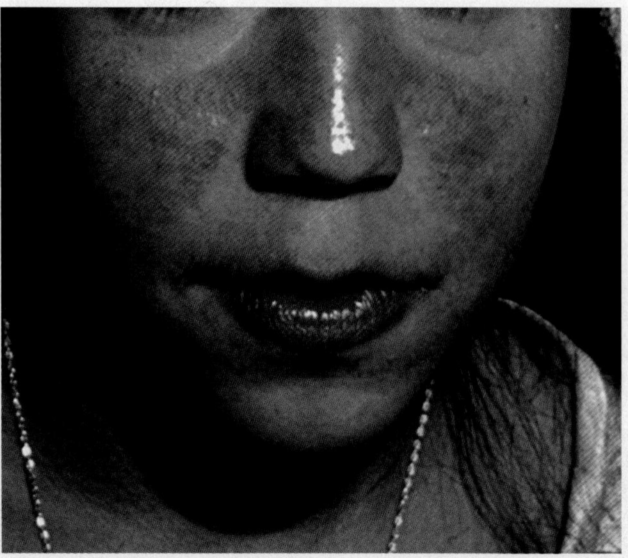

FIGURE 5.3. Systemic lupus erythematosus. This young girl has the classic "butterfly" rash of lupus. (Reprinted with permission from Goodheart HP. *Goodheart's Photoguide of Common Skin Disorders*. 2nd ed. Philadelphia, PA: Lippincott Williams & Wilkins, 2003.)

Diagnosis

Diagnosis is clinical and is based on the presence of at least 4 of the following 11 criteria established by the American College of Rheumatology:

- Malar rash.
- Discoid lupus rash.
- Photosensitivity.
- Oral or nasal mucocutaneous ulcerations.
- Nonerosive arthritis.
- Nephritis (proteinuria >0.5 g/day, cellular casts).
- Encephalopathy (seizures, psychosis).
- Pleuritis or pericarditis.
- Cytopenia.

Positive immunoserology confusing

- Positive ANA.
- Laboratory investigation of a patient with suspected SLE should include complete blood cell count, electrolytes, total protein, albumin, renal and hepatic panels, urinalysis, antinuclear antibodies (ANA, Anti-Ro, Anti-La, Scl-70, centromere, Jo-1, PM-Scl, histones, enzymes, tRNAs, and structural proteins), complement levels (C3 and C4 are low in SLE), and antiphospholipid antibody panels.

Points to Remember

- C3 and C4 are both usually depressed with active SLE disease.
- ANA is sensitive but not specific for SLE. Anti-Ro, Anti-La, and Anti-Sm antibodies are less sensitive but more specific for SLE.

Points to Remember

- In some children, acute SLE can be precipitated by a drug reaction. Agents most commonly implicated include hydralazine, isoniazid, penicillin, sulfonamides, and anticonvulsants. Drug-induced SLE is usually a self-limited disease and abates with withdrawal of the offending agent.
- A child born to a mother with SLE may develop a transient neonatal lupus-like syndrome within the first few days of life because of transplacental passage of maternal antibodies. Most infants are asymptomatic but findings may include cytopenias, malar erythema, and/or discoid lesions. One serious permanent sequelae is the development of in utero complete congenital heart block.

Management

- Glucocorticoids are the mainstay of the basic regimen and are used in higher doses for acute exacerbations. Intravenous pulse methylprednisolone may be indicated in acute exacerbations to avoid increasing the daily steroid prescription.
- Immunosuppressive agents such as azathioprine and/or cyclophosphamide are necessary adjunctive medications in some children.
- Hydroxychloroquine helps control photosensitive dermatitis and moderates glucocorticoid dosage.
- NSAIDs are useful in treating minor manifestations of SLE such as arthralgias and myalgias.
- Avoidance of triggers such as excessive sun exposure, unnecessary medications, and emotional stresses.
- Recognizing and treating infections early.
- Aggressive treatment of associated hypertension and renal disease.
- Dialysis and renal transplantation are indicated in patients with end-stage renal disease.
- Psychosocial support.

Juvenile Rheumatoid Arthritis

JRA is one of the most common chronic childhood illnesses and a leading cause of disability and blindness. The etiology is unknown, but it likely represents a spectrum of diseases of diverse pathogenesis rather than a single disorder. An immunogenetic basis is the underlying cause for some affected individuals. The mean age at onset is 1 to 3 years. Girls are affected at least twice as frequently as are boys. Classification of JRA is based on the recognition of three distinct types of disease: polyarthritis, oligoarthritis, and systemic disease (see Table 5.3).

Clinical Manifestations

- Constitutional symptoms include high-spiking fevers, fatigue, and/or weight loss.
- Arthritis is destructive and permanent; large joints are most commonly involved.
- Morning stiffness and pain after periods of inactivity are characteristic.
- Tenosynovitis.
- Rheumatoid nodules (usually over the tendons and/or pressure points).
- Uveitis is associated with the oligoarthritis and polyarthritis types.
- Additional features associated with systemic JRA include rash (nonpuritic, coincides with fevers see Fig. 5.4), hepatosplenomegaly, lymphadenopathy, pericarditis, hepatitis, pulmonary disease, and/or CNS disease.

Points to Remember

- Chronic uveitis associated with JRA is confined to children with polyarthritis or oligoarthritis. It is usually bilateral and often results in significant morbidity.

Diagnosis

- The classification criteria for JRA according to the American College of Rheumatology includes age of onset less than 16 years, clinical arthritis, duration of disease at least 6 weeks, and exclusion of other forms of juvenile arthritis.
- Laboratory findings may include the following:

TABLE 5.3

CLASSIFICATION OF TYPES OF ONSETS OF JUVENILE RHEUMATOID ARTHRITIS

Sign/Symptom of Onset	Polyarthritis	Oligoarthritis (Pauciarticular Disease)	Systemic Disease
Frequency of cases	30%	60%	10%
Number of joints involved	≥5	≤4	Variable
Female:male ratio	3:1	5:1	1:1
Systemic involvement	Moderate	Not present	Prominent
Occurrence of chronic uveitis	5%	5%–15%	Rare
Frequency of seropositivity			
Rheumatoid factors	10% (increases with age)	Rare	Rare
Antinuclear antibodies	40%–50%	75%–85%[a]	10%
Course	Systemic diseases generally mild; possible unremitting articular involvement	Systemic disease absent; major cause of morbidity in uveitis	Systemic disease often self-limited; arthritis is chronic and destructive in 50%
Prognosis	Guarded to moderately good	Excellent, except of eyesight	Moderate to poor

[a]In girls with uveitis.
Reprinted with permission from McMillan JA, Feigin RD, DeAngelis C, et al. *Oski's Pediatrics: Principles and Practice.* 4th ed. Philadelphia, PA: Lippincott Williams & Wilkins, 2006.

- Normocytic anemia.
- Elevated WBC and platelet counts.
- Elevated ESR and CRP.
- ANA seropositivity (present in 45% of children with JRA).
- Rheumatoid factor is positive in less than 10% of patients.
- Synovial fluid analysis reveals 10,000 to 20,000 WBC/mm^3.

- Radiographic changes may include the following:
  - Early changes include soft-tissue swelling, juxta-articular osteoporosis, and periosteal new-bone apposition.
  - Later findings include erosions and narrowing of the cartilaginous spaces.

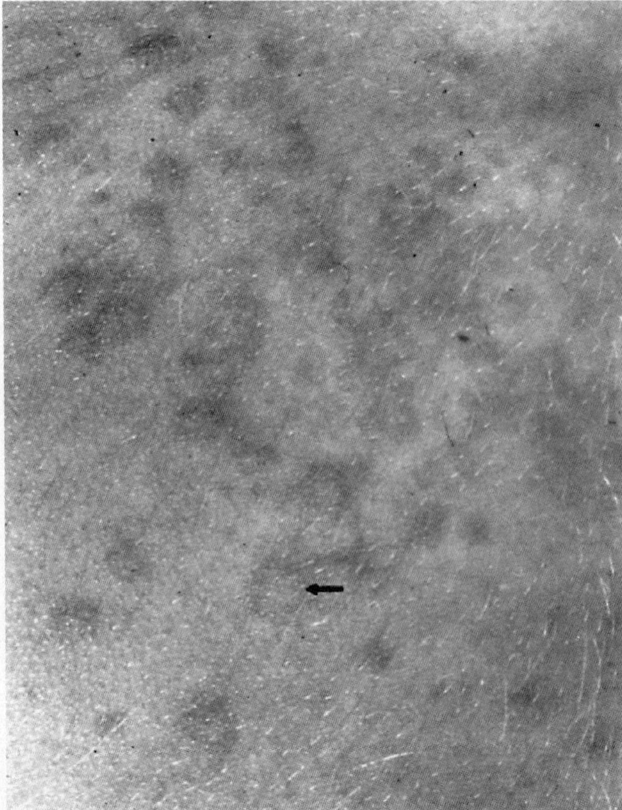

FIGURE 5.4. Rash of systemic-onset JRA. This 4-year-old girl presented with high-spiking fevers that occurred once a day, accompanied by a transient nonpruritic rash. The *arrow.* points to central clearing in a lesion. (Reprinted with permission from McMillan JA, Feigin RD, DeAngelis C, et al. *Oski's Pediatrics: Principles and Practice*. 4th ed. Philadelphia, PA: Lippincott Williams & Wilkins, 2006.)

TABLE 5.4

MANAGEMENT OF CHILDREN WITH JUVENILE RHEUMATOID ARTHRITIS

Medication program: suppression of inflammation
Nonsteroidal anti-inflammatory drugs
Hydroxychloroquine
Methotrexate
Glucocorticoid drugs
Immunosuppressive drugs
Preservation of function and prevention of deformities
Local and general rest
Physical therapy
Occupational therapy
Orthopedic surgery: preventive and reconstructive
Psychosocial development
Peer group relationships and schooling
Counseling of patients and families
Involvement of community agencies
Maintenance of adequate nutrition
Coordinated care

Reprinted with permission from McMillan JA, Feigin RD, DeAngelis C, et al. *Oski's Pediatrics: Principles and Practice.* 4th ed. Philadelphia, PA: Lippincott Williams & Wilkins, 2006.

Management

The management of children with JRA is outlined in Table 5.4.

Scleroderma

Scleroderma is a disorder in which excessive collagen accumulation leads to progressive hardening and tightening of connective tissue. The exact etiology is unknown. An immunologic basis is suspected. Genetic and environmental factors such as silica dust, industrial chemicals, and chemotherapy also likely play a role. It is four times more common in women than in men and is more common in African Americans and Native Americans than in whites. Scleroderma may be subdivided into localized and systemic forms. Localized scleroderma affects only the skin and can be further divided into morphea and linear forms. Systemic scleroderma is subclassified into diffuse and limited (CREST) forms when combining skin manifestations with effects on the internal organs and the vasculature.

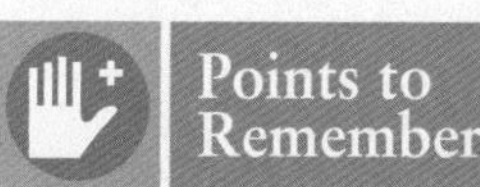

- An idiopathic angiitis is the basic lesion of systemic scleroderma and involves the lungs, heart, and kidneys in addition to the skin and GI tract.
- In patients with diffuse scleroderma, tightening and thickening of the skin is virtually universal at onset and becomes more generalized as the disease progresses.
- Swallowing dysfunction is present in 75% of patients with systemic scleroderma and is best characterized by a barium swallow examination (see Fig. 5.5).

Clinical Manifestations

- Localized scleroderma
  - Morphea scleroderma: thickened oval patches of skin with white center and purplish border.
  - Linear scleroderma: bands or streaks of indurated skin typically involving one or more extremities.
- Systemic scleroderma
  - Limited (CREST): calcinosis, Raynaud phenomenon, esophageal, abnormalities, sclerodactyly, and telangiectases.
  - Diffuse: see Table 5.5.

Diagnosis

- Diagnosis of localized scleroderma is based on the presence of characteristic skin findings.
- Diagnosis of systemic scleroderma is based primarily on clinical manifestations but is also aided by the presence of various antibodies including anti-Ro, anti-La, anti-microsomal, anti-centromere, and/or anti-Scl 70 antibodies.
- Skin biopsy revealing collagen deposition is helpful if diagnosis is uncertain.

Management

- NSAIDs are useful to relieve the musculoskeletal stiffness and aching; physical therapy is also useful for these symptoms.
- Raynaud phenomenon is managed with alpha-blocking agents or calcium-channel blockers and avoidance of triggers.

TABLE 5.5

CLINICAL MANIFESTATIONS IN CHILDREN WITH SYSTEMIC SCLERODERMA

Organ System	Frequency of Involvement (%)
Skin	
Digital arteries (Raynaud phenomenon)	75
Subcutaneous calcification	60
Telangiectases	30
Ulceration	30
Pigmentation	20
Musculoskeletal	
Contractures	75
Resorption of digital tufts	60
Muscle weakness	40
Muscle atrophy	40
Gastrointestinal tract	
Abnormal esophageal motility	75
Colonic sacculations	20
Duodenal dilatation	5
Pulmonary tract	
Abnormal diffusion	75
Abnormal vital capacity	70
Heart	
Electrocardiographic abnormalities	30
Cardiomegaly	15
Congestive failure	15

Reprinted with permission from McMillan JA, Feigin RD, DeAngelis C, et al. *Oski's Pediatrics: Principles and Practice.* 4th ed. Philadelphia, PA: Lippincott Williams & Wilkins, 2006.

- Angiotensin converting enzyme inhibitors are indicated for the treatment of associated hypertension.
- Treatment of associated GI problems (e.g., anti-GERD medications, surgical treatment of esophageal strictures).
- Ultraviolet light therapy may be of some benefit in treating skin lesions.
- Glucocorticoids are contraindicated as they may exacerbate small blood vessel disease and renal involvement.

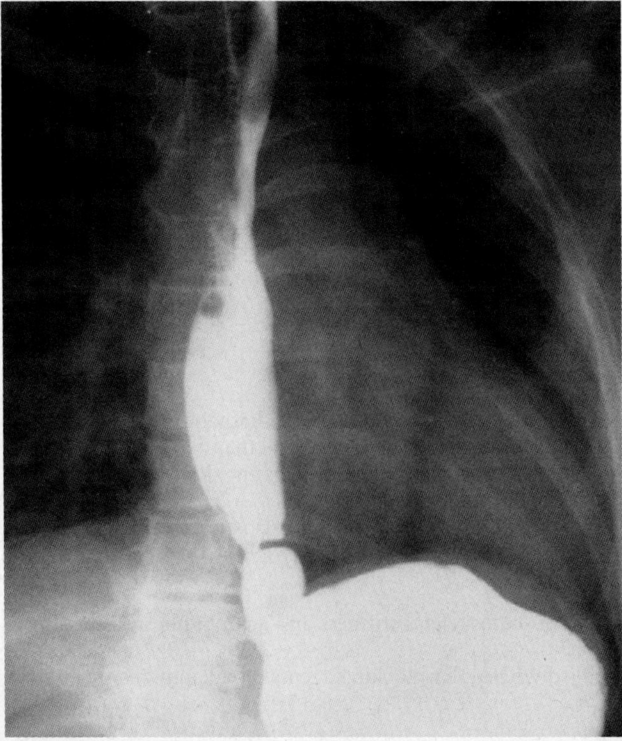

FIGURE 5.5. A barium swallow examination in the supine position of a 14-year-old girl who presented with severe dysphagia and scleroderma. The barium column collected in the esophagus, which was virtually without peristaltic movement. (Reprinted with permission from McMillan JA, Feigin RD, DeAngelis C, et al. *Oski's Pediatrics: Principles and Practice.* 4th ed. Philadelphia, PA: Lippincott Williams & Wilkins, 2006.)

TABLE 5.6

CLINICAL FEATURES ASSOCIATED WITH DERMATOMYOSITIS IN CHILDHOOD

Muscle weakness
- Proximal pelvic girdle (95%)
- Proximal shoulder girdle (75%)
- Neck flexors (60%)
- Pharyngeal muscles (30%)
- Distal muscles of the extremities (30%)
- Facial and extraocular muscles (5%)

Muscle contractures and atrophy (60%)
Muscle pain and tenderness (50%)
Skin lesions (85%)
- Heliotrope rash of eyelids
- Malar rash
- Subcutaneous and periorbital edema
- Periungual and articular rash (Gottron papules)

Raynaud phenomenon (20%)
Arthritis and arthralgia (25%)
Dysphagia, other gastrointestinal symptoms (10%)
Calcinosis (40%)
Pulmonary fibrosis (5%)
Constitutional symptoms
- Fatigue
- Malaise
- Weight loss
- Anorexia
- Low-grade fever

Adapted from McMillan JA, Feigin RD, DeAngelis C, et al. *Oski's Pediatrics: Principles and Practice*. 4th ed. Philadelphia, PA: Lippincott Williams & Wilkins, 2006.

Dermatomyositis

Dermatomyositis is a nonsuppurative inflammatory condition affecting striated muscle and skin. These multisystemic findings are accompanied early in the course by an immune-complex vasculitis and later by the development of calcinosis. It accounts for approximately 5% of all referrals to pediatric rheumatology clinics. It can present at any age but the onset is most common between 4 and 10 years of age. It is slightly more common in girls than in boys.

Points to Remember

- 85% of patients with dermatomyositis have at least one of the characteristic skin findings including heliotrope rash of eyelids and malar regions, Gottron papules, and/or nailbed telangiectasias (see Fig. 5.6). Dermatologic findings may be the first sign of disease or present later in the course.
- Progressive symmetric proximal muscle weakness is prominent in patients with dermatomyositis and may manifest as difficulty climbing stairs, inability to get up from the floor unaided (Gower sign), and/or difficulty combing hair.

Clinical Manifestations

Characteristic clinical features are shown in Table 5.6.

Diagnosis

- Acute onset of progressive, symmetric weakness of proximal limb-girdle muscles.
- Classic heliotrope rash and/or Gottron papules.
- Elevated serum muscle enzymes (e.g., CK, AST, aldolase).
- Electromyographic demonstration of myopathy and denervation.
- Muscle biopsy confirming inflammatory myositis.

Management

- Prednisone to decrease inflammation.
- Graduated rest, positioning and physical therapy.
- Immunosuppressive agents (e.g., methotrexate, cyclosporine A, cyclophosphamide) are indicated for disease with inadequate response to steroids.

Prognosis

- Seventy-five percentage of children with dermatomyositis have a uniphasic course that lasts 8 months to 2 years; remaining 25% continue to have acute exacerbations and remissions.
- Long-term survival is 90%; mortality is generally associated with pulmonary and GI tract complications.

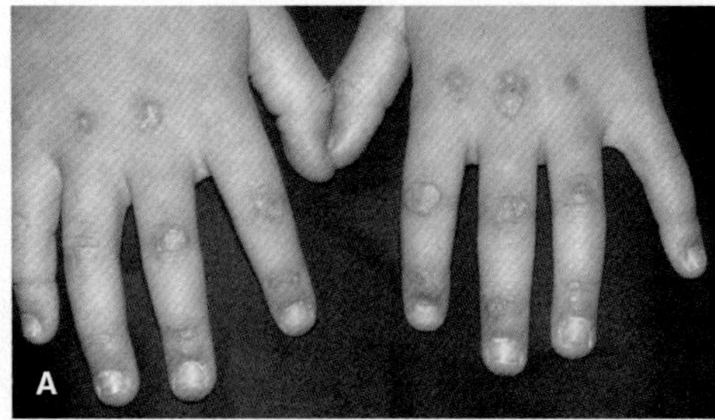

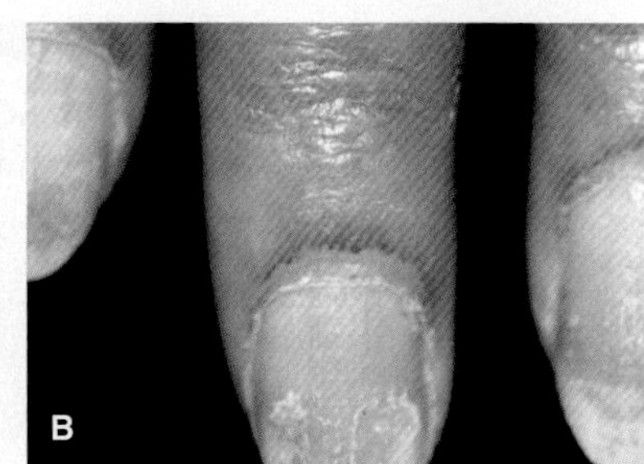

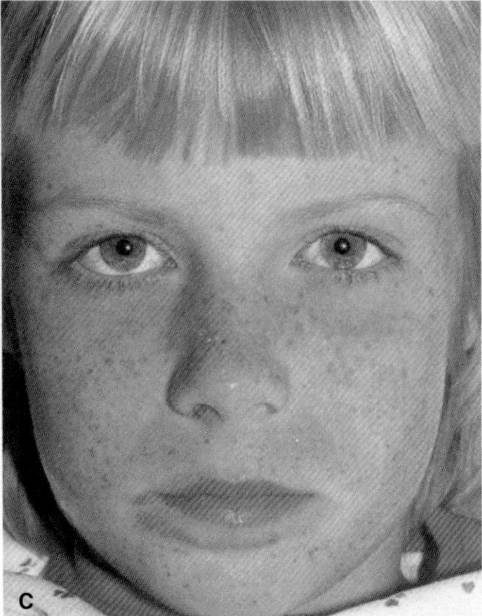

FIGURE 5.6. Characteristic dermatologic manifestations of dermatomyositis. Including (**A**) Gottron papules, (**B**) nailbed telangiectasias, and (**C**) heliotrope rash. Dermatomyositis. Heliotrope rash in a child. Note the characteristic serious expression. (**A**) and (**B**); Reprinted with permission from Goodheart HP. *Goodheart's Photoguide of Common Skin Disorders*. 2nd ed. Philadelphia, PA: Lippincott Williams & Wilkins, 2003. (**C**) Reprinted with permission from Ludwig S. *Visual Handbook of Pediatrics and Child Health: The Core*. Philadelphia, PA: Lippincott Williams & Wilkins, 2008.

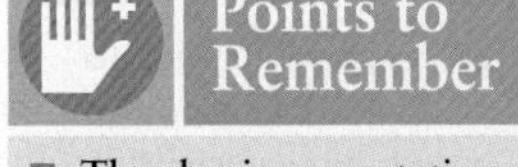

- **The classic presentation of HSP is a previously well child who develops malaise and low-grade fever followed by palpable purpura, colicky abdominal pain, and arthritis.**

VASCULITIC CONNECTIVE TISSUE DISEASES

Henoch-Schonlein Purpura

HSP is the most common vasculitis in children and peaks in children ages 4 to 7 years. It principally involves the skin, GI tract, joints, and kidneys. Although HSP is usually a self-limited illness, associated renal disease requires long-term follow-up and can result in significant morbidity. Males are more than twice as likely to be affected as females, and there is a higher incidence in Asians and whites compared with African Americans. Peak incidence is in the fall and spring.

Clinical Manifestations

- Classic skin finding is a palpable purpuric rash most prominent on the buttocks and lower extremities (see Fig. 5.7).
- Half of the patients have significant abdominal pain and may also have bloody stools, nausea, and vomiting.
- Increased risk of intussusception.
- Arthralgia or arthritis occurs in 65% to 85% of patients; nonmigratory; usually bilateral and symmetric; knees and ankles are more commonly affected than fingers and wrists; not associated with long-term joint damage.
- Renal involvement develops in 20% to 60% of patients; may be present at disease onset but may develop several months after other findings; may manifest as microscopic hematuria, gross hematuria, nephrotic syndrome, mild proteinuria, acute nephritis with hypertension, or rapidly progressive glomerulonephritis.

Points to Remember

- **Although renal involvement is the most feared complication of HSP, less than 1% of patients develop rapidly progressive glomerulonephritis.**

Diagnosis

- Diagnosis is primarily clinical.
- Adjunctive laboratory findings may include elevated ESR, elevated IgA, thrombocytosis, hematuria, and/or proteinuria.

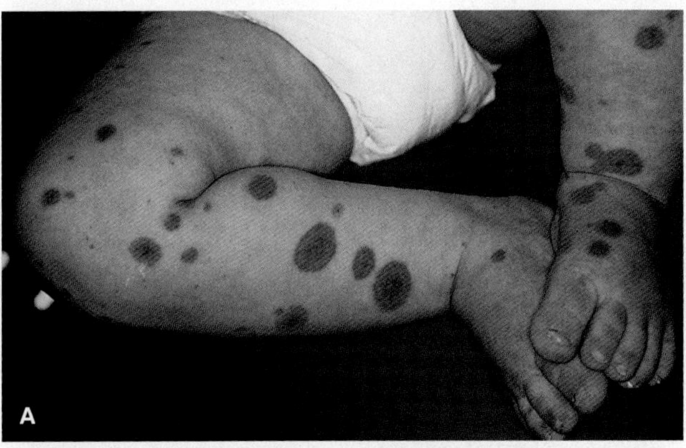

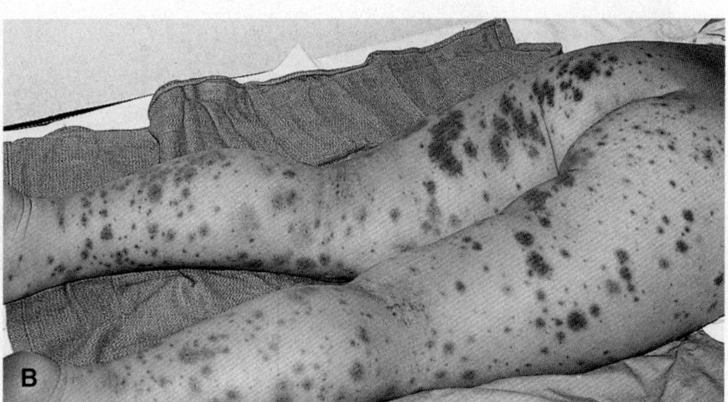

FIGURE 5.7. These two patients (**A**) and (**B**) have Henoch-Schonlein purpura, a form of vasculitis. The lesions are well demarcated and slightly raised. (Reprinted with permission from Fleisher GR, Ludwig S, Baskin MN. *Atlas of Pediatric Emergency Medicine*. Philadelphia, PA: Lippincott Williams & Wilkins, 2004.)

Points to Remember

- A child with HSP who has acute worsening of abdominal pain should be evaluated for intussusception.

Management

- HSP is typically a self-limited disease.
- NSAIDs are useful for associated arthralgias/arthritis.
- The role of corticosteroids is controversial but may provide some benefit in patients with severe abdominal pain and/or those with significant renal disease.

Points to Remember

- Hypersensitivity angiitis can develop as a hypersensitivity reaction to the administration of a therapeutic drug or in conjunction with a systemic illness such as serum sickness. Pulmonary and cutaneous findings (e.g., diffuse petechiae, palpable purpura) are common. Clinical course is variable but typically lasts several weeks. Glucocorticoids are indicated for severe disease.

Kawasaki Disease

Kawasaki disease is an acute febrile syndrome of vasculitis that occurs in children and has predilection for medium-sized arteries including the coronary arteries. The cause is unknown but evidence suggests an infectious agent or an immune response to an infectious agent. Eighty percentage of cases occur in children younger than 5 years, and 90% of cases involve children younger than 8 years. It is slightly more common in males than in females. In the United States, the incidence among Asian American children is three times higher than that in African American children and more than six times higher than that in white and Hispanic children. It is a self-limited illness but is associated with significant morbidity and mortality due to its cardiac sequelae.

Clinical Manifestations

Acute and subacute manifestations include the following (see Fig. 5.8):

- Fever for 5 or more days (typically >40°C).
- Irritability.
- Limbic sparing bilateral conjunctival injection.
- Nonsuppurative cervical lymphadenopathy.
- Rash (maculopapular, ill-defined erythematous plaques; primarily truncal).
- Pharyngeal injection, dry fissured lips, injected lips, and/or strawberry tongue.
- Edema of bilateral hands and feet.
- Arthritis, arthralgias.
- Abdominal pain.
- Hydrops of the gallbladder.
- Desquamation (typically occurs 2 to 3 weeks after onset of acute symptoms; particularly prominent in the periungual and diaper areas).
- Pancarditis (usually mild and self-limited).
- Coronary artery aneurysms (typically appear in subacute phase 11 to 25 days after onset).

Points to Remember

- The most serious complications of Kawasaki disease are cardiovascular and include aneurysms of the coronary arteries and other large arteries, aneurismal rupture, hemopericardium, myocarditis, coronary thrombosis, pericardial effusions, cardiac tamponade, mitral valve disease, and arrhythmias. Please refer to Chapter 4 for a more complete discussion.
- Desquamation is a constant feature of Kawasaki disease and typically occurs 2 to 3 weeks after the onset of acute symptoms.

Diagnosis

Diagnostic criteria include the presence of fever for 5 or more days and at least four of five of the following:

- Bilateral conjunctival injection.
- Pharyngeal injection, dry fissured lips, injected lips, and/or strawberry tongue.
- Erythema, edema, and/or desquamation of extremities.
- Rash.
- Cervical lymphadenopathy.

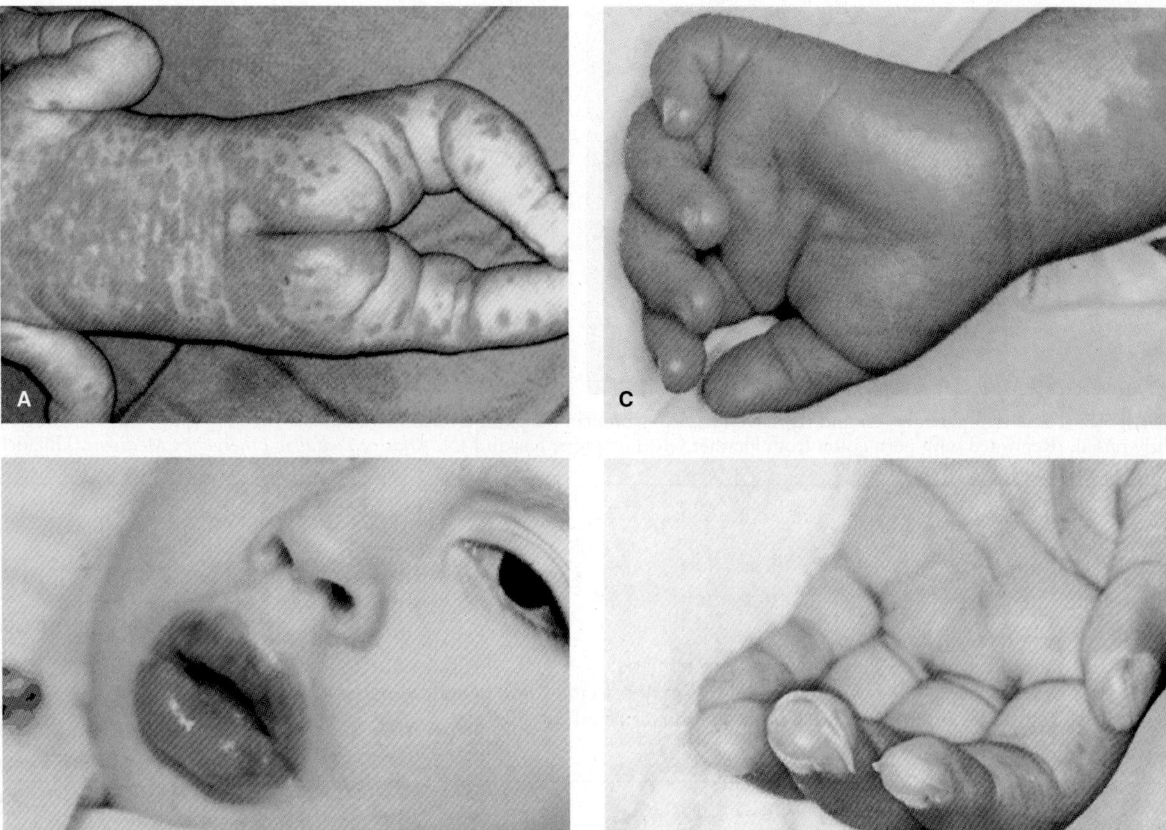

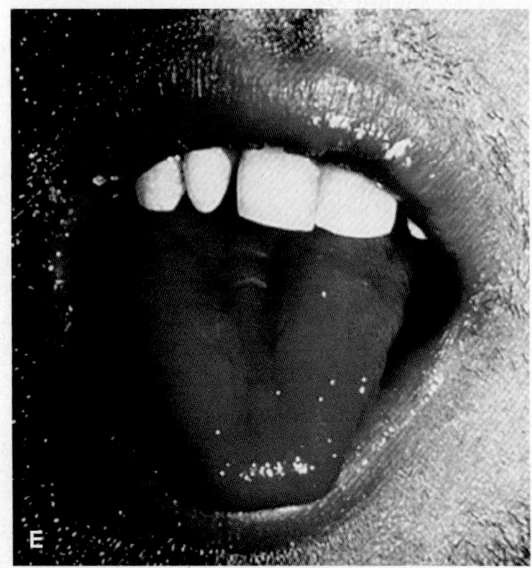

FIGURE 5.8. Kawasaki disease. (**A**) Rash of Kawasaki disease in a 7-month-old child on the fourth day of illness; (**B**) conjunctival injection, lip edema in a 2-year-old boy on the sixth day of illness; (**C**) erythema and edematous hand of a 1.5-year-old girl on the sixth day of illness; and (**D**) periungual desquamation in a 3-year-old child on the 12th day of illness. (**E**) Strawberry tongue. (**A**) to (**D**) Reprinted with permission from The Council on Cardiovascular Disease in Young, Committee on Rheumatic Fever, Endocarditis, and Kawasaki Disease. Diagnostic guidelines for Kawasaki disease. *Circulation*. 2001;103:335–336. (**E**) Reprinted with permission from Goodheart HP. *Goodheart's Photoguide of Common Skin Disorders*. 2nd ed. Philadelphia, PA: Lippincott Williams & Wilkins, 2003.)

Adjunctive laboratory markers may include the following:

- Elevated ESR and/or CRP.
- Leukocytosis with left shift.
  - Mild transaminitis.
  - Hypogammaglobulinemia.
  - Hyponatremia.
  - Hypophosphatemia.
  - Sterile pyuria.
  - Proteinuria.
  - Thrombocytosis (platelet counts ranging from 500,000 to 3 million/m^3; usually appears in second week of illness and peaks in third week).

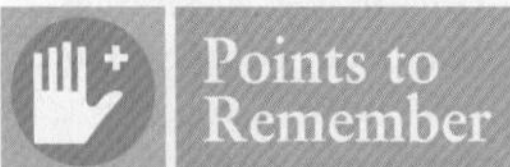

Points to Remember

- Thrombocytosis is a constant feature of Kawasaki disease and can be extreme. It is rarely present in the first week of illness and typically appears in the second week of illness.

Management

- The goals of treatment are to decrease the inflammatory response and to reduce the severity of the cardiovascular complications:

- IVIG reduces the risk of developing coronary artery aneurysms and should be given within 10 days of disease onset (earlier is better). It is usually given as a single dose, although subsequent doses may be needed for patients with refractory disease.
- High-dose aspirin is given initially and continued until 48 to 72 hours after resolution of fevers. Aspirin is then continued at lower doses for a minimum of 6 to 8 weeks to reduce the risk of thrombus formation (longer course is needed with persistent coronary manifestations).
- Use of steroids remains controversial but may be indicated for refractory disease.

- Long-term follow-up and serial echocardiograms are indicated for patients with coronary artery aneurysms.

Prognosis

Kawasaki disease is largely self-limited, but cardiovascular complications can result in long-term sequelae and death.

- Deaths in the acute phase of illness are rare but can result from pancarditis.
- Patients with coronary artery aneurysms are at increased risk of myocardial infarction related to thrombosis of aneurysms or stenosis of coronary arteries. Most infarctions occur within 1 year of illness without preceding signs or symptoms.

Polyarteritis Nodosa

PAN is a systemic vasculitis that can affect virtually every organ system and has a highly variable course. Although it most commonly presents in individuals in their 30s and 40s, it can present in childhood or adolescence. An association with hepatitis B infection has led to speculation of a causative role. Onset is usually insidious.

Clinical Manifestations

- Constitutional symptoms (e.g., fever, weight loss).
- Renal, GI tract, and cardiac disease can initially occur separately or together.
- Dermatologic findings (e.g., dermatitis, purpura, gangrene of distal extremities, livedo reticularis [Fig. 5.9], ulcers, erythematous, painful nodules).
- Neurologic abnormalities (e.g., peripheral neuropathy, seizures, cognitive dysfunction).

Diagnosis

- Diagnosis is established by the presence of three out of ten disease characteristics established by the American College of Rheumatology:
  - Weight loss of more than 4 kg.
  - Livedo reticularis.
  - Testicular pain and tenderness.
  - Myalgias, weakness, or leg tenderness.
  - Mononeuropathy or polyneuropathy.
  - Elevated diastolic blood pressure.
  - Elevated BUN or creatinine level.
  - Presence of hepatitis B surface antigen or antibody in serum.
  - Arteriogram demonstrating aneurysms or occlusions of the visceral arteries.
  - Biopsy of small- or medium-sized vessels containing granulocytes.

Management

- Glucocorticoids.
- Immunosuppressive agents (e.g., cyclophosphamide) are added in severe cases.

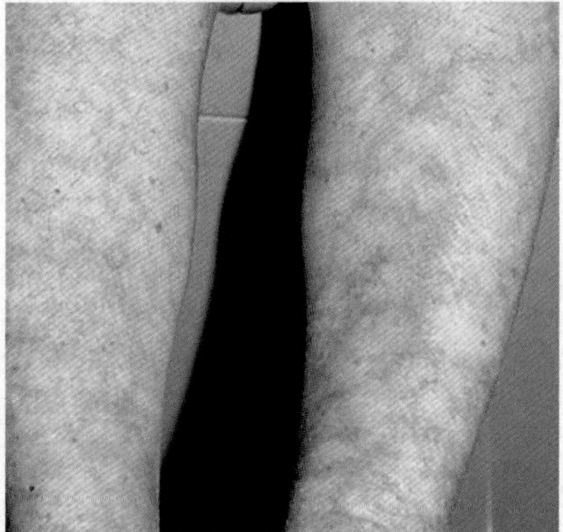

FIGURE 5.9. Livedo reticularis. (Reprinted with permission from Goodheart HP. *Goodheart's Photoguide of Common Skin Disorders*. 2nd ed. Philadelphia, PA: Lippincott Williams & Wilkins, 2003.)

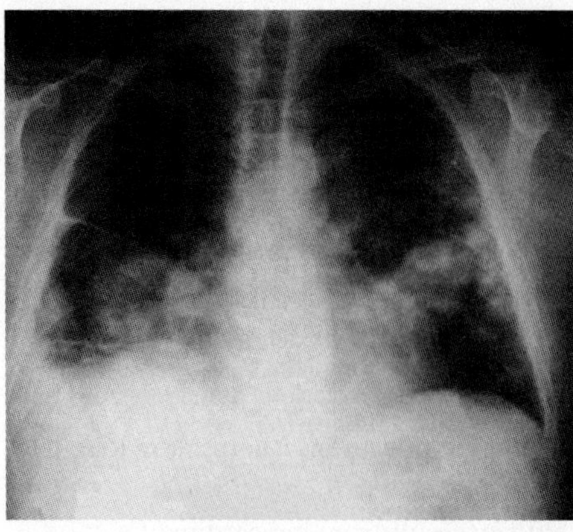

FIGURE 5.10. Wegener's granulomatosis (radiograph): granulomas in both lungs. (Reprinted with permission from *Stedman's Medical Dictionary*. 28th ed. Baltimore, MD: Lippincott Williams & Wilkins, 2005.)

Wegener's Granulomatosis

WG is a necrotizing granulomatous angiitis primarily involving the respiratory tract (e.g., sinuses, nasal passages, and lungs) and kidneys. It is extremely rare in children but has been described in patients of all ages. The cause of WG is unknown.

Clinical Manifestations

- Constitutional symptoms (e.g., fever, weight loss, fatigue).
- Involvement of the upper respiratory tract may present with rhinorrhea, sinopulmonary pain, mucosal ulceration, and/or epistaxis.
- Involvement of the lower respiratory tract may present with hemoptysis, shortness of breath, pleuritic chest pain, and/or recurrent pneumonias (Fig. 5.10).
- Glomerulonephritis.

Diagnosis

- Definitive diagnosis is via microscopic examination of a biopsy of the nasal mucosa, lung, or kidneys with granulomata and necrotizing vasculitis with leukocytic, lymphocytic, and giant-cell infiltration.
- Adjunctive laboratory markers may include elevated ESR and CRP levels, the presence of antineutrophilic antibodies (c-ANCA), elevated BUN and creatinine, proteinuria, and/or hematuria levels.

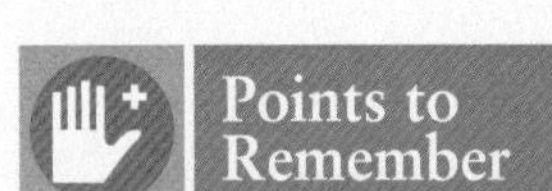

Points to Remember

- c-ANCA is positive in 80% to 95% of patients with WG.

Management

- Corticosteroids are the initial treatment of WG.
- Most patients also require additional immune modulators such as cytoxan, methotrexate, and/or rituximab.

Prognosis

Historically, death from renal or pulmonary disease occurred with only rare long-term survival but with treatment many now survive and experience remission and/or cure.

Churg-Strauss Syndrome

CS is a disorder leading to blood vessel inflammation, allergic granulomatosis, and allergic angiitis. Similar to many of the other vasculitides, the exact etiology of CS is unknown. An infectious trigger and genetic predisposition are suspected. Severity of disease is variable. There are typically three stages of presentation: allergic, hypereosinophilic, and vasculitic.

Clinical Manifestations

- Allergic stage: asthma, allergic rhinitis, sinusitis.
- Hypereosinophilic stage: constitutional symptoms (e.g., fever, night sweats), abdominal pain, GI bleeding.
- Vasculitic stage: shortness of breath, hemoptysis, hematuria, diarrhea, arthralgias, myalgias, rash.

Diagnosis

Diagnosis is based on the presence of four out of the following six findings:

- Asthma.
- Neuropathy.

- Recurrent sinusitis.
- Peripheral eosinophilia.
- Pulmonary lesions on chest x-ray or chest CT.
- Skin biopsy with extravascular eosinophils.

Management

- Corticosteroids.
- Cytoxan and other immune modulators.
- IVIG.

Behcet Syndrome

BS consists of a triad of recurrent uveitis, mucocutaneous ulcerations, and genital ulcerations. The basic pathologic lesion is a vasculitis of small- and medium-sized arteries and veins. It is thought to be autoimmune in etiology and can be associated with HLA-B5 and HLA-B27. Unlike almost all other autoimmune conditions, BS is more common in males than in females. The most common age of onset is between 18 and 40 years of age. Incidence is highest in individuals of Middle Eastern descent. Clinical course is highly variable. Active disease may span a period of a few weeks or extend to several years, and the typical pattern of involvement is characterized by frequent remissions and exacerbations.

Points to Remember

- **Approximately three-fourth of children with BS diagnosed younger than 2 years will have a nondestructive polyarthritis.**
- **Genital lesions in patients with BS are often initially misdiagnosed as herpetic lesions and are extremely painful.**

Clinical Manifestations

- Classic triad is recurrent uveitis, mucocutaneous aphthous ulcerations (see Fig. 5.11), and genital ulcerations.
- Other manifestations include deep vein thrombophlebitis, nondestructive polyarthritis, synovitis, erythema nodosum, colitis, ophthalmologic abnormalities (e.g., uveitis, optic neuritis, scleritis, retinal vasculitis), and/or CNS abnormalities (e.g., psychiatric disturbances, pseudotumor cerebri).

Diagnosis

- Diagnosis of BS is primarily clinical.
- Pathergy, the phenomenon in which superficial trauma reproduces typical cutaneous lesions, is an additional clinical clue that can be helpful in diagnosis.
- Adjunctive laboratory markers may include elevated ESR, hypergammaglobulinemia, positive HLA-B5 antibody, and/or positive HLA-B27 antibody.
- Biopsy of involved tissue demonstrates C3, C4, terminal components of the complement cascade, and fibrinogen deposits in vessel walls.

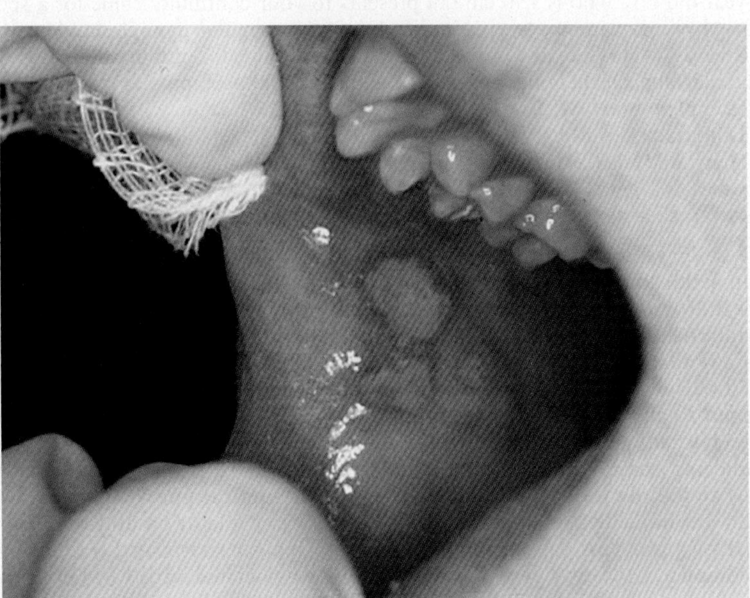

FIGURE 5.11. Mucocutaneous ulcerations in a patient with Behcet syndrome. (Reprinted with permission from Neville BW, Damm DD, White DK. *Color Atlas of Clinical Oral Pathology*. 2nd ed. Baltimore, MD: Williams & Wilkins, 1998.)

Management

- Immunosuppressive or alkylating agents may be indicated along with glucocorticoid drugs, especially in patients with CNS disease and/or uveitis.
- Arthritis is responsive to colchicines and interferon alpha.
- Thrombophlebitis is treated with antiplatelet agents and aspirin.

Takayasu Arteritis

Takayasu arteritis is a giant cell arteritis of unknown etiology that occurs predominantly in teenage girls and women younger than 40 years. Stenosis, occlusion, dilation, and aneurysm formation are confined to the aorta, its major branches, and the pulmonary arteries. It is more common in Asians, Latinos, blacks, and Sephardic Jews. The male to female ratio is 8:1.

Clinical Manifestations

- Onset is usually insidious.
- Course may be limited, lasting 3 to 6 months, or prolonged over many years.
- Constitutional symptoms include fever, fatigue, and anorexia.
- Signs of vascular insufficiency (e.g., renovascular hypertension, lightheadedness, visual changes, extremity weakness, stroke).
- Cardiac involvement may lead to aortic regurgitation and CHF.
- Chest pain and shortness of breath.

Diagnosis

- Diagnosis is suggested clinically and confirmed via magnetic resonance imaging (MRI)/magnetic resonance angiography and angiography.
- Adjunctive laboratory markers may include elevated ESR and CRP.
- Doppler ultrasound of the carotid and subclavian arteries may demonstrate changes in laminar flow.

Management

- Corticosteroids are the first-line treatment.
- NSAIDs are useful in managing the symptoms during the acute early phase of illness.
- Methotrexate and azathioprine are useful for patients who do not respond to corticosteroids or are maintained on steroids for prolonged periods of time.
- Aggressive management of associated hypertension.
- Anticoagulation therapy or antiplatelet agents may be required.
- Surgical stents and/or bypasses of affected vessels may be required.

QUESTIONS

1. A 15-year-old boy who is 190 cm tall presents to your continuity clinic for a sports physical. On physical examination, you notice long fingers, malar hypoplasia, dental crowding, ectopic lentis, pectus excavatum, an arm span to height ratio of more than 1.01 and a pansystolic murmur. Of the following, which is the most important next step in evaluation?
   a. Complete body MRI
   b. Echocardiogram
   c. Gene analysis of chromosome 15
   d. Chest CT
   e. No further workup is necessary

   Answer: b. Based on the clinical findings described in the vignette, this patient likely has Marfan syndrome. The differential diagnosis also includes homocystinuria and Loeys-Dietz syndrome, which can be phenotypically similar. An echocardiogram is the most important next step in the evaluation of this patient because mortality associated with Marfan syndrome is often due to associated cardiovascular abnormalities including aortic root dilation (predisposes to aortic root dissection and rupture) and mitral valve prolapse (predisposes to mitral regurgitation with risk of CHF and dysrhythmia). An initial echocardiogram at the time of diagnosis and subsequent yearly echocardiograms are indicated for all patients with Marfan syndrome to detect cardiovascular abnormalities and allow for appropriate medical and/or surgical intervention. Propranolol or losartan are indicated to slow the rate of aortic root dilatation and reduce the risk of aortic dissection. This patient should not be cleared for sports at this time.

   A complete MRI may reveal skeletal findings associated with Marfan syndrome but is not as urgent as an echocardiogram. Marfan syndrome is due to a mutation in the fibrilin gene on chromosome 15. Genetic testing is helpful to distinguish between Marfan syndrome and homocystinuria but is not urgent and is helpful only in some cases as there are a large number of separate causative mutations and related but distinct conditions (e.g., Ehlers-Danlos syndromes) can be caused by mutations in the same gene. A chest CT scan may reveal apical blebs associated with Marfan syndrome but is not as urgent as an echocardiogram.

2. A 5-year-old girl presents with a 1-month history of worsening fatigue, muscle aches, inability to rise from a chair or walk up stairs, headache, and weight loss. Her father notes that she used to participate in gymnastics and swimming lessons but is no longer able to participate in either activity. Initial laboratory testing reveals elevated CK and AST levels. ANA is negative. Which of the following set of skin findings would be consistent with a diagnosis of dermatomyositis in this patient?
   a. Maculopapular erythematous rash most prominent on the trunk and strawberry tongue
   b. Transient nonpuritic maculopapular rash that coincides with the presence of high fevers
   c. Purpuric lesions most prominent on the buttocks and bilateral lower extremities
   d. Heliotrope facial rash and gottron papules
   e. Cutaneous vesicular lesions in response to superficial trauma

Answer: d. This patient likely has dermatomyositis. This disorder most commonly presents in children between the ages of 4 and 10 years and is slightly more common in girls than in boys. Muscular findings associated with this disorder include proximal muscle weakness and myalgias. Systemic symptoms such as fatigue, weight loss, and low-grade fevers are also common. Dermatologic manifestations are present in 85% of patients and include heliotrope rash of eyelids and malar regions, Gottron papules, and/or nailbed telangiectasias. Dermatologic findings may be the first sign of disease or present later in the course.

A maculopapular rash most prominent on the trunk and the presence of a strawberry tongue are two of the clinical criteria used to establish a diagnosis of Kawasaki disease. A transient nonpuritic maculopapular rash that coincides with the presence of high fevers is characteristic of systemic JRA. Purpuric lesions most prominent on the buttocks and bilateral lower extremities are seen in HSP. Pathergy, the phenomenon in which superficial trauma reproduces vesicular cutaneous lesions, is associated with Behcet syndrome.

3. A 12-year-old boy with a past medical history significant only for asthma presents with nausea, vomiting, diarrhea, and diffuse muscle aches. On physical examination, he is noted to be jaundiced and is tender to palpation over his liver, which feels mildly enlarged. He also has a purplish, lacy rash on his lower extremities. During the course of his evaluation, he experiences an asthma exacerbation and is placed on a 5-day course of oral steroids. In addition to improvement of his breathing problems, he also notes improvement of his muscle aches and resolution of his rash. After completing the course of steroids, his myalgias and rash return and he also begins to experience paresthesias in his legs and feet. Which of the following is the most likely diagnosis in this patient?
   a. Polyarteritis nodosa
   b. Behcet syndrome
   c. Kawasaki disease
   d. Multiple sclerosis
   e. Reiter's syndrome

Answer: a. The patient in the vignette has the classic findings of PAN including myalgias, livedo reticularis, and a peripheral neuropathy. This diagnosis is further supported by the likely presence of a coexistent acute viral hepatitis infection, which is a known association with PAN and may play a causative role. The fact that his symptoms improved on steroids is also consistent with a diagnosis of PAN as steroids result in temporary improvement of the underlying inflammatory process.

4. A 15-year-old boy of Middle Eastern ancestry presents with recurrent oral and genital ulcers. After being erroneously diagnosed with herpes simplex virus infections, he is ultimately diagnosed with BS. Other than BS, which of the following connective tissue diseases is more common in males than in females?
   a. Takayasu's arteritis
   b. Juvenile rheumatoid arthritis
   c. Dermatomyositis
   d. Polyarteritis Nodosa
   e. Scleroderma

Answer: d. Of the conditions listed, polyarteritis nodosa is the only connective tissue disease other than BS that is more common in males than in females. Takayasu's arteritis, JRA, dermatomyositis, and scleroderma are all more common in females than in males.

5. A 12-year-old girl presents with multiple thickened patches of skin characterized by white centers and purplish borders. Testing reveals a positive ANA. The lesions are not painful and she is otherwise well. Which of the following diagnoses is the most likely etiology of this patient's skin findings?
   a. Linear scleroderma
   b. CREST syndrome
   c. Morphea scleroderma
   d. Diffuse scleroderma
   e. Sjogren's Syndrome

Answer: c. Scleroderma is a characterized by progressive hardening and tightening of connective tissue due to excessive collagen accumulation. Scleroderma is subdivided into localized (morphea and linear types) and systemic (limited and diffuse types) forms. The lesions in this patient are classic for localized morphea scleroderma. Localized linear scleroderma is characterized by bands or streaks of thickened skin typically involving the extremities. Patients with diffuse systemic scleroderma have generalized tightening and thickening of the skin most notable initially on the face. Patients with limited (also known as CREST) systemic scleroderma have thickening of the skin usually limited to the face, neck, and upper extremities.

Sjogren's syndrome is based on a triad of findings including (1) the sicca syndrome (dry eyes and dry mouth), (2) a connective tissue disease (usually SLE or scleroderma), and (3) high titers of autoantibodies (usually rheumatoid factors or ANAs). This patient does not meet the criteria for Sjogren's syndrome as she is not experience the sicca syndrome necessary for diagnosis.

6. A 12-year-old boy presents with hematuria and hemoptysis. His past medical history is significant for allergic rhinitis, chronic sinusitis, and recurrent epistaxis. ANA test result is positive. He is referred to a rheumatologist who diagnoses him with WG. His disease is refractory to treatment with steroids and he experiences only marginal benefit with cyclophosphamide. Which of the following clinical manifestations is this patient most likely to experience within the next 5 years?
   a. Spontaneous resolution of symptoms
   b. Development of secondary lymphoma
   c. End stage renal disease
   d. Pneumothorax
   e. Restrictive pulmonary disease

Answer: c. Wegener's granulomatosis is a rare disorder in children characterized by a necrotizing granulomatous angiitis involving the respiratory tract and the kidneys. Pulmonary disease may progress to hemorrhage, obstruction, atelectasis, and/or repeated episodes of infection. Most affected children have moderate to severe renal disease that will progress if untreated. Historically, death from renal or pulmonary disease was almost universal with only rare long-term survival. Treatment with glucocorticoids and immunosuppressive agents such as cyclophosphamide, however, have led to a dramatic improvement in prognosis. Given this patient's poor response to steroids and cyclophosphamide, however, his disease is likely to progress to end-stage renal disease and severe pulmonary manifestations.

7. Which of the following medications is most closely associated with drug-induced lupus?
   a. Erythromycin
   b. Hydrochlorothiazide
   c. Hydralazine
   d. Prednisone
   e. Diphenhydramine

Answer: c. Agents most commonly implicated in drug-induced lupus in children include hydralazine, isoniazid, penicillin, sulfonamides, and anticonvulsants. Drug-induced lupus is usually a self-limited disease and resolves with withdrawal of the offending agent. Prednisone is helpful for the treatment of more severe and/or prolonged cases. Erythromycin, hydrochlorothiazide, prednisone, and diphenhydramine are not closely associated with drug-induced lupus.

8. A 16-year-old girl who is 32 weeks pregnant presents with severe abdominal pain and vaginal bleeding. She is profoundly hypotensive and is ultimately found to have uterine rupture. After she is stabilized, you notice that she has a thin body habitus with somewhat unusual facial features including big eyes, a small chin, and a thin upper lip. Her skin is thin and fragile-appearing. Of the following, which is the most likely underlying diagnosis in this patient?
   a. Marfan syndrome
   b. Ehlers-Danlos syndrome type II

c. Loeys-Dietz syndrome
d. Ehlers-Danlos syndrome type IV
e. Homocystinuria

Answer: d. The EDSs are a heterogeneous group of disorders in which abnormalities of collagen production affect the skin, joints, and blood vessels. They are characterized by easy bruising, poor wound healing, joint hypermobility, characteristic facies, and hyperflexible skin. EDS type IV (also known as vascular type) is also associated with an increased risk of organ rupture. Uterine rupture in pregnant women with this disorder is a known and not uncommon complication and can be fatal.

Although Marfan syndrome, EDS type II, Loeys-Dietz syndrome, and homocystinuira share many common features with EDS type IV, they are not associated with an increased risk of uterine rupture.

9. A 3-year-old boy with a 6-day history of fever and irritability represents to his pediatrician with bilateral conjunctival injection; a maculopapular truncal rash; swelling of his hands and feet; and dry, red, cracked lips. He is admitted to the hospital for treatment of Kawasaki disease. Which of the following statements regarding Kawasaki disease is true?

a. It is most common in individuals of Eastern European descent.
b. Extreme thrombocytosis is an early marker of disease.
c. Desquamation of the hands, feet, and diaper area typically occurs 2 to 3 weeks after the onset of acute symptoms
d. 80% of cases occur in children between the ages of 5 and 8 years.
e. Associated coronary artery aneurysms place the patient at risk for subsequent myocardial infarctions, most of which occur 5 to 10 years after the acute disease

Answer: c. Kawasaki disease is an acute self-limited form of childhood vasculitis that has a predilection for the coronary arteries. Desquamation of the hands, feet, and diaper area typically occur 2 to 3 weeks after the onset of acute symptoms. Kawasaki disease is most common in individuals of Asian descent. Extreme thrombocytosis is a hallmark feature of the disease but is not usually present until 2 to 3 weeks after the onset of acute illness. Eighty percent of cases occur in children younger than 5 years and an additional 10% of cases occur in children between the ages of 5 and 8 years. The most feared complication of Kawasaki disease is coronary artery aneurysms. Most myocardial infarctions associated with coronary artery aneurysms due to Kawasaki disease occur within 1 year of the acute illness. Prompt treatment with IVIG and aspirin decreases the risk of developing coronary artery aneurysms.

SUGGESTED READINGS

Beighton P, De Paepe A, Steinmann B, et al. Ehlers-Danlos syndromes: revised nosology, Villefranche, 1997. Ehlers-Danlos National Foundation (USA) and Ehlers-Danlos Support Group (UK). *Am J Med Genet.* 1998;77:31–37.

Dietz HC, Cutting GR, Pyeritz RE, et al. Marfan syndrome caused by a recurrent de novo missense mutation in the fibrillin gene. *Nature.* 1991;352:337–339.

Judge DP, Dietz HC. Marfan's syndrome. *Lancet.* 2005;366:1965–1976.

Loeys B, Van Maldergem L, Mortier G, et al. Homozygosity for a missense mutation in fibulin-5 (FBLN5) results in a severe form of cutis laxa. *Hum Mol Genet.* 2002;11:2113–2118.

Loeys BL, Chen J, Neptune ER, et al. A syndrome of altered cardiovascular, craniofacial, neurocognitive and skeletal development caused by mutations in TGFBR1 or TGFBR2. *Nat Genet.* 2005;37:275–281.

Loeys BL, Schwarze U, Holm T, et al. Aneurysm syndromes caused by mutations in the TGF-beta receptor. *N Engl J Med.* 2006;355:788–798.

CHAPTER 6 ■ CRITICAL CARE AND EMERGENCY MEDICINE

JOAN H. DUNLOP

ABG	Arterial blood gas	ER	Emergency room
ALTE	Apparent life-threatening event	ET	Endotracheal
AMS	Altered mental status	GCS	Glasgow coma scale
ARDS	Acute respiratory distress syndrome	GI	Gastrointestinal
		Gtt	Drop
BP	Blood pressure	H	Hour
BSA	Body surface area	HIPAA	Health Insurance Portability and Accountability Act
BUN	Blood urea nitrogen		
CHF	Congestive heart failure	ICP	Intracranial pressure
CXR	Chest x-ray	IV	Intravenous
CBC	Complete blood count	LFTs	Liver function tests
CT	Computed tomography	OR	Operating room
EEG	Electroencephalogram	SVR	Systemic vascular resistance
EKG	Electrocardiogram	WBC	White blood cell

CHAPTER OBJECTIVES

For the purposes of board review, the "critical care" chapter will provide a summary of the following:

1. Initial management of common emergencies, including poisoning, shock, respiratory failure, trauma, and others
2. Basic emergency life support measures
3. Key points to the recognition of impending systemic failure.

COMMON EMERGENCIES

The following review of common pediatric emergencies is in no way intended to be comprehensive, but rather a summary of the material likely to appear on a board examination. In addition, some of the material reviewed in this section is also covered in depth in other chapters of the book.

Toxicology

Epidemiology

Ingestions and poisonings are a major source of pediatric morbidity and mortality.

- More than 50% of all poisonings occur in children under the age of 6.
- The most common forms of poison exposure/ingestion are cosmetics and personal care products, cleaning substances, analgesics, and foreign bodies.

Prevention

- Discussion regarding the safe storage of household cleaners, medications, and personal care items is a central part of anticipatory guidance during the health maintenance visits.
- Parents and caregivers should know how to contact their local poison control center.
- In emergency settings, an ingestion history is an important component of the history and physical exam, and in cases where ingestion is suspected, be sure to inquire about medications in the home. Always check for possible coingestions (e.g., aspirin and acetaminophen).

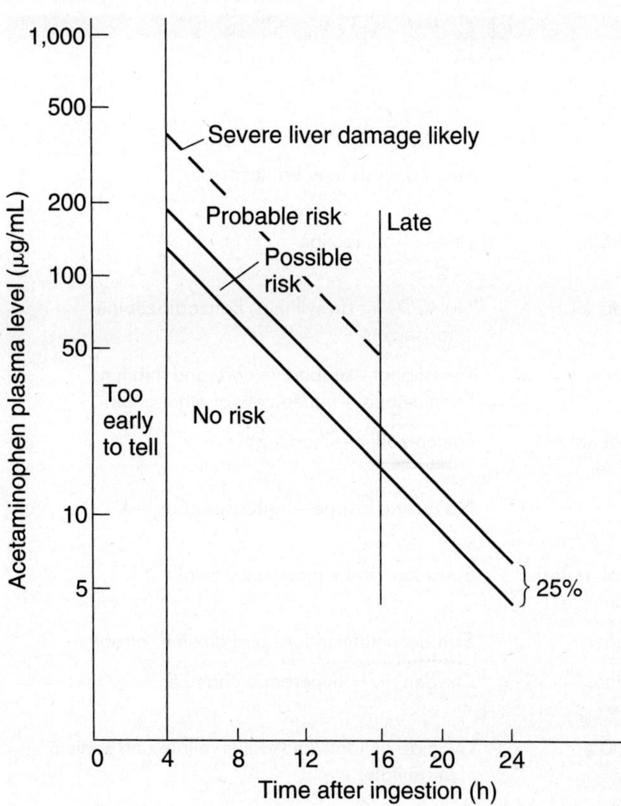

FIGURE 6.1. Nomogram. (Reprinted with permission from Helms RA, Quan DJ. *Textbook of Therapeutics: Drug and Disease Management*. Philadelphia: Lippincott Williams & Wilkins; 2006.)

Clinical Presentation

In general, this varies by ingestion; however, they can usually be categorized by their primary effect on the nervous system.

- Sympathomimetic symptoms—dilated pupils, agitated, wet mucous membranes, hyperactive bowel sounds, increased urination.
- Anticholinergic symptoms—dilated pupils, dry skin, confused, hypoactive bowel sounds, urinary retention, dry mouth.

See Tables 6.1 and 6.2 for specific presenting symptoms for various ingestions.

Points to Remember

- Measure acetaminophen levels at least 4 hours following ingestion. Use a nomogram to determine risk for hepatic toxicity (Fig. 6.1).

Treatment

- In general, treatment involves absorbing and/or flushing out the ingested substance. Specific treatments and antidotes are listed in Tables 6.1, 6.3 and 6.4.
- Gastric lavage is only indicated in specific situations. If the substance was ingested less than 60 minutes ago, is highly toxic, cannot be bound by charcoal, and does not put the patient at risk for aspiration or severe irritation upon efflux, only then is gastric lavage indicated.
- Consultation with your local poison control center is always recommended. Their expertise in toxicology can provide valuable additional information, i.e., which oral antidotes are neutralized by the administration of activated charcoal.

Points to Remember

- Syrup of ipecac and other emetics are no longer routinely recommended given the risk of aspiration.
- Some toxins not bound by charcoal include lithium, iron, and potassium. In most instances of overdose, however, activated charcoal (1 g/kg/dose) is used to absorb the drug if able to be given within 60 minutes of ingestion. This window of opportunity may be lengthened if a sustained-release preparation of a drug has been ingested.

Shock

Definition

Inadequate delivery of oxygen and nutrients to the tissues relative to their metabolic demand.

Etiologies

Etiologies include cardiogenic, hypovolemic, obstructive, and distributive etiologies. Hypovolemia is the most common cause of shock in children worldwide. Fluid loss due to diarrhea is the leading cause of hypovolemic shock.

TABLE 6.1

SPECIFIC POISONS AND TREATMENTS

Substance	Clinical Presentation	Specific Treatment
Nonsteroidal anti-inflammatory drugs	Gastrointestinal (GI) upset, GI bleeding, or asymptomatic	Renal dialysis may be necessary
Salicylates	Respiratory alkalosis, metabolic acidosis, AMS, tinnitus, wintergreen odor	Urine alkalinization
Tricyclic antidepressants	Seizure, arrhythmia, hypotension, decreased GI motility, dilated pupils	$NaHCO_3$ for arrhythmia, benzodiazepines for seizure
Ethanol/methanol	AMS, hypoglycemia, acidosis, afferent pupillary defect (methanol)	For ethanol—supportive care and thiamine For methanol—fomepizole or ethanol gtt
Ethylene glycol	AMS, anion gap metabolic acidosis, cranial nerve palsies and tetany, oxalate crystals in urine	Fomepizole or ethanol gtt
Hydrocarbons	Nausea and vomiting, choking/gagging—persistent cough	No gastric lavage—high aspiration risk
Caustics acids	Acid burns tend to be more superficial, alkali burns deeper; GI burns can occur with ingestion	Burns tend to be more superficial
Organophosphates	Hypersalivation, tearing, sweating, diarrhea	Skin decontamination, pralidoxime, atropine
Carbon monoxide	AMS, lethargy, cherry red mucous membranes, pulse ox can be normal, flu-like syndrome	Oxygen +/− hyperbaric chamber
Cyanide	Same as above but does not respond to 100% oxygen therapy	Cyanide antidote kit (sodium nitrite and sodium thiosulfate)
Acetaminophen	Vomiting, abdominal pain, elevated LFTs, oliguria	If <1 h since ingestion—activated Charcoal + *N*-acetylcysteine (NAC), otherwise IV NAC with close follow up of acetaminophen levels. NAC: Initial oral dose—140 mg/kg, then 70 mg/kg q 4 h × 17 doses
Iron	GI bleeding, anion gap metabolic acidosis, hyperglycemia; Symptoms can improve 6–72 h after ingestion, but multiorgan system failure may follow	Deferoxamine *15 mg/kg/h IV infusion until urine color clears or patient clinically well (not to exceed 6 g/24 h)*
Lead	Difficulty concentrating, tremor, headache, diffuse abdominal pain, constipation, seizure	2,3-dimercaptosuccinic acid
Opiates	AMS, pinpoint pupils, decreased GI motility, absent gag reflex	Naloxone (Narcan)
Theophylline	Sympathetic syndrome	Benzodiazepines for agitation or seizures, hyperpyrexia with cooling measures or sedation
Clonidine	AMS, hypotension, bradycardia	Naloxone
Phenothiazines	Neuroleptic malignant syndrome, depressed mental status, anticholinergic symptoms	Benztropine

Note: Animal/Human Bites as well as Rabies are discussed within the "infectious disease" chapter.
GI, gastrointestinal; AMS, altered mental status; LFTs, liver function tests; NAC, *N*-acetylcysteine; IV, intravenous.

TABLE 6.2

ETHANOL

Blood Alcohol Concentration (mg/dL)	Clinical Effect
100–150	Intoxication
150–200	Loss of muscle coordination
200–300	Decreased level of consciousness
300–500	Death

Note: Presentation of symptoms may vary depending on the patient's tolerance for alcohol.

TABLE 6.3

PLANTS, INSECTS AND REPTILES

Substance	Clinical Presentation	Specific Treatment
Foxglove	Digitalis effect—bradycardia, heart block, and hyperkalemia	
Jimsonweed	Belladonna effect	Benztropine
Mistletoe berries	Gastroenteritis, cardiovascular collapse	
Black widow	Black widow bite is generally painless but systemic reaction includes cramping, nausea and twitching, and hypertension	Specific antivenin exists for black widow bites.
Brown recluse spider	Bite is painful and causes extensive local necrosis	
Spider	Local reaction	Corticosteroids for inflammation, benzodiazepines for muscle relaxation
Snake (crotalid)	Localized bite marks, spreading hemorrhagic necrosis	CroFab antivenin: *Mild, 3–5 vials; moderate, 6–10 vials; severe, 10–20 vials* *Mix reconstituted antivenin in 1,000 mL Norman Saline over 4–6 h*

Clinical Presentation

- Hypotension is *not* required for a patient to be in shock. When shock is impending, compensatory mechanisms are activated to improve delivery of oxygen and nutrients to the tissues.
- Compensatory mechanisms include tachycardia, increased SVR, increased cardiac contractility, and increased venous tone. Thus the child's systolic BP may be normal, but pulse pressure may be narrowed if SVR is increased (as a compensatory measure in hypovolemic shock) or widened if SVR is decreased (as in distributive shock).
- When BP remains normal, the patient is in compensated shock.

Diagnosis

- Early recognition is key to preventing cardiac arrest and poor outcomes.
- Waiting for hypotension, and thus hypotensive shock, is inappropriate.
- Look for abnormalities in vital signs, specifically tachycardia.

Treatment

- Increase oxygenation and improve volume status. High flow oxygen is indicated in all children with shock.
- Attain vascular access to provide fluid resuscitation using 20 mL/kg of isotonic crystalloid.
- Vasoactive pharmacologic agents (i.e., pressors) can be used if shock persists despite adequate volume resuscitation.
- Volume resuscitation should be conservative (10 mL/kg) in cardiogenic shock; vasoactive agents may be used earlier in the course of treatment.
- Treat the underlying cause (e.g., bacterial infection in septic shock, CHF in cardiogenic shock) *after* basic therapy for shock has been implemented.

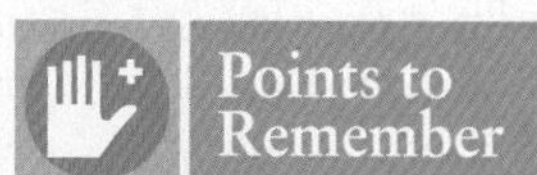

- **If IV access is difficult to attain after 60 seconds, interosseous access should be attempted.**

TABLE 6.4

COIN AND BATTERY INGESTIONS

Substance	Specific Treatment
Coins	Spontaneous passage of 25%–30% into the stomach in 8–16 h
Batteries	Should be removed without delay due to risk for pressure necrosis and low-voltage burn

Prevention

Early recognition of compensated shock will allow for correction of underlying causes and prevention of progression to hypotensive shock and cardiac arrest.

Respiratory Failure

Definition

A state of inadequate oxygenation and/or ventilation.

- Respiratory failure can quickly progress to respiratory arrest and cardiac arrest.
- In children, outcomes are more likely to be positive following isolated respiratory arrest.

Diagnosis

Clinical indicators include the following:

- Increased/decreased or no respiratory effort.
- Tachypnea and tachycardia (early).
- Bradypnea or apnea and bradycardia (late).
- Cyanosis.
- Poor distal air movement.
- Depressed mental status.

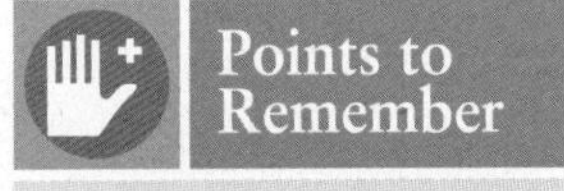

- ET tube size = (age + 16)/4

Treatment

For clinical presentation and treatment of specific conditions, see Table 6.5.

TABLE 6.5

RESPIRATORY EMERGENCIES

Condition	Pathophysiology	Presentation	Diagnostic Aids	Treatment
Acute asthma	Obstructive process, poor air exchange	Prolonged expiratory phase, wheezing	Hyperinflation on CXR	Bronchodilation, intubation only as last resort
Foreign body (also reviewed in "Gastrointestinal" chapter)	Inhaled foreign body acts as ball-valve usually in right mainstem bronchus	Wheeze or stridor, cough +/− fever	Decubitus or forced exhalation x-ray films showing air-trapping	Removal
Tension pneumothorax	Increasing pneumothorax prevents adequate oxygenation of opposite lung and decreased venous return	Deviated trachea, unilaterally absent breath sounds, hypotension	CXR (Fig. 6.2), transillumination	
Flail chest	Segment of chest wall separated from the rest of ribcage due to trauma, makes movement inadequate for ventilation	Paradoxical movement of segment of chest wall	CXR, evidence of steering wheel/handle bar impact	
Epiglottitis	Haemophilus influenzae	Tripoding (Fig. 6.3), drooling, stridor, fever	Toxic appearance, X-ray (Fig. 6.4) (not necessary if diagnosis clear)	Most experienced intubator in OR setting
Pulmonary embolus	Preventing perfusion to a ventilated area of lung	Tachypnea, hypoxia (depending on size), dyspnea	High resolution computed tomography, blood gas with arterial-alveolar gradient	Dissolution of clot (heparin gtt)

CXR, chest x-ray; OR, operating room.

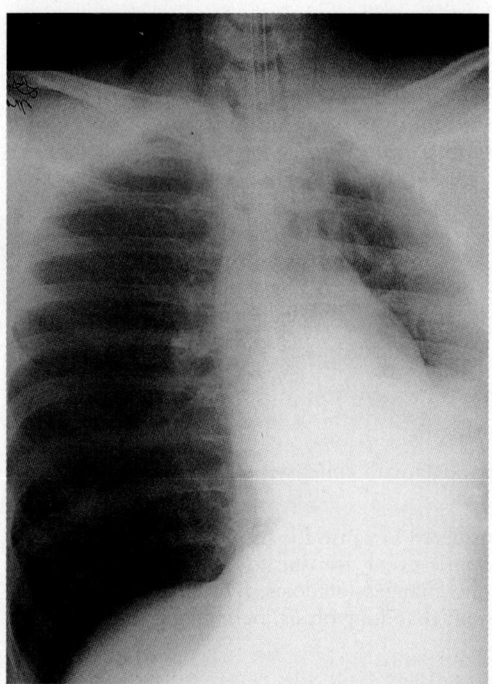

FIGURE 6.2. A right-sided tension pneumothorax displaces the heart to the left. (Reprinted with permission from Fleisher GR, Ludwig S, Baskin MN. *Atlas of Pediatric Emergency Medicine*. Philadelphia: Lippincott Williams & Wilkins; 2004.)

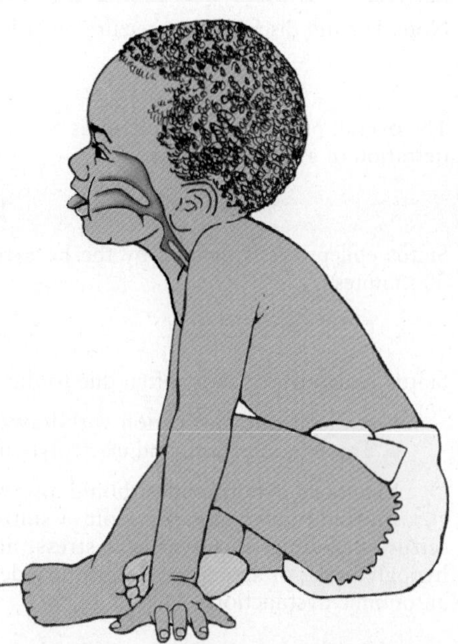

FIGURE 6.3. Characteristic posture of a child with acute epiglottitis—leaning forward on hands, in the "tripod" position, mouth open, tongue out, head forward and tilted up in a sniffing position in an effort to relieve the acute airway obstruction secondary to swollen epiglottis. (Reprinted with permission from Klossner NJ, Hatfield NT. *Introductory Maternity and Pediatric Nursing: Basis of Human Movement in Health and Disease*. 4th ed. Philadelphia: Lippincott Williams & Wilkins; 2005.)

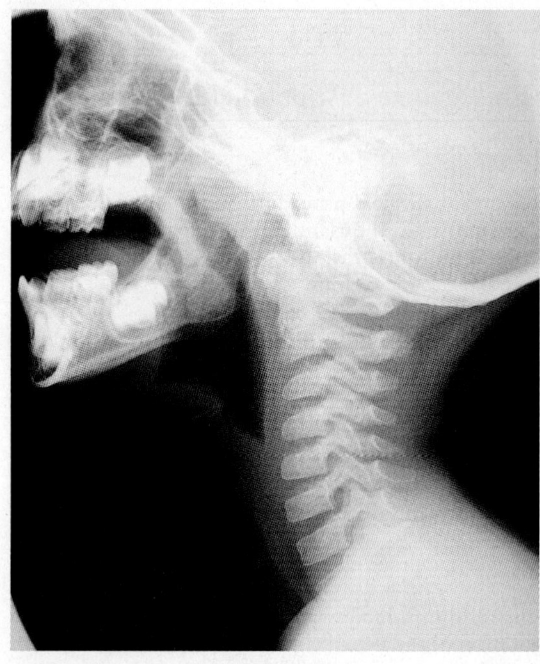

FIGURE 6.4. The patient has epiglottitis. The radiograph demonstrates a swollen epiglottis at the level of the hyoid bone, which is convex on both sides and appears in the shape of a thumbprint. Edema anterior to the epiglottis has obliterated the vallecula, which usually appears as an elongated black shadow. Note the marked swelling of the aryepiglottic folds, projecting inferiorly and posteriorly from the epiglottis and the arytenoid cartilages at the base of the folds. (Reprinted with permission from Fleisher GR, Ludwig W, Baskin MN. *Atlas of Pediatric Emergency Medicine*. Philadelphia: Lippincott Williams & Wilkins; 2004.)

Neurologic Emergencies: Status Epilepticus

Note: For full discussion of seizure disorders and management see the "Neurology" chapter.

Epidemiology

The overall prevalence of epilepsy is approximately 1%. Status epilepticus can occur as a manifestation of any seizure type.

Definition

Status epilepticus is defined by the occurrence of any epileptic seizure type lasting more than 30 minutes.

Etiology

Status Epilepticus is most often due to the following:

- Antiepileptic medication withdrawal in patients with epilepsy.
- Trauma, infection, and electrolyte imbalance.

Metabolic abnormalities should also be considered as cause for seizure.

Morbidity and sequelae from a status epileptic event are due to the systemic effects of seizure including cardiovascular stress, metabolic changes (acidosis, hypoxia, hyperkalemia, hypoglycemia, or azotemia), respiratory depression, rhabdomyolysis, pulmonary edema, and/or autonomic dysfunction.

Clinical Presentation

As stated above, the presence of seizure lasting 30 minutes or more, or multiple seizures without recovery to baseline totaling 30 minutes or more. These seizures can be clinically evident (e.g., generalized tonic-clonic) or subclinical.

Treatment

Evaluate airway, breathing, and circulation according to advanced life-support protocols. A benzodiazepine should be given. If ineffective, a fosphenytoin infusion is often the pharmacological step in management of status epilepticus. Phenobarbital may be used as an alternative to fosphenytoin in infants.

Laboratory studies: serum for glucose, electrolytes, antiepileptic drug levels (if directed by history), and BUN should be sent.

Prevention

Parents of children with known seizure disorder should be counseled to comply with prescribed medication and should also be trained to use rectal diazepam for breakthrough seizures.

Abdominal Surgical Emergencies: Appendicitis

Epidemiology

- Appendectomy is the most common emergent surgical procedure and the most common cause of an acute surgical abdomen. Seventy-seven thousand pediatric patient discharges annually are secondary to appendicitis and its complications.
- Appendicitis is most common in the second decade of life.

Clinical Presentation

- Classically, pain develops in the upper abdomen or periumbilical area and is associated with anorexia, nausea, or vomiting.
- Gradually, the pain migrates to the right lower quadrant.
- Diagnosis is more difficult as the history tends to be less clear in younger patients.
- Physical examination signs:
  - Fever—the most useful sign in the diagnosis of appendicitis.
  - Rebound tenderness.
  - Rovsing's sign—pressure in the left lower quadrant elicits pain in the right lower quadrant.
  - Psoas sign—pain on extension of the right hip (indicating a retrocecal appendix).
  - Obturator sign—pain on passive rotation of the flexed right thigh (indicating adjacent inflammation).

Diagnosis

- Physical exam findings as detailed above.
- WBC >10,000.
- Ultrasound or CT.
- Plain abdominal X-ray may show appendicolith on occasion.

Treatment

- Goal is appendectomy prior to appendiceal rupture.
- Antibiotics are indicated prior to surgery and can be discontinued if the appendix is found to be intact in the OR. A ruptured appendix requires broad spectrum antibiotic therapy effective against GI flora.

Allergic Emergency: Anaphylaxis

Epidemiology

In the United States, there are approximately 30,000 cases of food-induced anaphylaxis annually. The majority of these occur in adolescents and young adults. Food allergy is the most common cause of anaphylaxis, and results from IgE mediated reactions causing histamine release.

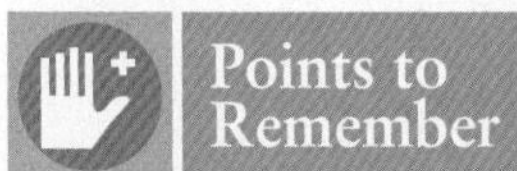

Points to Remember

- A second peak of histamine release and anaphylactic symptoms can occur at 8 hours.

Clinical Presentation

- Involves more than one organ system.
- Cutaneous manifestations are most common.
- Respiratory, gastrointestinal, and cardiovascular systems can also be involved.

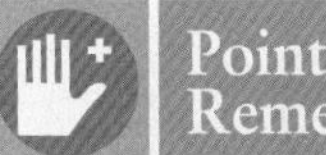

Points to Remember

- Anaphylactoid reactions, which are caused by direct mast cell degranulation rather than IgE, are similar to anaphylactic reactions and their treatment is the same.

Diagnosis

The diagnosis of anaphylaxis is based on the clinical presentation.

Treatment

Prompt treatment with intramuscular epinephrine 1:1,000 is the most important and urgent part of therapy. Antihistamines (H1 and H2 blockers) and corticosteroids are recommended to prevent later reactions. Patients should be observed for a second peak reaction for at least 8 hours. Supplemental oxygen and bronchodilators may be useful for respiratory symptoms.

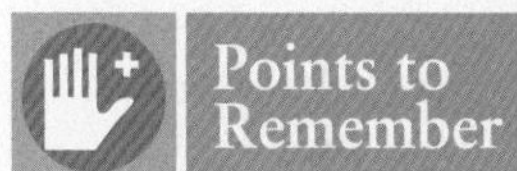

Points to Remember

- All patients with anaphylactic reactions should be prescribed an EpiPen and instructed on its use.

ALTE

ALTE refers to an episode that is of concern to the caregiver and is associated with a combination of apnea, color change, change in tone, choking, or gagging.

Epidemiology

The annual incidence of ALTE is approximately 0.5% to 0.6% per year.

Many underlying causes can produce an ALTE. Recent studies point to a higher incidence of future epilepsy among children with prior ALTE. Other diagnoses to consider are cardiac arrhythmias and/or malformations, gastroesophageal reflux, obstructive or central apnea, nonaccidental trauma, or metabolic disorders.

Treatment

Need for laboratory and radiologic studies depends on the results of a thorough history and physical examination.

Expanded examination could include CBC, electrolytes, swallow study, pH probe, EKG, EEG, sleep study, echocardiogram, head CT, and others. Further treatment is based on these findings.

Heat Exhaustion, Heatstroke

- Heatstroke is defined as T >40 with neurologic symptoms. Heatstroke is a serious illness with a relatively high incidence of mortality (12%).
- Heat exhaustion is temperature 38° to 40° without neurologic symptoms.

Epidemiology

It is particularly prevalent during hot and humid weather, and often seen among athletes and those working outdoors.

Clinical Presentation

Heat related illnesses stem from an inability to effectively cool the core body temperature. This can occur in situations where normal cooling reflexes are thwarted by the environment (e.g., hot, humid conditions) or internal factors (e.g., dehydration).

It is important to note that by the time the patient has presented for medical attention their temperature may have dropped slightly below the criteria, but this does not exclude the diagnosis of heatstroke/exhaustion.

Abnormalities on exam may include elevated temperature, tachycardia, normotension or hypotension, and lack of sweating. Heatstroke is associated with a collapse of normal sweating as a cooling measure, secondary to extreme dehydration.

End organ damage may be present, including hepatic and renal involvement and disseminated intravascular coagulation. Related lab abnormalities (elevated liver enzymes, BUN, and creatinine) may be seen.

Treatment

Management of fluid and electrolytes and reduction of core temperature. Simple evaporative cooling measures are used until temperature <39°. Supportive treatment of organ failure is provided.

Prevention

Athletes and those working outdoors must be provided adequate fluid/electrolytes. Coaches should be educated about early signs of heat-related illnesses as well as risk factors for heat-related illness, including the heat index.

Hypothermia

Hypothermia, a depression of core body temperature, requires treatment if body temperature falls below 35°C.

Epidemiology

Death from isolated hypothermia is relatively rare in the pediatric population. It is often associated with drowning injury.

Clinical Presentation

Hypothermia can present with central nervous system depression, cardiac arrhythmias, and renal failure.

Cardiac arrhythmias and EKG abnormalities can be present, including atrial fibrillation, J-waves (Fig. 6.5) (pathognomonic of hypothermia), PR, QRS, and QT elongation.

Treatment

Surface rewarming can be used in cases of hypothermia along with infusion and gastric lavage of warmed IV fluids. The fastest and most complete way to rewarm a patient is via surgical rewarming using bypass; however, the risks associated with this procedure are usually not warranted.

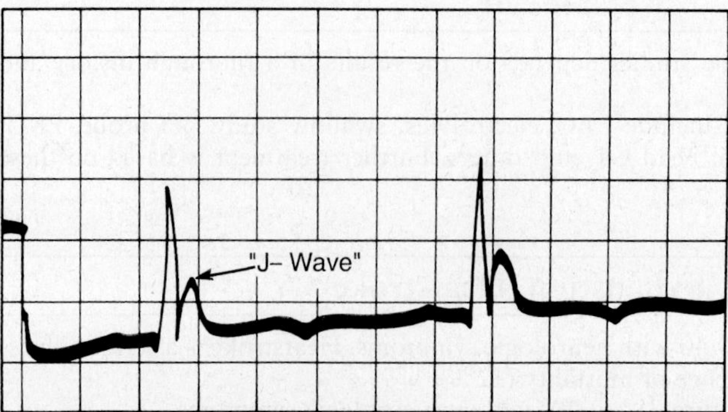

FIGURE 6.5. J-wave, pathognomonic of hypothermia. Rounded contour distinguishes it from an RSR' pattern. It may also be confused with a T wave with a short QT interval. (Reprinted with permission from Welton D, Mattox K, Miller R. Treatment of profound hypothermia. *JAMA.* 1978;240: 2291.)

Indications for Dialysis

Dialysis is an artificial replacement of lost kidney function used either in acute or chronic renal failure. For full discussion, see the "renal" chapter; for purposes of the boards, please commit to memory the indications for dialysis pertinent to the critical care/ER setting.

- Acidosis (due to renal insufficiency).
- Electrolyte imbalance (particularly hyperkalemia).
- Ingestion (particularly of substances not bound by activated charcoal such as alcohols, metals, and lithium).
- Fluid overload.
- Uremia.

TRAUMA

Epidemiology

Injury, both accidental and nonaccidental, is the most common cause of death and disability in childhood. More than 10,000 children die each year in the United States from serious injury.

Treatment

Management of pediatric trauma follows the ABCD (detailed below) algorithm laid out by the Advanced Trauma Life Support program (i.e., ATLS primary and secondary surveys).

1. Primary survey
   a) **Airway** management with cervical spine protection—Evaluate airway patency, identify airway compromise, secure definitive airway (if mental status is compromised, i.e., GCS score of <8, plan to intubate).
   b) **Breathing**—Assessment of oxygenation and ventilation. Expose the child's chest to assess chest wall excursion. Auscultate to verify gas flow. Percussion and visual inspection are performed to look for hemo- or pneumothorax, as well as injuries to the chest wall that may impede ventilation such as flail chest.
   c) **Circulation** with hemorrhage control—Evaluate the patient's hemodynamic status by observing the child's level of consciousness, skin color, and pulse. Identify external hemorrhage and control it with direct pressure.
   d) **Disability** (neurologic evaluation)—Perform a rapid evaluation including assigning a GCS score (see Table 6.6), pupillary reactivity and size, lateralizing signs, and spinal cord injury level.

TABLE 6.6

COMA SCALES

Glasgow Coma Scale		Modified Coma Scale for Infants
Eye Opening		
Spontaneous	4	Spontaneous
To speech	3	To speech
To pain	2	To pain
None	1	None
Verbal		
Oriented	5	Coos, babbles
Confused	4	Irritable
Inappropriate words	3	Cries to pain
Nonspecific sounds	2	Moans to pain
None	1	None
Motor		
Follows commands	6	Normal spontaneous movements
Localizes pain	5	Withdraws to touch
Withdraws to pain	4	Withdraws to pain
Abnormal flexion	3	Abnormal flexion
Abnormal extension	2	Abnormal extension
None	1	None

2. A head-to-toe secondary survey follows the primary survey and its interventions. Some caveats particularly for pediatric patients:
   a) **Head and neck**—Assess for signs of significant neurologic injury. Children's larger heads make head injury more likely. Similarly, they are more likely to sustain spinal cord injury without radiologic abnormality (SCIWORA).
   b) **Chest**—Children often sustain significant injury to the intrathoracic structures without evidence of thoracic skeletal trauma because of increased compliance of a child's ribcage.
   c) **Abdomen**—Be sure to evaluate for a seatbelt sign if history of a motor vehicle accident and bruising. The child's spleen and liver are more anterior and caudally located than those of adults, making them more injury-prone.

Head Trauma

Points to Remember

- The primary focus of treatment should be prevention of secondary brain injury by providing appropriate oxygenation and maintenance of sufficient BP to allow cerebral perfusion.

Epidemiology

Approximately 500,000 cases of brain injury occur annually in the United States.

Physical Examination

- Physical exam should include a thorough neurologic evaluation.
- Identification of pathognomonic bruising such as Battle sign (retroauricular ecchymosis) and raccoon eyes (periorbital ecchymosis) which raise suspicion for a basilar skull fracture.
- A unilateral dilated pupil, hemiparesis, or change in the level of consciousness are all concerning for rising ICP or further neurologic injury.

Diagnosis

- Head CT should be considered for any patient with concern for intracranial injury.
  - Subdural hematoma—Moon-shaped.
  - Epidural hematoma—Biconvex shaped.
- Any child younger than 12 months of age with any external head injury should have a head CT done to evaluate for intracranial injury.

Treatment

- Appropriate fluid resuscitation should be administered to maintain normovolemia in order to preserve cerebral perfusion pressure.
- Hyponatremia should be prevented as it can lead to cerebral edema.
- Hyperventilation leads to cerebral vasoconstriction and thus should only be used briefly for acute neurologic deterioration and concern for herniation.
- Mannitol can be used in a limited fashion as an osmotic diuretic to reduce ICP.

SPINAL CORD INJURY

Definition

- Neurogenic shock is caused by the disruption of descending sympathetic pathways to:
  - Vasculature—Loss of vasomotor tone, causing vasodilation.
  - Heart—Bradycardia or loss of compensatory tachycardia.
- Spinal shock—Immediately following injury, the cord may seem completely functionless, though some function may return at a later time.

Physical Examination

- Neurologic examination focused on determining a level of motor and/or sensory deficit will determine the level of injury and whether it is complete (motor and sensory loss) or incomplete.
- The neurologic level is the most caudal segment of the cord with normal function
  - Divided into sensory and motor.

Diagnosis

- Cervical spine radiographs should be obtained in patients with midline neck pain, palpation tenderness, neurologic deficits, or who are unable to confirm or deny pain or palpation tenderness because of age or AMS.

Management

- All patients with radiographic or neurologic evidence of injury should be immobilized and considered to have unstable spinal injuries.
- Persistent hypotension despite adequate fluid resuscitation should raise concern for neurogenic shock and the use of vasoactive agents should be considered.
- High dose steroids are administered to patients with nonpenetrating spinal cord injury.

BURNS

Clinical Presentation

Burns were formerly categorized by first, second, and third degree. More recently they are divided into shallow partial-thickness (second degree) and deep partial/full-thickness (third degree).

- Deep partial and full-thickness burns are insensate and dry. They can initially resemble superficial, partial-thickness burns.
- Superficial/shallow, partial-thickness burns are painful, red or mottled with a blistered/broken epidermis and weeping wetness.
- Chemical burns should be managed and classified as thermal burns; however, skin contamination is a necessary portion of wound management.
- Assess for indications of inhalation injury such as face burns, neck burns, singeing of the eyebrows and nasal hairs, carbon deposits in the oropharynx, carbonaceous sputum, and hoarseness.

Points to Remember

- Fluid management is of utmost importance in the initial and ongoing treatment of the burn patient, as fluid losses cause major morbidity and mortality.

Points to Remember

- The burn patient requires 2 to 4 mL isotonic crystalloid per kg per percent BSA affected by second and third-degree burns. Percentage body area is routinely estimated by using the Parkland formula.

Treatment

- The Parkland formula is used to estimate resuscitation fluids for burn patients
  - 2 to 4 mL × Patient's weight (in kg) × percent of BSA with second- and third-degree burns.
  - Half of the resuscitation fluid is given in the first 8 hours, then the second half is divided in the next 16 hours.
  - The rule of 9s is used to estimate BSA burned. Unique to the pediatric population is the child's proportionally larger head; thus special estimation charts are used for children (Fig. 6.6).
- Immediate airway support is required if there is any evidence for inhalational injury.
- Stridor is an indication for immediate ET intubation.
- Consider potential toxic inhalations such as carbon monoxide or cyanide.

Points to Remember

- The adult body is divided into anatomic regions that represent 9%, or multiples of 9%, of the total BSA. For example, each arm is 9%, the front of the torso is 18%, the back is 18%, and each leg is 18%.

For example, if a 20-kg, 6-year-old child sustains burns to one hands, both posterior thighs, and buttocks:

> BSA burned = 13.5%.
> (4% [posterior thigh] + 4% [posterior thigh] + 1.5% [hand] + 5% [buttocks]).
> Total fluid = 2 mL/kg × 20 kg × 13.5 = 540 mL.
> 270 mL given in the first 8 hours (~33 mL/h) in addition to maintenance fluids.
> 270 mL given in the subsequent 16 hours (~17 mL/h) in addition to maintenance fluids.

DROWNING AND NEAR DROWNING

Epidemiology

Drowning is a leading cause of death throughout the world. In the Unites States in 1998, it was the second leading cause of childhood accidental death.

The pathology associated with drowning is primarily due to hypoxic-ischemic and reperfusion injuries. Lung injury can lead to ARDS. Contrary to previous thinking, there are not major pathophysiologic differences between saltwater and freshwater drowning injuries.

Treatment

Rapid basic life support is key to decreasing hypoxia and ischemia. Hypothermia may be an element, and rewarming may be needed. Evaluate for potential traumatic injury (such as from diving or boating).

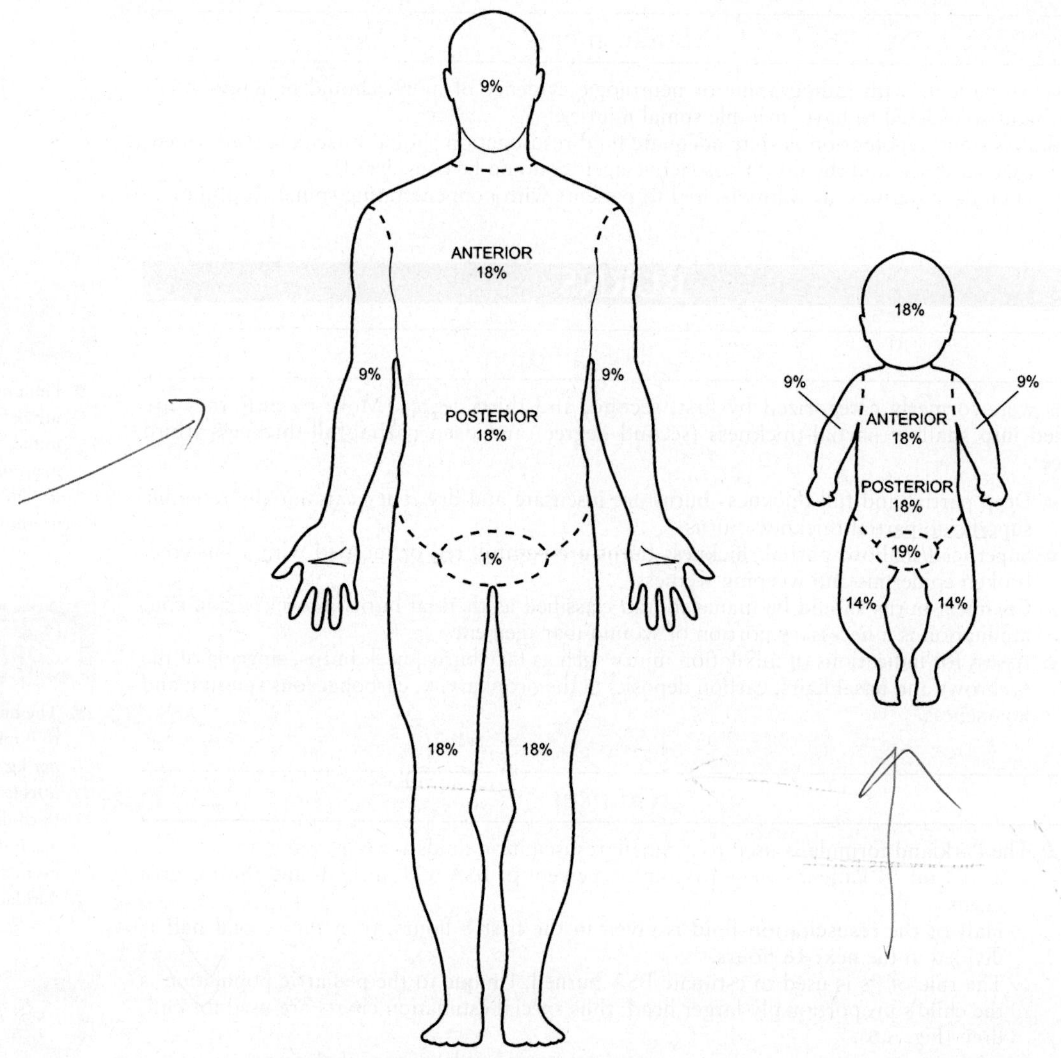

FIGURE 6.6. Rule of 9s. (Reprinted with permission from Mick NW, Peters JR, Egan D, et al. *Blueprints Emergency Medicine*. Philadelphia: Lippincott Williams & Wilkins; 2006.)

Prevention

The cornerstones of drowning prevention are adult supervision, proper pool fencing, and water safety education.

NONACCIDENTAL TRAUMA

Note: For further discussion of this topic please refer to the "growth and development" chapter.

Epidemiology

According to the Federal report, Childhood Maltreatment, the rate of childhood victimization in 2002 was 12.3/1,000

Clinical Presentation

- Nonaccidental trauma, or child abuse, can only be detected and diagnosed if the clinician has a high index of suspicion.
- Infants with depressed mental status with no known seizure disorder and no witnessed mechanism should have a retinal examination to look for signs of shaking.
- The distribution and shape of cutaneous findings often provide clues to diagnosis
  - Innocent bruising associated with activity usually appear over bony prominences.

- Electrical cords make omega-shaped loops, belts give U-shaped cuts, and belt buckles and hands may also produce distinguishable bruises.
- Nonaccidental immersion burns can produce a stocking-glove distribution.

Treatment

- Physicians have both a legal and ethical obligation to report suspected child abuse or neglect to the appropriate authorities, which in most jurisdictions is child protective services and the area police.
- Required reporting in all states supercedes privacy concerns mandated by laws such as HIPAA.
- Other treatment is centered at managing the sustained injury(s) and protecting the patient possibly through hospitalization if necessary.

SAMPLE BOARD REVIEW QUESTIONS

1. An afebrile 8-month-old infant with no significant past medical history presents with new onset seizure activity. An appropriate work up in the ER should include:
   a. Head CT to look for intracranial injury, resulting potentially from nonaccidental trauma
   b. EKG
   c. Neuromuscular testing
   d. Urine amino acids

   Answer: a. Although there may be cause to include EKG, metabolic laboratories, and neuromuscular testing in the workup of this child, given the risk of nonaccidental trauma in a child younger than 1 year of age and the potential immediate risk posed by intracranial injury, a CT would be an appropriate initial intervention.

Case for Questions 2 and 3

A 2-year-old boy has had fever and profuse watery diarrhea for 3 days. He has been refusing to take fluids by mouth. He presents to the emergency department lethargic with decreased urine output. The patient's vital signs are heart rate 150, respiratory rate 46, BP 100/60.

2. The most appropriate first intervention is:
   a. Checking an ABG to evaluate for acidosis
   b. Getting a CXR to check heart size
   c. Give antibiotics for presumed sepsis
   d. Give 20 cc/kg of isotonic crystalloid IV

   Answer: d. In cases of compensated shock, it is important to delineate that the first and most important intervention is treatment of shock. In this case, given the history, hypovolemia would be the most likely cause and fluids should be given without delay.

3. The sentence that most appropriately describes this patient's condition is:
   a. Normal vital signs
   b. Compensated hypovolemic shock
   c. Uncompensated hypovolemic shock
   d. Uncompensated distributive shock

   Answer: b. The patient has a normal BP, so his shock is currently compensated. The clinical history of volume loss points to hypovolemia as the most likely cause.

Case for Questions 4 to 6

A 13-year-old girl presents to the ER stating that she has taken a bottle (30 tablets) of extra strength Tylenol (500-mg tablets) 2 hours ago.

4. The most appropriate course of action would be:
   a. To perform abdominal ultrasound to look for a bezoar
   b. Check acetaminophen levels and LFTs immediately
   c. To wait until the 4-hour mark to check acetaminophen levels and LFTs
   d. To perform gastric lavage

   Answer: c. Imaging is not helpful in this case. Although you may be tempted to send acetaminophen levels and LFTs right away, these numbers are not able to be used with the nomogram and would not provide useful information. The patient's ingestion was too long ago for gastric lavage to be useful. The most appropriate course of action would be to keep the patient in the ER, and send levels at 4 hours.

5. Other lab tests you would want to include would be:
   a. CBC to look for long-standing anemia
   b. ABG to look for acidosis
   c. Heavy metal levels
   d. Serum aspirin level and urine drug screen to look for coingestions

Answer: d. Coingestions are quite common, and are an important part of the ingestion history. While aspirin levels and drug screen are not all-inclusive, they would detect some commonly coingested substances.

6. Upon further questioning, the patient reveals that she also took an overdose of her mother's antidepressant medication. What test should be performed immediately?
   a. EKG to look for QRS widening
   b. Head CT to look for signs of stroke
   c. Serum drug levels of the specific antidepressant
   d. Cardiac enzyme levels

Answer: a. Of the toxicities of antidepressants, the most feared is QRS widening associated with tricyclic antidepressants, which could quickly lead to arrhythmia-induced cardiac death. Head CT is not a sensitive indicator of stroke, and stroke is not commonly a cause of or a result of antidepressant ingestion. Serum drug levels are generally not useful in the ongoing management of this ingestion. Cardiac enzyme levels may be useful in ingestions where myocardial infarction results; however, this is not a typical toxicity of antidepressant ingestion.

7. A 20-month-old boy presents to the emergency department with depressed mental status. He has no known past medical history according to his grandparents, who accompany him. The boy is noted to have small, unresponsive pupils, and absent bowel sounds. His EKG, electrolytes, and glucose are normal. Which medication from his grandmother's list of prescribed medicines are you concerned that the patient may have ingested?
   a. A Calcium channel blocker
   b. A diuretic
   c. An opiate
   d. A beta-blocker

Answer: c. The small pupils (pinpoint) and absent bowel sounds point to an opiate-ingestion syndrome. A calcium channel blocker, diuretics, and beta-blockers should produce electrolyte or EKG changes if their levels are significant enough to cause depressed mental status.

Case for Questions 8 and 9

A 5-year-old is found unresponsive with an open bottle of his aunt's lithium tablets next to him.

8. What diagnostic testing would be most urgent in the setting of lithium ingestion?
   a. Urinalysis
   b. EKG
   c. LFT
   d. Glucose

Answer: b. Although in the long-term the other testing might be useful, the most important toxicity from lithium is cardiac. An EKG should immediately be obtained.

9. What interventions might decrease the child's lithium levels?
   a. Gastric lavage
   b. Whole bowel irrigation
   c. Activated charcoal
   d. Renal dialysis

Answer: d. Lithium is not bound by activated charcoal. Gastric lavage and whole bowel irrigation might decrease absorption of lithium tablets still in the GI tract, but will not decrease blood levels of lithium.

Case for Question 10

10. A 14-year-old girl is admitted to the intensive care unit after being rescued out of a burning house. She has deep and partial thickness burns covering approximately 8% of her body. She weighs approximately 50 kg. Assuming that she has not yet received any IV fluids, what are her fluid needs for the first 8 hours?
   a. 90 cc/h
   b. 180 cc/h
   c. 270 cc/h
   d. 400 cc/h

Answer: b. Using the Parkland formula, she requires between 400 and 800 cc of additional fluids during the first 8 hours (50–100 cc/h). You must add her maintenance fluid needs as well (90 cc/h). This puts you between 140–190 cc/h in the first 8 hours.

Case for questions 11 and 12

A 3-year-old boy presents to your office 1 hour after his mother witnessed him swallowing an AAA battery. He is asymptomatic and is playing happily. You order an X-ray, which shows the battery in the boy's stomach.

11. What advice would you give to the mother?
    a. The child needs to go to the emergency department of the local hospital to be evaluated for surgery
    b. Most batteries pass on their own so there is no further follow-up needed
    c. Because of the foreign body ingestion, the child must receive a tetanus booster
    d. A repeat X-ray is needed at the 8 to 16 hour mark to be sure the battery has passed through the stomach

Answer: d. The narrowest portion of the GI tract is the exit of the stomach at the pylorus. Given that the patient is currently asymptomatic and the ingestion was fairly recent, opportunity should be given for the battery to pass on its own.

12. The emergency department calls the next day to inform you that the mother brought her child to them for a second opinion. They tell you that a repeat X-ray showed the battery in the small intestine. They ask you how you would like to proceed. You tell them that:
    a. Since the patient has gone to see them for a second opinion, the decision is in their hands
    b. Because the battery has not yet been passed in stool, they should have surgery evaluate the patient
    c. The patient should be admitted for observation until the battery has been evacuated
    d. They can discharge the patient to home as the battery has already passed through the tightest juncture

Answer: d. The patient has passed the battery through the narrowest part of the GI tract, so there is no need for further concern.

Case for Questions 13 and 14

A 6-year-old girl with a known peanut allergy ingested a peanut butter cup at a friend's birthday party. Her mother calls you to report that the child is covered in hives. Over the phone, you hear the child wheezing audibly.

13. You instruct the mother to:
    a. Administer the child's home dose of epinephrine immediately, and call 911
    b. Drive to the ER immediately
    c. Give the child the steroids, diphenhydramine (Benadryl), and ranitidine that you had previously prescribed, and then bring her to the emergency department
    d. Give the child activated charcoal to bind the rest of the peanut allergen and then go to the emergency department

Answer: a. This child is having an anaphylactic reaction. It is appropriate to administer epinephrine immediately. The mother should call 911 to bring the child via the emergency medical services in case the child requires a second dose of epinephrine en route.

14. The local emergency department calls you 2 hours later to say that the child is doing great. She no longer has any urticaria or respiratory symptoms. They would like to discharge her home. You should:
    a. Agree to see the child immediately for follow-up
    b. Recommend that the child be observed for at least 8 hours given concerns for a second peak of the allergic reaction
    c. Ask that antibody levels be drawn now, as results are more accurate in the setting of an anaphylactic reaction
    d. Ask that the child be admitted and an allergy consult be obtained prior to discharge

Answer: b. Concern should be high for a second peak of the allergic reaction, particularly because respiratory distress was noted during the first reaction and the child should therefore not be immediately discharged. There is no evidence that antibody levels are more accurate in the setting of an acute allergic reaction and there is no indication for an allergy consult as the patient has a known peanut allergy with a clear response to the allergic trigger.

SUGGESTED READINGS AND REFERENCES

Dewolfe CC. Apparent life-threatening event: a review. *Pediatr Clin North Am.* 2005;52(4):1127–1146, ix.

Joint Task Force on Practice Parameters; American Academy of Allergy, Asthma and Immunology; American College of Allergy, Asthma and Immunology; Joint Council of Allergy, Asthma and Immunology. The diagnosis and management of anaphylaxis: an updated practice parameter. *J Allergy Clin Immunol.* 2005;115(3)(suppl 2):S483–S523.

Major P, Thiele EA. Seizures in children: determining the variation. *Pediatr Rev.* 2007;28:363–371.

McKiernan CA, Lieberman SA. Circulatory shock in children: an overview. *Pediatr Rev.* 2005;26(12):451–460.

Meyer RJ, Theodorou AA, Berg RA. Childhood drowning. *Pediatr Rev.* 2006;27(5):163–168.

http://www.poison.org/battery/ accessed July 22, 2010.

CHAPTER 7 ■ PEDIATRIC DERMATOLOGY

DAKARA RUCKER WRIGHT

AA	African American	PAS	Peroxidase-acid stain
BSA	Body surface area	PCR	Polymeric chain reaction
CALM	Café au lait macules	PDL	Pulsed-dye laser
CML	Chronic myelogenous leukemia	PWS	Port wine stain
CNS	Central nervous system	MEN	Multiple endocrine neoplasia syndrome
CSF	Cerebral spinal fluid	SSSS	Staphylococcal scaled skin syndrome
Ds	double stranded	SJS	Stevens–Johnson Syndrome
DVT	Deep vein thrombosis	Ss	Single stranded
EN	Epidermal nevus	TEN	Toxic epidermal necrolysis
GABHS	Group A beta hemolytic strep	TMP/SMX	Trimethoprim-sulfamethoxazole
GVHD	Graft versus host disease	TSST-1	Toxic Shock Syndrome Toxin
HPV	Human papillomavirus	UV	Ultraviolet
HSV	Herpes simplex virus	WBC	White blood cells
KOH	Potassium hydroxide		
LE	Lupus erythematosus		

CHAPTER OBJECTIVES

1. To describe primary dermatologic lesions and basic morphology
2. To distinguish basic neonatal eruptions, pigmented lesions, vascular lesions, hamartomas, diaper dermatitis, and papulosquamous conditions
3. To describe the etiology and clinical description of childhood exanthems/enanthems
4. To identify and manage common pediatric infectious disease that are present in skin
5. To identify common types of hair loss.

OVERVIEW

Most diagnoses in dermatology can be made by the clinical pattern and distribution of skin lesions. The history of disease and associated symptoms may be helpful. A skin biopsy is performed by shave or punch technique and is generally reserved for cases in which a clinical diagnosis cannot be made.

Proper description of skin lesions is very important in understanding dermatologic diagnosis and for communicating with dermatologists (Table 7.1).

TRANSIENT BENIGN CUTANEOUS LESIONS IN NEONATE

There are several benign rashes that can occur in the neonatal period. It is important to distinguish these rashes from the "newborn rashes you don't want to miss" detailed in the next section below. Commit to memory to the description of these common rashes as well as the typical time frame for eruption and resolution to hone in on the diagnosis during test day.

Transient Neonatal Pustular Melanosis

Presentation

- Small pustules with no underlying erythema present *at birth*.
- Ruptured pustules have a collarette of scale (may only see scale at birth), which then heals as hyperpigmented macules at the site of previous pustules.

TABLE 7.1

PRIMARY LESIONS AND DESCRIPTIONS

Lesion	Description
Macule	Circumscribed area of change in skin color without elevation or depression <1 cm diameter
Patch	Circumscribed area of change in skin color without elevation or depression >1 cm diameter
Papule	Solid, elevated, palpable lesion <0.5 cm diameter
Nodule	Solid, elevated, palpable lesion >0.5 cm diameter
Plaques	Elevated, plateau-like lesion usually formed by the confluence of papules
Vesicle	Fluid-filled blister <0.5 cm diameter
Bullae	Fluid-filled blister >0.5 cm diameter
Pustule	Blister filled with cellular debris, usually WBC, which gives the lesion a white or yellowish appearance
Cyst	Nodule or tumor filled with liquid or semisolid material. True cysts have an epithelial lining whereas pseudocyst is not lined
Wheal	The result of localized edema in the skin; pink or pale and usually rounded or flat-topped, sometimes with irregularly shaped margins; evanescent, lasting for <24 hours in any one place; invariably associated with pruritus
Telangiectasia	Superficial dilations of venules, capillaries, or arterioles; usually blanches with pressure
Lichenification	Thickening and darkening of the skin in which normal skin markings are accentuated; due to prolonged rubbing or scratching of the skin
Crusts	Accumulations of dried serum, blood, pus, or accumulated skin cells on the surface of a skin lesion
Scales	Flakes of skin composed of compact keratin; can be loose or adherent
Sclerosis	Thickened or indurated area of skin that has lost its normal elasticity; may be hypo- or hyperpigmented or both; lacks normal skin appendages such as hair and sweat glands
Erosion	Superficial epidermal loss with a moist base
Ulcer	Deep area of epidermal and dermal loss; can extend below the dermis
Fissure	Linear crack in skin surface that is narrow but not deep, usually are painful
Atrophy	Wasting of skin due to cell death and/or diminished cellular proliferation; skin surface appears depressed; skin is thin and translucent and wrinkles easily

Epidemiology

- Occurs in 5% of AA infants and more than 1% of white infants

Duration

- Pustules resolve within 1 to 2 days
- Hyperpigmented macules resolve over weeks to months

Key Feature

- Sterile pustules, *neutrophils* present on smear from pustule

Milia

Presentation

- One to 2 mm discrete white to yellowish papules (keratin-filled cysts) present *at birth*

Most Common Locations

- Cheeks, forehead, nose, and nasolabial folds

Epidemiology

- Common; occur in 40% to 50% of newborns

Duration

- Resolves spontaneously over several weeks

Key Feature

- Milia on the *hard palate* = "*Epstein pearls*" and on *gum line* = "*Bohn's nodules*" (seen in up to 85% of newborns).

Sebaceous Hyperplasia

Presentation

- Yellow-white follicular papules around nose and upper lips.

Epidemiology

- Fifty percent of term newborns.

Duration

- Resolves in first few weeks.

Key Feature

- Because of androgen stimulation *in utero*.

Erythema Toxicum Neonatorum

Presentation

- Initially erythematous blotchy macules that develop firm tiny white-yellow papules or pustules with irregular surrounding erythema on face, trunk, and extremities.
- Erythematous lesions may become confluent, usually not on palms and soles.

Epidemiology

- Common.
- Occurs in 21% to 40% of term newborns (rarely seen in preterm infants or low-birth-weight infants).

Duration

- Appears at *24 to 72 hours* of life, but new lesions can develop during the first 2 weeks of life.
- Resolves spontaneously in first few weeks of life.

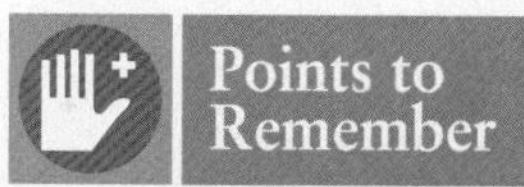

- **The differential diagnosis for erythema toxicum includes neonatal HSV infection and staphylococcal pustulosis.**

Key Feature

- Wright or Giemsa stain will show *eosinophils* with few neutrophils.

Miliaria Rubra (Prickly Heat)

Presentation

- Erythematous fine uniform papules in skin folds due to occluded eccrine ducts versus **miliaria crystalline**, which are tiny superficial vesicles, usually on head and neck.

Duration

- Presents at 1 to 2 weeks and resolves in 1 to 2 days.

Acne Neonatorum (Neo.natal Acne) Aka "Neonatal Cephalic Pustulosis"

Presentation

- Erythematous papules/pustules on cheeks, chin, and forehead.
- Comedonal lesions usually absent.

Duration

- First 30 days and lasts a few months.

Key Features

- *Pityrosporum* (*Malassezia*) may be etiologic trigger.
- *Neutrophils* and debris on smear.

Differential includes:
- Infantile Acne.
- Milia.

TABLE 7.2

BLUEBERRY MUFFIN RASH DIFFERENTIAL DIAGNOSIS

Extramedullary hematopoiesis
Congenital infection such as Rubella, CMV, Toxoplasmosis, and Parvovirus B19
ABO incompatibility such as twin–twin transfusion syndrome
Hemolytic disease of the newborn
Hereditary spherocytosis
Neoplastic hematopoiesis
Congenital Leukemia
Langerhans cell histiocytosis
Neuroblastoma
Rhabdomyosarcoma

Infantile Acne

Presentation

- Typical acneiform lesions on face consisting of comedones and papules, pustules, and/or nodules.

Duration

- Occurs later at 2 to 3 months.
- Usually resolves by 6 to 12 months of life.
- However, some cases can be persistent and may leave scarring.

Key Feature

- Because of androgen excess.

NEWBORN RASHES YOU DO NOT WANT TO MISS

- See differential for **"Blueberry Muffin Rash"** (Table 7.2) that signifies extramedullary hematopoiesis or malignant cutaneous infiltrates presenting as diffuse, multiple, dark erythematous to violaceous papules and nodules in a neonate or infant.
- Also see Table 7.3 for signs of occult spinal dysraphism.

TABLE 7.3

CUTANEOUS SIGNS OF OCCULT SPINAL DYSRAPHISM

Two or more spinal findings indicate a high risk for incomplete closure of the spinal axis
Lipomas
Hypertrichosis
Dimpling
Skin tags
Tails/pseudo-tails
Aplasia cutis
Hemangiomas
Dermoid cyst/sinuses
PWS (capillary malformations) and nevi less likely

Neonatal Impetigo

Presentation

- Superficial vesicles, pustules, or bullae on an erythematous base that easily ruptures, leaving denuded skin.

Duration

- Second or third day of life to second week.

Treatment

- Topical +/− oral if localized, oral if diffuse or ill and consider sepsis workup.

Key Feature

- See organisms on Gram's stain and positive culture.

Herpes Simplex (See "Infectious Diseases" Chapter for a Full Description) (Fig. 7.1)

Presentation

- Clustered vesicles on an erythematous base and eroded bullae that can leave scars.
- Lesions are usually concentrated on the head, particularly in areas of trauma, such as the site of placement of a scalp electrode.

Epidemiology

- Usually occurs during the second or third week of life.
- There are three commonly described forms of disease.

  Localized mucocutaneous disease (mean onset of 11 days of life).
  Disseminated HSV infection (60% have skin lesions).
  CNS HSV infection (60% have skin lesions).

Diagnosis

- Viral cultures of vesicles as well as from the eyes, mouth, and rectum.
- PCR of CSF.

Treatment

- IV acyclovir—because of the high morbidity and mortality associated with neonatal HSV infection, empiric treatment should be initiated without delay.

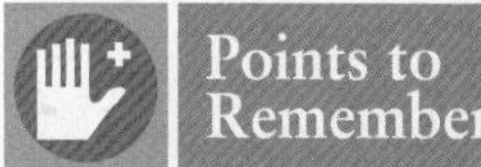

Points to Remember

- **Neonatal HSV should be suspected in any infant with vesicular lesions, whether grouped or scattered. Without treatment, 70% of infants with localized mucocutaneous HSV will develop disseminated disease.**

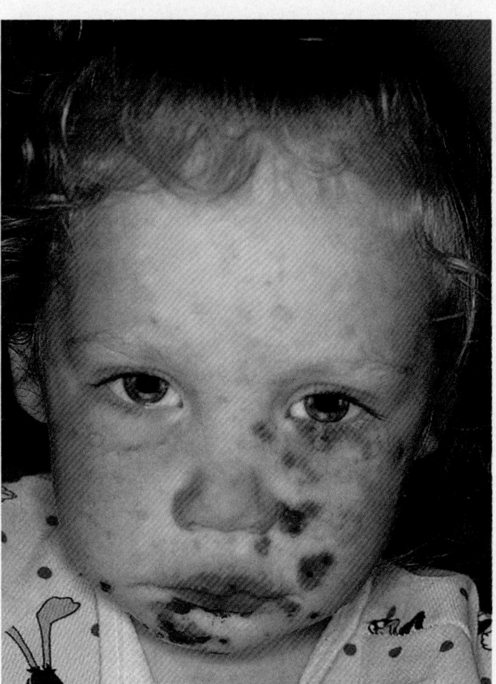

FIGURE 7.1. Patient showing dissemination of herpes simplex virus to the face. Fluorescein dye is dripping from the right eye after its instillation in an attempt to identify the typical dendritic ulcer seen with herpetic keratitis. (*Reprinted with permission from* Fleisher GR, Ludwig W, Baskin MN. *Atlas of Pediatric Emergency Medicine*. Philadelphia, PA: Lippincott Williams & Wilkins, 2004.)

Key Feature

- Most infants with neonatal HSV are born to mothers without a known history of genital herpes.
- HSV-2 is more common than HSV-1.

Congenital Candidiasis

Presentation

- Skin appears diffusely erythematous with scattered tiny papules, vesicles, and pustules usually on back, extensor surfaces, skin folds, palms, and soles.

Epidemiology

- Present at birth or within first 6 days of life.
- Rare disease that results from *in utero* candidal infection.
- In full-term infants, typically resolves over 1 to 2 weeks.

Diagnosis

- KOH preparation yields budding hyphae and pseudohyphae.

Treatment

- Topical or oral if localized, parenteral if disseminated or ill.

Key Feature

- May lead to *systemic/invasive candidiasis* in premature or very low-birth-weight neonates.
- Other risk factors for systemic disease include extensive invasive procedures.

Neonatal Candidiasis

Presentations

- Localized disease such as *diaper dermatitis* or *oral thrush*.
- Invasive dermatitis seen in extremely low-birth-weight neonates with extensive lesions and severe erosions.
- Systemic disease related to invasive procedures and infected indwelling devices.

Epidemiology

- Acquired infection from birth canal, present after 7 days of life.

Treatment

- Antifungal treatment may range from topical to parenteral therapy, depending on the condition of the patient.

Neonatal Varicella (Fig. 7.2)

Presentation

- Lesions are similar to those of varicella in older children, that is, crops of macules and papules developing into tear-drop vesicles with an erythematous base.

Epidemiology

- Rare condition that results from *in utero* infection 2 to 3 weeks prior to delivery.

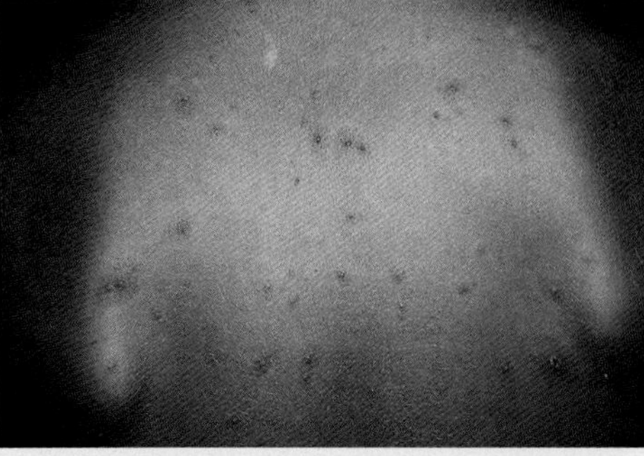

FIGURE 7.2. Vesicles and crusts typical of varicella (chicken pox). (*Reprinted with permission from* Goodheart HP. *Goodheart's Photoguide of Common Skin Disorders*, 2nd ed. Philadelphia, PA: Lippincott Williams & Wilkins, 2003.)

Diagnosis

- Suspected by a maternal history and confirmed via Tzanck preparation or culture.

Treatment

- Because disease can be fatal, any infant born to a mother who develops varicella 5 days before to 2 days after delivery should be treated with varicella-zoster immune globulin, and, if the infant develops clinical varicella, with intravenous acyclovir.

Points to Remember

- Tzanck preparation cannot differentiate between neonatal HSV and neonatal varicella; both reveal multinucleated giant cells.

Congenital Syphilis

Presentation

- *Early (birth to 2 years)*: symptoms and signs include sniffles, saddle nose, blisters, generalized papulosquamous eruption similar to 2° syphilis especially in the diaper area, perineal skin folds with linear scars, condyloma lata, petechiae, lymphadenopathy, and splenomegaly, and mental status changes consistent with neurosyphilis.
- *Late (>2 years)*: symptoms and signs include Hutchinson's teeth, mulberry molars, saber shins, gummas in bones, CNS lesions, perisynovitis, and keratitis.

PIGMENTED LESIONS (FIG. 7.3)

There are several pigmented lesions that commonly present in the neonatal period. Some of these lesions are external signs of systemic diseases, while others are benign. Familiarize yourself with descriptions of these nevi, macules, and spots detailed below.

Mongolian Spots

Presentation

- Blue-gray, brown, or blue-black patches.
- Most common location = lumbosacral area but may occur in other locations.

Epidemiology

- Present in more than 90% of AA, 80% of Asians, and 46% of Hispanics versus less than 10% of White.

Duration

- Present at birth; usually disappears by age 4 to 5 years.

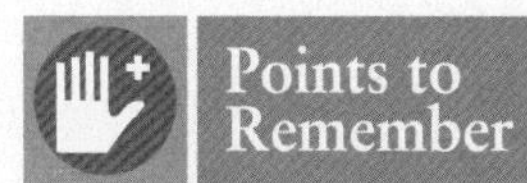

- Mongolian spots can be mistaken for bruising and child abuse; educate parents and document your examination!

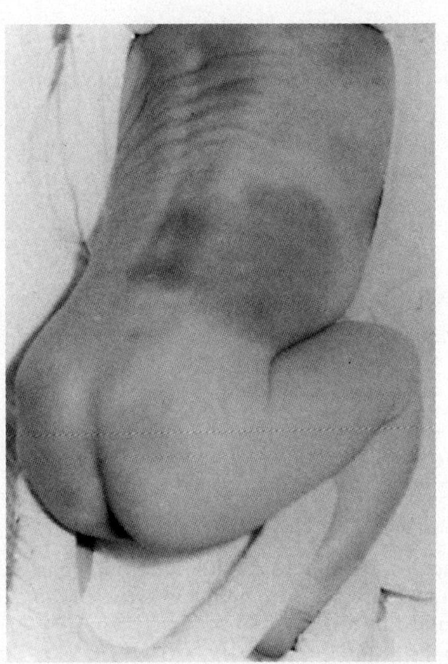

FIGURE 7.3. Pigmented lesions. (*Reprinted with permission from* McMillan JA, Feigin RD, DeAngelis C, et al. *Oski's Pediatrics: Principles and Practice*, 4th ed. Philadelphia, PA: Lippincott Williams & Wilkins, 2006.)

Café au lait

Presentation

- Uniformly pigmented tan to brown macules, usually hairless with distinct margins.
- Range in size from small to large (e.g., 20 cm) and can be present anywhere on the body.

Duration

- Present at birth or acquired within first few months.
- Present for life.

Key Feature

- If six or more macules more than 5 mm are present, you must rule out **Neurofibromatosis, type I (NF1)**.

Criteria

- At least two must be met:
  1. ≥6 CALMS larger than 5 mm before puberty and >15 mm postpuberty.
  2. Axillary or inguinal freckling.
  3. One plexiform neurofibroma (firm, brown plaque that feel like "bag of worms") or ≥2 neurofibromas.
  4. First degree relative with NF1.
  5. Optic glioma.
  6. ≥2 Lisch nodules.
  7. Sphenoid wing dysplasia of skull or thinning of the long bone cortex with or without pseudoarthrosis.

Management

- Routine head circumference measurement.
- Check blood pressure (due to risk of renovascular disease and anomalies).
- Ophthalmologic examination.
- Developmental monitoring.
- Neurology referral.

Congenital Nevus/Nevi

Presentation

- Tan to dark brown macules, papules, and large plaques.
- May have cobblestoned or verrucous surface with excess hair growth.

Epidemiology

- Large or giant congenital nevi greater than 20 cm have 4.5% to 10% risk of melanoma, usually within first 5 years of life.

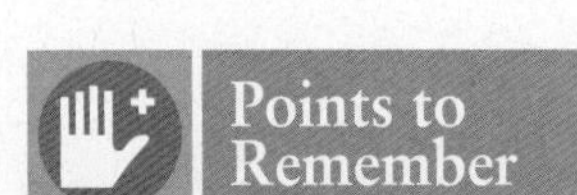

- The clinical signs of melanoma are ABCDE: asymmetry, border irregularity, color changes, diameter greater than 6 mm, enlarging or erosion.

Duration

- Present at birth or within the first year.
- Present for life.

Key Feature

- Lesions overlying the spinal column and skull or multiple satellite nevi can be associated with melanoma of the CNS.

Urticaria pigmentosa

Presentation

- Few-to-numerous red, tan, or gray discrete macules, papules, or nodules that may blister.
- Associated signs with dermatological eruption are rare but can include diarrhea, wheezing, widespread hives, flushing, hypotension, and fainting.

Key Features

- Because of accumulation of mast cells, lesions turn into hives when stroked (*Darier's sign*).

Prevention

- Avoid mast cell degranulators: opiates, alcohol, polymyxin B, amphotericin B.

VASCULAR LESIONS

Vascular lesions, when they appear in the neonate, are bound to prompt a long list of questions from anxious parents. Knowing which lesions require further investigation and treatment will serve you well both on examination day as well as in clinical practice.

Salmon Patch (Nevus Simplex)

Presentation

- Light pink macules composed of dilated dermal capillaries.
- Often located on eyelids (angels' kiss), glabella, nape of the neck (stork bite), upper lip, scalp, and overlying the spine.

Epidemiology

- The most common vascular lesions in infancy.
- Present in almost half of newborns.

Duration

- Present at birth.
- Facial lesions tend to fade over the first few years, whereas neck lesions often persist.

Port Wine Stain, also Known as Capillary Malformation (Fig. 7.4)

Presentation

- Dark reddish-to-purple-colored macule or patch, **present at birth.**

Most Common Location

- Head and neck.

Complications

- Because PWSs are permanent, they often become darker and thicker with time and may develop surface bleeding; children with significant PWS should be referred for PDL therapy.

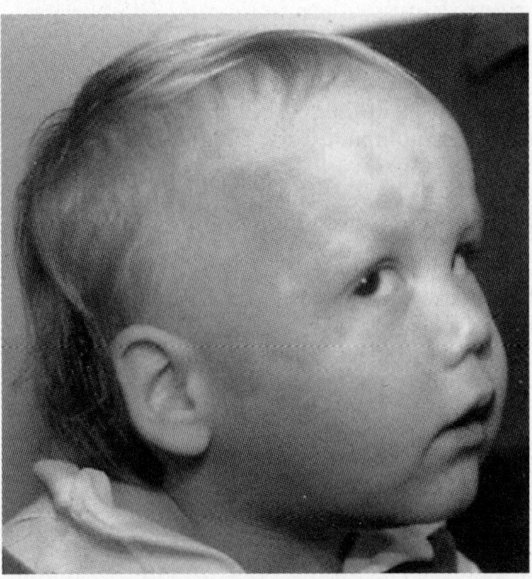

FIGURE 7.4. Port wine stain. (*Reprinted with permission from* McMillan JA, Feigin RD, DeAngelis C, et al. *Oski's Pediatrics: Principles and Practice*, 4th ed. Philadelphia, PA: Lippincott Williams & Wilkins, 2006.)

Points to Remember

- Infants with a PWS in the distribution of the trigeminal nerve are at risk for Sturge–Weber syndrome. This syndrome involves vascular malformations of the skin (PWS), ipsilateral leptomeningeal vessels (hypoxic injury, seizures, stroke, etc.), and ipsilateral eye findings (retinal detachment, glaucoma).

Associations

- **Sturge–Weber syndrome:** PWS involving the first ± (2nd, 3rd) branches of the trigeminal nerve (also high risk if involves upper and lower eyelids), seizures (leptomeningeal malformation), and glaucoma.
  1. V2 PWSs alone may rarely be associated with glaucoma or other ocular problems.
  2. V2 and/or V3 alone without V1 are not associated with SWS. Must have V1 involvement to have SWS.
- **Klippel-Trenaunay- Parkes-Weber syndrome:** large PWS involving the extremities associated with vascular malformations such as arteriovenous malformations or lymphatic malformations, venous varicosities, and hypertrophy. Most commonly affects the legs. Lesions may ulcerate and thrombophlebitis can occur. Risk of coagulopathy and pulmonary embolism.

Management

- Vascular laser, compression garments, pain control, and DVT prophylaxis.

Hemangioma

Points to Remember

- Hemangiomas are typically not present at birth unlike PWS. If extensive segmental lesion is on the face, you must rule out PHACES syndrome that includes imaging the brain and heart. Lesions in the distribution of a beard need to be evaluated for potential associated airway lesions with laryngoscopy. Multiple cutaneous hemangiomas may be associated with liver hemangiomas, watch for signs of congestive heart failure.

Presentation

- *Superficial hemangiomas* (strawberry hemangiomas) occur in the upper dermis and are bright red in color.
- *Deep hemangiomas* appear as subcutaneous nodules with bluish discoloration or telangiectasias.
- Most common location is head and neck.

Epidemiology

- Approximately 10% of White infants by 1 year (less prevalent in other races).
- More common in females and infants with low birth weight.
- Approximately 50% of hemangiomas resolve by the age of 5 and 90% by the age of 9 sometimes with residual fibrofatty tissue.

Duration

- Typically absent at birth, then appear at 2 to 3 weeks of age as an erythematous lesion with overlying telangiectatic vessels.
- Grow rapidly during the first 6 months of age, are stable in size between 6 and 12 months, then begin to regress between 12 and 18 months.

Treatment

- Often not necessary as 50% spontaneously resolve by the age of 5 and 90% by the age of 9.
- Complicated hemangiomas, including those that threaten vital structures, can be treated with oral prednisone, intralesional steroids, and, most recently, propranolol has been shown to be effective.

Complications (Rare)

- Erosion and secondary infection, especially on mucosal areas such as genital and oral.
- Bleeding.
- Multiple cutaneous hemangiomas may be associated with visceral hemangiomas (CNS, lungs, hepatic, and GI). Hepatic lesions may result in high-output cardiac failure or hemorrhage.
- Periorbital hemangiomas may lead to amblyopia.

Associations

- PHACES syndrome: *P*osterior fossa malformations (e.g., Dandy Walker), *H*emangioma (large segmental), *A*rterial anomalies, *C*oarctation of the aorta, *E*ye abnormalities (e.g., coloboma), *S*ternal Cleft or *S*upraumbilical raphe.
- Beard hemangiomas: Hemangiomas in the "beard" distribution on the jaw/neck can be associated with laryngeal hemangiomas and airway compromise.

Cutis Marmorata

- This is a benign common transient mottling present on extremities of children and young women.

BUMPS AND HAMARTOMAS

- Hamartomas are benign growths of cells or tissue.

Nevus Sebaceous

Presentation

- Yellowish-orange-brown plaque with cobblestone surface usually on scalp with alopecia.

Epidemiology

- Less than 1% chance of malignancy (basal cell carcinoma), which usually presents after puberty.

Key Feature

- Grows after puberty and becomes more warty.

Juvenile Xanthogranuloma

Presentation

- Yellowish-orange papules–nodules that can be one or multiple.

Epidemiology

- Less than 1% with ocular lesions.

Duration

- Erupt in first year of life.
- Present for life.

Key Feature

- *Rare associations with multiple lesions*: NF1 and CML.

Pyogenic Granuloma

Presentation

- Bright red-brown slightly raised pedunculated papule with a collarette of scale along base.

Duration

- May spontaneously resolve.

Key Feature

- There is a risk of bleeding and ulceration but NOT infection.

Differential Diagnosis

- **Spitz Nevus:** usually a benign, eruptive, smooth, dome-shaped tan-pink papule commonly on face or neck.

Epidermal Nevus (EN)

Presentation

- Brownish verrucous papules coalescing into plaques.
- Usually follows linear pattern (lines of Blaschko).

Duration

- Present at birth or become noticeable much later in childhood.

Key Feature

- Large lesions associated with **EN Syndrome**, one of the neurocutaneous syndromes.

Angiofibromas

Presentation

- Uniform flesh-colored to red papules over the nose and cheeks commonly mistaken for acne.

Key Feature

- Associations with MEN I and **Tuberous sclerosis.**
- The criteria needed to make the diagnosis of Tuberous sclerosis are listed below (see "Neurology" chapter for full discussion)
  1. **Major:** ≥3 hypomelanotic macules, connective tissue nevus (shagreen patch), periungual fibromas, retinal nodular hamartomas, subependymal astrocytomas, cardiac rhabdomyoma, renal angiomyolipoma or pulmonary lymphangiomyomatosis, cortical tubers.
  2. **Minor:** dental enamel pits, rectal hamartomas, bone cysts, gingival fibromas, nonrenal hamartomas, confetti hypopigmented skin lesions, and multiple renal cysts.

Points to Remember

- Definite Diagnosis of Tuberous sclerosis: *2 major or 1 major and 2 minor*

Subcutaneous Fat Necrosis of Newborn

- Localized subcutaneous nodules or plaques in healthy neonates during first week of life.
- Calcification may be associated with resolution.
- Follow for associated hypercalcemia for a few months after birth.

SCALY RASHES (PAPULOSQUAMOUS)

See Table 7.4 for differential diagnosis of "diaper dermatitis," rashes that can present in diaper area.

Pityriasis Rosea (Fig. 7.5)

Presentation

- Oval plaques composed of tiny papules covered with a fine, wrinkled scale.
- Lesions are typically concentrated on the trunk, while those on the back have their long axes parallel to the lines of skin stress, resulting in "Christmas tree" appearance.
- May or may not be pruritic.
- Fifty percent of cases begin with the appearance of a herald patch, a solitary erythematous patch, or plaque that precedes the generalized eruption by 1 to 2 weeks.

Duration

- May last several weeks to months and may reoccur.

Etiology

- Possibly due to human herpes virus type 6.

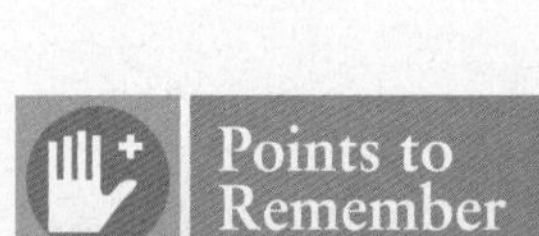

- **Because secondary syphilis can mimic Pityriasis rosea, testing for syphilis should be considered in sexually active patients.**

Epidemiology

- Most commonly affects teenagers and young adults.
- Usually occurs in the fall and spring and can occur in small epidemics.

Differential Diagnosis

- Secondary syphilis.
- Nummular eczema.
- Psoriasis.

Treatment

- If present, pruritus can be managed with an emollient containing menthol and phenol, a mild topical corticosteroid, or an oral antihistamine.
- Judicious exposure to sunlight may hasten the resolution of the eruption.
- Pityriasis rosea is not contagious and precautions are not necessary.

TABLE 7.4

DIAPER DERMATITIS

Type	Symptoms	Treatment
Irritant dermatitis	Scaly, erythematous rash with glazed skin surface. Present in covered areas and **spares skin folds.** Caused by chronic wetness, increased pH, and diarrhea	Frequent diaper changes, barrier creams, mild topical corticosteroid
Allergic contact dermatitis	Itchy erythematous small vesicles and papules with underlying erythema, leading to an eczematous eruption overlying areas of edema	Depends on contact allergen. Avoid allergen some of which can be topical agent, dye, elastic, or systemic agent
Candidal dermatitis	Beefy red moist patches with satellite papules/ pustules. **Involves folds** may extend onto perineum. May also have oral thrush. Antibiotic treatment may favor candidal overgrowth	Antifungal cream
Seborrheic dermatitis	Salmon to erythematous colored waxy patches and plaques with minimal scale (due to moisture) **in skin folds** or entire diaper area. **Not very itchy.** May involve scalp, face, and axillae	Emollients, ketoconazole cream, mild topical corticosteroid
Psoriasis	Well-demarcated pink to erythematous patches and plaques with minimal scale. **Involves skin creases** and gluteal cleft. May also involve scalp, trunk, and umbilicus	Topical vitamin D, mild topical corticosteroid, topical calcineurin inhibitors
Langerhans cell histiocytosis	Single-to-multiple yellowish-brown crusted papules, vesicles, nodules, erosions, or ulcerations with petechiae. **In skin folds,** trunk, scalp, and behind ears (seborrheic distribution)	Evaluate for multisystem disease. Lymphadenopathy
Jacquet's erosive dermatitis	Well-demarcated erosive to ulcerative papules and nodules. Multifactorial etiology with yeast, irritant dermatitis, and moisture	Frequent diaper changes. Barrier cream such as zinc oxide
Granuloma gluteale infantum	Oval red-purple granulomatous papules or nodules in perianal, perivulvar, or gluteal surfaces. Secondary to local irritation, maceration, and candida.	Avoid fluorinated steroids. Frequent diaper changes. Barrier creams
Acrodermatitis enteropathica	Crusted, scaling rash in perineal, perioral, and distal extremities. May have crusted vesicles or papules. Due to zinc deficiency. Disease includes diarrhea, failure to thrive, irritability, sparse hair, and recurrent candidal infections. Must be distinguished from **biotin deficiency and cystic fibrosis**	Zinc supplementation
Perianal streptococcus	Moist bright red rash **in perianal area and creases.** Yellowish sticky exudates at periphery ± small pustules in surrounding skin. Localized tenderness	Treat with systemic antistreptococcal antibiotics for at least 3–4 wk
Scabies	Nodular; burrows of mites under skin; usually associated with rash to other areas of the body	Permethrin 5% cream

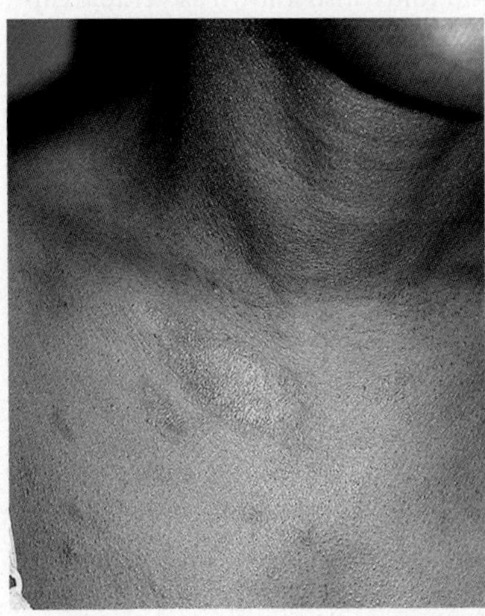

FIGURE 7.5. Pityriasis rosea. This patient has a herald patch on her chest. Other, smaller lesions can be seen. (*Reprinted with permission from* Goodheart HP. *Goodheart's Photoguide of Common Skin Disorders*, 2nd ed. Philadelphia, PA: Lippincott Williams & Wilkins, 2003.)

Atopic Dermatitis (Eczema)

Eczema is the most common skin condition of childhood. The exact etiology is unknown, but both genetics and the environment play a role. The underlying defect includes epidermal barrier dysfunction and immune dysregulation.

Presentation

- Erythematous, scaly pruritic patches that resolve with postinflammatory hypopigmentation (light patches) or hyperpigmentation (dark patches). Chronic lesions show lichenification (thickening of the skin and accentuation of skin lines).
- Distribution of lesions varies by age:
  1. Infants and toddlers: generalized distribution of lesions with involvement of the face, scalp, extremities, and trunk. Usually spares diaper area because of occlusion and moisture.
  2. Older children: concentrated in flexural areas (elbows, knees, wrists, ankles, etc.).
- Other clinical findings:
  1. Palms show hyperlinearity (increased creases).
  2. Generalized dry skin and scalp.
  3. Allergic shiners (darkening beneath the eyes).
  4. Keratosis pilaris.
  5. Ichthyosis vulgaris.
  6. Elevated IgE.
  7. Immediate skin test reactivity.

Duration

- Onset of symptoms below 1 year in 60% to 80% of affected children and before the age of 5 in 90% of cases.
- Course is chronic/relapsing, but 80% to 90% of affected patients experience resolution or improvement by adolescence.
- Symptoms are usually worse in the winter because of decreased humidity.

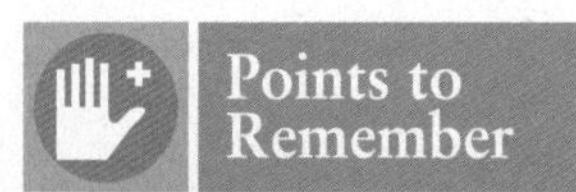

- Allergic march = eczema presents first, then asthma and allergic rhinitis.

Epidemiology

- Approximately 75% have family history of atopy—eczema, asthma, and allergic rhinitis.

Complications

- Most common complication is bacterial superinfection, usually caused by *Staphylococcus aureus*, heralded by increasing erythema and exudate. Treatment includes topical mupirocin, dilute bleach baths, and systemic antistaphylococcal antibiotics.
- Herpes simplex may spread rapidly and extensively over the entire skin surface (*Eczema herpeticum*); this disease can be severe and even fatal. Treat with oral acyclovir or valacyclovir.

Points to Remember

- Eczema usually spares the diaper area because of moisture. It is very itchy, whereas seborrheic dermatitis is not itchy and often involves the skin folds (axillae and inguinal creases).

Key Feature

- Rarely atopic dermatitis can be associated with an immunodeficiency such as Wiskott–Aldrich, hyper IgE, or Netherton syndrome.

Differential Diagnosis

- Psoriasis: usually not as itchy.
- Seborrheic dermatitis: not itchy, primarily exists in skin folds, also known as "cradle cap" on the scalp.
- Ichthyosis vulgaris: fish-like scales and dry skin.
- Scabies.
- Keratosis pilaris: not itchy, follicular scaly papules on cheeks, upper outer arms, and anterior thighs.

Points to Remember

- Only 5% of children with eczema also have food allergies that can rarely exacerbate their eczema. The most commonly implicated foods are eggs, milk, wheat, peanuts, soybeans, and fish.

Treatment

- Management is divided into daily management to prevent flares and treatment of exacerbations.
- Daily management is intended to hydrate the skin and control pruritus.
- Avoidance of irritants (fragrant soaps, detergents, etc.).
- Moisturizers (bland moistures such as petrolatum and thick creamy emollients).
- Short-term use of calcineurin inhibitors to avoid side effects due to prolonged topical corticosteroid use such as skin atrophy (they are commonly used on the face, in particular).

Exacerbations are treated with topical corticosteroids (to reduce inflammation), sedating antihistamines (to help with sleep), and antibiotics if a secondary infection is present.

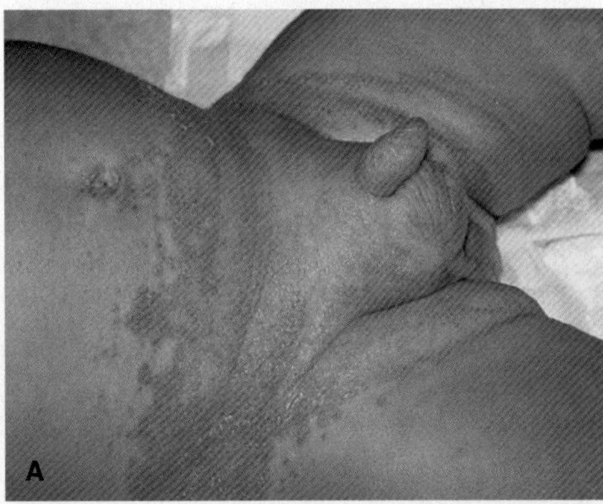

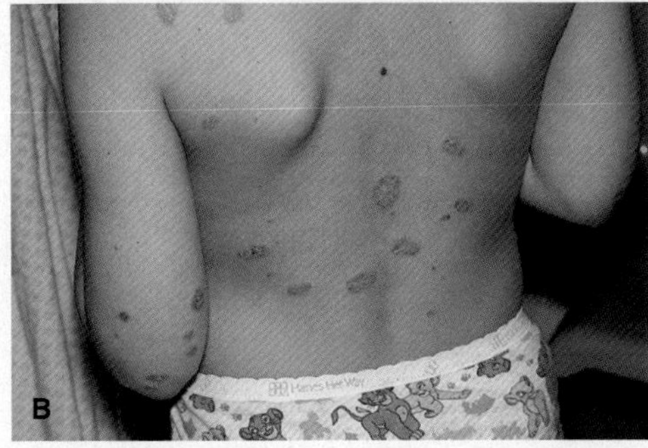

FIGURE 7.6. Psoriasis. (A) These plaques could easily be confused with a diaper rash or atopic dermatitis. (B) Guttate psoriasis. Thicker scale—actually plaques—than seen in Pityriasis rosea is noted. (*Reprinted with permission from* Goodheart HP. *Goodheart's Photoguide of Common Skin Disorders*, 2nd ed. Philadelphia, PA: Lippincott Williams & Wilkins, 2003.)

Psoriasis (Fig. 7.6)

The disease course is unpredictable and can be associated with arthritis. Onset of disease is before 16 years of age in 25% to 45% of patients, and there may be a positive family history

Presentation

- Lesions are well-demarcated erythematous papules or plaques covered with a silvery scale.
- Auspitz sign = removal of scale causes a bleeding point.
- Koebner phenomenon = appearance of lesions at sites of physical or thermal trauma.
- Distribution is symmetric; common sites include knees, elbows, eyebrows, ears, umbilicus, sacrum, and gluteal cleft.
- Other manifestations include: thick, adherent scale on the scalp; pitting, discolored, or thickened fingernails and toenails; and scaling and fissuring of palms and soles.

Differential Diagnosis

- Eczema.
- *Tinea corporis.*
- Seborrheic Dermatitis.
- Pityriasis Rosea.

Treatment

- Topical corticosteroids, calcipotriene (topical vitamin D), or tar preparations.
- Controlled exposure to sunlight.
- Severe disease can be treated with narrow-band UVB or PUVA (oral psoralen combined with UV light box) phototherapy, methotrexate, or biologic TNF inhibitors injections.

DISORDERS OF PIGMENTATION

Nevus Depigmentosus (Fig. 7.7)

Well-demarcated hypopigmented ("depigmentosus" is a misnomer) patch noted at birth or during infancy that persists; solitary, multiple, and segmental forms are also described.

Rare associations to rule out: Tuberous sclerosis and Hypomelanosis of Ito—swirls of hypopigmentation with associated neurologic disorders, that is, seizure, eye, or skeletal disorders.

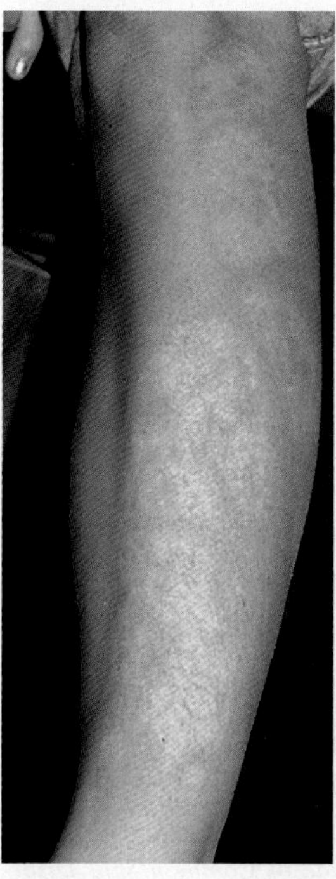

FIGURE 7.7. Nevus depigmentosus. This off-white linear hypomelanosis has been present since birth. It has enlarged commensurate with the patient's growth. (*Reprinted with permission from* Goodheart HP. *Goodheart's Photoguide of Common Skin Disorders*, 2nd ed. Philadelphia, PA: Lippincott Williams & Wilkins, 2003.)

Albinism

Inherited disorders of melanin synthesis that clinically presents as generalized absence or decrease of skin, hair, and iris pigmentation; ocular signs and symptoms include photophobia, photosensitivity, and nystagmus.

Management

- Diligent photoprotective measures, such as sunblock use (e.g., titanium dioxide or zinc oxide), sunglasses, and protective clothing, are imperative as patients have little-to-no melanin to protect skin cells from sunburn or skin cancer due to UVB and UVA.
- Monitor periodically for skin cancer.

Vitiligo

Acquired loss of pigmentation (rare congenital cases noted). The absence of melanocyte-pigment producing cells is thought to be due to autoimmune process.

Presentation

- Well-defined depigmented (ivory white or pink) macules and patches that range in size and distribution.

Treatment

- Phototherapy with narrow-band UVB, topical corticosteroids, topical calcineurin inhibitors, and camouflage with makeup.

Key Feature

- There are rare associations with alopecia and thyroid disease.

OTHER NONINFECTIOUS DERMATOLOGIC LESIONS

Urticaria (Hives)

Presentation

- Transient wheals with edematous center and erythematous halo that may be small and localized, large or generalized.
- If hives are present longer than 24 hours, it is not true *Urticaria*.

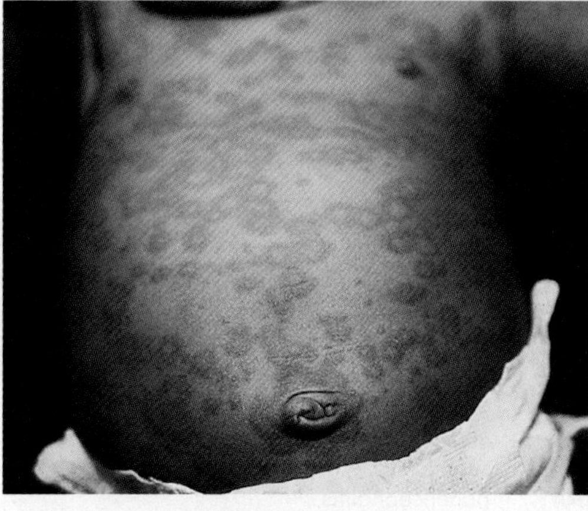

FIGURE 7.8. Erythema multiforme. (Courtesy of George A. Datto, III, MD.) (*Reprinted with permission from* Chung EK, Boom JA, Datto GA. *Visual Diagnosis in Pediatrics*. Philadelphia, PA: Lippincott Williams & Wilkins, 2006.)

- Acute *Urticaria* waxes and wanes for less than 6 weeks and is possibly due to viral infection, food, or drug.
- Chronic *Urticaria* waxes and wanes for months to years and is usually idiopathic, but a complete review of system and directed evaluation may be needed.

Key Feature

- Represents a type-I immediate hypersensitivity reaction.

Erythema Multiforme (Fig. 7.8)

Presentation

- Target lesions with predilection for extremities, especially the palms and soles.
- May also consist of mildly symptomatic mucosal lesions.
- If more extensive lesions are present, consider SJS.

Duration

- Lesions should resolve in 2 to 3 weeks but reoccurrences are common.

Key Feature

- Most cases of recurrent EM associated with herpes simplex.
- Lesion centers are dusky and may blister.

Acne

Etiology

- Because of combination of androgens, increased sebaceous gland activity, inflammatory response to *Propionibacterium acnes*, and keratin plugged pilosebaceous units.

Presentation

- Early lesions consist of open comedones (black heads) and closed comedones (white heads).
- Inflammatory lesions are erythematous papules, pustules, and nodulocystic lesions.
- May leave postinflammatory hyperpigmentation in darker-skinned persons and permanent scarring in all races.

Treatment

- Initially, topical benzoyl peroxide, topical retinoids, and topical antibiotics.
- Oral antibiotics and hormonal contraception for inflammatory lesions and flares with menstrual cycle.
- Isotretinoin for recalcitrant or nodulocystic disease.

INFECTIOUS RASHES AND INFESTATIONS

See Table 7.5 for childhood exanthems and other eruptions.

TABLE 7.5

CHILDHOOD EXANTHEMS

Disease	Age Group and Season	Cause	Rash	Systemic Symptoms	Comments
1st Disease—Measles (Rubeola)	In prevaccination era affected school-age children	Measles—Paramyxovirus (ssRNA)	Nonpruritic morbilliform rash that begins behind ears, spreads downward (**cephalocaudad**) **Koplik spots**—appear before rash. Blue-gray lesions on erythematous buccal mucosa. Fades within 2–3 d after the onset of rash	3 Cs: Cough, coryza, conjunctivitis High fever Complications: pneumonia, otitis media, diarrhea, postinfectious encephalomyelitis, subacute sclerosing panencephalitis, death	Rash lasts 4–7 d Vitamin A supplementation can decrease mortality especially in malnourished
2nd—Scarlet fever	1- to 10-y olds Fall, winter, spring	Group A beta-hemolytic streptococcus Toxin-mediated Can also get a staphylococcal scalded fever due to TSST-1	Sandpaper rash **Pastia's lines** (accentuation of rash in skin folds) Circumoral pallor **Strawberry tongue** (white then red) Petechiae on palate Desquamation after rash fades in 4–5 d	Sore throat, abrupt onset fever, headache, vomiting, malaise	Risk for acute rheumatic fever and glomerulonephritis Treat with penicillin
3rd—Rubella (German Measles)	Adolescents Spring	Rubella–Togavirus (ssRNA)	Confluent rose papules that begin centrally on face and spread acrally with rapid fading Red-purple macules on soft palate **(Forchheimer's spots)**	Mild prodrome, fever, malaise, cough, arthralgias **Posterior auricular/occipital adenopathy**	Rash resolves within 1–3 d Teratogenic-associated with congenital infection causing cataracts, deafness, cardiac (PDA)
5th—Fifth's Disease (Erythema Infectiosum)	5- to 15-y olds Winter/spring	Parvovirus B19	"**Slapped cheeks**" appears first 1–4 d then generalized lacy rash that lasts 4–9 d **Not contagious by the time rash appears** Rash waxes wanes several weeks with physical stimuli (temperature, sunlight)	Arthritis or arthralgias more common in adults	Aplastic crisis in sickle cell disease, other hemolytic anemias Possible fetal, death in all 3 trimesters, greatest in 2nd Hydrops fetalis—fetal ascites, pleural, and pericardial effusions, resulting from severe anemia
Papular–Purpuric Gloves and Socks Syndrome	Young adults Peaks spring/ summer in	**Parvovirus B19**	Purpuric macules and papules acrally with sharp demarcation along ankle and wrists Palatal erosions Intra-oral aphthae	Flu-like symptoms	Resolves in 2 wk
6th—Sixth's Disease/ Roseola Infantum (Exanthem subitum)	Usually by 3–5 y of age	Human herpes virus types 6 and 7 (**dsDNA**)	Rose-pink macules with halo on trunk, then spreads to extremities, neck, and face Red macules/streaks on soft palate Periorbital/eyelid edema	High fever for 3–5 d in otherwise well infant, then rash begins as fever ends Rash resolves over 1–3 d	Most common complication = seizures in association with fever

TABLE 7.5

CONTINUED

Disease	Age Group and Season	Cause	Rash	Systemic Symptoms	Comments
Varicella (Chicken pox)	1- to 14-y olds Late fall, winter, spring	Varicella (**dsDNA**)	Erythematous macules and papules -> vesicles on erythematous base "**Dewdrops on rose petals**" Lesions then crust over while new lesions develop over 3–4 d Lesions on scalp, face, or trunk then spread to extremities	Fever, malaise Pneumonia (esp. in immunocompromised)	Secondary bacterial infection of skin is the most common complication and may lead to scarring Pneumonitis more severe and common in adults Congenital varicella = hypoplastic limbs, scars, ocular, CNS disease Do not give aspirin to child with varicella -> Reye's syndrome
Mononucleosis	Young children and adolescents	Ebstein-Barr Virus (EBV) (**dsDNA**)	If accompanied by rash, it is morbilliform and involves on the trunk, upper extremities and spreads to entire body Periorbital edema	Fever, lymphadenopathy (LAD), sore throat, malaise, headache, hepatosplenomegaly (HSM)	Rash following beta-lactam antibiotics
Disease	**Age Group and Season**	**Cause**	**Rash**	**Systemic Symptoms**	**Other Info**
Hand Foot and Mouth	1- to 4-y olds Summer/Fall	Coxsackie A16, Enterovirus 71, other enteroviruses Picornaviruses (ssRNA)	Macules progress to gray, football-shaped vesicles/pustules on a red base Palms, soles, oropharynx	Fever for 12–24 h, anorexia, malaise;, abdominal pain, pneumonia, encephalitis, myocarditis occur rarely	Spontaneously resolves in 1 wk
Gianotti–Crosti syndrome (papular acrodermatitis of childhood)	1- to 6-y olds Any season	Possibly Hep B, EBV	Red-to-flesh colored papules or papulovesicles Face, buttocks, extremities. **Spares trunk**	Low-grade fever Mild LAD HSM	Resolves in few weeks to months Avoid steroid creams as may make rash worse
Kawasaki's disease (mucocutaneous lymph node syndrome)	6 mo to 6 y Winter/spring	Unknown	Polymorphous generalized exanthem Groin/palmoplantar tender erythema, edema followed by desquamation of perineum and digital skin	Criteria: 4 of 5 1. Fever 5 d >38.3° C 2. Rash 3. Nonexudative conjunctivitis 4. Strawberry tongue/ red fissured lips 5. Cervical adenopathy	Tx: Aspirin (80–100 mg) + IVIG (2 g/kg) Coronary aneurysm **Leading cause of acquired heart disease in children** Echo at baseline and at 6 wk
Henoch–Schonlein Purpura	2–11 y	Thought due to bacteria (e.g., GABHS) but unclear	Palpable purpuric papules and macules (vasculitis) Extensor surfaces and buttocks	Joint and abdominal pain Nephritis with hematuria	Glomerulonephritis IgA vasculitis Intussusception
Unilateral laterothoracic exanthem (Asymmetric periflexural exanthem)	1- to 5-y old Winter/spring	Unknown	Confluent pink macules and papules Unilaterally on axillae, arm, trunk. May spread bilaterally.	Fever, conjunctivitis, diarrhea, rhinopharyngitis, LAD	Spontaneous resolution in 3–8 wk

(continued)

TABLE 7.5

CONTINUED

Disease	Age Group and Season	Cause	Rash	Systemic Symptoms	Comments
Rocky Mountain Spotted	School-age Spring and summer	Rickettsia rickettsii Carried by wood tick (*Dermacentor andersoni*) in the western United States and *D. variabilis* in eastern United States	Discrete erythematous, blanching macules, and papules beginning in periphery and spreading centrally (**centripetally**) that evolve into petechial lesions Appears 3–5 d of illness	Prodrome usually within 14 d of tick bite: headache, GI upset, malaise, and myalgias Then fever and rash Photophobia and other neurologic sx	Rapid progression and high mortality rate if untreated Tx with doxycycline even if <8-y old

Impetigo

Impetigo is a common superficial skin infection caused most commonly by staphylococci and occasionally by streptococci. Impetigo may be in crusted (nonbullous) and/or bullous forms.

Nonbullous Impetigo

Presentation

- Begins with tiny vesicles that rupture, releasing serous fluid that dries and leads to the formation of a "honey-colored" crusts lesions tend to spread locally and can be located anywhere on the body, especially around the nose and at sites of skin breakdown (e.g., abrasions, excoriations, burns, lacerations).

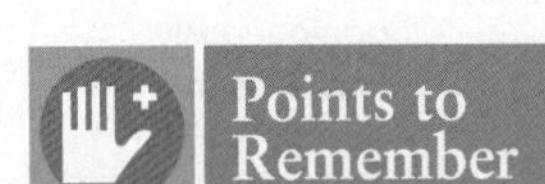

- Impetigo caused by *Streptococcus pyogenes* can lead to postreptococcal glomerulonephritis but NOT rheumatic fever!

Bullous Impetigo

Flaccid bullae that easily rupture leaving denuded erosions.

Etiology

- Most cases due to *S. aureus*.

Presentation

- Common in diaper area, face, and extremities.

Differential Diagnosis

- Immunobullous disorder.
- Staphylococcal-scalded skin syndrome.

Diagnosis

- Bacterial culture of the skin lesion or bullous fluid.

Treatment

- Impetigo that is localized can be treated topically with mupirocin.
- Impetigo that involves a large surface or multiple lesions should be treated with an oral agent active against *S. aureus* (cephalexin, dicloxacillin, clindamycin, or TMP/SMX, depending on the frequency of MRSA in the region).

SSSS Aka "Ritter's Disease"

Etiology

- Certain strains of *S. aureus* that produce exfoliative toxins.
- The toxins cause superficial intraepidermal cleavage, resulting in blister formation and skin sloughing.

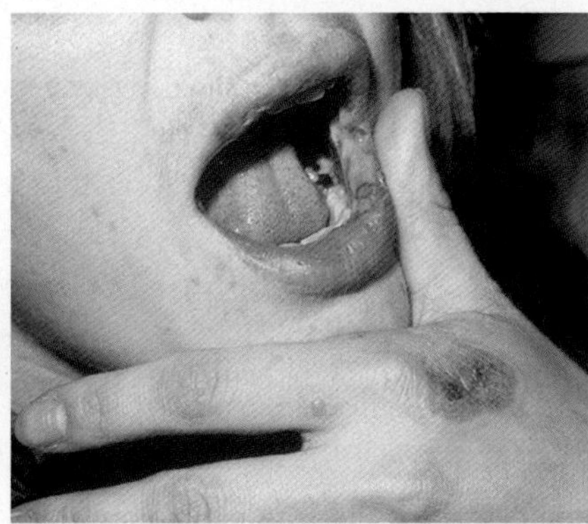

FIGURE 7.9. Stevens–Johnson Syndrome. Bullae and crusts are noted on the lips, and targetoid lesions are seen on the hand. (*Reprinted with permission from* Goodheart HP. *Goodheart's Photoguide of Common Skin Disorders*, 2nd ed. Philadelphia, PA: Lippincott Williams & Wilkins, 2003.)

Presentation

- SSSS initially presents with diffuse, painful cutaneous erythema, and edema, and *spares the mucosa.*
- Within 24 hours of initial skin changes, superficial blisters develop, followed by peeling of the skin, accentuated in flexors and perioral; bullae often develop in areas of trauma.

Differential Diagnosis

- Thermal burns.
- SJS (Fig. 7.9): fever, malaise, headache, and myalgias. Two mucosal sites of involvement, usually conjunctivae and mouth (*hemorrhagic crusting*). Less than 10% BSA with epidermal detachment. Can be caused by mycoplasma infection or medications.
- TEN: more than 30% BSA with sloughing skin. On clinical spectrum with SJS.
- Drug reaction: variable presentations but typically presents with coalescing macules and papules to generalized erythema (morbilliform).

Diagnosis

- If SSSS, identify and culture primary lesion.
- Most of skin eruption is sterile as blisters are toxin mediated.

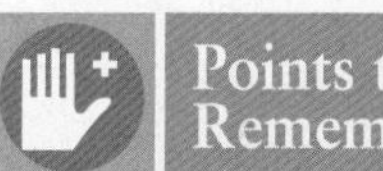

Points to Remember

- **Prognosis with SSSS is excellent in comparison with SJS and TEN because the skin separation in SSSS is intraepidermal and not deeper.**

Key Feature

- There is often a positive *Nikolsky's sign*: development of bullae in areas that are rubbed in lesional and nonlesional skin.

Treatment

- Mild cases can be treated with an oral antistaphylococcal antibiotic.
- More severe cases should be treated with IV antistaphylococcal antibiotics.

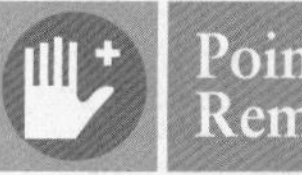

Points to Remember

- **Use a few drops of 10% to 20% KOH on skin scrapings to lyse epidermal cell walls and visualize fungal elements under light microscopy. Dermatophytes appear as branching septated filamentous (hyphae). Candida show pseudohyphae and budding. *Pityrosporum orbiculare* yeast (cause of *T. versicolor*) show short thick septated hyphae and various sized spore clusters (spaghetti and meatballs).**

SUPERFICIAL FUNGAL INFECTIONS

These are extremely common within the pediatric population; types include *Tinea versicolor*, dermatophytosis, and candidiasis. Terms for dermatophyte infections start with "*Tinea*," followed by the body site involved: *corporis*—body, *capitis*—scalp, *faciei*—face, *barbae*—beard, *pedis*—feet, *cruris*—groin, and *unguium*—nails. Of note, "onychomycosis" refers to dermatophyte or other types of fungal infections of the nails. Diagnosis is typically made either by KOH or fungal culture of skin scrapings from advancing edge of lesions

T. corporis Aka "Ringworm"

Etiology

- Most commonly *Trichophyton tonsurans* followed by *Microsporum canis* in young children and *Trichophyton rubrum* or *Trichophyton verrucosum* and others in older children.

Presentation

- Asymmetric erythematous sharply defined annular lesions with scaly slightly elevated vesicular, papular or pustular borders with clearer centers.
- Border advances as lesions spread.
- Can see single or multiple lesions that may or may not be itchy.

Differential Diagnosis

- Herald patch of Pityriasis rosea.
- Psoriasis.
- *Nummular eczema*: coin-shaped hyperpigmented eczematous macules/patches.
- *Contact allergic dermatitis*: delayed hypersensitivity reaction with weeping vesicles and bullae. Most common cause is poison ivy.
- *Contact irritant dermatitis*: nonimmune-mediated dermatitis that can occur in anyone. Irritants include: acids, soaps, detergents, water, fiberglass, and so on.
- *T. versicolor* (see below).
- Erythema migrans (Lyme disease).
- Granuloma annulare: annular lesions with raised border and no scale.
- LE.

Treatment

- Topical antifungal agents, such as ketoconazole, terbinafine, miconazole, and so on applied twice daily for 2 to 3 weeks.
- Systemic antifungals are used for widespread cutaneous infection or recalcitrant disease.

Tinea capitis

Epidemiology

- *T. tonsurans* is responsible for 90% of cases, followed by *M. canis*.
- Very common among AA children, M > F, especially those who are 3 to 7 years of age
- Asymptomatic carriage is also common.

Presentation

- "Black dot": one or more patches of hair loss with remnants of broken hair follicles.
- Seborrhea-like: widespread fine scaling of the scalp with less obvious hair loss.
- Kerion: inflammatory form with tender scattered fluctuant, erythematous, boggy nodules, indurated erythematous crusted plaques, pustules, and hair loss. Resembles bacterial abscesses (Fig. 7.10).
- Erythematous scaly patches of hair loss.

Occipital or posterior auricular lymphadenopathy is a common associated finding. When alopecia and cervical chain adenopathy is present, you must rule out *T. capitis*.

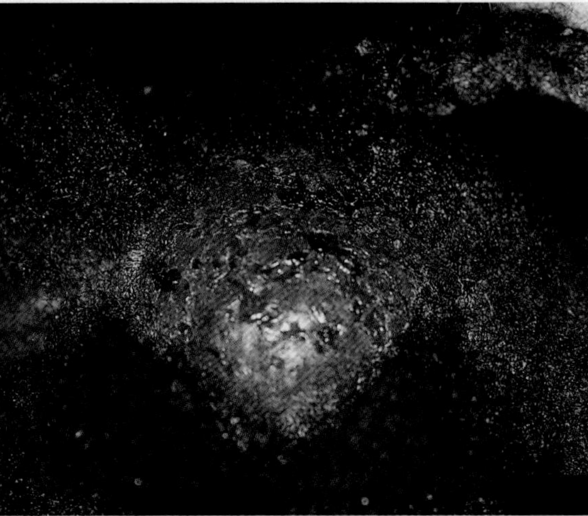

FIGURE 7.10. *Tinea capitis. T. capitis* may cause a variety of lesions of which a kerion is the most dramatic. As pictured here, kerions are elevated, boggy, exudative, and frequently covered by matted hair. (*Reprinted with permission from* Fleisher GR, Ludwig W, Baskin MN. *Atlas of Pediatric Emergency Medicine*. Philadelphia, PA: Lippincott Williams & Wilkins, 2004.)

Diagnosis

- KOH of scale scraping from area of hair loss or hair breakage reveals dermatophyte spores within hair shafts (endothrix) or spores coating outside of hair shaft (ectothrix) with surrounding septated hyphae from infected scalp skin cells.
- Clippings of broken hair or Q-tip/toothbrush moistened with tap water and rubbed onto areas of hair loss and scale; place into a sterile container or onto a fungal culture media for culture. Usually takes 7 days to 4 weeks to grow.

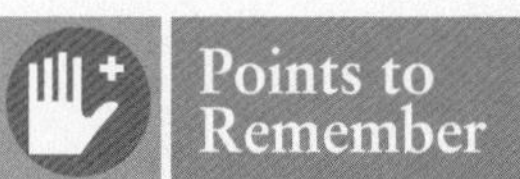

- **Higher doses and longer course duration usually required for griseofulvin microsized 20 to 25 mg/kg/d for 8 to 12 weeks. Do not forget to evaluate and treat close contacts. Wash fomites (sheets, pillowcases, hats, hair utensils in hot water).**
- ***T. capitis* MUST NOT be treated solely with topical antifungal agents. Oral therapy is needed to penetrate and kill spores in hair follicle.**
- **Kerions do not require drainage or antibiotic therapy. Prednisone adjuvant therapy may not be needed.**

Differential Diagnosis

- Seborrheic dermatitis or dandruff: look for scale on eyebrows, around nose, and in flexural creases.
- Eczema: look for clues elsewhere on body.
- Psoriasis: look for typical lesions on body, scale behind ears.
- Alopecia areata: typically does not have scale.
- Traction alopecia: if hair is pulled in tight hairstyles.
- Folliculitis.

Treatment

- Oral griseofulvin microsize/ultramicrosize (better absorption) or Terbinafine (Lamisil granules) are FDA-approved treatments.
- Selenium sulfide and ketoconazole shampoos may be used as adjuvant treatment and may decrease spore shedding.

Tinea pedis (Athlete's Foot) and *Tinea manuum*

Etiology

- *T. tonsurans* most common dermatophyte etiology in children.
- Also *T. rubrum*, *Trichophyton mentagrophytes*, and *E. floccosum*.
- Risk factors include: being an adolescent male, frequent moisture exposure, walking barefoot at swimming pools or in gyms.

Presentation

- Dry, dull erythema, scaling, and fissuring of hands/feet.
- Inflammatory blisters, particularly on sides of feet/hand, which may be painful and very pruritic.
- Maceration of the finger or toe webs often seen may become superinfected with bacteria Associated infections of nails (tinea unguium or onychomycosis) are common.

Key Feature

- "Two-foot, one-hand syndrome": *T. pedis* and *T. manuum* on one hand (spread of infection from feet to hand due to scratching).
- Possible "id reaction" on other parts of the body consisting of itchy eczematous dermatitis or vesicles on hands.

Differential Diagnosis

- Contact dermatitis: for example, to shoe leather or shoe rubber, in which case you would find more dorsal toe and feet involvement.
- Dyshidrotic eczema.
- Psoriasis.
- Palmer-plantar keratoderma (inherited keratin disorder).
- Juvenile Plantar Dermatoses (glazed red and scaly lesions on weight-bearing surfaces of feet due to friction and occlusion).

Treatment

- Topical antifungal for 2 to 4 weeks.
- May add wet compresses for vesicular infections.
- If toenails are involved, an oral antifungal is needed to treat nails and prevent reinfection.

Tinea Unguium or Onychomycosis

Etiology

- *T. rubrum*, *T. mentagrophytes*, and *E. floccosum*.
- Usually in association with *T. pedis* or *T. manuum*.
- The majority of patients have first-degree relative with onychomycosis.

Presentation

- Invasion of the distal portion of the underlying nail plate and nail bed, which may lead to lifting of the nail plate from the nail bed.
- Thickening of the toenail or fingernail with a yellowish discoloration.
- Usually does not involve all nails and may only involve one hand/foot.

Diagnosis

- KOH of underside of nail debris, fungal culture of nail clippings, and subungual debris.
- PAS stain of toenail clipping.

Treatment

- Topical antifungals are rarely effective due to poor penetration of nail plate. Usually need a systemic antifungal agent (Terbinafine PO for 6 weeks for fingernails and 12 weeks for toenails, which is more efficacious than griseofulvin). Must check liver function labs and a CBC if on terbinafine for more than 6 weeks.

Tinea cruris (Jock Itch)

Seen more in obese patients, male adolescents, or those who partake in vigorous physical activity with skin chafing of areas. Risk factors include: hot, humid weather, tight or wet clothing.

Etiology

- *T. mentagrophytes*, *E. floccosum*, or *T. rubrum*.
- May be due to autoinoculation from concurrent *T. pedis* infection.

Presentation

- Erythematous to brown patches with slightly raised scaly, vesicular or pustular borders, and central clearing involving inner thighs and groin. May also be on perianal or abdominal folds.
- May be unilateral or bilateral.
- Scrotum and labia majora usually are spared.

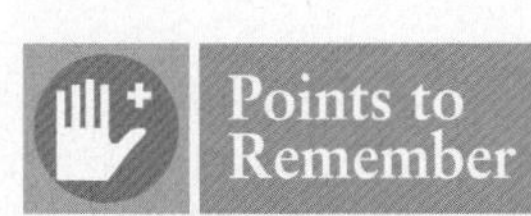

- *T. cruris* usually does not involve scrotum. If there is scrotal involvement with satellite pustules, think about candidiasis.

Diagnosis and Treatment

- Same as for *T. corporis*.

Intertrigo

Presentation

- Intense erythema of skin folds including axillae, neck, inframammary creases, or inguinal creases.

Etiology

- Moist warm conditions.
- May be due to *Candida* spp. or secondarily *S. aureus*.

Treatment

- Antifungal cream or powder, low-potency corticosteroid may also be needed.
- Keep skin dry.
- May need antibiotic if a bacterial cause is found.

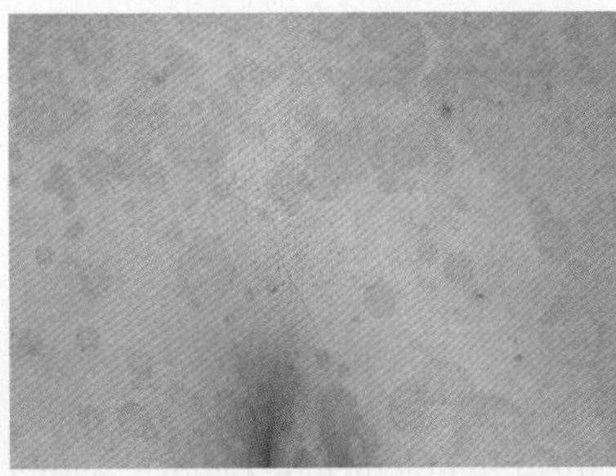

FIGURE 7.11. *Tinea versicolor.* This patient has light tan (faun-colored) *T. versicolor.* (*Reprinted with permission from* Goodheart HP. *Goodheart's Photoguide of Common Skin Disorders*, 2nd ed. Philadelphia, PA: Lippincott Williams & Wilkins, 2003.)

Tinea versicolor (Pityriasis versicolor) (Fig. 7.11)

Etiology

- Overgrowth of yeasts *Pityrosporum orbiculare* and *Pityrosporum ovale* (formerly *Malassezia furfur*), which are part of the normal skin flora.
- Therefore, lesions are not contagious.

Epidemiology

- Majority of cases present in adolescents.

Presentation

- Multiple oval macules and patches with fine powdery scale usually located on neck, proximal arms, upper back, and chest. May be slightly itchy.
- Minimal erythema that may be difficult to see in darker-skinned patients.
- Lesions may be hypo- or hyperpigmented. Hypopigmented lesions fail to tan like surrounding skin during sunlight exposure.

Diagnosis

- KOH of skin scrapings reveal hyphae and spores aka "spaghetti and meatballs".
- It is difficult to grow *Pityrosporum* yeast, so fungal culture is not helpful unless used to rule out other superficial fungal infections (dermatophytosis or candidiasis).

Treatment

- Wash areas with selenium sulfide shampoo or ketoconazole shampoo, leave on for 10 minutes, then rinse. Use daily for 2 weeks. Maintenance: use every other week or monthly.
- Topical antifungal creams for 2 to 4 weeks.
- Oral antifungal pills: various dosing regimens used. For example, ketoconazole 400 mg PO × 1 followed by physical activity to allow secretion of drug through sweat onto skin; delay shower for 10 to 12 hours, then repeat again in 1 × 4 weeks.

Key Feature

- Recurrences are common and return to normal pigmentation may take several months.

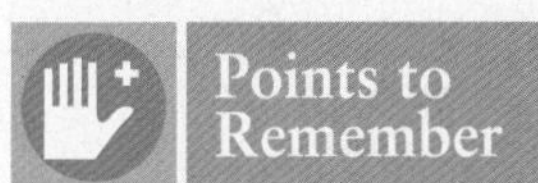

Points to Remember

- **"*Tinea*" *versicolor* is a misnomer. It is NOT due to dermatophyte fungal infection like *T. corporis*. It is caused by the yeast *P. orbiculare*.**

Molluscum Contagiosum

Etiology

- Caused by DNA poxvirus.
- Spread by autoinoculation or close contacts.

Epidemiology

- Very common.
- Lesions may last from months to years.

Presentation

- Classic lesions are pearly papules with central umbilication.
- Papules range in size from a pinhead to greater than 1 cm in diameter.

- Number of lesions may vary from a few to hundreds.
- Widespread lesions are more common in immunocompromised patients and also in patients with eczema.

Diagnosis

- Clinical.

Treatment

- No treatment is necessary.
- Possible treatments if lesions are distressing to the patient/family include removal with a curettage, topical cantharidin (must wash off in 2–4 hours), liquid nitrogen, and topical imiquimod.

Warts (Condyloma Acuminatum)

Etiology

- Warts are caused by over 70 different types of HPVs.
- Self-inoculation and spread to other people is common.

Presentation

- Several different types of warts:
  1. Common warts (verrucae vulgaris): rough skin-colored papules are usually round and often have tiny dark specks on the surface due to increased vessel proliferation from wart; often located on the hands; occasionally, common warts appear as a fingerlike projection and are called filiform warts.
  2. Plantar warts: occur on the plantar surface of the foot where pressure forces their growth inward, resulting in deep, painful lesions.
  3. Flat warts: tiny, flat-topped, skin-colored papules with a smooth surface that occur primarily on the face and dorsa of the extremities, may occur in the hundreds and coalesce to form plaques.
  4. Genital warts (condyloma acuminata): soft, flesh-colored to slightly pigmented papules that may be pedunculated; occur on the genitals and are sexually transmitted; usually caused by HPV 6 and 11 (infection due to types 16 and 18 results in high risk for anogenital cancers).

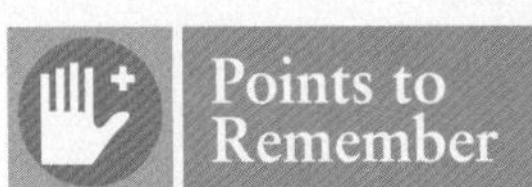

- Genital warts in a child should always raise the concern for sexual abuse; however, in children below 2 to 3 years, the infection can be acquired during vaginal delivery.

Treatment

Without treatment, warts usually last a few months to a few years. If the warts are not bothersome to the individual, treatment is not necessary.

Therapies (responses are variable):

- Options for common warts include salicylic acid 18% to 40%, cryotherapy (liquid nitrogen), and/or immune response enhancers (topical 5% imiquimod).
- Options for flat warts include all of the options for common warts and topical tretinoin.
- Genital warts often respond to the application of podophyllin 25% in tincture of benzoin applied at intervals of 1 to 3 weeks; other options include topical podofilox and imiquimod.
- Options for wart resistant to the above may include cantharidin (a blistering agent), immunotherapy with candida antigen, sensitization with squaric acid, PDL therapy, electrodesiccation, and/or surgical excision.

Pediculosis (Lice)

Etiology

- *Pediculus humanus capitis* (human **head** louse).

Presentation

- The usual manifestation of infestation with human head lice is the presence of the eggs firmly cemented to the hair shaft.
- The eggs hatch within 10 to 12 days.
- Usually results in pruritus of the scalp.

Key Feature

- Very contagious!.
- Lice are easily spread through close contact, combs, and clothing.

Pediculus humanus humanus (Human Body Louse)

Epidemiology

- Less common than head lice.
- Live in the seams of clothing and feed on the skin.

Presentation

- Produce small, red papules and wheals.

Pediculus pubis (Crabs)

Epidemiology

- Usually sexually acquired.

Presentation

- In young children, in addition to clinging to pubic hair, pubic lice can also attach to body hair and nits may be found in the eyelids.
- Very pruritic.

Diagnosis

- Scrape area with #15 blade, place on slide with mineral oil, apply cover slip and look for lice via microscope.

Treatment

- **Head lice:** first-line treatment is permethrin 1% cream; alternative treatments include pyrethrins, malathion (only treatment that is ovicidal). Lindane cream is NOT used as a treatment in the United States because of its associated neurotoxicity; symptomatic family members and close contacts should also be treated.
- **Body lice:** Permethrin 5% for 8 to 14 hours; rid clothing and bedding of lice and eggs via washing at high temperatures or dry cleaning; mattresses should be sprayed with a pediculicide.
- **Pubic lice:** Permethrin 1% to affected areas for 10 minutes; alternatives include pyrethrin, lindane. Repeat in 7 to 10 days; wash clothing and bedding; if eyelids are involved, petrolatum, applied several times daily may be effective.

Papular *Urticaria* (Fig. 7.12)

Papular *Urticaria* is a common disorder caused by hypersensitivity to insect bites.

Etiology

- Fleas are the most common cause, but papular *Urticaria* can also result from bites of mosquitoes, lice, and mites.

Presentation

- Classic lesions are papules with an erythematous flare that occur in crops; a visible central punctum representing the site of the insect's bite may be present.
- Lesions are intensely pruritic.

Duration

- Each crop of papules lasts several days but recurrences may occur over several months.

Key Feature

- Secondary bacterial infections from excoriations are common.

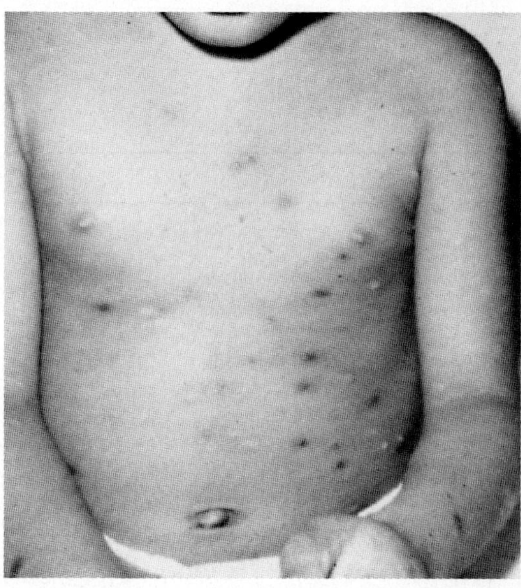

FIGURE 7.12. Papular *Urticaria*. (*Reprinted with permission from* McMillan JA, Feigin RD, DeAngelis C, et al. *Oski's Pediatrics: Principles and Practice*, 4th ed. Philadelphia, PA: Lippincott Williams & Wilkins, 2006.)

Points to Remember

- **Intense, unremitting pruritus that is often worse at night is a classic feature of scabies.**

Treatment

- Eliminate the biting insects from the child's environment and prevent insect bites; if elimination is impossible, reduce the child's exposure by appropriate clothing and insect repellent.
- Treat acute lesions with topical steroids, topical antipruritic agents containing pramoxine, camphor or menthol, and/or oral antihistamines.
- Secondary bacterial infections should be treated with antibiotics.

Points to Remember

- **Acropustulosis of infancy is also very itchy. Onset birth to 2 years. Recurrent discrete vesiculopustular lesions typically on palms and soles. Lesser number on dorsal hands, feet, wrists, and ankles. Resolves in 2 to 3 years.**

Scabies

Scabies is an infestation with the mite, *Sarcoptes scabiei.* The female mites burrow into the skin and deposit eggs, and then a rash is produced as the body becomes sensitized to the mite and its products.

Presentation

- Lesions are intensely pruritic, erythematous papules, nodules, and/or linear burrows; vesicles and pustules are occasional seen as well; secondary excoriation is common because of the intense pruritus.
- Distribution varies by age.
- Infants: generalized lesions involving the trunk, diaper area, extremities (palms/soles), and head.
- Children and adolescents: lesions are concentrated in the interdigital spaces, wrists, axillae, and at the belt line; males commonly have involvement of the genital area.
- Complications: secondary bacterial infection.

Points to Remember

- **Even after effective treatment, the pruritus of scabies often takes a week or more to resolve.**

Diagnosis

- Identification of the mite and/or or eggs in a scraping from one of the lesions in oil.

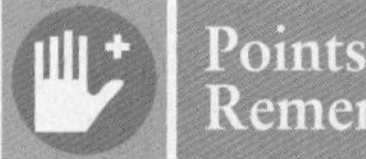

Points to Remember

- ***T. capitis* is the most common cause of localized hair loss in children.**

Treatment

- Five percent permethrin cream applied topically to the body from head to toe, left on for 8 to 14 hours, then rinsed off; a second treatment 7 to 10 days after the initial treatment is recommended to kill hatched eggs.
- All asymptomatic family members and close contacts should receive of a single treatment at the time the index case is initially treated to prevent cycles of reinfection.
- All clothing and bedding should be washed to prevent reinfection.

HAIR LOSS (SEE TABLE 7.6)

TABLE 7.6

COMMON HAIR DISORDERS IN CHILDREN

	Definition	Clinical Manifestations	Treatment	Miscellaneous
Alopecia areata	Unknown but autoimmune process is suspected	Well-circumscribed round or oval patches of complete or relatively complete hair loss (nonscarring) Lesions tend to appear rapidly and can be single or multiple. Hair loss may involve eyebrow and eyelashes Exclamation point hair can be seen Scalp appears normal without scale, erythema, or scarring Pitting of the nails is a common associated finding	Topical and intralesional corticosteroids, anthralin, contact sensitizing agents, topical tacrolimus, topical minoxidil, phototherapy Systemic corticosteroids have been used but hair falls out again when steroids are discontinued. Not recommended	Course is unpredictable; 90% of children will regrow hair within 1 y; recurrences are common "Alopecia totalis" = loss of all scalp hair "Alopecia universalis" = loss of all body hair
Trichotillomania	Twisting or pulling out one's own hair including eyebrows and eyelashes	Irregular and bizarre patches of alopecia, hair of different lengths Scalp usually appears normal, although petechiae may be seen	Difficult Address any underlying psychological issues SSRIs	Trichotillomania can be a habit, especially in young children; a response to stress, or in post puberty, evidence of a more severe psychological problem
Traction alopecia	Hair loss secondary to prolonged tension on the hair shaft, usually from cornrows or braids	Hair loss at the margins of the scalp or as oval or linear areas in part lines. May see pustules where hair is pulled	Hair styles with less tension on hair shaft. Rule out bacterial folliculitis	Permanent hair loss may result if pressure is maintained for a long time
Telogen effluvium	A stressful event causes follicles in the anagen (or growing) phase to be converted to the telogen (or resting) phase Inciting factors include febrile illnesses, drug reactions, and delivery of a baby Hair loss begins ~2 to 3 mo after the inciting event	Diffuse hair loss Gentle hair pull test reveals >7 telogen hair (hair with bulb)	No treatment is necessary Avoid stressful events that can include: illness, dieting, thyroid disease, pregnancy	Hair returns to normal by ~5 mo *Anagen effluvium-sudden arrest of cell division in hair matrix. Ex. chemotherapy induced*
Androgenic Alopecia	Hair thinning due to increased androgens	Hair thinning commonly in vertex and bitemporal areas. In females, frontal hair line is preserved, see widened part at vertex. Increased telogen hair	Minoxidil 2% or 5% solution or 5% foam Oral contraception Spironolactone	

SAMPLE BOARD REVIEW QUESTIONS

1. A 10-year-old healthy girl with the history of an erythematous rash on her cheeks 4 days ago without fever presents to your office. On physical examination, she has an erythematous reticulated rash on her extremities and trunk. She denies itch or prolonged sun exposure. The most likely diagnosis is:
   a. Lupus erythematosus
   b. Erythema multiforme
   c. Erythema infectiosum
   d. Roseola infantum

   Answer: c. Erythema infectiosum is characterized by a "Slapped cheeks" appearance or an erythematous rash on cheeks, which is followed 1 to 4 days later by a generalized lacy reticulated rash lasting for 4 to 9 days. There are usually no systemic symptoms. LE can present with erythematous rash on cheeks, as well as nose and forehead in a "butterfly" pattern that is exacerbated by sun exposure. Patients with LE tend to have other systemic symptoms such as arthralgias and myalgias. The body rash of systemic LE is not reticulated but typically annular scaly erythematous patches. *Erythema multiforme* is a rash that consists of targetoid lesions with a dusky tone or a blister in the center. *Roseola infantum*: begins with high fever followed by exanthema of rose-pink macules with halo on trunk, extremities, neck, and face.

2. A mother brings in her 4-month-old infant who is irritable with diarrhea and presents with a nonpruritic scaly crusted rash around his mouth, nose, eyes, and diaper area. He has just been weaned off breast milk and his mother is concerned that he may have a milk allergy. Which of the following diagnoses should you consider first?
   a. Milk protein allergy
   b. Acrodermatitis enteropathica
   c. Eczema
   d. Contact dermatitis

   Answer: b. The clinical description is of *acrodermatitis enteropathica* that can be seen in two settings—days to weeks after birth in the bottle-fed infant and shortly after weaning in breast-fed infants. Zinc supplementation results in correction of skin lesions. *Milk allergy* or other food allergy may also present with diarrhea and rash but does not have skin lesions primarily around the facial orifices and the diaper area. *Eczema* can present in the diaper area but is not as involved as other parts of body because of the moisture and occlusion from diapers. One key to clue of eczema is pruritus; if infant is not scratching or has no excoriations, than probably not eczema. *Irritant contact dermatitis* can be due to irritation from diarrhea in diaper area and from foods irritating the mouth, and *allergic contact dermatitis* can be from an allergen such as in the elastic from diapers, food dyes, fragrances, and so on. It usually is itchy and does not occur only in setting of weaning off breast milk.

3. A 4-year-old boy has a 3-month history of recurrent very itchy bumps on arm and legs. No one else in the household is affected. On physical examination, you note clusters of erythematous papules in groups of three on his extremities. The remainder of the skin examination is normal. Which of the following is the most likely diagnosis?
   a. Papular *Urticaria*
   b. Scabies
   c. Gianotti–Crosti syndrome
   d. Bacterial folliculitis

   Answer: a. *Papular Urticaria* is a hypersensitivity to insect bites, commonly fleas, which presents as small urticarial papules in groups or clusters; these tend to be very itchy and recurrent in nature. The group of three refers to the "breakfast, lunch, and dinner" pattern of the papules. *Scabies* also cause itchy papules with burrows. Lesions are typically located under arms, umbilicus, diaper area, and finger web spaces. Usually several household members are affected. *Gianotti–Crosti* presents with red-to-flesh colored papules or papulovesicles on the face, buttocks, and extremities and spares the trunk. It usually is not itchy and does not reoccur. *Bacterial folliculitis* does not present in groups of three, it has a follicular base but does not tend to be very itchy.

4. A 3-month-old has a hemangioma on the jaw that has doubled in size since birth; he now presents with a new strange cry. Your next important step is which of the following?
   a. Intralesional corticosteroid therapy
   b. Vincristine therapy
   c. A referral to ENT for endoscopy
   d. Observation; this is normal growth pattern for hemangiomas

Answer: c. Refer to *ENT for endoscopy*. Hemangiomas on the jaw, also referred to as "beard hemangiomas," can be associated with laryngeal hemangiomas, stridor, and airway compromise. Although intralesional corticosteroids may help flatten the cutaneous hemangioma, laryngeal lesions must be ruled out first via direct visualization. *Vincristine* is used as second-line agent to treat symptomatic or complicated hemangiomata, but further evaluation is needed before considering. *Observation* is not appropriate as laryngeal lesions large enough to cause stridor can lead to airway compromise without intervention.

5. A 1-month old presents with a PWS on the temple and ipsilateral lower eyelid, which extends to the cheek. What is the most important next step in management?
   a. PDL therapy
   b. Systemic corticosteroids
   c. Skull radiographs
   d. Ophthalmologic examination

Answer: d. *Ophthalmologic examination*. For PWS involving the V1 distribution, you must evaluate for eye abnormalities associated with Sturge–Weber syndrome. PWS in the V2 distribution alone may also be associated with glaucoma or other ocular problems. *Skull radiographs* are not the proper modality to evaluate for leptomeningeal lesions of Sturge–Weber syndrome; rather a CT or MRI should be performed. *PDL* is used to lighten PWS, but evaluation for underlying eye abnormalities should be performed first. *Systemic corticosteroids* are not part of the management of PWS.

6. When SJS is due to a drug reaction, what is the typical time frame for lesions of SJS to appear after a drug is started?
   a. 48 hours
   b. 1–3 weeks
   c. 3 days
   d. Within minutes

Answer: b. *1–3 weeks*.

7. For the past several months, a 9-year-old healthy girl has complained of a slightly itchy rash. Physical examination reveals well-demarcated erythematous plaques with silvery scale on her elbows and lower back. She has adherent scale along her hairline. No other skin lesions were present. Which of the following is the most likely diagnosis?
   a. Pityriasis rosea
   b. *T. corporis* and *capitis*
   c. Psoriasis
   d. Nummular eczema

Answer: c. *Psoriasis*. The lesions are well-demarcated, erythematous papules or plaques covered with a silvery scale typically on elbows, knees, and lower back. Patients also may have a thick adherent scale along the hairline. *Tinea corporis* presents typically with asymmetric, erythematous, sharply defined annular lesions with scaly, slightly elevated vesicular, papular or pustular borders with clearer centers. It is not specifically in the distribution listed above. The hallmarks of *T. capitis* are alopecia, broken hair, or localized to diffuse scale, not typically a thick adherent scale along the hairline. *Nummular eczema* would be more pruritic and would include ill-defined, scaly, coin-shaped lesions, not necessarily in the distribution described. *Pityriasis rosea* presents with oval lesions with powdery scale along skin lines in a "Christmas tree" pattern on chest and back.

8. A 7-year old complains of a tender lump on the scalp. On physical examination, he has minimal scale and broken hair in the area. He has no known drug allergies. Which of the following is the appropriate therapy?
   a. Selenium sulfide shampoo
   b. Topical ketoconazole 2%
   c. Oral griseofulvin
   d. Oral cephalexin

Answer: c. *Oral griseofulvin*. The description is most consistent with a diagnosis of *T. capitis*, and the only effective treatment is a systemic antifungal such as griseofulvin. Selenium sulfide and topical ketoconazole can help decrease spore shedding but will not kill the infecting dermatophyte within the hair follicles and hair shaft. Oral cephalexin will not treat *T. capitis*. It may treat folliculitis but folliculitis typically presents with perifollicular pustules on the scalp.

9. A 16-year-old AA healthy girl with acne reports no improvement with an over-the-counter benzoyl peroxide wash. She reports fairly regular menstrual periods. Physical

examination reveals several whiteheads and blackheads on cheeks and chin with significant postinflammatory hyperpigmented macules. Her back and chest are clear. She has no known drug allergies. What is the best treatment?

a. Topical retinoid
b. Oral antibiotic
c. Topical antibiotic
d. Fading cream

Answer: a. *Topical retinoid* is the best treatment for comedonal acne, and it also helps with residual pigmentation. A *fading cream* alone will not stop the comedonal lesions that result in the postinflammatory hyperpigmentation. An *oral antibiotic* could be added to the topical retinoid if monotherapy is not effective or used if lesions were more inflammatory. A *topical antibiotic* is not the best treatment for comedones and will not help improve hyperpigmentation.

10. What is the most common cause of SJS in the pediatric population?

a. *Mycoplasma pneumonia*
b. HSV
c. Amoxicillin
d. TMP/SMX

Answer: a. *M. pneumonia* is the most common cause of SJS in pediatric patients. HSV is associated with recurrent erythema multiforme. TMP/SMX is the most common drug-associated cause of SJS. Penicillins can also cause SJS, but this is not the most common cause in the pediatric population.

11. You are caring for a 2-year-old boy who presented with painful, erythematous skin with large bullae and skin sloughing. He has yellow crusting around the skin of the mouth and nose. A culture is taken from one of the flaccid blisters. What results would expect from that culture?

a. It would grow *S. aureus*
b. It would be sterile
c. It would grow *S. pyogenes*
d. It would grow *M. pneumoniae*

Answer: b. *Sterile*. This child most likely has SSSS. The skin findings in this condition are caused by a toxin produced by phage II *S. aureus*. The causative bacterium is not present in the bullous fluid but rather is often present on distant skin or mucosal sites. *S. pyogens* can cause scarlet fever, which is also toxin mediated, but bullous lesions are not present. *M. pneumoniae* is associated with SJS, which presents with targetoid lesions and mucosal involvement in two sites. The clinical description is more consistent with SSSS. Moreover, you cannot culture *M. pneumonia* from the skin lesions in patients with SJS.

12. Identify the most likely diagnosis for a rash with the following description: erythematous macules with edematous rings and violaceous centers or central blisters most prominently concentrated on the extremities with only mild erosions to the lips.

a. SJS
b. Erythema multiforme
c. SSSS
d. Erythema migrans

Answer: b. *Erythema multiforme*. *SJS* is diagnosed when there are two mucosal sites involved and less than 10% BSA with targetoid lesions. Mucosal lesions are typically severely affected. *SSSS* does not involve mucosal surfaces, although crusting may be noted on skin around the nose and mouth. Bullous lesions are present. *Erythema migrans*, which involves an expanding erythematous border with central clearing, is a cutaneous sign of Lyme disease.

13. *T. versicolor* is most often due to:

a. *T. tonsurans*
b. *P. orbiculare*
c. *M. canis*
d. Human herpes viruses 6 and 7

Answer: b. *P. orbiculare* is a dimorphic yeast, not a dermatophyte. "Tinea" in *T. versicolor* is a misnomer. *T. tonsurans* and *M. canis* are dermatophytes that can cause *T. capitis* as well as other superficial fungal infections. *Human herpes viruses 6 and 7* (HHV 6 and 7) cause roseola infantum.

14. Which of the following antibiotics is most commonly associated with SJS?

a. TMP/SMX
b. Azithromycin
c. Amoxicillin
d. Tetracycline

Answer: a. *TMP/SMX (Bactrim)* is the most common drug associated with SJS. The other choices have been much less commonly associated with this condition.

15. A 1-day-old infant is diagnosed with transient neonatal pustular melanosis. You perform a smear from one of the lesions and expect to see:

a. Neutrophils
b. Eosinophils
c. No cells
d. *S. aureus*

Answer: a. *Neutrophils* can be seen on smear. *Eosinophils* are seen in a smear from erythema toxicum neonatorum. *S. aureus* can cause pustules in the newborn but is not the cause of transient neonatal pustular melanosis.

SUGGESTED READINGS

Eichenfield LF, Frieden IJ, Esterly NB. *Neonatal Dermatology*. 2nd ed. Philadelphia, PA: Elsevier, Inc, 2008.
Paller AS, Mancini AJ. *Hurwitz Clinical Pediatric Dermatology*. 3rd ed. Philadelphia, PA: Elsevier, Inc, 2006.

CHAPTER 8 ■ DYSMORPHOLOGY

HILARY TINKEL VERNON

AS	Angelman syndrome
ASD	Atrial septal defect
AV	Atrioventricular
BWS	Beckwith-Wiedemann syndrome
CATCH-22	DiGeorge syndrome: cardiac abnormalities, abnormal facies, thymic aplasia, cleft palate, hypocalcemia, 22q11 deletion
CHARGE	Coloboma, heart malformation, choanal atresia, retardation of growth and/or development, genital anomalies, and ear anomalies
CNS	Central nervous system
DNA	Deoxyribonucleic acid
GU	Genitourinary
IUGR	Intrauterine growth restriction
MELAS	Mitochondrial myopathy, encephalopathy, lactic acidosis, and stroke
MERRF	Myoclonic epilepsy associated with ragged red fibers
NF	Neurofibromatosis
NTD	Neural tube defect
OI	Osteogenesis imperfecta
VACTERL	Vertebral defects, anal atresia, cardiac defects, tracheo-esophageal fistula, renal malformations, and limb defects
VSD	Ventricular septal defect
WAGR	Wilms tumor, aniridia, genitourinary abnormalities, and mental retardation
WPW	Wolff-Parkinson-White

CHAPTER OBJECTIVES

1. To understand chromosome structure and how alterations in structure lead to disease
2. To understand and recognize patterns of inheritance of genetic disorders
3. To know the inheritance patterns, clinical manifestations, diagnosis, and treatment of important genetic disorders.

MOLECULAR GENETICS

Chromosome Arrangement

Genetic material consists of double-helical DNA arranged into chromosomes. There are an estimated 25,000 genes in the human genome. The mitochondria of cells also contain their own DNA, which encodes for 13 protein encoding genes responsible for some of the mitochondrial function.

Humans have 23 sets of paired chromosomes for a total of 46. The first 22 pairs, called autosomes, are labeled by their number. The other pair, the sex chromosomes, is labeled by XX (female) or XY (male). One of each of the 22 autosomes and one X chromosome are derived from the mother, and one of each autosome and either an X or Y chromosome are derived from the father. A chromosome has a long arm, called the q arm, and a short arm, called the p arm. The arms are separated by the centromere.

The process by which a human cell with 46 chromosomes divides to create identical daughter cells (which also have 46 chromosomes) is called mitosis. The chromosomes duplicate themselves, line up along the mitotic plate with their duplicate pair, and then separate into two individual, identical daughter cells.

Meiosis is the process by which cells with 46 chromosomes divide in order to form daughter cells with 23 chromosomes. The cells with 23 chromosomes are sex cells, either a sperm or an egg, which provide half of the chromosomes to the human zygote. Meiosis takes place in two cell divisions: meiosis I, during which recombination, or crossing over occurs,

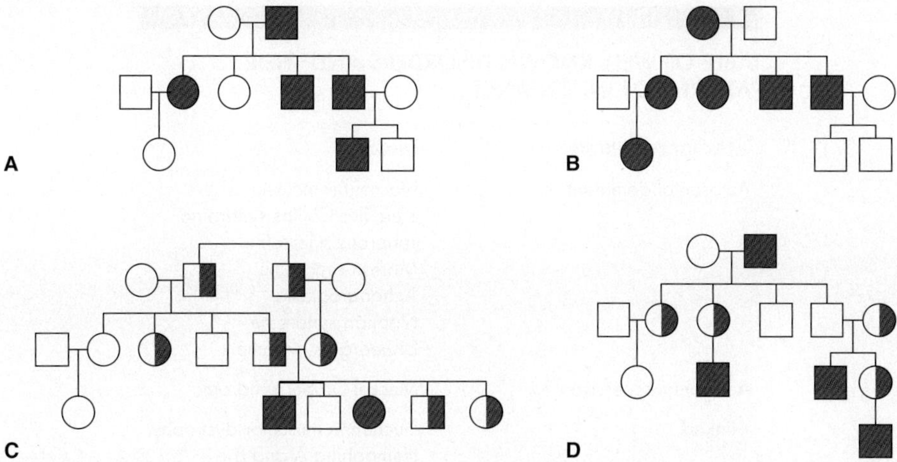

FIGURE 8.1. Patterns of inheritance. (A) Autosomal dominant inheritance. (B) Mitochondrial inheritance. Note the passage of the disease phenotype only from mother to child. (C) Autosomal recessive inheritance. Children born to consanguineous parents (indicated by the double line) are more likely to have an autosomal disease. (D) X-linked inheritance.

and meiosis II. One sperm with 46 chromosomes undergoing meiosis results in four cells, each with 23 chromosomes.

Inheritance Patterns

Genetic disorders can be inherited through several mechanisms: autosomal recessive, autosomal dominant, X-linked, mitochondrial or multifactorial inheritance. Figure 8.1 shows the pedigrees for common inheritance patterns.

- **Autosomal recessive**—An abnormal copy of each gene on an autosome has to be inherited from each parent in order to cause disease; an individual with one abnormal copy and one normal copy is called a carrier and is usually asymptomatic; thus, a child born to two parents who are both carriers has a one in four chance of having the disease, a two in four chance of being a carrier, and a one in four chance of inheriting two normal genes.
- **Autosomal dominant**—One abnormal copy of a gene on an autosome is sufficient to cause disease; there is a one in two chance that an affected parent will pass the disease to his or her child.
- **X-linked disease**—The disease causing mutation is located on the X chromosome; an affected father will pass the mutation on to all of his daughters but none of his sons; an affected mother will pass the mutation on to half of her daughters and half of her sons; all males inheriting the mutation are affected since they have only one copy of the X chromosome; females are variably affected since although they have two copies of the X chromosome, there is random inactivation of one X chromosome in every cell.
- **Mitochondrial inheritance**—A mutation in the mitochondrial DNA is inherited in a dominant manner from the mother, since only the egg cell donates mitochondria to the zygote; thus, a mother will pass the disease to all of her children.
- **Multifactorial inheritance**—The process by which a disease develops via a combination of mechanisms including both genetic (one or more contributing genes) and environmental factors.
- Common genetic disorders and their patterns of inheritance are shown in Table 8.1.

Anticipation and Imprinting

Two other important concepts to understand are anticipation and imprinting.

- **Anticipation**—Certain diseases become more severe in ensuring generations via a process known as anticipation. In this process, deleterious repeated nucleotide sequences actually expand from generation to generation.
- **Imprinting**—Some disease-causing mutations cause a different phenotype depending on whether they are inherited from the mother or the father. This is known as imprinting.

Chromosome and Gene Abnormalities

There are multiple potential mechanisms that lead to chromosome and gene abnormalities.

TABLE 8.1

TABLE OF WELL-KNOWN DISORDERS AND THEIR PATTERNS OF INHERITANCE

Inheritance Pattern	Diseases
Autosomal dominant	Neurofibromatosis Treacher Collins syndrome Tuberous sclerosis Marfan syndrome Achondroplasia Noonan syndrome DiGeorge syndrome
Autosomal recessive	Meckel-Gruber syndrome
X-linked	Duchenne muscular dystrophy Hemophilia A and B Alport syndrome Fragile X syndrome
Mitochondrial inheritance	MELAS MERRF Leigh syndrome
Multifactorial	Cleft lip and palate Neural tube defects

MELAS, Mitochondrial myopathy, encephalopathy, lactic acidosis, and stroke; MERRF, Myoclonic epilepsy associated with ragged red fibers.

- **Aneuploidy**—An abnormal total number of chromosomes, i.e. one extra (47 chromosomes), or one less (45 chromosomes).
- **Structural abnormalities**—A balanced translocation occurs when pieces of chromosomes switch places with each other, but there is no change in the total content of DNA; an unbalanced translocation is when a translocation occurs in an unequal manner and pieces of chromosome are either missing or are in triplicate.
- **Contiguous gene syndrome**—Deletion of small parts of a chromosome resulting in the loss of several genes causing a predictable phenotype.
- **Single gene disorder**—A change in the sequence of a particular gene, such as a nucleotide deletion, insertion, or alteration, leading to a single gene disorder.
- **Uniparental disomy**—Two maternal or two paternal copies (rather than one of each) of an imprinted gene are inherited.
- **Mosaicism**—An individual has two distinct cell lines, each with their own chromosomes.

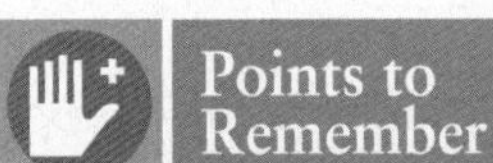

Points to Remember

- Features seen in a newborn can be combinations of malformations and deformations. For example, a child with Potter sequence has agenesis of the kidneys (a malformation), and therefore oligohydramnios due to lack of fetal urine. The oligohydramnios leads to flattened facies (deformation).

Malformations and Deformations

There are multiple mechanisms by which an abnormal feature can develop in a fetus.

- A **malformation** is an abnormal feature caused by an abnormality in the baby's genetic makeup. For example, a flattened occiput in a child with Down syndrome is a malformation.
- A **deformation** is caused by factors external to the developing fetus causing altered structural development. For example, oligohydramnios can cause arthrogryposis, or contraction of the extremities, due to space constraints in the uterus. The position of the fetus in the uterus can also lead to deformations. A fetus that is breech, for example, is more likely to develop hip subluxation. A **disruption** is when normal fetal structures are permanently damaged. For example, amniotic bands can cause digit or limb amputation.

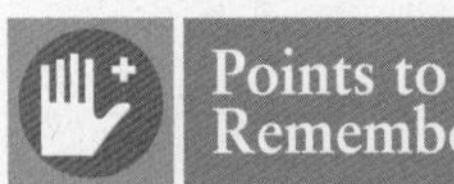

Points to Remember

- Every child with suspected trisomy 21 should have a karyotype. This not only confirms the diagnosis but also has implications for recurrence; there is a much higher chance for recurrence in a sibling when a familial unbalanced translocation is the causative factor for the Down syndrome.

ANEUPLOIDIES

Trisomy 21 (Down Syndrome)

Trisomy 21, or Down syndrome, is a condition in which there is an extra copy of chromosome 21. The majority of cases are a full trisomy, usually caused by **nondisjunction** in meiosis I in the egg. About 3% of cases are caused by an **unbalanced translocation** between chromosome 21 and another chromosome. Seventy-five percent of these translocations are new in the affected child,

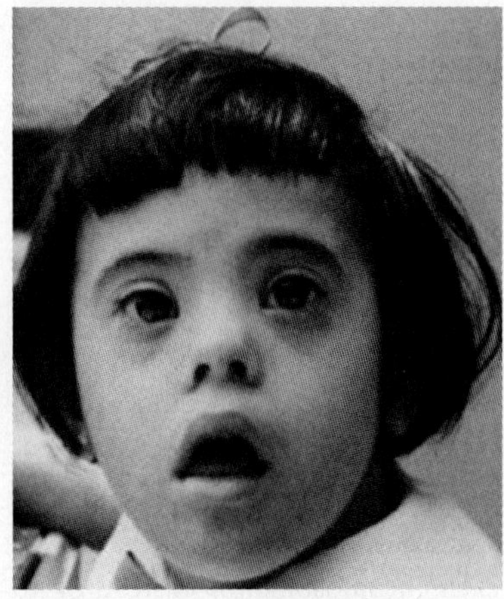

FIGURE 8.2. A child with trisomy 21. (Reprinted with permission from McMillan JA, Feigin RD, DeAngelis C, et al. *Oski's Pediatrics: Principles and Practice*. 4th ed. Philadelphia: Lippincott Williams &Wilkins; 2006.)

and 25% of these cases are familial (the parent has a balanced translocation). In the remaining cases, there is mosaicism, with one cell line with the normal number of chromosomes, and one cell line with trisomy 21.

There is a **maternal–age-related increase** in aneuploidy including Down syndrome. For example, the risk of a 20-year-old mother giving birth to a child with Down syndrome is about 1/1,500, whereas the risk of a 35-year-old mother giving birth to a child with Down syndrome is about 1/355.

Points to Remember

- **Mothers with advanced age may opt for more stringent prenatal screening and testing (i.e., amniocentesis) due to their increased risk of having a fetus with aneuploidy.**

Clinical Manifestations

- Characteristic facies include epicanthal folds, upslanting palpebral fissures, flat nasal bridge, and small ears (Fig. 8.2).
- Cardiac malformations (particularly **AV canal defects**).
- Mental retardation.
- Short stature.
- Bowel abnormalities (e.g., duodenal atresia, Hirschsprung's disease).
- Flattened posterior skull (brachycephaly).
- Brushfield spots (iris hamartomas).
- Single palmar crease, fifth finger clinodactyly.
- Wide space between first and second toes.
- Hypothyroidism.
- Leukemia.
- Early-onset Alzheimer disease.

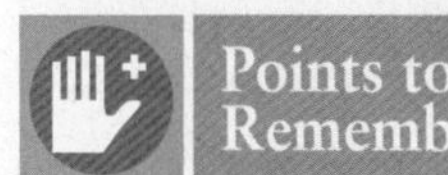

Points to Remember

- **The "double bubble" sign on abdominal X-ray or ultrasound refers to the appearance of bowel when it is affected by duodenal atresia.**

Trisomy 13 (Patau Syndrome)

Trisomy 13 syndrome, also known as Patau Syndrome, is an aneuploidy in which there is an extra copy of chromosome 13. The incidence is about 1 in 5,000 to 12,000 live births. More than three-fourths of the cases result from chromosomal nondisjunction, and advanced maternal age is associated with an increased risk. As is seen in trisomy 21, some cases are due to unbalanced chromosomal translocation between chromosome 13 and another chromosome, and 5% of cases are mosaic. Survival is very limited, but about 5% of children born with trisomy 13 live beyond 1 year of age. Survivors have severe mental retardation.

Clinical Manifestations

- Microcephaly.
- Cutis aplasia of the scalp.
- Microphthalmia.
- Cleft lip and/or palate.
- **Flexed and overlapping fingers.**
- Cardiac malformations.
- Holoprosencephaly.
- Omphalocele.
- Kidney defects.

Trisomy 18 (Edwards Syndrome)

Trisomy 18, or Edwards syndrome, occurs in approximately 1 in 3,000 to 7,000 live births. Most cases are caused by maternal nondisjunction, and advanced maternal age is associated with

Points to Remember

- It can be helpful to remember the differences in clinical findings between trisomy 13 and 18 by thinking of trisomy 13 as having more features consistent with "midline" defects. For example, features of Trisomy 13 include cutis aplasia, holoprosencephaly and omphalocele, which are all "midline" defects.

increased risk. Although survival is very limited, between 5% and 10% of children with trisomy 18 live beyond 1 year of age. Survivors have severe mental retardation.

Clinical Manifestations

- Hypotonia, low birth weight.
- Clenched hands with overlapping digits.
- Cardiac defects.
- **Rocker-bottom feet.**
- Microcephaly.
- Hernias.
- Small chin.

Triploidy

Triploidy is a **lethal** condition in which a fetus has three of each chromosome (69 instead of 46 chromosomes). Most pregnancies in which the fetus has triploidy end in spontaneous miscarriage or stillbirth. Those infants who are born alive usually die shortly after birth. Infants have abnormal placentas (small or cystic), severe IUGR, and multiple birth defects, including heart defects, NTDs, craniofacial abnormalities, and other birth defects.

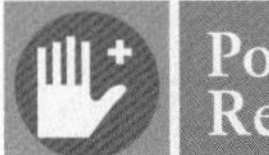

Points to Remember

- Aneuploidies involving sex chromosomes are generally milder in phenotype than aneuploidies of the autosomes.

Turner Syndrome

Turner syndrome results when a female has a single X chromosome and absence of all or part of the second sex chromosome (X or Y). Turner syndrome occurs in 1% to 2% of all pregnancies, but most of these spontaneously abort in the first trimester. The incidence of Turner syndrome is about 1 in 2,000 to 5,000 female live births. **Intelligence is generally normal**, although there can be associated learning disabilities.

Points to Remember

- Sometimes girls with Turner syndrome are not recognized until they present with primary amenorrhea in adolescence.

Clinical Manifestations

- Small size, **short stature.**
- **Premature ovarian failure** ("streak ovaries").
- Renal abnormalities.
- Heart defects (e.g., **coarctation of the aorta,** bicuspid aortic valve).
- Webbed neck, low hairline, and low-set ears (Fig. 8.3).
- Lymphedema (seen in newborns).
- Cubitus valgus (increased carrying angle of the arms).
- Shield chest with widely spaced nipples.

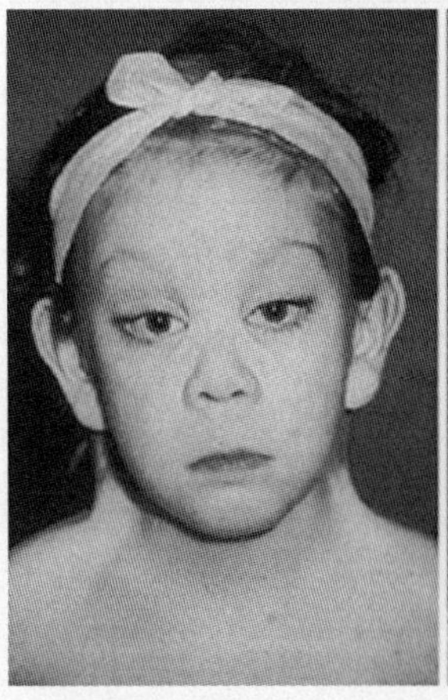
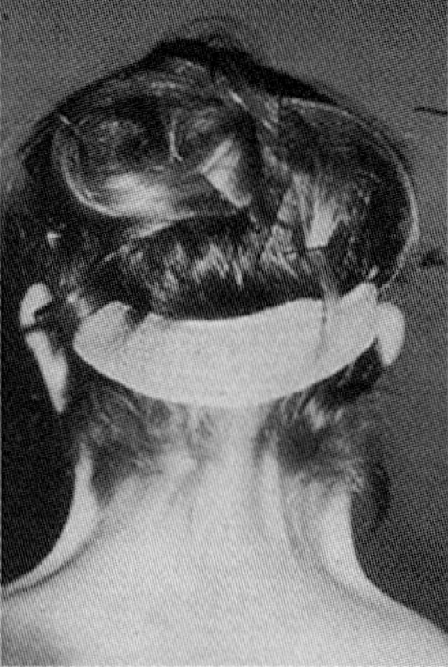

FIGURE 8.3. A child with Turner syndrome. Note the webbing of the neck. (Reprinted with permission from McMillan JA, Feigin RD, DeAngelis C, et al. *Oski's Pediatrics: Principles and Practice.* 4th ed. Philadelphia: Lippincott Williams &Wilkins; 2006.)

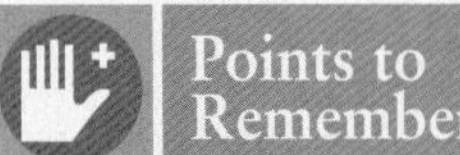

Points to Remember

- Males with Klinefelter syndrome do not have obvious facial dysmorphism.

Klinefelter Syndrome

Klinefelter syndrome is caused by an extra X chromosome in a male, resulting in a 47, XXY karyotype. It is the most common aneuploidy of the sex chromosomes, with a prevalence of 1 in 500 males. Intelligence ranges from below to above normal, but certain learning disabilities are associated with Klinefelter syndrome including difficulties with expressive language.

Clinical Manifestations

- **Small testicular size** (the most common clinical feature).
- Sparse body hair.
- Gynecomastia.
- **Eunuchoid body habitus.**
- Infertility.

Points to Remember

- Infertility is common in men with Klinefelter syndrome, but many affected men are able to have biological children via assisted reproductive technology.

CONTIGUOUS GENE SYNDROMES

Small parts of a chromosome can be deleted resulting in the loss of several genes causing a predictable phenotype known as a contiguous gene syndrome.

DiGeorge Syndrome

DiGeorge syndrome results from a **deletion of chromosome 22q11.** This deletion leads to abnormal development of the third and fourth pharyngeal pouches and results in thymic hypoplasia and T-cell immunodeficiency.

Points to Remember

- CATCH-22 is a pneumonic to help remember the findings of DiGeorge syndrome—cardiac abnormalities, abnormal facies, thymic aplasia, cleft palate, hypocalcemia, 22q11 deletion.

Clinical Manifestations

- Absent thymus and **T cell-immunodeficiency.**
- Parathyroid hypoplasia and **hypocalcemia,** which can cause seizures and tetany.
- **Congenital heart disease** (conotruncal abnormalities and outflow tract abnormalities, including interrupted aortic arch and tetralogy of Fallot, are most common but pulmonary atresia and VSD are also seen).
- Abnormal facies and palate abnormalities (cleft lip/palate, velopalatal insufficiency).

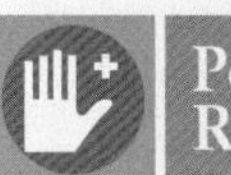

Points to Remember

- The facial appearance of patient's with Wolf-Hirschorn Syndrome has been described as a "greek–helmet-like" appearance.

Wolf-Hirschorn Syndrome

Wolf-Hirschorn syndrome results from deletion of one copy of chromosome 4p16. Clinical features include pre- and postnatal growth retardation, mental retardation dysmorphic facies (protruding eyes, hypertelorism, high nasal bridge, mental retardation and maxillary hypoplasia [Fig. 8.4]), congenital heart defects (e.g., ASD, VSD and others), midline defects, and seizures.

WAGR

WAGR syndrome results from deletion of one copy of chromosome 11p13. The chromosomal region that is deleted contains several genes including the *WT1* gene thought to be responsible for the susceptibility to Wilms tumor (which is seen in about 60% of patients) and GU abnormalities, and the *PAX6* gene, thought to be responsible for the aniridia.

Miller-Dieker Syndrome

Miller-Dieker syndrome is caused by the deletion of several genes on chromosome 17p. Features of this syndrome include **lissencephaly** (smooth brain, without gyri), facial dysmorphism (high

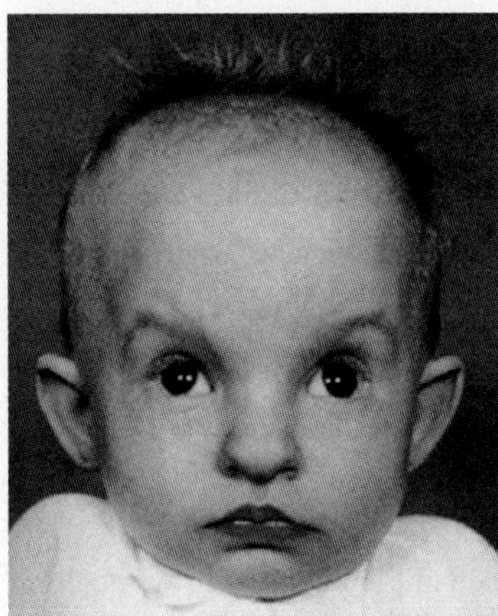

FIGURE 8.4. A child with Wolf-Hirschorn syndrome. Note the widely spaced eyes (hypertelorism) and high nasal bridge. (Reprinted with permission from McMillan JA, Feigin RD, DeAngelis C, et al. *Oski's Pediatrics: Principles and Practice*. 4th ed. Philadelphia: Lippincott Williams &Wilkins; 2006.)

forehead, bitemporal narrowing, short nose), and other anomalies. Deletion or mutation in the *LIS1* gene in this region causes isolated lissencephaly.

Clinical Features

- Mental retardation.

Smith-Magenis Syndrome

Smith-Magenis syndrome is usually due to a deletion of chromosome 17p11.2. Clinical manifestations include mental retardation, speech delay, **self-injurious behavior,** and sleep disturbance. Facial dysmorphisms include synophrys (unibrow), brachycephaly, frontal bossing, and tented upper lip. There can additionally be hearing loss and **tooth agenesis.**

Williams-Beuren Syndrome (Williams Syndrome)

Williams-Beuren syndrome is caused by a deletion on one copy of chromosome 7q11.

Clinical Manifestations

- Mild to moderate mental retardation.
- Heart abnormalities (**supravalvular aortic stenosis,** peripheral pulmonic stenosis).
- Short stature.
- Facial dysmorphism (puffy eyes, flat midface, epicanthal folds).
- Hyperacusis.
- Infantile hypercalcemia.
- **Cocktail personality** and **aptitude for music.**

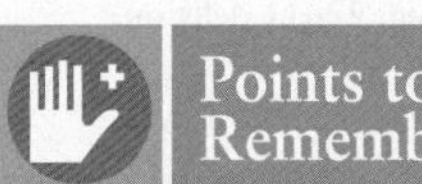
Points to Remember

- Children with Williams syndrome are often described as having a "cocktail personality," because they are often friendly with strangers, have verbal skills which exceed their visuospatial skills, and have a strong aptitude for music.

X-LINKED DISORDERS

A family history in which there are affected males in multiple generations and in which there are **skipped generations** (in which an unaffected female passes the altered gene to her male offspring) offers an important clue to the presence of an X-linked disease. Examples of X-linked disorders include Duchenne type muscular dystrophy, hemophilia, and Alport syndrome. These diseases are discussed briefly in Table 8.2, and are more extensively discussed in other chapters.

TABLE 8.2

COMMON X-LINKED DISORDERS

	Defect	Clinical Characteristics
Duchenne muscular dystrophy	Mutations in dystrophin gene leading to lack of the dystrophin protein	Progressive muscular weakness, wheelchair bound by ~10 y of age
Hemophilia A and B	A—deficiency in factor VIII B—deficiency in factor IX	Prolonged bleeding, bruising, joint and muscle hemorrhage
Alport syndrome	Defect in basement membrane of kidney glomerulus, 85% are caused by mutation in *COL4A5* gene	Nephritis with hematuria and proteinuria (90% advance to end-stage renal disease by age 40 y), sensorineural hearing loss, retinopathy

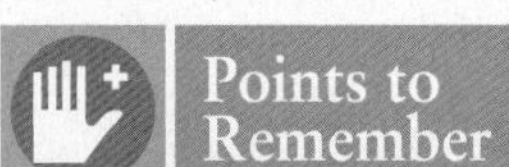
Points to Remember

- Becker muscular dystrophy is a form of X-linked muscular dystrophy that is milder than Duchenne and is caused by a reduction in the amount or function of the dystrophin protein.
- Female carriers of Alport syndrome can also be affected, with about 10% advancing to end-stage renal disease by age 40.

DISORDERS OF IMPRINTING

In disorders of imprinting, the clinical presentation of disease differs depending on whether the gene is inherited from the mother or the father. The most well-known examples are the Prader-Willi syndrome and AS. Prader-Willi syndrome results from loss of paternally inherited genes on chromosome 15q and AS results from the loss of the maternally inherited genes on chromosome 15q.

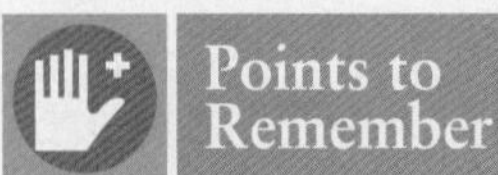
Points to Remember

- Prader-Willi results from the loss of paternally inherited genes. AS results from loss of maternally inherited genes.

Prader-Willi Syndrome

In 75% of cases of Prader-Willi syndrome, the paternally inherited genes are deleted, resulting in only one copy of the responsible genes; in 20% of cases the paternal copy of 15q is deleted and replaced by a second copy of the maternal chromosome 15q, resulting in two copies of the responsible genes, but both copies are inherited from the mother (**uniparental disomy**).

Clinical Manifestations

- Infantile **hypotonia,** poor feeding, and failure to thrive.
- Eventual **hyperphagia** and obesity with onset around the toddler years.
- Hypogonadism, small hands and feet, and short stature.
- Intelligence ranges from low-normal to moderate mental retardation.

Angelman Syndrome

AS has more severe clinical manifestations than Prader-Willi syndrome, including severe mental retardation and seizures.

Clinical Manifestations

- Developmental delay, lack of speech, **mental retardation.**
- Abnormal gait.
- Seizures.
- Acquired microcephaly (normal head circumference at birth, with onset of microcephaly in the toddler years).
- Hypopigmentation.

Beckwith-Wiedemann Syndrome

BWS results from disruption of a region of imprinted genes on chromosome 11p15. There are multiple possible mechanisms that disrupt this region.

Clinical Manifestations

- Macrosomia, hemihyperplasia, macroglossia.
- Organomegaly often leading to **omphalocele.**
- Neonatal **hypoglycemia.**
- Ear lobe pits.
- Predisposition to develop embryonal tumors (e.g., Wilms tumor, hepatoblastoma).

ANTICIPATION

In the process known as anticipation, deleterious repeated nucleotide sequences increase in number from generation to generation and are inherited in an **autosomal dominant manner.** The **expanded repeated sequences** can cause both increased severity of disease as well as earlier onset of disease. Friedreich's ataxia, fragile X syndrome, and myotonic dystrophy are all diseases that have anticipation as their underlying mechanism. Myotonic dystrophy and Friedreich's ataxia are described in greater detail in Chapter 18.

Fragile X Syndrome

Fragile X syndrome is caused by lack of function of the *FMR1* gene on chromosome X. The gene is not functional due to the repeated nucleotide sequence in it. Males are most severely affected, but females can be variably affected based on the percentage of inactivation of the abnormal X chromosome.

Clinical Manifestations

- Mental retardation (moderate to severe), possible autism.
- **Macro-orchidism** (postpubertal).
- Long face, large ears, large jaw.

DISORDERS OF MITOCHONDRIAL INHERITANCE

Disorders of the mitochondria have multiple possible inheritance mechanisms. This is because some of the proteins of the mitochondria are encoded by genes that are entirely processed from gene to protein within the mitochondria. Diseases caused by mutations in these genes are always inherited from the mother, and there is 100% penetrance, although there can be variable expressivity. The disease expression and severity is affected by **heteroplasmy** (the variation in the mitochondrial contents from cell to cell). Thus, depending on the distribution of mitochondria in various organ systems, individuals can be affected by these diseases in very different ways, and variation can occur over time within the same individual. Examples of diseases inherited from the mitochondria include MELAS and MERRF.

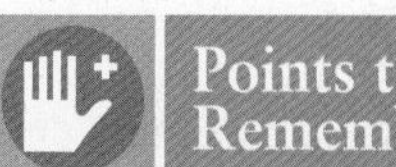

Points to Remember

- Not all of the proteins of the mitochondria are encoded by genes in the mitochondria. Some mitochondrial proteins are encoded by genes located in the nucleus; therefore, disease involving these genes can be inherited in an autosomal dominant or autosomal recessive manner.

MERRF

MERRF is characterized by myoclonus, followed by seizures, ataxia, weakness, and eventually dementia. Early childhood development is usually normal. Other features can include hearing loss, short stature, optic atrophy, pigmentary retinal changes, abnormal fat distribution, and cardiomyopathy with **WPW syndrome.** In the serum, lactate and pyruvate are moderately elevated at rest and increase after activity.

MELAS

MELAS is characterized by **stroke-like episodes,** basal ganglia infarctions, and calcifications. Other features include diabetes mellitus, thyroid dysfunction, and other endocrinologic abnormalities. **Hearing loss** is also a common feature. As with MERRF, lactate and pyruvate are elevated, and increase after exercise.

Leigh Syndrome

Leigh syndrome is a disease resulting in lactic acidemia, most commonly caused by defects in oxidative phosphorylation. It causes focal brain lesions and severe, early-onset neurodegeneration.

DISORDERS OF MULTIFACTORIAL INHERITANCE

NTDs and cleft lip/palate are examples of defects that have both genetic and environmental contributions.

Cleft Lip With or Without Cleft Palate

Cleft lip with or without cleft palate occurs in about 1 in 2,000 live births. About 20% to 50% of these cases are associated with known genetic syndromes. There are likely multiple genes that interact with each other and with environmental factors that lead to clefting. Clearly, there are important genetic causative factors, since 30% of affected individuals have a family history of cleft lip/palate, and offsprings and siblings of affected individuals have an increased risk compared to the general population.

Neural Tube Defects

NTDs are among the most common birth defects, with an incidence of 1 to 2 per 100 births. Both environmental and genetic factors contribute to the development of NTDs. One of the most important environmental factors is maternal intake of **folic acid.** Folic acid supplementation before and during pregnancy decreases the risk of NTDs by 50% to 70%. Genetic factors are thought to play about a 60% role in causing NTDs. The risk of a couple having a second affected child with an NTD is three to five fold over the general population. However, the number and identity of the NTD-related genes is unknown.

AUTOSOMAL DOMINANT DISORDERS

Neurofibromatosis

NF is a disease caused by disruption of the *NF1* gene and is inherited in an autosomal dominant manner. About half of the cases of NF are caused by de novo mutations. A more thorough discussion of NF is included in Chapter 18.

Clinical Manifestations

- **Multiple café au lait spots.**
- Axillary and/or inguinal freckling.
- Neurofibromas.
- Iris Lisch nodules.
- Scoliosis, plexiform neurofibromas, CNS gliomas, and malignant peripheral nerve sheath tumors can be present.

Tuberous Sclerosis

Tuberous sclerosis is an autosomal dominant disorder caused by mutations in either the *TSC1* or *TSC2* genes. Tuberous sclerosis is discussed more extensively in Chapter 18.

Clinical Manifestations

- Skin lesions including **ash leaf spots** (hypomelanotic macules), facial angiofibromas, shagreen patches, and ungual fibromas.
- Brain lesions (cortical tubers, subependymal nodules, seizures).
- Kidney lesions (angiomyolipomas, cysts).
- Heart lesions (**rhabdomyomas**).

Treacher Collins Syndrome

Treacher Collins syndrome is an autosomal dominant disorder of craniofacial development which occurs with an incidence of 1 in 50,000 live births.

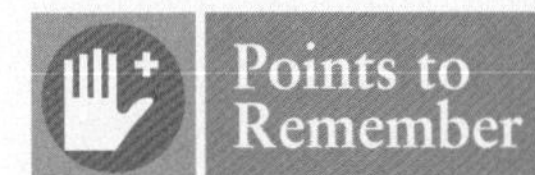

- **Individuals with Treacher Collins syndrome can have airway compromise due to micro/retrognathia.**

Clinical Manifestations

- Midface hypoplasia, **micrognathia.**
- Small and/or misshapen ears, conductive hearing loss.
- Cleft palate.
- **Intelligence is normal.**

Marfan Syndrome

Marfan syndrome is an **autosomal dominant** disorder of connective tissue caused by a mutation in the gene encoding for fibrillin, leading to abnormal TGF-β (transforming growth factor-β) signaling. The birth incidence is around 1 in 9,800. About one quarter of cases arise from new mutations. Marfan syndrome is discussed more extensively in Chapter 5.

Clinical Manifestations

- Progressive aortic dilatation, which can lead to aortic dissection.
- Mitral valve prolapse or mitral incompetence.
- Eye findings, including myopia and lens dislocation.
- Skeletal features, including joint laxity, arachnodactyly, and scoliosis.

Cornelia de Lange Syndrome

Cornelia de Lange syndrome is inherited most often in an autosomal dominant manner, though almost all cases are new mutations.

Clinical Manifestations

- Malformations of the upper extremities.
- **Synophrys (unibrow)**, arched eyebrows, **long eyelashes,** and microcephaly.
- Mental retardation, autistic and self-destructive behavior.
- Cardiac septal defects.
- Hearing loss.
- Myopia.
- Cleft palate.
- GU abnormalities (cryptorchidism or hypoplastic genitalia)
- Congenital diaphragmatic hernias.

CHARGE Syndrome

CHARGE syndrome is a multisystem disorder whose name is also an acronym by which the clinical features can be remembered. CHARGE stands for coloboma, heart malformation, choanal atresia, retardation of growth and/or development, genital anomalies, and ear anomalies. Rhombencephalic dysfunction and hypoplasia of the semicircular canals are also frequently seen. Most cases of CHARGE syndrome are sporadic, and two-thirds of cases are due to a mutation on chromosome 8.

	A	*a*
A	*AA*	*Aa*
a	*Aa*	*aa*

FIGURE 8.5. "*A*" represents the wild-type allele, and "*a*" represents the mutant allele. A child born to two parents with achondroplasia has a 25% chance of inheriting two wild-type alleles ("*AA*") resulting in an individual with average stature, a 50% chance of inheriting one mutant allele ("*Aa*") resulting in achondroplasia, and 25% chance of inheriting two mutant alleles from each parent ("*aa*"), resulting in neonatal lethality.

Achondroplasia

Achondroplasia is caused by a specific mutation in the *FGFR3* gene and is inherited in an autosomal dominant manner. It occurs in 1 in 10,000 to 30,000 live births, and more than 80% cases are the result of a de novo mutation.

Clinical Manifestations

- Short stature and rhizomelia (disproportionately short proximal arms and legs).
- Macrocephaly.
- Facial features such as frontal bossing and midface hypoplasia.
- Cervicomedullary compression.
- **Normal intelligence.**

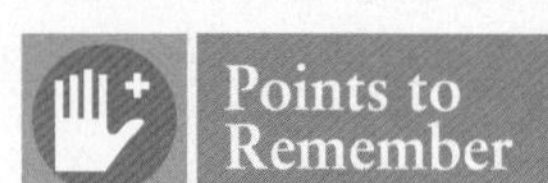

- Cervicomedullary compression can lead to neurologic deficits.

When a child is born to two parents affected with achondroplasia, there is a 25% chance of that child inheriting two mutant copies of the gene (Fig. 8.5). This is not compatible with survival.

Osteogenesis Imperfecta

OI is a group of disorders in which there is a **wide range of severity** ranging from lethality in the newborn period (OI type II) to mild predisposition to fracturing in adulthood. OI types I to V are inherited in an autosomal dominant manner, and OI type VII is inherited in an autosomal recessive manner.

Clinical Manifestations

Clinical manifestations depending on the type of OI:

- Fractures of varying ages and stages of healing, **wormian bones,** vertebral compression fractures, and osteopenia.
- Abnormal dentition including brown or gray teeth and weak teeth.
- Progressive hearing loss.
- **Blue-colored sclerae** and ligamentous laxity.

Noonan Syndrome

Noonan syndrome is a multiple congenital anomaly syndrome characterized by congenital heart disease, chest wall abnormalities, and other features. Four causative genes have been identified, and each independently causes Noonan syndrome.

Clinical Manifestations

- Cardiac anomalies (e.g., **pulmonary valve stenosis,** often with dysplasia, ASDs and VSDs, branch pulmonary artery stenosis, tetralogy of Fallot and **hypertrophic cardiomyopathy**).
- Short stature.
- Broad or webbed neck.
- Shield-shaped chest with low-set nipples.
- Coagulation disorders and lymphatic abnormalities.
- Mild mental retardation in up to one-third of individuals.

AUTOSOMAL RECESSIVE DISORDERS

Meckel-Gruber Syndrome

Meckel-Gruber syndrome is characterized by **renal cysts,** CNS abnormalities (encephalocele, Dandy-Walker malformation, hydrocephalus), liver abnormalities (biliary duct dysplasia and liver cysts), and postaxial polydactyly.

MISCELLANEOUS DISORDERS

Vacterl

There are many syndromes in which an underlying genetic cause is strongly suspected but no causative gene has been discovered. One such clinical presentation is known as the VACTERL association. The name is an acronym that stands for the most prominent clinical features: vertebral defects, anal atresia, cardiac defects, tracheo-esophageal fistula, renal malformations, and limb defects. Facial dysmorphisms, learning disabilities, and growth abnormalities are common.

Goldenhar Syndrome

Goldenhar syndrome, also known as hemifacial microsomia or oculoauriculovertebral syndrome, is a disorder that involves the **first and second branchial arch derivatives.** Most cases are sporadic but autosomal dominant inheritance is occasionally seen. There is a wide range of clinical presentations.

Clinical Manifestations

- Craniofacial asymmetry.
- Ocular dermoid growths.
- Unilateral ear deformities ranging from pits and tags to anotia.
- Additional features, including cardiac defects, vertebral defects, and CNS defects.

SAMPLE BOARD REVIEW QUESTIONS

1. A 4-year-old child is seen in your office. She is very friendly and has a strong aptitude for music. She has an IQ of 70. She has a history of supravalvular aortic stenosis that was repaired in infancy. She was also noted to have hypercalcemia as an infant. What chromosome abnormality is most likely in this patient?
   a. Trisomy 21
   b. Deletion of chromosome 7q11
   c. Deletion of chromosome 17p11.2
   d. Monosomic for the X chromosome
   e. Deletion of chromosome 5p

   Answer: b. This patient most likely has Williams syndrome, which is caused by a deletion of chromosome 7q11. Patients with Williams syndrome are often referred to as having "cocktail party" personalities due to their strength of verbal skills which are out of proportion to their visuospatial skills. They often have an aptitude for music. There is an association with congenital heart disease, especially supravalvular aortic stenosis. Idiopathic hypercalcemia of the newborn is seen in 15% of cases.

2. You are seeing a 15-year-old patient who has multiple café au lait spots and a history of a plexiform neuroma. What other clinical manifestations would be consistent with a diagnosis of NF type 1?
   a. Axillary freckling
   b. Bilateral vestibular schwannomas
   c. Conotruncal cardiac anomaly
   d. 2,3 toe syndactyly
   e. Ash leaf spots

   Answer: a. Diagnostic criteria for NF type 1 include the following: six or more café au lait macules, two or more neurofibromas of any type or one plexiform neurofibroma, freckling in the axillary or inguinal region, an optic glioma, two or more iris hamartomas, and osseous lesions such as sphenoid dysplasia and a first degree relative with NF1. Bilateral vestibular schwannomas are seen in NF type 2.

3. A 5-year-old child with a known genetic syndrome comes to your office for a routine check-up. As an infant he was very hypotonic and had failure to thrive. However, once he entered the toddler years he became hyperphagic. Physical examination at this visit reveals an obese child with small hands and feet. He has moderate mental retardation. Which of the following types of genetic abnormalities is responsible for this patient's genetic syndrome?
   a. A deletion of the paternal copy of chromosome 15q resulting in maternal uniparental disomy
   b. A deletion of the maternal copy of chromosome 15q resulting in paternal uniparental disomy
   c. A mitochondrial deletion passed from the mother
   d. Deletion of chromosome 12q
   e. Translocation between chromosome 5p and 1p

Answer: a. This child has Prader-Willi syndrome, which is caused by disruption of the paternal copy of chromosome 15q. This area of the genome is imprinted; certain genes are expressed in a parent-of-origin-specific manner. If the maternal copy of chromosome 15q is disrupted, the child would have AS.

4. You are called to see a 2-day-old newborn baby in the nursery. She has excess skin at the back of her neck and widely spaced nipples. You are concerned about a possible diagnosis of Turner syndrome. What physical finding would be consistent with anomalies seen in Turner syndrome?
   a. Bilateral hip clicks
   b. Asymmetric Moro reflex
   c. Reduced femoral pulse
   d. Lack of red reflex bilaterally
   e. Periumbilical abdominal mass

Answer: c. Reduced femoral pulses would be consistent with coarctation of the aorta, which is the most common cardiac anomaly seen in Turner syndrome.

5. A baby boy is born with an omphalocele. Upon further examination he has an enlarged tongue and bilateral ear pits. He also has hypoglycemia that is difficult to control. Based on the most likely genetic diagnosis, what medical surveillance will this child require throughout his early childhood?
   a. Annual brain magnetic resonance imaging
   b. Abdominal ultrasound every three months
   c. Annual measurement of homocysteine levels
   d. Echocardiogram every 6 months
   e. Annual hearing screen

Answer: b. This child most likely has BWS. Children with this syndrome are prone to embryonal tumors such as Wilms tumor and hepatoblastoma. They should have an abdominal ultrasound every 3 months for the first 8 years of life, as well as α-fetoprotein measurements.

6. A 15-year-old boy with a known genetic diagnosis is seen in your office for well-child care. He has macro-orchidism, a long face with large ears and a large jaw. He has mental retardation and some autistic features. His mother has a history of premature ovarian failure. What is the mechanism of inheritance of this syndrome?
   a. X-linked
   b. Autosomal recessive
   c. Autosomal dominant
   d. Mitochondrial
   e. Multigenic

Answer: a. This child has fragile X syndrome. This is an X-linked mental retardation syndrome. It is caused by a triple repeat in the *FMR1* gene. This triplet repeat can be unstable once it is of a certain size and can expand from one generation to the next. Women who carry the premutation are prone to premature ovarian failure.

7. The genetic mutation that causes the above child's syndrome is:
   a. A point mutation
   b. An expanded triplet nucleotide repeat
   c. An unbalanced translocation
   d. An extra chromosome
   e. A contiguous gene deletion

Answer: b. This child has fragile X syndrome, an X linked mental retardation syndrome. It is caused by a triple repeat in the *FMR1* gene. This triplet repeat can be unstable once it is of a certain size and can expand from one generation to the next.

8. You see an 8-year-old child for well-child care in your office. He has no health complaints at this time. He is very tall and thin and has long fingers. He also has a pectus excavatum, flat feet, and very lax joints. You send him for an ophthalmology exam and find that he has bilateral partially dislocated lenses. What is the most important diagnostic test for him to undergo at this time?
   a. An echocardiogram to examine for a VSD
   b. A renal ultrasound to look for renal cysts
   c. An echocardiogram to examine aortic root diameter
   d. An abdominal ultrasound to look for liver tumors
   e. A renal ultrasound to look for hydronephrosis

Answer: c. This child likely has Marfan syndrome, which is a connective tissue disorder caused by mutations in the fibrillin 1 gene. The major source of morbidity and mortality in these patients is due to cardiovascular manifestations. These manifestations include dilation of the aortic root, which can rupture or dissect. The size of the aortic root should be measured regularly, with surgical repair indicated when the diameter reaches a critical size. At this age, measurement of the aortic root will help to confirm the diagnosis as well as provide a baseline for future measurements.

9. A baby is stillborn. He has bilateral renal agenesis. There was severe oligohydramnios during the pregnancy. The facial features of this child are flattened, and there are bilateral clubfeet. The flat facial features are an example of which of the following?
   a. Malformation
   b. Disruption
   c. Teratogen
   d. Placental abnormality
   e. Deformation

Answer: e. The flattened facial features are due to intrauterine space constraints caused by the lack of amniotic fluid (caused by the renal agenesis). A deformation is caused by factors external to the developing fetus causing altered structural development.

10. You see a child in your office with MELAS. She has a history of lactic acidemia with multiple strokes. She also has hearing loss and hypothyroidism. Based upon the mechanism of inheritance of this disease, how are her parents affected?
   a. Her mother or father is affected since this is an autosomal dominant disease
   b. Neither of her parents is affected since this is an autosomal recessive disease
   c. Her mother is affected since this is a mitochondrial disease
   d. Her father is affected since this is a Y-linked disease
   e. Neither parent is affected since this is caused by a virus

Answer: c. MELAS is inherited through the mitochondrial DNA. Only the mother passes mitochondria to the offspring. The mother can be mildly or severely affected depending on the percentage of affected mitochondria she has (heteroplasmy).

11. Which of the following syndromes has mental retardation as one of its features?
   a. Achondroplasia
   b. Treacher Collins
   c. OI
   d. Marfan syndrome
   e. Miller-Dieker syndrome

Answer: e. Miller-Dieker syndrome is a disease which has lissencephaly (smooth brain, cerebral gyri are absent or abnormally large) as one of its major features. These children have severe mental retardation.

12. You see a child in clinic with a known genetic mutation in the *FGFR3* gene. He has macrocephaly, midface hypoplasia, and short stature. He has normal intelligence, and is doing well in school. What else would you expect to find on his physical exam?
   a. Short torso compared to limb length
   b. Short proximal limbs
   c. Normal arm length, but short leg length
   d. Café au lait spots
   e. Extra digits

Answer: b. This child has achondroplasia, which has rhizomelia (shortening of the proximal limbs) as it's cardinal feature.

13. A newborn baby has the following features: microcephaly, cutis aplasia of the scalp, microphthalmia, and cleft palate. Further diagnostic workup reveals a tetralogy of Fallot and holoprosencephaly. What is the most likely diagnosis?
   a. Trisomy 18
   b. Trisomy 21
   c. Trisomy 13
   d. Monosomy X
   e. Trisomy 17

Answer: c. This child most likely has trisomy 13. Additional clinical features include flexed and overlapping fingers, polydactyly, and hernias. Survival is in general very limited, but about 5% of children born with trisomy 13 live beyond 1 year of age. Survivors have severe mental retardation.

14. You see a child in your office with history of a conotruncal cardiac anomaly, which has been repaired. He also had seizures as an infant due to hypocalcemia. He has nasal speech and a repaired cleft palate. What is his most likely genetic abnormality?
   a. Deletion of chromosome 22q11
   b. Deletion of chromosome 5p
   c. Point mutation in the *FGFR3* gene
   d. Deletion of chromosome 4p16
   e. Deletion of chromosome 7q11

Answer: a. This child most likely has DiGeorge syndrome, which is caused by a deletion of chromosome 22q11. Conotruncal cardiac anomalies are the most common, but outflow tract anomalies can also be seen. Additional features include absent thymus and T cell immunodeficiency, and increased risk for psychiatric disorders.

15. A couple decides that they want to have a second child. Their first child has a recessive disease. What is the chance that the second child will be a carrier for this disease?
   a. 25%
   b. 100%
   c. 30%
   d. 50%
   e. 75%

Answer: d. Each parent is a carrier for this disease (they each have one normal and one abnormal copy of the gene in question). They each have a 50% chance of passing the abnormal gene to every offspring. There is a 25% chance that the offspring will have the disease (two abnormal copies of the gene), a 50% chance that they will carry the disease (one normal and one abnormal copy if the gene), and a 25% chance of having two normal copies of the gene.

SUGGESTED READINGS

Jones K. *Smith's Recognizable Patterns of Human Malformation*. Philadelphia: Elsevier; 2005.

Moeschler JB, Shevell M, and the Committee on Genetics. Clinical genetic evaluation of the child with mental retardation or developmental delays. *Pediatrics*. 2006;117:2304–2316.

CHAPTER 9 ■ EAR, NOSE, AND THROAT

JOSEPH B. CANTEY

AAP	American Academy of Pediatrics	EBV	Epstein-Barr virus
AOM	Acute otitis media	ENT	Ear, nose, and throat
BAER	Brainstem auditory evoked response	GERD	Gastroesophageal reflux disease
		HIV	Human immunodeficiency virus
CHL	Conductive hearing loss	OME	Otitis media with effusion
CMV	Cytomegalovirus	PPD	Purified protein derivative
CT	Computed tomography	SNHL	Sensorineural hearing loss

CHAPTER OBJECTIVES

1. To understand the major etiologies and appropriate initial management of hearing loss in children
2. To review the proper management of common congenital malformations of the upper airway, including abnormalities of the external ear and cleft lip and/or palate
3. To review the clinical manifestations, differential diagnosis, and management of infants with laryngomalacia
4. To review the epidemiology, clinical manifestations, diagnosis, and management of otitis externa, acute otitis media, and otitis media with effusion
5. To understand the etiologies, clinical manifestations, and appropriate management of patients with mastoiditis, sinusitis, and parotitis
6. To understand the epidemiology, clinical manifestations, diagnosis, and management of cervical lymphadenitis and deep neck infections (e.g., retropharyngeal and peritonsillar abscesses) in children.

NONINFECTIOUS DISORDERS OF THE EARS, NOSE, AND THROAT

Hearing Loss

Neonates are born with fully functional auditory systems that can distinguish sounds of different amplitudes, pitch, and frequency. Although infants do not gain the ability to generate specific words until approximately 1 year of age, receptive auditory stimulation is critical for the attainment of verbal milestones. Failure to promptly identify and manage infants and children with hearing loss can result in severe deficits in both verbal and social development. The AAP recommends universal newborn hearing screening, as well as periodic hearing screening for well children through adolescence.

Points to Remember

- **The initial evaluation of a child with language delay should always include a hearing test.**

Etiologies of Hearing Loss

Hearing loss can be genetic or acquired.

Genetic hearing loss can occur as an isolated condition or can be one feature of a more complex disorder. Table 9.1 provides a brief summary of genetic conditions associated with hearing loss that have distinguishing characteristics beyond hearing loss.

Etiologies of acquired hearing loss include perinatal and postnatal causes:

- Perinatal causes of hearing loss include low birth weight, hypoxia or asphyxia, hyperbilirubinemia, mechanical ventilation, ototoxic medications (e.g., aminoglycosides, loop diuretics) meningitis, and perinatal infections (e.g., congenital CMV, congenital rubella).

Points to Remember

- **Congenital CMV is the leading infectious cause of acquired hearing loss in children. Hearing loss is often present at birth but can develop and/or become clinically significant later in childhood, emphasizing the need for ongoing screening.**

TABLE 9.1

GENETIC CONDITIONS ASSOCIATED WITH HEARING LOSS

	Inheritance	Additional Features
Neurofibromatosis I	Autosomal dominant	Café-au-lait spots, optic gliomas
Neurofibromatosis II	Autosomal dominant	Café-au-lait spots, acoustic neuromas
Treacher–Collins	Autosomal dominant	Malar hypoplasia, cleft palate, retrognathia
Alport syndrome	Autosomal dominant	Nephritis and renal failure
Waardenburg syndrome	Autosomal dominant	White/gray forelock, synophrys (unibrow)
Usher syndrome	Autosomal recessive	Retinitis pigmentosa, vestibular dysfunction
Pendred syndrome	Autosomal recessive	Goiter, ±hypothyroidism
Jervell and Lange–Nielson syndrome	Autosomal recessive	Prolonged QT interval

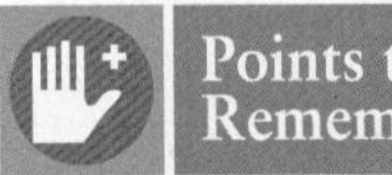

Points to Remember

- Sensorineural hearing loss is the most common readily identifiable sequelae of bacterial meningitis, with deafness present in approximately 31% of pneumococcal meningitis cases, 10% of meningococcal meningitis cases, and 6% of Hib meningitis cases. Hearing loss occurs early in the course of illness and, if present, will be evident by the time of hospital discharge—thus, all infants and children with bacterial meningitis should have a hearing test before or soon after hospital discharge.

- Acquired causes of hearing loss after the perinatal period include meningitis, recurrent middle-ear infections, longstanding otitis media with effusion, and noise-induced hearing loss.

Conductive Versus Sensorineural Hearing Loss

- Conductive hearing loss (CHL) results when obstruction of the outer ear, impedance of the normal compliance of the tympanic membrane, or structural middle-ear pathology precludes sound from being received by the cochlea. Causes of CHL include stenotic or atretic ear canals, cerumen impaction, foreign bodies, otitis externa, otitis media, chronic middle-ear effusions, tympanic perforation, and tympanosclerosis. Audiometric testing in CHL reveals a discrepancy between air conduction (poor) and bone conduction (normal).
- Sensorineural hearing loss (SNHL) results from damage to or malformation of the vestibulocochlear nerve (CNVIII) tract or cochlea. Causes of SNHL include meningitis, ototoxic drugs, congenital infections, perinatal hypoxia, and hereditary conditions. Audiometric testing in SNHL reveals similarly poor results with both air and bone conduction. Electrophysiologic testing with the brainstem auditory evoked response (BAER) test can help localize the lesion.

Diagnosis

Diagnosis of suspected hearing loss begins with a comprehensive history and physical examination, with particular attention paid to perinatal and family history, dysmorphic physical findings, and thorough inspection of the ears, auditory canals, and tympanic membranes. Even in the presence of a suggestive history and physical examination, however, formal audiometric testing is needed to identify the degree and location of impairment.

Audiometry can be behavioral (measuring children's responses to auditory stimuli, such as looking for sounds or completing a task) or electrophysiologic (responses are measured regardless of the patient's participation). Types of audiometric testing are shown in Table 9.2.

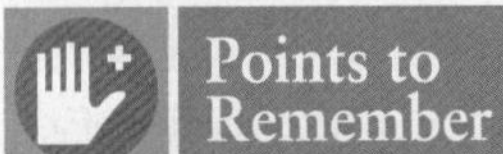

Points to Remember

- Patients with osteogenesis imperfecta are at risk for developing conductive hearing loss.
- The etiology of CHL is more likely to be identified on physical examination than SNHL, and the majority of causes are either medically or surgically treatable.

Management

- CHL is usually receptive to medical or surgical intervention. For example, chronic middle-ear effusions can be drained with tympanostomy tubes, and cerumen can be disimpacted under direct visualization.
- SNHL presents more of a challenge as damage is more likely to be permanent regardless of etiology. Efforts to treat SNHL include various amplification devices and cochlear implants.

Congenital Malformations of the External Ear

Congenital anomalies of the external ear are usually distinct from malformation of the middle and inner ear. Anomalies range from complete absence of the external ear (anotia), to a hypoplastic ear (microtia), to a specific deformity (e.g., ear pits or tags). These malformations are usually corrected by plastic surgery. Ear pits or tags have classically been associated with other systemic malformations, particularly renal anomalies, and may be seen in systemic dysmorphology syndromes. However, in a well-appearing infant with an otherwise normal physical examination, renal ultrasonography and/or or further work-up is not indicated in the setting of ear tags or pits alone.

TABLE 9.2

TYPES OF AUDIOMETRIC TESTING

Test	Type	Description	Ages
Behavioral observation	Behavioral	Measures child's response to lateral sounds, including change in suck, widening of eyes, or attempts to localize sound	<6 mo
Visual reinforcement	Behavioral	Reinforces attempts to localize sound with reward of animation or toy for correct responses	6 mo to 3 y
Conditioned play	Behavioral	Conditions child to complete task in response to auditory stimuli	3–5 y
Conventional audiometry	Behavioral	Child raises hand on side of stimulus; requires cooperation	~5 y on
Tympanometry	Electrophysiologic	Not technically a hearing test; measures compliance of tympanic membrane	Any
Otoacoustic emissions	Electrophysiologic	Measures electrical response of cochlear hair cells to sound stimulus; measures cochlear function but not CN VIII function	Any
Brainstem auditory evoked response (BAER)	Electrophysiologic	Measures action potentials from cochlea to brainstem; often requires sedation and cannot be interpreted in setting of neurologic dysfunction	Any

Cleft Lip and/or Palate

Cleft lip and/or palate occurs in approximately 1 in 750 children. A combination of cleft lip and cleft palate is more common than isolated occurrences of either. Collectively, two-thirds are associated with other dysmorphisms and/or known syndromes and one-third occur as an isolated finding. The risk of recurrence varies widely between isolated clefts and inherited or syndromic clefts. In the case of isolated clefts, the risk of a similar anomaly for a first-degree relative of an affected individual is 2% to 4%.

Infants with cleft palates are at risk for feeding difficulties and may require special nipples for bottle feeding and/or orthodontic devices to facilitate breast-feeding. Attention to growth is critical. These patients are also at risk for recurrent episodes of acute otitis media secondary to Eustachian tube obstruction. Depending on the severity of the cleft lip or palate, definitive surgical management can range from single-stage correction to extensive serial correction over years.

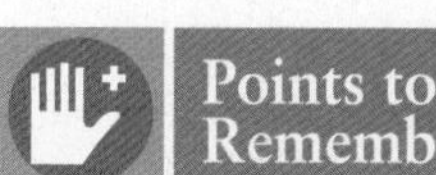

Points to Remember

- **Cleft palate without cleft lip is more likely to be associated with other congenital anomalies than either cleft lip alone or cleft lip with cleft palate.**

Laryngomalacia

Laryngomalacia is the prolapse of the epiglottis, aryepiglottic folds, or arytenoid cartilages due to poor neurologic control, redundant laryngeal soft tissue, or inadequate cartilaginous support. It is a common cause of chronic and/or recurrent stridor in infants and is almost always noticed within the first few weeks or months of life. Most cases are mild and resolve spontaneously by the age of 12 months.

Clinical Manifestations

- Intermittent stridor exacerbated by crying, supine positioning, and upper respiratory infections.
- More severe laryngomalacia can be associated with feeding difficulties, failure to thrive, cyanosis, and/or apnea.
- There is an association between laryngomalacia and GERD in some infants.

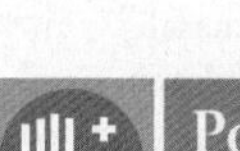

Points to Remember

- **Laryngomalacia is a common cause of chronic and/or recurrent stridor in infants. The differential diagnosis for laryngomalacia includes subglottic stenosis, vocal cord paralysis, and tracheomalacia.**

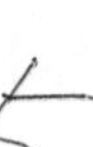

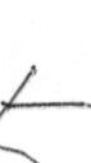

Diagnosis

- The diagnosis can be made in most cases on the basis of an office examination complemented by fiberoptic laryngoscopy.
- Direct visualization of the airway via direct laryngoscopy and bronchoscopy or flexible fiberoptic bronchoscopy is only indicated for more severe or atypical cases of laryngomalacia.

Management

- Ninety percent of patients with laryngomalacia will experience spontaneous resolution by the age of 12 months.
- Medical management of any associated GERD.
- Surgical intervention via supraglottoplasty or tracheotomy is indicated for severe cases associated with respiratory compromise and/or failure to thrive.

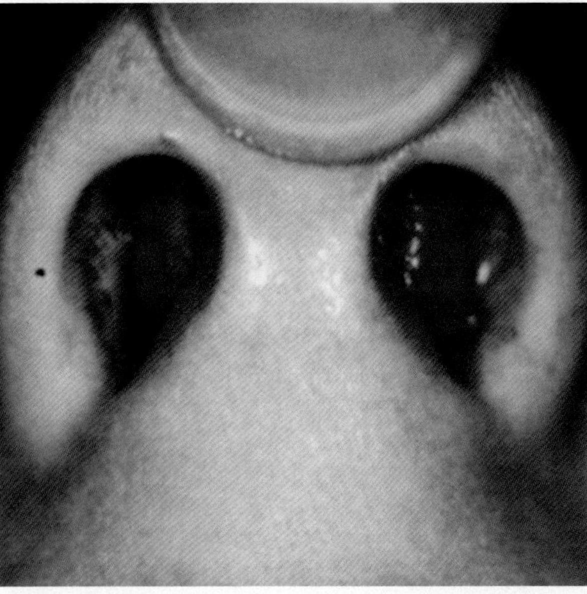

FIGURE 9.1. Bilateral septal hematomas. (*Used with permission from* Handler SD, Myer CM. Atlas of ear, nose and throat disorders in children. Ontario, Canada: BC Decker; 1998:52.)

Nasal Septal Hematoma

Nasal septal hematomas are a rare but potentially serious complication of nasal trauma. The rich vascular supply of the nose allows for pooling and collection of the blood between the cartilage of the nose and the perichondrium. Progressive swelling and pressure on the feeding arteries from the hematoma can lead to irreversible avascular necrosis of the nasal cartilage.

Clinical Manifestations

- Nasal septal hematomas classically present within a few days of the trauma with nasal obstruction and pain.
- Examination of the nasal septum reveals a swollen, boggy mucosa with swelling over the hematoma site (Fig. 9.1).
- Bilateral lesions are much more common than unilateral ones.

Diagnosis

- Direct visualization on physical examination.

Management

- Immediate otolaryngology consultation for incision, drainage, and packing to relieve the pressure and prevent permanent deformation of the nasal airway.
- Empiric antibiotics are commonly prescribed because the pooled blood provides a portal of entry for bacteria. Coverage should include *Staphylococcus aureus*, group A streptococcus, *Streptococcus pneumoniae*, *Moraxella catarrhalis*, and *Haemophilus influenzae*.

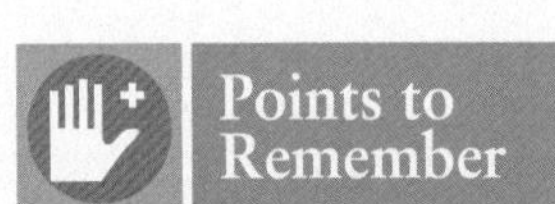

Points to Remember

- Nasal polyps can be associated with any condition leading to chronic inflammation of the nasal passages. In children, nasal polyps are often associated with asthma and cystic fibrosis.

INFECTIOUS DISORDERS OF THE EARS, NOSE, AND THROAT

The Common Cold

Common colds are a frequent reason for outpatient visits to general pediatric clinics and emergency rooms. On average, children have six to eight colds per year. The peak incidence is in the second 6 months of life and remains persistent until the second decade of life. Over 200 viruses have been identified as causative organisms, many of which belong to the rhinovirus family. Several of the viruses that cause common colds are also capable of causing lower tract disease (e.g., influenza, parainfluenza, RSV, human metapneumovirus).

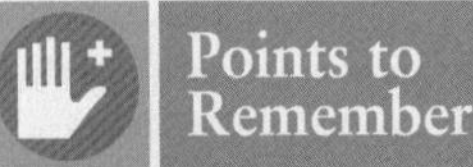

Points to Remember

- The differential diagnosis for rhinorrhea should include infectious causes, allergic causes, and foreign body impaction.

Clinical Manifestations

- Pharyngitis, sneezing, cough, nasal congestion, and rhinitis are classic symptoms.
- Fever is more common in younger children and is usually low grade.
- Illness duration is usually 6 to 7 days but can be as long as 2 weeks.
- Complications include otitis media, sinusitis, or lower respiratory tract illness.

Diagnosis

- Diagnosis is clinical.
- Laboratory work and imaging are not indicated for routine common colds.

Management

- Treatment of the common cold is supportive and primarily focuses on ensuring adequate hydration; supportive care for infants may include gentle bulb suctioning and/or nasal saline drops to relieve nasal obstruction.
- Over-the-counter cough and cold medicines are NOT beneficial and can be harmful, especially in infants and toddlers.

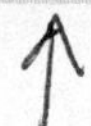

Points to Remember

- The Food and Drug Administration (FDA) has banned all over-the-counter cough and cold medicines in children under 2 because of lack of efficacy and potential harm.

Otitis Externa

Otitis externa (i.e., "swimmer's ear") is the infection of the epithelial lining of the external auditory canal. *Pseudomonas aeruginosa* and *S. aureus* are the most common causative pathogens.

Clinical Manifestations

- Otalgia with manipulation of the tragus or pinna.
- Erythema, edema, and drainage of the external auditory canal.
- Complications include cellulitis and abscess formation.

Diagnosis

- Visual inspection via otoscopy.

Management

- Topical antibiotic drops with anti-pseudomonas and anti-staphylococcal activity.
- Topical steroids (e.g., dexamethasone) are added to some antibiotic formulations.
- Pain control with NSAIDS.

Points to Remember

- Otalgia and purulent otorrhea can be seen with otitis externa, AOM with perforation, and foreign body impaction. Careful otoscopic examination is needed for differentiation.

Acute Otitis Media (AOM)

AOM is one of the most common infections of childhood. It is often preceded by an upper respiratory tract infection. Peak incidence is between 6 months and 3 years of age, by which time 80% of children have had at least one episode. Two-thirds of cases of AOM are due to bacterial infections. Common pathogens include *S. pneumonia*, nontypeable *H. influenzae*, and *M. catarrhalis*.

Clinical Manifestations

- Acute onset of otalgia.
- Fever.
- Irritability.
- Severe complications are rare but include mastoiditis, labyrinthitis, osteomyelitis, facial nerve paralysis, epidural and subdural abscess, meningitis, and lateral sinus thrombosis
- Otoscopic findings consistent with AOM include erythema and/or bulging of the tympanic membrane, loss of normal landmarks, and decreased mobility with insufflation (Fig. 9.2B).

Points to Remember

- Otalgia is an important feature of AOM but can also be due to Eustachian tube dysfunction associated with a viral upper respiratory tract infection or referred pain from infectious or noninfectious conditions of the tonsils, adenoids, teeth, or pharynx.

Diagnosis

- Diagnosis is clinical and is based on the presence of symptoms and findings on otoscopy.

Management

- Antimicrobial therapy for AOM has increasingly come into question, particularly in well-appearing, older children. The AAP supports "watchful waiting" for 48 to 72 hours as an option in select cases. In an otherwise healthy child with nonsevere illness and adequate follow-up, a period of watchful waiting is an option for patients who are at least two years old (Table 9.3).

Points to Remember

- Watchful waiting is NOT an option for infants less than 6 months of age, patients between 6 months and 2 years of age in whom the diagnosis is certain, and patients with underlying risk factors for severe or recurrent infection (e.g., trisomy 21, cleft palate).

TABLE 9.3

AAP RECOMMENDATIONS ON THE MANAGEMENT OF AOM

	Severe Illness[a]	Nonsevere Illness
<6 mo	Treat	Treat
6 mo to 2 y	Treat	Treat if certain of diagnosis
>2 y	Treat	Watchful waiting possible

[a]Severe illness = fever >39°C and/or moderate-to-severe otalgia.

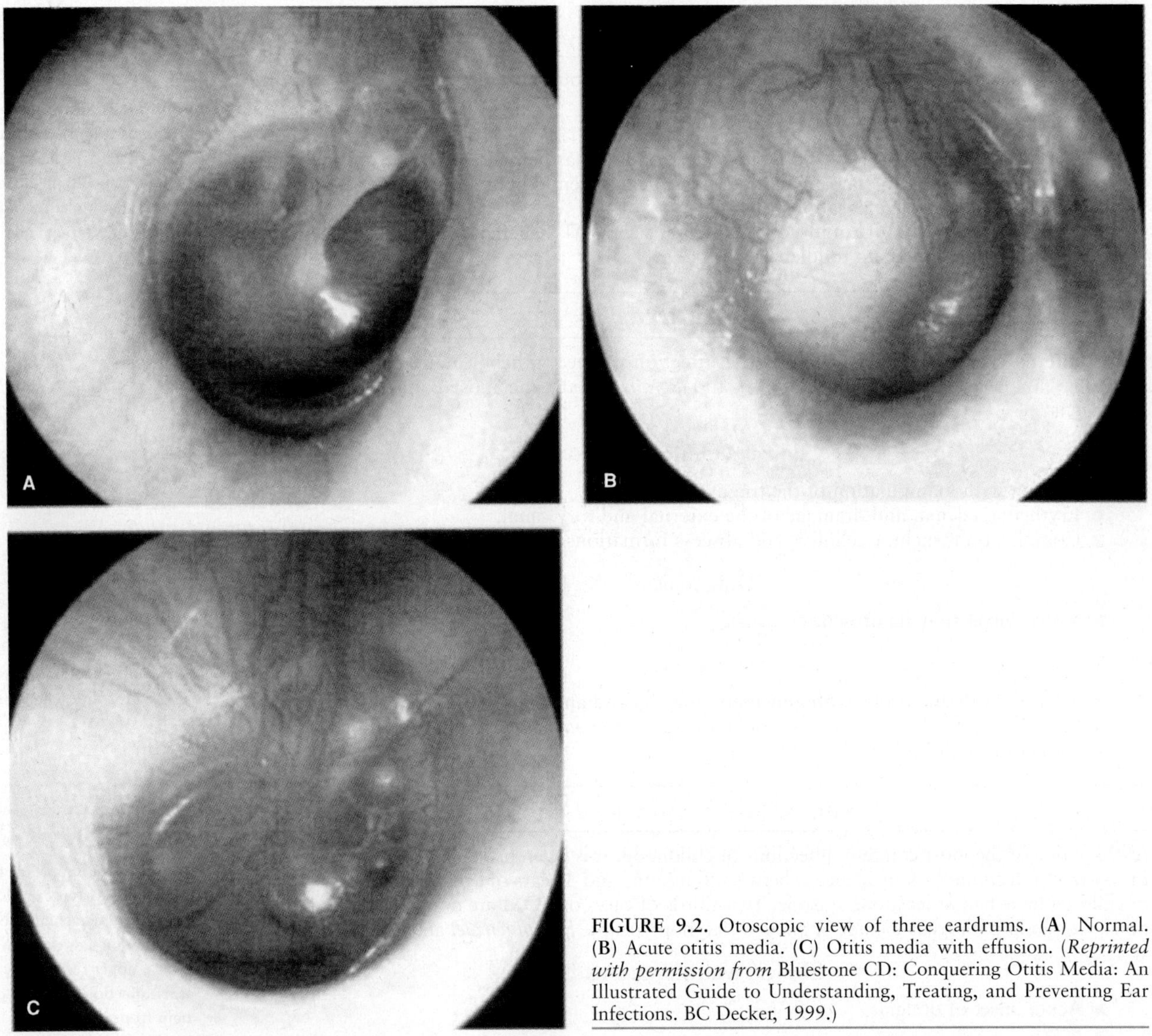

FIGURE 9.2. Otoscopic view of three eardrums. (**A**) Normal. (**B**) Acute otitis media. (**C**) Otitis media with effusion. (*Reprinted with permission from* Bluestone CD: Conquering Otitis Media: An Illustrated Guide to Understanding, Treating, and Preventing Ear Infections. BC Decker, 1999.)

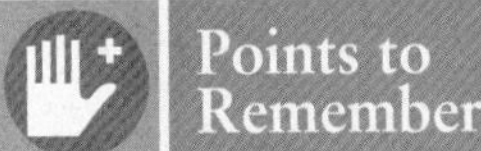

- Recurrent AOM is common. Anatomic malformations, particularly those involving mid-face hypoplasia or increased flexibility or tortuosity of the Eustachian tube, can predispose to recurrent fluid collections in the middle ear that may then become infected. Myringotomy and tympanostomy tube placement is one treatment option for children with recurrent AOM.

- High-dose amoxicillin or amoxicillin-clavulanate are first-line therapies for patient who require antibiotics. Macrolides can be used for penicillin-allergic patients.

Otitis Media with Effusion (OME)

OME is a common diagnosis in children and often occurs following an episode of AOM. Approximately 10% of children with AOM will have a subsequent middle-ear effusion that lasts for 3 months or longer.

Clinical Manifestations

- OME is often asymptomatic but can be associated with a feeling of fullness in the affected ear and/or conductive hearing loss.
- Pneumatic otoscopy reveals an opaque tympanic membrane with visible fluid behind the membrane but without inflammation (see Fig. 9.2C).

Diagnosis

- Visual inspection via otoscopy.

Management

- Most cases of OME will resolve without specific intervention and without permanent sequelae.

- OME that is persistent or associated with significant symptoms (e.g., hearing loss) warrants intervention; the role of antimicrobial therapy is controversial; definitive treatment is via myringotomy and tympanostomy tube placement.

Points to Remember

- Of the four paired paranasal sinuses, the ethmoid, maxillary, and sphenoid sinuses are present at birth. The frontal sinuses begin to form after the first birthday but generally do not become clinically important until around 10 years of age.

Mastoiditis

Local spread of an episode of acute otitis media can result in infection of the ipsilateral mastoid air spaces or mastoiditis. This represents one of the rare but serious complications of AOM. Common causative organisms for acute mastoiditis include *S. pneumoniae*, *H. influenzae*, group A streptococcus, and *S. aureus*. Chronic mastoiditis is often polymicrobial and is most commonly caused by anaerobic bacteria and Gram-negative bacilli (including *P. aeruginosa*). *Mycobacterium tuberculosis* is a rare but important cause of chronic mastoiditis.

Clinical Manifestations

- Fever.
- Otalgia.
- Postauricular swelling, tenderness, and redness with external ear displaced inferiorly and anteriorly (Fig. 9.3).
- Complications include meningitis, brain abscess, epidural abscess, subdural empyema, venous sinus thrombosis, subperiosteal abscess, facial-nerve paralysis, jugular venous thrombosis, and internal carotid artery erosion and hemorrhage.

Points to Remember

- Children with mastoiditis almost always have a concomitant AOM on the ipsilateral side.

Diagnosis

- Classic mastoiditis can be a clinical diagnosis.
- Confirmatory plain films or computed tomography (CT) scans of the mastoid area reveal coalescence of the air cells or evidence of sclerosing osteomyelitis.

Management

Medical Management

- Initial empiric therapy for acute mastoiditis should include broad-spectrum coverage with vancomycin and a third-generation cephalosporin.
- Initial empiric therapy for chronic mastoiditis should include broad-spectrum coverage with vancomycin and a third-generation cephalosporin in addition to anti-*pseudomonal* and anaerobic coverage.
- Long-term antimicrobial therapy should be tailored by microbiologic diagnosis of tympanocentesis fluid or selected on the basis of results of culture of middle-ear fluid or fluid drained from the mastoid itself.

Surgical Management

- Lack of appropriate response to medical therapy or development of complications necessitates mastoidectomy and possibly other surgical interventions.

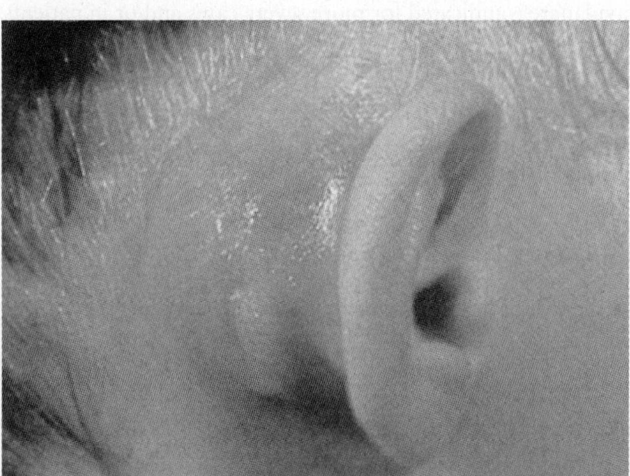

FIGURE 9.3. Postauricular swelling, tenderness, and redness associated with mastoiditis. Also note the inferior and anterior displacement of the ear. (*Reprinted with permission from* McMillan JA, Feigin RD, DeAngelis C, et al.: Oski's Pediatrics: Principles and Practice, 4th ed. Philadelphia: Lippincott Williams & Wilkins, 2006.)

TABLE 9.4

IMPORTANT COMPLICATIONS OF SINUSITIS

Orbital	Bone	Intracranial
Preseptal cellulitis	Frontal osteomyelitis (Pott's puffy tumor)	Epidural abscess
Orbital cellulitis	Maxillary osteomyelitis	Subdural empyema
Orbital abscess		Venous sinus thrombosis
Optic neuritis		Meningitis
		Intracerebral abscess

Points to Remember

- Approximately 5% of all upper respiratory infections are complicated by acute sinusitis—many of these, however, do not come to medical attention.

Points to Remember

- Patients with uncomplicated acute sinusitis should improve within 48 to 72 hours of appropriate antibiotic therapy. Failure to do so warrants careful reevaluation.

Sinusitis

Obstruction of the relatively small draining ostia of the sinuses can lead to accumulation of secretions followed by superinfection. The ethmoid and maxillary sinuses are the most common sites of sinusitis in young children. Frontal sinusitis is almost exclusively seen in adolescents and adults. The most common risk factors for sinusitis in children are viral upper respiratory tract infections and allergic rhinitis. Common infecting organisms mirror those of acute otitis media (e.g., *S. pneumoniae*, *H. influenzae*, and *M. catarrhalis*). Sinusitis due to anaerobes, *S. aureus*, and fungal pathogens is less common but does occur.

Clinical Manifestations

- Typical presentation of acute sinusitis is nasal discharge, congestion, and cough that persists beyond 10 days without improvement and is often associated with fevers, facial pain, periorbital edema, and/or headache.
- A less common presentation of acute sinusitis is a more acute presentation with fever above 39°C, copious purulent nasal discharge, and/or marked facial pain.
- Chronic sinusitis is distinguished from acute sinusitis by the presence of symptoms lasting longer than 4 weeks and often has a more subacute presentation.
- Physical examination may reveal evidence of facial tenderness and/or periorbital edema but is neither sensitive nor specific for diagnosing sinusitis.
- Complications of sinusitis can be severe and are shown in Table 9.4.

Diagnosis

- Acute uncomplicated sinusitis can be diagnosed by history and physical examination.
- CT scan is sensitive for sinusitis but lacks specificity so is only indicated when the diagnosis is uncertain and in cases of severe, chronic, and/or complicated sinusitis.

Management

Medical Management

- A 10- to 14-day course of empiric antibiotic therapy is appropriate for uncomplicated acute sinusitis.
  - High-dose amoxicillin is the preferred treatment for mild-to-moderate sinusitis.
  - High-dose amoxicillin/clavulanate is indicated for more severe cases and/or in patients with risk factors for resistance.
  - PCN allergic patients can be treated with third-generation cephalosporins or Macrolides.
- Three to four weeks of appropriate antibiotic therapy may be necessary for chronic sinusitis.
- Decongestants and antihistamines are often used as adjunctive therapy but have not been studied adequately to establish effectiveness.

Surgical Management

- Surgical puncture and drainage of the sinuses via a transnasal route may be necessary in patients who fail to respond to empiric treatment, severely immunosuppressed patients, and patients with life-threatening complications such as orbital cellulitis or intracranial spread.

Parotitis

Inflammation of the parotid gland in children is usually viral in etiology but can also be due to bacterial infection and noninfectious causes (Fig. 9.4).

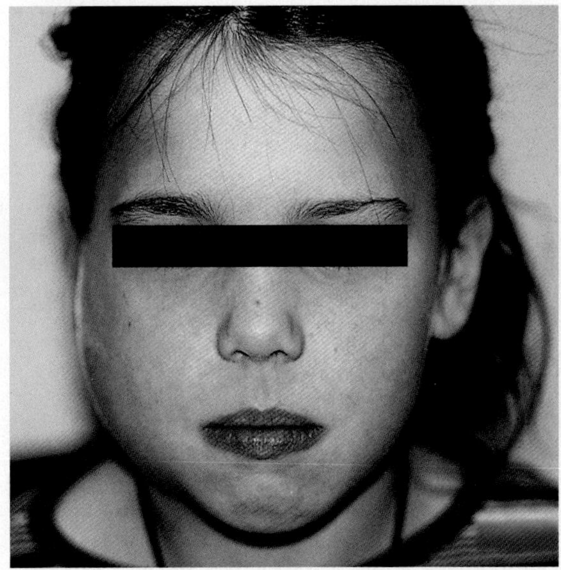

FIGURE 9.4. Parotitis. An 8-year-old girl with a 1-day history of right cheek swelling. The swollen area at the angle of the mandible was warm and tender. (*Reprinted with permission from* Fleisher GR, Ludwig W, Baskin MN. Atlas of Pediatric Emergency Medicine. Philadelphia: Lippincott Williams & Wilkins, 2004.)

Viral Parotitis

Viral parotitis is classically associated with mumps but can also be seen with parainfluenza, influenza, coxsackie viruses, echoviruses, and EBV. Viral parotitis typically follows a brief prodrome of constitutional symptoms (e.g., fever, headache, anorexia, malaise) and manifests as tender enlargement of the parotid gland. Absence of redness and warmth of the overlying skin is typical. It often starts on one side but ultimately involves both sides in 75% of cases. Typical duration of swelling is 7 to 10 days. Diagnosis is clinical as amylase may or may not be elevated. Management is largely supportive consisting of analgesics and a soft diet.

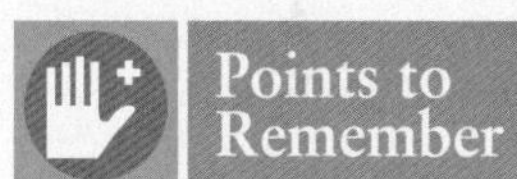

Points to Remember

- **HIV is a rare but important cause of viral parotitis in children.**

Bacterial Parotitis

Bacterial parotitis is rare in children. When it does occur, it is often due to stasis of secretions in the parotid gland because of dehydration or an abnormality of the Stensen duct. Abnormalities of the Stensen duct can be congenital or acquired (e.g., stone). The most common pathogen is *S. aureus*. Less common causes include streptococcal species, enteric Gram-negative bacilli, *H. influenzae*, and oral anaerobes. Children with bacterial parotitis are usually highly febrile and ill-appearing with a swollen, hot, tender, erythematous parotid gland. It is almost always unilateral. Purulent secretions are often able to be expressed via the Stensen duct. Management is via IV antibiotics and analgesics. Antibiotic therapy should be guided by Gram stain and culture of secretions. Incision and drainage is indicated in cases refractory to medical management.

Noninfectious Parotitis

Any child with chronic and/or recurrent parotitis should be evaluated for potential noninfectious causes of parotitis. Noninfectious causes of parotitis include obstruction of the Stensen duct by a stone or anatomic abnormality, autoimmune disease (e.g., SLE), granulomatous disease (e.g., sarcoid), lymphoma, drug-induced parotitis, and heavy metal exposure.

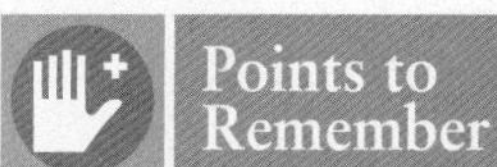

Points to Remember

- **Any firm or nontender nodes, especially those in the posterior triangle or supraclavicular region, should raise suspicion for lymphoma or other neoplasm. Generalized lymphadenopathy should raise suspicion for a more systemic process such as HIV, leukemia, or tuberculosis.**

Cervical Lymphadenitis

Acute infection of the cervical lymph nodes is a relatively common occurrence in pediatrics. It is important to note, however, that the most common cause of cervical lymph node enlargement is drainage of a remote infection in the head and neck rather than primary infection of the lymph node itself. Acute versus subacute adenitis is differentiated by the presence of symptoms for less than or greater than 2 weeks, respectively. Seventy-five percent of cases of acute cervical lymphadenitis are due to infection with *S. aureus* or group A streptococcus. Subacute cervical lymphadenitis is more commonly caused by viral processes (e.g., EBV, CMV, adenovirus), *Bartonella henselae*, nontuberculous mycobacteria, and *M. tuberculosis*. Most children presenting with cervical lymphadenitis are between the ages of 1 and 4 years.

Clinical Manifestations

- Unilateral, painful lymph node enlargement (typically 2–7 cm in size) (Fig. 9.5).
- Overlying warmth and erythema are present to varying degrees.
- Systemic symptoms are usually absent or mild.

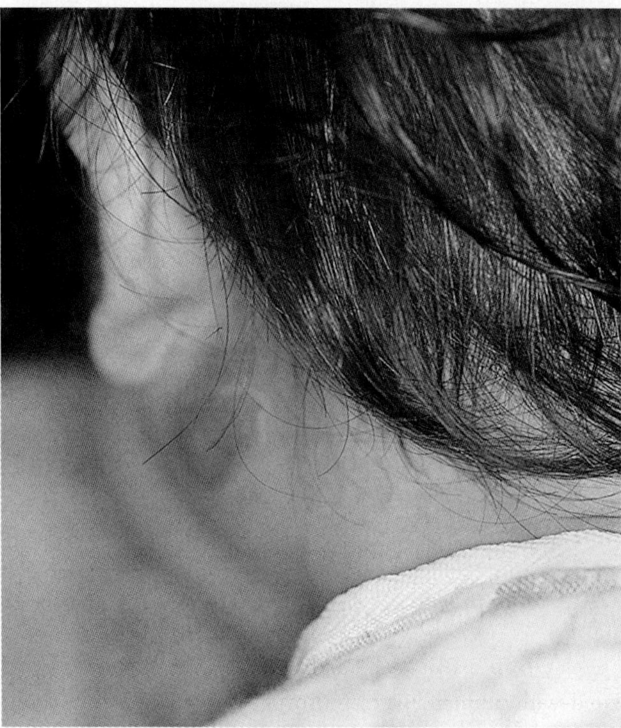

FIGURE 9.5. Mycobacterial lymphadenitis. This young girl, who had recently returned from India, presented with an inflamed lymph node and additional signs of systemic disease. An excisional biopsy showed caseating granulomas. (*Reprinted with permission from* Fleisher GR, Ludwig W, Baskin MN. Atlas of Pediatric Emergency Medicine. Philadelphia: Lippincott Williams & Wilkins, 2004.)

Diagnosis

- Largely clinical.
- Ultrasound and/or CT with contrast are indicated only in severe and/or refractory cases when abscess formation is suspected.

Management

- Empiric antibiotic therapy with amoxicillin/clavulanate or clindamycin is appropriate for acute uncomplicated cervical adenitis.
- In children with more severe or refractory cases, needle aspiration should be done to identify an organism; the aspirate should be sent for Gram stain and aerobic as well as anaerobic culture, fungal culture, and mycobacterial testing; a Mantoux PPD should be placed and serologies sent for EBV, CMV, *B. henselae*, HIV, Toxoplasmosis, and/or *Francisella tularensis*; a biopsy of the lymph node should be obtained for staining and microscopy.
- Surgical incision and drainage should be performed for patients with cervical lymphadenitis associated with abscess formation.

Retropharyngeal Abscess

A potential space exists between the middle and deep layers of cervical fascia in infants and young children. Local spread of organisms into this potential space can lead to a retropharyngeal abscess. The retropharyngeal space fully regresses by early puberty and is no longer clinically significant. Thus, retropharyngeal abscesses occur at a mean age of 4 years and are rare in older children and adolescents. Most retropharyngeal abscesses occur following an episode of cervical adenitis. Retropharyngeal abscesses are often polymicrobial with both aerobic and anaerobic pathogens being present. The predominant organisms are group A streptococcus, *S. aureus*, and oropharyngeal anaerobic bacteria.

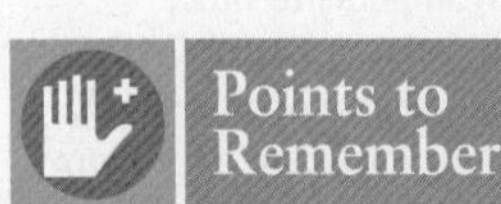

- Widening of the prevertebral soft tissue more than 7 mm at C2 (approximately one-half vertebral body) or 14 mm at C6 (approximately 1 whole vertebral body) is suggestive of retropharyngeal inflammation.

Clinical Manifestations

- Insidious onset.
- Often follows a mild antecedent infection.
- Fever.
- Restricted range of motion of neck; preferred position is often with hyperextension.
- Ipsilateral tender lymphadenopathy.
- Stridor due to airway obstruction.

Diagnosis

- Lateral plain films of the neck, with the neck extended and in a true lateral position, may demonstrate widening of the prevertebral soft tissue (Fig. 9.6).
- Neck CT with IV contrast is highly sensitive and specific.

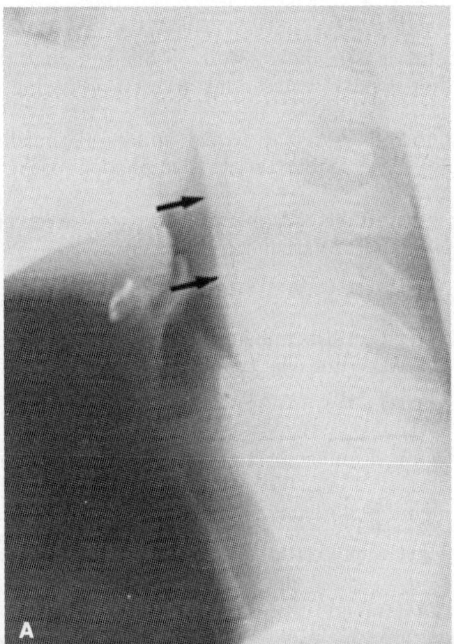

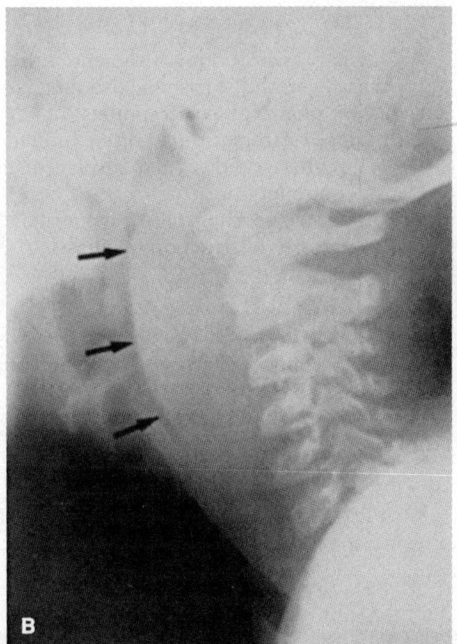

FIGURE 9.6. Retropharyngeal space. (A) Normal lateral cervical view. (B) Expansion of prevertebral soft tissues by retropharyngeal abscess. (Courtesy of Dr. A. Weber, Massachusetts Eye and Ear Infirmary, Boston, MA. *Reprinted from* Gorbach SL, Bartlett JG, Blacklow NR: Infectious Diseases, 3rd ed. Philadelphia: Lippincott Williams & Wilkins, 2003.)

Management

- Empiric IV antibiotics with ampicillin/sulbactam or clindamycin.
- Surgical drainage is indicated for children who fail to improve on IV antibiotics or have large abscesses at the time of diagnosis.

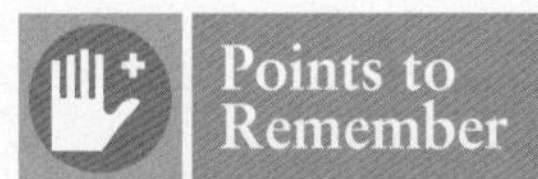

- **Approximately one-third of children with small retropharyngeal abscesses improve with IV antibiotics alone.**

Peritonsillar Abscess

Peritonsillar abscesses are the most common deep neck infection in children and the most common sequelae of acute tonsillitis. They occur most commonly during adolescence but can rarely occur in young children. The most common pathogens include group A streptococcus and other streptococcal species, *S. aureus*, and oral anaerobes.

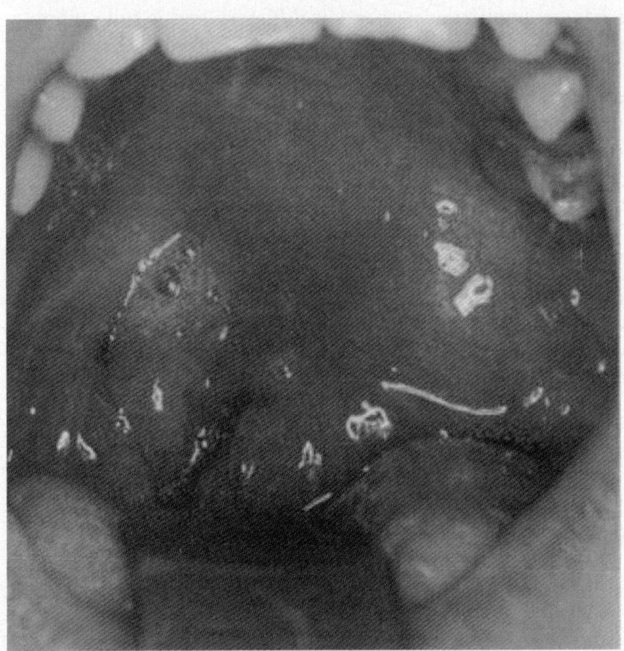

FIGURE 9.7. Peritonsillar abscess. Note the erythema and swelling on the left and the right deviation of the uvula. (Courtesy of Seth Zwillenberg. *Reprinted from* Chung EK, Boom JA, and Datto GA. Visual Diagnosis in Pediatrics. Philadelphia: Lippincott Williams & Wilkins, 2006.)

Clinical Manifestations

- Classic presentation is with acute onset of throat pain more severe on one side than the other, fever, chills, trismus, drooling, and "hot potato" voice; a history of a preceding or current pharyngitis is common.
- Physical examination is often limited by trismus but may reveal unilateral tonsillar swelling/mass with uvular displacement (Fig. 9.7); tender cervical lymphadenopathy is also commonly present.
- Complications: rupture of peritonsillar abscess into the parapharyngeal space can lead to acute airway obstruction, mediastinitis, sepsis, and/or vascular compression.

Diagnosis

- Unless an obvious swollen mass is clearly seen on physical examination, a CT scan of the neck with IV contrast is necessary to differentiate severe peritonsillar cellulitis from true abscess.

Management

- Drainage, either by needle aspiration or surgical drainage, is an essential aspect of treating peritonsillar abscess.
- Appropriate adjunctive antibiotic therapy includes clindamycin or ampicillin/sulbactam.

Table 9.5 summarizes important differences between retropharyngeal and peritonsillar abscesses.

TABLE 9.5

RETROPHARYNGEAL VERSUS PERITONSILLAR ABSCESS

	Retropharyngeal Abscess	Peritonsillar Abscess
Age of patient	Infants and young children	Adolescents
Typical origin of infection	Cervical adenitis	Tonsillitis
Onset	Insidious	Acute
Microbiology	Often polymicrobial with both aerobes and anaerobes	Usually due to a single aerobic organism
Medical vs surgical treatment	Many resolve with medical management alone	All require drainage via needle aspiration or surgery in addition to medical management

SAMPLE BOARD REVIEW QUESTIONS

1. A 4-year-old male presents with a 3-day history of fever, difficulty swallowing, and refusal to move his neck. He has no significant past medical history and is fully immunized. On physical examination, he is alert and anxious but is nontoxic. His neck is hyperextended, and he refuses to turn it laterally in either direction. Visualization of his tonsils and posterior pharynx are unremarkable. Pulmonary, cardiac, and abdominal examinations are normal. Which of the following radiologic findings is most consistent with this patient's presentation?
   a. Subglottic stenosis on PA x-rays of the neck
   b. Edema and enlargement of the epiglottis on lateral x-rays of the neck
   c. Foreign body in the trachea on PA and lateral chest x-rays
   d. Widening of the prevertebral space on lateral x-rays of the neck

   Answer: d. This patient has a classic presentation for a retropharyngeal abscess. The most sensitive and specific way to diagnose a retropharyngeal abscess is CT scan of the neck with IV contrast. X-rays can be normal but widening of the prevertebral space on lateral x-rays of the neck is suggestive of retropharyngeal abscess. Subglottic stenosis (steeple sign) on PA x-ray of the neck is the classic x-ray finding for viral croup. Edema and enlargement of the epiglottis (thumbprint sign) on lateral x-ray of the neck is classic for epiglottis.

2. You are seeing a 2-month-old full-term male for his well-child check. He is exclusively breast-fed and is gaining weight well. Physical examination in your office is normal, but his mother is concerned because he breathes funny when he gets upset and makes a funny noise on inspiration. The only other time she's noticed the same noise is when he's

congested and is laid on his back, but it improves with repositioning on his tummy. Which of the following responses is most appropriate regarding the likely course in this infant?

a. The early age of his presentation indicates more severe pathology that will likely require surgical intervention via supraglottoplasty
b. The early age of his presentation likely indicates more severe disease pathology that will likely require surgical intervention via tracheostomy
c. This condition is likely to get progressively worse over the first 12 to 18 months of life and then gradually improve without intervention. It is likely to resolve completely by 3 to 4 years of age
d. This condition is likely to improve over time without intervention. It is likely to resolve completely by 12 months of age.

Answer: d. This patient has laryngomalacia. The inspiratory noise described in this vignette is stridor. The most common cause of chronic and/or recurrent stridor in infancy is laryngomalacia. The description of the stridor getting worse with agitation, concurrent viral upper respiratory illnesses, and supine positioning is classic as is improvement with prone positioning. Laryngomalacia is usually clinically apparent in the first few weeks or months of life and improves over time such that 90% of patients will experience spontaneous resolution by 12 months of age. Supraglottoplasty and tracheostomy are surgical options reserved for severe cases of laryngomalacia. Of note, anticipatory guidance regarding the importance of supine positioning during sleep in infancy should be reinforced with this mom as it has been shown to decrease the risk of sudden infant death syndrome.

3. A 13-year-old male is brought to your clinic by his mother who is concerned about his hearing. She reports that over the past few months he has not seemed like he hears well. She initially attributed it to normal teenage behavior as her son had passed all of his hearing tests as an infant and young child and had always seemed to hear well. She became alarmed, however, when she found out that her father did not become deaf until he was a teenager. She did not know him well because he died in his early 40s from kidney problems. You are not able to do a hearing test in your office, but you decide to do a urinalysis because of the interesting family history. Urinalysis reveals specific gravity of 1.001, negative glucose, negative ketones, 2+ protein, negative leukocyte esterase, negative nitrite, 2 to 3 WBC/hpf, 40 RBC/hpf, and 0 to 1 epithelial cells/hpf, and no bacteria. Which of the following conditions is the most likely etiology in this patient?

a. Waardenburg syndrome
b. Jervell and Lange-Nielsen syndrome
c. Alport syndrome
d. Congenital CMV infection

Answer: c. This patient has Alport syndrome. Alport syndrome is characterized by hematuria, proteinuria, progressive renal failure, sensorineural hearing loss, and ocular lesions. Affected male patients typically have severe disease, whereas the course in female patients tends to be mild. The most common form of Alport syndrome is X-linked. Deafness occurs in the majority of male patients but is not a universal finding. Hearing loss is not present at birth but is clinically apparent in most males by adolescence. Persistent microscopic hematuria is present in affected males during the first 2 decades of life. Episodes of gross hematuria occur frequently, usually appearing a few days after the onset of an upper respiratory infection. In male patients, the risk of developing ESRD by age 40 is 90%.

4. A 7-year-old female presents with a 2-day history of progressive ear pain. She is afebrile and otherwise well. On physical examination, she has severe otalgia with manipulation of the pinna. There is no postauricular swelling. Otoscopy demonstrates an erythematous, edematous canal with purulent drainage. You are not able to visualize the tympanic membrane because of the edema and drainage. She denies any history of trauma or foreign body impaction. She has had this problem several times in the past, usually during the summer. Which of the following is the most appropriate initial management for this patient?

a. A period of observation only because she is above 2 years, does not have severe disease, and is otherwise healthy
b. High–dose oral amoxicillin
c. Topical steroids
d. Topical antibiotics with anti-pseudomonal and anti-staphylococcal activity with or without topical steroids

Answer: d. This patient has a classic case of otitis externa. Otalgia with manipulation of the pinna and an erythematous, edematous external auditory canal with purulent drainage are cardinal features of otitis externa. Otitis externa is often related to swimming and/or trauma. The differential diagnosis for otalgia and purulent drainage also include acute otitis media with tympanic membrane perforation and foreign body ingestion, but these are less likely etiologies in this patient. Appropriate management for otitis externa includes topical antibiotics with anti-pseudomonal and anti-staphylococcal activity. Topical steroids are an adjunctive therapy added to some topical antibiotic formulations but are not sufficient on their own. A period of observation only is appropriate for patients with acute otitis media who are above 2 years, do not have severe disease, and are otherwise healthy. High-dose oral amoxicillin is a first-line medication for cases of acute otitis media in which antibiotics are indicated.

5. A 14-year-old girl presents with a 6-day history of fever and sore throat. She was seen by her pediatrician 4 days ago and treated with penicillin without improvement. Her throat has become so painful that she is unable to swallow her own secretions. Physical examination is limited by trismus, but you are able to partially visualize a right tonsillar mass with deviation of the uvula to the left. CT scan with IV contrast demonstrates a right peritonsillar abscess. Which of the following is the most important part of the management of peritonsillar abscess?

a. Drainage via needle aspiration or surgery
b. Trial of empiric IV penicillin
c. Trial of empiric IV clindamycin or ampicillin/sulbactam
d. Trial of empiric high dose oral amoxicillin

Answer: a. The most important part of the management of peritonsillar abscess is drainage of the abscess. In more than 90% of cases, this can be accomplished via needle aspiration. If needle aspiration is unsuccessful, intraoral surgical incision and drainage or acute tonsillectomy is indicated. Antibiotics are an important adjunctive treatment for peritonsillar abscess but do not eliminate the need for drainage.

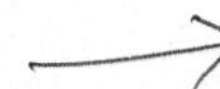

6. A 15-year-old male presents to urgent care with a 4-day history of headache, fever, and vomiting. Review of systems is positive for 2 to 3 weeks of preceding cough, congestion, and rhinorrhea. Past medical history is significant for asthma and allergies. Immunizations are up to date. On physical examination, the patient is febrile and ill-appearing but has a nonfocal examination. He does not have any nuchal rigidity or meningeal signs. His lungs are clear to auscultation bilaterally and breathing is unlabored. Initial laboratories demonstrate a WBC 19,000 with 83% PMNs and an elevated CRP of 16. Which of the following is the most appropriate next step in the diagnostic evaluation of this patient?

a. Chest x-ray
b. Lumbar puncture
c. X-rays of the sinuses
d. Head CT

Answer: d. This patient has sinusitis complicated by an intracranial abscess. This diagnosis can be confirmed with a head CT that includes imaging of the sinuses and intracranial space. Sinusitis should be suspected in any patient with rhinorrhea, cough, and congestion that lasts beyond 10 days. It is also usually associated with the development of fevers and headache. Allergic rhinitis is a risk factor for sinusitis. CT scan is not necessary in all cases of suspected sinusitis, but the severity of this teenage boy's complaints, including his ill appearance and history of vomiting, suggest that he may have an intracranial complication. Other serious complications of sinusitis include orbital cellulitis, osteomyelitis, and venous sinus thrombosis.

7. A 9-year-old male presents to the emergency room with a 3-week history of swollen cervical lymph nodes. His parents delayed seeking care as they recently immigrated from Honduras and do not have health insurance. On physical examination, he has a 2.5 cm tender left anterior cervical node and a 1.5 cm tender right anterior cervical node. Which of the following features is more suggestive of cervical lymphadenitis due to bacterial infection other than mycobacteria?

a. Bilateral distribution
b. Subacute onset
c. Age above 4
d. Focal tenderness

Answer: d. Although 75% of cases of acute cervical lymphadenitis are due to infection with *S. aureus* or group A streptococcus, infectious cervical lymphadenitis can also be caused by viruses, fungi, and atypical bacteria. Mycobacterial infection is an important consideration in high-risk patient populations. Cervical lymphadenitis due to Mycobacteria typically has a subacute to chronic onset, occurs in all age groups, can be unilateral or bilateral, and lacks focal tenderness. Cervical lymphadenitis due to bacterial infection typically has an acute onset, is most common in children 1 to 4 years of age, is unilateral, and has focal tenderness.

8. A 17-year-old male presents with sore throat, fever, shortness of breath, and neck pain and is ultimately diagnosed with Lemierre syndrome. Which of the following statements about Lemierre syndrome is true?

a. The most common causative organism is *Fusobacterium necrophorum*
b. Most cases are preceded by pharyngitis
c. Septic thrombophlebitis of the internal jugular vein predisposes to widespread septic emboli
d. All of the above

Answer: d. Lemierre syndrome is a rare but serious complication of peritonsillar abscess. Anaerobic bacteria flourish within the crater of the abscess and infection spreads to the adjacent internal jugular vein, creating a septic thrombophlebitis and placing the patient at risk for widespread septic emboli. The most common causative organism in Lemierre syndrome is the anaerobic bacterium *F. necrophorum.*

9. Mastoiditis usually results as a complication of which of the following infections?

a. Parotitis
b. Sinusitis
c. Acute otitis media
d. None of the above

Answer: c. Mastoiditis is almost always associated with a ipsilateral acute otitis media. The classic examination finding is postauricular erythema, tenderness, and swelling with superior and lateral displacement of the external ear. Other serious but rare complications of acute otitis media include labyrinthitis, osteomyelitis, facial nerve paralysis, intracranial abscess, meningitis, lateral sinus thrombosis, and otitic hydrocephalus.

10. A 7-month-old male presents with fever and a left-sided cervical abscess. He is the product of a full-term uncomplicated pregnancy and delivery. He was admitted at 2 months of age for a buttocks abscess due to infection with *Serratia marcescens.* His symptoms fail to respond to appropriate empiric IV antibiotics so an incision and drainage of the lesion is performed. No anatomic abnormalities are noted on imaging or during the procedure. An intraoperative wound culture grows *Staphylococcus epidermidis.* Review of family history is significant for a maternal uncle who died during childhood from pneumonia. Which of the following underlying conditions best explains this patient's presentation?

a. Chronic granulomatous disease
b. Branchial cleft cyst
c. Heterotaxy associated with functional asplenia
d. Munchausen syndrome by proxy

Answer: a. This patient's presentation could be explained by chronic granulomatous disease. Chronic granulomatous disease (CGD) is a disorder of intracellular microbial killing of catalase-positive organisms due to impaired oxidative burst. Patients with CGD typically present with abscesses, ulcerative stomatitis, and/or episodes of pneumonitis that are unusually severe, recurrent, or caused by unusual organisms. *S. aureus* is the most common infecting agent in patients with CGD. Other common pathogens include *Escherichia coli*, klebsiella, Enterobacter species, *S. marcescens*, salmonellae, and pseudomonas. The fact that this patient is now returning with an abscess due to *S. epidermidis* should raise the concern of an underlying immunodeficiency as this is an unusual cause of infection in a healthy host in the absence of an indwelling catheter. The prior episode of infection with *S. marcescens* also supports this diagnosis. The family history of an uncle who died in childhood of pneumonia may or may not be relevant to the patient but does raise the concern for an X-linked disease. Although autosomal recessive and autosomal dominant forms of CGD do exist, 70% of cases are X-linked. Diagnosis of CGD is most commonly established via nitroblue tetrazolium (NBT) dye test.

SUGGESTED READINGS

American Academy of Pediatrics. Hearing assessment in infants and children: recommendations beyond neonatal screening. *Pediatrics* 2003;111(2):436–440.

American Academy of Pediatrics Subcommittee on Management of Acute Otitis Media. Diagnosis and management of acute otitis media. *Pediatrics* 2004;113:1451.

Declau F, Boudewyns A, Van den Ende J, et al. Etiologic and audiologic evaluations after universal neonatal hearing screening: analysis of 170 referred neonates. *Pediatrics* 2008;121(6):1119–1126.

Gregg RB, Wiorek LS, Arvedson JC. Pediatric audiology: a review. *Pediatr Rev* 2004;25(7):224–233.

Paradise JL, Dollaghan CA, Campbell TF, et al. Otitis media and tympanostomy tube insertion during the first three years of life: developmental outcomes at the age of four years. *Pediatrics* 2003;112:265.

Sininger YS, Doyle KJ, Moore JK. The case for early identification of hearing loss in children. *Ped Clin Nor Amer* 1999;46(1):1–14.

Suslak L, Desposito F. Infants with cleft lip/cleft palate. *Pediatr Rev* 1988;9(10):331–334.

CHAPTER 10 ■ ENDOCRINOLOGY

MICHELLE B. DUNN

17-OHP	17-α-hydroxyprogesterone	GnRH	Gonadotropin-releasing hormone
21-OH	21-hydroxylase	HbA1C	Hemoglobin A1C
ACTH	Adrenocorticotropic hormone	hCG	Human chorionic gonadotropin
APECED	Autoimmune polyendocrinopathy–candidiasis–ectodermal dystrophy syndrome	IBD	Inflammatory bowel disease
BMP	Basic metabolic panel	IGF	Insulin-like growth factor
BUN	Blood Urea Nitrogen	IGFBP3	Insulin-like growth factor binding protein 3
CBC	Complete blood cell count	LH	Leuteinizing hormone
CRH	Corticotropin-releasing hormone	MIS	Mullerian inhibiting substance
CRP	C-reactive protein	MRI	Magnetic resonance imaging
DHEA	Dehydroepiandrosterone	NICU	Neonatal intensive care unit
DHEAS	DHEA sulfate	PTH	Parathyroid hormone
DKA	Diabetic ketoacidosis	SGA	Small for gestational age
DHT	Dihydrotestosterone	SRY	Sex-determining region of the Y chromosome
ESR	Erythrocyte sedimentation rate	T3	Triiodothyronine
FISH	Fluorescent in situ hybridization	T4	Thyroxine
FSH	Follicle-stimulating hormone	TRH	TSH-releasing hormone
GI	Gastrointestinal	TSH	Thyroid-stimulating hormone
GH	Growth hormone	VSD	Ventricular Septal Defect
GHRF	Growth hormone releasing factor	WIC	Women, Infants, and Children Program

CHAPTER OBJECTIVES

1. Understand normal sexual differentiation and identify common causes of ambiguous genitalia
2. Identify etiologies of poor growth
3. Recognize normal puberty and the proper evaluation for both delayed and precocious puberty
4. Know the signs, symptoms, and laboratory values associated with hypo- and hyperthyroidism
5. Recognize the laboratory findings and clinical signs of hypoparathyroidism and pseudohypoparathyroidism
6. Identify the symptoms and causes of hypo- and hypercalcemia
7. Explain the etiology of rickets
8. Understand the pathogenesis and treatment of type 1 diabetes
9. Know how to recognize and treat DKA
10. Explain the difference between type 1 and type 2 diabetes pathogenesis and treatment
11. Recognize metabolic syndrome in children and know how to screen for its consequences.

SEX DIFFERENTIATION

Normal Prenatal Development

Without the influence of multiple events during development, a fetus becomes female (Table 10.1). To develop into a male, a fetus must have the action of the SRY. The fetus starts out with

TABLE 10.1

REQUIREMENTS FOR MALE DEVELOPMENT

Requirement	Presence	Absence
SRY	Bipotential gonad becomes a testis Wolfian ducts develop into vas deferens, epididymis, and seminal vesicles	Ovary develops Mullerian ducts become fallopian tubes, uterus, and upper third of vagina
MIS	Mullerian ducts regress	Wolfian ducts involute
Testosterone	Differentiates male internal and external genitalia	Ambiguous genitalia
DHT	Forms scrotum and penis	Ambiguous genitalia

DHT, dihydrotestosterone; MIS, mullerian inhibiting substance; SRY, sex-determining region of the Y chromosome.

a bipotential gonad. In the presence of SRY, this differentiates into a testis; without it, it becomes an ovary. Two X chromosomes, not just the absence of SRY, are necessary for the ovary to differentiate normally. Without a second X chromosome, streak gonads occur, though the child otherwise has normal internal and external female genitalia. A fetus has both mullerian ducts (which develop into the fallopian tubes, uterus, and the upper third of the vagina) and wolffian ducts (which develop into the vas deferens, epididymis, and the seminal vesicles). The testicles secrete MIS, which leads to regression of the mullerian structures. Male differentiation also requires testosterone and gonadotropin release by the pituitary gland. Testosterone must be converted to DHT by the enzyme 5-α reductase, and target organs must respond appropriately to androgens.

Ambiguous Genitalia

If ambiguous genitalia is suspected, it is important to establish whether there are palpable gonads in the scrotum or inguinal canal. Palpable gonads generally are testicles and make a Y chromosome likely. A karyotype is an essential part of the initial evaluation for ambiguous genitalia, since the genetic sex helps determine the origin of the disorder.

Male Pseudohermaphroditism

Male pseudohermaphrodism describes genetic males (XY karyotype) with ambiguous genitalia. It can have many causes, including defects in adrenal production of androgens, lack of testicular testosterone synthesis, or failure of target tissues to respond to androgens.

Diagnosis: Measure testosterone and DHT levels. There are many enzymatic defects which can block testosterone biosynthesis in either the testes or the adrenal gland. An hCG stimulation test (where testosterone levels are measured after several days of hCG treatment) determines if the Leydig cells of the testes can produce testosterone. If failure of testosterone biosynthesis is suspected, various testosterone precursors can be measured to determine the origin of the enzymatic block.

Treatment: Steroid replacement can be given depending on which pathway is blocked.

5-α-Reductase deficiency: Inadequate conversion of testosterone to DHT leads to normal internal genitalia but ambiguous external genitalia, including cryptorchidism, microphallus, and hypospadias. Patients can have some virilization at puberty with increase in penile size and pubic hair development from higher levels of testosterone.

Diagnosis: A ratio of testosterone to DHT greater than the normal value of five.

Androgen insensitivity of target tissues can be partial or complete. Complete androgen insensitivity is generally not suspected in infancy, as the child appears phenotypically female. Patients present in adolescence with normal breast development, little pubic hair growth, and amenorrhea.

Diagnosis: Partial androgen resistance is suspected when a patient with ambiguous genitalia has normal or high levels of testosterone. If the infant does not have improved penile length with a trial of IM testosterone, the diagnosis can be confirmed with genetic testing of a tissue biopsy.

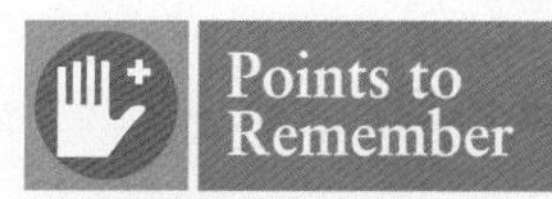

- **Complete androgen insensitivity presents in adolescence; partial presents at birth.**

Other rarer causes of male pseudohermaphroditism include absent or defective testes, XY gonadal dysgenesis, and true hermaphrodism (where both ovarian and testicular tissue are present). MRI is generally necessary to delineate which internal structures are present and guide sexual assignment.

Female Pseudohermaphroditism

Female pseudohermaphroditism refers to genetic females (XX karyotype) who have undergone virilization. *Virilization* occurs when the fetus is exposed to excessive androgens. The patient can

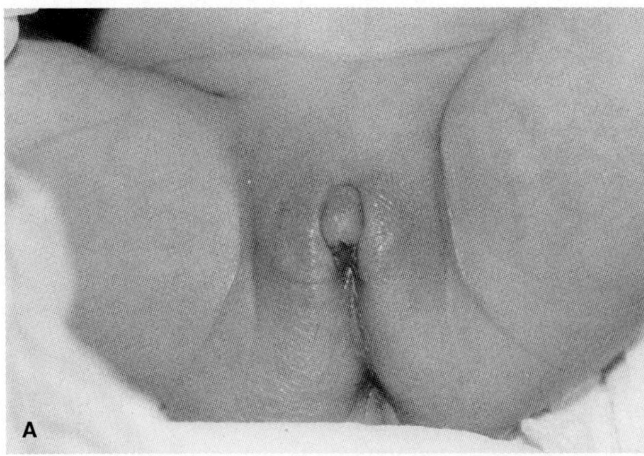

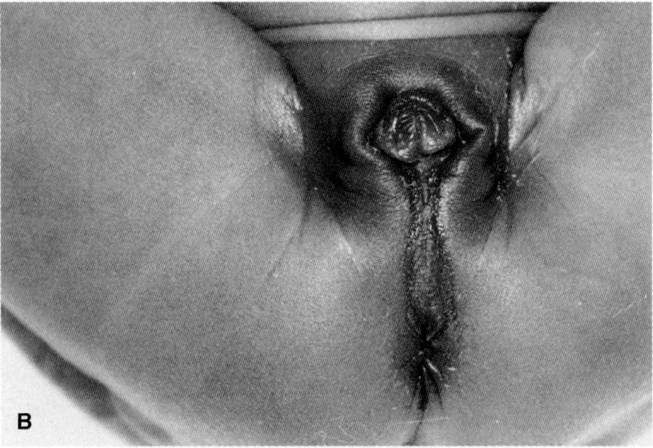

FIGURE 10.1. Ambiguous genitalia in female pseudohermaphrodites with congenital adrenal hyperplasia. Both cases exhibit enlargement of the clitoris, posterior fusion of the vaginal orifice, and development of rugae of the labia majora. **(A)** Female infant with salt-losing 21-OH deficiency, whose ambiguous genitalia were not detected at the time of her newborn physical examination. **(B)** Female infant with 11-β-hydroxylase deficiency. (Reprinted with permission from McMillan JA, Feigin RD, DeAngelis C, et al. Oski's Pediatrics: Principles and Practice, 4th ed. Philadelphia, PA: Lippincott Williams & Wilkins, 2006.)

have either clitoromegaly (clitoral length >1 cm) or posterior labial fusion, or both. Because MIS is not present, the internal genitalia (ovaries, uterus, and upper third of the vagina) are normal (Fig. 10.1). **Female pseudohermaphroditism is generally due to congenital adrenal hyperplasia or maternal exposure to exogenous androgens.** Sources of maternal androgens include use of progestins during pregnancy, ovarian or adrenal tumors, and maternal congenital adrenal hyperplasia.

Congenital adrenal hyperplasia is a group of autosomal recessive disorders with an enzymatic deficiency in one of the steps necessary to synthesize cortisol. The result is hyperplasia of the adrenal glands, high levels of ACTH, and increased production of the adrenal steroids which do not require the deficient enzyme. **The most common cause of congenital adrenal hyperplasia is 21-OH deficiency**, which causes excess of adrenally produced androgens, especially androstenedione. Rarer causes of congenital adrenal hyperplasia include 11-α-hydroxylase deficiency and 3-β-hydroxysteroid dehydrogenase deficiency.

21-Hydroxylase deficiency causes virilization of female infants and can cause aldosterone deficiency in either sex. Approximately 75% of affected infants have aldosterone deficiency, causing salt wasting. **Congenital adrenal hyperplasia typically presents as a sick infant with ambiguous genitalia or an ill phenotypically male infant.** The symptoms of hypoglycemia, weakness, hypotension, and electrolyte abnormalities usually do not occur until 4 to 10 days of age and may not appear for as long as 4 weeks.

Diagnosis: Elevation of serum 17-OHP levels. Equivocal results can be supplemented with an ACTH stimulated 17-OHP level.

Treatment: Hydrocortisone and fludrocortisone replacement. Sick patients may require aggressive fluid and electrolyte management in addition to stress dose hydrocortisone. Adequacy of glucocorticoid dosing can be assessed via 17-OHP level. Stress dose steroids are needed during illness or other times of stress. Surgery may be required on the female genitalia depending on the degree of virilization.

A milder form of 21-OH deficiency, **nonclassic 21-OH deficiency**, typically presents in later childhood, at puberty, or as an adult with signs of androgen excess. These can include early pubic and axillary hair, acne, hirsutism, hairline recession, and amenorrhea.

Diagnosis: High morning 17-OHP levels.

Treatment: Glucocorticoid therapy is used to suppress overproduction of adrenal androgens.

GROWTH

Normal Physiology

The pituitary gland's release of GH is regulated by the hypothalamus. GHRF stimulates GH secretion, and somatostatin inhibits it. Various neurotransmitters control hypothalamic hormone release in response to external factors, such as sleep, exercise, and stress. The pituitary releases GH in bursts, which fluctuate throughout the day. The largest release occurs in early sleep. Somatomedins, also called IGFs, mediate the effects of GH. The main actor is IGF-1, the majority of which is produced in the liver. IGF-1 acts on target tissues to cause linear growth. IGF-1 and GH cause negative feedback at both the pituitary gland and the hypothalamus. Defects can occur anywhere in the hormonal axis, including mutations in GH, the GHRF receptor, various transcription factors, or the GH receptor. Response to GH therapy can differentiate those with GH resistance.

Short Stature

Short stature is defined as **height less than 2 standard deviations (SD) below the mean.** Calculating growth velocity is necessary when evaluating for growth disorders. Growth rates are affected by the timing of puberty.

A common reason for crossing percentiles may be **adjustment to genetic growth potential.** This is the case when an infant "finds his curve," since birth weight and length are not necessarily correlated with genetic height potential. If the decline in growth does not go below the genetically anticipated potential, and the growth velocity is normal, the child likely does not need further evaluation.

Points to Remember

- Red Flags: Children below the third percentile for height, who are crossing percentiles downward, or whose growth velocity is less than 4 cm a year.

Familial (genetic) short stature: Patients have normal growth rate, normal bone age, and normal pubertal growth spurt. Their predicted height corresponds to that of their parents.

Constitutional growth delay: A delayed growth pattern, with a 2- to 4-year lag in height, bone age, and pubertal development causing a crossing of percentiles in early adolescence. These children have delayed epiphyseal fusion, usually resulting in a normal final height. This growth pattern is more frequent in boys and tends to run in families. If the growth velocity and predicted height are normal, no further evaluation is needed (Fig. 10.2).

Points to Remember

- Genetic short stature: bone age = chronological age

Poor growth as a result of chronic disease: Common in cases such as renal disorders (renal tubular acidosis, renal insufficiency), gastrointestinal (IBD, celiac disease, other malabsorption), cardiac dysfunction, or other chronic illnesses. **Chronic medications**, such as glucocorticoids and stimulants, can stunt growth. Children with **inborn metabolic errors, chromosomal abnormalities, skeletal dysplasias, and dysmorphic syndromes** (Turner, Prader–Willi, and Noonan syndromes) also can have poor growth.

Small for gestational age children: Defined as less than 2 SD below mean for gestational age. May have poor postnatal growth. Approximately 15% fail to catch up with their peers by age 2.

Points to Remember

- Constitutional delay: bone age < chronological age

Growth problems can stem from **nutritional deficiencies** of various origins, including from GI pathology, psychosocial problems, or an eating disorder. **Psychosocial factors** such a stressful home environment can cause poor growth.

Endocrine causes of short stature: Include excess glucocorticoids, hypothyroidism, GH deficiency, pseudohypoparathyroidism, and poorly controlled diabetes. **Excess glucocorticoids**, which can come from exogenous or endogenous sources, result in short stature with low growth rate, delayed bone age, and cushingoid features ("moon" facies, centripetal obesity, dorsal fat pad, and proximal muscle weakness). With removal of the glucocorticoid source, catch up growth occurs, but final adult height can be compromised. **Hypothyroidism** leads to decreased linear growth with increased weight gain and delayed bone age. Growth improves with thyroid replacement.

Growth hormone deficiency: Can be idiopathic, organic, or familial. It may occur alone or with other pituitary hormone deficiencies. Affected children usually have short stature, poor growth, delayed bone age, and can be overweight. Fasting hypoglycemia and micropenis in boys may also be present.

Causes of GH deficiency include congenital abnormalities, trauma, central nervous system (CNS) infection, vascular abnormalities, radiation, and infiltrative processes. Pituitary abnormalities can be associated with other midline defects. GH insensitivity or resistance can also exist.

Craniopharyngiomas are the most common tumors associated with pituitary and hypothalamic deficiencies. Children may have headaches, visual abnormalities, growth failure, and diabetes insipidus. Diagnosis is made via imaging. Treatment requires surgical excision and possible radiation therapy, followed by hormone replacement.

Evaluation of Poor Growth

- Thorough history, including growth and puberty patterns in family members, the child's gestational age, birth size, nutritional status, and symptoms of organ dysfunction.
- Examination of the growth curve is essential to look at growth velocity and for characteristic patterns.
- The physical examination includes accurate height and weight, assessment of visual fields and optic nerves, teeth, thyroid size, and a search for features of chronic disease, dysmorphic features, and disproportionate growth.
- Laboratory and radiology tests should include bone age, CBC, ESR, CRP, BMP, thyroid studies, karyotype for girls, IGF-1, IGFBP-3, and a celiac screen. Pharmacological GH deficiency testing can be done if needed. Classical GH deficiency is diagnosed based on failure of adequate GH release on two different pharmacologic tests.

Treatment

GH therapy is approved for GH deficiency, chronic renal insufficiency, Turner syndrome, Prader–Willi syndrome, SGA infants who have not caught up by 2 years of age (if other causes

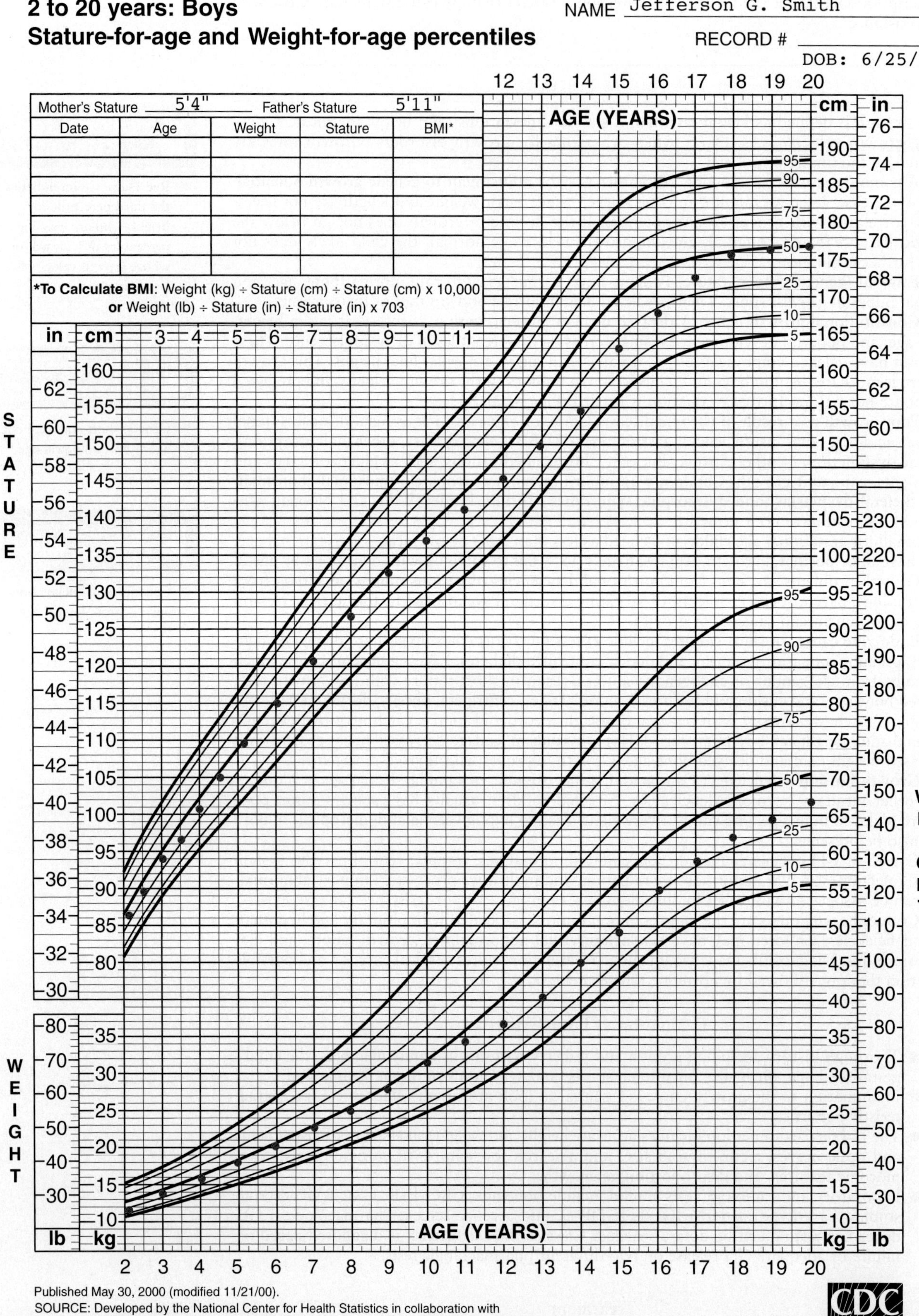

FIGURE 10.2. Constitutional growth delay. The patient's height percentile falls during early adolescence, but then catches up when he enters his late growth spurt.

of growth failure are excluded), and idiopathic short stature (approved by Food and Drug Administration in 2003 for height 2.25 SD below the mean with a **predicted height less than 63 inches for boys or 59 inches for girls**). GH therapy is NOT appropriate for familial short stature. GH hormone replacement is given subcutaneously 6 to 7 days a week. Side effects include insulin resistance, mild sodium and water retention, and anti-GH antibodies, none of which tend to be clinically significant. There is no increase in rates of leukemia or other cancers. In boys with severe constitutional delay, testosterone can be given for 4 to 6 months bearing in mind that this will increase growth, bone age, and induce puberty.

Tall Stature

Tall stature is defined as **height 2 SD above the mean.** Most patients have familial (genetic) tall stature and have normal growth velocity and bone age. Syndromes associated with tall stature are Marfan, Klinefelter, XYY, homocystinuria, and cerebral gigantism. Obesity can cause excessive growth, as can hyperthyroidism.

GH excess (pituitary gigantism) is rare and causes an increased linear growth rate. The usual culprit is a pituitary GH-producing tumor or a GH-releasing factor producing tumor in the hypothalamus or elsewhere. Precocious secretion of sex hormones causes increased linear growth but also **results in earlier closure of epiphyseal plates and advanced bone age, which can stunt adult height.** In cases of excessive predicted adult height, sex steroids can be used to stop growth.

PUBERTY

Normal Physiology

Prior to puberty, the hypothalamic–pituitary–gonadal axis is inhibited by some yet unknown mechanism. As puberty begins, GnRH pulses from the hypothalamus increase. GnRH rise increases the frequency and amount of LH and FSH release from the pituitary gland. Circulating LH and FSH stimulate the testes to produce testosterone or the ovaries to release estrogen, resulting in the development of secondary sex characteristics. Concurrently, the adolescent growth spurt occurs. The control mechanisms connecting puberty and growth acceleration are not completely understood.

Puberty in the Female

- Begins between ages 8 and 13 years and is completed in an average of 4.2 years.
- **Thelarche** (breast budding) is the first sign of pubertal development in 90% and occurs at an average of 10.5 years of age in Caucasians and 9.5 years of age in African Americans.
- Approximately 6 months after thelarche, **adrenarche** (development of pubic hair denoting activation of the hypothalamic–pituitary–adrenal axis) occurs.
- **Menarche** generally occurs 2.3 ± 1.0 years after thelarche.
- United States average age of menarche is 12.43 years.
- Higher body mass index (BMI) correlates with earlier menarche.
- **Linear growth acceleration** occurs soon after thelarche, generally at Tanner stage 3 for breast development.
- Growth velocity decreases after menarche, and growth is completed at an average bone age of 15 years.

Puberty in the Male

- Commences between ages 9 and 14 years and is usually completed in 3.5 years.
- First visible sign of puberty in most boys is **testicular enlargement** (>2.5 cm), which occurs at an average age of 11.5 years.
- **Adrenarche** follows about 6 months later with the development of pubic hair.
- Facial hair, voice deepening, and the production of sperm start at approximately Tanner stage 3 to 4.
- **Pubertal growth spurt** begins relatively later than in girls, at approximately genital Tanner stage 4. The period of growth acceleration also lasts longer than in girls, completing at a bone age of 17.

Precocious Puberty

Traditionally defined as sexual development in boys prior to 9 years of age and girls prior to 8 years of age. However, in girls, precocious puberty is now defined as development prior to 6 years of age in African Americans and before 7 years of age in other races.

Points to Remember

- Prepubescent males with bilaterally enlarged testicles almost always have central precocious puberty.

Central Precocious Puberty

True or central precocious puberty occurs when **early hypothalamic GnRH secretion occurs.** This is usually idiopathic in females, but more likely secondary to another process in males and necessitates further investigation. The main pathologic cause of precocious puberty is a CNS lesion, the most common of which is a hypothalamic hamartoma. Rarer causes include neurofibromas, gliomas, hydrocephalus, trauma, and postinfectious changes. **Findings of central precocious puberty** include accelerated linear growth; advanced bone age; and pubertal levels of LH, FSH, estradiol, and testosterone. Since hormone levels fluctuate, diagnosis may require a GnRH stimulation test. Precocious sexual development may occur with severe untreated hypothyroidism, but in contrast, these children have poor growth and may have a delayed bone age.

Treatment: Long acting GnRH agonists, generally as a monthly intramuscular injection. This halts the progression of sexual development, growth acceleration, and advancement of the bone age. Decision to treat precocious puberty is based on age at diagnosis, likely compromise to adult height, and social factors.

Gonadotropin-Independent Precocious Puberty

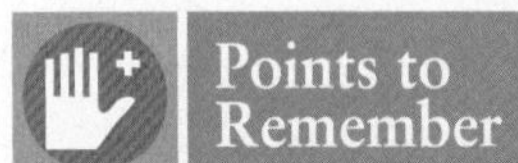

Points to Remember

- McCune–Albert syndrome: includes cafè au lait spots, polyostotic fibrous dysplasia, and precocious puberty.

Precocious puberty can occur independently of pituitary gonadotropins for a variety of reasons. In girls, these include exogenous estrogens (creams, pills), estrogen-producing tumors of the ovary or adrenal gland, ovarian cysts, and McCune–Albright syndrome.

In boys, precocious puberty may result from exogenous sources, such as topical androgens, adrenal enzymatic deficiencies, testicular tumor, familial Leydig cell hyperplasia, HCG-producing tumors, and adrenal tumors. **Clinical findings** include virilization, increased linear growth, and normal sized testes for age. A testicular tumor causes a difference in size between the testes. **Treatment** involves removing the source of excess androgens, or in the case of adrenal enzyme deficiency, treating with glucocorticoid replacement.

Premature Adrenarche

- Causes pubic and axillary hair development and axillary odor in the absence of other pubertal changes (testicular or breast enlargement) or virilization.
- Usually occurs between 6 and 8 years of age.
- Growth velocity and bone age can increase, but generally are within 2 **SD** of the mean.
- Puberty tends to ensue at a normal age.
- Can be caused by mild 21-OH deficiency which can be detected by ACTH stimulation test.

Premature Thelarche

- Defined as development of breast tissue without other signs of puberty.
- Patients do not develop pubic hair or have increased linear growth velocity.
- Occurs commonly (incidence estimated at 20.8 cases per 100,000 patient years), generally between 1 and 4 years of age.
- Can be unilateral or bilateral and generally does not progress beyond Tanner stage 3.
- Estrogen levels are generally prepubertal or mildly increased.
- Breast tissue usually regresses within 6 months to 6 years.

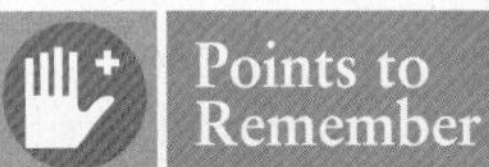

Points to Remember

- Differential diagnoses of pathologic gynecomastia:
  - Klinefelter syndrome
  - Partial androgen insensitivity
  - Partial blocks in testosterone biosynthesis
  - Hyperthyroidism
  - Adrenal or testicular tumor
  - Liver disease or tumor
  - Chronic illness
  - Illicit and therapeutic drugs.

Gynecomastia

- Pubertal (physiologic) gynecomastia occurs in approximately 40% of boys.
- Breast enlargement usually starts during Tanner stages 2 to 3, lasting approximately 2 years, and can be unilateral or asymmetric.
- May have increased ratios of estrogen to testosterone.
- **Important to distinguish between physiologic and pathologic gynecomastia.** Clues to pathologic origin of gynecomastia include history (onset before or after puberty, rapid progression, nipple discharge, drug use) or physical exam suggestive of underlying condition (>4 cm of breast tissue, small testicles, testicular mass, abnormal neurologic exam, eunuchoid body habitus).
- Severe cases are sometimes treated with tamoxifen, aromatase inhibitors, or surgery.

Delayed Puberty

Defined as no signs of puberty in girls by age 13 years or boys by age 14 years. Arrest of pubertal development also requires investigation. **If LH and FSH levels are high, there is likely a primary gonadal problem. If LH and FSH levels are low or normal, the cause of delayed puberty is likely a central hormonal abnormality or chronic disease.**

Primary Gonadal Delayed Puberty

Elevated gonadotropin (LH, FSH) levels indicate gonadal failure, since the pituitary lacks negative feedback from sex steroids (estrogen, testosterone). Common causes of gonadal failure are chemotherapy, radiation therapy, and autoimmune failure. Evaluation for other causes requires a karyotype.

Persons born with an XY karyotype with **androgen insensitivity syndrome** develop breasts, but never grow sexual hair or have menarche. Those with an XY karyotype and **complete 17-α-hydroxylase deficiency** have no secondary sexual characteristics, since they cannot form any sex steroids. If a phenotypic girl has partial androgen insensitivity or partial 17-α-hydroxylase deficiency, they can have some androgen effect, causing ambiguous genitalia as a neonate or virilization at puberty.

Turner syndrome (45X karyotype) generally causes lack of breast development, since ovaries usually fail prior to puberty. Girls with Turner syndrome do develop sexual hair, since adrenal androgens are not affected. Many patients are mosaic for this condition. (See chapter 12 "Genetics" for further discussion.)

Klinefelter syndrome patients (XXY) generally have gynecomastia and small testes as well as a eunuchoid body habitus (tall with a slim build and long limbs). (See chapter 12 "Genetics" for further discussion.)

Treatment: Replacement of sex steroids. For boys, testosterone injections can be given. In girls, conjugated estrogens are started and gradually increased to induce breast development for 1 to 2 years. Next, monthly cycles with estrogen and a progestin are started to induce menses. Oral contraceptive pills can be used for long-term treatment.

Normal or Low Gonadotropin Levels and Delayed Puberty

Constitutional delay is the most common cause of delayed puberty with normal or low gonadotropin levels. This can generally be diagnosed by physical examination and history and treated with reassurance. In seriously affected boys, short-term intramuscular testosterone can be considered.

Kallmann syndrome occurs secondary to lack of fetal GnRH neuron migration causing hypogonadotropic hypogonadism. Patients can have anosmia or hyposmia. A GnRH stimulation test can help differentiate this condition from constitutional delay.

Diagnosis: Evaluation of a possible organic cause for delayed puberty with normal or low gonadotropins requires imaging of the CNS. A prolactin-secreting adenoma can cause gonadotropin deficiency. Primary LH and FSH deficiency is associated with other pituitary hormone deficiencies such as GH deficiency. Uncorrected hypothyroidism can also delayed pubertal development.

Hypogonadotropic delayed puberty and growth failure may be caused by any ***chronic disease***. In evaluation for delayed puberty, it is important look at a patient's nutritional status and for evidence of undiagnosed conditions such as IBD or the female athletic triad. Several syndromes such as Prader–Willi and Laurence–Moon–Biedl can cause delayed puberty.

Treatment: In patients with hypogonadotropic pubertal delay, puberty can be induced and maintained with exogenous estrogen or testosterone. Gonadotropin injections can help with fertility problems.

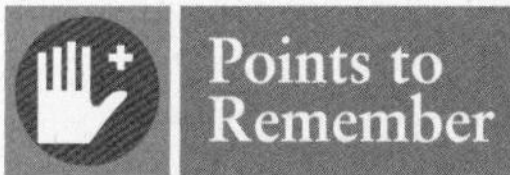

- **Female athletic triad: amenorrhea, disordered eating, and osteoporosis/penia.**

THYROID

Normal Physiology

TSH secreted by the pituitary gland stimulates the thyroid gland to take in iodine and synthesize T4 and T3. TRH secreted by the hypothalamus stimulates the pituitary to produce TSH. T4 exists in the blood stream in a free form (unbound) as well as bound to T4-binding globulin and other proteins. The free portion of T4 is biologically active, and it enters cells and is converted to T3. T3 is three to four times more potent than T4. T3 and T4 stimulate increased oxygen consumption, protein synthesis, and metabolism in the cell.

Hypothyroidism

Etiology: In children, hypothyroidism is either congenital (present at birth) or acquired. It is categorized by cause as primary (resulting from a defect in the thyroid gland itself) or central (stemming from failure of stimulation by the hypothalamus or pituitary grand). Familial dysfunction, generally acquired via autosomal recessive inheritance, only accounts for 10% to 15% of cases congenital hypothyroidism. Incidence of congenital hypothyroidism increases in areas of iodine deficiency. Sporadic cases are two times more common in girls than in boys; but in familial forms, sex distribution is equal.

Acquired hypothyroidism is an autoimmune process (**Hashimoto thyroiditis**) in the majority of cases. This is more common in females, and can occur on its own, in association with other autoimmune diseases (type 1 diabetes, Addison disease, vitiligo, etc.) and other disease processes, such as Down syndrome. **Other causes of hypothyroidism are as follows:** drug induced (from antithyroid drugs or lithium), iodine deficiency, irradiation, surgical excision, and subacute thyroiditis.

Box 10.1 Signs and Symptoms of Congenital Hypothyroidism

Large fontanelles	Prolonged jaundice
Umbilical hernia	Constipation
Macroglossia	Lethargy
Mottled, dry skin	Difficulty feeding
Hypotonia	Cool skin (hypothermia)
Abdominal distention	Sleeps through the night (newborn Hoarse cry period)
Respiratory distress	Goiter (rare)

Signs, Symptoms, and Consequences

See Box 10.1 for signs and symptoms of congenital hypothyroidism.

If hypothyroidism is untreated beyond 3 months of age, risk of intellectual impairment and poor growth increases.

Symptoms of acquired hypothyroidism vary based on age of onset (Box 10.2).

Usually, onset of hypothyroidism after 3 years of age does not compromise adult intelligence. However, untreated hypothyroidism can impair growth, elevate serum cholesterol, decrease school performance, and lead to slipped capital femoral epiphysis. Once hypothyroidism is treated, most clinical symptoms improve; however, a long period without treatment can compromise adult height.

Diagnosis: It is important to measure the concentration of free T4 in the blood, since many factors (including pregnancy, estrogen, and anticonvulsants) can affect T4-binding globulin and thus the total T4 concentration. **A low free T4 level for age is diagnostic of hypothyroidism.** If TSH is elevated with a low free T4, then primary hypothyroidism exists. A normal or low TSH in conjunction with a low free T4 generally indicates a central (hypothalamic or pituitary) cause. Testing for titers of thyroid peroxidase antibodies and thyroglobulin antibodies can confirm autoimmune thyroiditis. Children who have high risk for hypothyroidism, such as those with Down syndrome, diabetes, or a strong family history of autoimmune thyroid disease, should have serum TSH measured annually.

Treatment: Hypothyroidism is easily treated with **levothyroxine**. The dose must be individually tailored by monitoring TSH and free T4. As age increases, the amount of levothyroxine required per kilogram of weight decreases. Certain medications, such as iron and calcium, can inhibit absorption of levothyroxine, as can any disease causing intestinal malabsorption. In these cases, serum free T4 levels need to be followed closely, and drug doses adjusted accordingly.

Hyperthyroidism

Etiology: More than 95% of childhood cases of hyperthyroidism are caused by diffuse thyroid hyperplasia (Graves disease). **Graves disease** is an autoimmune disorder most commonly seen in

Box 10.2 Signs and Symptoms of Acquired Hypothyroidism

Short stature, decreased growth velocity	Lethargy
Obesity, myxedema	Delayed reflex return
Goiter (primary hypothyroidism)	Bradycardia
Delayed skeletal and dental age	Delayed puberty
Cold intolerance	Abnormal menses
Constipation	Precocious puberty (rare)
Dry, cool skin	Muscular pseudohypertrophy (rare)
Thinning of hair	Galactorrhea (rare)*

*Hypothalamic thyroid-releasing hormone stimulates problem release from the posterior pituitary. In primary hypothyroidism, increased thyroid-releasing hormone may produce hyperprolactinemia and galactorrhea.

Box 10.3 Signs and Symptoms of Hyperthyroidism

Goiter	Proptosis
Anxiousness, nervousness	Heat intolerance
Tachycardia	Increased growth velocity
Widened pulse pressure	Diarrhea
Increased appetite	Sleep disturbances
Weight loss or gain	Fatigue
Tremor	

adolescence and is six to eight times more prevalent in girls than boys. Autoantibodies to the thyroid's TSH receptors stimulate the gland to produce excessive T4. Graves disease can be familial and may be associated with other autoimmune diseases, including type 1 diabetes, Addison disease, myasthenia gravis, and vitiligo. Newborns of mothers with a history of Graves disease may develop newborn thyrotoxicosis from maternal antibodies crossing the placenta. On occasion, hyperthyroidism can occur in the early phase of autoimmune thyroiditis (Hashimoto thyroiditis). Other causes include a functional thyroid nodule, pituitary resistance to inhibition by T4, TSH-secreting pituitary adenoma, and factitious hyperthyroidism from ingestion of thyroid hormone.

Signs, Symptoms, and Consequences

For signs and symptoms of hyperthyroidism, see Box 10.3 and Figure 10.3. Clinical manifestations of hyperthyroidism are also referred to as thyrotoxicosis.

Diagnosis: Elevated free T4 with a low TSH. T3 is also elevated. Autoantibodies to the TSH receptor occur in 95% of patients.

Treatment: Graves disease can be treated with oral medication, radioiodine ablation therapy, or surgical excision. **Antithyroid medications** (propylthiouracil and methimazole) decrease production of thyroid hormone by the thyroid and block its effects. Propylthiouracil inhibits conversion of T4 to the more active T3 and crosses the placenta less than methimazole.

Radioiodine therapy consists of iodine-131 given orally, which induces thyroid gland cell death. The treatment is successful over 90% of the time. Hypothyroidism results in 40% to 80% of treated patients. Radioiodine treatment is gaining favor in adolescents and older children as experience and safety data increase.

Surgical treatment for hyperthyroidism involves either **subtotal or total thyroidectomy** and is generally reserved for those patients who fail medical management, have large goiters, or have severe ophthalmopathy. Cure rate is 90%, but the surgery carries risks of hypoparathyroidism, recurrent laryngeal nerve damage, and hypothyroidism.

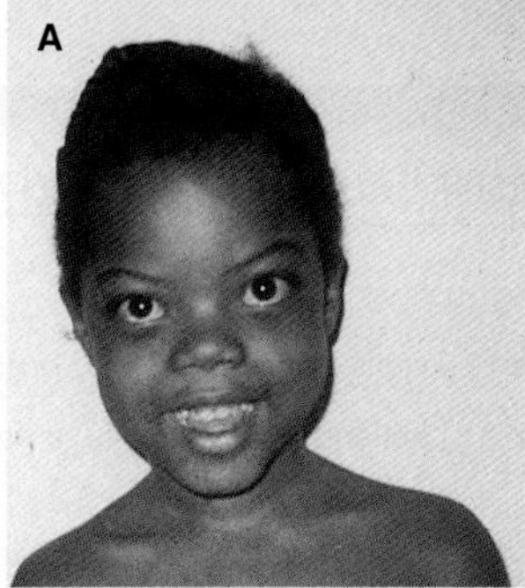

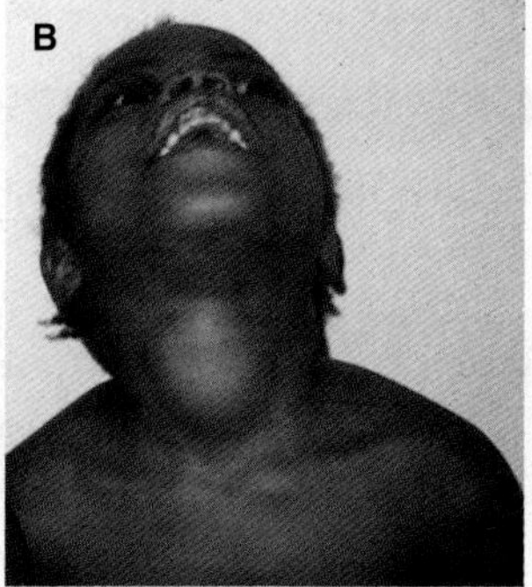

FIGURE 10.3. Hyperthyroidism thyrotoxicosis (Graves disease) occurs in approximately 2 per 1,000 children younger than 10 years. Affected children exhibit hypermetabolism and accelerated linear growth. Facial characteristics shown in this 6-year-old girl are (**A**) "staring" eyes (not true exophthalmos, which is rare in children) and (**B**) an enlarged thyroid gland (goiter). From Bickley LS, Szilagyi P. *Bates' Guide to Physical Examination and History Taking*. 8th ed. Philadelphia, PA: Lippincott Williams & Wilkins, 2003.

Box 10.4 Causes of Thyromegaly

Diffuse
Hashimoto thyroiditis
Thyrotoxicosis
  Graves disease
Thyroiditis
  Thyroid-stimulating hormone–secreting adenoma
  Pituitary resistance to thyroid hormone
Goitrogen exposure
Dyshormonogenesis
Iodine deficiency (endemic)
Idiopathic (simple) goiter
Acute, subacute thyroiditis

Nodular
Hashimoto thyroiditis
Thyroid cyst
Thyroid adenoma
Hyperfunctional (hot)
Hypofunctional (cold)
Thyroid carcinoma
  Papillary
  Follicular
  Mixed papillary or follicular
  Anaplastic
  Medullary
Nonthyroidal masses
  Lymphadenopathy
  Branchial cleft cyst
  Thyroglossal duct cyst

Thyroid Enlargement

Differential

For a complete differential of thyromegaly, see Box 10.4. The most common cause of enlarged thyroid gland (goiter) in children is **Hashimoto thyroiditis** (chronic lymphocytic thyroiditis). The gland becomes enlarged when the thyroid is infiltrated with lymphocytes and plasma cells. A simple or colloid goiter is an enlarged thyroid gland which is not caused by lymphocytic infiltration. It is usually asymptomatic. Graves disease (diffuse toxic goiter) also can cause an enlarged thyroid gland.

Acute suppurative thyroiditis is a rare cause of a large thyroid. Patients have a tender thyroid gland and are febrile. The most commonly implicated organisms are *Streptococcus pyogenes*, *Staphylococcus aureus*, and *Streptococcus pneumonia*. **Subacute thyroiditis** can be painful (subacute granulomatous thyroiditis) or asymptomatic (subacute lymphocytic thyroiditis). Subacute granulomatous thyroiditis typically follows an upper respiratory tract infection or other viral prodrome and is generally thought to have a viral etiology. Associated viruses include mumps, adenovirus, Epstein–Barr, influenza, and enteroviruses. Subacute lymphocytic thyroiditis patients may have an autoimmune etiology. Patients may present with symptoms of hyperthyroidism for up to 2 months, followed by euthyroidism or a short hypothyroid phase.

Diagnosis

See Table 10.2 for clinical strategies for differentiating causes of thyromegaly.

TABLE 10.2

CLINICAL FINDINGS ASSOCIATED WITH DIFFERENT CAUSES OF THYROID ENLARGEMENT

Condition	Clues to Diagnosis
Hashimoto thyroiditis	Nontender, firm, usually symmetric with a granular surface
Colloid goiter	Incidental finding, patients are usually asymptomatic and euthyroid
Graves disease	Symptoms of hyperthyroidism, elevated T4, and suppressed TSH
Acute thyroiditis	Leukocytosis, elevated ESR, painful thyroid exam. A fine needle aspirate reveals purulent material
Subacute granulomatous thyroiditis	Euthyroid or transiently hyperthyroid, no leukocytosis
Subacute lymphocytic thyroiditis	Symptoms of thyrotoxicosis w/increased T4. Distinguished from Graves with low radioiodine uptake on thyroid scan

TSH, thyroid-stimulating hormone.

Thyroid Nodules

Differential: Many solitary thyroid nodules result from benign tumors such as follicular adenomas. Colloid nodules are also common. A **thyroglossal duct cyst** consists of remnants of the embryonic thyroid gland, as it migrates from the base of the tongue to its position in the neck. It usually presents as a mobile, midline swelling in the neck, which is nontender unless it is acutely infected. A lateral location occurs in a minority of cases. Lymphocytic thyroiditis may cause a thyroid nodule. Malignancy of the thyroid is rare in children but is more common in females, and previous radiation of the neck greatly increases risk. **Papillary adenocarcinoma** is the most common type of thyroid malignancy in childhood. It tends to grow slowly and metastasize to local lymph nodes. **Follicular carcinoma** can also occur and is more likely to invade into blood vessels and spread to the lung and bone. **Medullary thyroid carcinoma** is associated with multiple endocrine neoplasia (MEN) types 2a and 2b.

Diagnosis: Diagnostic studies for delineation of a thyroid nodule include thyroid function tests, radionucleotide uptake and scan, ultrasound, and fine needle aspiration. In most cases, patients are euthyroid, but lymphocytic thyroiditis may cause hypothyroidism. Most malignant lesions are "cold" on **radionucleotide scanning**, but a majority of "cold" nodules are benign. **Ultrasound** can differentiate between cystic and solid lesions. Malignancies are most commonly solid. **Fine needle aspiration** is useful for obtaining pathology and avoiding unnecessary surgery if the nodule appears benign. Immediate surgery is indicated if the nodule is rapidly growing or associated with adjacent lymphadenopathy.

PARATHYROID

Normal Physiology

The parathyroid gland produces PTH. PTH targets osteoblastic cells in bone and renal tubular cells. In the bone, PTH indirectly activates osteoclasts to increase resorption of mineralized bone, which increases calcium and phosphorous in the blood. PTH activates proximal and distal tubule cells in the kidney to promote resorption of calcium and inhibit resorption of phosphorous, raising blood levels of calcium and decreasing phosphate. PTH also stimulates production of 1-α,25-dihydroxy vitamin D in the kidney. Changes in blood concentration of ionized calcium control PTH release. Lower calcium stimulates PTH release, and higher calcium inhibits the parathyroid from releasing PTH.

Hypoparathyroidism

Hypoparathyroidism causes hypocalcemia and usually hyperphosphatemia. Hypocalcemia can cause seizures, numbness, Chvostek sign, Trousseau sign, laryngospasm, bronchospasm, and prolonged QT. (See "Treatment" discussed later in the chapter.)

Autoimmune hypoparathyroidism can occur alone or as part of APECED syndrome. **Neonatal hypocalcemia** (early first 3 days, late after 5th day) results from agenesis or hypoplasia of the parathyroid glands, as part of the constellation of features associated with chromosome 22q11 mutations. There are multiple other known causes of hypoparathyroidism, including familial forms and infiltrative causes, for example, copper (Wilson disease) or iron (chronic transfusion therapy). A rare cause is autosomal dominant hypoparathyroidism, which results from increased function of the calcium sensing receptor of the parathyroid gland. This condition can also cause hypomagnesemia and hyperphosphatemia. **Hypoparathyroidism can be treated with vitamin D**, though patients need to be monitored for hypercalciuria.

Points to Remember

- **Chvostek sign is positive if tapping on the facial nerve causes the upper lip to twitch.**
- **Trousseau sign occurs when a blood pressure cuff is inflated above the systolic blood pressure for three minutes and muscle spasm in the hand is seen.**

Pseudohypoparathyroidism

Refers to a group of disorders where the bone and kidney are resistant to PTH, resulting in hypocalcemia, hyperphosphatemia, and increased concentrations of PTH.

Albright hereditary osteodystrophy refers to patients with PTH resistance and certain **characteristic physical findings**, including obese body habitus, round face, joint deformities, short metacarpal and metatarsal bones of the fourth and fifth digits, and hypoplastic dental enamel. A majority of patients also have mental retardation. These patients usually are not recognized in infancy and are typically diagnosed in the preschool age group. Patients with this phenotype who lack PTH resistance use to be referred to as having "pseudo-pseudohypoparathyroidism," but this term is no longer used. Now Albright hereditary osteodystrophy is used to describe the physical constellation of symptoms regardless of the presence of PTH resistance.

Pseudohypoparathyroidism is differentiated from hypoparathyroidism as a cause of hypocalcemia by an elevated PTH concentration in the former. The disorder is treated with 1,25-dihydroxyvitamin D (calcitriol) and calcium supplementation. Patients must have blood calcium and urine calcium levels followed closely to avoid hypercalciuria.

Points to Remember

- **MEN1 involves neoplasia of the pancreas, tumors of the anterior pituitary gland, and parathyroid gland hyperplasia. This autosomal dominant disorder always manifests hyperparathyroidism, but the other complications are less common. MEN2A causes medullary carcinoma of the thyroid, pheochromocytoma, and hyperparathyroidism.**

Hyperparathyroidism

Etiology: Hyperparathyroidism usually results from parathyroid adenomas, parathyroid gland hyperplasia, and chronic renal disease. Parathyroid gland hyperplasia is associated with MEN types 1 and 2 (MEN1 and MEN2).

Neonatal severe hyperparathyroidism is rare and is caused by loss of function of calcium sensing receptor located on chromosome 3.

Clinical Manifestations: Hyperparathyroidism causes hypercalcemia, resulting in muscle weakness, paralysis, hyporeflexia, constipation, anorexia, nausea, polyuria, polydipsia, nephrocalcinosis, bradycardia, and reduced QT interval.

Treatment: Hyperparathyroidism usually requires **subtotal parathyroidectomy** for correction.

CALCIUM AND PHOSPHATE METABOLISM

Normal Physiology

The level of calcium in the blood is regulated via PTH, vitamin D, and calcitonin. A majority of the body's calcium store is in the bone. Much of the calcium in the blood is bound by proteins, mainly albumin. Only the ionized portion of the calcium in the blood is physiologically active. Acidosis decreases the amount of calcium bound to protein, thus increasing the amount of free calcium. **PTH** increases calcium resorption from bone and the kidney, decreases phosphate resorption from the kidney, and stimulates renal activation of vitamin D.

Vitamin D is obtained from diet and sunlight. Sunlight starts formation of vitamin D from a precursor, which then requires activation steps in the liver (to 25-hydroxyl vitamin D) and kidney (to 1-α,25-hydroxy vitamin D). Vitamin D stimulates calcium resorption in the kidney as well as calcium and phosphate absorption in the intestines. **Calcitonin**, which is secreted by C cells in the thyroid gland, is stimulated by an acute increase in blood calcium levels. It inhibits osteoclast activity in the bones, decreasing calcium and phosphate levels.

Hypocalcemia

Etiology: Hypocalcemia is seen frequently in neonates. Early neonatal hypocalcemia occurs in the first 3 days of life, and late neonatal hypocalcemia occurs after 5 days of life. Preterm infants can have hypocalcemia from decreased PTH secretion. Asphyxia can cause hypocalcemia. Infants of diabetic mother can become hypocalcemic secondary to hypomagnesemia from maternal urinary magnesium loss. Hypomagnesemia impairs PTH secretion and action. Late neonatal hypocalcemia can occur from a high phosphate diet, hypoparathyroidism, or hypomagnesemia.

Childhood hypocalcemia can result from any process causing calcium malabsorption or resorption. Renal and liver dysfunction can lead to hypocalcemia from impaired activation of vitamin D. Medications, including calcitonin and bisphosphonates, can cause hypocalcemia. A defect in the calcium sensing receptor leads to the parathyroid gland not sensing hypocalcemia and not releasing PTH, resulting in hypocalcemia.

Signs and Symptoms: Hypocalcemia can cause seizures, numbness, Chvostek sign, Trousseau sign, laryngospasm, bronchospasm, and prolonged QT.

Diagnosis: A low PTH level suggests hypoparathyroidism. High PTH levels suggest vitamin D deficiency or pseudohypoparathyroidism. Magnesium and creatinine should also be measured.

Treatment: In an acutely ill patient, IV calcium should be given with careful cardiac monitoring until the patient stabilizes. If hypomagnesemia is the etiology, magnesium must be replaced. Long-term management depends on the etiology and usually requires both supplemental calcium and vitamin D replacement.

Hypercalcemia

Etiology

- Hyperparathyroidism, as already described.
- Hypercalcemia can also occur iatrogenically, especially in patients receiving parenteral nutrition, when they receive too much calcium or vitamin D.
- Idiopathic infantile hypercalcemia, which usually resolves by 1 year of age and has several different mechanisms.
- Williams syndrome, which is caused by an elastin gene mutation on chromosome 7.
- Granulomatous disorders, such as tuberculosis, sarcoidosis, and neonatal subcutaneous fat necrosis.
- Hypophosphatemia increases vitamin D synthesis, which can cause hypercalcemia.

Points to Remember

- **Williams syndrome: Patients may have distinctive facial features, supravalvular aortic stenosis, and developmental delay with a "cocktail party" personality**

TABLE 10.3

LABORATORY VALUES FOR CAUSES OF HYPERCALCEMIA

Cause	Phosphate	PTH	Vitamin D
Hyperparathyroidism	Low	High	
Iatrogenic		Low	Low
Idiopathic infantile hypercalcemia		Low	Normal
Granulomatous diseases		Low	High
Hypophosphatemia		Low	High
Hypophosphatasia		Low	Low
Williams syndrome		Low	Normal
Vitamin A intoxication		Low	Low

PTH, parathyroid hormone.

- Hypophosphatasia is an autosomal recessive disorder which results in undermineralized bones and hypercalcemia.
- Excessive vitamin A.

Signs and Symptoms: Muscle weakness, paralysis, hyporeflexia, constipation, anorexia, nausea, polyuria, polydipsia, nephrocalcinosis, bradycardia, and decreased QT interval.

Diagnosis: Table 10.3 details how to differentiate causes of hypercalcemia based on laboratory values.

Treatment: In an acutely ill child, fluid resuscitation and the use of furosemide diuretics lowers calcium. Adjunctive therapy with glucocorticoids (which decrease intestinal absorption of calcium), calcitonin, dialysis, and bisphosphonates (limited data in children) can be considered. Long-term therapy involves a low calcium and vitamin D diet with careful monitoring.

Rickets

Rickets is weakening of the bones, generally seen as an effect of low levels of active vitamin D. The process has multiple etiologies.

Etiology

- **Vitamin D Deficiency:** Classically occurs in breast-fed infants who are dark skinned and do not get enough sunlight exposure or vitamin D supplementation. It can also occur in rapidly growing children, such as low-birth-weight infants and adolescents. Congenital rickets results when pregnant mothers are significantly vitamin D deficient. Any disease process with intestinal malabsorption can lead to Vitamin D deficiency, including celiac disease, cystic fibrosis, and pancreatitis.
- **X-Linked Hypophosphatemic Rickets (Vitamin D Resistant Rickets or Familial Hypophosphatemia):** Caused by defective proximal tubular reabsorption of phosphates and impaired conversion of 25-dihydroxy-D3 to 1,25-dihydroxy-D3. The condition has an X-linked dominant inheritance.
- **Vitamin D–Dependent Rickets:** Results from reduced activity of 1-α-hydroxylase, which converts 25-dihydroxy-D3 (calciferol) to the active form, 1,25-dihydroxy-D3. It can also be caused by end organ resistance to calcitriol.
- **Renal:** Renal disease causes rickets via secondary hyperparathyroidism, inhibition of vitamin D stimulation by hyperphosphatemia, and lack of vitamin D activation by the kidney.

Signs and Symptoms

- In infants, hypocalcemia from vitamin D deficiency can cause seizures and tetany.
- Can present with hypotonia, failure to thrive, widened cranial sutures, frontal bossing, and craniotabes.
- Older children may have bowlegs, kyphosis, widened wrists, a rachitic rosary, developmental delay, delayed dentition, and pelvic deformities.
- Vitamin D–resistant rickets patients develop bowed legs, but generally lack other clinical features.

Diagnosis: Radiographs of wrists, knees, and shoulders reveal widened distal metaphyses with cupping and fraying as well as osteopenia (Fig. 10.4). Table 10.4 details how to differentiate the type of rickets based on laboratory values.

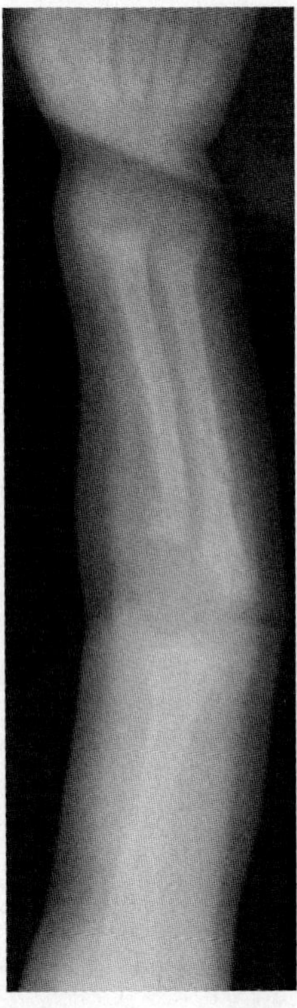

FIGURE 10.4. Radiographic findings in rickets of the upper extremity. Rickets in an 11-month-old boy breast-fed since birth. Radiograph of the upper extremity shows profound demineralization of the skeleton, with frayed, irregular cupping of the end of the metaphysis and poorly defined cortex. Note the retardation of skeletal maturation. From Fleisher GR, Ludwig S, Baskin MN. *Atlas of Pediatric Emergency Medicine*. Philadelphia, PA: Lippincott Williams & Wilkins, 2004.

Treatment: Initial management involves correcting the calcium and phosphorous levels. This may require an intravenous calcium drip. Supplementation with vitamin D is also started. Bones start healing in 1 to 2 weeks. Once x-rays show completed healing, vitamin D dose can be lowered. Both vitamin D–resistant and vitamin D–dependent rickets require oral phosphate supplementation and high doses of 1,25-dihydroxy-D3.

Hypophosphatemia

Etiologies

- Decreased intestinal absorption caused by vitamin D deficiency, malabsorption, or phosphate binding antacids.
- Increased renal excretion occurs from hyperparathyroidism, vitamin D deficiency, diuretics, and hyperglycemia or ketosis.
- A shift from extracellular to intracellular compartments, which occurs secondary to insulin.

Signs/Symptoms: Irritability, muscle weakness, myalgias, paresthesias, and in severe cases rhabdomyolysis. Chronic hypophosphatemia can cause rickets.

Treatment: Phosphorus replacement, either oral or intravenous.

TABLE 10.4

LABORATORY VALUES IN RICKETS

Type of Rickets	25-OH Vitamin D	1,25-$(OH)_2$ Vitamin D	PTH	Calcium	Phosphorous
Vitamin D deficiency	Low	Normal or high	High	Low	Low
Vitamin D resistant	Normal	Normal or low	Normal or high	Normal	Low
Vitamin D dependent	Normal	Low	Normal or high	Normal or low	Low

PTH, parathyroid hormone.

TABLE 10.5

CAUSES OF ADRENAL INSUFFICIENCY

Primary Adrenal Insufficiency	Secondary Adrenal Insufficiency
Congenital adrenal hyperplasia Autoimmune adrenal insufficiency (Addison disease) Adrenal hemorrhage Adrenal resistance to adrenocorticotropic hormone Adrenoleukodystrophy Isolated defects in mineralocorticoid synthesis Infections (tuberculosis, fungal, HIV)	Hypothalamic or pituitary dysfunction from tumors, surgery, or radiation Withdrawal from glucocorticoid therapy Insufficient replacement of glucocorticoids in a patient with known adrenal dysfunction

ADRENAL GLAND

Normal Physiology

The adrenal gland secretes three categories of hormones, glucocorticoids, mineralocorticoids, and androgens. **Glucocorticoid** secretion is controlled by ACTH release from the pituitary gland, which occurs in response to CRH from the hypothalamus. Cortisol inhibits the release of CRH and ACTH via negative feedback of both the pituitary and hypothalamus. **Glucocorticoids regulate metabolism, have anti-inflammatory effects, and protect the body during stress.**

The most potent mineralocorticoid is aldosterone. **Aldosterone** production is stimulated by angiotensin II in response to renin release by the kidney. Renin release occurs in response to decreased renal blood flow or low blood pressure. **Mineralocorticoids regulate extracellular fluid volume and potassium metabolism by stimulating the kidney to reabsorb sodium and excrete potassium.**

DHEA, DHEAS, and androstenedione are the primary **adrenal androgens.** Androstenedione can be converted peripherally to testosterone. Adrenal androgen regulation is not completely understood. Increased androgen secretion begins with adrenarche, which generally occurs with early signs of puberty.

Points to Remember

- **Two polyglandular autoimmune syndromes: Type I includes Addison disease, hypoparathyroidism, and chronic mucocutaneous candidiasis, and type II includes Addison disease, thyroid disease, and insulin dependent diabetes.**

Points to Remember

- **Hyperpigmentation is most commonly seen on the backs of the hands, elbows, and knees, and on the buccal mucosa.**

Adrenal Insufficiency

Etiology: Adrenal insufficiency can be either primary (resulting from dysfunction in the adrenal gland) or secondary (stemming from hypothalamic or pituitary dysfunction or adrenal suppression from exogenous glucocorticoid therapy). Table 10.5 details the causes of both primary and secondary adrenal insufficiency. Autoimmune primary adrenal insufficiency is known as Addison disease.

Signs and symptoms: Failure of the adrenal gland to produce aldosterone or cortisol can be life threatening. **Cortisol deficiency causes weakness, hypoglycemia, hypotension, and shock.** More subacute symptoms include fatigue, weight loss, abdominal pain, vomiting, anemia, eosinophilia, and hyperpigmentation. See Box 10.5 for a complete list of symptoms of adrenal insufficiency.

Box 10.5 Signs and Symptoms of Adrenal Insufficiency

- Glucocorticoid deficiency
  - Fasting hypoglycemia
  - Increased insulin sensitivity
  - Decreased gastric acidity
  - Gastrointestinal symptoms (e.g., nausea, vomiting)
  - Fatigue
  - Headaches
- Mineralocorticoid deficiency
  - Muscle weakness
  - Weight loss
  - Fatigue
  - Nausea, vomiting, anorexia
  - Salt craving
  - Hypotension
  - Hyperkalemia, hyponatremia, acidosis
- Androgen deficiency (in older children and adults)
  - Decreased pubic and axillary hair
  - Decreased libido
- Increased proopiomelanocortin cleavage products
  - Hyperpigmentation due to melanocyte stimulation

Box 10.6 Causes of Cushing Syndrome

ACTH Independent
Iatrogenic (e.g., glucocorticoid therapy)
Adrenocortical tumors (e.g., adenoma, mircinoma, micronodular disease)

ACTH Dependent
Hypothalamic CRH-producing tumor
Pituitary ACTH-producing tumor
Ectopic CRH-producing tumor (e.g., pancreas, lung)
Ectopic ACTH-producing tumor (e.g., lung, bronchus, gut)
Iatrogenic (e.g., ACTH therapy)
Increased serotonin levels (e.g., idiopathic)

ACTH, adrenocorticotropic hormone; CRH, corticotropin-releasing hormone.

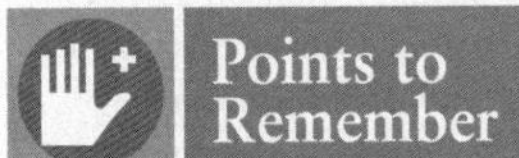

Points to Remember

- **ACTH stimulation test: a cortisol level is drawn before and after a dose of ACTH is given to measure adrenal response.**

Diagnosis: Suggested by the combination of hyponatremia, hyperkalemia, and hypoglycemia. Further evidence of glucocorticoid insufficiency requires a low cortisol level, with increased ACTH. An ACTH stimulation test may be needed to confirm the diagnosis. A low aldosterone level in setting of increased renin level confirms mineralocorticoid insufficiency.

Treatment: In an acutely ill child, treatment includes volume resuscitation, glucose, glucocorticoid replacement with IV hydrocortisone, and correction of hyperkalemia. Patients require frequent glucose and electrolyte monitoring. Once stabilized, **maintenance glucocorticoid dose is calculated based on the child's surface area.** The **dose must be increased during times of stress,** such as illness and surgery, and parents must be trained to give IM hydrocortisone if the patient cannot tolerate oral doses during an illness. **Mineralocorticoid is replaced with oral fludrocortisone.**

Glucocorticoid Excess

Etiology: Cushing syndrome, the clinical effect of elevated glucocorticoids, can occur with endogenous production of excess cortisol or from exogenous steroids. Endogenous causes include adrenal tumors, adrenal hyperplasia, and ACTH-producing tumors (Box 10.6). **Cushing disease** refers specifically to excess glucocorticoid from an ACTH-producing pituitary adenoma. Cushing disease occurs nine times more commonly in females than males.

Signs and symptoms: Box 10.7 details clinical features of glucocorticoid excess.

Diagnosis: Glucocorticoid excess can be suspected when an obese child has poor height velocity. Bone age is usually delayed. Excessive cortisol secretion is confirmed with a 24-hour urine-free cortisol level. A midnight free cortisol level compared with an 8:00 AM cortisol level

Box 10.7 Clinical Features of Hypercortisolism

Obesity with violaceous striae (generalized in infants, truncal in older children with moon facies or buffalo hump)
Decreased height velocity (short stature, delayed bone age)
Plethora, increased hematocrit
Easy bruising
Hypertension
Osteoporosis
Glucose intolerance
Poor wound healing
Increased frequency of infections
Renal stones, hypercalciuria
Weakness, muscle wasting (unusual in infants)
Depression or other psychiatric symptoms

can demonstrate an increased ratio, showing loss of the normal circadian rhythm of cortisol stimulation. Once excess cortisol secretion is confirmed, the etiology requires elucidation. A high-dose dexamethasone suppression test and CRH stimulation test can help differentiate Cushing disease from other causes of glucocorticoid excess. Patients with Cushing disease have an exaggerated response to CRH, with a large increase in both ACTH and cortisol. In patients with ectopic ACTH secretion, no response is seen.

MRI with gadolinium is only about 50% sensitive in finding pituitary adenomas. Sampling blood ACTH levels in the petrosal sinuses bilaterally after administration of CRH may be necessary to find out on which side of the pituitary an adenoma is located. MRI of the abdomen can be used to find adrenal adenomas.

Treatment: In children with Cushing syndrome from excess administration of glucocorticoids, the only treatment is decreasing these drugs if possible. In Cushing disease, cure is possible with transsphenoidal resection of the pituitary adenoma. Drug therapy with medications which inhibit steroid production in the adrenal gland can be used if surgery fails. Radiation therapy can be used, but it can cause hypopituitarism.

TYPE 1 DIABETES

Epidemiology: Type 1 diabetes occurs in 15 to 17 per 100,000 children in the United States with approximately 13,000 children and adolescents diagnosed each year. It has equal prevalence in males and females. Incidence is bimodal, with peaks between 4 and 6 years and in early puberty (10 to 14 years old). Risk of developing diabetes is increased with a positive family history (Box 10.8).

Pathogenesis: Type 1 diabetes occurs when the insulin-producing beta cells in the pancreas are destroyed via T cells and autoantibodies after an environmental stimulus. Genetic factors predispose patients to develop type 1 diabetes. The triggering environmental factor may be a virus, a food, or a toxin.

Diagnosis: Defined as fasting glucose level of more than 126 or random glucose level of more than 200 with symptoms. Clinical evidence of hyperglycemia includes polydipsia, polyuria, hyperphagia, and weight loss. Several antibodies are markers for type 1 diabetes, including islet cell antibodies, insulin autoantibodies, antibodies against glutamic acid decarboxylase, and tyrosine phosphatase IA-2 or ICA512.

Treatment: Type 1 diabetes requires therapy with insulin. The goal of therapy is to tightly regulate blood glucose by trying to use insulin physiologically. Multiple preparations of insulin with varying durations of action and time to peak activity are available. The most commonly used types are regular insulin (which is short acting), rapid-acting insulins (aspart and lispro), and insulin glargine, a long-acting product without a peak. The necessary amount of insulin needed for basal control, carbohydrate coverage, and hyperglycemic correction factor is estimated based on weight (approximately 1 unit/kg/day) and is adjusted as needed based on blood sugar.

Goals of therapy: Target hemoglobin A_{1C} (HbA_{1C}) is generally less than 8 for school-age children and less than 7.5 for adolescents. Targets are higher for younger children because they are more susceptible to hypoglycemia.

Complications: DKA is the presenting symptom in 25% to 40% of new onset type 1 diabetics. DKA may present with vomiting, dehydration, abdominal pain, abnormal breathing (Kussmaul respirations), and decreased level of consciousness. Glucose is elevated, ketones are in the urine, and the blood pH is acidotic. Patients require fluid resuscitation, intravenous insulin, and electrolyte correction. Once resuscitation is begun, there is a risk for cerebral edema, a major cause of morbidity and mortality in DKA. Symptoms of this include headache, lethargy, seizures, pupillary changes, decreased heart rate, and increased blood pressure.

Long-term effects: Diabetes causes **both microvascular and macrovascular complications,** leading to multiple end-organ effects such as diabetic retinopathy, renal impairment, peripheral neuropathy, poor wound healing, and cardiac disease. Consistent control of blood sugar can lower the risk of these complications.

Associated conditions: Children with type 1 diabetes are at increased risk for other autoimmune endocrine diseases, especially hypothyroidism and celiac disease. Screening is recommended annually.

Box 10.8 Risk of Developing Type 1 Diabetes if One Sibling is Affected

Identical twins: <50%	HLA haploidentical: 1 in 20
HLA identical: 1 in 5	HLA nonidentical: 1 in 100

Health Supervision

- Review glucose levels and HbA_{1C} every 3 months.
- Height and weight plotted.
- Blood pressure monitoring and aggressive treatment of hypertension.
- Assess lower extremities for peripheral neuropathy.
- Urine microalbumin should be checked once a year after 5 years of diabetes or once puberty starts.
- Yearly screening for thyroid dysfunction and celiac disease.
- Fasting lipid panel drawn every few years and aggressively treat hyperlipidemia to help lower cardiac risk factors.
- Diabetics require a dilated funduscopic examination yearly after they have had diabetes for 5 years to assess for diabetic retinopathy.

TYPE 2 DIABETES

Epidemiology: Type 2 diabetes incidence in children has been increasing along with the rise in obesity. Rates vary by ethnicity and location, and are highest in Native Americans, Asians, Mexican Americans, and African Americans. Many patients with type 2 diabetes have a family history of the disease, pointing to a genetic predisposition.

Pathophysiology: Although type 1 diabetes results from autoimmune destruction of the pancreas, type 2 diabetes has a more heterogeneous etiology. Insulin resistance, the failure to respond to normal levels of insulin, is the first step toward the development of type 2 diabetes. The pancreas responds by increasing its secretion of insulin to maintain euglycemia. When the pancreas can no longer meet the need for more insulin, hyperglycemia results.

Diagnosis: Fasting glucose level of more than 126, a random glucose level of more than 200 in the presence of symptoms, or a 2-hour blood sugar of more than 200 on a glucose tolerance test. Patients frequently are overweight and may have acanthosis nigricans, a marker of insulin resistance. Determining whether a patient has type 1 or type 2 diabetes can be difficult. Having detectable levels of insulin and c-peptide indicate type 2 diabetes. A lack of autoantibodies typical of type 1 diabetes is helpful in the diagnosis, as is a family history and signs of insulin resistance (Table 10.6).

Therapy: The goal is to achieve near normoglycemia measured by fasting glucose and HbA_{1C} and to decrease long-term complications. **First-line therapy is lifestyle modification to produce weight loss and increased insulin sensitivity.** Many children have significant hyperglycemia at diagnosis and may require insulin therapy at least temporarily to improve glycemic control. The **first-line oral drug is metformin** (approved for children older than 10 years), which decreases hepatic glucose production and enhances insulin sensitivity. The thiazolidinediones (rosiglitazone and pioglitazone) improve peripheral insulin sensitivity but are rarely used in children. Aggressive control of dyslipidemia and hypertension in type 2 diabetics is recommended to help decrease risk of cardiac disease and renal dysfunction. Type 2 diabetics require monitoring for the same end-organ complications, such as retinopathy and nephropathy, as type 1 diabetic patients.

Screening: Overweight children older than 10 years (BMI >85%) or who have started puberty should be screened for diabetes (fasting blood sugar) if they have two additional risk factors. These risk factors include a family history of type 2 diabetes in a first or second degree relative, having a high-risk race or ethnicity (Hispanic, Native American, African American, or Asian), or signs of insulin resistance (acanthosis nigricans, polycystic ovarian syndrome, hypertension, or dyslipidemia). Screening should be repeated every 2 years.

TABLE 10.6

CHARACTERISTICS SUGGESTIVE OF TYPE 1 VERSUS TYPE 2 DIABETES AT PRESENTATION

	Type 1	Type 2
Polydipsia and polyuria	Present for days to weeks	Absent, or present for weeks to months
Ethnicity	Caucasian	African American, Hispanic, Native American, Asian
Weight	Weight loss more common	Obese
Other findings		Acanthosis nigricans
Family history	Negative	Positive
Insulin or C-peptide level	Low	High
Ketoacidosis	More common	Less common
Autoantibodies	Positive	Less common

METABOLIC SYNDROME

Definition: The definition of metabolic syndrome (insulin-resistance syndrome or syndrome X) in children is debated. In adults, metabolic syndrome consists of abdominal obesity (based on waist circumference) and at least two of the following factors: high triglycerides, low high-density lipoprotein (HDL), hypertension, and elevated fasting blood sugar. In children, the International Diabetes Federation defines metabolic syndrome as the combination of abdominal obesity (waist circumference greater than 90th percentile for age), insulin resistance (elevated fasting blood sugar), dyslipidemia (elevated triglycerides and decreased HDL), and hypertension. Children with central obesity and at least two of the other associated findings are classified as having the metabolic syndrome. Controversy exists over using BMI versus waist circumference for the definition of obesity. The cutoff for elevated fasting glucose varies between 100 and 110 depending on author opinion.

Screening: Overweight children (BMI >85%) should undergo screening for other findings of the metabolic syndrome, including blood pressure, fasting glucose, and a fasting lipid panel.

Complications: Metabolic syndrome increases the risk of type 2 diabetes and coronary artery disease. Obesity increases the risk for many other problems, such as obstructive sleep apnea, asthma, slipped capital femoral epiphysis, Blount disease, steatohepatitis, and gallbladder disease. Females with obesity are at a high risk of developing polycystic ovarian syndrome, leading to irregular periods, acne, hirsutism, and infertility. Obese children also may have poor self-image and are at risk for depression.

Management: One of the first steps in combating metabolic syndrome is aggressive weight management via improved diet and increased exercise. If lifestyle modifications are unsuccessful and lipid levels are above age-based cutoffs, lipid lowering drugs may be required. Hypertension also should be treated first with lifestyle modifications, followed by drug therapy if this fails to lower blood pressure.

SAMPLE BOARD REVIEW QUESTIONS

1. You are called to evaluate a 2-hour-old female infant in the newborn nursery. Apgars were 8 and 9, and the infant has been already successfully breast-fed. The nurse in the nursery noted that the infant has an enlarged clitoris and posterior fusion of the labia majora. The rest of the physical exam is normal. Maternal history reveals no medical problems and no medications taken during pregnancy except for prenatal vitamins. What laboratory tests are needed to establish the most likely diagnosis?
   a. Chromosomal analysis and skeletal survey
   b. Electrolytes and glucose
   c. Chromosomal analysis and 17-OHP level
   d. Chromosomal analysis and testosterone level
   e. Maternal toxicology screen and pelvic ultrasound

   Answer: c. The most likely diagnosis in a presumed virilized female infant without known exposure to exogenous androgens is congenital adrenal hyperplasia cause by 21-OH deficiency, which is diagnosed by an elevated 17-OHP level. Chromosomal analysis is necessary to determine the genetic sex. Female pseudohermaphrodism can also be caused by exposure to exogenous androgens, from maternal medications or tumor. An infant with congenital adrenal hyperplasia needs close monitoring of glucose and electrolytes, but salt wasting usually does not occur in the first week of life, and electrolyte abnormalities do not establish a definitive diagnosis.

2. The parents of an overweight 10-year-old boy (BMI >95% for age) in your practice express concern that their son could have a "glandular" problem causing his obesity. They admit that he does not enjoy sports and prefers to play video games. However, his parents do not understand his weight gain when he eats the same diet as the rest of the family. They also think he has less energy than his siblings. Exam reveals a well-appearing child with a weight greater than the 97th percentile and height in the 75th percentile. He is noticeably overweight, with acanthosis nigricans on his neck and a few striae on his abdomen. What additional information about his growth would help you determine whether an endocrine disorder is a likely cause of his body habitus?
   a. His history of decreased energy
   b. The presence of acanthosis nigricans and striae
   c. Lack of obesity in the rest of the family
   d. A reduction in height growth not concordant with weight overgrowth
   e. A family history of hypothyroidism

   Answer: d. Children with endocrine disorders causing obesity, including hypothyroidism, Cushing syndrome, and GH deficiency, have poor linear growth. If this child previously had tracked along the 97th percentile for height, and then had decreased growth velocity and height percentile, this could indicate an underlying problem. Screening laboratory work would include a TSH, free T4, IGF-1, IGFBP-3, screening for any underlying medical problems suggested by history and physical examination, and urine cortisol level if Cushing syndrome in suspected. Decreased energy, acanthosis nigricans, and striae are all nonspecific for endocrine problems.

3. A 3.5-year-old girl presents to your practice after moving from out of state. Her mother is 63 inches tall, and her father is 71 inches tall. Their daughter's weight and height are below the third percentile. Weight for height is in the 25th percentile. Her parents report that she was 6 lb 7 oz baby born at 39 weeks without complications. She was admitted once at age 6 weeks with respiratory syncytial virus bronchiolitis. Otherwise, her parents report that she has always been healthy and developmentally appropriate. Examination reveals a pleasant 3-year-old girl with no obvious dysmorphic features. Recent laboratory work from her previous pediatrician showed normal CBC, CMP, thyroid studies, tissue transglutaminase, IGF-1, IGFBP3, ESR, and CMP. A bone age done 2 months ago was 36 months. What test is needed to complete for the evaluation of her poor growth?
   a. Serologic testing for IBD
   b. Karyotype
   c. Urine cortisol level
   d. GH stimulation test
   e. None-reassurance is all that is required

Answer: b. Evaluation of a female with short stature requires a karyotype to look for possible Turner syndrome. Though girls with Turner syndrome often have widely spaced nipples, low hairline, and widened carrying angle, these findings may not be present. Screening labs did not show elevated inflammatory markers, which would indicate possible IBD. The child has no physical findings of Cushing syndrome, so a urine cortisol is not necessary. GH stimulation test may be required if GH deficiency is suspected, though normal IGF-1 and IGFBP-3 levels make this less likely. Reassurance and no further testing is not appropriate until all the indicated testing is done and is normal, at which point idiopathic short stature can be diagnosed.

4. During a routine physical examination, a 14-year-old boy confesses that he gets teased in school for being so short. His parents keep reassuring him that he will soon "hit his growth spurt," but he is not convinced and thinks something is wrong. On examination, his height is in the 10th percentile and his weight is in the 5th to 10th percentile. Examining his growth chart, you find that he tracked along the 50th percentile until the last 18 months, when his growth seemed to slow down. His genitals and pubic hair are Tanner stage 2. What is the most appropriate response to his concern?
   a. Referral to a psychologist for counseling to build his self-esteem
   b. Reassurance that he will eventually grow
   c. Screening lab work and a bone age x-ray
   d. Testosterone injections monthly for 3 months
   e. Follow-up exam in 1 year to track his progress

Answer: c. The most likely explanation for this child's decrease in height percentile is constitutional growth delay. However, his poor growth velocity over the past 18 months and crossing of percentiles deserves at least a screening laboratory workup for thyroid dysfunction, GH deficiency, underlying chronic illness, etc. A careful physical exam is needed to look for signs of chronic disease, such as anal skin tags or mouth ulcers. A delayed bone age with normal lab work would indicate constitutional growth delay. His growth and sexual development could then be followed closely (every 3 to 6 months) to track his growth velocity. Testosterone injections could be considered in a severe case of constitutional delay/delayed puberty. Follow up in 1 year is not soon enough to closely follow his growth.

5. The mother of one of your clinic patients is concerned that her 12-year-old daughter has not started to develop breasts. She says that in her family everyone had menarche by the age of 12. She is worried that her daughter might have something wrong with her. She says her daughter eats a well balanced diet and is generally healthy. On exam, the child is in the 25th percentile for height and 10th to 25th percentile for weight. She is nondysmorphic and well appearing. She has Tanner 2 breast development and Tanner 2 pubic hair. What is the proper response to your patient's mother's concerns?
   a. Referral to endocrinology for delayed puberty
   b. Karyotype, bone age, LH, FH, and estradiol measurement
   c. Reassurance that her daughter has started puberty and close follow up
   d. Referral to GI for workup of occult GI disease
   e. Administration of conjugated estrogens to help start breast development.

Answer: c. Delayed puberty in females is considered no pubertal development by the age of 13. This patient has started to develop both breast and pubic hair, and thus has started puberty within the proper time frame. As long as her growth and physical exam are normal, there are no concerns. Her mother needs to be reassured that her development is normal. Her growth and pubertal development should be followed closely, and she can be referred to an endocrinologist if concerns arise.

6. A 5-year-old girl has developed breast budding bilaterally. Her mother brings her to the pediatrician for evaluation. She has 3 cm of breast tissue on the right and 2 cm on the left. How will you determine whether she has benign premature thelarche or precocious puberty?
   a. If she has pubic hair, then this is precocious puberty; otherwise, she has premature thelarche
   b. Since she has bilateral breast enlargement, this is more likely precocious puberty than premature thelarche
   c. The patient can be followed every 6 months to see if the breast development regresses or progresses to tell the difference
   d. If she has accelerated growth velocity, advanced bone age, and pubertal levels of LH, FSH, and estradiol, this is likely precocious puberty
   e. If estrogen level is increased, this is likely precocious puberty

Answer: d. Precocious puberty is diagnosed when the patient has accelerated growth, advanced bone age, and pubertal levels of the gonadotropins and estrogen. In girls, this is generally idiopathic. If gonadotropin levels are prepubertal and growth velocity is normal for age, this is likely premature thelarche and can be monitored closely. Precocious puberty can be treated with long-acting GnRH agonists. In premature thelarche, estrogen levels may be mildly elevated.

7. A 15-year-old girl is brought into your clinic by her mother for her yearly physical examination. Mother reports she has been generally healthy, but since school started this year, she has had an "attitude change." Her grades are not as high as the previous year, and she has gotten in trouble for falling asleep in school. When interviewed alone, the patient denies drug use, symptoms of depression, or psychological stress. She complains of chronic fatigue despite sleeping at least 9 hours a night and trouble concentrating. What physical exam findings and laboratory results would support a diagnosis of primary hypothyroidism?
   a. Increased weight, elevated heart rate, low TSH, and high free T4
   b. Increased weight, low heart rate, low TSH, and low free T4
   c. Decreased weight, high heart rate, low TSH, and high free T4
   d. Increased weight, low heart rate, high TSH, and low free T4
   e. Decreased weight, low heart rate, high TSH, and low free T4

Answer: d. An increase in weight and low pulse can be found in patients with hypothyroidism. Primary hypothyroidism indicates dysfunction of the thyroid gland itself, which causes low T4 and an elevated TSH. Secondary hypothyroidism originates from dysfunction of the hypothalamus or pituitary gland and would cause low T4 in the setting of an inappropriately low TSH.

8. A 5-year-old girl with Down syndrome (trisomy 21) presents to your office for her annual physical exam. Other than a history of a VSD repaired at the age of 7 months, she has not had any significant health problems. Mother reports her daughter is thriving in her special education kindergarten class. When you plot her height on a Down syndrome growth chart, you note that she is now at the 10th percentile for height and 75th for weight, whereas she had previously been tracking at the 25th for height and 50th for weight. What must you check before attributing her increasing BMI to diet and lack of exercise?
   a. TSH and free T4
   b. Echocardiogram to make sure her VSD has not reopened
   c. Tissue transglutaminase and antiendomysial antibody (IgA)
   d. Urine free cortisol
   e. Bone age, IGF1, and IGFBP3

Answer: a. Children with Down syndrome are at increased risk for developing hypothyroidism and require regular screening. This could account for decrease in height percentile with increased weight. Celiac disease generally would cause poor weight gain. Cushing syndrome could cause weight gain with poor growth, but this is less common than hypothyroidism. GH deficiency also can cause these findings but is not as common as hypothyroidism.

9. A 1-month-old male infant presents to the emergency room with a generalized tonic clonic seizure at home which lasted approximately 5 minutes. He is currently sleeping in his mother's arms. On exam, his vital signs and weight are normal for age. The only notable finding on exam is a heart murmur. Labs reveal an electrolyte abnormality, and head CT is negative. Mother states her child is formula fed. He was diagnosed with a heart murmur at birth, and she was supposed to follow up with a pediatrician and a heart specialist, but she has been unable to make it to any of the appointments secondary to transportation issues. If the baby's formula is being properly prepared and his vitamin D level is normal, what diagnostic test would you want to do?
   a. Chromosomal analysis for possible trisomy 21
   b. Head MRI for possible periventricular leukomalacia
   c. FISH for 22Q11
   d. Leg films to look for bowing
   e. Liver function tests

   Answer: c. Hypocalcemia is a common cause of seizures in infants. Vitamin D–deficiency rickets can lead to hypocalcemia. This is most common in dark skinned, exclusively breast-fed babies. 22q11 can cause cardiac defects and hypocalcemia secondary to hypoplasia of the parathyroid glands. It is diagnosed via FISH analysis for the specific deletion.

10. A 1-week-old, 38 week gestational age male infant is in the NICU for aortic stenosis diagnosed on prenatal echo and poor feeding. The cardiologists have made the decision that the child can wait until he is older for cardiac repair, since he appears to have adequate systemic blood pressures. However, the baby is taking PO feeds very poorly and is requiring a majority of his feeds via NG tube. Labs have persistently shown hypercalcemia, despite adequate hydration and discontinuing parenteral nutrition. What diagnosis would explain his cardiac anomaly and hypercalcemia?
   a. Down syndrome
   b. 22Q11 deletion
   c. Prader–Willi syndrome
   d. CHARGE association
   e. Williams syndrome

   Answer: e. Williams syndrome, caused by an elastin gene mutation, is associated with hypercalcemia in neonates, supravalvular aortic stenosis, and mental retardation.

11. An 18-month-old male presents for an initial visit to a new primary care office. The family moved into the area about 9 months ago, but his insurance just recently became active. On exam, he is noted to have bowed legs and is not yet walking. Mother admits to giving her child whole milk a few times, but he "didn't like it." He mostly drinks water and juice. When the family moved to the area, it took some time to find the WIC office. Mother says she only could afford a small amount of formula during this time, so her child received about 8 oz of formula a day from 9 months until 1 year. What is the proper treatment for this condition?
   a. Referral to orthopedics for bracing and possible osteotomies
   b. Calcium and vitamin D supplementation with laboratory monitoring
   c. Nutritional counseling
   d. Switching to soy milk
   e. Referral to nephrology for renal replacement therapy

   Answer: b. Initially, this child will need measurement of calcium, phosphorus, and 1,25-vitamin D levels to confirm vitamin D–deficiency rickets. Initial therapy involves replacing both calcium and vitamin D. Patients may also require phosphorous replacement. Maintenance therapy generally consists of lower doses of vitamin D.

12. An 8-year-old girl presents to the emergency department with abdominal pain and lethargy for several days. She has no significant past medical history and has not had any fever. Triage assessment reveals an ill appearing child with mild diffuse abdominal pain. Initial vitals are temperature of 36.3, heart rate of 167, respiratory rate of 30, and blood pressure of 74/39. She is rushed to a room, and IV access is obtained. A normal saline bolus is started. Initial glucose is 43 and potassium is 5.7. In addition to giving her a bolus of dextrose, what other medication should be given?
   a. Ceftriaxone, once blood cultures are drawn
   b. Albumin
   c. Phenylephrine
   d. Hydrocortisone
   e. Glucagon

Answer: c. With hypotension, hypoglycemia, and hyperkalemia, this is likely adrenal crisis. Treatment should include stress-dose steroids. Sepsis also is on the differential, and antibiotics would certainly be advisable until diagnosis is confirmed.

13. A 4-year-old girl has recently been diagnosed with type 1 diabetes after a 2-week history of thirst and secondary enuresis. Her parents bring her to her first endocrinology appointment after hospital discharge. Mother is 6 months pregnant and has multiple questions regarding her daughter's health and that of her future child. Which of the following is a true statement regarding her unborn child.

a. Prenatal testing is available
b. Siblings of children with diabetes need frequent blood sugar monitoring
c. Keeping her child at a healthy weight can prevent the development of diabetes
d. Her child has a less than 1% lifetime risk of developing diabetes
e. Her child is at increased risk of diabetes, but screening in the absence of symptoms is not recommended

Answer: e. Having a first-degree relative with type 1 diabetes does increase the risk of developing the disease. However, there is no prenatal testing available, and there is no recommended screening protocol.

14. A 5-year-old boy presents to the emergency room with a two day history of abdominal pain and emesis. His parents report that he started vomiting with PO fluids and complaining about his stomach the day prior to presentation. Now he refuses to get out of bed and has been sleeping most of the day. Initial vitals are temperature of 37.2, pulse rate of 157, respiratory rate of 34, and blood pressure of 96/45. Mucous membranes are dry. It is difficult to get him to wake up and answer questions. He complains of diffuse abdominal pain on palpation, but he has negative psoas and obturator signs. Bedside glucometer reading is "high." What principles of fluid management must you remember when resuscitating this child.

a. Give 20 to 40 cm^3/kg normal saline boluses, and then start fluids with potassium and phosphorous to make up fluid deficit over 24 to 48 hours
b. Obtain a CT scan of his abdomen to look for a steroid-secreting tumor
c. Give up to 80 cm^3/kg in initial boluses, and then start fluids with electrolyte replacement to correct 75% of fluid deficit in the first 12 hours
d. Once initial labs return, if he is hyponatremic, start 2% saline
e. If his initial BUN and creatinine are elevated, start fluids at one-third calculated maintenance and replace urine output cubic centimeter for cubic centimeter.

Answer: a. A child in DKA can present with severe dehydration from osmotic diuresis, emesis, and poor PO. Hyperglycemia can cause hyponatremia and prerenal azotemia. It is important to start resuscitation immediately and bolus isotonic fluids. However, you do not want to correct his water deficit or hyperglycemia too quickly, since this can lead to cerebral edema.

15. A 12-year-old African American girl presents for her annual physical examination. On exam, her BMI is greater than the 95th percentile for age, and she has acanthosis nigricans. What screening test is recommended?

a. Fasting insulin level
b. Fasting glucose level
c. Serum c-reactive protein
d. Complete blood count
e. Thyroid studies

Answer: b. Fasting glucose level to screen for type 2 diabetes is appropriate in overweight children older than 10 years or who have started puberty and have two additional risk factors for diabetes. Being African American and having markers of insulin resistance (acanthosis nigricans) gives this patient two risk factors. Fasting glucose level of more than 126 qualifies as having diabetes.

SUGGESTED READINGS

Aggoun Y. Obesity, metabolic syndrome, and cardiovascular disease. *Pediatr Res*. 2007;61:653–658.

Anhalt H, Neely EK, Hintz R. Ambiguous genitalia. *Pediatr Rev*. 1996;17:213–220.

August G. Treatment of adrenocortical insufficiency. *Pediatr Rev*. 1997;18:59–62.

Burgert T, Markowitz M. Understand and recognizing pseudohypoparathyroidism. *Pediatr Rev*. 2005; 26:308–309.

Diamantopoulos A, Bao Y. Gynecomastia and premature thelarche: a guide for practitioners. *Pediatr Rev*. 2007;28:e57–e67.

Foley T. Hypothyroidism. *Pediatr Rev*. 2004;25:94–100.

Graham EA. Economic, racial, and cultural influences on the growth and maturation of children. *Pediatr Rev*. 2005;26:284–288.

Gundakaram A, Varma S. Index of suspicion. *Pediatr Rev*. 2005;26:257–263.

Hannon TS, Gungor N, Arsianian SA. Type 2 diabetes in children and adolescents: a review for the primary care provider. *Pediatr Ann*. 2006;35:880–887.

Hopwood NJ, Keich RP. Thyroid masses: approach to diagnosis and management in childhood and adolescence. *Pediatr Rev*. 1993;14:481–487.

Joiner TA, Foster C, Shope T. The many faces of vitamin D deficiency rickets. *Pediatr Rev*. 2000;21:296–302.

Kaufman FR. Type 1 diabetes mellitus. *Pediatr Rev*. 2003;24:291–299.

Kokotos F. Hyperthyroidism. *Pediatr Rev*. 2006;27:155–157.

Lenore L. Congenital adrenal hyperplasia. *Pediatr Rev*. 2000;21:159–170.

Nesmith JD. Type 2 diabetes mellitus in children and adolescents. *Pediatr Rev*. 2001;22:147–152.

Ornstein RM, Jacobson MS. Supersize teens: the metabolic syndrome. *Adolesc Med Clin*. 2006;17:565–587.

Rodd C, Goodyear P. Hypercalcemia of the newborn: etiology, evaluation, and management. *Pediatr Nephrol*. 1999;13:542–547.

Rosen D. Physiologic growth and development during adolescence. *Pediatr Rev*. 2004;25:194–200.

Schneider MB, Brill SR. Obesity in children and adolescents. *Pediatr Rev*. 2005;26:155–162.

Sethuraman U. Vitamins. *Pediatr Rev*. 2006;27:44–55.

Singh J, Moghal N, Pearce SHS, et al. The investigation of hypocalcemia and rickets. *Arch Dis Child*. 2003;88:403–407.

Umpaichitra V, Bastian W, Castells S. Hypocalcemia in children: pathogenesis and management. *Clin Pediatr*. 2001;40:305–312.

CHAPTER 11 ■ FLUIDS & ELECTROLYTES

KATHERINE S. DAHAB AND ASHLEY HALL SHOEMAKER

ADH	Antidiuretic hormone	ICU	Intensive care unit
ACTH	Adrenocorticotropic hormone	IO	Intraosseous
ATN	Acute tubular necrosis	IV	Intravenous
CAH	Congenital adrenal hyperplasia	IVF	Intravenous fluids
CNS	Central nervous system	NICU	Neonatal intensive care unit
CXR	Chest x-ray	ORS	Oral rehydration solution
DDAVP	1-desamino-8-D-arginine vasopressin	PRBC	Packed red blood cells
		PTH	Parathyroid hormone
DI	Diabetes insipidus	RTA	Renal tubular acidosis
ECF	Extracellular fluid	SIADH	Syndrome of inappropriate antidiuretic hormone
EKG	Electrocardiogram		
FISH	Fluorescent in situ hybridization	TPN	Total parenteral nutrition
GI	Gastrointestinal	UTI	Urinary tract infection
ICF	Intracellular fluid		

CHAPTER OBJECTIVES

1. Review the composition of body fluids and the major ions within them
2. Review normal acid–base physiology
3. Identify the primary causes of acidosis or alkalosis in clinical scenarios
4. Review etiologies, clinical manifestations, and management of hypernatremia, hyponatremic, hyperkalemic, hypokalemia, hypercalcemia, and hypocalcemia
5. Recognize clinical signs and symptoms of dehydration
6. Review etiologies and management of isotonic, hyponatremic, and hypernatremic dehydration.

BODY FLUID COMPOSITION

The cell membrane separates intracellular and extracellular fluid and maintains differential solute compositions within each compartment. Table 11.1 shows the solute concentrations for plasma (ECF = plasma + interstitial fluid) and for ICF.

Extracellular Plasma Composition

- Na^+ is the major extracellular cation and osmole.
- K^+, Ca^{2+}, and Mg^{2+} are minor extracellular cations.
- Electroneutrality is maintained by balancing the cations with Cl^- and HCO_3^- anions, negatively charged plasma proteins, and organic acids.

Intracellular Fluid Composition

- K^+ is the major intracellular cation and osmole.
- Phosphorus is the primary intracellular anion and balances the K^+ to maintain electroneutrality within the cell.

The Balancing Act of Fluids

- The actual solutes in ICF and ECF are different, but the total solute concentrations are similar due to osmosis
  - A change in the concentration of solute in one compartment creates a new osmotic gradient, and water shifts between the ECF and ICF to correct the gradient.

TABLE 11.1

SOLUTE COMPOSITION OF PLASMA AND INTRACELLULAR FLUID

	Extracellular Plasma (mEq/L)	Intracellular Fluid (mEq/L)
Na^+	140	10
K^+	4	150
Ca^{2+}	5	3
Mg^{2+}	2	26
Cl^-	110	3–5
HCO_3^-	24–26	10
Phosphorus	2	95
Organic acids	6	15
Proteins	16	5–6

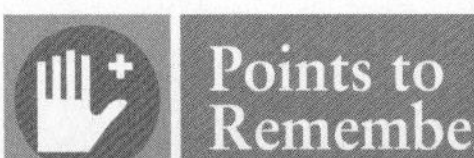
Points to Remember

- IV mannitol is an osmotic diuretic that is useful in the treatment of elevated intracranial pressure. Mannitol increases the osmolality of the ECF, causing water to flow from the ICF (brain) to the ECF (blood). This leads to a net decrease in ICF volume, helping to decrease brain edema and lower intracranial pressure.
- Children with nephrotic syndrome and marked hypoalbuminemia have increased movement of water from the intravascular space (plasma) to the interstitial space secondary to a decreased intravascular oncotic pressure. This is known as "third spacing" and clinically presents as ascites and peripheral edema. Despite the appearance of fluid overload, these children may actually have intravascular dehydration.

- ECF is divided into interstitial fluid and plasma via the vascular capillary bed
  - Unlike the cell membrane, the capillary bed is freely permeable to Na^+, K^+, and glucose.
  - The capillary bed is NOT permeable to plasma proteins; thus, proteins determine the oncotic pressure of the interstitial space and the plasma and influence the osmotic gradient within the ECF.

ACID–BASE PHYSIOLOGY

Several mechanisms exist to maintain arterial blood pH between 7.35 and 7.45. This pH allows enzyme systems to function properly and maintains normal cell membrane permeability.

Acid–base regulation mechanisms include:

1. Extra- and intracellular buffers (instant first line of defense against pH changes).
2. The lungs have the capacity to help compensate for primary metabolic disorders, and the kidneys have the capacity to help compensate for primary respiratory disorders.
3. Therapeutic correction of underlying factors causing acid–base abnormality.

The carbonic acid–bicarbonate buffering system is the most important buffering system in the body. It is represented by the following equation and provides a framework for thinking about acid–base disorders and regulatory mechanisms.

$$HCO_3^- + H^+ \leftrightarrow H_2O + CO_2$$

By definition, acidemia is pH less than 7.36 and alkalemia is pH more than 7.44.

The lungs play a major role in acid–base balance by regulating the carbon dioxide tension in the blood.

- Increased ventilation blows off more CO_2, shifting the HCO_3-carbonic acid buffer system to the right and causing a respiratory alkalosis. This can be a primary problem or a compensatory response to a primary metabolic acidosis.
- Decreased ventilation blows off less CO_2, shifting the HCO_3-carbonic acid buffer system to the left and causing a respiratory acidosis. This can be a primary problem or a compensatory response to a primary metabolic alkalosis.

The kidneys have two main functions in acid–base balance.

- Regulate plasma HCO_3^- concentration by controlling HCO_3^- reabsorption and by regenerating HCO_3^- used to buffer endogenously produced H^+ (under normal conditions, this allows the kidneys to maintain an extracellular HCO_3^- concentration of 22 to 26 mEq/L).
- Effect net H^+ excretion in the form of titratable acids and NH_4^+.

Table 11.2 lists the body's expected compensatory changes to acidosis or alkalosis.

Acid–Base Disorders

Respiratory Acidosis

- A primary respiratory acidosis is defined as a primary rise in plasma CO_2 tension leading to a decrease in blood pH. Important causes of a primary respiratory acidosis are shown in Table 11.3.

TABLE 11.2

EXPECTED COMPENSATORY CHANGES TO ACIDOSIS OR ALKALOSIS

Underlying Process	Initial Change	pH	Expected Compensation
Respiratory acidosis (acute)	Increased $PaCO_2$	Decreased (<7.40)	1 mEq/L increase in HCO_3^- for every 10 mm Hg rise in $PaCO_2$
Respiratory acidosis (chronic)	Increased $PaCO_2$	Decreased (<7.40)	4 mEq/L increase in HCO_3^- for every 10 mm Hg rise in $PaCO_2$
Respiratory alkalosis (acute)	Decreased $PaCO_2$	Increased (>7.40)	1–3 mEq/L decrease in HCO_3^- for every 10 mm Hg fall in $PaCO_2$
Respiratory alkalosis (chronic)	Decreased $PaCO_2$	Increased (>7.40)	2–5 mEq/L decrease in HCO_3^- for every 10 mm Hg fall in $PaCO_2$
Metabolic acidosis	Decreased HCO_3^-	Decreased (<7.40)	$PaCO_2$ decreased by 1–1.5 × the fall in HCO_3^-
Metabolic alkalosis	Increased HCO_3^-	Increased (>7.40)	$PaCo_2$ increased by 0.25–1 × the rise in HCO_3^-

- A respiratory acidosis can also be a compensatory mechanism for a primary metabolic alkalosis. In response to a high pH, the renal tubular cells increase H^+ secretion which leads to both the generation of new HCO_3^- and the urinary excretion of NH_4^+ and Cl^-.

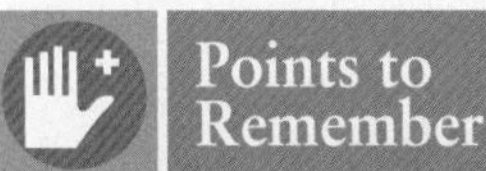

- **Aspirin overdose causes a primary respiratory alkalosis followed by the development of a primary metabolic acidosis.**

Respiratory Alkalosis

- A primary respiratory alkalosis is defined as a primary decrease in plasma CO_2 tension leading to an increase in blood pH. This situation is achieved by an increase in alveolar ventilation since total body metabolic CO_2 production is constant. Important causes of a primary respiratory alkalosis are shown in Table 11.4.
- A respiratory alkalosis can also be a compensatory mechanism for a primary metabolic acidosis. In response to a low pH, the kidney will decrease the secretion of H^+ into tubular fluid which in turn will lead to a diuresis of HCO_3^-. The kidney will also decrease the rate of ammonium excretion and thus decrease the generation of new HCO_3^-.

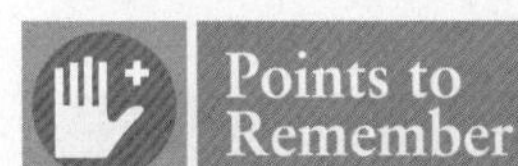

- **Respiratory compensation for metabolic disorders is rapid—the effects on pH begin within minutes.**

Metabolic Acidosis

A primary metabolic acidosis is defined as a drop in blood pH characterized by a primary decrease in plasma HCO_3^- concentration. Metabolic acidosis can be classified as a normal anion

TABLE 11.3

IMPORTANT CAUSES OF PRIMARY RESPIRATORY ACIDOSIS

Upper or Lower Airway Obstruction
- Aspiration
- Bronchospasm
- Laryngeal edema

Suppression of Respiratory Center
- Sedatives
- Hypnotics
- CNS injury

Hypoventilation due to Neuromuscular Disease
- Myasthenia gravis
- Muscular dystrophy
- Guillian–Barre syndrome
- Botulism

Lung or Thoracic Wall Abnormalities
- Severe scoliosis
- Pneumothorax
- Pneumonia
- Smoke inhalation
- Pulmonary edema due to heart failure
- Pulmonary embolism
- Chronic lung disease

CNS, central nervous system.

TABLE 11.4

IMPORTANT CAUSES OF PRIMARY RESPIRATORY ALKALOSIS

CNS Abnormality
Head trauma
Brain tumor
Fever
Anxiety, panic attack
Decreased Oxygen Delivery
Anemia
Shock
Hyperventilation due to Drugs
Salicylates
Methylxanthines
Iatrogenic
Mechanical hyperventilation

CNS, central nervous system.

gap metabolic acidosis or an increased anion gap metabolic acidosis. In children, a normal anion gap is less then 14 to 16. The anion gap is calculated by the following equation:

$$\text{Anion gap (mEq/L)} = Na^+ - (Cl^- + HCO_3^-)$$

Normal Anion Gap Metabolic Acidosis

- In children, a primary normal anion gap metabolic acidosis is usually caused by GI loss of HCO_3^- or impaired renal excretion as shown in Table 11.5.
- A normal anion gap metabolic acidosis can also be a compensatory response to a primary respiratory alkalosis.

Points to Remember

- Increased production of organic acids due to inborn errors of metabolism is a rare, but important, cause of metabolic acidosis and should be considered in any infant presenting with an anion gap metabolic acidosis.

Increased Anion Gap Metabolic Acidosis. An increased anion gap metabolic acidosis is almost always secondary to an increase in unmeasured anion. Etiologies can be remembered by the pneumonic "MUDPILES" and are shown in Table 11.6.

Metabolic Alkalosis

A primary metabolic alkalosis is defined as an increase in the blood pH due to an increase in the plasma HCO_3^- concentration. Important causes of a primary metabolic alkalosis are shown in Table 11.7.

Clinical Case Vignette

A 4-week-old, exclusively breast-fed male infant presents to your clinic with the chief complaint of persistent vomiting for the past 2 days. His mother describes the emesis as projective and nonbilious. He has not had any associated fevers or diarrhea. He has been slightly fussier than normal and has had less wet diapers than normal but continues to show interest in breastfeeding. His abdomen is soft, nontender, and nondistended but reveals a small palpable mass in the midepigastric area with visible peristaltic waves.

The above case illustrates pyloric stenosis. Pyloric stenosis usually presents between 1 and 12 weeks of age with nonbilious projectile emesis. Risk factors include male sex, first born, and

TABLE 11.5

IMPORTANT CAUSES OF NORMAL ANION GAP METABOLIC ACIDOSIS

Gastrointestinal Loss of HCO_3^-
Diarrhea
Enteric fistulas
Enterostomies
Impaired Renal Excretion of Acid
Type I RTA
Hyperaldosteronism

RTA, renal tubular acidosis.

TABLE 11.6

IMPORTANT CAUSES OF INCREASED ANION GAP METABOLIC ACIDOSIS

M	Methanol	Ingestion
U	Uremia	Renal failure leading to retention of H^+ and anions (sulfate, phosphate, urate)
D	Diabetic ketoacidosis (DKA)	New onset or poorly controlled type I diabetes
P	Paraldehyde or phenformin	
I	Iron or isoniazid	Ingestion
L	Lactic acid	Usually caused by hypoperfusion due to sepsis, heart failure, and/or dehydration; can also result from mitochondrial disorders
E	Ethylene glycol	Ingestion
S	Salicylate (aspirin)	Ingestion

positive family history. Classic physical exam findings include a palpable "olive" in the epigastric area or right upper quadrant and/or visible peristalsis. These findings, however, may or may not be present and diagnosis should be confirmed via ultrasound. The classic electrolyte abnormality is a hypochloremic, hypokalemic metabolic alkalosis. Fluid and electrolyte abnormalities should always be addressed before proceeding with surgical pyloromyotomy.

TABLE 11.7

IMPORTANT CAUSES OF PRIMARY METABOLIC ALKALOSIS

GI Loss of H^+
- Vomiting
- Diarrhea with a high Cl^- content

Renal Loss of H^+
- Diuretics
- Laxative abuse

Loss of Cl^- in Excess of HCO_3^- Loss
- Cystic fibrosis

Net Addition of HCO_3^- or its precursors
- Mineralocorticoid excess (e.g., hyperaldosteronism, Cushing syndrome, etc.)

ELECTROLYTE DISORDERS

Hypernatremia

Hypernatremia is defined as a serum sodium more than 145 mEq/L. In children, hypernatremia is usually due to a deficit of water rather than an excess of salt.

Etiology

- Excessive salt intake (dietary or parenteral).
- Total body water deficit
  - Diabetes insipidus (see separate section later).
  - GI losses.
- Burns.

Clinical Manifestations

Hypernatremia is usually well tolerated and clinical effects may not be evident until serum sodium is above 160 mEq/L.

Symptoms can include:

- Agitation.
- Irritability.

- Lethargy.
- Tachypnea.
- Increased tone.
- Brisk reflexes.
- Myoclonus.
- Chorea.
- Doughy skin.

Complications of severe hypernatremia include rhabdomyolysis, intracranial hemorrhage, and venous sinus thrombosis.

Treatment

Life-threatening cerebral edema can occur if hypernatremia is corrected too rapidly due to the brain's inability to quickly extrude idiogenic osmoles that have accumulated during the period of hypernatremia. Thus, the serum sodium should be corrected no faster than 1 mEq/h or 15 mEq/24 hours.

Diabetes Insipidus

DI is an important cause of hypernatremia. The body's normal response to hypernatremia is to release ADH, thus holding on to free water and decreasing serum osmolality. ADH secretion results in a high urine osmolality. In DI, however, the body cannot release ADH normally (central DI) or cannot respond normally to ADH (nephrogenic DI). Thus, the urine osmolality in DI is inappropriately low (specific gravity <1.010).

Etiology

- Central DI (lack of ADH secretion).
- Brain tumor.
- Head trauma.
- Cerebral infection.
- Idiopathic (>25% of cases in children).
- Nephrogenic DI (renal tubular resistance to ADH).
- Hereditary (90% X-linked, presents in infancy).
- Renal damage leading to loss of the concentration gradient.
- Vesicoureteral reflux.
- Sickle cell disease.
- Pyelonephritis.
- Decreased renal responsiveness.
- Drugs (e.g., lithium, amphotericin B).
- Electrolyte abnormalities (e.g., hypokalemia, hypercalcemia).
- Infiltrative diseases (e.g., sarcoidosis).

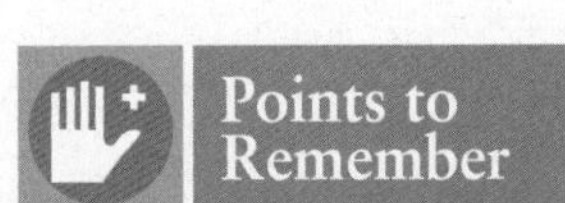

- **Without unlimited access to free water, patients with DI will develop hypernatremic dehydration.**
- **Infants with DI often present with failure to thrive, irritability, fever, and constipation. If hypernatremic dehydration is severe, seizures may occur.**

Clinical Manifestations

Patients with DI are unable to concentrate their urine and without free access to water quickly develop hypernatremic dehydration.

Other symptoms of DI include:

- Polydipsia
- Polyuria.
- Nocturia.
- Fever.
- Failure to thrive.
- Constipation.
- Vomiting.
- Irritability.

Diagnosis

A water deprivation test is used for diagnosis of DI. Patients are not allowed to eat or drink and their weight, urine osmolality, serum osmolality, and serum sodium are measured. A diagnosis of DI is made if the patient loses 3% to 5% or more of their body weight or has a 10 mOsm/kg or more increase in serum osmolality above baseline while urine specific gravity remains less than 1.010.

After establishing the diagnosis of DI, DDAVP is administered. If the urine osmolality increases to more than 450 mOsm/kg, the patient has central DI. If the urine osmolality remains less than 200 mOsm/kg, the patient has nephrogenic DI.

Treatment

DI is treated with unrestricted access to free water. Central DI can be treated with DDAVP. A low salt diet and thiazide diuretics can help by causing chronic volume depletion and promoting proximal tubular reabsorption of water.

TABLE 11.8

ETIOLOGIES OF HYPONATREMIA

	Serum Osmolality	Urine Sodium	Causes
Hypervolemic hyponatremia	Low	Low	Nephrotic syndrome Liver failure Heart failure Renal failure
Euvolemic hyponatremia	Low	Normal to high	SIADH Water intoxication Renal failure
	Normal to high	Normal	Hyperglycemia Mannitol infusion Pseudo-hypernatremia (lab error due to hyperproteinemia or hyperlipidemia)
Hypovolemic hyponatremia	Low	Low	GI losses Burns Cystic fibrosis Chronic diuretic use
		High	Adrenal insufficiency ATN Acute diuretic use

ATN, acute tubular necrosis; GI, gastrointestinal; SIADH, syndrome of inappropriate antidiuretic hormone.

Hyponatremia

Hyponatremia is defined as a serum sodium less than 130 mEq/L. In children, hyponatremia usually develops due to underlying conditions that impair the kidney's ability to excrete free water.

Etiology

Etiologies of hyponatremia separated by volume status are shown in Table 11.8.

Points to Remember

- **In a patient with hyperglycemia, total body sodium is often normal despite low serum sodium. Correct the serum sodium by adding 1.6 mEq/L for every 100 mg/dL serum glucose of more than 180 mg/dL.**

Clinical Manifestations

Symptoms of hyponatremia include the following:

- Nausea.
- Headache.
- Confusion.
- Myalgias.
- Seizures.
- Nausea/vomiting.
- Depressed deep tendon reflexes.

Complications of severe hyponatremia include cerebral herniation with seizures, respiratory arrest, dilated pupils, and decorticate posturing.

Points to Remember

- **Children are at increased risk of symptomatic cerebral edema, possibly due to their higher brain to skull size ratio creating less room for brain expansion as well as an impaired ability to regulate brain cell volume.**

Treatment

In patients without life-threatening complications, the goal of treatment is to increase serum sodium by no more than 1 mEq/L/h. Rapid correction of hyponatremia can lead to cerebral demyelinating lesions with confusion, quadriplegia, and pseudobulbar palsy. Hypertonic saline should only be used if the patient is symptomatic and the risk of cerebral edema outweighs the risk of cerebral demyelinating lesions.

Clinical Case Vignette. A 3-year-old male presents with a 1-week history of eye swelling. One month ago at his well child visit, his weight was 15 kg. Today he weighs 18 kg and is afebrile with normal vital signs. On exam, he has periorbital edema, 2+ pitting edema of his lower extremities, and a nontender, tympanic, distended abdomen. A urinalysis is obtained and is significant for a specific gravity of 1.030, 4+ proteinuria, trace hematuria, and no glucosuria. A comprehensive metabolic panel is normal except for sodium 130 mEq/L and albumin 1.5 g/dL. Urine sodium concentration is low at 5 mEq/L.

The above case illustrates nephrotic syndrome, a cause of hypervolemic hyponatremia. Nephrotic syndrome, liver failure, congestive heart failure, and renal failure are all edematous states with subsequent circulatory volume depletion. Intravascular volume depletion leads to

ADH release and thirst with a resultant dilutional hyponatremia. It is characterized by a serum osmolality of less than 280 with a urine osmolality of more than 100 and low urine sodium (<25 mEq/L), as the kidneys try desperately to hold on to both sodium and water.

Clinical Case Vignette. A 4-week-old female infant is brought in by ambulance with generalized seizures. She was born full term after an uncomplicated pregnancy with a birth weight of 3.1 kg. She takes 3 ounces of cow's milk formula every 3 hours without difficulty. There is no preceding history of illness, fever, or trauma. Today her weight is 3.4 kg, temperature 35.5°C, heart rate 150 beats per minute, and respiratory rate 12 breaths per minute. While you are securing an airway, the initial lab work returns revealing a serum sodium of 116 mEq/L. A 3 mL/kg bolus of 3% saline leads to resolution of the seizures. Further history reveals that the parents were diluting the infant's formula due to financial concerns. The infant shows adequate weight gain and a normal serum sodium after 2 days of feeding with appropriately prepared formula.

Water intoxication due to inappropriate formula preparation is a common cause of seizures in infants younger than 6 months. Infants rely on formula for their caloric needs and will accept a low-solute formula to the point of water intoxication. They may present with seizures, lethargy, and/or poor feeding. This is a form of euvolemic hyponatremia similar to psychogenic polydipsia in psychiatric patients. It is characterized by low serum and urine osmolality. It will correct rapidly and spontaneously via free water diuresis after normal feedings begin.

Clinical Case Vignette. A 12-year-old male is admitted to the ICU with fever, hypotension, petechiae, and altered metal status. He is treated empirically with IV ceftriaxone and vancomycin for presumed meningitis. On hospital day 3, he is noted to have decreasing urine output. On exam, his heart rate is 85, his mucous membranes are moist, he has good skin turgor, and there is no peripheral edema. His lab test results are significant for sodium 126 mEq/L, serum osmolality 270 mEq/L, urine osmolality 600 mEq/L, and urine sodium 25 mEq/L. He is diagnosed with SIADH, and his IVF rate is decreased to restrict his fluid intake.

SIADH is a diagnosis of exclusion. It can be caused by drugs (e.g., vincristine, cyclophosphamide, carbamazepine), malignancies (e.g., neuroblastoma, brain tumors), pulmonary disorders (e.g., tuberculosis, Legionella pneumonia), and CNS disorders (e.g., infection, hydrocephalus, postoperative). SIADH is treated with fluid restriction. If a patient is symptomatic and rapid correction is needed, it is acceptable to use hypertonic saline and loop diuretics.

Points to Remember

- 98% of total body potassium is stored in the ICF, and 75% of those stores are in muscle tissue.

Hyperkalemia

Hyperkalemia is defined as a serum potassium greater than 6.5 mEq/L. Because the kidneys are responsible for 90% of potassium excretion, renal failure is one of the most important causes of hyperkalemia.

Etiology

Etiologies of hyperkalemia are shown in Table 11.9.

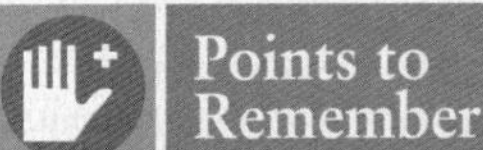

Points to Remember

- Hemolysis of the lab specimen can lead to a report of hyperkalemia, especially in newborns with labs obtained via heel sticks. Always send a stat repeat K to confirm hyperkalemia in a patient not expected to have hyperkalemia.

Clinical Manifestations

- Weakness (lower extremities > upper extremities).
- Nausea.
- Decreased deep tendon reflexes.
- Paresthesias.
- Arrhythmias (Fig. 11.1).
- EKG changes associated with potassium level 7 to 8 mEq/L: peaked T waves, decreased amplitude and widening of P waves, PR prolongation, and widened QRS complex.
- EKG changes associated with potassium level more than 8 mEq/L: Sine wave pattern as QRS complex merges with T wave, followed by ventricular fibrillation.

TABLE 11.9

ETIOLOGIES OF HYPERKALEMIA

Increased Intake	Impaired Renal Excretion	Transcellular Movement
Iatrogenic (e.g., PRBC, IVF, TPN)	Drugs (e.g., amiloride)	Cell damage (e.g., tumor lysis syndrome, rhabdomyolysis)
	Renal tubular damage (e.g., RTA, sickle cell disease)	Insulin deficiency
	Aldosterone deficiency (e.g., Addison disease, CAH)	Metabolic acidosis

CAH, congenital adrenal hyperplasia; IVF, intravenous fluids; PRBC, packed red blood cells; RTA, renal tubular acidosis; TPN, total parenteral nutrition.

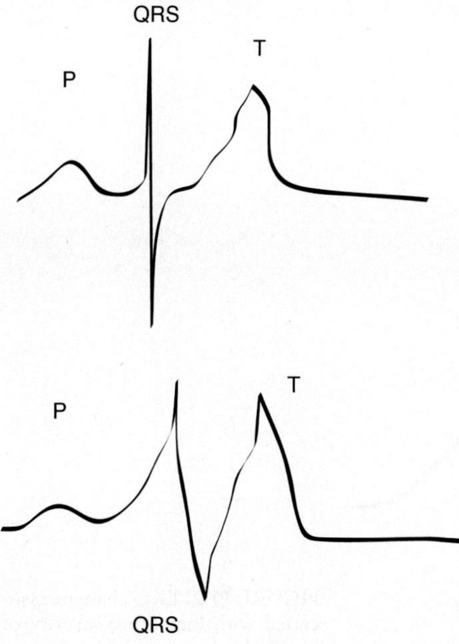

FIGURE 11.1. EKG changes associated with increasing severity of hyperkalemia.

Treatment

Treatment of hyperkalemia depends on the severity of hyperkalemia, presence of symptoms, EKG findings, and the host. Treatment strategies include

- Discontinue all exogenous forms of potassium (e.g., IVFs, TPN, PRBC).
- Polystyrene sulfonate (Kayexalate) to increase GI excretion of potassium.
- Furosemide to increase urinary excretion of potassium.
- Calcium gluconate to stabilize cardiac cell membrane.
- Bicarbonate, nebulized albuterol, and/or insulin can be used as temporizing agents to drive potassium into the cells.
- Dialysis to remove potassium from the blood stream.

Clinical Case Vignette. A 1-week-old, full-term male infant is brought to the emergency room for lethargy, poor feeding, and vomiting. His birth weight was 3.3 kg, current weight is 2.8 kg, heart rate 180 beats per minute, respirations 60 breaths per minute, blood pressure 65/48. Peaked T waves are noted on the cardiorespiratory monitor. Immediate fluid resuscitation is begun with normal saline. A bedside blood glucose is 40 mg/dL and the patient receives a D10 bolus. Although an EKG is being obtained to further evaluate the peaked T waves, the lab calls to report serum sodium of 123 mEq/L and serum potassium of 7.9 mEq/L. You suspect salt-wasting adrenal crisis and administer stress dose hydrocortisone (100 mg/m^2).

CAH is most commonly caused by 21-OH-deficiency, leading to the inability to convert 17-OH-progesterone to 11-deoxycortisol, a precursor of cortisol. Seventy-five percent of patients are also unable to convert progesterone to 11-deoxycorticosterone, a precursor of aldosterone. This results in elevated ACTH levels, adrenal hyperplasia, and overproduction of androgens that do not require the missing enzyme. Female patients often present at birth with ambiguous genitalia from increased androgen production. Male patients appear normal at birth but can present with a salt-wasting crisis (hyponatremia, hyperkalemia, hypoglycemia, and hypotension) or precocious puberty. Treatment is with hydrocortisone and fludrocortisone. Stress doses of hydrocortisone are required during times of physiologic stress (fever, vomiting). Of note, stress dose hydrocortisone has sufficient glucocorticoid and mineralocorticoid activity.

Hypokalemia

Hypokalemia is defined as a serum potassium less than 3.5 mEq/L. The resultant increase in the difference between ICF and ECF potassium leads to hyperpolarization of membranes and prolongation of action potentials and the refractory period.

Etiology

- Decreased potassium intake (rare!).
- Decreased GI absorption of potassium (e.g., pica with clay ingestion).

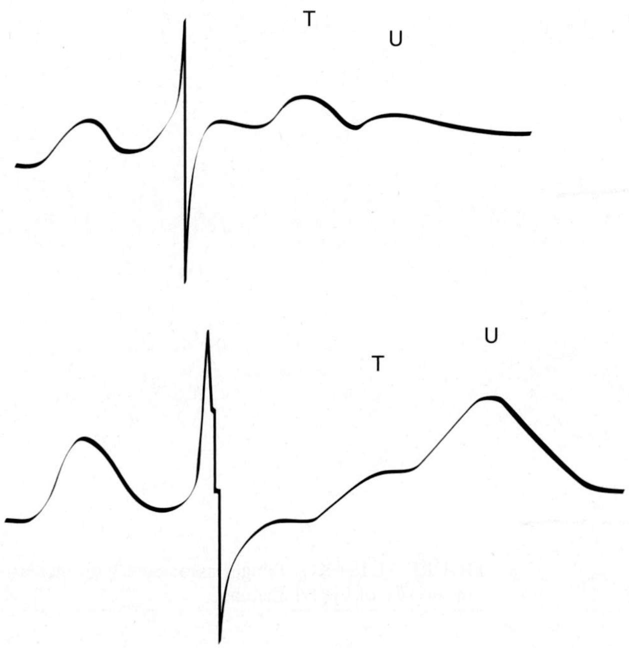

FIGURE 11.2. EKG changes associated with increasing severity of hypokalemia.

- Urinary potassium loss
  - Elevated aldosterone states (e.g., hypovolemia, adrenal tumors, Cushing syndrome, ingestion of licorice, Barter syndrome).
  - Metabolic alkalosis.
  - Osmotic diuresis.
  - Type 1 and 2 RTAs.
  - Hypomagnesium.
  - Thiazide and loop diuretics.
  - Gitelman syndrome.
- Intracellular shift (β_2-agonists, caffeine, insulin).

Clinical Manifestations

- Muscle weakness (lower extremities > upper extremities).
- Tetany.
- Muscle cramping.
- Ileus.
- Arrhythmias (primarily in patients with underlying cardiac disease; healthy patients are rarely affected) (Fig. 11.2).
- Initial EKG changes include depressed ST segments, decreased T-wave amplitude, and increased U-wave amplitude.
- Severe hypokalemia leads to increased width and amplitude of P waves, PR interval prolongation, and widening of QRS complex.

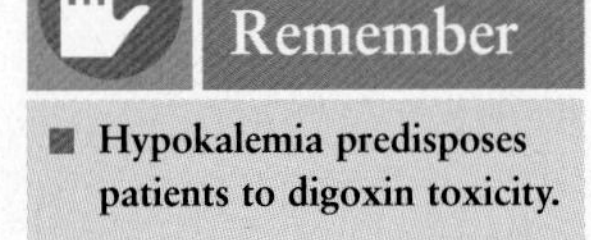
Points to Remember

- **Hypokalemia predisposes patients to digoxin toxicity.**

Treatment

- Symptomatic hypokalemia and/or hypokalemia with EKG changes should be treated with IV potassium chloride (1 mEq/kg up to 20 mEq over 1 hour).
- Asymptomatic patients with normal EKGs can be repleted with oral supplements or by adding 20 to 40 mEq/L KCl to their IVFs.

Hypercalcemia

Points to Remember

- **Hypoalbuminemia is one example of a condition where the total calcium level is "normal" despite true hypercalcemia → always check an iCa!**

Hypercalcemia is defined as serum calcium more than 12 mg/dL. Because ionized calcium rather than total calcium is physiologically relevant; however, an ionized calcium should always be checked as well.

Serum calcium is regulated by dietary intake, urinary excretion, vitamin D, and PTH. PTH causes an increase in the conversion of 25-hydroxyvitamin D to the active form (1,25-dihydroxyvitamin D/calcitriol), increased bone resorption of calcium, decreased urinary excretion of calcium, and increased urinary excretion of phosphorous. Calcitriol in turn causes increased intestinal absorption of phosphorous and calcium as well as bone and renal calcium absorption.

TABLE 11.10

ETIOLOGIES OF HYPERCALCEMIA

Mechanism	Etiology	PTH	Vitamin D	Calcium	Phosphorous
Primary hyperparathyroidism	Parathyroid adenoma Multiple endocrine neoplasia type I or II Benign familial hypocalciuric hypercalcemia	High	High	High	Low
Constitutively active PTH receptor	Jansen metaphyseal chondrodysplasia	Low	High	High	Low
Elevated vitamin D levels (increases intestinal absorption of calcium and phosphorous)	Excess intake of vitamin D Subcutaneous fat necrosis in infants Sarcoidosis Hypophosphatemia	Low	High	High	High (except in hypophosphatemia)
Excessive calcium intake	Especially with parenteral nutrition	Low	Low	High	Normal/high
Increased bone resorption	Malignancies Immobilization	Low	Low to normal	High	Variable

Etiology

Etiologies of hypercalcemia are shown in Table 11.10.

Clinical Manifestations

- Confusion.
- Depression.
- Nephrogenic DI.
- Vomiting.
- Nephrocalcinosis.
- Pancreatitis.
- Constipation.
- Arrhythmias.

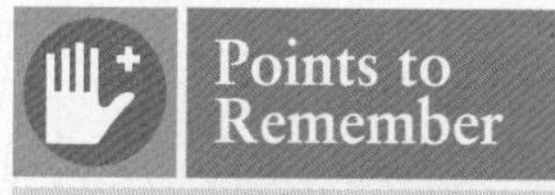

- **The symptoms of hypercalcemia can be remembered as "bones, stones, groans, and psychiatric overtones."**

Treatment

- Hydration with normal saline (dilutes serum calcium levels and causes calciuria which further increases kidney calcium excretion).
- Loop diuretic further increases urinary calcium excretion.
- Glucocorticoids block vitamin D activity and decrease serum vitamin D levels.
- Calcitonin and bisphosphonates block bone resorption and subsequent calcium release.
- Hemodialysis or parathyroidectomy may be needed in extreme cases.

Hypocalcemia

Hypocalcemia is defined as serum calcium less than 8.0 in newborns and less than 8.8 mg/dL in children. Because ionized calcium rather than total calcium is physiologically relevant, it is important to check the ionized calcium level to confirm hypocalcemia.

Etiology

Etiologies of hypocalcemia are shown in Table 11.11.

Clinical Manifestations

- Tetany.
- Paresthesias.
- Prolonged QTc.
- Rickets.
- Laryngospasm.
- Seizures.

TABLE 11.11

ETIOLOGIES OF HYPOCALCEMIA

Mechanism	Etiology	PTH	Vitamin D	Calcium	Phosphorous
Primary hypoparathyroidism	Early neonatal hypocalcemia (transient) Suppression from maternal hyperparathyroidism DiGeorge syndrome X-linked Autoimmune polyglandular syndrome (associated with Addison disease and mucocutaneous candidiasis)	Low	Low	Low	High
Secondary hypoparathyroidism	Hypomagnesemia (causes decreased release of and responsiveness to PTH)	Normal to low	Low	Low	Normal to high
End organ resistance to PTH	Pseudohypoparathyroidism including Albright's hereditary osteodystrophy	High	Low	Low	High
Hyperphosphatemia	Infants fed cow's milk Tumor lysis syndrome Laxatives and enemas Rhabdomyolysis	Normal to high	Low	Low	High
Low vitamin D levels	Inadequate intake with little sun exposure Malabsorption of fat soluble vitamins Medications that increase P450 and vitamin D metabolism (phenobarbital and phenytoin) Renal osteodystrophy	High	Low	Normal to low (once skeletal calcium depleted)	Low, except high in renal osteodystrophy (kidneys cannot adequately excrete phosphorous)
Lack of 1-α-hydroxylase (kidney enzyme that converts vitamin D to calcitriol)	Vitamin D–dependent rickets type 1	High	Low calcitriol	Low	Low
End-organ resistance to vitamin D	Vitamin D–dependent rickets type 2 (also have alopecia)	High	High	Low	Low
Binding of calcium	Fat released from omentum in pancreatitis Citrate in blood products	Variable	Variable	Low	Low
Inadequate calcium intake	Strict vegetarians Premature infants	High	High	Low	Low

PTH, parathyroid hormone.

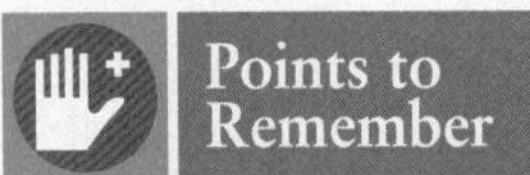

Points to Remember

- If hypocalcemia is due to the binding of calcium to substances such as phosphorous, citrate, or fat, calcium replacement should be conservative as the patient is at risk for hypercalcemia.

Treatment

- Symptomatic patients:
  - IV calcium gluconate (these patients should be monitored closely because bradycardia and tissue injury from calcium extravasation can occur).
  - Correction of any underlying hypomagnesemia or vitamin D deficiency.
  - Thiazide diuretics (decrease urinary calcium excretion).
- Asymptomatic patients:
  - Oral calcium replacement (oral calcium should not be given with meals because phosphorous decreases intestinal absorption of calcium).

Clinical Case Vignette. An infant is transferred to the NICU for seizures on day of life 2. Serum calcium is low at 6 mg/dL and seizures resolve after administration of IV calcium gluconate. On exam, the patient is noted to have a bulbous nose, low set ears, long fingers, and a II/VI left upper sternal border systolic murmur. A CXR reveals decreased pulmonary vascular markings and no thymic shadow. An echocardiogram reveals that the infant has tetralogy of fallot. FISH for 22q11 deletion is positive and the infant is diagnosed with DiGeorge syndrome.

DiGeorge syndrome is caused by a deletion in chromosome 22 that results in dysgenesis of the third and fourth pharyngeal pouches causing thymic and parathyroid hypoplasia. Congenital heart disease is also common. Thymic hypoplasia leads to varying degrees of lymphopenia and immunodeficiency. Hypoparathyroidism leads to hypocalcemia, particularly in the neonatal period and during times of stress. Supplementation with calcitriol and calcium is often necessary to maintain normal calcium levels.

Points to Remember

- If available, the best way to clinically assess the degree of dehydration is to evaluate for acute weight loss.
- Hypotension is a late sign of dehydration and indicates hypovolemic shock. Tachycardia is an earlier sign of dehydration.

DEHYDRATION

Dehydration is a common problem in infants and young children due to frequent GI illnesses, high surface to volume ratio, and inability to communicate the need for fluids. The best way to clinically assess the degree of dehydration is to evaluate for acute weight loss. If this information is not available, several other clinical parameters are also useful (see Table 11.12).

General Treatment Strategies:

- Patients with severe dehydration require rapid IV or IO fluid resuscitation.
- Initial resuscitation should be with isotonic fluid (e.g., normal saline); most patients can tolerate up to three 20 cm^2/kg boluses without developing fluid overload (e.g., congestive heart failure, pulmonary edema) but patients with underlying cardiac or renal disease may require more gentle fluid resuscitation; fluid resuscitation beyond the first 60 cm^2/kg should be with colloid.
- After the emergency phase of fluid resuscitation, the restoration phase should take place; fluids are repleted over the next several hours or days.
- Patients with mild or moderate dehydration can be managed with ORS. The goal is to use a solution that will replace fluids and electrolytes without leading to an osmotic diuresis. The World Health Organization ORS consists of 90 mEq/L sodium, 20 mEq/L potassium, 80 mEq/L chloride, 30 mEq/L citrate, and 111 mEq/L glucose.
- Administer 60 to 80 cm^2/kg of ORS over the first 4 hours and then switch to formula (or age-appropriate liquids for older children) with the goal of 150 cm^2/kg over the next 24 hours. Infants who are breast-fed should be breast-fed throughout the rehydration process to maintain maternal milk supply and because of the immunologic benefits of breast milk.
  - Vomiting patients can usually be treated successfully with ORS by giving small volumes (5 to 10 cm^2) every 5 minutes. Antiemetics can be given if needed.
  - If the patient has diarrhea, ongoing stool losses should be replaced with ORS at a 1:1 ratio.

Points to Remember

- Despite numerous studies showing efficacy and the successful use of ORS in other countries, ORS has not been readily adopted in the United States.
- Except in cases of severe enteropathy, lactose intolerance, or malnutrition, lactose free or diluted formula is not recommended for patients with diarrheal illnesses.
- Early feeding is an important part of recovery from gastroenteritis. Highly specific diets such as the BRAT diet (bananas, rice, applesauce, and toast) are too restrictive. The best advice is for patients to avoid foods high in simple sugars (e.g., jello, soda) because the osmotic load may worsen the diarrhea.

Isotonic Dehydration

Isotonic dehydration occurs when sodium and free water are proportionally decreased. It is common in patients with mild-to-moderate dehydration, particularly in patients with a short diarrheal illness. Treatment should proceed as described earlier.

TABLE 11.12

CLINICAL EVALUATION OF THE SEVERITY OF DEHYDRATION

	Mild	Moderate	Severe
% Weight Loss			
Infant	<5	10	15
Child	<3	6	9
Physical Exam			
Behavior	Consolable	Irritable	Lethargic
Blood pressure	Normal	Orthostatic	Hypotensive
Mucous membranes	Normal	Dry	Parched/crack
Tears	Present	Decrease	Absent
Eyes	Normal	Deep set	Sunken
Skin turgor	Normal	Decrease	Tenting
Fontanels	Flat	Slightly depressed	Sunken
Capillary refill	Normal	3–5 s	>5 s
Urine output	Normal	Decreased	Anuric

Reprinted with permission from McMillan JA, Feigin RD, DeAngelis C, et al. *Oski's Pediatrics: Principles and Practice*. 4th ed. Philadelphia, PA: Lippincott Williams & Wilkins, 2006.

Hyponatremic Dehydration

Hyponatremic dehydration occurs when sodium loss exceeds free water loss.

Etiology

- Nonrenal causes (urine sodium <10 mEq/L)
  - GI losses.
  - Severe burns.
  - Cystic fibrosis.
  - Chronic diuretic use.
- Renal causes (urine sodium >20 mEq/L)
  - Acute diuretic use.
  - Acute tubular necrosis.
  - Polycystic kidney disease.
  - Adrenal insufficiency.

Clinical Manifestations

Compared with isotonic dehydration, hyponatremic patients become symptomatic quickly due to intravascular volume depletion. Severe hyponatremia can also lead to cerebral edema as described in the previous section on hyponatremia.

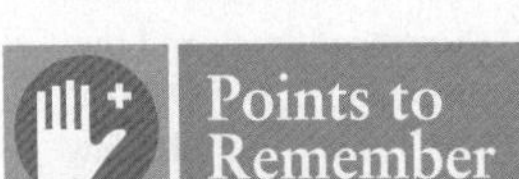

Points to Remember

- **Rapid correction of serum sodium can lead to cerebral demyelinating lesions.**
- **Hypertonic saline should only be used for patients with significant neurologic symptoms.**

Treatment

- Initial treatment should aim to restore circulating blood volume with isotonic fluid (e.g., normal saline).
- After initial fluid replacement, hypotonic fluids should be used to slowly correct the serum sodium. Once the patient is euvolemic, vasopressin will turn off and the body can excrete excess water while holding on to sodium, thus helping to correct the hyponatremia.
  - Goal: sodium correction of 0.5 mEq/L/h, maximum 10 to 12 mEq/L over 24 hours.
  - The following formulas are helpful in determining the appropriate IVF and rate:
    - Serum Na deficit = 0.7 × weight (140 − serum Na).
    - Serum Na change with 1 L of IVF = Na content of IVF (mEq/L) − serum Na/(0.6 × weight (kg) +1).

Points to Remember

- **Concentrated urine and a low urine sodium in a patient with hypernatremic dehydration indicates that the patient has extrarenal fluid losses (e.g., GI loss, burns).**
- **Diabetes insipidus can lead to hypernatremic dehydration from renal water loss if the patient does not have adequate access to free water and an intact thirst.**

Hypernatremic Dehydration

Hypernatremic dehydration occurs when free water loss exceeds sodium loss.

Etiology

- Nonrenal causes (hypertonic urine, urine sodium <10 mEq/L)
  - GI losses.
  - Severe burns.
  - Side effect of charcoal administration.
- Renal causes (isotonic or hypotonic urine, urine sodium >20 mEq/L)
  - Osmotic diuresis.
  - Postobstructive diuresis.
  - DI.

Clinical Manifestations

Compared with isotonic dehydration, patients with hypernatremic dehydration may be asymptomatic due to preserved extracellular volume. Skin often takes on a doughy consistency. Severe cases can cause brain shrinkage and tearing of bridging vessels.

Points to Remember

- **Patients with hypernatremic dehydration are often severely dehydrated before becoming symptomatic due to initial preservation of the extracellular volume.**

Treatment

- Initial treatment should aim to restore circulating blood volume
  - If serum sodium is less than 175 mEq/L, use isotonic fluid (e.g., normal saline).
  - If serum sodium is more than 175 mEq/L, normal saline (154 mEq/L) will actually be a hypotonic fluid. In this situation, 3% normal saline (513 mEq/L) should be added to make a fluid that is no more than 10 to 15 mEq/L lower than the serum sodium.
- After initial resuscitation, treatment goals include:
  - Replacing free water deficit plus maintenance requirements over 48 hours.
  - Goal sodium correction of 0.5 mEq/L/h (maximum of 15 mEq/L/day) because bringing down the sodium too rapidly can result in cerebral edema.
  - The following formula is helpful in determining the appropriate IVF rate:
    - Free water deficit = 0.7 × wt (kg) [1 − current Na/desired Na].

SAMPLE BOARD REVIEW QUESTIONS

1. A 2-month-old male infant is brought to emergency room because of 3 days of vomiting and diarrhea. He was born full term without complications and is fed cow's milk formula. His weight is 5 kg, temperature 100.9°F, heart rate 189 beats per minute, respirations 45 breaths per minute, and blood pressure 68/52. Physical examination is significant for an irritable infant with a sunken fontanelle, doughy skin, and capillary refill of 3 seconds. You obtain IV access, send basic labs, and administer a 20 cm^2/kg normal saline bolus for the patient's obvious dehydration. Although the bolus is running, you receive a call from the lab for a panic value. The patient's sodium is 169 mEq/L, potassium is 5.1 mEq/L, chloride is 139 mEq/L, and bicarbonate is 10 mEq/L. Of the following, which is the best management strategy for this patient's dehydration?
   a. Continue initial resuscitation with normal saline and then replace the remaining deficit over the next 48 hours
   b. Stop the normal saline bolus and begin resuscitation with 3% saline
   c. Stop the normal saline bolus and begin resuscitation with a mixture of normal saline and 3% saline to equal 165 mEq/L
   d. Continue with normal saline resuscitation, then rehydration over 12 hours
   e. Stop the normal saline bolus and begin rehydration over 48 hours

   Answer: a. Hypernatremic dehydration is treated by first resuscitating the patient with an isotonic fluid until cardiovascular status is stable, and then replacing the remaining free water deficit over 48 hours. Normal saline is the appropriate isotonic fluid unless the serum sodium is more than 175 mEq/L, in which case 3% saline should be added to create a fluid with sodium concentration no more than 10 mEq/L lower than the serum sodium. The goal should be to decrease serum sodium by 0.5 mEq/L/h (maximum of 15 mEq/L/day) because bringing down the sodium too rapidly can result in cerebral edema.

2. You receive a call from the pharmacy to notify you that one of your patients in the NICU received parenteral nutrition that contained an inappropriately high concentration of potassium due to a pharmacy error. While you wait for the results of a stat potassium level you obtain an EKG to look for signs of hyperkalemia. Which of the following EKG findings are suggestive of hyperkalemia?
   a. Flat T waves
   b. Prominent U waves
   c. Flat P waves
   d. Depressed ST segments
   e. Prolonged QTc

   Answer: c. Hyperkalemia leads to peaked T waves, wide and flat P waves, PR prolongation, widened QRS complex, and eventually a sine wave pattern. Hypokalemia is associated with flat T waves, depressed ST segments, and a prominent U wave. Hypocalcemia is associated with prolongation of the QTc interval.

3. A 7-month-old exclusively breast-fed African American male infant presents for well child care. Although prescribed vitamin supplements, his mother has never given him the vitamins because she is breast-feeding him and thought vitamin supplementation was unnecessary for breastfeeding infants. Physical examination is significant for widening at the wrists and palpable bumps along his ribcage. Which of the following lab values are consistent with a diagnosis of nutritional vitamin D deficiency in this patient?
   a. High PTH, low calcium, high phosphorous, low 25-OH-vitamin D
   b. Low PTH, high calcium, high phosphorous, low 25-OH-vitamin D
   c. High PTH, normal calcium, high phosphorous, low 25-OH-vitamin D
   d. High PTH, low calcium, low phosphorous, low 25-OH-vitamin D
   e. High PTH, low calcium, low phosphorous, normal 25-OH-vitamin D

   Answer: d. 25-OH-vitamin D is found in fish, fortified milk, and infant formulas but is low in breast milk. The AAP recommends supplementing vitamin D in breast-fed babies beginning at birth. Vitamin D is converted into the active form, 1-,25-OH-vitamin D (calcitriol) in the kidney. Vitamin D deficiency leads to decreased absorption of calcium and phosphorous in the kidneys. This leads to a low serum phosphorous level and eventually a low serum calcium level. Initially, calcium levels will be maintained through bone resorption. Low calcium and vitamin D levels stimulate the secretion of PTH, leading to elevated PTH levels.

4. A 13-year-old girl with Addison disease has had 3 days of vomiting and has been unable to take her medications. She presents to the emergency room where she is lethargic, hypotensive, and continues to vomit. Her lab test results are significant for sodium 117 mEq/L, potassium 7.9 mEq/L, bicarbonate 12 mEq/L. Hyponatremia places her at risk for which of the following complications?

a. Cerebral demyelinating lesions
b. Cerebral edema
c. Cerebral hemorrhage
d. Rhabdomyolysis
e. Venous sinus thrombosis

Answer: b. Hyponatremia can lead to cerebral edema and subsequent herniation. Children are more susceptible than adults. Rapid correction of hyponatremia may cause cerebral demyelinating lesions due to rapid fluid shifts out of the cell. Rhabdomyolysis, venous sinus thrombosis, and cerebral hemorrhage from tearing of bridging vessels are all complications of hypernatremia, not hyponatremia.

5. A 9-year-old girl is in the PICU recovering from surgery to remove a newly diagnosed brain tumor. She seems to be recovering well until postoperative day 3 when she experiences a seizure. Lab test results are remarkable for a serum sodium of 115 mEq/L. Which of the following other laboratory values would you expect in this patient?
   a. Increased urine osmolality, increased serum osmolality
   b. Decreased urine osmolality, decreased serum osmolality
   c. Increased urine osmolality, normal serum osmolality
   d. Decreased urine osmolality, increased serum osmolality
   e. Increased urine osmolality, decreased serum osmolality

   Answer: e. Hyponatremia in a patient who has recently had brain surgery is most likely due to SIADH. Hyponatremia occurs because of inappropriate retention of fluid. Thus, patients with SIADH have inappropriately concentrated urine despite low serum osmolality.

6. A 3-year-old female child is admitted for a water deprivation test due to new onset polydipsia and polyuria. Initial workup demonstrated a normal glucose and negative urine ketones. She has a history of two febrile UTIs, no other past medical history, and she has been growing along the 50th percentile for weight and height. During the test, she loses 4% of her body weight. Her serum sodium is 150 mEq/L, serum osmolality is 300 mOsm/kg, and urine osmolality is 100 mOsm/kg. After administration of DDAVP, urine osmolality is 150 mOsm/kg. Which of the following is the most likely diagnosis in this patient?
   a. Psychogenic polydipsia
   b. Nephrogenic DI secondary to vesicoureteral reflux
   c. Hereditary nephrogenic DI
   d. Idiopathic central DI
   e. SIADH

   Answer: b. Polydipsia and polyuria in a patient in whom a diagnosis of diabetes mellitus has been excluded should raise concern for DI. A diagnosis of DI is confirmed by a water deprivation test revealing a 3% to 5% weight loss, elevated serum osmolality, and low urine osmolality. After a diagnosis of DI has been established, DDAVP can be administered to differentiate between central and nephrogenic DI. In central DI (lack of ADH secretion), the urine osmolality will increase to more than 450 mOsm/kg after the administration of DDAVP. In nephrogenic DI (renal tubular resistance to ADH), the urine osmolality will remain less than 200 mOsm/kg as is the case in this patient. The most likely etiology of nephrogenic DI in this patient is renal damage from vesicoureteral reflux leading to loss of the concentration gradient and an inability to respond to ADH.

7. Which of the following symptoms is consistent with hypercalcemia?
   a. Confusion
   b. Seizures
   c. Depressed reflexes
   d. Tetany
   e. Fever

   Answer a. Symptoms of hypercalcemia can be remembered with the phrase "stones, bones, groans, and psychiatric overtones." Patients may appear confused or depressed. They may develop nephrocalcinosis and are at risk for nephrogenic DI. Gastrointestinal symptoms include pancreatitis, constipation, and vomiting.

SUGGESTED READINGS

Feld LG, Kaskel FJ, eds. *Fluid and Electrolytes in Pediatrics: A Comprehensive Handbook*. New York, NY: Humana Press, 2010.

Hellerstein S. Fluid and electrolytes: clinical aspects. *Pediatr Rev*. 1993;14(3):103–115.

Crocetti M, Barone MA, eds. *Oski's Essential Pediatrics*, 2nd ed. Philadelphia, PA: Lippincott Williams & Wilkins, 2004:18–22.

Zhou P, Markowitz M. Hypocalcemia in infants in children. *Pediatr Rev*. 2009;30(5):190–192.

CHAPTER 12 ■ GASTROENTEROLOGY

ARVIND IYENGAR SRINATH

AIDS	Acquired immunodeficiency syndrome	LDH	Lactate dehydrogenase
ALT	Alanine aminotransferase	LES	lower esophageal sphincter
ANA	Anti-nuclear antibody	LFTs	Liver function tests (AST, ALT)
AOM	Acute otitis media	LLQ	Left lower quadrant of the abdomen
AFP	Alpha-fetoprotein	LKM	Anti-liver kidney microsomal antibody
AG	Aminoglycoside	LMP	Last menstrual period
ALF	Acute liver failure	LUQ	Left upper quadrant of the abdomen
ALTE	Apparent life-threatening event	MEN	Multiple endocrine neoplasia
AST	Aspartate aminotransferase	MRCP	Magnetic resonance cholangiopancreatography
AXR	Abdominal x-ray	MRI	Magnetic resonance imaging
BMP	Basic metabolic panel	MVC	Motor vehicle collision
CBC	Complete blood count	NEC	Necrotizing enterocolitis
CF	Cystic fibrosis	NG	Nasogastric
CL	Chlamydia	NJ	Nasojejunal
CMP	Comprehensive metabolic panel	NPO	Nothing by mouth (nil per os)
CMV	Cytomegalovirus	NS	Normal saline
Coags	Coagulation studies (PT, PTT)	NSAIDs	Nonsteroidal anti-inflammatory drugs
CRP	C-reactive protein	OG	Orogastric
CT	Computed tomography	OR	Operating room
DIOS	Distal intestinal obstruction syndrome	PCN	Penicillin
DKA	Diabetic ketoacidosis	PTC	Percutaneous transhepatic cholangiography
EBV	Epstein–Barr virus	PID	Pelvic inflammatory disease
EKG	Electrocardiogram	PUD	Peptic ulcer disease
ERCP	Endoscopic retrograde cholangiopancreatography	PRBC	Packed red blood cells
ESLD	End-stage liver disease	PT	Prothrombin time
ESR	Erythrocyte sedimentation rate	PTT	Partial thromboplastin time
FQ	Fluoroquinolones	RDW	Red blood cell distribution width
GAS	Group A streptococcus	ROS	Review of systems
GC	Gonococcal infection (gonorrhea)	RLQ	Right lower quadrant of the abdomen
GER	Gastroesophageal reflux	RUQ	Right upper quadrant of the abdomen
GERD	Gastroesophageal reflux disease	SBP	Spontaneous bacterial peritonitis
GI	Gastrointestinal	SLE	Systemic lupus erythematosus
GVHD	Graft-versus-host disease	SMA	Superior mesenteric artery
hCG	Human chorionic gonadotropin	STD	Sexually transmitted disease
HPF	high-powered field	TEF	Tracheoesophageal fistula
HIDA	Hepatobiliary iminodiacetic acid	TMP-SMX	Trimethoprim-sulfamethoxazole (Bactrim)
HLH	Hemophagocytic lymphohistiocytosis	TPN	Total parenteral nutrition
HSV	Herpes simplex virus	UA	Urinalysis
HTN	Hypertension	UC	Ulcerative colitis
HUS	Hemolytic uremic syndrome	U/S	Ultrasound
IBD	Inflammatory bowel disease	UTI	Urinary tract infection
ICP	Intracranial pressure	VIP	Vasoactive intestinal peptide
INR	International normalized ratio	VZV	Varicella zoster virus
IV	Intravenous		
IVFs	Intravenous fluids		

CHAPTER OBJECTIVES

1. To know the differential diagnosis for and approach to common GI complaints including vomiting, diarrhea, constipation, abdominal pain, GI bleeding, rectal pain, and hematemesis
2. To know various congenital abnormalities of the GI tract—their presenting symptoms, diagnosis, and management
3. To know the common disorders associated with each part of the GI tract—their presenting symptoms, diagnosis, and management.

Points to Remember

- **Don't forget to think about inborn errors of metabolism in young infants with vomiting, especially those who are ill appearing—ask about consanguinity and look for metabolic acidosis, hypoglycemia, hyperammonemia, and/or ketosis.**
- **Elevated ICP from intracranial hemorrhage due to nonaccidental trauma can present with vomiting in an infant and is something you never want to miss.**

VOMITING

Vomiting is a common complaint in infants and children that can occur from pathology within or outside of the GI system. It often reflects a relatively benign underlying process but can be a symptom of serious and/or life-threatening disease. The most common cause of vomiting in children is viral gastroenteritis. GER/GERD is a very common cause of vomiting in infants. Table 12.1 shows common and important causes of vomiting according to age.

Approach to Vomiting

1. Complete history focusing on duration and frequency of symptoms, quality of emesis (bilious vs. nonbilious), diet history, growth pattern, history of preceding trauma, possibility of ingestion, LMP, ill contacts, family history, past medical history, and prior surgical history.

TABLE 12.1

AGE-SPECIFIC COMMON AND/OR IMPORTANT CAUSES OF VOMITING

	Infant (0–1 y)	Child (1–12 y)	Adolescent (>12 y)
Infectious	Gastroenteritis UTI/pyelonephritis Meningitis/encephalitis	Gastroenteritis UTI/pyelonephritis Meningitis/encephalitis Hepatitis	Gastroenteritis UTI/pyelonephritis Meningitis/encephalitis PID Hepatitis
Inflammatory	Appendicitis	Appendicitis, Pancreatitis	Appendicitis, Pancreatitis
Metabolic	Inborn errors of metabolism	Inborn errors of metabolism	
Endocrine	Congenital adrenal Hyperplasia	DKA	DKA
Allergic	Milk protein intolerance	Celiac disease	Celiac disease
Obstructive	Pyloric stenosis Duodenal atresia Enteric duplication Ileus Malrotation with volvulus Hirschsprung disease	Intussusception Appendicitis Adhesions (postsurgical) Foreign body IBD Ileus Annular pancreas Duodenal hematoma (trauma)	Appendicitis Adhesions (postsurgical) IBD Ileus Bezoar Annular pancreas Duodenal hematoma (trauma)
Neurologic (increased ICP)	Hydrocephalus Intracranial hemorrhage Intracranial mass lesion	Intracranial hemorrhage Intracranial mass lesion Pseudotumor cerebri	Intracranial hemorrhage Intracranial mass lesion Pseudotumor cerebri
Miscellaneous	GER/GERD HTN	Psychologic Toxic ingestion Cyclic vomiting Abdominal migraine SMA syndrome HTN	Psychologic Toxic ingestion Pregnancy Nephrolithiasis Cholecystitis Cyclic vomiting Abdominal migraine Bulimia SMA syndrome HTN

DKA, diabetic ketoacidosis; GER, gastroesophageal reflux; GERD, gastroesophageal reflux disease; HTN, hypertension; IBD, inflammatory bowel disease; ICP, intracranial pressure; PID, pelvic inflammatory disease; SMA, superior mesenteric artery; UTI, urinary tract infection.

ROS should focus on the presence of fever, abdominal pain, diarrhea, headaches, neck pain, dysuria, altered mental status, and/or change in urine output.

2. Complete physical examination with special attention given to overall appearance, temperature, heart rate, blood pressure, abdominal distention/tenderness/masses, bowel sounds, neurologic abnormalities, and hydration status.
3. Initial labs depend on the suspected etiology (and are not always needed) but may include BMP/CMP, CBC, UA, urine culture, ESR, CRP, amylase, lipase, toxicology screen, urine hCG, celiac studies, and/or CSF analysis and culture.
4. Useful imaging studies depend on the suspected etiology but may include AXR, abdominal/renal/hepatic U/S, upper GI series, abdominal CT, and/or head CT.

Points to Remember

- Bilious emesis should always raise concern for obstruction distal to the ampulla of Vater. However, repeated episodes of vomiting can lead to bilious emesis in the absence of obstruction.
- Bilious emesis in a neonate should be assumed to be malrotation with volvulus until proven otherwise. Workup via upper GI series with small bowel follow-through and get a STAT surgical consult.

Clinical Case Vignette

A 4-day-old full-term infant presents with two episodes of bilious emesis. Physical exam is remarkable for a fussy infant with a tense abdomen. He is slightly tachycardic but is otherwise hemodynamically stable with good perfusion. You establish IV access and obtain an emergent upper GI series which confirms your suspicion of malrotation with volvulus. The surgeons take the patient to the OR and perform a Ladd's procedure. They are able to save the entire bowel, and the patient has an uneventful postoperative course with full recovery.

DIARRHEA

Acute Diarrhea

Acute diarrhea is defined as diarrhea lasting less than 2 weeks. In otherwise healthy children, acute diarrhea is almost always infectious. Transmission is usually from person to person via the fecal-oral route or via the ingestion of contaminated food or water. Viral, bacterial, and parasitic causes of acute gastroenteritis are shown in Table 12.2.

Points to Remember

- Severe abdominal pain and tenesmus are indicative of involvement of the large intestine and rectum.
- Acute bloody diarrhea with signs of colitis is likely indicative of a bacterial pathogen.

Approach to Acute Diarrhea

1. Complete history focusing on duration of symptoms, quality and quantity of stool, presence of blood in the stool, hydration status, recent dietary exposure, travel history, sick contacts, child-care attendance, exposure to pets/animals, water source, recent antibiotic use, possible ingestions, and associated symptoms such as fever, abdominal pain, and vomiting.
2. Complete physical examination with special attention given to overall appearance, temperature, heart rate, blood pressure, abdominal distention/tenderness/masses, bowel sounds, and hydration status.
3. If the patient is significantly dehydrated, a BMP should be obtained. Stool studies should be considered if the patient is ill appearing or febrile, the diarrhea is bloody, or the history suggests an etiology for which specific treatment is indicated. Stool studies may include stool fecal leukocytes (high sensitivity and positive predictive value for bacterial gastroenteritis), hemoccult, gram stain, bacterial culture, ova/parasites, rotavirus antigen, and/or *C. diff* toxin and assay.
4. Treatment: Supportive care is the cornerstone of therapy for all causes of acute gastroenteritis and entails ensuring adequate hydration and fluid management. Mild and moderate dehydration should be managed with oral rehydration therapy. IV hydration may be necessary for severe dehydration. Correct any associated electrolyte abnormalities. Specific antimicrobials and antiparasitic agents are indicated in select cases as shown in Table 12.2. Antidiarrheal agents should NOT be used in children with suspected bacterial diarrhea.

Points to Remember

Toddler's diarrhea

- Common cause of diarrhea in toddlers 1–3 yrs old of unknown etiology
- 2 or more loose, voluminous stools/day at least 4 days a week
- Not associated with failure to thrive
- Treatment: reduce total fluid intake to 90 mL/kg/day and minimize high fructose-containing juices

Chronic Diarrhea

Chronic diarrhea is defined as diarrhea lasting more than 2 weeks. Several of the infectious etiologies that cause acute diarrhea can also cause chronic diarrhea. When evaluating a patient with chronic diarrhea, however, there are many important noninfectious etiologies to consider. These are shown in Box 12.1.

Approach to Chronic Diarrhea

1. Complete history focusing on duration of symptoms, quality and quantity of stool, presence of blood in the stool, hydration status, recent dietary exposure, travel history, sick contacts, family history, exposure to pets/animals, water source, recent antibiotic use, and associated symptoms such as fever, abdominal pain, vomiting, fatigue, rash, and weight loss.

TABLE 12.2

INFECTIOUS CAUSES OF ACUTE DIARRHEA

	Distinguishing Features	Treatment
Viruses		
Rotavirus	■ Most common cause of diarrhea in hospitalized children <5 y ■ Seasonal (winter–spring) ■ Vomiting usually occurs early in course	Supportive
Noroviruses	■ Outbreaks (e.g., day care centers) ■ 12–48 h incubation period ■ 1–2 d recovery	Supportive
Adenovirus	■ Most serotypes cause respiratory tract infections but some cause gastroenteritis	Supportive
Bacteria		
Campylobacter jejuni	■ Bloody diarrhea ■ Sources: raw poultry, unpasteurized milk, untreated water, feces from infected animals	Supportive (TMP-SMX, macrolide or FQ)
Salmonella species	■ Bloody diarrhea ■ Sources: poultry, reptiles ■ Can be associated with bacteremia, sepsis, and/or meningitis (especially in infants)	Supportive ([a]ceftriaxone)
Shigella species	■ Bloody diarrhea ■ Often associated with significant tenesmus ■ Can be associated with seizures	Supportive (Azithromycin, [a]FQ)
Yersinia enterocolitica	■ Bloody diarrhea ■ Source: handling of raw pig intestines (chitterlings), undercooked pork, contaminated water, contact with infected animals	Supportive ([a]TMP-SMX, AG, FQ, ceftriaxone or doxycycline)
Enterotoxigenic *Escherichia coli*	■ Traveler's diarrhea ■ Source: contaminated water, fruit, vegetables	Supportive (FQ or [a]ceftriaxone)
Enterohemorrhagic *Escherichia coli*	■ Bloody diarrhea ■ Source: undercooked beef, contact with infected animals, unpasteurized milk ■ *E. coli* H157:07 can be associated with HUS	Supportive Avoid antibiotics as they may increase risk of HUS
Bacillus cereus	■ Self-limited vomiting, diarrhea ■ Source: reheated rice	Supportive
Staph aureus	■ Self-limited vomiting, diarrhea ■ Occurs within 12–72 h of exposure ■ Most common cause of food poisoning	Supportive
Vibrio cholerae	■ Secretory diarrhea ■ Source: untreated water ■ Raw shell fish	Supportive ([a]doxycycline)
Clostridium difficile	■ Bloody or nonbloody diarrhea ■ Associated with recent antibiotic use ■ Infants <1 y are often asymptomatically colonized	[a]Oral metronidazole or oral vancomycin
Parasites		
Giardia lamblia	■ Fatty, greasy, smelly stools ■ Abdominal cramping ■ Source: unclean water (camping, well water)	Metronidazole
Entamoeba histolytica	■ Source: soil ■ Often associated with peripheral eosinophilia ■ Can lead to liver abscess	Mebendazole
Cryptosporodium	■ Secretory diarrhea ■ Source: soil, contaminated water ■ Common in immunocompromised patients	Nitazoxanide

[a]Treatment options for severe disease and/or immunocompromised patients.
AG, aminoglycoside; FQ, flouroquinolones; HUS, hemolytic uremic syndrome.

Box 12.1 Noninfectious Causes of Chronic Diarrhea

Malabsorptive disorders (e.g., cystic fibrosis, celiac disease)
Immunodeficiency (e.g., HIV)
Hirschsprung disease
VIPoma
Acrodermatitis enteropathic (zinc deficiency)
Abetalipoproteinemia
Intractable diarrhea of infancy
Inflammatory disorders (e.g., IBD)
Cholestatic conditions
Toddler's diarrhea
Irritable bowel syndrome

2. Complete physical examination with special attention given to overall appearance, temperature, heart rate, blood pressure, abdominal distention/tenderness/masses, bowel sounds, hydration status, and skin exam.
3. Laboratory evaluation should be guided by the history and physical exam and based on the differential diagnosis. As described in the evaluation of acute diarrhea, a BMP should be obtained in any patient who is significantly dehydrated and consideration should be given to sending stool studies. Other potentially useful labs include CBC, CRP, ESR, CMP, stool trypsin, fecal elastase, fecal fat test, stool pH and Clinitest, serum IgA, and celiac markers, and a sweat test.
4. Further evaluation including hydrogen breath test for carbohydrate malabsorption, endoscopy with biopsy, ERCP, liver biopsy, and abdominal imaging may be warranted on an individual basis.

CONSTIPATION

Constipation is characterized by hard stool, painful stooling, and/or less than three stools per week.

There are multiple causes of chronic constipation in children as shown in Table 12.3.

Regardless of the underlying etiology, chronic constipation can lead to multiple problems including abdominal/rectal pain, encopresis (involuntary leakage of stool around retained stool), rectal fissures, urinary incontinence, UTIs, ureteral obstruction, rectal prolapse, bacterial overgrowth, social exclusion, depression, and/or anxiety.

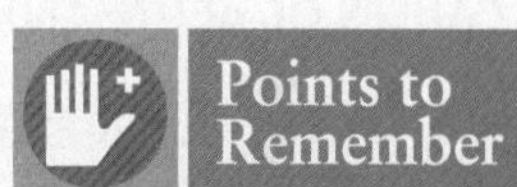

- Functional fecal retention is the most common cause of chronic constipation in children.
- Patients with irritable bowel syndrome can have diarrhea and/or constipation.

Approach to Constipation

1. Complete history focusing on duration of symptoms, previous stooling pattern, diet, fluid intake, growth pattern, medication use, family history, and associated symptoms such as abdominal/rectal pain, rectal bleeding, weight gain/loss, vomiting, encopresis, urinary patterns, psychosocial stressors, fatigue, cold intolerance, and neurologic abnormalities.
2. Complete physical exam with special attention given to overall appearance, abdominal distention/tenderness/masses, bowel sounds, perianal inspection, rectal examination, spinal abnormalities, and neurologic exam.

TABLE 12.3

DIFFERENTIAL DIAGNOSIS OF CHRONIC CONSTIPATION IN CHILDREN

Functional	Neurologic	Obstructive	Endocrine	Medicinal
Functional fecal retention	Spinal cord defects	Mass/tumor	Hypothyroidism Hyperparathyroidism	Narcotics Lead intoxication
Irritable bowel syndrome	Hirschprung disease		Pheochromocytoma	Iron use Laxative abuse/tolerance

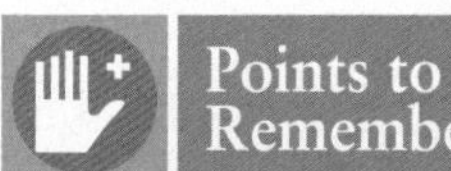

- Constipation due to functional fecal retention often starts in infancy during diet transitions (breast milk → formula → cow's milk, baby foods → table foods).
- Recurrent, small pellet stools represent incomplete evacuation while infrequent, massive stools are due to functional fecal retention.
- Signs of constipation due to a distal GI obstruction include abdominal distention, narrow stool caliber, and lack of encopresis.

3. Routine labs are not indicated in every patient with constipation and should be guided based on the history and physical exam.
4. Routine imaging is not indicated in every patient. AXR, abdominal CT, and/or spinal MRI may be indicated in select patients.
5. Treatment depends on the underlying etiology. Management of chronic constipation due to functional fecal retention includes three phases: (1) complete evacuation of colon via use of oral stool softeners, (2) sustained evacuation via a regular stooling schedule, high-fiber diet, and oral stool softeners, and (3) weaning of stool softeners as rectal tone recovers with continued stooling schedule and dietary management.

Clinical Case Vignette

A mother brings her 6-year-old daughter to your clinic because of a long-standing constipation since the age of 3 years that is initially palliated then quickly refractory to short courses of stool softeners. She is toilet trained but frequently has loose stool in her underwear. Examination is remarkable for a well-appearing girl with a mildly distended abdomen, normoactive bowel sounds, palpable stool in the left lower quadrant, and hard stool in the rectal vault. The rest of her physical exam is normal. You correctly diagnose her with functional fecal retention. You start her on a high dose of oral stool softener and educate the patient and her mother about the importance of establishing a stooling routine. Once she starts stooling normally and not having fecal soiling, you plan to wean her medications as tolerated and continue behavioral intervention.

ABDOMINAL PAIN

Acute Abdominal Pain

Acute abdominal pain can be the result of pathology within or outside of the GI tract. Important GI causes of acute abdominal pain in infants and children are summarized in Table 12.4. Non-GI causes of acute abdominal pain are listed in Table 12.5.

TABLE 12.4

GI CAUSES OF ACUTE ABDOMINAL PAIN IN INFANTS AND CHILDREN

	Risk Factors	Location and Quality	Other Distinguishing Features
Pancreatitis	Gallstones, trauma, abnormal pancreatic anatomy	Acute onset epigastric pain with radiation to the back and/or LUQ	Almost always associated with nausea, vomiting, and anorexia
Cholecystitis	Obesity, hemolytic disease	Recurrent episodes of RUQ pain	Symptoms exacerbated by fatty foods
Intestinal obstruction	Adhesions from prior abdominal surgery, abnormal anatomy (malrotation), IBD, hernias, malignancy	Pain is usually constant and generalized	Distention, obstipation, and emesis are variably present; obstruction distal to the ampulla of Vater may result in bilious emesis; bowel sounds are hyperactive earlier in the course then become hypoactive
Perforated peptic ulcer	*H. pylori* infection, high intake of spicy foods	Acute burning epigastric pain ± radiation to the back	Associated with hematemesis and/or melena
Appendicitis	Most common in teenagers but can present at any age	Periumbilical pain with subsequent localization to the RLQ	Almost always associated with anorexia; vomiting and fever also often present; peritoneal signs may or may be not be present; pain improves after rupture
Intussusception	Most common in toddlers	Intermittent episodes of severe generalized abdominal pain; lethargy may be a prominent finding	"Sausage-shaped" palpable RUQ mass may be present; "currant jelly stools" are a late finding
Gastroenteritis	Common in all age groups	Periumbilical pain, gradual onset	Associated with diarrhea and vomiting
Esophagitis	GERD, caustic ingestion, immunodeficiency	Burning epigastric pain; pain with swallowing	Infectious etiologies in immunocompromised patients include candida, HSV, and CMV

CMV, cytomegalovirus; GERD, gastroesophageal reflux disease; HSV, Herpes simplex virus; IBD, inflammatory bowel disease; LUQ, left upper quadrant of the abdomen; RLQ, right lower quadrant of the abdomen; RUQ, right upper quadrant of the abdomen.

TABLE 12.5

NON-GI CAUSES OF ACUTE ABDOMINAL PAIN IN INFANTS AND CHILDREN

Renal	Metabolic	Gynecologic/Testicular
Pulmonary	Cardiac	Miscellaneous
Pyelonephritis	Testicular torsion	Myocardial ischemia
Nephrolithiasis	Ovarian torsion PID Ectopic pregnancy	Myocarditis Aortic dissection
Metabolic	Pulmonary	Miscellaneous
DKA	Pneumonia	Anaphylaxis
Uremia	Pulmonary embolism	Toxic ingestion
Adrenal insufficiency Porphyria	Pleuritis	Abdominal migraine Psychosocial Narcotic withdrawal Splenic rupture Vasculitis

DKA, diabetic ketoacidosis; PID, pelvic inflammatory disease.

Points to Remember

- In addition to the causes of acute abdominal pain in normal hosts, neutropenic enterocolitis (typhlitis), GVHD, CMV, and fungal infections should be considered in immunocompromised patients with acute abdominal pain.
- Don't forget about non-GI causes of acute abdominal pain!

Approach to Acute Abdominal Pain

1. Complete history focusing on duration of symptoms, quality and location of pain, previous episodes, personal/family history, medication use, history of trauma, and the presence of associated symptoms including fever, vomiting (bilious vs. nonbilious), hematemesis, change in stool pattern or quality, urinary symptoms, chest pain, and shortness of breath. Adolescent females should always be asked about sexual activity and LMP.
2. Complete physical exam with special attention given to overall appearance, abdominal distention/tenderness/masses, bowel sounds, perianal inspection, rectal examination, flank tenderness, and cardiopulmonary exam.
3. Routine laboratory tests are not indicated in every patient with acute abdominal pain and should be guided based on the history and physical exam. Useful lab tests may include a CBC, CMP, amylase, lipase, ESR, CRP, UA, urine culture, urine hCG, GC/CL studies, and/or cardiac enzymes.
4. Imaging depends on the suspected etiology and may include AXR, abdominal CT, abdominal U/S, pelvic U/S, testicular U/S, upper GI series, and/or barium or air-contrast enema.
5. An EKG should be obtained if a cardiac etiology is suspected. Endoscopy with biopsy may be indicated if esophagitis and/or gastritis are suspected.

Points to Remember

- Giving a patient with severe acute abdominal pain morphine DOES NOT interfere with your ability to establish the correct diagnosis.

Chronic Recurrent Abdominal Pain

Chronic and/or recurrent abdominal pain is not a specific diagnosis but rather describes a heterogeneous group of disorders. Major causes of chronic and/or recurrent abdominal pain in children are shown in Box 12.2.

Functional abdominal pain is the most common cause of chronic and/or recurrent abdominal pain in children and deserves special mention. Functional abdominal pain is a diagnosis of exclusion in which there is no evidence of an inflammatory, anatomic, metabolic, or neoplastic

Points to Remember

- Almost all of the causes of chronic abdominal pain can present acutely as an exacerbation.

Box 12.2 Major Causes of Chronic and/or Recurrent Abdominal Pain in Children

Functional abdominal pain	Reflux esophagitis
Lactose intolerance	*Helicobacter pylori* gastritis
Simple constipation	Peptic ulcer disease
Musculoskeletal pain	Mesenteric lymphadenitis
Parasitic infection	Inflammatory bowel disease

Note: Above etiologies are listed in order of prevalence.

TABLE 12.6

FUNCTIONAL ABDOMINAL PAIN DISORDERS IN CHILDREN

	Characteristics and Features
Functional dyspepsia	■ Persistent/recurrent pain in the upper abdomen superior to umbilicus ■ Not relieved by defecation ■ Not associated with a change in frequency and/or form of stool
Irritable bowel syndrome	■ Abdominal pain that usually improves with defecation ■ Associated with a change in the frequency and/or form of stool
Childhood functional abdominal pain	■ Episodic or continuous abdominal pain ■ Some loss of daily activity ■ Associated with other somatic complaints such as headache, limp pain, or difficulty sleeping ■ Insufficient criteria for other functional abdominal pain disorders
Abdominal migraine	■ Paroxysmal episodes of intense, acute periumbilical pain that lasts ≥1 h ■ Intervening periods of usual health lasting weeks to months ■ Pain interferes with normal activities ■ Pain associated with anorexia, nausea, vomiting, headache, and/or photophobia

process that explains the symptoms. The Rome III Criteria categorizes functional abdominal pain into four different disorders as shown in Table 12.6.

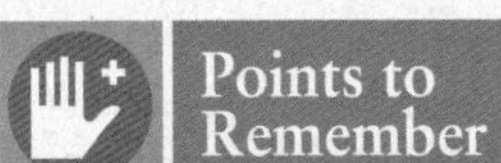

Points to Remember

- NG lavage can be used to help confirm the level of the bleed—the aspirate will be clear with lower GI bleeds and bloody with upper GI bleeds.
- The hematocrit is NOT a reliable indicator of acute blood loss. The best indicator of significant acute blood loss is orthostasis.
- Occult GI bleeding results in iron deficiency and is often detected by anemia associated with a low MCV and elevated RDW.
- Not everything that looks like blood is! Red food coloring, fruit punch, red candy, and beets can mimic the appearance of hematemesis and/or hematochezia while bismuth, iron, spinach, blueberries, grapes, and licorice can turn the stool dark and be mistaken for melena. Always confirm the presence of blood with a guaiac test!

Approach to Chronic and/or Recurrent Abdominal Pain

1. Complete history focusing on duration and pattern of symptoms, quality and location of pain, personal/family history, diet history, impact on daily life, change in stool pattern, relationship to stooling, and associated symptoms. Signs and symptoms suggestive of organic disease rather than functional abdominal pain are shown in Box 3.
2. Complete physical exam with special attention given to overall appearance, abdominal distention/tenderness/masses, bowel sounds, perianal inspection, rectal examination, skin findings, evaluation of the oral cavity, and joint exam.
3. Routine lab tests are not indicated in every patient with chronic abdominal pain and should be guided based on the history and physical exam. Useful screening labs may include a CBC, CMP (glucose, LFTs, bilirubin, etc.), ESR, and CRP.
4. Imaging studies depend on the suspected etiology and may include AXR, abdominal CT, and/or abdominal U/S.

GASTROINTESTINAL BLEEDING

Upper verses lower GI bleeding is differentiated based on whether the source is above or below the ligament of Trietz. Hematemesis (vomiting blood) and melena (black and tarry stools) are usually signs of upper GI bleeding, while hematochezia (bright red blood per rectum) usually indicates a lower GI bleed. Occult blood loss can occur with upper or lower GI bleeds. Severe GI bleeding is a life-threatening emergency as the patient can quickly develop hypovolemic shock. The differential diagnosis for GI bleeding based on presentation is given in Table 12.7.

Box 12.3 Signs and Symptoms Suggestive of Organic Disease in Patients with Chronic and/or Recurrent Abdominal Pain

Growth deceleration	GI bleed
Weight loss	Dysphagia
Unexplained fevers	Unexplained rashes
Pain radiating to back	Nocturnal symptoms
Bilious emesis	Arthritis
Hematemesis	Anemia/pallor
Oral ulcers	Delayed puberty
Chronic diarrhea	

TABLE 12.7

DIFFERENTIAL DIAGNOSIS OF GASTROINTESTINAL BLEEDING BASED ON PRESENTATION

Hematemesis and/or Melena	Hematochezia	Occult GI Blood Loss
Swallowed blood (e.g., epistaxis, dental work, etc.)	Milk-protein allergy	Esophagitis
Esophagitis	Intestinal ischemia (NEC)	Gastritis
Gastritis	Meckel diverticulum	
PUD	Vasculitis (e.g., HSP)	Acid peptic disease
Mallory–Weiss tear	Sloughed polyp	Eosinophilic gastroenteritis and/or colitis
Esophageal varices	Intestinal or colonic ulcer	Celiac disease
Vascular malformations	Colitis—infectious vs. IBD	Inflammatory bowel disease
	Vascular malformation	
	Anal fissure	

IBD, inflammatory bowel disease; NEC, necrotizing enterocolitis; PUD, peptic ulcer disease.

Approach to Gastrointestinal Bleeding

1. Complete history focusing on duration, quantity, and location of bleeding; quality of bleeding (e.g., clots, color, etc.), personal/family history, GERD symptoms, nose bleeds, medication use, and associated symptoms including weight loss, abdominal pain, fever, change in stool pattern, and/or vomiting.
2. Complete physical exam with special attention given to overall appearance, heart rate, blood pressure, perfusion, abdominal distention/tenderness/masses, and rectal examination.
3. Initial lab tests may include CBC, Coags, LFTs, ESR, CRP, stool guaiac, and/or stool studies. A type and screen should be done in all patients with moderate or severe bleeding. The Apt test is useful in neonates with apparent GI bleeding to investigate the possibility of swallowed maternal blood.
4. Imaging studies should be based on the suspected etiology and may include AXR, upper GI series, abdominal U/S, abdominal CT, and/or angiography.
5. Further workup may include upper endoscopy and/or colonoscopy (to locate and evaluate the source of bleeding), a Meckel's scan, and/or a tagged red blood cell scan.
6. Emergent treatment for severe GI bleeds includes volume resuscitation (NS, PRBC) and airway protection; definitive treatment of GI bleeding depends on underlying etiology.

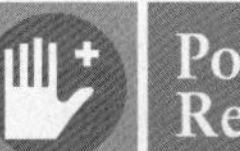

Points to Remember

- Intestinal bleeding is a LATE sign of acute intestinal obstruction.
- The most common causes of bloody stools in infants younger than 6 months are milk protein allergy and rectal fissure.
- A toddler with abdominal pain and a lower GI bleed should be assumed to have intussusception until proven otherwise.
- Meckel's diverticulum classically presents as large volume painless GI bleeding in a toddler.

Clinical Case Vignette

A 15-year-old female gymnast presents to the ER with hematemesis and epigastric pain. She is pale but has stable vital signs and is nontoxic. Initial labs are remarkable for a microcytic anemia. NG lavage did not clear and endoscopy revealed an antral gastric ulcer. Upon further questioning, you learn that the patient has had multiple gymnastic-related injuries and uses high doses of ibuprofen regularly. You hospitalize her and keep her NPO with several days of IV pantoprazole. Once her exam improves and she is tolerating PO, she is sent home on oral iron and a proton-pump inhibitor and counseled about avoidance of NSAIDs.

RECTAL PAIN

Rectal pain is a relatively uncommon complaint in children and when present often represents organic pathology. The differential diagnosis for rectal pain in children is shown in Box 12.4.

Points to Remember

- Perianal dermatitis due to GAS is a relatively common cause of rectal pain in toddlers and school-age children. It presents with perianal erythema, pain, and pruritus. Diagnosis should be confirmed via rapid strep test and/or culture. Treatment is with a 10-day course of PCN.
- Think about pinworm infection in a preschool or school-age child with perianal pruritus!

Approach to Rectal Pain

1. Complete history focusing on the quality of pain, associated symptoms including rectal bleeding, diarrhea, constipation, and fever, personal/family history, and travel history. Patients should also be asked about voluntary or involuntary anal intercourse and/or the possibility of a foreign body.
2. Complete physical exam with special attention given to the rectal exam looking for dermatitis, fissures, mucosal friability, rectal fullness, palpable masses, localized tenderness, and/or hemorrhoids.
3. Initial labs depend on the suspected etiology and may include rapid strep test and culture, GC/CL studies, tape test (pinworm), CBC, CRP, and ESR.
4. Further evaluation may include AXR, pelvic CT, and/or colonoscopy/sigmoidoscopy.

Box 12.4 Differential Diagnosis of Rectal Pain in Children

Hemorrhoids
Anal fissure
Infections
  GAS dermatitis
  Bacterial abscess
  Pinworms
Foreign body
  Self-inflicted
  Sexual abuse
Rectal prolapse
  Cystic fibrosis
Inflammatory
  Proctitis (e.g., trauma, STDs, infection)
  IBD ± perianal fistula
Neoplasm
Trauma

GAS, group A streptococcus; IBD, inflammatory bowel disease; STDs, sexually transmitted diseases.

Clinical Case Vignette

A 3-year-old male who attends daycare presents with a 2-week history rectal itching. His exam is remarkable for mild perianal excoriations but is otherwise normal. The tape test is positive for parasitic eggs. The patient is given one dose of mebendazole for presumed Enterobius vermicularis *(pinworm) infection. Follow-up 2 weeks later denotes resolution of symptoms.*

HEPATOMEGALY

In general, normal liver size is defined as extension less than 3.5 cm below the right costal margin in newborns and less than 2 cm in children. Liver size can also be assessed clinically by assessing the span of dullness to percussion with a normal span being 4 to 5 cm in infants and 6 to 8 cm in older children. Hepatomegaly, enlargement of the liver, can result from a variety of mechanisms and represents a wide array of pathology. Causes of hepatomegaly in infants and children are grouped together by mechanism and shown in Table 12.8.

TABLE 12.8

MECHANISMS AND CAUSES OF HEPATOMEGALY IN INFANTS AND CHILDREN

Mechanism	General Conditions	Causes in Infants	Causes in Children
Inflammation	Infections Toxins Drugs Autoimmune	■ Maternal medications ■ Tylenol ingestion ■ Sepsis ■ Viral hepatitis ■ Congenital infections (CMV, toxoplasmosis) ■ TB	■ Tylenol ingestion ■ Obesity ■ Parasitic infections ■ Sepsis ■ Viral hepatitis ■ Autoimmune hepatitis ■ TB
Inappropriate storage	Glycogen Lipids Fats Metals Abnormal Proteins	■ Maternal diabetes ■ Metabolic disorders ■ Glycogen storage diseases	■ Wilson disease
Infiltration	Tumors Cysts Extramedullary hematopoiesis	■ Metabolic disorders ■ Leukemia/lymphoma ■ Hepatoblastoma ■ HLH	■ Leukemia/lymphoma ■ Hepatocellular cancer ■ HLH
Vascular congestion	Suprahepatic Intrahepatic	■ Congestive heart failure ■ Portal vein thrombosis	■ Congestive heart failure ■ Portal vein thrombosis
Cholestasis	Biliary obstruction	■ Biliary atresia ■ TPN cholestasis	■ Choledochal cysts ■ Cystic fibrosis
Miscellaneous		■ Malnutrition	

CMV, cytomegalovirus; HLH, hemophagocytic lymphohistiocytosis; TPN, total parenteral nutrition.

Approach to Hepatomegaly

1. Complete history focusing on perinatal and birth history, growth pattern, developmental milestones, diet, medication use, travel history, personal/family history, and associated symptoms including weight loss/gain, abnormal stooling pattern, skin problems, mental status changes, neurologic abnormalities, and easy bruising or bleeding.
2. Complete physical exam with special attention given to assessing the size and consistency of the liver and looking for dysmorphic features, jaundice, edema, skin changes, lymphadenopathy, splenomegaly, and signs of malnutrition.
3. Initial labs generally include a CBC, CMP (specifically to look at glucose, LFTs, total bilirubin, direct bilirubin, albumin, and total protein), and coags. Further labs on a case-by-case basis may include viral studies, NH3, lactic acid, pyruvic acid, acylcarnitine profile, plasma amino acids, urine organic acids, AFP, triglycerides, sweat test, LDH, uric acid, ceruloplasmin, and urine copper.
4. Abdominal U/S is the initial imaging study of choice. Further studies may include abdominal CT, MRI, cholangiography, and HIDA scan.
5. Liver biopsy and/or bone marrow biopsy are indicated in select cases depending on the suspected etiology.

A schematic approach to the evaluation of hepatomegaly is shown in Figure 12.1.

Clinical Case Vignette

A 17-year-old female presents to the clinic with a 2-week history of jaundice, nausea, and foul-smelling diarrhea. There is no history of recent travel, no medications, no mental status changes, and no history of bleeding/bruising. On exam, the patient is nonobese, tachycardic, has a II/VI systolic ejection murmur at the LLSB radiating to the LUSB, liver edge is palpable 3 cm below the costal margin, and the patient has 1+ nonpitting edema in the lower extremities. Lab workup is remarkable for normal ALT/AST, direct bilirubin 26 mg/dL, albumin 2.5, and INR 2.9. She is immediately referred to the ER. Further laboratory workup is remarkable for positive ANA and antismooth muscle antibodies, negative anti-LKM antibodies. Subsequent percutaneous liver biopsy is remarkable for piecemeal necrosis and cirrhosis. She is diagnosed with ALF secondary to type I autoimmune hepatitis and is started on corticosteroids.

Points to Remember

- Classic signs of liver disease seen in adults including spider angiomas, xanthomas, and palmar erythema are rare in children.
- ALT is more specific for hepatocellular injury than AST.
- Tests of true liver function include albumin and PT.
- Radionuclide scanning (HIDA scan) is useful in infants to distinguish biliary atresia from neonatal hepatitis. In biliary atresia, hepatic uptake of radionuclide is normal but there is no excretion into the intestines. In neonatal hepatitis, hepatic uptake of radionuclide is impaired but excretion into the intestines is normal.
- Cholangiography allows direct visualization of the intra- and extrahepatic biliary tree.

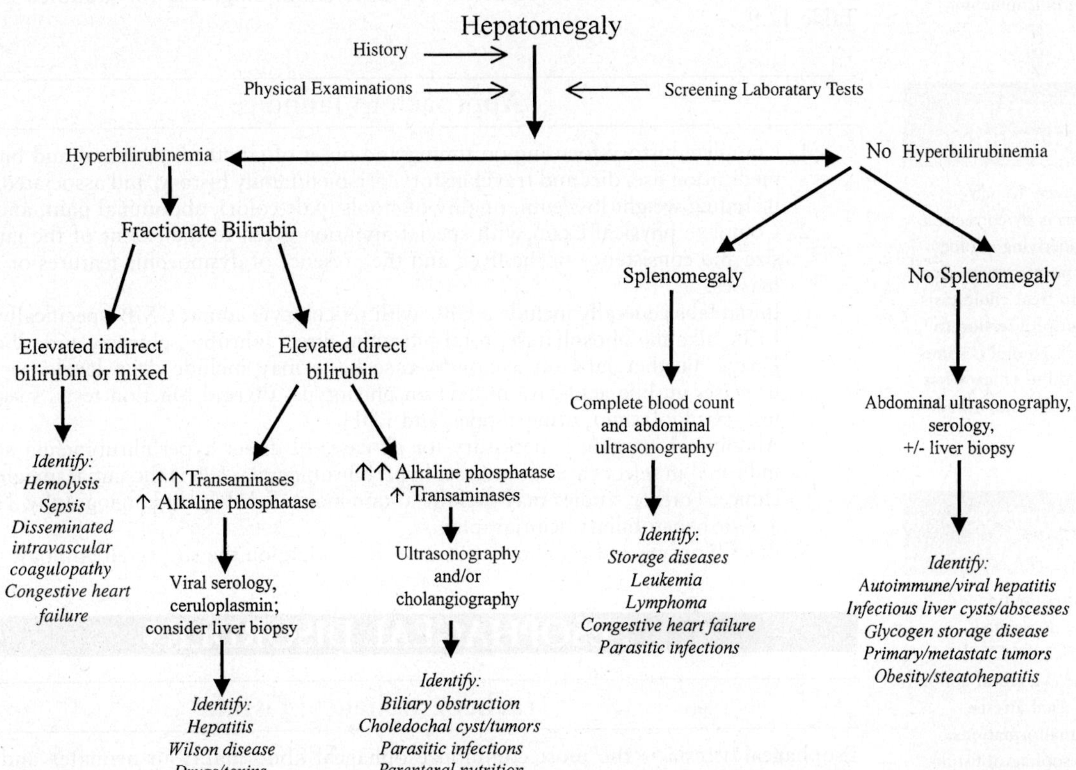

FIGURE 12.1. Diagnostic algorithm for child with hepatomegaly. (Reprinted with permission from Wolf AD, Lavine JE. Hepatomegaly in neonates and children. *Pediatr Rev.* 2000;21:303–310.)

TABLE 12.9

IMPORTANT CAUSES OF HYPERBILIRUBINEMIA

Direct/Conjugated Hyperbilirubinemia		Indirect/Unconjugated Hyperbilirubinemia
Extrahepatic	**Intrahepatic**	
■ Congenital abnormalities of the extrahepatic biliary tract (e.g., biliary atresia, choledochal cyst) ■ Obstructive gallstones ■ Abdominal masses	■ Congenital abnormalities of the intrahepatic biliary tract (e.g., Alagille syndrome) ■ Membrane transport and secretion disorders ■ Total parenteral nutrition ■ Hepatocellular disease (e.g., viral hepatitis, Wilson disease, autoimmune hepatitis) ■ Inborn errors of metabolism (e.g., Dubin–Johnson syndrome) ■ Sepsis ■ Drug-induced cholestasis ■ Alpha-1 antitrypsin deficiency	■ Gilbert disease ■ Hemolytic anemia ■ Neonatal physiologic jaundice ■ Breast milk jaundice ■ Hepatocellular damage (e.g., viral hepatitis) ■ Crigler–Najjar syndrome ■ Cystic fibrosis ■ Hypothyroidism

Points to Remember

- Clinical manifestations of direct hyperbilirubinemia include jaundice, pruritus, and pale stools.
- The most common cause of an indirect hyperbilirubinemia in a nonneonate is Gilbert disease, a benign disorder of mildly impaired bilirubin conjugation found in 5% to 10% of the population.
- Viral hepatitis is associated with both a direct and indirect hyperbilirubinemia.

JAUNDICE

Jaundice is the yellowish discoloration of the skin and mucous membranes due to hyperbilirubinemia. Hyperbilirubinemia can be divided into direct/conjugated hyperbilirubinemia and indirect/unconjugated hyperbilirubinemia. Direct hyperbilirubinemia results when bile cannot flow normally from the liver into the biliary system and then into the intestine. This functional obstruction (also called cholestasis) can result from intrahepatic or extrahepatic processes. Indirect hyperbilirubinemia results from increased red blood cell turnover or disorders of impaired conjugation. The differential diagnosis for jaundice is shown in Table 12.9.

Points to Remember

- The only way to halt cholestasis is by correction of the underlying etiology. There is no proven medical therapy to treat cholestasis or prevent progression to cirrhosis. Ursodiol is sometimes used but efficacy has not been well established.

Approach to Jaundice

1. Complete history focusing on timing and onset of jaundice, perinatal and birth history, medication use, diet and travel history, personal/family history, and associated symptoms including weight loss/gain, quality of stools (pale color), abdominal pain, and pruritus.
2. Complete physical exam with special attention given to the extent of the jaundice, the size and consistency of the liver, and the presence of dysmorphic features or abdominal masses.
3. Initial labs generally include a CBC with reticulocyte count, CMP (specifically to look at LFTs, alkaline phosphatase, total bilirubin, direct bilirubin, glucose, and albumin), and Coags. Further labs on a case-by-case basis may include drug levels, viral studies, urine/serum bile acids, α_1-antitrypsin phenotype, thyroid function tests, sweat chloride test, ceruloplasmin, urine copper, and LDH.
4. Abdominal imaging is necessary for all cases of direct hyperbilirubinemia and may be indicated in select cases of indirect hyperbilirubinemia. U/S is the initial imaging study of choice. Further studies may include abdominal CT, MRI, cholangiography, HIDA scan, and/or hepatobiliary scintigraphy.
5. Liver biopsy is indicated in select cases depending on the suspected etiology.

Points to Remember

- The most common syndrome associated with TEFs is VACTERL syndrome (Vertebral abnormalities, Anal atresia, Cardiac malformations, Tracheoesophageal fistula, Renal anomalies, and Limb abnormalities).

ESOPHAGEAL DISORDERS

Tracheoesophageal Fistula

Esophageal atresia is the most common esophageal abnormality in neonates and is almost always associated with a TEF. The most common type of TEF is a proximal blind esophageal pouch with a fistula connecting the distal esophagus to the trachea (see Fig. 12.2). Half of patients with TEFs have other associated congenital abnormalities.

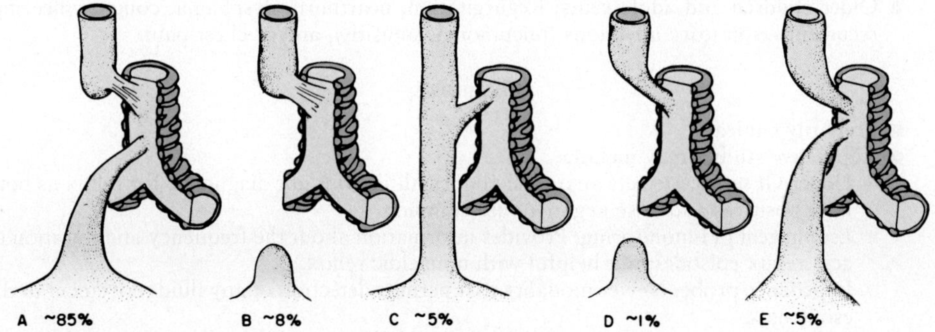

FIGURE 12.2. Schematic pictures of various types of TEFs and their relative frequencies. (Reprinted with permission from McMillan JA, Feigin RD, DeAngelis C, et al. *Oski's Pediatrics: Principles and Practice*. 4th ed. Philadelphia, PA: Lippincott Williams & Wilkins, 2006.)

Clinical Manifestations

- Usually presents at birth or in early infancy with copious oral secretions, respiratory distress exacerbated by feeding, and/or aspiration.
- Half of patients have a maternal history of polyhydramnios.

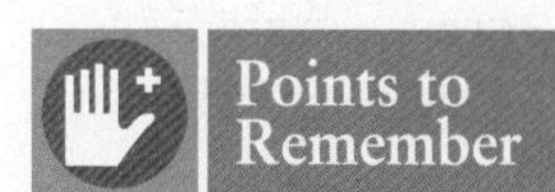

- **Think about a TEF in any infant with coughing/choking during feeds!**

Diagnosis

- Most TEFs will be picked up by the inability to pass an NG/OG tube into the stomach; x-ray demonstrates the NG/OG coiled in the esophagus.
- Esophagrams and/or bronchoscopy can be used to diagnose TEFs not associated with esophageal atresia.

Treatment

- Surgical correction.

Achalasia

Achalasia is a loss of LES relaxation leading to high resting LES pressure and absent or nonperistaltic esophageal contractions. The etiology is unknown. Only 5% of cases occur in children younger than 5 years.

Clinical Manifestations

- Vomiting, regurgitation, and dysphagia.
- Dysphagia first occurs with solids then also with liquids as the disease progresses.
- Aspiration, recurrent pneumonias.

Diagnosis

- Gold standard is manometry.
- Upper GI may show characteristic "bird's beak" appearance with tapering of esophagus.

Treatment

- Balloon dilation or surgical myotomy of LES.

Gastroesophageal Reflux Disease

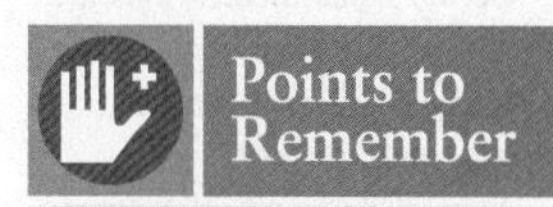

- **Most infants outgrow reflux symptoms by 12 months of age.**

It is important to distinguish between GER and GERD. GER is simply the passage of gastric contents into the esophagus and can be physiologic in infants. GERD is when a patient is symptomatic from and/or experiences complications of GER. GERD is more common in premature infants than in term infants. Risk factors for GERD in older children and adolescents include obesity, tobacco/alcohol/drug use, anatomic abnormalities (e.g., hiatal hernia), and neurologic impairment.

Clinical Manifestations

- **Infants:** Recurrent vomiting, poor weight gain, irritability, Sandifer syndrome, stridor, recurrent wheezing, recurrent respiratory infections (e.g., pneumonia, AOM), and/or ALTE (apparent life-threatening episode).

Points to Remember

- Sandifer syndrome is a rare but classic phenomenon in infants with GERD and refers to stereotypic repetitive stretching and arching movements.

Points to Remember

- A baby who "spits up" but is otherwise in no distress and is growing appropriately is a "happy refluxer" with GER (not GERD) and does not need treatment.

Points to Remember

- Traditional reflux therapy of semisupine posture in an infant seat or swing is detrimental rather than beneficial and is no longer recommended.

Points to Remember

- Inadequately treated severe GERD can lead to esophageal strictures, Barrett's esophagitis, and/or adenocarcinoma.

Points to Remember

- Two other types of esophagitis important to know about are corrosive esophagitis and pill esophagitis. Corrosive esophagitis results from the ingestion of caustic substances. Pill esophagitis occurs when medications are taken with inadequate fluids and the pill temporarily lodges in the esophagus. Doxycycline and other tetracycline derivatives are common causes. Both pill esophagitis and corrosive esophagitis cause odynophagia and retrosternal pain. Treatment is supportive with antacids and a bland liquid diet until symptoms resolve.

- **Older children and adolescents:** Regurgitation, heartburn, dysphagia, cough, wheezing, recurrent respiratory infections (pneumonia, sinusitis), and/or chest pain.

Diagnosis

- Primarily clinical.
- Adjunctive studies may include:
  - **Upper GI series:** Detects anatomic abnormalities, but not diagnostic for reflux as both false positives and false negatives are common.
  - **Esophageal pH monitoring:** Provides information about the frequency and duration of acid reflux episodes; not helpful with nonacidic reflux.
  - **Impedance probe:** Newer modality that permits detection of any fluid movement in the esophagus.
- **Endoscopy:** Detects anatomic abnormalities and GERD-related esophagitis.

Treatment

- Lifestyle changes
  - **Infants:** Thickening feeds, more frequent small volume feeds.
  - **Older children and adolescents:** Weight loss, diet modification, avoidance of alcohol/tobacco/drugs.
- Pharmacologic treatment for patients with more severe disease and/or disease refractory to life-style changes.
  - Acid reduction via antacids, H_2 antagonists, or proton pump inhibitors.
  - Metoclopramide is a prokinetic agent commonly used to treat GERD although efficacy not well established and there are many side effects of prolonged use.
- Surgical treatment vis Nissen fundoplication is a last resort for refractory GERD; continuous feeds via a gastronomy or jejunostomy tube are also used in severe cases.

Eosinophilic Esophagitis

Eosinophilic esophagitis is a form of food allergy that predominantly affects the esophagus. It is characterized by extensive eosinophilic infiltration of the esophagus and occurs mostly in males. It can occur at any age.

Clinical Manifestations

- Vomiting, chest/epigastric pain, strictures, dysphagia.
- Associated conditions include atopy and food allergies.

Diagnosis

- May see peripheral eosinophilia and increase IgE levels.
- Confirmation via endoscopy with biopsy with more than 15 to 20 eosinophils/hpf.

Treatment

- Elimination of inciting foods.
- Topical nonabsorbable corticosteroids.

Infectious Esophagitis

Infectious esophagitis is characterized by infection-related esophageal inflammation. It occurs almost exclusively in immunocompromised patients, especially in patients with HIV/AIDS. The most common pathogens are candida, HSV, and CMV. VZV, *diphtheria*, and other types of bacterial pathogens are rare causes.

Clinical Manifestations

- Fever, dysphagia, odynophagia, and retrosternal pain.
- Candidal esophagitis is often associated with oral candidiasis (visible white plaques).

Diagnosis

- If oral lesions are visible and consistent with candidal infection, a trial of presumptive treatment with oral fluconazole is reasonable.
- If etiology is unclear, endoscopy with biopsy is indicated.

Treatment

- Depends on underlying pathogen.

Esophageal Perforation

Esophageal perforation is a rare but serious phenomenon associated with significant morbidity and mortality. It is usually iatrogenic (e.g., endoscopy, NG/OG tube placement, suctioning) but occasionally results from a sudden increase in esophageal pressure from vomiting (Boerhaave syndrome) or blunt trauma.

Clinical Manifestations

- Acute onset of severe epigastric/retrosternal pain and dysphagia.
- Ill-appearance with fever, tachycardia, abdominal pain, and/or crepitus.

Diagnosis

- Cervical spine and CXR showing retrosternal free air and pneumomediastinum.
- If x-rays are normal but there is a high degree of suspicion, obtain an esophagram with water-soluble contrast.

Treatment

- Medical management including NPO, gastric drainage, and broad-spectrum IV antibiotics may be adequate for small esophageal tears in otherwise stable patients.
- Larger esophageal perforations require emergent surgical repair.

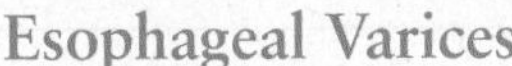

Esophageal Varices

Rupture of esophageal varices is an important cause of morbidity and mortality in patients with portal HTN.

Clinical Manifestations

- Acute onset of hematemesis and/or melena.

Diagnosis

- Confirmation via endoscopy.

Treatment

- Preventive measures for known varices include sclerotherapy and β-blockers.
- Acute management of variceal bleeding includes (in order)
  - ABCs (airway protection, volume resuscitation with PRBCs).
  - Pharmacologic treatment with octreotide.
  - Endoscopic sclerotherapy, band ligation, and/or thrombin injection.
  - Mechanical intervention with Sengstaken-Blakemore tube.
- Patients with severe and/or recurrent episodes of esophageal variceal bleeding may require surgical management with portosystemic shunt and/or liver transplantation.

GASTRIC DISORDERS

Pyloric Stenosis

Pyloric stenosis is a condition that develops postnatally in the first weeks of life in which hypertrophy of the pyloric muscle leads to gastric outflow obstruction. The peak age of onset is ~3 weeks of age, but it can present as early as 1 week or as late as 5 months. Risk factors include male gender, first-born, White race, positive family history, and erythromycin exposure.

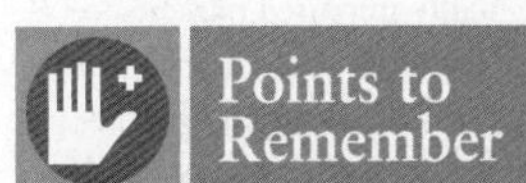

- **Erythromycin use in neonates is associated with increased incidence of pyloric stenosis.**

Clinical Manifestations

- Progressive nonbilious postprandial projectile vomiting.
- Classic physical exam findings are a palpable pyloric "olive" in the RUQ and visible peristaltic waves; these findings are variably present.

Diagnosis

- Diagnosis via pyloric U/S or upper gastrointestinal series.
- Classic electrolyte finding is hypochloremic, hypokalemic metabolic alkalosis; electrolytes are also often normal.

Treatment

- Acute management is to correct fluid and electrolyte abnormalities.
- Definitive surgical treatment with pyloromyotomy.

Gastric Volvulus

Gastric volvulus is a surgical emergency that occurs when the stomach rotates around itself and causes an obstruction. This occurs when one of the ligaments tethering the stomach to the peritoneum is stretched or absent.

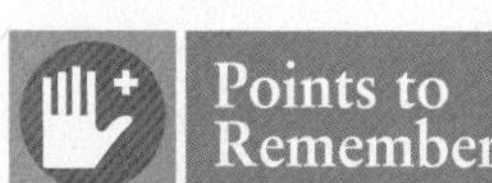

Points to Remember

- Risk factors for *H. pylori*–associated gastritis include low socioeconomic status, household crowding, and poor hygiene.
- The gold standard for diagnosis of *H. pylori* infection is gastric biopsy. Noninvasive tests include stool antigen testing and urease breath test (low specificity).

Clinical Manifestations

- Acute onset of severe epigastric pain, intractable retching and emesis.
- Inability to pass NG/OG tube into stomach.

Diagnosis

- AXR.

Treatment

- Emergent surgery (delay in treatment can lead to intestinal ischemia).

Peptic Ulcer Disease

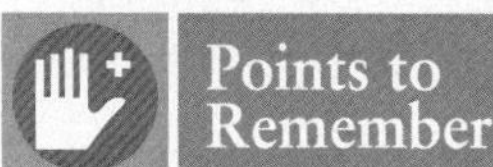

Points to Remember

- Zollinger–Ellison syndrome is a severe form of refractory PUD due to autonomous gastrin secretion by a gastrinoma and is often associated with MEN type I. It is characterized by recurrent, multiple, atypically located ulcers and treated with proton pump inhibitors ± octreotide to inhibit tumor growth.
- Bezoars are an accumulation of exogenous matter in the stomach or intestine. They usually occur in females with underlying personality disorders, patients with dysmotility disorders, and neurologically impaired patients. They can present with symptoms of intestinal obstruction, a palpable mass, and/or malnutrition. Diagnosis is via endoscopy. Treatment is via endoscopic removal.

PUD affects the stomach and/or duodenum and may be associated with inflammation. Primary PUD occurs in healthy children and is usually chronic, associated with *Helicobacter pylori*, and duodenal in origin. Secondary PUD is usually gastric and is caused by an underlying disorder including hypergastrinemia and Zollinger–Ellison syndrome.

Conditions predisposing to PUD include alcohol use, caffeine, and/or tobacco use, gastrostomy tubes, NSAIDS, burn injuries, and/or systemic illnesses.

Clinical Manifestations

- Epigastric pain
  - **Gastric ulcers**: Pain worsens with meals, especially with spicy foods, caffeine.
  - **Duodenal ulcers**: Pain improves with meals.
- Complications include hemorrhage, perforation, and/or obstruction (scarring).

Diagnosis

- Endoscopy with biopsy.

Treatment

- Life-style changes including avoidance of inciting substances and/or foods.
- Proton pump inhibitors.
- Treatment of *H. pylori* with clarithromycin + amoxicillin/metronidazole.
- Surgical therapy for severe and/or refractory cases; options include vagotomy, pyloroplasty, and antrectomy.

SMALL AND LARGE INTESTINES

Congenital Anatomical Abnormalities

Points to Remember

- Suspect duodenal atresia in a neonate with Down syndrome with bilious emesis in the first 24 hours of life.

Duodenal Atresia

Duodenal atresia is often associated with Down syndrome, congenital heart disease, TEF, malrotation, and/or renal anomalies but can also be an isolated abnormality.

Clinical Manifestations

- Presents in the neonatal period with bilious emesis, abdominal distension, and/or failure to pass meconium.
- 50% of patients have a maternal history of polyhydramnios during pregnancy.

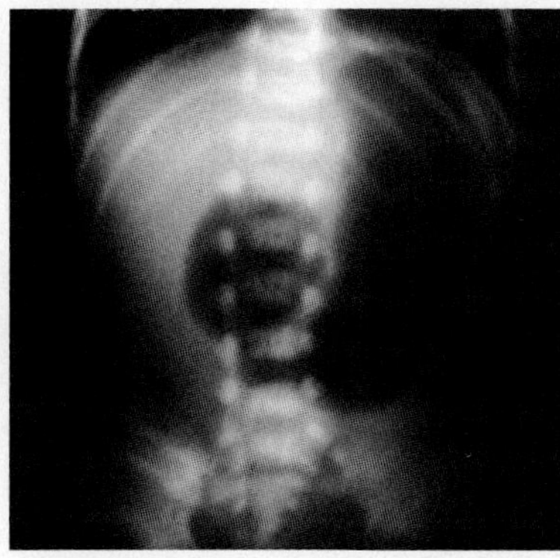

FIGURE 12.3. Classic radiographic appearance of duodenal atresia. There is a double bubble of gas in the stomach and proximal duodenum, with no gas in the distal intestinal tract. Reprinted with permission from Michael W. Mulholland, Ronald V. Maier, et al. *Greenfield's Surgery Scientific Principles And Practice*. 4th ed. Philadelphia, PA: Lippincott Williams & Wilkins, 2006.

Diagnosis

- Double-bubble sign on upright AXR (see Fig. 12.3).

Treatment

- NG decompression, NPO, fluid/electrolyte corrections.
- Surgical reanastomosis.

Malrotation

Malrotation is a developmental abnormality in which incomplete rotation of the midgut places the cecum in the RUQ and fixes the mesentery on a narrow base. The small bowel is at increased risk for twisting on the pedicle of mesentery (i.e., volvulus) which compromises bowel vascularity and may lead to ischemia and necrosis. Presentation is most common in early infancy and more than 90% of clinically significant cases present in the first year of life, although it can present at any age.

Clinical Manifestations

- Most cases of malrotation present with volvulus with acute onset of bilious emesis, abdominal pain, and/or abdominal distention.
- Some patients with malrotation present with more subtle signs of chronic intermittent intestinal obstruction and others remain asymptomatic throughout life.

Points to Remember

- **Any infant presenting with bilious emesis should be assumed to have malrotation with volvulus until proven otherwise and should be treated as a surgical emergency.**

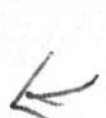

Diagnosis

- AXR is useful to look for volvulus and/or intestinal obstruction.
- Definitive diagnosis is via upper GI series with small bowel follow-through.

Treatment

- Malrotation with volvulus is a life-threatening surgical emergency. Delay in treatment can lead to bowel ischemia and necrosis, which can result in the need for extensive bowel removal and short gut syndrome. Definitive surgical procedure is the Ladd procedure.

Meckel Diverticulum

Meckel diverticulum is a remnant of the embryonic yolk sac that results from failure of the omphalomesenteric/vitelline duct to involute. It occurs in 1% to 3% of the population, is more common in males than in females, and typically presents in patients younger than 2 years. Most of these anomalies contain ectopic gastric mucosa which secrete acid, leading to ulceration and bleeding of the adjacent intestinal mucosa.

Points to Remember

- **Rule of 2's for Meckel diverticulum:**
  - **2% of infants**
  - **2 inches in size**
  - **2 feet from ileocecal valve**
  - **Detected in patients younger than 2 years**

Clinical Manifestations

- Painless rectal bleeding (hematochezia); GI bleeding can be minor and intermittent or severe and life-threatening.
- Can present with intussusception or volvulus.

Diagnosis

- Meckel's scan (Technetium-99 m pertechnetate radionuclide scan).

Treatment

- Surgical excision.

Points to Remember

- The most common lead point in an older child with intussusception is a Meckel diverticulum.
- Henoch–Schonlein purpura can be complicated by intussusception.

Points to Remember

- The classic triad of colicky abdominal pain, vomiting, and bloody stools only occurs in 10% of children with intussusception.

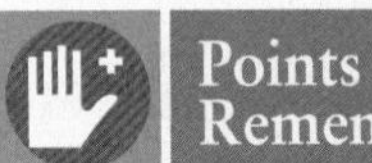

Points to Remember

- Air or contrast enemas are BOTH diagnostic and therapeutic for intussusception.

Acquired Intestinal Obstructions

Intussusception

Intussusception is the telescoping of one segment of bowel into another, causing luminal obstruction and compression of the mesenteric vessels. Without prompt intervention, intestinal ischemia and infarction develop. Intussusception is most common in infants and toddlers 3 months to 3 years of age and is usually idiopathic or related to hypertrophied Peyer patches following a viral illness. Intussusception in an older child should raise the suspicion of a specific lead point such as a Meckel diverticulum, lymphoma, or polyp.

Clinical Manifestations

- Episodes of severe abdominal pain, extreme irritability, and/or bilious emesis alternating with periods of lethargy.
- "Current jelly stools" are due to sloughing of bowel mucosa and are a late finding.
- Physical exam findings include abdominal tenderness and abdominal distention; a RLQ sausage-shaped mass may be palpable.

Diagnosis

- Gold standard is an air or contrast enema.
- A "target" or "crescent" sign on AXR or abdominal U/S is useful in some cases (Fig. 12.4).

Treatment

- Most cases of intussusception can be reduced via air or contrast enema.
- Surgical treatment is indicated for refractory cases.
- Observation for 24 to 48 hours is key, as recurrence can occur.

Ileus

An ileus is characterized by the absence of intestinal peristalsis without evidence of mechanical obstruction. Etiologies include infection, gut manipulation (surgery), metabolic abnormalities (e.g., hypercalcemia, hypokalemia, acidosis, uremia), and medications (e.g., loperamide, narcotics).

Clinical Manifestations

- Abdominal pain and/or distention.
- Vomiting.
- Lack of or minimal bowel movements and hypoactive or absent bowel sounds.

Diagnosis

- AXR with diffusely dilated bowel with or without air-fluid levels.

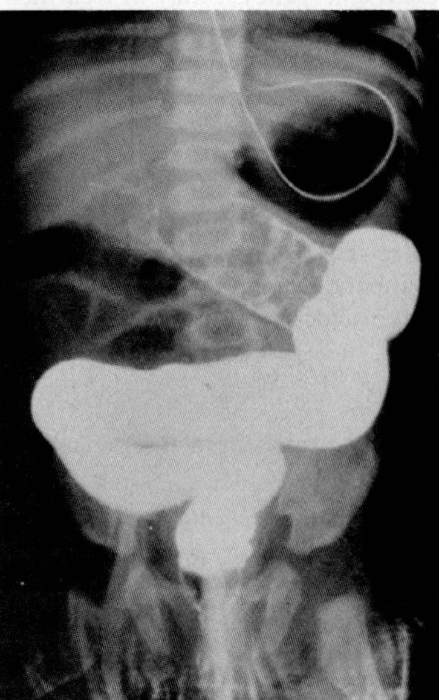

FIGURE 12.4. Barium enema study showing the coiled-spring pattern of barium around the intussusceptum in the transverse colon. (Reprinted with permission from McMillan JA, Feigin RD, DeAngelis C, et al. *Oski's Pediatrics: Principles and Practice*. 4th ed. Philadelphia, PA: Lippincott Williams & Wilkins, 2006.)

Treatment

- Depending on the underlying condition, most self-resolve with time.
- NG decompression can help relieve symptoms.

Points to Remember

- Incarcerated or strangulated inguinal hernias can also cause intestinal obstruction.
- DIOS is an important phenomenon in CF patients characterized by recurrent episodes of partial/complete intestinal obstruction due to thick intestinal contents.

Duodenal Hematoma

Blunt trauma to the epigastric area can result in a duodenal hematoma and intestinal obstruction. Examples of scenarios in which blunt trauma can cause duodenal hematomas include MVCs, bicycle handlebar injuries, nonaccidental trauma, and assault.

Clinical Manifestations

- Usually presents 2 to 3 days after the original injury with epigastric pain and progressive, intractable vomiting.
- Concomitant risk of pancreatitis.

Diagnosis

- Upper GI series with "coiled-spring appearance".
- Abdominal CT.

Treatment

- Bowel rest with NG decompression, NPO, and TPN until obstructive symptoms resolve (usually 7 to 10 days).
- Surgery is rarely indicated but may be necessary in cases with duration of more than 2 weeks.

Superior Mesenteric Artery Syndrome

SMA syndrome is a rare but serious problem that occurs when the SMA collapses onto and compresses the duodenum. Rapid weight loss can lead to loss of the SMA's posterior fat pad, which predisposes the patient to SMA syndrome, especially when in the supine position.

Clinical Manifestations

- Vomiting and severe abdominal pain.

Diagnosis

- Upper GI series with small bowel follow-through revealing cutoff of duodenum to the right of midline.

Treatment

- Conservative treatment is appropriate in most cases and includes improved nutrition (oral feeds, TPN, and/or NJ feeds) and prone or lateral positioning.
- Refractory and/or severe cases require surgery.

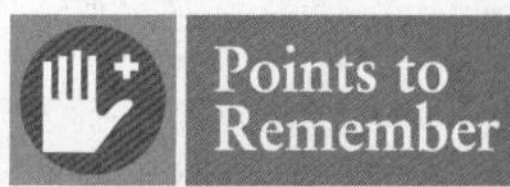

Points to Remember

- Think about SMA syndrome in an adolescent who starts vomiting after being in a body cast for orthopedic surgery.

Miscellaneous Infectious Processes

Small Intestinal Bacterial Overgrowth

Small intestinal bacterial overgrowth can result from conditions that alter normal defenses such as partial bowel obstruction, motility disorders, diabetes mellitus, short bowel syndrome, intestinal duplications, and immunodeficiency.

Clinical Manifestations

- Bloating, constipation, diarrhea, and flatulence.
- Can be associated with malabsorption and vitamin deficiency.

Diagnosis

- Breath tests (lactulose-hydrogen; glucose-hydrogen) are helpful in some cases.
- Gold standard for diagnosis is duodenal aspirate with 10^5 CFU/mL or more colonic flora.

Treatment

- Correct underlying condition.
- Cycle antibiotics (e.g., rifaximin, metronidazole).

Inflammatory Processes

Inflammatory Bowel Disease

IBD includes Crohn's disease and UC. They are chronic, relapsing inflammatory diseases of the bowel. Although Crohn's disease and UC share many common features, several features allow differentiation of the two disorders. A comparison of Crohn's disease and UC is shown in Table 12.10.

Diagnosis

- Lab findings may include elevated ESR and CRP and anemia.
- Imaging studies including upper GI series and abdominal CT may be helpful.
- Gold standard for diagnosis is endoscopy/colonoscopy/sigmoidoscopy to visualize gross pathology and confirm diagnosis with biopsy.

Treatment

- Crohn's disease (depends on disease location and severity)
  - Medical therapy includes steroids, mesalamine, sulfasalazine, azathioprine, methotrexate, and infliximab (in order of increasing disease severity).
  - Surgical resection for refractory and/or severe localized disease; surgical intervention is also often necessary for strictures and fistulas.
- UC
  - Medical therapy is similar to Crohn's disease.
  - Surgical colectomy is curative for severe and/or refractory disease.

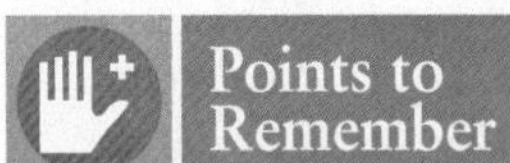

Points to Remember

- Consider celiac disease in a toddler who presents with constitutional symptoms, weight loss, and worsening abdominal bloating and diarrhea associated with bread products.

Celiac Disease

Celiac disease is an immune-mediated enteropathy caused by sensitivity to dietary gluten. Gluten proteins are found in wheat and related grains such as rye and barley. Celiac disease most commonly presents in patients 2 to 3 years old but can present at any age. It is more common in females and in patients with a first-degree relative with the disease. Associated conditions include type I diabetes, Down syndrome, Turner syndrome, autoimmune thyroiditis, and IgA deficiency.

TABLE 12.10

COMPARISON OF CROHN'S DISEASE AND ULCERATIVE COLITIS

Feature	Crohn's disease	Ulcerative Colitis
Epidemiology	■ Affects males and females equally ■ Bimodal age of onset with peaks in 2nd/3rd decades and again in 6th decade ■ Twice as common as UC	■ More common in females ■ Bimodal age of onset with peaks in 2nd/3rd decades and again in 6th decade
Clinical presentation	■ Diarrhea, abdominal pain, nausea, vomiting, (GI bleeding less common than in UC) ■ Fever, weight loss, anemia, growth failure ■ Extraintestinal manifestations	■ Diarrhea, hematochezia, abdominal cramps ■ Fever, weight loss, anemia, growth failure
Site of disease	Mouth to anus (ileocolic = most common)	Colon (may have some ileal involvement, i.e., "backwash ileitis")
Pattern of disease	Discontinuous (skip) regions	Continuous
Gross pathology	Strictures, fistulas, fissures, serosal fat, "cobble-stoning"	Diffuse continuous inflammation
Histology	Transmural inflammation, noncaseating granulomas	Mucosal and submucosal inflammation, crypt abscesses
Perianal disease (tags, fissures, abscesses)	Common	Rare
Extraintestinal involvement	Common ■ Spondyloarthropathy ■ Aphthous ulcers ■ Erythema nodosum ■ Pyoderma gangrenosum ■ Uveitis ■ Primary sclerosing cholangitis	Rare ■ Pyoderma gangrenosum and primary sclerosing cholangitis are more common in UC than in Crohn's disease
Toxic megacolon	No association	Strong association
Risk for cancer	Increased	Greatly increased
Perinuclear antineutrophil	Uncommon	Common cytoplasmic antibodies (pANCA)

GI, gastrointestinal; pANCA, perinuclear staining antineutrophil cytoplasmic antibody; UC, ulcerative colitis.

TABLE 12.11

INTESTINAL MANIFESTATIONS OF CELIAC DISEASE

Symptoms (in Order of Prevalence)	Signs (in Order of Prevalence)
Failure to thrive, weight loss	Height <25th percentile
Diarrhea	Body weight <25th percentile
Irritability	Wasted muscles
Vomiting	Abdominal distention
Anorexia or excessive appetite	Edema
Foul-smelling, bulky stools	Finger clubbing
Abdominal pain and/or distention	
Rectal prolapse	

Note: Nonintestinal manifestations of celiac disease include osteopenia/osteoporosis, short stature, delayed puberty, anemia, arthritis, hepatitis, dermatitis herpetiformis, dental enamel hypoplasia, brain calcifications, and neurologic symptoms.

Clinical Manifestations

- Intestinal manifestations of celiac disease are shown in Table 12.11.

Diagnosis

- Elevated levels of tissue transglutaminase are very specific for celiac disease but can be falsely negative in cases of IgA deficiency; antigliadin antibodies are NOT useful because of low sensitivity and low specificity.
- Definitive diagnosis requires small intestinal biopsy revealing villous atrophy.

Treatment

- Lifelong gluten-free diet results in complete resolution of symptoms.

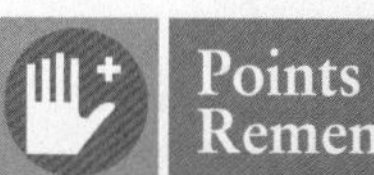

Points to Remember

- Autoimmune enteropathy is often misdiagnosed as celiac disease and consists of antienterocyte antibodies leading to similar symptoms. Classic case scenario is a patient who is diagnosed with celiac disease but fails to respond to gluten-free diet.

Malabsorptive Syndromes

Malabsorptive syndromes can be caused by loss of specific transporters, enzymes, or lack of intestinal surface area.

Clinical features of malabsorption include diarrhea, steatorrhea, abdominal distention, flatulence, and poor growth. Depending on the extent and location of disease, malabsorption can also lead to vitamin deficiencies.

Diagnosis depends on the specific suspected etiology, but almost all malabsorptive syndromes are associated with an elevated fecal fat content.

Selected malabsorptive syndromes are shown in Table 12.12.

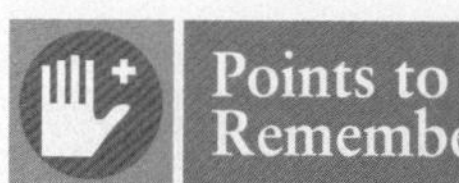

Points to Remember

- Most water is reabsorbed in the colon, vitamin B12 in distal ileum, and carbohydrates, protein, and water-soluble vitamins in proximal small intestine.

Lactose Intolerance

Lactose intolerance is one of the most common causes of malabsorption in children and young adults. Congenital lactase deficiency is almost unheard of, and acquired lactase deficiency is very rare in children younger than 4 to 6 years.

Clinical Manifestations

- Abdominal pain and/or distention following ingestion of lactose-containing foods.
- Diarrhea is usually not present initially but can develop over time.

Diagnosis

- Establishing a diagnosis of lactase deficiency is difficult because the laboratory tests (breath hydrogen production, lactose tolerance test) are too sensitive and false positives are very common.
- The best way to establish the diagnosis is by symptomatic improvement with initiation of a lactose-free diet and exacerbation of symptoms with reintroduction of lactose-containing foods.

Treatment

- Lactose-free diet (some patients can tolerate low–lactose-containing foods since lactose intolerance is dose related).

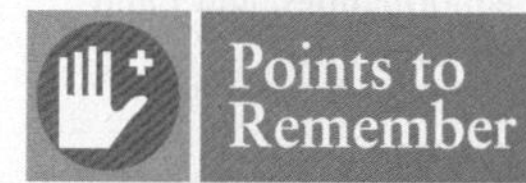

Points to Remember

- Despite many parents reporting a history of lactose intolerance in their infants, congenital lactase deficiency is extremely rare.

TABLE 12.12

SELECTED MALABSORPTIVE SYNDROMES

	Specific Etiologies	Comments
Food-induced enteropathies	■ Celiac disease ■ Milk protein intolerance ■ Eosinophilic enteropathy	Treatment is mainly removal of inciting agent
Infection-induced enteropathies	■ Parasitic infections (giardia, cryptosporidium, etc.) ■ Bacterial overgrowth ■ Tropical sprue ■ Postinfectious enteropathy	
Congenital enteropathies	■ Microvillus inclusion disease ■ Tufting enteropathy ■ Congenital enzyme deficiencies (e.g., Wolman disease, lactase deficiency, enterokinase deficiency, sucrose-isomaltase deficiency, etc.) ■ Congenital bile acid malabsorption	Theses are all extremely rare conditions Note that congenital lactase deficiency is extremely rare
Autoimmune enteropathy		Often confused with IBD and celiac disease until biopsies return or patient does not respond to treatment
Short-bowel syndrome	■ Most cases are due to bowel resection secondary to ischemic injury from NEC, malrotation, trauma, etc. ■ Congenital causes include multiple atresias, gastroschisis, etc.	Degree of malabsorption depends on the length and specific part of small intestine removed and whether or not the ileocecal valve is present
Miscellaneous	■ Malnutrition ■ Radiation enteritis ■ Exocrine pancreatic insufficiency (e.g., cystic fibrosis)	

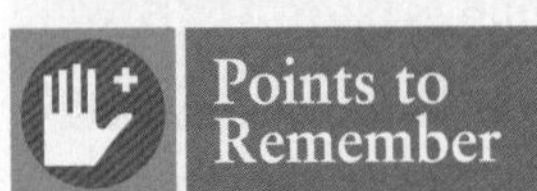
Points to Remember

■ VACTERL syndrome describes a spectrum of defects including Vertebral abnormalities, Anal atresia, Cardiac defects, Tracheoesophageal fistula, Radial dysplasia, Renal abnormalities, and Limb abnormalities.

ANUS AND RECTUM

Imperforate Anus

Imperforate anus is a rare congenital abnormality of the GI tract with an incidence of 1/5000 live births. Half of patients with imperforate anuses have other associated anomalies. Fistulas between the distal rectum and perineum or urogenital tract are common. Treatment is via diverting colostomy for high/intermediate lesions and serial anal dilation for low lesions.

Hemorrhoids

Hemorrhoids are rare in children but can occur and should be included in the differential diagnosis for any child presenting with rectal pain and/or hematochezia. Risk factors for hemorrhoids in children include constipation and portal HTN. Treatment for internal hemorrhoids (above dentate line) involves correction of the underlying etiology, sclerosis therapy, and/or band ligation. Treatment for external hemorrhoids involves reassurance and proper anal hygiene.

Pilonidal Disease

Pilonidal disease occurs due to chronic infection in a cyst underneath the skin near the buttock crease. Some pilonidal cysts are congenital and others form when a trapped hair stimulates a foreign body reaction. When the cyst becomes infected and forms an abscess, this leads to further exacerbation and extension of the previous cyst. Treatment can range from medical management with warm soaks and antibiotics to surgical incision and drainage and/or marsupialization.

Anal Fissure

Anal fissures in children are usually a consequence of constipation or inflammatory disorders such as IBD. Symptoms include painful defecation with streaks of bright red blood on stool surface. Diagnosis is clinical and treatment is aimed at underlying etiology.

Rectal Prolapse

Rectal prolapse is usually idiopathic but can be associated with infections, malnutrition, IBD, CF, and chronic constipation. It is usually painless until it becomes chronic and/or ulcerated. Treatment involves correcting the underlying condition, manual reduction, and (if refractory) linear cauterization.

Hirschsprung Disease

Hirschsprung disease results from abnormal migration of neural crest cells leading to an aganglionic section of bowel beginning at the anus and progressing proximally. This results in a functional distal bowel obstruction with enlargement of the normal bowel proximal to the affected bowel. It usually presents in the neonatal period with failure to pass meconium but should be considered in older patients with long-standing and/or refractory constipation. Diagnosis is via suction biopsy, and treatment usually involves surgical resection of the aganglionic segment followed by reanastomosis of the normal proximal bowel to the rectum.

APPENDIX

Appendicitis

Appendicitis is one of the most common causes of acute abdomen in children and should be high on the differential diagnosis of any child presenting with severe abdominal pain. The peak incidence in children is 10 to 12 years of age, but it can occur at any age.

Clinical Manifestations

Symptoms

- Abdominal pain (usually starts periumbilically then migrates to RLQ).
- Nausea, vomiting, and anorexia.
- Fever.

Signs

- RLQ tenderness (± rebound; usually at McBurney's point 2/3 of the way between the umbilicus and anterior superior iliac spine).
- Rovsing's, psoas, and obturator signs are helpful if present but have low sensitivity.
- Rovsing's sign: palpation of LLQ leads to pain in RLQ.
- Psoas sign: pain on extension of the right hip (seen with retrocecal appendicitis).
- Obturator sign: pain on internal rotation of the right hip (seen when the inflamed appendix lies in the pelvis).

Diagnosis

- Diagnosis is primarily clinical.
- Helpful lab studies include elevated WBC, ESR, and CRP.
- If the diagnosis is unclear, helpful imaging studies include abdominal CT with contrast and/or abdominal U/S.

Treatment

- Emergent appendectomy is the treatment for nonperforated appendicitis; most patients are also treated with a short course of an IV second-generation cephalosporin.
- If perforation has already occurred and the patient is hemodynamically stable, patients are typically treated with broad-spectrum IV antibiotics (ampicillin, metronidazole, and gentamicin/clindamycin) and percutaneous drainage of abscess if present. Interval appendectomy after the inflammation has lessened was previously strongly advocated but is currently under debate.

Points to Remember

- The perforation rate for appendicitis in infants is 50% compared with 10% in the general population because of delayed diagnosis.

Points to Remember

- In almost all cases of appendicitis, pain precedes the onset of nausea/vomiting/anorexia.
- The "hamburger sign" refers to the fact that patients with appendicitis usually do not want to eat and even their favorite food doesn't sound good to them—if they're hungry, it's probably NOT appendicitis!

Points to Remember

- Imaging studies in patients with suspected appendicitis are most helpful when the diagnosis is unclear, especially in female adolescent patients in whom it is often difficult to clinically differentiate RLQ pain from appendicitis versus ovarian pathology.
- If an inflamed appendix presses on the bladder, the bladder can become inflamed and urinalysis may demonstrate WBCs and RBCs—don't let a "positive" urinalysis fool you if everything else points to appendicitis!

Points to Remember

- If the diagnosis of appendicitis is delayed beyond 36 to 48 hours, the perforation rate exceeds 65%. Symptoms usually decrease after perforation as the body "walls off" the infectious process. If appendiceal perforation leads to peritonitis, however, the child has worsening abdominal pain and quickly becomes septic.

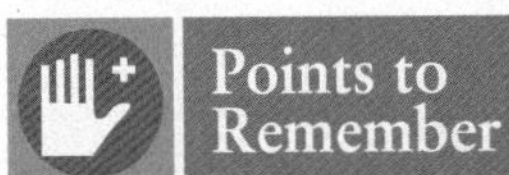

Points to Remember

- Exocrine pancreatic function tests:
  - Direct stimulation with secretin and cholecystokinin
  - Malabsorption: fecal elastase or 72-hour fecal fat
  - Serum trypsinogen

EXOCRINE PANCREAS

Anatomical Abnormalities

Pancreas Divisum

Pancreatic divisum is the most common congenital pancreatic anomaly and is due to lack of fusion of the ducts of the dorsal and ventral pancreatic buds. This leads to an abnormal drainage system through a small accessory duct of Santorini, which leads to relative outflow obstruction and predisposes to recurrent pancreatitis. Treatment is with duct stenting and/or sphincterectomy.

Annular Pancreas

Annular pancreas is due to incomplete rotation of the ventral pancreatic bud. It is associated with maternal polyhydramnios, Down syndrome, intestinal atresia, imperforate anus, and malrotation. Presentation is usually as bowel obstruction, pancreatitis, or biliary colic. Treatment is duodenojejunostomy.

Pancreatitis

Acute Pancreatitis

Acute pancreatitis is defined as an isolated episode of pancreatitis with complete resolution. Pancreatitis occurs when some type of insult causes activation of proenzymes within the pancreas leading to autodigestion and further activation and release of active proteases. Etiologies of acute pancreatitis in children are shown in Table 12.13.

Clinical Manifestations

- Continuous mid-epigastric pain radiating to the back.
- Anorexia and vomiting.
- Fever.
- Complications include hemorrhagic pancreatitis and pancreatic pseudocysts.

Diagnosis

- Any two of the following:
  - Lipase of more than 3× normal limit (amylase is less specific).
  - Clinical symptoms as above.
  - Radiographic evidence of pancreatic inflammation.
- Abdominal U/S and CT are useful in diagnosing complications of pancreatitis.

Treatment

- Most cases improve with expectant management in 2 to 4 days including NPO, IVFs, and IV analgesics.
- Follow clinical response and serial amylase/lipase measurements; reintroduce enteral diet slowly.

Chronic/Recurrent Pancreatitis

Children with chronic or recurrent pancreatitis warrant investigation for one of the underlying predisposing conditions shown in Table 12.13. Initial lab investigation may include serum lipid, calcium, phosphorus, and total and direct bilirubin. Depending on the suspected etiology, useful imaging studies may include abdominal U/S, CT, and/or MRCP/ERCP. Treatment of acute exacerbations of chronic pancreatitis is the same as for acute pancreatitis. More definitive treatment depends on the underlying etiology.

TABLE 12.13

ETIOLOGIES OF ACUTE PANCREATITIS IN CHILDREN

	Examples
Idiopathic	
Infections	Enteroviruses, EBV, hepatitis A/B, influenza, mycoplasma, mumps
Trauma	Blunt abdominal trauma, child abuse
Drugs and toxins	Acetaminophen, alcohol, corticosteroids, valproic acid, furosemide
Obstructive	Pancreatic divisum, annular pancreas, biliary tract malformations, gall stones
Systemic disease	Cystic fibrosis, diabetes mellitus, organic academia, SLE, hyperlipidemia
Hereditary	

DISORDERS OF PANCREATIC INSUFFICIENCY

Schwachman–Diamond Syndrome

Schwachman–Diamond syndrome is an autosomal recessive disorder characterized by pancreatic insufficiency, neutropenia, metaphyseal dysostosis, failure to thrive, and short stature. Patients suffer recurrent pyogenic infections and are at an increased risk of myelodysplastic syndrome and AML. Treatment of pancreatic insufficiency includes enzyme replacement therapy.

Cystic Fibrosis

Eighty-five percent to 90% of CF patients have pancreatic insufficiency by 1 year of age and require enzyme replacement therapy.

Pancreatic Tumors

Pancreatic tumors are very rare in children and include pancreatoblastomas, pancreatic adenocarcinomas, cystadenomas, rhabdomyosarcomas, and VIPomas. For the purpose of the boards, VIPoma is the most important to remember. VIPomas are non–α-cell pancreatic tumors that secrete VIP. They present with watery diarrhea and a hypokalemic metabolic acidosis. Diagnosis is via increased serum VIP. Treatment is via resection and/or octreotide.

Points to Remember

- **Meperidine is sometimes used to treat the pain associated with pancreatitis instead of morphine because of the concern for exacerbation of sphincter of Oddi dysfunction with morphine, but this is NOT well supported in the literature.**
- **Pancreatic pseudocysts are a rare potential complication of pancreatitis that should be considered with prolonged pancreatitis. Fifty percent of patients will have a palpable mass. U/S is the first option for diagnosis. Drainage is warranted if pseudocyst is more than 6 cm diameter.**

HEPATOBILIARY DISEASES

General Signs and Symptoms of Liver Disease

- Hepatomegaly.
- Ascites.
- Dermatologic: jaundice, pruritus, spider angiomas, palmar erythema, xanthomas.
- Easy bruising and/or bleeding.
- Anorexia and/or malaise.
- Encephalopathy.
- Esophageal varices.
- Pale stools.
- Pruritus.

Because many drugs are metabolized in the liver, patients with liver dysfunction have altered metabolism of certain medications and require special dosing.

Points to Remember

- **Dermatologic findings of liver dysfunction are not as prominent in children as they are in adults.**

Laboratory Markers of Liver Disease

- Hepatocellular injury
  - Elevated AST and ALT (ALT is more specific for liver injury than AST).
- Hepatic synthetic dysfunction
  - Prolonged PT/INR.
  - Hypoalbuminemia.
  - Hypoglycemia.
- Hepatic clearance dysfunction
  - Hyperammonemia.
- Cholestasis
  - Direct hyperbilirubinemia.
  - Elevated GGT.

Points to Remember

- **Patients with impaired hepatic synthetic function are coagulopathic because several of the clotting factors are dependent on vitamin K produced by the liver. Of the vitamin K–dependent factors, Factor VII has the shortest half-life and so is the most specific for liver injury.**

Diseases of Hepatocellular Injury

Viral Hepatitis

Viral hepatitis is one of the most commonly encountered liver diseases in children and is the most common cause of ALF in children. Please see Chapter 16 for a full discussion of viral hepatitis.

Autoimmune Hepatitis

Autoimmune hepatitis accounts for approximately 20% of cases of chronic hepatitis. It typically has an insidious onset but can also present with acute hepatic failure. The type I form is most common in young women ages 15 to 25 years and is associated with other immunologic disorders including thyroiditis, IBD, arthritis, rash, and hemolytic anemia. Type II usually occurs in young children.

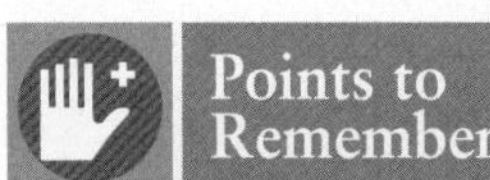

- Autoimmune hepatitis can present similarly to acute viral hepatitis and should be included in the differential diagnosis of any patient presenting with acute hepatitis.

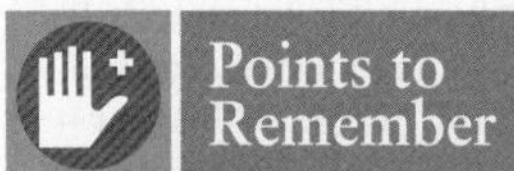

- 20% to 30% of patients with autoimmune hepatitis don't have autoantibodies on presentation.

Clinical Manifestations
- Nausea and vomiting.
- Jaundice.
- Weakness and malaise.
- Behavioral changes.

Diagnosis
- Elevated transaminases (usually 500 to 1,000 IU).
- Hypergammaglobulinemia.
- 70% of patients have positive ANA and anti–smooth-muscle antibodies; anti–liver-kidney antibodies are elevated in a subset of patients.
- Liver biopsy demonstrates inflammation of hepatic lobules and portal areas.

Treatment
- First-line treatment is corticosteroids ± azathioprine.
- Options for patients with refractory disease include cyclosporine A, tacrolimus, and/or mycophenolate mofetil.
- Patients who progress to ESLD require liver transplantation.

Prognosis
- More than 75% rate of remission in 1 to 3 months but many will relapse.
- Can recur in transplanted liver.

Wilson Disease

Wilson disease is an autosomal recessive degenerative disorder of copper metabolism. It typically presents between adolescence and age 40 years with hepatic, neurologic, and/or psychiatric manifestations. Hepatic manifestations are more common in females and in patients who present during childhood and adolescence. Neuropsychiatric manifestations are more common in patients who present as adults.

Clinical Manifestations
- Hepatic
  - Asymptomatic hepatomegaly.
  - Subacute or chronic hepatitis.
  - Fulminant hepatic failure.
- Neuropsychiatric
  - Behavioral changes.
  - Deterioration in school or job performance.
  - Abnormal speech (e.g., slurred speech, severe dysarthria).
  - Tremors and/or dystonia.
- Miscellaneous
  - Kayser–Fleischer rings.
  - Hemolytic anemia.
  - Fanconi syndrome.

Diagnosis
- Low serum ceruloplasmin.
- Elevated serum and/or urine copper.
- Serum alkaline phosphatase and aminotransferase levels are usually elevated but can be disproportionately low with fulminant disease.
- Liver biopsy for histologic changes and copper content is diagnostic.

Treatment
- Chelation therapy with penicillamine or triethylene tetramine dihydrochloride.
- Restrict daily copper intake.
- Zinc to impair copper absorption.
- Liver transplant if severe.

Prognosis
- Without treatment, Wilson disease is uniformly fatal.
- Patients who present with fulminant ALF have a poor prognosis.
- With early detection and proper treatment, most patients do well but response to therapy is variable.

Reye Syndrome

Reye syndrome is an acute encephalopathy and fatty degeneration of the viscera including the liver. The exact etiology of Reye syndrome is unknown, but it is believed to be associated with aspirin use in children with viral infections including influenza and varicella.

Clinical Manifestations

- Usually presents within 1 week after recovery of a viral illness.
- Initial phase consists of vomiting, irritability, and/or lethargy.
- Some patients go on to develop delirium, stupor, seizure, coma, and/or death from brainstem herniation.
- Mild hepatomegaly may be present.

Diagnosis

- Abnormal labs may include elevated LFTs, elevated NH3, prolonged PT, and/or hypoglycemia.
- Liver biopsy demonstrates elevated triglyceride content, diffuse fatty infiltration of hepatocytes with minimal inflammatory changes, and abnormal mitochondria.

Differential Diagnosis

- Includes CNS infections, salicylate and other drug toxicity, urea cycle disorders, disorders of fatty acid oxidation, and organic acidemias.

Treatment

- Supportive.

Nonalcoholic Steatohepatitis

Steatohepatitis (fatty infiltration of the liver) in children is most commonly associated with obesity and type II diabetes. It is usually asymptomatic and picked up on laboratory work obtained for another reason or on screening labs for obese patients. AST:ALT ratio is usually less than 1. Hepatomegaly may or may not be present. Diagnosis is via liver U/S or biopsy. Treatment is via weight loss through diet and exercise.

Tyrosinemia

Hereditary tyrosinemia is an autosomal recessive condition that results from deficient activity of fumarylacetoacetate hydrolase and causes progressive multisystem disease affecting the liver, kidneys, and peripheral nervous system.

Clinical Manifestations

- Symptoms begin in infancy and include jaundice, failure to thrive, and/or hepatosplenomegaly.
- Some patients develop liver failure by 1 year of age while others have acute hepatic crises precipitated by intercurrent illness.
- Increased risk of hepatocellular carcinoma.

Diagnosis

- Elevated serum tyrosine ± methionine.
- Elevated serum AFP.
- Tyrosine metabolic products excreted in urine (elevated urine succinylacetone).

Treatment

- Dietary modifications (limit phenylalanine, tyrosine, methionine).
- Medical management with tyrosine degradation inhibitor.
- Liver transplantation for hepatocellular carcinoma and/or acute or chronic liver failure.

α_1-Antitrypsin Deficiency

Homozygous deficiency of α_1-antitrypsin deficiency is associated with neonatal cholestasis and with childhood and adulthood cirrhosis. Diagnosis is via genetic testing. Most patients ultimately require liver transplantation, which is curative.

Drug-Induced Liver Disease

Drug-induced liver disease is less common in children than in adults and often presents with nonspecific symptoms. It can occur as a known side effect of a medication or due to accidental or nonaccidental overdose. Acetaminophen is the most common offending agent. Treatment is primarily supportive including withdrawal of the offending agent. *N*-acetylcysteine is a specific antidote available for acetaminophen toxicity. Selected hepatotoxic drugs and their patterns of injury are shown in Table 12.14.

TABLE 12.14

PATTERNS OF HEPATIC DRUG INJURY

Drug	Disease
Acetaminophen	Centrilobular necrosis
Valproic acid	Microvesicular steatosis
Isoniazid	Acute hepatitis
Sulfonamides, phenytoin	General hypersensitivity
Methotrexate	Fibrosis
Chlorpromazine, erythromycin, estrogens	Cholestasis
Ceftriaxone	Biliary sludge
Oral contraceptives, anabolic steroids	Hepatic adenoma or hepatocellular carcinoma

Miscellaneous Liver Diseases

Portal Hypertension

Portal HTN is defined as an elevation of portal pressure more than 10 to 12 mm Hg. It can be due to extrahepatic obstruction (e.g., portal vein thrombosis) or intrahepatic obstruction (e.g., hepatocellular disease, cirrhosis, Budd–Chiari syndrome, veno-occlusive disease, Alagille syndrome). It can also be idiopathic.

Clinical Manifestations

- Abdominal pain and distention.
- Splenomegaly.
- Esophageal varices.
- Ascites.

Diagnosis

- Portal vein cavernous transformation via U/S.

Treatment

- Treatment of underlying disease.
- Medications to decrease portal pressure (β-blockers, vasopressin).
- Surgical portosystemic shunt and/or liver transplantation.
- Treat complications (e.g., esophageal varices).

Ascites and Spontaneous Bacterial Peritonitis

Ascites is fluid accumulation in the peritoneal cavity. Causes of ascites in children include liver failure, heart failure, protein losses, malnutrition, infectious, chylous, dysfunctional ventriculoperitoneal shunts, hypothyroidism, and malignancy. The most worrisome life-threatening complication of ascites is SBP. The most common organism associated with SBP is *Escherichia coli,* followed by *Klebsiella* then streptococcal species. Broad-spectrum empiric antibiotic coverage with IV cefotaxime should be initiated while awaiting identification of organism.

Fulminant Hepatic Failure

Fulminant hepatic failure is a clinical syndrome characterized by acute, severe impairment of liver synthetic, excretory, and detoxifying functions. In children, criteria for diagnosis include:

- Biochemical evidence of acute liver injury AND.
- No evidence of chronic liver disease AND.
- Hepatic-based coagulopathy defined as
  - PT more than 15 seconds or INR more than 1.5 not corrected by vitamin K in the presence of clinical hepatic encephalopathy OR.
  - APT more than 20 seconds or INR more than 2 regardless of the presence of clinical hepatic encephalopathy.

Forty percent to 50% of cases of fulminant hepatic failure are idiopathic. Known etiologies include ingestions, infections, and other causes of hepatocellular injury.

Treatment

- Supportive measures include
  - **Neurologic:** Avoid sedatives, limit protein intake, lactulose, invasive ICP monitoring, ensure cerebral perfusion if cerebral edema.
  - **Respiratory:** Intubation to prevent aspiration possibly reduce cerebral edema via hyperventilation.
  - **Gastrointestinal:** Antacids, glucose control.
  - **Renal:** Avoid hypovolemia (risk hepatorenal syndrome).
  - **Hematology:** Vitamin K, FFP, plasmapheresis, platelets.
- Liver transplantation.

Prognosis

- Varies with inciting disease but overall mortality is ~70% without transplant.

Systemic Diseases Associated with Liver Disease

Several systemic diseases can be associated with hepatocellular and/or cholestatic liver disease (see Table 12.15).

Biliary Disease

Malformation of the Biliary Tract

Biliary Atresia

Biliary atresia is atresia or hypoplasia of any portion of the extrahepatic biliary system. The etiology is unknown but it is believed to be an acquired disorder rather than a consequence of abnormal fetal development.

Clinical Manifestations

- Jaundice in an otherwise seemingly healthy infant in the first few months of life.

Diagnosis

- Laboratory data reveals elevated total and direct bilirubin, elevated transaminases, and an elevated GGT.
- A hepatobiliary scan demonstrates lack of excretion of tracer from liver into the intestinal tract.
- Definitive diagnosis is via liver biopsy demonstrating bile duct proliferation and a widened portal area.

Treatment

- Initial treatment is via a Kasai procedure (portoenterostomy).
- 80% of patients eventually require liver transplantation.

Points to Remember

- Biliary atresia is the most common cause of cholestasis in nonpremature infants 0 to 3 months of age and is the single most common pediatric etiology requiring liver transplantation.

Points to Remember

- Conditions associated with hydrops of the gallbladder include hemoglobinopathies, Kawasaki disease, prolonged fasting, and systemic infections.
- Murphy's sign: pain with inspiration when pressure is placed on RUQ
- Charcot's triad: fever, jaundice, and right upper quadrant pain
- Reynold's pentad: fever, jaundice, right upper quadrant pain, hypotension, and altered mental state
- Gallstones are much rarer in children than in adults and are usually associated with an identifiable risk factor such as hemolytic disease, hypercholesterolemia, obesity, CF, and biliary tract malformations.
- 42% of patients with sickle cell disease will have gallstones by the age of 18.
- Patients with distal obstructions from gallstones can have concomitant pancreatitis.

TABLE 12.15

SYSTEMIC DISEASES ASSOCIATED WITH LIVER DISEASE

	Liver Manifestations
Inflammatory bowel disease	Primary sclerosing cholangitis, portal hypertension, cirrhosis, biliary carcinoma
Obesity	Nonalcoholic fatty liver disease
Bone marrow transplant	GVHD, veno-occlusive disease
Sickle cell disease	Gall stones, hemosiderosis (chronic transfusions)
Cystic fibrosis	Cholestasis, hepatic steatosis, focal biliary cirrhosis
Collagen vascular disease	Hepatocellular injury

GVHD, graft-versus-host disease.

Alagille Syndrome

Alagille syndrome is an autosomal dominant disorder characterized by intrahepatic bile duct paucity and facial (triangular shaped), ocular (posterior embryotoxon), cardiac (pulmonary valve stenosis, peripheral pulmonic stenosis, and other defects), vertebral arch (butterfly vertebrae), and/or renal abnormalities. 15-50% of cases are due to a spontaneous mutation. The severity of liver disease is variable—some patients have very mild liver disease while others develop liver failure and require transplantation in the first year of life. Treatment is primarily supportive.

Choledochal Cyst

Choledochal cysts are congenital cystic dilations of parts of the biliary tract. They usually present in the first 6 years of life and are four times more common in females than in males. There are five major types of choledochal cysts. Type I is the most common and is the dilation of the common bile duct. Type V is an autosomal recessive condition also known as Caroli disease and consists of intrahepatic bile duct cysts.

Points to Remember

- In addition to being at increased risk for colorectal cancer, patients with Peutz–Jegher syndrome are also at increased risk for breast and gynecologic malignancies and patients with familial adenomatous polyposis are at increased risk for hepatoblastoma, thyroid cancer, and cholangiocarcinoma.

Clinical Manifestations

- Jaundice, abdominal pain, vomiting, acholic stools, hepatomegaly, and/or RUQ mass.
- Increased risk of cholangiocarcinoma.

Diagnosis

- U/S, hepatobiliary scan, ERCP, and/or MRCP.

Treatment

- Excision of cyst and a choledochojejunostomy and cholecystectomy.

Acquired Biliary Disease

Acquired biliary diseases and their characteristics are shown in Table 12.16.

TABLE 12.16

ACQUIRED BILIARY DISEASE

	Definition	Signs and Symptoms	Diagnosis	Treatment
Hydrops of the gall bladder	Gall bladder distension that is NOT due to calculi or inflammation	RUQ pain with palpable mass	Ultrasound	Supportive care
Cholelithiasis	Stone in the gall bladder	Nonobstructing gallstones are often asymptomatic	Ultrasound	Anticipatory guidance
Biliary colic	Gallstone impaction in cystic or common bile duct (choledocholithiasis)	Recurrent colicky RUQ pain worsened by fatty foods	Ultrasound, ERCP, or MRCP	Removal of stone and cholecystectomy
Cholecystitis	Gall bladder inflammation due to obstruction, trauma, infection, or autoimmune disease	RUQ/epigastric pain, nausea, vomiting, fever, jaundice, Murphy's sign	Ultrasound, CT, or HIDA scan	NPO, antibiotics, pain control, and cholecystectomy
Ascending cholangitis	Bacterial infection of obstructed common bile duct usually due to stricture or stones	Charcot's triad, Reynold's pentad	Ultrasound, ERCP, or PTC	NPO, antibiotics, stone removal or dilation via ERCP vs. PTC
Primary sclerosing cholangitis	Inflammation and subsequent fibrosis of hepatobiliary system; (occurs in <10% of IBD pts; mainly ulcerative colitis) (rare in childhood)	Abdominal pain, fever, jaundice, pruritus, hepatomegaly ± splenomegaly	Labs: direct hyperbilirubinemia, transaminitis, ↑ serum Ig, + ANA, antismooth muscle Ab Imaging: "beaded appearance" of biliary tree on ERCP	None—liver transplant not curable Poor prognosis due to increased risk of cholangiocarcinoma *(50% 10–12 y survival)*

ERCP, endoscopic retrograde cholangiopancreatography; HIDA, hepatobiliary iminodiacetic acid; MRCP, magnetic resonance cholangiopancreatography; PTC, percutaneous transhepatic cholangiography; RUQ, right upper quadrant of the abdomen.

TUMORS AND MALIGNANCIES OF THE GI TRACT

Polyposis Syndromes Associated with Colorectal Cancer

Familial polyposis syndromes and their characteristics are shown in Table 12.17. All patients with familial polyposis syndromes need regular surveillance with colonoscopies due to the increased oncogenic risk. Consideration should also be given for prophylactic proctocolectomy.

TABLE 12.17

FEATURES OF INHERITED POLYPOSIS SYNDROMES ASSOCIATED WITH COLORECTAL CANCER

	Pattern of Inheritance	Polyp Histology and Distribution	Average Age of Onset	Clinical Manifestations	Risk of Colorectal Cancer (%)
Familial adenomatous polyposis	Autosomal dominant	Adenomas in large intestines	2nd decade	Rectal bleeding, abdominal pain, bowel obstruction	100
Gardner syndrome	Autosomal dominant	Adenomas in small and large intestines	2nd decade	Rectal bleeding, abdominal pain, bowel obstruction	100
Peutz–Jeghers syndrome	Autosomal dominant	Hamartomas in small and large intestines	1st decade	Rectal bleeding, abdominal pain, intussusception, mucosal pigmentation of lips	40
Juvenile polyposis	Autosomal dominant	Hamartomas and rarely adenomas in small and large intestines	1st decade	Rectal bleeding, abdominal pain, intussusception	10–50

Lymphomas

Lymphomas are the most common gastrointestinal tract malignancy in children. Predisposing conditions include AIDS, ataxia-telangiectasia, Wiskott–Aldrich syndrome, agammaglobulinemia, severe combined immunodeficiency syndrome, bone marrow or solid organ transplantation, and long-standing celiac disease. Any part of the GI tract can be involved. Intestinal lymphomas often present with abdominal pain, abdominal mass, change in bowel habits, and/or systemic symptoms. Intestinal lymphomas can also present acutely with intussusception.

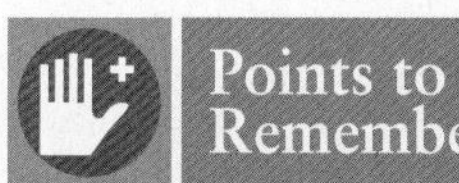

- **Consider intestinal lymphoma in a child older than 2 years presenting with intussusception.**

Carcinoid Tumors

Carcinoid tumors are low-grade malignancies of intestinal enterochromaffin cells. The most common location is the appendix. They are often found incidentally during an appendectomy. Carcinoid tumors outside of the appendix usually metastasize to the liver and produce carcinoid syndrome, which consists of diarrhea, vasomotor disturbances, bronchoconstriction, and/or right heart failure. Diagnosis is via elevated urine serotonin metabolite—5-hydroxyindoleacetic acid (5-HIAA). Treatment consists of palliation with somatostatin analogs followed by surgical resection.

GASTROINTESTINAL MANIFESTATIONS OF CYSTIC FIBROSIS

CF has several important gastrointestinal manifestations, most of which are due to inspissated secretions. These are listed in Table 12.18.

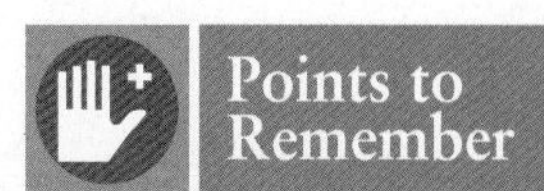

- **Meconium ileus in a neonate is almost always associated with CF.**

TABLE 12.18

GASTROINTESTINAL COMPLICATIONS OF CYSTIC FIBROSIS

Intestines	
■ Meconium Ileus	■ Occurs in 20% of newborns with CF ■ Presents as delay in passage of meconium and bowel obstruction ■ Diagnosis via AXR, contrast enema
■ DIOS	■ Distal intestinal obstruction syndrome
■ GERD	■ Manifests as regurgitation and FTT in infants and dysphagia, epigastric pain, and blood loss in older patients
Pancreas	
■ Pancreatic exocrine deficiency	■ Loss of enzyme activity leads to intestinal malabsorption of fats, proteins, and to a lesser extent, carbohydrates ■ Complete loss of enzyme activity is seen in 85%–90% of patients ■ Presents as poor weight gain, abdominal distention, and fatty stools ■ Treatment is via enzyme replacement
■ Diabetes	■ 40% of CF patients have some degree of carbohydrate intolerance ■ 15%–20% of CF patients >18 y old have insulin-dependent diabetes
Nutrition and Metabolism	
■ Vitamin and mineral deficiencies	■ Malabsorption of fat-soluble vitamins A, D, E, K due to pancreatic insufficiency ■ Coagulopathy due to hypoprothrombinemia and vitamin K deficiency
■ Edema and hypoproteinemia	■ Secondary to pancreatic deficiency ■ Associated findings include hepatomegaly, transaminitis, rash, and anemia
■ Salt loss	■ "Salty taste" of skin ■ May develop dehydration with massive salt depletion with GI illnesses
Hepatobiliary	
■ Focal biliary cirrhosis	■ Pathognomonic for CF ■ Present in 25% of patients; may present as early as age 3 d ■ Wide spectrum of severity—asymptomatic to hepatic failure
■ Primary sclerosing cholangitis	■ Present in one-third of adult patients
■ Portal hypertension	■ Present in 1%–2% of adults ■ Manifests as esophageal varices and hypersplenism
Gallbladder	
■ Gall stones	■ Present in one-third of adult patients

SAMPLE BOARD REVIEW QUESTIONS

1. A 3-month-old male infant presents with a 2-day history of multiple episodes of nonprojectile emesis which was nonbilious initially but has now become slightly bilious. His stools have also been more watery than normal, but he is otherwise well. He has been afebrile and is still playful. He is drinking well and has normal urine output. On physical examination, he is well-appearing, has a normal abdominal exam, and appears well hydrated. What diagnostic study is indicated at this time?
   - a. Abdominal U/S
   - b. Upper GI series
   - c. AXR
   - d. No further workup

   Answer: d. Bilious emesis should always raise the concern for intestinal obstruction and demands a complete history and physical examination. Even in the absence of obstruction, however, repeated vomiting can lead to reflux of duodenal contents into the stomach and emesis that progressively becomes bilious in nature. This patient likely has viral gastroenteritis. This diagnosis is supported by the presence of vomiting and watery stools in an otherwise well-appearing infant with a benign abdomen who is still tolerating PO.

No further diagnostic studies are indicated at this time. His parents should be educated on the natural history of viral gastroenteritis, the importance of ensuring adequate hydration, and signs and symptoms of dehydration.

An abdominal U/S would be indicated if there was concern for pyloric stenosis. The peak age of onset of pyloric stenosis is ~3 weeks of age, but it can present as early as 1 week or as late as 5 months. The key part of the history in infants with pyloric stenosis is progressive nonbilious postprandial projectile vomiting. An upper GI series would be indicated if there was concern for malrotation. Bilious emesis in a neonate should be assumed to be malrotation with volvulus until proven otherwise. Patients with malrotation, however, will have tender, distended abdomens and are usually more ill-appearing. The emesis is bilious from the onset. An AXR can be useful for many types of intestinal obstruction but is not useful for patients with viral gastroenteritis.

2. You are the primary care pediatrician caring for a 10-year-old boy who presents to you for his annual physical exam. His mother is concerned because the patient's 10-year-old twin brother was recently diagnosed with *H. pylori* gastritis as part of a workup for chronic abdominal pain. Your patient does not complain of any gastrointestinal complaints and has a normal physical exam. Which of the following is the best plan of care for your patient in regard to his likely exposure to *H. pylori* infection?
   a. No evaluation or intervention at this time
   b. Diagnostic evaluation via stool *H. pylori* antigen testing and urease breath test
   c. 7-day prophylactic course with pantoprazole, clarithromycin, and amoxicillin
   d. 14-day empiric treatment course with pantoprazole, clarithromycin, and amoxicillin

   Answer: a. *H.* pylori is a relatively common infection that is often acquired in childhood and can persist into adulthood. Infection can be asymptomatic or symptomatic. Symptoms are very nonspecific. Some patients experience a brief illness with epigastric pain, nausea, and/or vomiting with spontaneous resolution while others experience more chronic symptoms with chronic abdominal pain and other symptoms of gastritis. Treatment is only for symptomatic patients and includes a 7- to 14-day course of pantoprazole, clarithromycin, and amoxicillin or a 7- to 14-day course of bismuth subsalicylate + metronidazole + tetracycline + proton pump inhibitor/H_2-blocker. Your patient is currently asymptomatic and, although he is at risk for infection, currently requires no further evaluation or treatment.

3. A 12 yo boy with multiple fractures from a motor vehicle collision has had a complicated postoperative course after undergoing a spinal fusion 40 days ago and remains hospitalized. You are consulted by the surgeons because the patient has developed nausea, abdominal pain, nonbilious emesis, and inability to tolerate oral or NG feeds. He has been treated with antiemetics without any improvement. His stools have been normal. His exam is limited because he is immobilized in a body cast, but he appears neurologically intact and his only complaints are abdominal pain and nausea. A head CT and AXR obtained by the surgeons a couple of days ago when his symptoms developed were both normal. You suggest a trial of NJ feedings, which the patient tolerates well. What is the most likely diagnosis?
   a. Elevated ICP secondary to complications from the spinal fusion
   b. SMA syndrome
   c. Impaired intestinal motility secondary to narcotics
   d. Viral gastroenteritis

   Answer: b. This patient has been hospitalized for a long period of time and has likely lost a great deal of weight due to increased metabolic rate and inadequate nutrition. This puts him at risk for SMA syndrome which can account for his current symptoms of abdominal pain, nausea, emesis, and inability to tolerate oral or NG feeds. SMA syndrome occurs when the SMA loses its posterior fat pad and supine positioning causes it to collapse onto and compress the duodenum. It is usually diagnosed empirically with resolution of symptoms when feeds are given in a way which bypasses the duodenum. An upper GI is indicated when the diagnosis is unclear and will demonstrate abrupt duodenal cutoff to the right of the midline. Treatment consists of improved nutrition (NJ feeds and/or TPN), prone or lateral positioning, and prokinetics. Surgery is indicated in refractory cases.

4. An 18-month-old female child is diagnosed with Meckel's diverticulum after extensive workup for lower gastrointestinal bleeding. Her parents are reluctant to have the lesion

surgically excised. In explaining the risks of not removing the lesion, you explain to them that which of the following are potential complications of an unresected Meckel's diverticulum?

a. Diverticulitis
b. Intussusception
c. Volvulus
d. All of the above

Answer: d. Meckel's diverticulum is a remnant of the omphalomesenteric duct and is a cause of painless rectal bleeding in infants and toddlers. Acid secretion via gastric mucosa in the Meckel's diverticulum leads to ulceration of adjacent normal ileal mucosa. The bleeding can be mild and intermittent or severe and life-threatening. The "Rule of 2's" is helpful to remember important characteristics of Meckel's diverticula: they occur in 2% of the population, are most commonly detected in patients younger than 2 years, are on average 2 inches in size, and are usually located 2 feet from the ileocecal valve. Diverticulitis, intussusception (the diverticulum acts as a lead point), and volvulus are common sequelae of untreated diverticula.

5. A 14-year-old female is referred to your GI clinic by her pediatrician because of poor weight gain, chronic abdominal pain, nonbloody diarrhea, and the rash shown in Figure 12.5. Labs sent by her pediatrician are notable for a mild normocytic anemia, normal electrolytes, slightly elevated ESR of 31, anti-tissue transglutaminase antibody negative, normal IgG and IgM, undetectable IgA, negative pANCA (perinuclear staining antineutrophil cytoplasmic antibody), and negative stool studies looking for infectious pathogens. An AXR was done previously and was normal. What is the next most appropriate step in the management of this patient?

a. Upper endoscopy with small bowel follow-through and biopsies
b. Hydrogen breath test
c. Empiric lactose elimination from diet with follow-up in 2 weeks
d. 1-week course of empiric metronidazole

Answer: a. The patient's symptoms and particularly her rash (dermatitis herpetiformis) are consistent with celiac disease. Celiac disease can present at any age but often presents during adolescence with nonspecific symptoms such as fatigue, abdominal pain, diarrhea, and bloating. Diagnosis is usually made via the presence of anti-tissue transglutaminase antibody. Because this is an IgA antibody, however, it will not be detectable in patients with IgA deficiency as is the case with this patient. Thus, diagnosis of celiac disease in patients with IgA deficiency requires small intestinal biopsy. Biopsy findings consistent with celiac disease include villous atrophy, crypt elongation, decreased villous/crypt ratio, and increased intraepithelial lymphocytes.

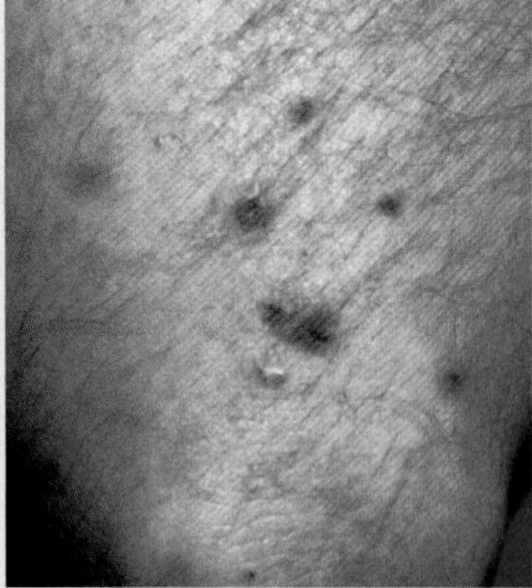

FIGURE 12.5. Pruritic, symmetric, grouped vesicles on an erythematous base are seen on the elbows and knees. (Courtesy W. Witmer. Reprinted with permission from Elder AD, Elenitsas R, Johnson BL, et al. *Synopsis and Atlas of Lever's Histopathology of the Skin*. Philadelphia, PA: Lippincott Williams & Wilkins, 1999.)

6. A previously healthy 1-year-old male infant presents to your office with a several day history of painful defecation and low grade fever. Physical examination is remarkable for a small perianal fistula draining scant purulent material. The patient's parents are concerned that the patient has an underlying condition contributing to this problem.

Family history is unremarkable. What do you tell them and what is your plan of action?

a. The child likely has IBD. He will need upper endoscopy and colonoscopy. The fistula itself necessitates a 10-day course of clindamycin in addition to wide excision/drainage
b. The child likely has an immunodeficiency. In addition to CBC with smear, he will need HIV testing and immunologic workup. The fistula itself necessitates a 10-day course of clindamycin in addition to wide excision/drainage
c. This is a relatively common condition in infants and children less than 2 year old and usually self resolves without treatment by the age of 2
d. This is a relatively common condition in infants and children less than 2 year old. The fistula itself necessitates a 10-day course of clindamycin in addition to wide excision/drainage

Answer: c. Perianal fistulas are relatively common in otherwise healthy infants and children younger than 2 years. Symptoms typically include low-grade fevers and mild rectal pain. An abscess can develop in the area and then drain through the fistula. Because the fistula allows the abscess to drain and heal on its own, antibiotics and/or surgical drainage are not usually necessary. The process can take place over several weeks. If the patient experiences severe and/or persistent symptoms, a fistulotomy may be indicated although there is still remains a 20% risk of recurrence.

Patients older than 2 years with perianal fistulas and/or abscesses often have a predisposing condition such as an immunodeficiency (e.g., AIDS, leukemia, diabetes mellitus), Crohn's disease, or prior rectal surgery. Symptoms are more severe and they require antibiotics as well as surgical manipulation.

7. A 3-year-old female with a long history of chronic constipation presents with rectal pain and the following findings on physical exam (Fig. 12.6). Which of the following is the most appropriate way to manage this patient?

a. Aggressive medical treatment of constipation and surgical removal of the mass
b. Aggressive medical treatment of constipation and 10-day course of clindamycin and metronidazole.
c. Attempt manual reduction and schedule follow-up colonscopy within 2 weeks
d. Aggressive medical treatment of constipation and attempt at manual reduction of the mass

Answer: d. Rectal prolapse (Fig. 12.6) is often idiopathic but can be due to multiple predisposing factors including chronic constipation, parasitic infections, malnutrition, diarrhea, IBD, pertussis, Ehlers–Danlos syndrome, neural tube defects, CF, and chronic constipation. It is most common in children between 1 and 5 years of age but can occur at any age. If severe, the chronic exteriorization leads to congestion and edema, ulceration, and rectal pain (as described for this patient). In this case, the patient's chronic constipation is the most likely underlying etiology and must be treated aggressively. Manual reduction of the rectal prolapse should be attempted (toilet paper wrapped around the provider's finger allows gentle pressure to be applied to the prolapsed segment of bowel; toilet paper adheres to mucosa, allowing release of finger; paper is later expelled when softened). If manual reduction is unsuccessful, linear cauterization may be necessary.

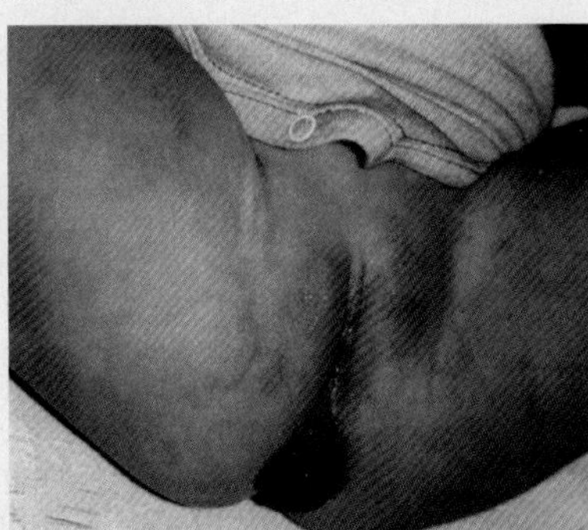

FIGURE 12.6.

8. A 17-year-old adopted male with an unknown family history is diagnosed with familial adenomatous polyposis syndrome via colonscopy as part of an evaluation for rectal bleeding, abdominal pain, and constipation. You explain to your patient and his adoptive family that this diagnosis places him at significant risk of malignancy. Which of the following options is most consistent with the current recommendations regarding surveillance and/or prophylactic colectomy for your patient?
   - a. No surveillance needed. Prophylactic colectomy within the next 3 to 6 months
   - b. Surveillance colonoscopy every 6 to 12 months. Prophylactic colectomy by age 20
   - c. Surveillance colonoscopy every 6 to 12 months. Timing of prophylactic colectomy is controversial
   - d. Surveillance colonoscopy every 5 years. Prophylactic colectomy by the age of 40.

Answer: c. Familial adenomatous polyposis syndrome is an autosomal dominant condition due to mutation of the APC tumor suppressor gene on chromosome 5. Average age of onset is 16 years (range 8 to 34 years). Polyps may be asymptomatic or cause symptoms such as hematochezia, cramps, and/or obstructive symptoms. It is important to note that the symptoms do not correlate with degree of dysplasia. Diagnosis is made via family history (absent in this patient's case), testing for APC gene mutation, and more than 5 colonic polyps. There is a significant risk of malignant degeneration of polyps, especially those located in the colon, and surveillance colonoscopies are critical to early detection and treatment of premalignant and malignant lesions. Current recommendations are for surveillance colonoscopies every 6 to 12 months. The timing of prophylactic colectomy is controversial.

9. A 2-year-old female presents to her pediatrician for a well-child check and is noted to have hepatomegaly. U/S raises suspicion for a choledochal cyst and the diagnosis is confirmed via MRCP. Which of the following is a potential complication of the patient's condition?
   - a. Cholangiocarcinoma
   - b. Malrotation
   - c. Cirrhosis
   - d. All of the above

Answer: d. Choledochal cysts are congenital dilatations of the biliary tract. They are diagnosed via U/S, MRCP, or ERCP. Treatment is surgical excision ± hepatic lobectomy depending on their size. Excision is necessary since choledochal cysts can potentially be cancerous, lead to malrotation, and/or result in cholestasis leading to cirrhosis.

10. A 14-year-old obese female is diagnosed with pancreatitis. She is admitted to the hospital, made NPO, maintained on IVFs, and treated with IV analgesics. On hospital day 3, she has is afebrile without abdominal pain and has not vomited in the past 24 hours. Her amylase is decreasing but her lipase continues to remain elevated and has not decreased since admission. She is hungry and asking for something to eat. What is the most appropriate response to her request?
    - a. Start her on a regular diet and monitor her labs and clinical status closely
    - b. Start her on a clear liquid diet then advance her diet as tolerated
    - c. Continue her NPO status until her amylase and lipase have normalized
    - d. Continue her NPO status until after cholecystectomy since she is obese and likely has gallstone pancreatitis

Answer: b. Start her on a clear liquid diet then advance her diet as tolerated. Acute pancreatitis typically presents with abdominal pain (continuous, midepigastric and periumbilical, radiates to back) and vomiting with or without fever. Acute pancreatitis is diagnosed with elevated serum lipase (elevated serum amylase is less specific). Initial treatment consists of NPO, electrolyte correction, MIVF, and IV analgesics. NG decompression may be helpful in cases with severe vomiting. The use of prophylactic antibiotics is controversial and they are used only in severe cases to prevent or treat associated infected pancreatic pseudocysts. Biliary stones and/or sludging is one of the most common causes of acute pancreatitis, and this patient is at risk of gallstones because of her obesity. This patient will need to be worked up for gallstones, but even if present, does not need an urgent cholecystectomy. If she is found to have gallstones, cholecystectomy can be scheduled electively as she is at small risk for recurrence of gallstone pancreatitis. Patients can begin refeeding once their clinical symptoms are improved and their amylase is decreasing. Lipase remains elevated for 8 to 14 days so should not be used as a marker of a patient's readiness to begin enteral feeds. When refeeding is initiated in

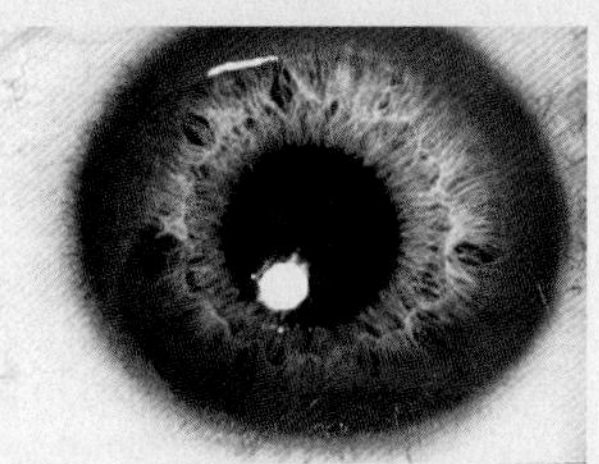

FIGURE 12.7.

patients with resolving pancreatitis, a clear liquid diet with advancement as tolerated is most appropriate.

11. A 14-year-old female with a history of recently diagnosed seizures presents to you for routine follow-up. She reports that her seizures are well controlled on valproic acid. On physical examination, you note the following findings (Fig. 12.7). Her vision is 20/20 in both eyes and her neurologic exam is within normal limits. Her abdominal exam is remarkable for a liver edge 2 cm below the costal margin. As part of her workup and monitoring, you order a CMP with LFTs and a valproic acid level. What additional testing is indicated at this time?
    a. Serum ceruloplasmin and serum and urine copper
    b. Antiactin, antinuclear, and antimitochondrial antibodies
    c. Viral hepatitis panel
    d. α_1-Antitrypsin phenotype
    e. All of the above

Answer: a. This patient has Kayser–Fleischer rings (Fig. 12.7) noted on exam, which are a characteristic finding in patients with Wilson disease. Wilson disease can present with hepatic and/or neurologic manifestations, and this patient's newly diagnosed seizure disorder could also be a manifestation of Wilson disease. Wilson disease, a disorder of copper metabolism, is diagnosed via low serum ceruloplasmin and elevated serum and urine copper. Although Kayser–Fleischer rings can also be present in patients with cirrhosis of other etiologies (including autoimmune hepatitis; viral hepatitides and α_1-antitrypsin phenotype; and drug toxicity since the patient is on a potentially hepatotoxic medication, as mentioned in the other answer choices), they are most commonly associated with Wilson disease, a diagnosis which is further supported by the patient's neurologic symptoms. If studies for Wilson disease are negative, other causes of liver dysfunction should be further investigated.

12. A 16-year-old male with α_1-antitrypsin deficiency and chronic liver failure presents with fevers, rigors, and abdominal pain. You note ascites on exam and perform a diagnostic paracentesis. Gram stain of the fluid is remarkable for Gram (+) cocci in chains. You suspect pneumococcal peritonitis and promptly start the patient on IV antibiotics after drawing a blood culture. Which of the following is most consistent with what you expect for the rest of the patient's peritoneal fluid analysis?

	Total Protein (g/dL)	Ascites:Plasma Protein Ratio	Ascitic: Plasma LDH	Serum:Ascites Albumin (g/dL)	WBC Cells/mm^3
A	2.3	0.3	0.5	1.5	50
B	2.3	0.8	1.0	0.5	600
C	2.3	0.3	1.0	1.5	300
D	2.3	0.8	0.3	0.5	600
E	None of the above				

Answer: b. The peritoneal fluid in patients with peritonitis reflects an exudative process, with elevated total protein, an elevated ascites:plasma protein ratio, elevated ascites:plasma LDH, low serum:ascites albumin, and WBC >5,000 with >50% PMNs. In patients with hypoproteinemia from liver dysfunction such as the patient described above, however, the total protein in the peritoneal fluid may be lower than expected despite an exudative process. Thus, the findings in **B** are most consistent with exudative peritoneal fluid as expected for a patient with peritonitis. Table 12.19 demonstrates characteristics of transudative and exudative peritoneal fluid analysis.

13. A 15-year-old male presents to the ED with acute onset of chest pain and increased work of breathing. His mother reports that he went out with his friends "binge drinking" the night prior and vomited multiple times in the morning. On physical examination, the

TABLE 12.19

CHARACTERIZATION OF TRANSUDATIVE VERSUS EXUDATIVE PERITONEAL FLUID

	Transudative	Exudative
	Clear/straw-colored	Turbid/cloudy
Total protein (g/dL)	<2.5–3.0 or less than half plasma protein	>3.0 g/dL (maybe less in pts. with hypoproteinemia)
Ascites:plasma protein ratio	<0.5	>0.5
Ascites:plasma LDH	<0.6	>0.6
Serum:ascites albumin (g/dL) (invalid if ascitic fluid albumin <1)	>1.1	<1.1
WBC (cells/mm^3)	<250–300; <33% PMN	>500; >50% PMN
Gram stain/Cx	No organisms	Organisms (need 10–20 mL of fluid)

patient is significantly distressed and appears very uncomfortable. His vital signs are notable for a temperature of 37.3, respiratory rate of 28, blood pressure of 140/90, heart rate of 110, and SaO_2 of 98% on room air. His lungs are clear to auscultation bilaterally and his breathing is unlabored. His heart beat is regular without any murmurs, rubs, or gallops and capillary refill is brisk. His abdominal is soft and nontender. The base of his neck is tender to palpation with subcutaneous crepitus. You are concerned for esophageal perforation secondary to increased esophageal pressure from vomiting. You obtain STAT cervical and chest x-rays which are normal. You are still concerned for esophageal perforation so obtain an esophagram with water-soluble contrast, which is also read as normal. What is the next most appropriate step in the management of this patient?

a. Discharge home on an H_2 blocker for presumed GERD with close outpatient follow-up by his pediatrician
b. Send a urine toxicology screen to look for drugs of abuse
c. Obtain a chest/esophageal U/S
d. Obtain an esophagram with barium

Answer: d. Esophageal perforation is a rare but serious condition in children. The most common etiologies of esophageal perforation include blunt trauma (e.g., motor vehicle accidents, gunshot wounds, child abuse), iatrogenic trauma (e.g., endoscopy, NG tube placement, excessive suctioning), and Boerhaave syndrome. Boerhaave syndrome is a rare complication of sudden increased esophageal pressure due to vomiting, coughing, or straining. Symptoms begin acute and include pain, neck tenderness, dysphagia, subcutaneous crepitus, and possible fever and tachycardia. Diagnosis is usually made by seeing a widened mediastinum or paracervical free air on cervical spine and chest x-ray. Normal x-rays, however, do not rule out the diagnosis and further investigation is needed in cases with high suspicion. An esophagram with water-soluble contrast is typically the next step in diagnosis. Water-soluble contrast is preferable to barium contrast for the initial esophagram because of the risk of inflammatory mediastinitis with barium contrast in the setting of perforation. Esophagram with water-soluble contrast, however, misses more than 30% of cervical esophageal perforations and, if negative, a subsequent barium study is needed if the degree of suspicion is high enough. Endoscopy and chest CT can also be helpful when the diagnosis is uncertain. An U/S is not useful. Discharge home without further evaluation in the setting of suspected esophageal perforation is not appropriate as a missed diagnosis could be life threatening. A urine toxicology screen to look for drugs of abuse may be helpful in the overall evaluation of the patient but is not the most urgent next step.

14. A 5-month-old female infant who you have cared for since birth presents with a several week history of spitting up after feeds. There have not been any formula changes. The vomiting is not particularly forceful and the emesis is nonbilious and nonbloody. She appears comfortable when she feeds without excessive fussiness or arching. ROS is negative for increased work of breathing, fevers, diarrhea, or constipation. Her growth percentiles have consistently been in the 50% to 75% for length, weight, and head circumference. Her physical examination is normal. The patient's uncle is a pediatrician and wrote her a prescription for omeprazole. Her parents want to get your opinion before starting her on the medication. Which of the following is the most appropriate advice to give to her parents at this time?

a. Your daughter is showing signs of GERD, and omeprazole is an appropriate first-line treatment.
b. Your daughter is showing signs of GERD and does warrant treatment, but an H_2 blocker such as ranitidine is a more appropriate first-line treatment. Omeprazole is reserved for patients who are refractory to H_2 blockers.
c. Your daughter is showing signs of GER but does not need medical treatment at this time. Her signs and symptoms are consistent with physiologic reflux.
d. Your daughter's signs and symptoms are more consistent with a viral gastritis rather than GERD. The symptoms are likely to resolve on their own within the next few days. As long as she is staying well hydrated, no specific intervention is needed.

Answer: c. It is important to distinguish between GER and GERD. GER is simply the passage of gastric contents into the esophagus and can be physiologic in infants. GERD is when a patient is symptomatic from and/or experiences complications of GER (e.g., poor weight gain, excessive irritability, recurrent aspiration pneumonias, stridor, wheezing).

This patient has GER but does not have GERD. She is spitting up but is otherwise well. She is not excessively fussy with feeds and is growing well. Physiologic GER is common in infants and is a benign condition that typically resolves within the first year of life. Physiologic GER does not require medications. Supportive care includes feeding the infant with smaller more frequent feeds and burping in the middle of feeds. Keeping the patient upright for ~30 minutes after each feed has historically been included in "reflux precautions," but there is no evidence to support it and it is no longer recommended.

Infants with GERD as opposed to physiologic GER do warrant medical therapy in addition to supportive measures. The first-line medication for GERD is a histamine-2-receptor-antagonist (i.e., H_2 blocker) such as ranitidine. If the patient is refractory to ranitidine, then a proton-pump inhibitor such as omeprazole is appropriate.

15. A 2-year-old male child presents to your clinic with diarrhea. For the past 6 weeks, he has been having four to five large, loose stools per day. The stools are light brown in color and there has been no obvious blood in them. He does not express any discomfort with stooling. There have been no recent dietary changes. He has good oral intake, has not had any associated emesis, abdominal pain, or fevers, and is acting appropriately. There is no significant travel or family history. His physical examination is normal and his weight and height continue to be at the 75% for age. Which of the following is the most appropriate response to give his parents?

a. Your son likely has toddler's diarrhea due to disaccharide intolerance. He should thus be switched to lactose-free milk. His symptoms will resolve in 2 to 3 days.
b. Your son likely has toddler's diarrhea due to a chronic parasitic infection. He will be prescribed a 10-day course of metronidazole. His symptoms will resolve in 2 to 3 days.
c. Your son likely has toddler's diarrhea. The exact cause is unknown, but it is likely due to excess fluid intake, large amounts of high fructose-containing juices, and/or too little dietary protein. You should reduce his total fluid intake, decrease his high fructose-containing juice intake, and increase his protein intake. His symptoms will resolve in about 2 to 3 weeks.
d. Your son likely has toddler's diarrhea. The exact cause is unknown, but it is likely due to excess fluid intake and/or large amounts of high fructose-containing juices. You should reduce his total fluid intake, decrease his high fructose-containing juice intake, and increase his fat intake. His symptoms will resolve in about 2 to 3 days.

Answer: d. This patient likely has toddler's diarrhea, a relatively common condition that most affects children between the ages of 1 and 3 years. Diagnosis is primarily clinical and is based on noting ≥2 loose, nonbloody, voluminous stools per day for at least 4 weeks in an otherwise healthy toddler who continues to grow and develop appropriately. Toddler's diarrhea is a diagnosis of exclusion and should only be made after ruling out other causes of diarrhea (e.g., infection, IBD, celiac disease). Most other causes of diarrhea can be ruled out clinically by taking a thorough personal and family history and doing a complete physical examination. Adjunctive laboratory and/or imaging studies should be obtained to rule out other conditions if necessary. The exact etiology is not known but it is thought that excessive fluid intake, particularly high fructose-containing juices, plays a role in its pathogenesis.

Thus, treatment is aimed at reducing total fluid intake to 90 mL/kg/day, decreasing high fructose-containing juices (e.g., apple juice, pear juice), and increasing dietary fat (to slow motility) to ~40% of daily calories/day. With appropriate dietary management, symptoms typically resolve in 2 to 3 days.

16. A 5-week-old ex/38 week male is being evaluated in the gastroenterology clinic for cholestasis. He was the product of an uncomplicated pregnancy and delivery. All maternal serologies were negative. He is described by his parents as a vigorous feeder, and he has demonstrated appropriate weight gain. Family history is noncontributory. Your differential diagnosis is broad, and you decide to continue your workup by ordering an abdominal U/S and a HIDA scan. What findings on clinical history, abdominal U/S, and HIDA scan are more consistent with biliary atresia rather than neonatal hepatitis?

- **a.** Full-term gestation, enlarged liver, and pale stools. Abdominal U/S with "triangular cord sign" at porta hepatis. HIDA scan with rapid uptake into the liver but no excretion into the intestine.
- **b.** Preterm gestation, enlarged liver, and pale stools. Abdominal U/S with "triangular cord sign" at porta hepatis. HIDA scan with slow uptake into the liver but excretion into the intestine.
- **c.** Full-term gestation, liver edge 1 cm below costal margin, and normal stool pigment. Abdominal U/S with "triangular cord sign" at porta hepatis. HIDA scan with rapid uptake into the liver but no excretion into the intestine.
- **d.** Preterm gestation, enlarged liver, and pale stools. Abdominal U/S with biliary sludging. HIDA scan with rapid uptake into the liver but no excretion into the intestine.

Answer: a. Biliary atresia consists of atresia or hypoplasia of any portion of the extrahepatic biliary system. The etiology is unknown, but it is thought to be an acquired disorder. The classic history is that of a full-term thriving infant who develops jaundice at 3 to 6 weeks of age. Unlike in neonatal hepatitis, patients with biliary atresia have normal birthweight, an enlarged and firm liver, and absent stool pigment. Although U/S may be normal in patients with biliary atresia, the classic finding is "triangular cord sign" at the porta hepatis. A HIDA scan with rapid uptake of tracer into the liver but no excretion into the intestine is consistent with biliary atresia. In neonatal hepatitis, HIDA scan findings include slow uptake of tracer in the liver with normal excretion into the intestine.

17. A mother brings her 6-year-old daughter to your clinic with a long-standing history of constipation since the age of 3 years that is initially palliated then quickly refractory to short courses of stool softeners. She is toilet trained but frequently has loose stool in her underwear. Physical examination is remarkable for a well-appearing child with a mildly distended abdomen, normoactive bowel sounds, palpable stool in the left lower quadrant, and hard stool in the rectal vault. Given the most likely diagnosis, which of the following is the most appropriate management strategy?

- **a.** Start the patient on a high dose of oral stool softener, and ask her mother to implement a stooling routine with her. Once her stool becomes loose and frequent and the fecal soiling has stopped, wean the stool softener to lower but regular doses. Continue behavioral interventions, and eventually wean off the stool softener as tolerated.
- **b.** Start the patient on rectal suppositories until her stool becomes loose and frequent and the fecal soiling has stopped. Wean the suppositories as tolerated, and begin behavioral interventions once stooling is regular.
- **c.** Start the patient on oral stool softeners. Consult pediatric gastroenterology for rectal suction biopsy and possible barium enema.
- **d.** Start the patient on a course of oral steroids. Consult pediatric gastroenterology for upper endoscopy and colonoscopy.

Answer: a. The most likely diagnosis in this patient is functional fecal retention. This is a common condition in young children and is usually behaviorally mediated. The child begins to hold stool due to inattentiveness, embarrassment of going to the bathroom, or an inconsistent stooling routine. The stool stays in the rectum longer and more water is absorbed from it, thus making the stool harder and more painful to pass through the anus. This contributes to the child's desire to hold the stool for as long as possible and further exacerbates the problem. Fecal soiling results when stool proximal to the impacted stool begins leaking around the impaction. Although patients may show some initial response to short courses of stool softeners, symptoms reoccur and are quickly refractory to this intervention.

The most important part of treatment for functional fecal retention is behavior modification with implementation of a regular stooling schedule. Adjunctive medical treatment consists of three phases: (a) complete evacuation, (b) sustained evacuation, and (c) weaning from intervention. In the complete evacuation phase, high dose stool softeners are used to clear the impacted stool and continued until stools are regular and loose. It is unadvisable to use anything per rectum, since the patient is likely aversive to manipulation of this area due to tenderness and irritation from previous traumatic passage of hard stool and such intervention may discourage the child from cooperating with the stooling schedule. In the sustained evacuation stage, stool softeners are titrated down to reach a soft stool consistency. In the weaning from intervention stage, the patient is eventually weaned off stool softeners. Continuing implementation of a regular stooling schedule is critical for long-term success.

Consultation with pediatric gastroenterology for rectal suction biopsy and possible barium enema would be indicated to further evaluate for Hirschsprung disease. Although Hirschsprung disease should be considered in the evaluation of children with chronic constipation, it is much less common than functional fecal retention and is inconsistent with the physical examination finding of hard stool palpable within the rectal vault.

Consultation with pediatric gastroenterology for upper endoscopy and colonoscopy would be indicated to further evaluate for IBD. The lack of abdominal pain, constitutional symptoms, diarrhea, and bloody stools argues against the diagnosis of IBD in this patient. Furthermore, functional fecal retention is much more common than IBD, especially in a young child.

18. A full-term newborn male is diagnosed with a high level imperforate anus. The surgical team has already consulted and is planning on creating a diverting colostomy within the next 72 hours. Your attending would like to know what further diagnostic evaluation is indicated in this patient. Which of the following answers is correct?

- **a.** Echocardiogram, esophagogram, skeletal survey, and renal U/S
- **b.** Renal U/S and spinal MRI
- **c.** Chromosomal analysis
- **d.** No further evaluation is needed

Answer: a. Imperforate anus is an abnormal division of the cloaca into urogenital and rectal portions that occurs around 4 to 6 weeks of gestation. An accompanying fistula between the distal rectum and the perineum or urogenital tract is common. The incidence of imperforate anus is 1:5,000. It can be an isolated abnormality, but half of affected patients have other abnormalities such as congenital heart disease, TEF, bony abnormalities, and renal malformations. Two important syndromes associated with imperforate anus are VATER syndrome (vertebral, anal, tracheal, esophageal, radial, and renal abnormalities) and VACTERL syndrome (vertebral, anal, cardiac, tracheal, esophageal, renal, and limb abnormalities). Thus, every infant with an imperforate anus should be screened for other anomalies with an echocardiogram, esophagogram, skeletal survey, and renal U/S. If other abnormalities are present, consideration should be given to obtaining a genetic consultation and chromosomal analysis. A spinal MRI is not useful in the evaluation of this patient.

19. A 16-year-old Asian female presents to you with chronic recurrent abdominal pain that occurs primarily after ingestion of dairy products. You suspect lactose intolerance and suggest a trial of a lactose-free diet. Her mother has a friend who was tested for lactose intolerance via a "breath test" and asks you about the utility of a breath test to help with the diagnosis in her daughter. Which of the following is the most accurate response?

- **a.** The lactose intolerance hydrogen breath test is very sensitive but has low specificity for the diagnosis of lactose intolerance. Thus, it will overdiagnose lactose intolerance.
- **b.** The lactose intolerance hydrogen breath test is very sensitive but has low specificity for the diagnosis of lactose intolerance. Thus, it will underdiagnose lactose intolerance.
- **c.** The lactose intolerance hydrogen breath test is very specific but has low sensitivity for the diagnosis of lactose intolerance. Thus, it will overdiagnose lactose intolerance.
- **d.** The lactose intolerance hydrogen breath test is very specific but has low sensitivity for the diagnosis of lactose intolerance. Thus, it will underdiagnose lactose intolerance.

Answer: a. Lactose intolerance is a relatively common condition that can be genetic or multifactorial in etiology. In the genetic form of lactose intolerance, lactase activity starts to decrease around 4 to 6 years and the patient becomes symptomatic when the amount of enzyme activity becomes insufficient. Although many parents report lactose intolerance in infants, it is important to note that congenital lactase deficiency is extremely rare. Symptoms of lactose intolerance include abdominal pain, bloating, and/or diarrhea following the ingestion of dairy products. The best way to diagnose lactose intolerance is via a 2-week trial of a lactose-free diet followed by reintroduction of a lactose-containing diet. If symptoms improve on the lactose-free diet and then reoccur when lactose is reintroduced, a diagnosis of lactose intolerance is made. The lactose intolerance hydrogen breath test is rarely helpful, as it is very sensitive but has low specificity for the diagnosis of lactose intolerance. Thus, it will overdiagnose lactose intolerance. The mainstay of treatment for lactose intolerance is dietary restriction of lactose. Of note, however, because lactose intolerance is dose related, low-lactose containing foods such as cheese can be reintroduced as tolerated and may preclude the need for calcium supplementation.

SUGGESTED READINGS

Abi-Hanna A, Lake AM. Constipation and encopresis in childhood. *Pediatr Rev*. 1998;19(1):23–30.

Boyle JT. Gastrointestinal bleeding in infants and children. *Pediatr Rev*. 2008;29(2):39–52.

D'Agata ID, Balistreri WF. Evaluation of liver disease in the pediatric patient. *Pediatr Rev*. 1999;20(11):376–390.

Feldman M, Friedman LS, Brandt LJ, et al. *Feldman: Sleisenger & Fordtran's Gastrointestinal and Liver Disease*. 8th ed. Maryland Heights, MO: W.B. Saunders, 2006.

McMillan JA, Feigin RD, DeAngelis CD, et al. *Oski's Pediatrics, Principles & Practice*, 4th ed. 2006.

Michail S. Gastroesophageal reflux. *Pediatr Rev*. 2007;28(3).

Wolfe AD, Levine JE. Hepatomegaly in neonates and children. *Pediatr Rev*. 2000;21(9):303–310.

CHAPTER 13 ■ METABOLISM

HILARY TINKEL VERNON

ALDP	Adrenoleukodystrophy protein	LCHAD	Long-chain 3-hydroxyacyl-CoA dehydrogenase deficiency
ASD	Atrial septal defect	LV	Left ventricle
AV	Atrioventricular	MCAD	Medium-chain acyl-CoA dehydrogenase deficiency
BBB	Blood-brain barrier	ML	Mucolipidoses
BCAA	Branched-chain amino acid	MPS	Mucopolysaccharidoses
BCKD	Branched-chain amino acid alpha-ketoacid dehydrogenase	MSUD	Maple syrup urine disease
CDG	Congenital disorder of glycosylation	NKH	Nonketotic hyperglycinemia
CPS1	Carbamoyl phosphate synthetase I	NPO	Nothing by mouth (nil per os)
CSF	Cerebrospinal fluid	NTBC	(2-[2-Nitro-4-triflouro-methylbenzoyl]-1-3-cyclohexan-edione)
EEG	Electroencephalogram	OTC	Ornithine transcarbamylase
ERT	Enzyme replacement therapy	PAH	Phenylalanine hydroxylase
FAH	Fumarylacetoacetase	PKU	Phenylketonuria
GALT	Galactose-1-phosphate uridyl transferase	SLOS	Smith-Lemli-Opitz Syndrome
GP	Glycoproteinoses	VLCAD	Very-long-chain acyl-CoA dehydrogenase deficiency
GSD	Glycogen storage disease	VSD	Ventricular septal defect
IEM	Inborn error of metabolism	WBC	White blood cell
IV	Intravenous		

CHAPTER OBJECTIVES

1. To understand newborn screening and common presenting signs of IEMs
2. To understand the classifications of IEMs
3. To know the descriptions of the important IEMs and their major clinical manifestations.

INTRODUCTION

IEMs are deficiencies of the biochemical processes of the body. Most often there is a disruption of a single enzyme or transport system, which causes an accumulation of a precursor molecule and/or a deficiency of the product molecule. Pathology can occur through intoxication from excessive precursor molecule, disruption of energy metabolism, or more complex disruptions of entire molecular processing pathways. Most of these disorders are inherited in an **autosomal recessive** manner, but X-linked, mitochondrial, and autosomal dominant inheritance patterns can also be found. IEMs can be organized into groups depending on the metabolite or metabolic process that is disrupted, for example, amino acid metabolism or catabolism, carbohydrate synthesis or breakdown, fat metabolism, etc.

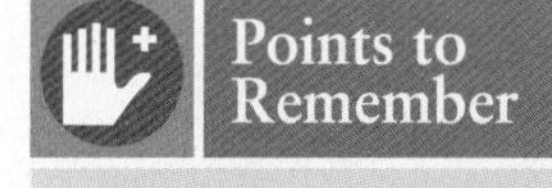

- **Most IEMs are autosomal recessive disorders—always ask about a family history of consanguinity!**

Newborn Screening

Newborn screening programs vary widely from state to state. At a minimum, every state screens for galactosemia, PKU, hemoglobin S, hemoglobin C, congenital hypothyroidism, and congenital adrenal hyperplasia.

Clinical Presentations

IEMs have varied clinical presentations. They can present dramatically in the newborn period with neurological deterioration (coma or lethargy), seizures, or hypotonia. They can present

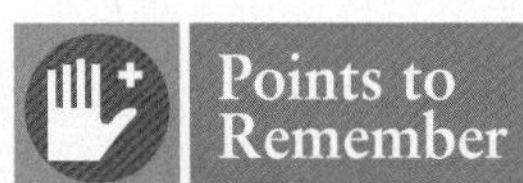

Points to Remember

- **Consider an IEM in a neonate presenting with a sepsis-like picture.**

later in life from childhood to adulthood with recurrent symptomatic episodes such as altered mental status, coma, or ataxia. They can present with chronic and/or progressive symptoms such as failure to thrive, developmental delay, static encephalopathy, or progressive muscle weakness. The same IEM can have a mild presentation in one patient and a severe presentation in another. The severity of presentation is often related to the amount of functional enzyme or transporter present.

Physical Examination Findings

Performing a detailed physical examination can help to identify specific disorders, as some IEMs have unique physical findings such as abnormal urine odor, skin pigmentation, and urine color. Table 13.1 describes important physical findings found in specific IEMs.

TABLE 13.1

PHYSICAL FINDINGS OF INBORN ERRORS OF METABOLISM

Finding	Disorders
Hair, sparse	Biotinidase deficiency, Menkes disease
Hair, kinky	Menkes disease
Hirsutism	GP, ML, MPS
Photosensitization	Porphyrias
Coarse facies (Fig. 13.1)	GP, ML, MPS
Macrocephaly	Canavan, glutaric acidemia I, GP, ML, MPS
Microcephaly	CDG, leukodystrophies, PKU, maternal PKU syndrome
Cataracts	Fabry disease, alpha-mannosidase deficiency, Niemann-Pick disease, SLOS, Zellweger
Cherry-red macular spots	GM1 and GM2 gangliosidoses, Krabbe disease, Niemann-Pick disease
Corneal clouding	GP, ML, MPS
Kayser-Fleischer rings (Fig. 13.2)	Wilson disease
Marfanoid appearance	Homocystinuria
Port wine urine	Porphyrias
Maple syrup urine odor	Maple syrup urine disease
Mousy urine odor	PKU
Sweaty feet urine odor	Isovaleric academia

CDG, carbohydrate-deficient glycoprotein syndrome; GP, glycoproteinoses; GSD, glycogen storage disease; ML, mucolipidoses; MPS, mucopolysaccharidoses; PKU, phenylketonuria; SLOS, Smith-Lemli-Opitz syndrome.

Laboratory Findings

It is essential to order the correct laboratory studies when attempting to diagnose an IEM. The initial evaluation of every infant or child suspected of having an IEM should include at minimum a complete blood cell count, chemistry panel, glucose, **blood gas, ammonia, lactate**, and urinalysis. See Table 13.2 for descriptions of laboratory findings found in specific IEMs.

DISORDERS OF AMINO ACID METABOLISM

Disorders of amino acid metabolism include tyrosinemia, homocystinuria, NKH, MSUD, and PKU.

Phenylketonuria

Classic PKU results from a deficiency of the PAH enzyme, which is responsible for converting phenylalanine into tyrosine. Other forms of PKU can be caused by deficiencies in the synthesis of biopterin, which is required for the PAH enzyme to function properly. PKU is inherited in an autosomal recessive manner and has an overall prevalence of 1 in 13,500. The clinical phenotype correlates directly with the level of phenylalanine.

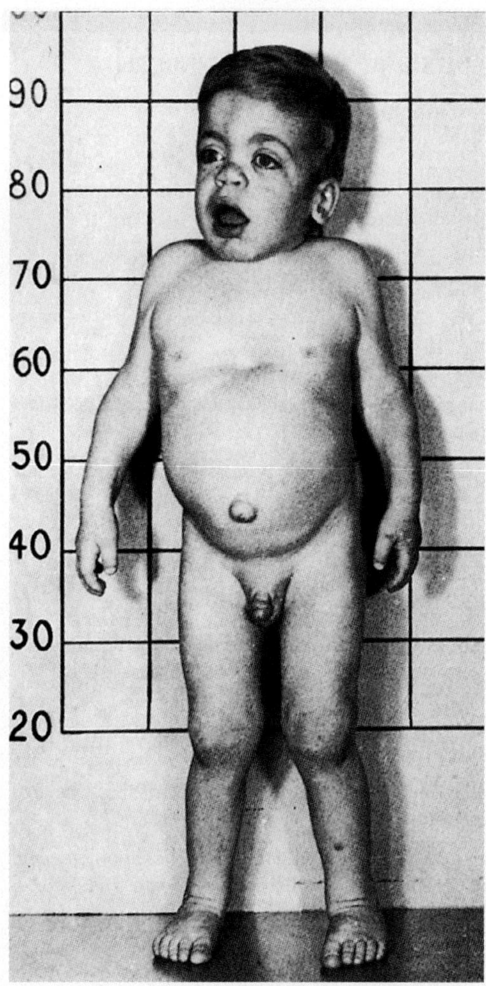

FIGURE 13.1. Hurler syndrome in a 4-year-old boy. The patient demonstrates the unusual coarse facies, depressed bridge of the nose, open mouth, and large tongue. The hands are spade-like, the abdomen protrudes, and an umbilical hernia is present. (Courtesy of Dr. V.A. McKusick, Johns Hopkins Hospital, Baltimore, MD.)

Clinical Manifestations of Untreated PKU

- Eczema.
- Hypopigmentation.
- Seizures.
- Limb spasticity.
- Mousy odor.
- Severe mental retardation.

Treatment

- **Phenylalanine-restricted diet** in infancy, ideally continued throughout lifetime.
  - Proper adherence to diet results in excellent outcome and normal intelligence.
- More recently, a synthetic form of biopterin has become clinically available and allows further liberalization of diet in some patients.

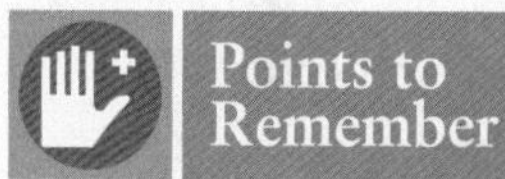

- **Women of childbearing age with PKU must maintain strict adherence to their diet because of the teratogenic effects of elevated phenylalanine. Infants born to mothers with uncontrolled PKU can have microcephaly, growth retardation, developmental delay, and congenital heart disease.**

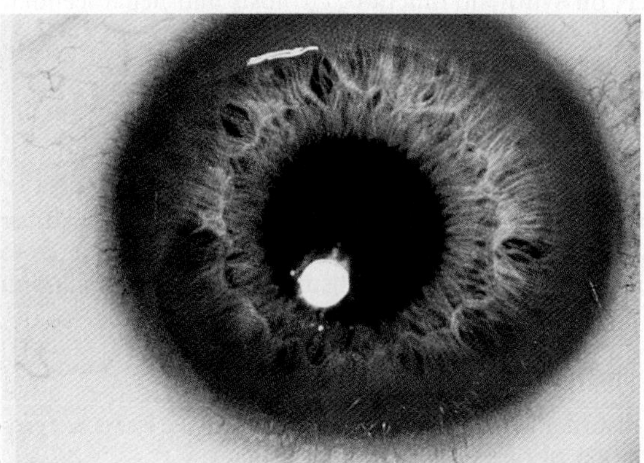

FIGURE 13.2. Kayser-Fleischer ring. Very few rings are this pronounced. (From Tasman W, Jaeger E. *The Wills Eye Hospital Atlas of Clinical Ophthalmology*. 2nd ed. Philadelphia, PA: Lippincott Williams & Wilkins, 2001.)

TABLE 13.2

ABNORMAL COMMON LABORATORY TEST RESULTS THAT SUGGEST AN INBORN ERROR OF METABOLISM

Finding	Disorders
Pancytopenia	Organic acidemias, Gaucher disease, Pearson syndrome (mitochondrial disorder)
Thrombocytopenia	Gaucher disease, other lysosomal storage disorders with splenomegaly
Hemolytic anemia	Disorders of pyrimidines
Defective T- and B-cell function	Adenosine deaminase deficiency
Acidosis	Organic acidemias, amino acidemias, mitochondrial disorders of energy production
Lactic acidosis	Mitochondrial disorders, organic acidemias, glycogen storage disease type I (GSD I)
Elevated ammonia	Urea cycle defects, organic acidemias, mitochondrial fatty acid oxidation disorders
Increased anion gap	Organic acidemias
Hypoglycemia	Mitochondrial fatty acid oxidation disorders, GSDs, pyruvate carboxylase deficiency, hereditary fructose intolerance
Elevated uric acid	GSD I, purine disorders
Low uric acid	Purine disorders
Hematuria	Disorders with renal stones, methylmalonic acidemia, vitamin B_{12} activation defects
Ketonuria	Organic acidemias, amino acidemias, mitochondrial fatty acid oxidation defects, glycogen storage disorders
Myoglobinuria	Mitochondrial fatty acid oxidation defects, mitochondrial myopathies
Urine reducing substance	Galactosemia, hereditary fructose intolerance

Tyrosinemia

There are five known inherited disorders of tyrosine metabolism. We will address tyrosinemia types I and II in this chapter.

Tyrosinemia Type I

Tyrosinemia type I, also known as **hepatorenal tyrosinemia**, results from a deficiency of the FAH enzyme. It has an incidence of 1 in 12,000–100,000. Toxicity is thought to occur from accumulation of metabolites proximal to the FAH enzyme step. There can be acute, subacute, and chronic forms of this disease, which can vary even within the same family.

Clinical Manifestations

- Liver: **liver failure with early effects on synthetic function**, cirrhosis and hepatocellular carcinoma.
- Kidney: proximal renal tubular dysfunction leading to **hypophosphatemic rickets.**
- GI: failure to thrive and abdominal crises.
- Neurologic: paresthesias, seizures, and paralysis.

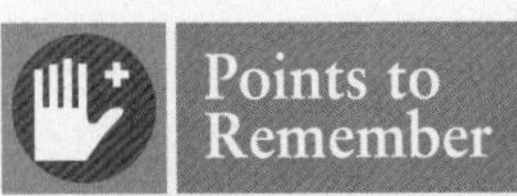

Points to Remember

- **The liver is the most commonly affected organ in tyrosinemia type I.**
- **Because of liver synthetic dysfunction, coagulation is often disproportionately abnormal compared to other tests of liver function.**

Treatment

- Traditionally centered around dietary restriction of tyrosine and phenylalanine with or without liver transplantation; however, the drug NTBC is now used in some patients to create a block upstream of the pathway of tyrosine metabolism, leading to accumulation of less toxic metabolites.

Tyrosinemia Type II

Tyrosinemia type II is an **oculocutaneous** disorder. It results from deficiency of the enzyme tyrosine aminotransferase, leading to accumulation of tyrosine and phenolic acids.

Clinical Manifestations

- Eye: photophobia, decreased tear production, corneal ulceration, and scarring.
- Skin: crusted, hyperkeratotic lesions most commonly found on the palms and soles.
- Neurologic: seizures, behavioral abnormalities, developmental delay.

Treatment

- Dietary restriction of tyrosine and phenylalanine.

Maple Syrup Urine Disease (MSUD)

MSUD results from deficient activity of the BCKD complex and occurs in approximately 1 in 200,000 births. It derives its name from the **sweet smelling urine** of affected patients. Deficiency of this enzyme leads to accumulation of the BCAAs including leucine, isoleucine, and valine. Much of the toxicity is related to the elevated level of leucine, which is neurotoxic.

Clinical Manifestations (Vary According to Level of Functional Enzyme Present)

- Severe forms present in infancy with **lethargy,** vomiting, hypotonia, seizures, and/or death.
- Patients with intermediate levels of enzyme can present during childhood or adulthood with episodic neurologic decompensation, often when the patient is undergoing catabolic stress during an intercurrent illness.
- Chronic progressive forms of MSUD exist and can present with gradual neurologic problems including seizures and developmental delay.

Diagnosis

- Elevated levels of the BCAAs in serum.
- Ammonia, lactate, and bicarbonate are often normal.

Treatment

- Restriction of intake of the BCAAs.

Homocystinuria

Homocystinuria is an autosomal recessive condition classically caused by cystathionine beta-synthase deficiency. This enzyme is responsible for metabolizing homocysteine to cystathionine. Pyridoxine is a cofactor for this enzyme. The reported incidence varies from 1 in 344,000 worldwide to 1 in 65,000 in Ireland.

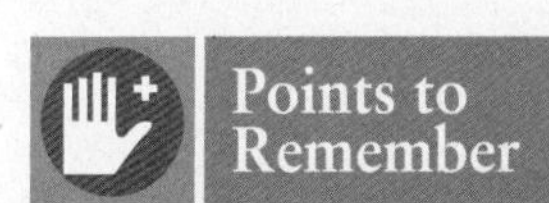

- **Up to 50% of patients with untreated homocystinuria will have a vascular event by the age of 30 years.**

Clinical Manifestations

- Mental retardation.
- Eye lens dislocation.
- **Marfanoid body habitus.**
- Osteoporosis.
- Acute vascular **thrombosis.**

Treatment

- 50% of patients will respond to pyridoxine supplementation.
- Other treatment modalities include methionine-restricted, cystine-supplemented diet and administration of betaine, which serves as a methyl donor in the conversion of homocysteine to methionine.

Nonketotic Hyperglycinemia

NKH results from defects in the glycine cleavage system.

Clinical Manifestations (Depend on Severity of Defect)

- Classic NKH presents in the neonatal period with lethargy, apnea, hypotonia, and seizures; EEG shows **a burst suppression pattern**; patients who survive past the neonatal period have severe developmental delay.
- Later onset form of NKH can present after the neonatal period and show varying neurologic symptoms.

Diagnosis

- CSF glycine to plasma glycine ratio greater than 0.08 is diagnostic of NKH.
- Ketosis and acidosis are not seen.

Treatment

- Sodium benzoate and dextromethorphan may help to reduce seizure activity and increase arousal in some patients.
- **Depakote should be avoided** since it can raise CSF glycine levels.

DISORDERS OF PROTEIN/NITROGEN METABOLISM (UREA CYCLE DEFECTS)

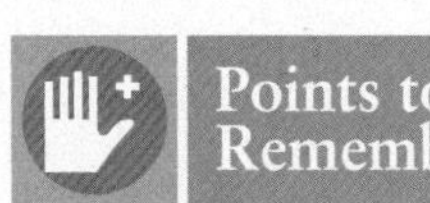

Points to Remember

- The finding of hyperpnea in urea cycle defects is important since it can cause a respiratory alkalosis in the setting of an apparent metabolic decompensation.
- Because of its X-linked inheritance, females with OTC deficiency have a varied picture depending on the amount of functional enzyme present and can range from mildly affected to severely affected.

In normal individuals, excess nitrogen is converted into urea, which is excreted in the urine by a process known as the urea cycle. A defect in this cycle will lead to abnormal nitrogen metabolism, and an **elevation in ammonia**, which at high levels is neurotoxic. Excess nitrogen is also stored as glutamine and glycine, which are also elevated in these disorders. All disorders of the urea cycle are inherited in an autosomal recessive manner, except OTC deficiency, which is inherited in an X-linked manner.

Clinical Manifestations (Vary According to the Specific Enzyme Involved and the Amount of Residual Enzyme Activity)

- Infants with severe disease can present acutely with poor feeding, lethargy, vomiting, irritability, **hyperpnea**, and hypotonia.
- Moderate forms can present in infancy with failure to thrive and/or developmental delay.
- Milder forms can present during childhood with episodic encephalopathy triggered by intercurrent metabolic stress, or more chronically with developmental delay.
- Arginase deficiency can present with **spastic diplegia.**

Diagnosis

The specific deficient enzyme in a patient with a suspected urea cycle defect can be identified by examining the patterns of urine organic acids and plasma amino acids.

- CPS1 deficiency: normal urine orotic acid, low to undetectable levels of plasma citrulline; elevated plasma ammonia, glutamine and glycine.
- OTC deficiency has a profile similar to CPS 1 deficiency except that there is also a large amount of orotic acid found in the urine.
- Citrullinemia (deficient argininosuccinate synthetase): elevated levels of plasma and urine citrulline; elevated plasma ammonia, glutamine and alanine; mildly elevated orotic acid; reduced plasma argininosuccinic acid.
- Arginase deficiency: mild to moderate hyperammonemia.

Treatment

- Acute treatment during crisis periods is centered around reducing the levels of ammonia by dialysis and IV medications designed to provide alternative mechanisms of nitrogen excretion, such as **sodium benzoate** and **phenylbutyrate.**
- Chronic management involves protein restriction, treatment with sodium benzoate and phenylbutyrate for alternate nitrogen excretion, and support during times of intercurrent illness, which can lead to metabolic crisis.

Prognosis

- The outcomes for the urea cycle defects generally depend on the amount of residual enzyme, timely treatment in times of crisis, and previous and ongoing levels of hyperammonemia.
- Patients who have been subjected to extremely high levels of ammonia have very poor neurologic outcomes.

DISORDERS OF ORGANIC ACID METABOLISM

Disorders of organic acid metabolism include propionic acidemia, isovaleric acidemia, methylmalonic aciduria, and glutaric aciduria.

Propionic Acidemia, Isovaleric Acidemia, and Methylmalonic Aciduria

These are disorders that involve metabolism of one or more of the BCAAs and are all inherited in an autosomal recessive manner.

Clinical Manifestations

- Each can present with a severe neonatal form with metabolic decompensation, an acute or intermittent later onset form, or a chronic form with failure to thrive and developmental delay.
- Patients with isovaleric acidemia are often described as having a peculiar body odor reminiscent of **sweaty feet.**
- Patients with propionic acidemia and methylmalonic aciduria are susceptible to acute and chronic cerebral events leading to **basal ganglia** abnormalities, renal tubular acidosis, pancreatitis, and cardiomyopathies.

Diagnosis

- Patients with metabolic decompensation can have an anion gap metabolic acidosis, ketonuria, and hyperammonemia; hyper, hypo-, and normoglycemia can all be seen.
- Both the **acylcarnitine profile** and **urine organic acid profile** are essential in making a diagnosis.

Treatment

- Protein restriction.
- Carnitine supplementation (provides alternate methods of propionic acid and methylmalonic acid secretion).
- Support during times of intercurrent illness.
- There are B_{12} responsive forms of methylmalonic aciduria, and every patient should be tested for responsiveness.

Glutaric Aciduria Type 1

Glutaric aciduria type 1 is due to a deficiency in glutaryl-CoA dehydrogenase leading to abnormal metabolism of L-lysine, L-hydroxylysine, and L-tryptophan.

Clinical Manifestations

- Infants with glutaric aciduria are susceptible to **basal ganglia** infarcts, dyskinesia, and dystonia, as well as cerebellar and frontotemporal atrophy. The frequency of infarcts decreases dramatically with age.
- Infants can present with macrocephaly even before metabolic decompensation occurs.

Diagnosis

- Elevated levels of glutaric acid in the urine or CSF.
- Abnormal acylcarnitine profile.
- Patients do not generally have hypoglycemia, acidosis, or hyperammonemia.

Treatment

- Lysine and tryptophan restricted diet.
- Carnitine supplementation.
- Support during intercurrent illnesses.

Points to Remember

- **Subdural hematomas can be seen in glutaric aciduria and can be mistaken for nonaccidental trauma.**

DISORDERS OF FATTY ACID METABOLISM

Defects in fatty acid oxidation lead to **defective energy production during fasting.** Long-chain free fatty acids are esterified in the cell cytosol and then enter the mitochondria as fatty acylcarnitines. Medium- and short-chain fatty acids are able to enter the mitochondria directly. They then undergo beta oxidation, which shortens the fatty acids until they become acetyl-CoA, which is then used to make **ketone bodies.** Some of the energy released during fatty acid oxidation is used to make ATP via the respiratory chain. Fatty acids are a preferred energy source for the myocardium. These disorders are all inherited in an **autosomal recessive** manner. Plasma acylcarnitine profile, urine acylglycines, and urine organic acids are helpful in making the diagnosis of a fatty acid oxidation defect.

MCAD is the most common fatty acid oxidation disorder, occurring in approximately 1 in 15,000 births. During prolonged fasting, the liver is unable to utilize medium-chain fatty acids for energy. Hypoglycemia develops, but urine ketones remain inappropriately low. Lethargy and seizures can progress to coma and death if an exogenous source of **glucose** is not provided. There is a high mortality rate for patients presenting with their first crisis.

VLCAD can present with cardiomyopathy, rhabdomyolysis, muscle weakness, and/or coma in times of fasting.

LCHAD is strongly associated with maternal HELLP (hemolytic anemia, elevated liver enzymes, low platelet count) syndrome during pregnancy. It can present with hypoglycemia, lethargy, hypotonia, and/or cardiomyopathy.

DISORDERS OF CARBOHYDRATE METABOLISM

Disorders of carbohydrate metabolism include hereditary fructose intolerance, galactosemia, and the GSDs.

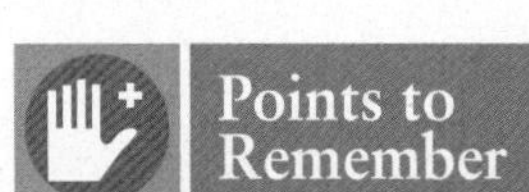

- **Infants who have unrecognized galactosemia in crisis may improve when placed on IV fluids and made NPO, but decompensate again when lactose-containing formula is reintroduced.**

Galactosemia

Galactosemia is a result of deficient GALT. Most patients present in the first or second week of life with hepatomegaly, **jaundice**, vomiting, hypoglycemia, hypotonia, and cataracts. Neonates can also present with ***Escherichia coli*** sepsis. Treatment includes a **lactose-free diet** throughout life. However, despite this treatment, patients are often still affected by developmental delay and hypergonadotrophic hypogonadism, thought to be due to endogenous production of galactose from glucose. Diagnosis is made by measuring the level of GALT or galactose 1 phosphate in blood cells, which can be done via a blood spot on the newborn screening card.

Hereditary Fructose Intolerance

Hereditary fructose intolerance results from a defect of fructose 1,6-bisphosphate aldolase. When patients are exposed to fructose, they can have gastrointestinal symptoms with nausea and

TABLE 13.3

CLASSIFICATION OF GLYCOGEN STORAGE DISORDERS

Type	Enzyme or Metabolic Process Affected	Major Organ Involvement	Clinical Features
0	Glycogen synthetase	Liver	Hypoglycemia, ketosis, no hepatomegaly
Ia	Glucose-6-phosphatase (von Gierke disease)	Liver, kidney	Hypoglycemia, hepatomegaly, growth retardation, lactic acidosis
II	Lysosomal alpha-glucosidase (Pompe disease)	Muscle, generalized	Myopathy, cardiomyopathy, hepatomegaly; death in infancy; ERT recently available, which extends life expectancy
III	Debrancher (Cori disease)	Liver, muscle	Mild Ia, cirrhosis, ketosis, myopathy, cardiomyopathy
IV	Brancher (Andersen disease)	Liver, muscle	Hepatomegaly, cirrhosis ± myopathy ± cardiomyopathy; failure to thrive and death in childhood
V	Muscle phosphorylase (McArdle disease)	Muscle	Weakness, cramps, myoglobinuria, atrophy
VI	Hepatic phosphorylase (Hers disease)	Liver	Hepatomegaly
VII	Muscle phosphofructokinase (Tarui disease)	Muscle, RBC	Weakness, cramps, myoglobinuria ± mild hemolytic anemia
VIII	Loss of activation of phosphorylase	Liver, brain	Hepatomegaly, progressive central nervous system dysfunction
IXa-1	Phosphorylase kinase (PK), alpha-liver subunit	Liver, RBC, WBC	Hepatomegaly, ketosis

cAMP, cyclic adenosine monophosphate; ERT, enzyme replacement therapy; RBC, red blood cell; WBC, white blood cell.

vomiting, seizures, and coma. Liver failure and proximal renal tubule defects can be seen. A chronic form can also develop leading to growth failure and chronic renal and liver damage. Treatment includes a **fructose- and sucrose-free diet;** once this is instituted, most patients do well.

Glycogen Storage Disorders

The glycogen storages disorders are a large class of disorders that cause defects in glycogen production or utilization. They primarily present with either muscle or liver abnormalities or both. Table 13.3 shows the specific enzyme defects and their clinical presentations.

DISORDERS OF CHOLESTEROL BIOSYNTHESIS

Smith-Lemli-Opitz Syndrome (SLOS)

SLOS is the most well-known disorder of cholesterol biosynthesis and is caused by defects in 3beta-hydroxysterol-delta7-reductase. Affected patients have a range of manifestations from learning disabilities and behavioral abnormalities to severe neonatal malformations leading to death. A frequent finding in patients with SLOS is syndactyly of the second and third toes. Other physical features include heart defects (ASD, VSD, AV canal), kidney malformations, microcephaly, brain malformations such as agenesis of the corpus callosum, polydactyly, and gastrointestinal malformations.

CONGENITAL DISORDERS OF GLYCOSYLATION

CDGs are a recently recognized group of disorders that result in abnormally glycosylated proteins. These disorders have a wide spectrum of clinical presentations, often with multiorgan system dysfunction. They can be divided into N-glycosylation defects (the more common defects) or O-glycosylation defects, depending on where the glycan group is attached to the protein. There are more than 20 identified CDGs.

Clinical Manifestations

- N-glycosylation disorders present with a wide range of clinical features including seizures, hypotonia, microcephaly, and immunodeficiency.
- O-glycosylation disorders also present with a wide range of clinical features including muscle-eye-brain disease (Walker-Warburg syndrome), a form of limb girdle muscular dystrophy, and hyperphosphatemic familial hypercalcinosis.

Points to Remember

- **An interesting clinical feature that can be associated with CDGs is inverted nipples.**

Treatment

The only currently treatable CDG is CDG-Ib (phosphomannose isomerase deficiency); it can be successfully treated with administration of mannose.

Diagnosis

Transferrin is a glycoprotein and will show an abnormal electrophoresis pattern if glycans are not attached properly. This can help identify many but not all CDGs.

PEROXISOMAL DISORDERS

Peroxisomal disorders can result from deficiency of a single enzyme within the organelle leading to accumulation of toxic substrate or from disrupted biogenesis of the entire organelle. Diagnosis is made by examining products of various peroxisomal functions, including findings of an abnormal very-long-chain fatty acid profile, abnormal plasmalogen synthesis, and deficiency of alpha oxidation of phytanic acid.

ALDP Protein Defects

Defects in the protein ALDP lead to abnormal fatty oxidation of very-long-chain fatty acids in the peroxisome. It can manifest with various clinical presentations including X-linked **adrenoleukodystrophy** (a childhood onset neurodegenerative disease), **childhood Addison**

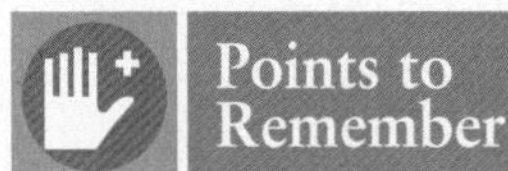

Points to Remember

- **Relatively milder peroxisome biogenesis disorders include neonatal adrenoleukodystrophy and infantile Refsum disease.**

disease, and **adrenomyeloneuropathy** (an adult onset somatosensory and pyramidal tract degenerative disease). There is some evidence that administration of Lorenzo's oil (oleic acid and erucic acid) when given in the presymptomatic state may have some benefit to patients. Stem cell transplantation can also stabilize the disease if performed in the presymptomatic phase.

Zellweger Syndrome

Zellweger syndrome is a severe disease caused by defects in one of various genes that lead to disruption of biogenesis of the entire peroxisome. Patients manifest facial dysmorphism, large

TABLE 13.4

LYSOSOMAL STORAGE DISORDERS

Disorder and Enzyme Deficiency	Clinical Presentation	Outcome and Treatment
MPS I (Hurler, Hurler/Scheie, Scheie) Alpha-L-iduronidase[a]	■ Facial dysmorphism ■ Hepatosplenomegaly (Fig. 13.3) ■ Cataracts ■ Cardiomyopathy ■ Pulmonary disease ■ Neurologic decline (severe in Hurler; none in Scheie) ■ Dysostosis multiplex (complex bone disease)	ERT is available for MPS I but does not cross blood-brain barrier (BBB) so will not correct/prevent CNS disease. Stem cell transplantation is the only way to prevent neurologic decline but has variable success.
MPS II (Hunter syndrome) Iduronate-2-sulfatase[a]	■ Facial dysmorphism ■ Airway obstruction ■ Skeletal deformity ■ Cardiomyopathy ■ Neurological decline	ERT is available but does not cross BBB so will not correct/prevent CNS disease. (X-linked)
Gaucher disease type I acid beta-glucosidase[a]	■ Hepatosplenomegaly ■ Cytopenias ■ Skeletal disease ■ Bone marrow biopsy shows large blue histiocytes (Gaucher cells)	ERT is available. (More common in Ashkenazi Jews)
Fabry disease Alpha-galactosidase[a]	■ Renal: glomerular sclerosis, tubular atrophy, interstitial fibrosis, ESRD ■ GI: achalasia, vomiting, etc. ■ Cardiac: LV dysfunction, atherosclerosis ■ Neuro: decreased sweating, acroparesthesias, pain crises, strokes	ERT is available. Life expectancy of affected men is approximately 50 y without ERT. Female carriers are variably affected. (X-linked)
Neimann-Pick disease type A Acid sphingomyelinase[a]	■ Infantile onset ■ Failure to thrive ■ Hepatosplenomegaly ■ Macular cherry red spot ■ Respiratory abnormalities ■ Neurologic deterioration ■ Bone marrow biopsy shows sea-blue histiocytosis	Supportive treatment. (More common in Ashkenazi Jews)
Tay-Sachs disease Hexosaminidase A[a]	■ Normal at birth ■ Cherry-red spots in macula seen as early as 3 mo of age. ■ Hypotonia and developmental regression are seen at approximately 6 mo of age ■ Spasticity, blindness, seizures, and macrocephaly by 1 year of age.	Supportive treatment Most children die between 3 and 4 years of age. (More common in Ashkenazi Jews)

[a]Denotes the deficient enzyme for each disorder.
ESRD, end-stage renal disease; GI, gastrointestinal; LV, left ventricle; ERT, enzyme replacement therapy; MPS, mucopolysaccharidose.

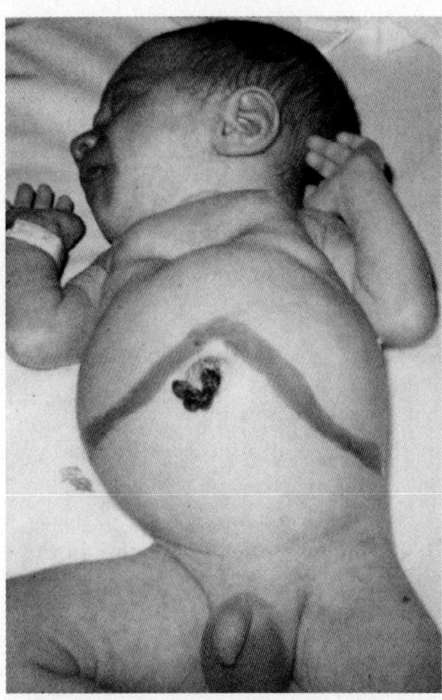

FIGURE 13.3. Abdominal distention resulting from massive hepatosplenomegaly in infant. Note the distention is more prominent in the upper abdomen. (From Fletcher MA. *Physical diagnosis in Neonatology*. Philadelphia, PA: Lippincott-Raven Publishers, 1998:354.)

anterior fontanelle, hypotonia, **bony calcific stippling of joints,** liver dysfunction, and early death.

DISORDERS OF ENERGY METABOLISM

Disorders of energy metabolism include disorders of **mitochondrial energy production** defects and disorders of **gluconeogenesis.** They are often quite severe and refractory to treatment, although as with most other IEMs there can be a spectrum of presentations. **Lactic acidemia** and/or elevated CSF lactate is a feature of many, but not all, of these disorders. Elevated lactate can also be accompanied by an alteration in the lactate to pyruvate ratio signifying an altered cellular redox state. Defects in the respiratory chain can have a wide range of clinical presentations ranging from **Leigh syndrome** to fatal neonatal lactic acidemia. Unfortunately, there is not sufficient treatment available for these disorders, and treatment is primarily supportive.

DISORDERS OF LYSOSOME METABOLISM

Functions of cellular organelles can be disrupted by accumulation of a toxic substance within the organelle or malformation/lack of formation of the entire organelle. Disorders of lysosome metabolism include the mucopolysaccharidoses, the lipidoses, and the ML. The mucopolysaccharidoses result from a deficiency of degradation of acid mucopolysaccharides leading to lysosomal accumulation and include Hunter, Hurler, and Sanfilippo disease. The lipidoses include mannosidosis, I-cell disease, and sialidosis. The ML include Niemann-Pick, Krabbe, Fabry, Gaucher, and Tay-Sachs disease. Characteristics of the major lysosomal storage disorders are shown in Table 13.4.

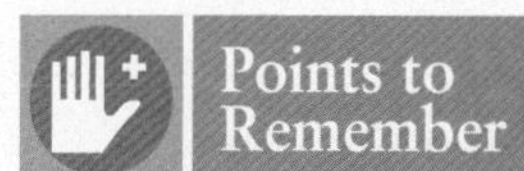

Points to Remember

- **Unlike patients with Hurler syndrome, patients with Hunter syndrome do not have cataracts.**

SAMPLE BOARD REVIEW QUESTIONS

1. A 2-year-old child is brought to your office because her parents are concerned that she is not meeting her speech and language developmental milestones. Physical examination is significant for hepatomegaly, coarse facial features, and gingival hypertrophy. The most likely laboratory abnormality is:
   - **a.** Abnormal urine organic acid profile
   - **b.** Lactic acidemia
   - **c.** Increased lactate to pyruvate ratio
   - **d.** Abnormal plasma amino acids
   - **e.** Mucopolysaccharides in the urine

Answer: e. This child likely has a lysosomal storage disorder, more specifically a mucopolysaccharidoses. This family of diseases results from a deficiency of degradation of acid mucopolysaccharides leading to lysosomal accumulation. The degradation of heparan sulfate, dermatan sulfate, keratan sulfate, or chondroitin sulfate, alone or in combination, may be involved, depending on the specific enzyme affected. These excess products are excreted in the urine.

2. You send the child described in (1) for further diagnostic workup including an ophthalmologic examination. If this child has abnormal ophthalmologic findings, which of the following is most likely?
   a. Cataracts
   b. Lens dislocation
   c. Morning glory anomaly
   d. Coloboma
   e. Aniridia

Answer: a. Cataracts are a finding in some of the mucopolysaccharidoses including Hurler syndrome.

3. You are called to evaluate an infant who was apneic and began seizing shortly after birth and required intubation. The infant appears to be nondysmorphic. The mother of this child noticed increased fetal hiccups while in utero. An EEG showed a burst suppression pattern. The diagnostic test of choice to prove the most likely diagnosis is:
   a. CSF to plasma glycine ratio
   b. CSF lactate
   c. Urine organic acids
   d. Urine amino acids
   e. Renal ultrasound

Answer: a. This child most likely has NKH. A burst suppression pattern on the EEG and apnea should raise high suspicion for this disease. This diagnosis is made by a drawing simultaneous plasma and CSF amino acids. A CSF glycine to plasma glycine ratio greater than 0.08 is diagnostic. Mothers with infants who have NKH often note increased fetal hiccups, which continue after birth.

4. A 2-year-old previously healthy child presents to your emergency department unresponsive. The history given by the parents is that the child had a 1-day history of gastroenteritis with vomiting, diarrhea, and refusal to eat. Urinalysis had a specific gravity of 1.015 and was negative for glucose, ketones, bacteria, nitrites, leukocyte esterase, and white blood cells. The metabolic panel was remarkable for Na of 138 mEq/L, Cl of 112 mEq/L, K of 3.6 mEq/L, CO_2 of 12 mEq/L, glucose of 15 mg/dL, and a blood urea nitrogen of 32 mg/dL. What biochemical abnormality is likely the cause of this child's neurologic decompensation?
   a. Abnormality in the urea cycle
   b. Abnormality in fatty acid oxidation
   c. Abnormality of BCAA metabolism
   d. Abnormality of lysosome storage
   e. Abnormality of neurotransmitter production

Answer: b. This child likely has a disorder of fatty acid oxidation, such as MCAD. The combination of hypoglycemia without ketonuria should raise the suspicion for this family of disorders. When fasting, these patients are not able to utilize fatty acids for energy production. These patients are unable to produce ketones because of incomplete metabolism of fatty acids, the complete breakdown of which would normally result in ketone production.

5. The method of prevention of further episodes of crisis in the child described in (4) is:
   a. High-fat diet
   b. Low-protein diet
   c. Avoidance of fasting
   d. Lactose-free diet
   e. Elemental diet

Answer: c. The goal of treating children with disorders of fatty acid oxidation is to avoid fasting and the need to use fatty acids for fuel. Children with these disorders should be seen promptly for medical intervention in times of intercurrent illness if oral feeds are not tolerated.

6. You see a 3-month-old child who was apparently normal at birth but whose parents now have concerns about reduced muscle tone. The child is globally hypotonic and underweight. She also appears to have an enlarged tongue. A chest x-ray shows an enlarged

heart, and EKG shows biventricular hypertrophy. What is the likely cause of this child's heart disease?

a. Hurler syndrome
b. Galactosemia
c. McArdle's disease
d. Pompe disease
e. Gaucher disease

Answer: d. This child likely has Pompe disease, which is a GSD caused by deficiency of lysosomal alpha-glucosidase. Pompe disease causes myopathy, cardiomyopathy, and hepatomegaly because of buildup of glycogen storage in these organs. The enlarged tongue is caused by buildup of glycogen storage products in the tongue muscle. The natural course of this disease is death in infancy due to the cardiac disease.

7. A 2-week-old former full-term infant who was doing well for the first few days of life now presents to your emergency department with persistent vomiting. Laboratory testing reveals conjugated hyperbilirubinemia. Further urine testing shows reducing substances in the urine. The most likely abnormality on the newborn screen is:

a. Elevated levels of phenylalanine
b. Reduced levels of biotinidase enzyme activity
c. Reduced activity of GALT enzyme
d. Elevated levels of C4 substances on acylcarnitine profile
e. Abnormal hemoglobin electrophoresis

Answer: c. This child likely has classical galactosemia. The newborn screen will detect elevated levels of galactose, and based on this further testing will show reduced activity of GALT enzyme, the enzyme deficiency responsible for classical galactosemia. An interesting note about testing for urine reducing substances is that both glucose and lactose will give a positive test. Therefore, the test is considered to be suspicious for galactosemia if there is positive urine reducing substances but no glucose.

8. The child described in (7) is at higher risk than a normal infant for sepsis caused by what organism?

a. *E. coli*
b. *Salmonella*
c. *Haemophilus influenzae*
d. Group B *Streptococcus*
e. Measles

Answer: a. An infant presenting with *E. coli* sepsis should raise suspicion for galactosemia. The reason for the increased risk in galactosemia is unknown. Infants presenting with *E. coli* sepsis should be tested for galactosemia.

9. Upon reintroduction of oral feeds after recovery in the child described in (7), what is the most appropriate formula?

a. High-calorie cow's milk–based formula
b. Soy-based formula
c. Standard-calorie cow's milk–based formula
d. Low iron infant formula
e. Elemental formula

Answer: b. Infants with galactosemia cannot tolerate lactose and should receive a soy-based formula. Elemental formulas are expensive and unnecessary in this case.

10. A 2-week-old former full-term infant with no prenatal risk factors presents to your emergency department with altered mental status. The complete blood cell count with differential is unremarkable, and there are no signs of trauma. The metabolic panel is remarkable for: Na of 138 mEq/L, Cl of 112 mEq/L, K of 3.6 mEq/L, CO_2 of 15 mEq/L, glucose of 65 mg/dL, and a blood urea nitrogen of 19 mg/dL. Ammonia and lactate levels are normal. Upon obtaining urine for a urinalysis, the nurse comments that the urine has an unusually sweet odor. The laboratory abnormality expected is:

a. Metabolic acidosis with anion gap
b. Abnormal urine organic acids with elevation in methylmalonic acid
c. Elevated ammonia levels
d. Abnormal plasma amino acids with elevation in the BCAAs
e. Unbalanced translocation of chromosomes 5 and 12

Answer: d. This child likely has MSUD. This is an abnormality in the branched-chain alpha-keto acid dehydrogenase enzyme responsible for the metabolism of leucine, isoleucine, and valine. This is seen only on plasma amino acids, and all other laboratory studies to detect metabolic abnormalities may be unrevealing.

11. A 4-month-old infant presents to your office with developmental regression. On physical examination, he has an increased startle response. Ophthalmologic examination shows a cherry red spot on the macula, and enzyme testing reveals lack of hexosaminidase A enzyme. The inheritance pattern of the gene responsible for this disease is:

a. Both the mother and father have one normal copy and one mutant copy of the gene
b. The mother has a mutant copy of this gene encoded in her mitochondrial DNA
c. The father has one mutant and one normal copy of the gene, and the mother has two normal copies of the gene
d. Both parents have two normal copies of the gene
e. Both parents have two mutant copies of the gene

Answer: a. This child has Tay-Sachs disease. This is inherited in an autosomal recessive manner, in which one mutant copy of each gene has to be inherited from each parent for the disease to manifest in the offspring.

12. What effective medical therapy is available to treat the disease in the child described in (11)?

a. Protein-restricted diet
b. Enzyme replacement therapy with hexosaminidase A enzyme
c. Supportive care only
d. Fat-restricted diet
e. Supplementation with oleic and erucic acid

Answer: c There is no effective medical therapy that can reverse or halt the neurologic decline associated with Tay-Sachs disease. The only medical therapy is supportive care including nutritional support, respiratory care, and antiepileptics.

13. A 14-year-old previously healthy girl is seen in the emergency department for change in mental status associated with a viral gastroenteritis. Her laboratory tests are as follows: urinalysis had a specific gravity of 1.015, and was positive for large ketones and negative for glucose, bacteria, nitrites, leukocyte esterase, or white blood cells. The metabolic panel was remarkable for: Na of 138 mEq/L, Cl of 112 mEq/L, K of 3.6 mEq/L, CO_2 of 15 mEq/L, glucose of 65 mg/dL, and a blood urea nitrogen of 6 mg/dL and a creatinine of 0.8 mg/dL. Ammonia concentration was 210 μmol/L. The likely causative underlying disease is:

a. Ornithine transcarbamylase (OTC) deficiency
b. Late onset maple syrup urine disease
c. Medium-chain Acyl-CoA Dehydrogenase deficiency (MCAD)
d. Gaucher disease
e. Phenylketonuria

Answer: a. OTC deficiency is a urea cycle disorder and has an X-linked inheritance pattern. Females are variably affected and can present any time during their lifetime. The combination of hyperammonemia, lack of anion gap, ketonuria, and a low blood urea nitrogen should suggest a urea cycle disorder.

14. A tall and thin 20-year-old patient is seen in your office. He has an IQ of 65. He has a history of eye lens dislocation. Plasma amino acids are significant for a very high homocysteine level and a low methionine level. What medical complication has a high likelihood of manifesting in this patient?

a. Hyperammonemia and increased intracerebral pressure
b. Hyperleucinemia and increased intracerebral pressure
c. Cherry red spot on the macula
d. Acute vascular thrombosis and stroke
e. Pulmonary hypertension

Answer: d. This patient has homocystinuria, which carries with it a risk of up to 50% of having a vascular event by the age of 30 years.

15. Zellweger syndrome and childhood adrenoleukodystrophy are due to defects in what cellular organelle?

a. Lysosome
b. Mitochondria
c. Peroxisome
d. Endoplasmic reticulum
e. Ribosome

Answer c. Defects in the protein ALDP lead to abnormal fatty oxidation of very-long-chain fatty acids in the peroxisome and cause adrenoleukodystrophy. Zellweger syndrome is caused by defects in the biogenesis of the entire peroxisome, and there are various causative genes.

SUGGESTED READINGS

Levy PA. Inborn errors of metabolism: part 1: overview. *Pediatr Rev*. 2009;30:131–138.
Levy PA. Inborn errors of metabolism: part 2: specific disorders. *Pediatr Rev*. 2009;30:e22–e28.
Staretz-Chacham O, Lang TC, LaMarca ME, et al. Lysosomal storage disorders in the newborn. *Pediatrics*. 2009;123:1191–1207.
Scriver CR, Sly WS, Childs B, et al. eds. *The Metabolic & Molecular Bases of Inherited Disease*. 8th ed. New York, NY: McGraw-Hill, 2001.

CHAPTER 14 ■ GROWTH & DEVELOPMENT

SABRINA R. VINEBERG

AAP	American Academy of Pediatrics	MBP	Munchausen-by-proxy
ADHD	attention-deficit/hyperactivity disorder	MR	Mental retardation
CBC	Complete blood count	NOS	Not otherwise specified
CD	Conduct disorder	OCD	Obsessive compulsive disorder
CMV	Cytomegalovirus	ODD	Oppositional defiant disorder
CNS	Central nervous system	PDD	Pervasive developmental disorder
CP	Cerebral palsy	PEDS	Parents' Evaluation of Developmental Stages
CRP	C reactive protein	PKU	Phenylketonuria
CSF	Cerebrospinal fluid	PPD	Purified protein derivative
DQ	Developmental quotient	PTSD	Posttraumatic stress disorder
ESR	Erythrocyte sedimentation rate	REM	Rapid eye movement
FTT	Failure to thrive	SSRI	Selective serotonin reuptake inhibitor
GAD	Generalized anxiety disorder		
GI	Gastrointestinal	TCA	tricyclic antidepressant
ICP	Intracranial pressure	UA	urinalysis
IQ	Intelligence quotient	UTI	Urinary tract infection
LFT	Liver function test	VCUG	Voiding cystourethrography

CHAPTER OBJECTIVES

1. To understand the factors contributing to normal childhood growth, how to properly assess growth, and to recognize when growth is abnormal
2. To understand how to assess development in children
3. To recognize when development is abnormal and to understand the classic features, diagnosis, and treatment of major developmental abnormalities
4. To understand behavioral and psychosocial issues that can affect development in children of different ages
5. To understand how external and societal factors can influence child development.

INTRODUCTION

A thorough knowledge of human growth and development is fundamental to anyone working within the discipline of Pediatrics. The fact that children change so much as they grow and learn is what makes studying them and caring for them so exciting. The summary of topics reviewed below will help you to recognize the difference between normal and abnormal growth and development. To this end, the chapter has been organized into the following headings:

- Growth and its measurements.
- FTT.
- Development.
- Sensory and communication disorders.
- CP.
- MR.
- Autism spectrum disorders.

In addition, it is important to have a basic understanding of the behavioral and psychosocial issues common to each age group, as well as the specific external influences and events that have an impact on child development. These subjects are also reviewed within this chapter. At the close of the chapter you will find a question section to help solidify your knowledge base of these areas through practice.

GROWTH AND ITS MEASUREMENTS

There are several ways that growth is assessed and defined in infants, children, and adolescents. This section includes not only a discussion of these measurements, which include height, weight, and head circumference, but also clinical scenarios in which abnormal growth should be identified.

Linear Growth and Weight

- Adequacy of growth is determined by comparison to other children of the same age; therefore, height (*length in infants and toddlers*) and weight should be measured and plotted at every health supervision visit.
- Causes for:
  - *Short stature*: malnutrition, chronic illness, endocrine disorders, syndromes associated with dwarfism, familial short stature.
  - *Tall stature*: genetic disorders, neurologic syndromes, pituitary abnormalities.
  - *Underweight*: similar to short stature.
  - *Overweight*: often due to exogenous factors (overeating) and associated with increased height. Can also be a result of genetic syndromes such as Prader-Willi and Bardet-Biedl syndrome.

Points to Remember

- For a full review of these topics refer to the Endocrine chapter.
- If a child is overweight as a result of an endocrine abnormality, they will usually have *decreased* height for age.

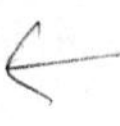

Growth Velocity

- Healthy infants may initially lose up to 10% of their birth weight but should regain birth weight by 10 to 14 days, and then gain approximately 30 grams per day for the first month.
- Average birth weight is 3.5 kg (approximately 7.5 lb).
- After 2 months, growth velocity slows to approximately 20 grams per day.
- By the age of 3 years, growth velocity slows to about 3 inches and 4 to 6 lb per year and remains relatively stable until puberty.

Points to Remember

- Birth weight generally doubles by 5 months, triples by 12 months
- Birth length increases by 50% by the age of 1 year, doubles by the age of 4 years
- Normal head growth is 1 cm per month for the first 6 months, 0.5 cm per month from 6 to 12 months

Prematurity

- Very low-birth-weight infants may lose up to 12% to 15% of their birth weight, and may take up to 20 days to regain birth weight.
- Catch-up growth may take up to 8 weeks or more, often requiring parenteral and enteral nutrition with caloric intake of 120 to 140 kcal/kg/day.

Head Growth

- Head circumference should be measured in all children younger than 2 years.
- Abnormal head size or head growth can be congenital or acquired, and the degree of associated neurologic deficit is related to the etiology of the abnormal head size.

Microcephaly

- *Definition*: head circumference 2 standard deviations below the mean: approximately 35 cm for girls and 36 cm for boys.
- *Etiologies*: include early closure of sutures, chromosomal abnormalities, intrauterine infection, metabolic disorder, perinatal insult.
- *Associated anomalies* may include agyria, lissencephaly, and schizencephaly.

Macrocephaly

- *Definition*: head circumference 2 standard deviations above the mean.
- *Etiologies*: many potential causes and syndromes that predispose children to macrocephaly including hydrocephalus, metabolic disorder, neurocutaneous syndromes, glycogen/lysosomal storage diseases. Genetic factors may predispose to macrocephaly—check parental head size.

Hydrocephalus

- *Definition*: Excess CSF within the ventricles. Hydrocephalus may cause increased ICP and loss of brain tissue.
- There are two types of hydrocephalus:
  - *Noncommunicating*: block with in ventricular system.
  - *Communicating*: block outside ventricular system.

- Hydrocephalus is most commonly related to impaired CSF absorption or obstruction of CSF flow but can rarely be related to increased CSF production.
- *Etiologies*: include congenital malformations (myelomeningocele with Chiari malformation, Dandy-Walker malformation), arachnoid cysts or tumors, intrauterine or postnatal infections (rubella, CMV, toxoplasmosis, syphilis, bacterial infection), and intraventricular hemorrhage in premature infants.
- *Physical examination*: findings in infants include bulging fontanelle, splayed cranial sutures, and impaired upward gaze.

Breast Hypertrophy

- Breast hypertrophy can be normal at birth (boys and girls) because of the presence of maternal hormones but should regress within 6 months.
- Premature thelarche:
  - *Definition*: breast enlargement without development of nipples or areola.
  - Premature thelarche can occur in girls 1 to 4 years of age and may be unilateral. There is no associated linear growth or hair development. Girls should have normal bone age. Close follow-up recommended because it may be difficult to distinguish this condition from the onset of precocious puberty.
  - Pubertal gynecomastia is breast hypertrophy that occurs, not uncommonly, in boys Tanner stage 2 to 3. It may be unilateral. It is related to an increased estradiol to testosterone ratio. Pubertal gynecomastia is managed by providing reassurance to patient and family.

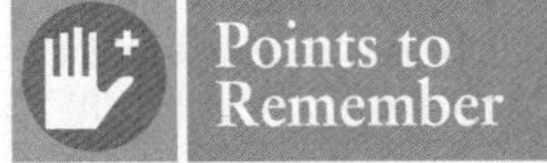

- **Breast hypertrophy is also discussed in the Endocrine and Adolescent Medicine chapters**

Conditions associated with abnormal growth: Multiple disorders and chronic diseases are associated with abnormal growth (see Table 14.1).

TABLE 14.1

CONDITIONS ASSOCIATED WITH ABNORMAL GROWTH[a]

GI disorders
Short bowel syndrome
Inflammatory bowel disease (Crohn disease/ulcerative colitis)
Celiac disease
Cystic fibrosis (malabsorption due to pancreatic insufficiency)
Endocrine disorders
Thyroid disease
Growth hormone deficiency
Panhypopituitarism
Genetic syndromes associated with abnormal growth patterns
Overgrowth/obesity
Bardet-Biedl syndrome
Beckwith-Wiedemann syndrome
Carpenter syndrome
Cohen syndrome (obesity, hypotonia, prominent incisors)
Prader-Willi syndrome
Sotos syndrome
Weaver syndrome (accelerated growth and maturation, macrosomia, craniofacial anomalies, camptodactyly)
Tall stature
Homocystinuria
Klinefelter syndrome
Marfan syndrome
XYY syndrome
Short stature
Achondroplasia/hypochondroplasia
Bloom syndrome
Jeune syndrome
Mucopolysaccharidoses (Hunter and Hurler syndromes)
Noonan syndrome
Opitz syndrome
Robinow syndrome
Russell-Silver syndrome
Rubinstein-Taybi syndrome
Seckel syndrome (severe short stature, microcephaly, prominent nose)
Turner syndrome

[a]For further review of these topics, please refer to individual chapters.
GI, gastrointestinal.

FAILURE TO THRIVE

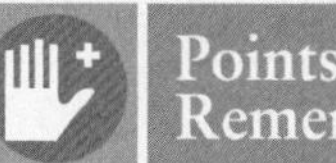

Points to Remember

- **Children with trisomy 21 grow at different rates than other children. As a result, there are special growth charts for use in children with trisomy 21.**

FTT, while often used as a diagnosis, is usually a "sign" of another problem or underlying medical condition. The term is used to describe children who fail to gain weight adequately in childhood. Although there is often no organic etiology for FTT, an underlying cause may be found in a small percentage of children. A brief review of FTT is provided below.

Definition

Weight less than 5th *percentile on more than one occasion or weight below 80% of ideal body weight for age*. In severe cases of FTT, linear growth and head circumference may be affected as well. FTT is most common in children younger than 2 years, but older children can be affected as well.

Predisposing Factors

These include low birth weight, intrauterine growth retardation, prematurity, multiple birth, and chronic illness or frequent intercurrent illness.

Etiologies (see Table 14.2)

- Etiologies are either organic or environmental/psychosocial, with the majority of cases of FTT being due to environmental/psychosocial factors. Twenty-five percentage of cases, however, can be attributed to a combination of both.
- When considering an organic etiology:
  - If only weight is affected, consider a primary GI disorder.
  - If weight and height are affected, consider a primary endocrine disorder or severe nutritional problem.
  - If weight, height, and head circumference are affected, consider a primary neurologic disorder or systemic disease.

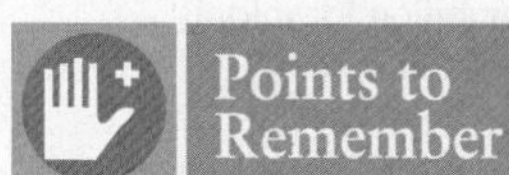

Points to Remember

- **When weight, height, and head circumference are all affected in a child with FTT, the etiology can be attributed to organic disease 70% of the time.**

Evaluation

Evaluation of a child with suspected FTT should include the following:

- *Observation* of child/caregiver interaction and interaction between parents/caregivers.
- A detailed *nutritional history* including duration of feeding, quantity and type of food, avoidance of specific foods or textures, and stool pattern/consistency.
- *Psychosocial history*: number of caretakers; who lives in the home; employment and financial status; presence of family stress; and maternal factors including maternal age, planned versus unplanned pregnancy, family support, and presence of postpartum depression.
- *Accurate measurements* of weight, height, and head circumference.
- A complete *developmental assessment* and identification of any delays.
- Look for *signs of neglect* (see *Child Maltreatment* section for more information).
- *Laboratory studies* to consider, depending on risk factors and physical examination findings—CBC, electrolytes, UA, ESR/CRP, LFTs, HIV, PPD, sweat test.
- When considering an organic etiology as the cause for FTT, look for signs of:
  - *Genetic syndromes*: dysmorphic features.
  - *Neurologic/CNS dysfunction*: hypotonia/spasticity.
  - *Pulmonary, cardiac, GI disorder*: frequent respiratory infections, swallow dysfunction or gastroesophageal reflux, evidence of malabsorption.

Treatment/Prognosis

- Goal of treatment is to enable catch-up growth. Nutritional requirements in children with FTT should be based on expected weight not actual weight.
- Severe malnutrition can predispose to malabsorption or electrolyte abnormalities during refeeding; therefore, these children should be hospitalized.
- If no weight is gained in 4 to 6 weeks and no underlying organic etiology is discovered, consider nasogastric supplementation.
- Prognosis is generally good with multidisciplinary involvement and close follow-up but 25% to 60% of infants with FTT will remain small for age.

TABLE 14.2

CAUSES OF FAILURE TO THRIVE

Inadequate Caloric Intake		Inadequate Appetite or Inability to Eat Large Amounts	Inadequate Caloric Absorption: No Weight Gain during Refeeding; Increased Losses	Increased Caloric Requirements
Weight Gain During Refeeding	**No Weight Gain During Refeeding**			
Inappropriate feeding technique Disturbed mother/child relationship[a] Inappropriate nutrient intakc (excess fruit juice consumption, factitious food allergy, inadequate quantity of food, inappropriate food tor age, neglect, inappropriate preparation of formula, food fads) Inappropriate parental knowledge of correct nutrition for infants and children	Psychosocial problems[a] Maternal/infant dysfunction, economic deprivation Mechanical problems (adenoidal hypertrophy, dental lesions, vascular slings) Insufficient lactation in mother Cleft palate Nasal obstruction Sucking or swallowing dysfunction (CNS, neuromuscular, esophageal motility problems) Regurgitation (gastroesophageal reflux) Malformation (posterior urethral valves) Congenital syndromes (alcohol, phenytoin, drugs) Generic syndromes (Turner, trisomies 21,18,13)	Psychosocial problems (apathy)[a] Cardiopulmonary disease Hypotonia (muscle weakness) Anorexia of chronic infection (chronic sinusitis) or immune deficiency diseases (HIV infection or AIDS) Endocrine disorders (hypothyroidism, diabetes insipidus) CNS tumors Genetic syndromes Metabolic conditions (lead toxicity, iron deficiency, zinc deficiency) Anemia Chronic constipation Disturbance in appetite and satiety	Psychosocial problems (refeeding diarrhea, intercurrent illnesses, hepatitis, rumination, regurgitation)[a] Malabsorption—diarrhea (lactose intolerance, cystic fibrosis, cardiac disease, malrotation, inflammatory bowel disease, milk allergy, parasites, celiac disease) Vomiting or "spitting up" or diarrhea (gastroenteritis, congenital adrenal hyperplasia) Intestinal tract obstruction (pyloric stenosis, hernia, malrotation, intussusception, chalasia) Biliary atresia/cirrhosis CNS problems—increased intracranial pressure (subdural hematoma) Chronic metabolic problems (hypercalcemia, storage diseases, and inborn errors of metabolism such as galactosemia, methylmalonic acidemia, renal tubular acidosis, diabetes mellitus, adrenal insufficiency) Necrotizing enterocolitis or short bowel syndrome	Hyperthyroidism Cerebral palsy Malignancy Chronic systemic disease (juvenile rheumatoid arthritis) Chronic systemic infection (UTI, HIV, tuberculosis, toxoplasmosis) Chronic respiratory insufficiency (bronchopulmonary dysplasia, cystic fibrosis) Congenital or acquired heart disease Anemia Toxins (lead)

[a]Environmental causes are the most common source of problems.
CNS, central nervous system; HIV, human immunodeficiency virus, UTI, urinary tract infection.

DEVELOPMENT

It is crucial for all pediatricians, regardless of practice area, to have a thorough understanding of normal child development. This allows us to not only counsel parents about normal behavior, but also to alert them to abnormalities that may require further investigation. A child's development is influenced by multiple factors, including family, culture, and community. This section provides an overview on assessing development, a review of key developmental milestones, and a discussion of abnormal development. Specific developmental abnormalities, such as MR and CP, are discussed in more detail in later sections of this chapter.

Assessing Development

- The role of the pediatrician includes monitoring of development, detection and diagnosis of abnormal development, and coordination of developmental services and specialists.
- There are five major streams of development:
  - Visual-motor.
  - Language (cognitive).
  - Motor.
  - Social.
  - Adaptive.
- Development is assessed through screening tools (e.g., PEDS, Ages and Stages). These should not be used to make a definitive diagnosis, but rather to help determine which children require further evaluation.

Points to Remember

- Developmental milestones should be assessed at every well-child visit.

Points to Remember

- When assessing development in premature infants:
  - Use the original due date, not actual birth date, to calculate the age of the infant (i.e., a 32-week preemie at 12 weeks of age would be expected to have the milestones of a 1-month old, not a 3-month old).
  - Most premature infants catch-up by 2 years of age, so no need to correct after this point.

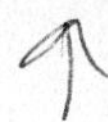

Intelligence Testing

- The *Wechsler Scale* is used most commonly for intelligence testing. There are separate tests for preschool, school-aged, and adult patients. This tool produces scores for verbal IQ, performance IQ (measures perception, visual-motor coordination, problem solving), and full-scale IQ.
- The *Bayley Scales of Infant Development* is used for testing in infants and can be used for infants as young as 1 month of age.

Measures of Academic Achievement

- *Peabody Individual Achievement Test* measures reading recognition and comprehension, spelling, general information, and math. There is a separate subtest for written expression.
- *Woodcock-Johnson Psycho-Educational Battery* includes tests of cognitive ability and achievement (reading score, math score, measure of writing ability, knowledge of science, social studies, humanities).
- *Wechsler Individual Achievement Test* measures basic reading, mathematics and numeric operations, spelling, reading comprehension, listening comprehension, and oral and written expression.

Developmental Milestones (see Table 14.3)

Abnormal Development

Developmental Delay

It is quantified using *DQ*. DQ = developmental age/chronological age × 100. DQ is calculated separately for different streams of development. Delay is defined as *performance considerably below average (DQ <75) within a given stream.*

Developmental Deviancy

Atypical development within a single stream, in other words, milestones out of sequence. This may be a sign of a CNS abnormality. An example of developmental deviancy is a child who walks before crawling. Such a child may have mild central hypotonia as an etiology for this deviancy.

Developmental Dissociation

Development in one stream occurring at a rate that is significantly different from development in other streams. An example of developmental dissociation is seen in autism, where there is abnormal social development while motor milestones are often normal.

Developmental "Red Flags" (see Table 14.4)

TABLE 14.3

NORMAL DEVELOPMENTAL MILESTONES

	Gross Motor	Fine Motor	Language (Expressive and Receptive)	Cognitive/Social/Adaptive
Birth to 2 mo	Presence of primitive reflexes Holds head up momentarily	Fixes and follows slow moving targets Hands closed	Crying, short vowel sound, guttural noises Startles Turns to sound (bell or voice)	Visual preference for human face
2–4 mo	Head up 45° then 90° Weight on forearms when prone	Follows past midline (180°) Bats at objects Brings hands to midline by 4 mo Hands open	Cooing, long vowel sounds	Social smile Vocalizing Associates sounds with particular people and objects by 4 mo
4–6 mo	Weight on hands with arms extended Sits with support or propping Rolls (first prone to supine, then supine to prone)	Reaches with both hands Puts objects in mouth	Raspberries Laughs and squeals Orients to voice	Follows the path of an object that is dropped Smiles at mirror Excites at sight of food
6–9 mo	Sits without support Creeps and crawls Bears weight with support May pull to stand by 9 mo	Unilateral reach Rakes with all fingers Transfers object from one hand to the other Rotates hand while holding object	Simple consonant babbling, imitates sound Recognizes own name	Stranger anxiety Separation anxiety Enjoys mirror
9–12 mo	Moves to sitting position independently Pulls to stand Cruises Walks independently	Crude pincer with thumb opposite several fingers to fine pincer with thumb and index finger by 12 mo Points with index finger Turns pages of a book Uses cup Cooperates with dressing	"Mama," "Dada" nonspecific at first, then specific, usually has first word by 12 mo Understands "no" Recognizes objects by name Follows one-step commands with gestures	Object permanence Peek-a-boo and patty cake (10 mo) Waves "bye-bye" (10 mo) Makes postural adjustments with dressing (12 mo)
15 mo	Walks well Runs Pivots Walks backwards Creeps up stairs Can sit in chair	Stacks two blocks Uses spoon Removes shoes	Four to six words Knows some body parts Follows one-step command w/o gesture	Parallel play Hugs parents Indicates desires by pointing
18 mo	Walks up stairs with help or rail Throws ball Squats (21 mo)	Builds tower of three to four blocks Scribbles spontaneously Imitates strokes on paper Uses spoon for solids without spilling Removes most clothes	Ten or more words Combines two words Points to at least five body parts Begins to name body parts Follows two-step commands	Beginning of interest in toilet training Beginning of magical thinking/symbolic play Imitates household chores
24 mo	Runs well Jumps with two feet Stands on one foot briefly Kicks ball Up and down stairs, two feet per step	Builds tower of four to six blocks Copies vertical line Uses spoon and fork Puts on some clothes with help Turns pages singly Place pieces in formboard puzzles	50+ word vocabulary, uses "I," "me," and "mine", two- to three-word phrases 25%–50% of speech understandable to strangers Follows commands with two actions/two objects	Helps to undress Listens to stories with pictures

(continued)

TABLE 14.3

CONTINUED

	Gross Motor	Fine Motor	Language (Expressive and Receptive)	Cognitive/Social/Adaptive
36 mo	Goes up the stairs one foot at a time Rides tricycle Balances on one foot	Builds tower of eight to ten blocks Copies a circle May be able to copy a cross by 3.5 y Eats neatly Dresses independently	900 words, 5–8 word sentences 75% of speech understandable Knows first and last name, age, and sex Uses "I" and other pronouns (around 30 mo) Asks "why" Understands concepts like "cold," "tired," "hungry"	Cooperative play, sharing
4 y	Skips Hops on one foot Climbs Catches a ball in both hands	Copies a cross Cuts with scissors Draws person with head and one other body part	Understands and verbalizes concepts of size, numbers, shapes Counts to five Identifies four colors Ask "why," "when," and "how" questions; tells a story Speech 100% understandable	Able to follow rules of more complex games by 4.5 y Imaginative play
5 y	Skips rope Jumps from height and lands on feet Skates and swims	Copies a square Prints first name Ties shoelaces Draws a person with six body parts	Follows a series of three simple instructions Reads a few letters Tells meaning of familiar words	Domestic role playing Plays board or card games
6 y	Rides a bike	Copies a horizontal diamond	Learns to understand rules of syntax and grammar Learns to read Expresses feelings and thoughts	

TABLE 14.4

DEVELOPMENTAL "RED FLAGS"

Age	Missed Milestones Requiring Intervention
2 mo	Lack of visual fixation No social smile
4–6 mo	Fails to track person or object No steady head control No response/turn to sound or voice
6 mo	Decrease/absence of vocalizations
9–12 mo	Fails to sit independently Lack of babbling with consonant sounds
18 mo	Fails to walk independently Does not seek shared attention to object/event with caregiver
24 mo	No single words
36 mo	No three word sentences Cannot follow simple commands
>3 y	Speech unintelligible Dependence on gestures to follow commands

SENSORY AND COMMUNICATION DISORDERS

Abnormal development has many causes, among them problems with vision and hearing. Deviation from normal development often comes to attention when children are unable to communicate as would be expected for their age. This section will provide a review of sensory disorders including hearing impairment and visual impairment and a discussion of language and communication disorders.

Points to Remember

- For more information on hearing and vision screening tests, please refer to Preventive Pediatrics, Biostatistics, & Ethics chapter.

Hearing Impairment

- Hearing impairment is identified using a hearing screen. The purpose of identifying hearing impairment is to prevent speech and language delay, which can have significant long-term behavioral, emotional, and educational consequences.

Etiologies

- *Congenital*: infections (e.g., CMV, rubella), chromosomal disorders, maternal drug use during pregnancy, prematurity.
- *Acquired*: perforated tympanic membrane, otitis media with effusion, cholesteatoma, tympanosclerosis, ototoxic drugs.
- Red flags for the presence of hearing impairment include the following:
  - Inattentiveness.
  - Talking inappropriately loudly at all times.
  - Volume turned excessively high on TV or radio.
  - Difficulty in the classroom.
- It is important to distinguish *sensorineural* hearing loss from *conductive* hearing loss. Mixed forms of hearing loss can occur as well.

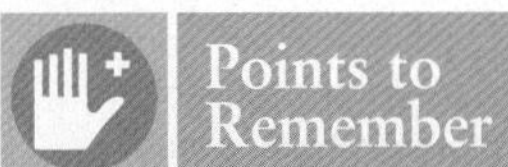

Points to Remember

- Conductive hearing loss: no transmission of sound waves from external ear to cochlea
- Sensorineural hearing loss: no transmission of signal to brainstem.

Treatment

The use of hearing aids and assistive listening devices is beneficial both in and out of the classroom. Placement of children with hearing impairment at the front of the classroom may further optimize learning.

Visual Impairment

- Signs of visual impairment in children are often unrecognized by family members or even by the children themselves; therefore, early screening and detection by the pediatrician is crucial.
- Signs, symptoms, and behaviors often associated with visual impairment and uncorrected refractive errors in children include the following:
  - Frequent eye rubbing, squinting, blinking.
  - Torticollis.
  - Frequent closing or covering of one eye.
  - Holding books very close to the face, sitting very close to the TV.
  - Complaints of pain, blurry vision, double vision, headaches, fatigue.
  - Photophobia or tearing.
  - Problems with hand-eye coordination.

Strabismus

- *Definition*: ocular misalignment.
- Intermittent strabismus can be normal until 6 months of age. Persistent strabismus will lead to eventual suppression of the image from the deviated eye in an effort to prevent diplopia. Undiagnosed/untreated strabismus will eventually lead to amblyopia.

Points to Remember

- Pediatric glaucoma and cataracts can lead to amblyopia and vision loss if undetected and untreated.
- For more information about visual impairment please refer to Ophthalmology chapter.

Amblyopia

Definition: *loss of visual acuity*, often from disuse (untreated strabismus or refractive error much greater in one eye than the other). Amblyopia becomes harder to treat as children get older and delay of/lack of input to neurons in the visual cortex has been prolonged.

Glaucoma

Can be congenital or acquired. Signs and symptoms include corneal clouding or enlargement, tearing, ocular injection, photophobia, and blepharospasm.

Cataracts

One-third of cataracts are congenital. Screening for congenital cataracts consists of evaluation for the presence of red reflex with an ophthalmoscope at birth. Significant infantile cataracts require immediate surgical intervention.

Language Delay and Communication Disorders

Language delay is the most sensitive indicator of possible MR and communication disorders. It is also a risk factor for future learning disability and poor academic performance. Fifty percentage of children with language delay will also have delays in other areas. Of note, language delays can also occur as the result of a poor linguistic environment.

Epidemiology

The prevalence of language and speech delays in preschool children is about 15% often with some overlap. In school-aged children with no obvious neurological defects, the prevalence of language and speech disorders is 2% to 3% and 4% to 6%, respectively.

Etiologies

Etiologies for language delay include the following:

- Hearing impairment.
- MR.
- Autism spectrum disorder.
- Structural/anatomic abnormalities.
- Elective mutism.
- Child abuse/neglect.

Evaluation

Evaluation must include the following:

- *Medical history*—prematurity, previous use of aminoglycosides or other ototoxic drugs, known CNS insult or injury.
- *Family history* of speech delay or hearing impairment.
- *Developmental history and screening* including use of specific language screening instruments such as Early Language Milestone (ELM) and Clinical Linguistic Assessment Measurement (CLAM). These instruments help to differentiate between receptive, expressive, mixed language disorders.
- *Behavioral history*—may help to elicit signs of autism.
- *Hearing screen* and *physical examination.*

Expressive Language Disorder

- *Definition*: deficit in expressive language skills such as *fluency*, *syntax*, or *word retrieval*, or a *difficulty in learning new words*. These deficits may be developmental or due to neurologic injury.
- *Red flags* for an expressive language disorder include pointing at objects instead of naming them, using immature grammar, or having disorganized speech.

Mixed Receptive Expressive Language Disorder

In addition to problems with expressive language, these children have difficulty *discriminating sounds* and *understanding words and phrases*. They appear to have difficulty understanding instructions, respond to questions inappropriately, and exhibit poor memory skills.

Stuttering: Impairment in Fluency of Speech

Stuttering can vary in severity and will resolve spontaneously by adolescence in 60% of cases. It is often exacerbated by stress and accompanied by facial or hand tics.

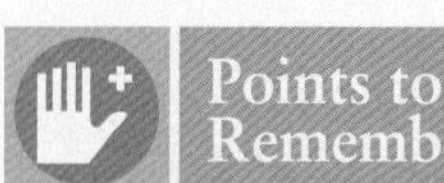

Points to Remember

- **All suspected communication disorders should be referred to speech/language pathologist for formal assessment and treatment, which may include referral to neurologist if indicated.**

Phonological Disorder

In this disorder, children are unable to produce speech sounds that are age-appropriate. Children may lisp, substitute one letter/sound for another, and omit sounds. It is important to distinguish developmentally appropriate abnormalities from true phonological disorder, as most of these abnormalities may be present at some point during normal language development.

CEREBRAL PALSY

CP is the most common movement disorder of childhood, with reported prevalence rates of 1 to 6 per 1,000. Risk factors for CP include birth asphyxia, prematurity, and intrauterine growth retardation; however, it is believed that antenatal events, rather than events related to labor and delivery, actually account for most cases. CP is often associated with other deficits. The types of CP and associated abnormalities are discussed in more detail below.

Definition

Disorder of movement and posture resulting from a CNS insult or anomaly. *Cause is static*, but manifestations can change over time. Progressive neurologic disorders do not cause CP.

Types of CP

- *Spastic*—topographic classification of spastic CP includes the following:
  - Hemiplegia.
  - Diplegia.
  - Spastic quadriplegia.
  - Bilateral hemiplegia.
- *Extrapyramidal*—can be further classified into athetoid, rigid, ataxic, dystonic, and mixed forms.
- CP can also be classified according to severity, which is assessed by the DQ (see Table 14.5).

Diagnosis by Age

CP should ideally be diagnosed by 12 months of age; however, significant motor delay can be identified at any age. For each age group, there are specific findings that should raise concerns for this diagnosis.

- Birth to 6 months
  - CP is difficult to diagnose in infants because early presentations are subtle. Signs include hypotonia, feeding difficulties, adductor tightness making diaper changes difficult, and behavior disturbance (increased colic, impaired periodicity).
  - Look for decreased movement or asymmetric movement, either generalized or in specific limbs. Children may also have signs of increased tone such as scissoring of the lower limbs.
- 6 to 18 months
  - Delayed acquisition of motor milestones is the basis for diagnosis in this age group.
  - Look for persistence of primitive reflexes.

TABLE 14.5

EXPANDED CLASSIFICATION OF CEREBRAL PALSY

Rates of Motor Development	Motor Signs	Associated Dysfunction
Minimal normal: MQ 75–100 Qualitative abnormalities only	Subtle, transient abnormalities of tone Persistence, exaggeration of some primitive reflexes to a mild degree Soft signs reflected as clumsy or awkward motor performance	Communicative disorders Specific learning disabilities ADHD
Mild: MQ 50–74	Transient abnormalities of tone Occasional "hard" signs Persistent primitive reflexes; delayed postural responses Soft signs may be present to functionally important degree (i.e., tremor, synkinesis, poor coordination)	Communicative disorders Specific learning disabilities ADHD
Moderate: MQ 40–50 Assisted ambulation May need bracing Usually does not require assistive devices Pharmacotherapy or nerve blocks may be used	Traditional neurologic findings Many exaggerated obligatory primitive reflexes, some obligatory Postural responses delayed or absent	Mental retardation Communicative disorders Specific learning disabilities Seizures ADHD+ Stereotypic behaviors
Severe, profound: MQ <35 Wheelchair mobility Usually requires bracing, assistive devices, and surgery	Traditional neurologic signs predominate Obligatory primitive reflexes Absent postural reponses	Mental retardation Seizures ADHD++ Stereotypic behaviors

ADHD, attention-deficit hyperactivity disorder; MQ, motor quotient.
Modified from McMillan JA, Feigin RD, DeAngelis C, et al. *Oski's Pediatrics: Principles and Practice*. 4th ed. Philadelphia, PA: Lippincott Williams & Wilkins, 2006.

Comorbidities Associated With CP (Percentage of Children With Comorbidity)

- MR or other learning disabilities/communication disorders (60%).
- Deafness (10%).
- Strabismus (50%).
- Oral-motor dysfunction.
- Seizure (30% to 40%).
- Behavioral disturbance (decreased attention, impulsivity, distractibility).

Treatment

- Aim of treatment is to maximize function and enhance/optimize communication through physical, speech, and occupational therapy.
- Physical therapy and medications (such as intrathecal baclofen, diazepam) are used to help normalize tone.
- Surgery and bracing help prevent, minimize, or correct deformities.

MENTAL RETARDATION

MR, now commonly known as intellectual disability, is a term used to describe significant deficits in cognition. The degree of cognitive delay is most commonly delineated by the IQ; however, it is important to recognize that many other factors influence a child's cognitive behavior and should be taken into account when assessing and treating children with MR. This section will review definitions, diagnosis, treatment, and prognosis of MR.

Definitions

MR is defined as a static encephalopathy. The three components required for diagnosis are *cognitive delay*, *impaired adaptive behavior*, and *onset younger than 18 years*. Children with MR have an IQ that is more than 2 standard deviations below the mean. The majority of individuals with MR (approximately 85%) fall into the mildly delayed range. These individuals have an IQ of 50 to 69 and may be capable of economic independence. Patients with moderate delay (IQ of 35 to 49) are often capable of supported employment and community living. Individuals with severe or profound delay (IQ <34) usually require group home versus institutional placement (Fig. 14.1)

Screening and Diagnosis

- The Pediatrician plays a vital role in early identification of patients with MR. Clinicians must integrate data from specific tests, assessment of developmental milestones, neurobehavioral observations, and parental concerns when considering this diagnosis.
- Although motor development may be normal in patients with MR, 50% to 75% of patients will also have CP or other degree of motor dysfunction (clumsiness, ataxia, tremor). As is the case in Rett's syndrome, motor deterioration may occur over time.

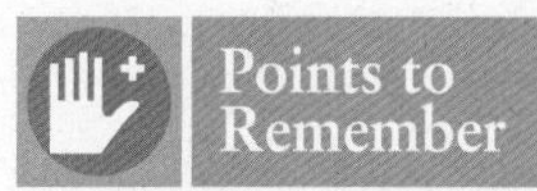

- The most sensitive early marker of MR is impaired language development.

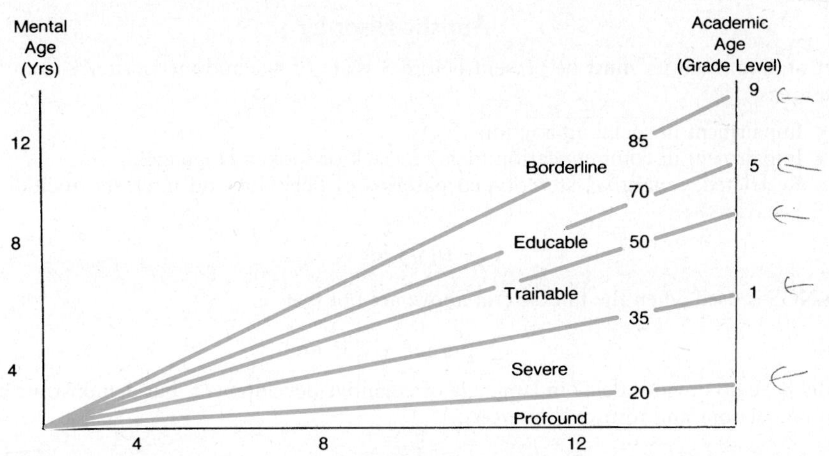

FIGURE 14.1. Levels of academic achievement to be expected with different degrees of intellectual disability at successive ages. (Reprinted with permission from McMillan JA, Feigin RD, DeAngelis C, et al. *Oski's Pediatrics: Principles and Practice*. 4th ed. Philadelphia, PA: Lippincott Williams & Wilkins, 2006.)

- Moderate to severe MR is usually obvious early in development, but milder delays are more difficult to diagnose and may not become evident until the child enters school.
- *Evaluation* should include the following:
  - Familial history, genetic history, prenatal and perinatal history, and detailed developmental history (plateau vs. regression of milestones).
  - Physical examination to identify dysmorphic features or malformations.
  - Formal psychometric testing.
  - Genetic testing and neuroimaging if indicated.
  - Hearing and visual testing.

Treatment and Prognosis

- Multidisciplinary follow-up through medical and educational systems is crucial.
- Coexisting behavioral disorders must be treated as well.
- Children can switch developmental curves over time (accelerate development or plateau with time). In addition, MR and learning disability can coexist, making prognosis more difficult to predict.
- Prognosis depends on degree of impairment. Outcomes are easier to predict in children with lower IQ.
- Failure to self-feed and/or ambulate independently is associated with decreased longevity.

AUTISM SPECTRUM DISORDERS

There has been a great deal of controversy in recent years surrounding the seemingly alarming rate at which children are being diagnosed with autism spectrum disorders, and the possible etiologies for the apparent increase in prevalence of these conditions. Although research is ongoing in this area and it may take awhile before anyone truly understands what causes these disorders, an understanding of the current criteria for diagnosis and ongoing management of children with autism spectrum disorders is an important part of pediatrics.

Definitions and Diagnostic Criteria

PDDs are a group of disorders defined by developmental difficulties across multiple developmental streams. Patients with PDD have impairments in social interaction and personal communication, often with a restricted pattern of interests and activities. Behavior in these children deviates from that which is expected for the child's mental age.

Abnormalities are often present in infancy but not usually recognized until at least the second year of life and include abnormalities of posture and motor behavior such as jumping, hand flapping, and unusual body postures.

Children with PDD often have unusual responses to sensory inputs and an absence of emotional reactions.

According to *DSM-IV*, PDDs include autistic disorder, Rett syndrome, childhood disintegrative disorder, Asperger syndrome, and PDD NOS.

Autistic Disorder

Onset of abnormalities must be present before 3 years of age and meet criteria from three different areas:

- Impairment in social interaction.
- Impairment in communication (delay or lack of spoken language).
- Restricted, repetitive, stereotyped patterns of behavior and interests (including motor behaviors).

PDD NOS

PDD NOS is used when the full criteria above are not met.

Asperger Syndrome

Usually have no obvious delay in language or cognitive development, but demonstrate abnormal social interactions and restricted interests.

Childhood Disintegrative Disorder

Normal development followed by loss of previously acquired skills. This loss of skills is persistent.

Rett Syndrome

This condition occurs in females. Children appear to be developing normally until 6 to 18 months and then undergo a plateau of head growth, development of stereotypic hand movements and ataxia, and loss of social and gross motor skills. These girls may develop seizures and profound MR.

Epidemiology

- The current prevalence for autism spectrum disorders in children aged 3 to 10 years is approximately 1:110 or 9 per 1,000 children (www.cdc.gov/autism) with a male to female ratio of 4:1 (National Center on Birth Defects and Developmental Disabilities).
- The apparent increase in prevalence/incidence may be due to increased recognition and diagnosis of children previously diagnosed as mentally retarded, etc. and not to actual increase in number of children with these disorders.

Points to Remember

- There are no data to support a relationship between vaccines, thiomersal, or infections and development of PDD.
- Screening for autism spectrum disorders should be completed in the medical home at 18, 24, and 30 months of age.

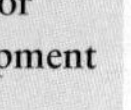

Etiology

- Sibling and twin studies are suggestive of a genetic etiology for PDD. Siblings of children with PDD have a 50-fold increased risk for learning disability.
- PDDs are neurodevelopmental disorders. Studies show evidence of brain abnormalities beginning in prenatal period.

Treatment

- Goals of treatment include promotion of language development, social interaction, and lifelong learning.
- Pharmacotherapy is often used when behaviors (e.g., self-injurious) affect the progress of other therapeutic interventions. Many parents seek complementary alternative medical therapy. Although the specifics are unlikely to be tested on the boards, it may be important to know that melatonin has been used to treat sleep disorders in autistic children.
- Behavioral approaches attempt to minimize aggression and self-injury while encouraging recognition of social cues.

BEHAVIORAL AND PSYCHOSOCIAL ISSUES: INFANT/TODDLER/PRESCHOOL

During each stage of development, children are confronted with novel situations and engage in new behaviors as they grow and learn new skills. Although many of these behaviors can be developmentally appropriate at certain ages, it is important to recognize when they become pathologic and be prepared to manage them in such instances. This section will also review events and milestones that should be part of normal infant development, and how future growth and behavior can be affected if they are disrupted.

Infant-Parent Attachment

Definition

Permanent affective two-way bond connecting parent and child that develops over first 1 to 2 years of life. There is an important period for bonding over the first hours and days of life, and this is enhanced by skin-to-skin contact. Bonding is important but not essential for forming attachments, as evidenced by the fact that adopted children can become securely attached to their adoptive parents. Secure attachments are important for the future cooperative relationship between parents and child, and play an important role in a child's ability to form future relationships. Proper attachments also produce children who are happier, more outgoing, have increased self-esteem, and are more motivated in the preschool years and beyond. Establishment of consistent routines and avoidance of overstimulating activities are important elements in the formation of secure infant-parent attachment.

Colic

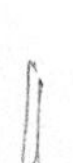

Normal crying peaks around 6 to 8 weeks of age, and usually last 2.5 to 3 hours daily. Crying is often worse in the evening and at night. It improves around 3 months of age as infants become better able to deal with sensory stimuli.

Definition

Colic is defined as crying for at least 3 hours per day, at least 3 days per week for at least 3 weeks.

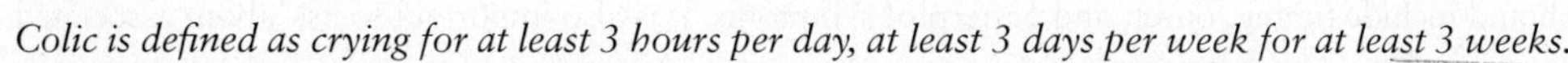

Colic can be associated with increased gas/burping, "pulling up" of the legs and inconsolability. It usually improves by 4 months of age, but may persist up to 6 months.

Treatment of Colic

There are many different techniques that may help calm a colicky baby. These include the following:

- Swaddling.
- White noise/shushing.
- Rocking or gentle swinging.
- Pacifier/sucking.

Habits and Abnormal Behaviors

Young toddlers frequently engage in self-soothing behaviors that include *thumb-sucking, rocking, head-banging* (especially before bedtime), and *masturbating*. These behaviors usually emerge around 12 to 18 months of age and often resolve/extinguish by the age of 4 years. These habits can be considered developmentally normal if they are intermittent and do not interfere with other activities. However, if they are associated with other neurologic abnormalities or developmental delay, further evaluation may be warranted.

Temper Tantrums

Usually begin around 12 months and are related to frustration over the child wanting something that they cannot have or wanting to do something that they are developmentally unable to do. They are often related to the child trying to gain independence.

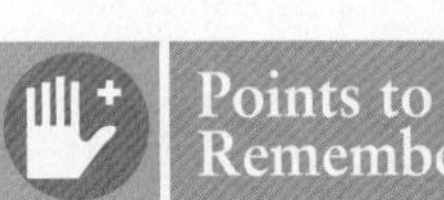

Points to Remember

- Tantrums are not usually intended as "attention seeking."
- Methods for dealing with tantrums include ignoring them and helping the child find other ways to deal with frustration and emotions.
- In children older than 3 years "time outs" can be used to remove the child from the situation and give them a chance to calm down. Excessive attention can reinforce negative behavior.

Breath-holding Spells

- *Definition: involuntary breath-holding that leads to a brief period of unconsciousness and is usually triggered by anger, confrontation, fear, or pain.* They are most common between 6 and 18 months but may persist up to 4 to 6 years. Spells usually resolve in 30 to 60 seconds, but some children may jerk or have brief seizures associated with the spells. The episodes are often very frightening to parents even though they are usually benign. There are two types of breath-holding spells:
  - *Cyanotic spells*: associated with red or blue-purple color change. Cyanotic spells are often related to anger or frustration and may occur after a period of intense crying.
  - *Pallid spells*: associated with the child suddenly becoming pale and limp, sometimes in the absence of crying. Pallid spells often result from being frightened or startled and may be followed by a period of sleepiness.
- *Etiology*: Primarily behavioral, however, there is an association between breath-holding spells and iron deficiency anemia.
- *Treatment*: For true breath-holding spells, it is important not to reinforce the behavior; parents should make sure that the child is in safe place and ignore the behavior.

Toilet Training and Associated Abnormalities

There are several signs that indicate readiness for toilet training. These include the child being able to express that the diaper is soiled or that they need to urinate or have a bowel movement. This usually occurs between 18 to 24 months, but many children are still in diapers at 2.5 to 3 years of age. Positive feedback is far more effective than punitive measures in ensuring the success of toilet training.

Points to Remember

- Daytime (diurnal) enuresis is abnormal after the age of 4 years; nocturnal enuresis is abnormal after the age of 6 years.

Enuresis

- *Definitions*: In *primary enuresis* the child has never had period of being continent for at least 6 months. *Secondary enuresis* occurs after period of being dry for at least 6 months.
- Only 10% of children with enuresis have underlying medical condition (see Table 14.6).

Nocturnal Enuresis

Epidemiology: A family history of nocturnal enuresis is common—children have a 44% chance of nocturnal enuresis if one parent wet the bed and a 70% chance if both parents wet the bed, which suggests a genetic component.

Other nonorganic etiologies include small bladder capacity, poor arousal from sleep, and high nocturnal urine production.

Diagnosis should focus on medical, developmental, and family history. Problem-specific history should include timing, onset, and pattern of symptoms. It is also important to ask about associated

TABLE 14.6

DIFFERENTIAL DIAGNOSIS OF ENURESIS

Diagnostic Categories of Differential Diagnosis	Examples
Increased urinary output	Diabetes mellitus, diabetes insipidus, sickle-cell disease, excessive water intake
Increased bladder irritability	Urinary tract infection, constipation, pregnancy, bladder spasm
Structural problems	Ectopic ureter, epispadias (females), partial urethral valves, and thickened bladder wall (males)
Abnormal sphincter control	Spinal cord abnormalities, sphincter weakness, neurogenic bladder

symptoms (frequency, urgency, polydipsia), force of stream, bowel habits (constipation, encopresis), or signs of UTI.

Physical examination should include the following:

- Complete neurologic examination.
- Back examination (look for sacral dimple, tuft).
- Signs of constipation on abdominal examination (palpable stool mass) and rectal examination (tags or fissures).

Laboratory tests: Urinalysis (specific gravity, glucose, signs of infection)

Treatment:

- *Behavioral therapy*—alarm systems are the most effective over the long term (70% to 80% success), but require motivation because parents must awaken with the child when alarm goes off. These are most successful in children aged 7 years or older. Other choices include motivational therapy (sticker charts, rewards), decreased fluid intake at bedtime, and hypnotherapy.
- *Pharmacologic therapy*—desmopressin acetate (**DDAVP**) is available as a nasal spray or oral medication and works by decreasing urine production for up to 7 hours. There are few side effects, but it is only 40% to 60% effective, and symptoms often relapse after stopping the medication. The other available option is imipramine, but it is rarely used because of its side effects (headache, abdominal pain, mood swings, risks of toxicity), because it is only 30% to 50% effective, and because of the high relapse rate (60%).

Diurnal Enuresis

Epidemiology: Affects 3% to 4% of children aged 4 to 12 years with a male to female ratio of 1:2.

Diagnosis: History and physical examination are similar to nocturnal enuresis, and urinalysis should be performed. Further diagnostic workup may include ultrasound, VCUG, urodynamics.

Etiology: The most common cause for isolated diurnal enuresis is *bladder spasm*.

Treatment: Behavioral (frequent reminders to use bathroom or alarms) or pharmacologic (oxybutynin hydrochloride) especially in cases of neurogenic bladder.

Encopresis

Definition: incontinence of stool or passage of stool into inappropriate places in children older than 4 years of age (chronologically or mentally). Symptoms cannot be explained by the use of laxatives or an underlying medical condition.

Constipation with overflow incontinence is a subtype of encopresis where child leaks stool around a hard fecal mass. It accounts for 90% of encopresis. In these children, the rectum is often so distended that stretch receptors that usually signal the need to defecate are ineffective, and the child is unaware of the need to stool until after soiling occurs.

Diagnosis:

- *History* should include bowel patterns from birth to help rule out Hirschsprung disease, as well as medical/surgical and developmental histories (including toilet training history), and any history of abuse or trauma.
- *Problem-focused history* including present bowel habits (frequency of stooling into toilet vs. accidents, stool consistency, presence/absence of urge to defecate) and urinary habits (enuresis, UTI can be associated with constipation).
- *Physical examination* should include rectal examination looking for anal fissures (can cause pain and stool withholding), tags (inflammatory bowel disease), absent anal wink (neurologic abnormality).

- *Imaging*: an abdominal x-ray may be helpful in assessing the degree of constipation or fecal impaction present.

Treatment: *must* include both medication and behavioral interventions.

- Initial bowel clean-out should include oral medication and enemas/suppositories. This may be done as an outpatient.
- Ongoing medications and a behavioral plan are necessary to prevent reaccumulation of stool and recurrence of encopresis.
- Medication options include lactulose, polyethylene glycol (polyethylene glycol 3350 [Miralax]), or mineral oil. Chronic use of stimulant laxatives should be avoided.
- Establishing scheduled times to sit on the toilet is essential until the urge to defecate redevelops. This may take 6 to 9 months.

BEHAVIORAL AND PSYCHOSOCIAL ISSUES: SCHOOL AGE

As children get older and enter a formal learning environment, they are faced with new situations and challenges. It is during the elementary school years that most learning disorders and problems with attention become apparent. In addition, it is not uncommon for symptoms of certain emotional disorders and disorders of conduct and behavior to develop in children in this age group, some of which may persist into adulthood. This section will also review sleep disorders of childhood.

School Difficulties

Learning Disorders

- *Diagnosis* assumes academic performance significantly below that which is expected for intellectual potential and compared with children of the same age, either in reading, mathematics, written expression, or a combination of these (learning disorder NOS). The child's learning difficulties cannot be related to a sensory deficit, and the child must have had appropriate educational opportunities.
- The most common learning disorder is an isolated *reading disability* more commonly known as *dyslexia*.
  - *Definition*: Dyslexia is a lifelong disorder that may include difficulty sounding out words and identifying words (decoding), reading comprehension, and reading speed. Many children with dyslexia will also have difficulty with written composition.
  - *History*: There is often a family history of reading disorder/dyslexia.
  - *Treatment* is multidisciplinary and often dependent on the child's school system. Treatment includes speech/language therapy and academic accommodations such as untamed tests, reductions in required reading, and use of visual cues for learning.

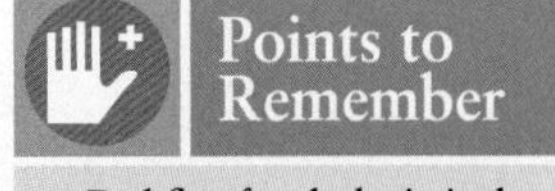

- Red flag for dyslexia is the inability to read words by first grade.
- Reversals [b and d] in writing can be normal in children through 7 years of age.

ADHD

ADHD consists of symptoms of hyperactivity, impulsivity, and difficulty staying on-task. These symptoms are worse when the child is faced with nonpreferred tasks. In addition to problems with concentration, children may exhibit difficulty with executive functions such as planning and organization. There are three subtypes of ADHD, *predominantly inattentive*, *predominantly hyperactive/impulsive*, and *combined type*.

- *Epidemiology:*
  - There is an estimated prevalence of 3% to 5% in school-aged children.
  - ADHD is often associated with learning disorders or other psychiatric disorders.
- *Etiologies* may include environmental factors (infection, lead exposure, prenatal drug/alcohol/tobacco exposure) and genetic factors.
- *Diagnosis*: evaluation must include medical, developmental, family, and social history in addition to standardized questionnaires that should include information from multiple sources (parents, teachers of multiple subjects).
  - Children with the predominantly inattentive type of ADHD are more likely to present with school difficulty. Those children who are hyperactive are more likely to be diagnosed at a younger age due to behavioral problems.
- *Differential diagnosis:*
  - Genetic disorders.
  - Toxic exposures such as lead.
  - Neurologic/neurodegenerative disorders. Sudden onset of symptoms or developmental regression may suggest a neurologic disorder.
- *Treatment* is multidisciplinary and includes behavioral therapy, academic modifications, and pharmacotherapy.
  - Behavior therapy includes positive reinforcement and consistency.

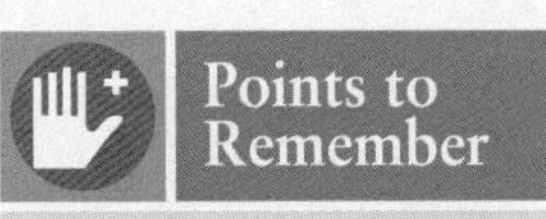

- Symptoms of ADHD must be present before the age of 7 years and must be present in more than one setting.

- Academic accommodations can include untimed tests, limitations in the amount of assigned homework, an extra set of textbooks to be kept at home, and a homework/assignment calendar.
- Stimulant medications include *methylphenidate* (Ritalin, Concerta) or *amphetamine* (Adderall). These are effective in more than 70% of children but may be associated with adverse effects such as appetite suppression, insomnia, and rebound exacerbation of symptoms. The adverse effects can often be minimized through dose titration.
- Other pharmacologic options include nonstimulant medications such as *norepinephrine reuptake inhibitors* (atomoxetine [Strattera]) or medications that are effective at treating comorbid depression such as *TCAs*, *clonidine*, or *bupropion*.

Points to Remember

- What is the difference between a 504 plan and an IEP or Individual Education Plan? The 504 plan allows for special accommodations for children with disabilities, often allowing them to remain in "mainstream" classrooms. An IEP, however, is intended for students requiring specialized instruction, usually provided within a separate classroom setting.

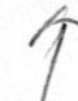

EMOTIONAL DISORDERS: SCHOOL AGE

Many emotional disorders can present in childhood, and most of these are anxiety disorders. Whether or not emotional behavior is appropriate or pathologic depends on the intensity and duration of symptoms and the settings in which these symptoms occur. Although some childhood emotional disorders are precursors to anxiety and mood disorders in adulthood, many will resolve as the child ages. A brief overview of several of the emotional disorders of childhood is presented here.

Separation Anxiety Disorder and School Refusal

Separation Anxiety Disorder

Fear related to separation that is persistent and interferes with normal developmental tasks leading to impairment in relationships. In children, separation anxiety disorder is commonly manifested as school refusal.

Epidemiology

Going to school marks the first prolonged separation from parents/primary caretakers for the majority of children and is often when the symptoms of separation anxiety disorder first becomes apparent. Separation symptoms are more common in girls.

Diagnosis

In younger children, separation anxiety disorder may present only as separation anxiety. In older children and adolescents there are often other psychiatric illnesses, stressors, or emotional disturbances that contribute to school refusal. These include depression, low self-esteem, loss of a school friend, death in the family, and bullying at school. Onset is often acute in young children and more gradual in adolescents.

School Refusal

This may manifest as:

- Reluctance or total refusal to go to or remain in school.
- Anxiety/panic attacks when forced to go to school.
- Somatic complaints.

Treatment

Treatment includes family therapy and facilitating rapid return to school, with an understanding that relapses may occur with new emotional or family stress.

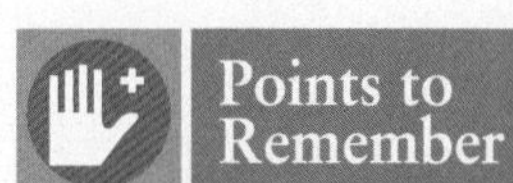

Points to Remember

- Specific phobias that develop early in childhood may resolve without therapy.

Specific Phobia

This is a *marked or persistent fear of a specific object or situation*, where exposure to the object or situation leads to anxiety. In order for a diagnosis of specific phobia to be made, avoidance of the stimulus must interfere with normal activity and relationships. Specific phobias can include fear of animals, fear of natural events such as thunder, and fear of situations (elevators, crowds, heights). *Treatment* is usually behavioral and can involve direct exposure to the stimulus or gradual desensitization.

Social Phobia

This is defined as *avoidance of contact with unfamiliar people that is severe enough to interfere with normal social functioning*. Children may appear shy/socially withdrawn and anxious with even minimal contact with strangers.

Epidemiology

Onset is usually at early school age. Social phobia may be part of an adjustment disorder or GAD.

Etiology

Social phobia may be due to a persistence of the stranger anxiety that is typically present in infants and toddlers but resolves in most children.

Social Phobia

This can be a manifestation of a speech/language delay or disorder. These children try to avoid situations that would involve speaking to people who are unknown to them.

Treatment

Treatment is behavioral with an emphasis on increasing assertiveness and improving self-esteem.

Obsessive Compulsive Disorder (OCD)

OCD consists of *obsessional thoughts and compulsive activities that interfere with normal activity and cause patient distress.* Obsessional thoughts may interfere with school and relationships, and the anxiety caused by these thoughts is often temporarily reduced by compulsive activities.

Epidemiology

Symptoms may begin in childhood or adolescence. The presentation of OCD is often earlier in boys. Children with OCD often develop symptoms of depression as well.

Treatment

Treatment includes behavioral therapy and more recently use of SSRIs.

Generalized Anxiety Disorder (GAD)

GAD is defined by *excessive or unrealistic anxiety or worry.* Children may focus unnecessarily on anticipated future problems. The onset of GAD may be gradual or sudden, and symptoms are often worse with increased stress.

Differential Diagnosis

This includes mixed anxiety disorder, attention deficit disorder, adjustment disorder, and psychotic or mood disorder.

Treatment

Treatment includes individualized therapy and psychotropic drugs such as anxiolytics and SSRIs.

DISRUPTIVE BEHAVIOR DISORDERS: SCHOOL AGE

The term disruptive behavior disorders is used to describe a group of disorders that are characterized by behavior that is more disruptive to others than to the person initiating it. As a result, the child with the disorder may not experience a significant amount of distress related to their condition. The most common disruptive behavior disorders are discussed below.

Oppositional Defiant Disorder (ODD)

ODD consists of hostile, negative, and defiant behavior toward authority figures without violating basic rights of others. Children with ODD must have significant impairment in social or academic functioning for a diagnosis to be made.

Epidemiology

- ODD is more common in males, and may be diagnosed as early as 3 years of age.
- Children with ODD suffer from poor insight, low self-esteem, labile mood, and bad temper. Symptoms of ODD may be present only at home and not in school.
- ODD may evolve into CD when the child is older.

Conduct Disorder (CD)

CD is defined as *repetitive, persistent behavior that violates other people's basic rights and age-appropriate social rules, causes social, occupational, and academic dysfunction and occurs in several settings*. In addition, *behavior does not seem to cause any distress to the patient*, and patient does not seem affected by distress caused to others.

Behaviors fall into four groups:

- Behaviors that result in harm to people or animals.
- Behavior that results in property loss or damage.
- Deceitful behavior or theft.
- Serious violation of parental and school rules.

Epidemiology

CD occurs more frequently in males. These children often have a history of difficult temperament from a very young age, early antisocial behavior, and may have previous diagnosis of ODD. CD can be childhood-onset (symptoms present before the age of 10 years) or adolescent-onset.

Risk factors for CD include the following:

- Parent psychiatric illness or criminal behavior.
- Poor parent-child relationship or children placed outside home at early age (lack of proper attachment and bonding).
- High family stress.
- Low socioeconomic status.

Treatment

These patients require psychiatric care. Family therapy is often useful.

Prognosis

In CD prognosis is usually poor and is related to the age of onset of symptoms, family/social circumstances, and the presence/absence of antisocial personality traits.

SLEEP DISORDERS: SCHOOL AGE

Sleep disorders in children fall into two categories: dyssomnias and parasomnias. While dyssomnias refer to problems with the amount and quality of sleep, parasomnias refer to disturbing events that occur when the child is sleeping. Below is a brief description of sleep disturbances in children that fall within these categories.

Dyssomnias

Insomnia

Insomnia is defined as *difficulty initiating and maintaining sleep* or *not feeling rested after adequate sleep*. It is often *associated with symptoms of daytime fatigue or irritability*. Insomnia may occur in conjunction with other mental health disorders and may have an organic etiology such as a medical condition or a psychoactive drug.

Hypersomnias

Hypersomnias result in *excessive daytime sleepiness and prolonged transition to awake state after sleep* that *interferes with social activities, relationships, and school*. This *occurs after an apparently normal amount of sleep*. There are several different hypersomnias:

- *Sleep apnea*: Pauses in respiration lead to frequent brief arousals and restless movements during sleep.
  - *Epidemiology*: Sleep apnea accounts for approximately 50% of hypersomnia cases.
  - *Predisposing factors* include large tonsils or adenoids, maxillofacial abnormalities, hypothyroidism, and obesity.
  - Sleep apnea can lead to decreased school performance, headaches, changes in mood and personality, and even development of pulmonary hypertension in severe cases.

Kleine-Levin Syndrome

This syndrome consists of recurrent episodes of excessive sleepiness that may last days to weeks, primarily in teenage boys. It is associated with binge eating and weight gain, hypersexuality, and mood disorders.

Narcolepsy

- *Diagnosis*: Usually brought to medical attention when teachers complain that the child is falling asleep during class, although "naps" may be short enough to go unrecognized by others.

- Narcolepsy is associated with vivid auditory or visual hallucinations during transitions between awake and asleep states (hypnagogic and hypnopompic). Patients may be hesitant or afraid to go to sleep as a result.
- Patients also experience *cataplexy* (episodic loss of muscle tone initiated by strong emotions) and *sleep paralysis* (paralysis while falling asleep/waking).

Circadian Rhythm Disorders

In these disorders, a child's sleep-wake cycle is not consistent with normal day-night routine.

Sleep-Wake Schedule Disorder

There is a lack of synchronization between the individual's internal circadian rhythm and the normal sleep-wake cycle, which leads to trouble falling asleep at night and difficulty waking in the morning.

Delayed Sleep Phase Type

For these children, onset of sleep can be:

- *Advanced*—child falls asleep early, wakes in middle of night.
- *Delayed*—sleep occurs late, waking in the middle of the day (adolescents are particularly vulnerable to this).
- *Disorganized*—random patterns of sleeping and waking.
- *Frequently changing*—often related to travel and frequent changing of time zone.

Parasomnias

These are *abnormal events* that occur during sleep or on threshold between wakefulness and sleep. Emotional disturbance is the primary complaint in parasomnias (vs. sleepiness in dyssomnias).

Nightmare Disorder

- *Definition*: Frightening dreams that lead to frequent awakenings.
- *Epidemiology*: Peak incidence between the age of 3 and 6 years. The majority of children outgrow nightmare disorder.
- In nightmare disorder the *child complains about the event*. On awakening, the child may be tearful, agitated, and anxious. The dream is usually recalled, especially immediately upon awakening.
- Nightmares occur during REM sleep, primarily during the second half of the night.

Sleep Terror Disorder

- *Definition*: Repeated episodes of abrupt awakening that often begin with a scream. In these episodes, the child sits up abruptly with signs of intense anxiety (dilated pupils, perspiration, tachycardia, tachypnea) but is unresponsive and difficult to arouse/awaken.
- *Epidemiology*: Peak incidence between ages 4 and 12 years, often with a family history.
- Febrile illness can be a predisposing factor; there can be increased frequency of sleep terrors during times of stress.
- In sleep terror disorder, the *parent complains about the event*. In almost all cases, the child has no memory of the event.
- Episodes occur during non-REM sleep, usually during the first third of the night. They are accompanied by delta activity on EEG (stage 3 and 4 sleep).
- Children with sleep terrors may develop sleepwalking as they get older and must be protected from injury.
- *Treatment*: Main therapy is educating family.

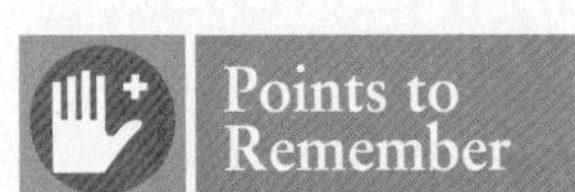

- **The child complains about nightmare disorder, whereas the parent complains about sleep terror disorder**

Sleepwalking

Sleepwalking consists of complex movements that lead to leaving the bed and walking, without being conscious of the event or remembering it.

- *Epidemiology*: Peak onset at 6 to 12 years of age. Sleepwalking is more common among first-degree relatives and is more common in boys than in girls.
- Like sleep terrors, sleepwalking occurs in non-REM sleep, usually during the first third of night and is accompanied by delta activity on EEG (stage 3 and 4 sleep).
- Episodes may last up to 30 minutes and can include opening doors, eating, getting dressed, and going to the bathroom. The child may return to bed prior to awakening or fall asleep in another place. In addition, children may talk in their sleep. During the episodes, the individual is unresponsive and very difficult to awaken. Sleepwalkers must be protected from injury.
- Treatment: Safeguard the environment against possible injury to the child during a sleepwalking event, reduce stress, and potentially introduce an afternoon nap.

BEHAVIORAL AND PSYCHOSOCIAL ISSUES: OLDER CHILD/ADOLESCENT

As children approach adolescence and adulthood, they are once again faced with new challenges and expectations as they seek new privileges and responsibilities. Changing relationships with family members and peers bring about demands that in some individuals can lead to stress and anxiety. Below is a brief review of some of the behavioral and psychiatric disorders that can present in older children and adolescents.

Points to Remember

- **Please refer to the Adolescent Medicine, Gynecology, Mental Health, and Substance Abuse chapter for more information about these topics.**

Depression

Definition

Depressed mood and loss of interest or pleasure. Other symptoms of depression include the following:

- Low self-esteem.
- Excessive guilt.
- Difficulty concentrating and problems with school performance.
- Social withdrawal.
- Psychomotor retardation.
- Fatigue and increased sleeping.
- Decreased appetite and weight loss.
- Irritability.
- Suicidal ideation/preoccupation with death.

Associated Symptoms

Depression may also be associated with somatic symptoms such as headache, abdominal pain, or chest pain, all of which may lead to multiple medical evaluations. Younger children may cry for "no reason," become withdrawn, act out, show signs of increased aggression.

Spectrum of Disorders

- *Grief response* is a normal and expected reaction to personal loss, although unresolved bereavement places the child or adolescent at risk for later depression.
- *Adjustment disorder with depressed mood*—symptoms lead to impairment in social function and are due to a specific stressor such as illness, school change, parental separation, or divorce. The symptoms usually resolve within 6 months.
- *Dysthymic disorder*—the symptoms of dysthymic disorder are similar to major depressive disorder but not as severe or long-lasting. Symptoms may be persistent or intermittent but must be present for at least 1 year for a diagnosis of dysthymic disorder to be made.
- *Major depressive disorder*—children must have at least one major depressive episode, no manic or hypomanic episodes and no other disorder that can explain the depressive symptoms.
  - *Major depressive episode* is characterized by at least 2 weeks of symptoms, which are present most of the day nearly everyday. There must be depressed mood and/or decreased interest or pleasure. Other symptoms are listed above in section (A).

Risk Factors

- Family member with depression or other mood disorder.
- Victims of abuse and/or neglect.
- Loss of a parent, particularly before the age of 11 years (most common risk factor).
- Parental physical or mental illness.
- Chronic illness.

Treatment

Treatment requires multifaceted approach to address multiple causes of depression, with the goal of reducing disability and allowing the child/adolescent to function. Treatment includes psychotherapy and pharmacotherapy (SSRIs, TCAs). Many children will have recurrence of symptoms.

Points to Remember

- **Attempted suicide is three times more common in females. Completed suicide is five times more common in males.**

Suicide

Prior to suicide the child/adolescent often communicates suicidal thoughts or intent and suicidal methods. These children have often had previous contact with a psychiatrist.

Points to Remember

- Asking a patient about suicidal thoughts will not increase the likelihood that they will attempt suicide or "plant ideas" about suicide.

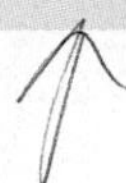

Risk Factors

- Depression, bipolar disorder, schizophrenia, or other psychiatric condition.
- Frequent discipline problems.
- Drug abuse.
- Social isolation.
- Psychiatric illness in the family.
- Previous suicide attempt.
- Chronic illness.

Treatment

Treating the underlying illness is the most important factor in preventing future suicide attempts. Depressed adolescents on SSRIs must be monitored closely because of increased risk for suicide attempts (see Points to Remember).

Points to Remember

- FDA issued a "Black Box" warning in 2004 related to the use of antidepressants in children and adolescents with major depressive disorder after analysis of several short-term placebo-control trials showed a significant increased risk of suicidal thinking and behavior. The warning is applied to most drugs used to treat depression in children and adolescents, including but not limited to SSRIs and TCAs.

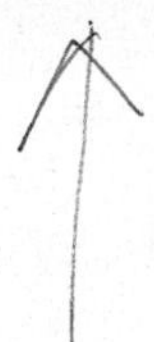

Somatoform/Conversion Disorders

Somatization is defined as *symptoms with no evidence of pathophysiology* for which patient seeks medical attention.

Somatoform Disorders

Severe symptoms that require intervention but are not due to other psychiatric diagnosis. *Child believes symptoms to be real.* Disorders include the following:

- *Somatization disorder*—multiple somatic complaints.
- *Conversion disorder*—motor or sensory symptoms that would suggest neurologic disorder when no disorder is actually present. For example, right upper arm paralysis that appears to resolve when patient is asleep.
- *Pain disorder*—pain often linked to psychological symptoms.
- *Hypochondriasis*—preoccupation with illness.
- *Body dysmorphic disorder*—preoccupation with an imagined defect in appearance.

Epidemiology

Overall prevalence in the pediatric/adolescent population is 2% to 10%. These disorders are often preceded by a stressful life event, and symptoms usually resolve within 1 year.

Presentation

Patients commonly present with neurologic complaints, but with symptoms that do not follow normal anatomic patterns. Complaints include dizziness, weakness, paresthesias, pseudoseizures, and paralysis.

Differential Diagnosis

- *Factitious disorder*—patient is faking symptoms for secondary gain.
- *Munchausen syndrome by proxy*—parent inventing/falsifying medical history.
- Somatic symptoms associated with other psychiatric conditions such as depression, anxiety disorders.

Medical Evaluation

In these patients medical evaluation should be done quickly to avoid secondary gain.

Treatment

Treatment includes reassurance, behavioral treatments, and pharmacologic management if indicated. It may require collaboration between the pediatrician and mental health professionals. It is important to try to give child an "out," or a chance to give up the symptoms on their own.

Psychotic Disorders

Psychotic disorders are diagnosed most commonly in adolescence/young adulthood. They are very difficult to diagnose in childhood. Both genetic and environmental factors play a role. These disorders can be associated with incoherent thinking, delusions and hallucinations, and major behavioral changes.

Schizophrenia

Characteristic features of schizophrenia include *disordered thinking*, *delusional beliefs* (often paranoid), *hallucinations* (usually auditory), and *abnormal speech or movements* (catatonia, agitation, mutism, echolalia). There are associated negative symptoms as well including flat affect, lack of motivation or energy.

- Onset may be abrupt or gradual, course can be remitting or chronic.
- *Epidemiology*: 12-fold risk of schizophrenia if parent or sibling is affected.
- *Treatment* includes psychiatric care/rehabilitation, family counseling, and neuroleptic medication.
- Prognosis is poor in more than 75% of patients.

Delirium

Delirium is defined by disturbances of consciousness, attention, behavior, perception and thinking, memory, and the sleep-wake cycle. Delirium is often associated with visual and auditory hallucinations. Symptoms have fluctuating intensity. Patients are disoriented, with abnormal or absent response to normal environmental stimuli. Treatment is often aimed at identification and management of any underlying disorders.

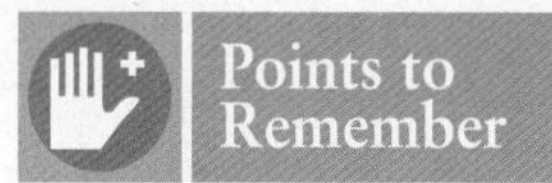

- **Delirium can be due to drug ingestion in children.**

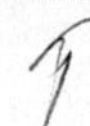

Bipolar Disorder

Bipolar disorder is associated with a significant disturbance of mood with abnormalities in thought and perception. Bipolar disorder consists of both *depressive* and *manic* or *hypomanic* episodes. During manic episodes patients exhibit *elevated mood, pressured speech, irritability, flight of ideas, decreased sleep, and disinhibited behavior*. These episodes may also be associated with psychotic symptoms.

- *Treatment*: Patients may require hospitalization. Initial treatment may include neuroleptic medication, mood stabilizers, and ongoing psychotherapy.

EXTERNAL INFLUENCES ON DEVELOPMENT/ BEHAVIOR: CHILD MALTREATMENT

Millions of cases of suspected child abuse and/or neglect are reported every year in the United States and approximately one-third of these cases are substantiated. Children who are victims of abuse and neglect are at increased risk for medical problems, such as FTT, and also for many of the behavioral and developmental abnormalities discussed earlier in this chapter. Because of this, pediatricians must be able to recognize the risk factors and manifestations of child maltreatment and abuse.

Physical Abuse

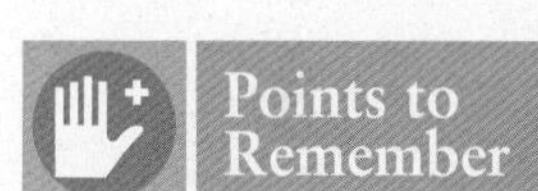

- **It is very difficult to tell the age of a bruise on the basis color alone**

Risk Factors

Risk factors for physical abuse include the following:

- *Parental characteristics* (depression, drug use).
- *Child characteristics* (difficult temperament, chronic disability).
- *Family/society characteristics* (social isolation, stress, chaotic family, low education or socioeconomic status).

Manifestations of Abuse

- *Bruises/contusions* are more likely to be intentional below the age of 6 months, and accidental bruising becomes more common as infants become more mobile.
  - Bruises on bony prominences are more likely to be nonintentional, whereas those on dorsal surfaces are more likely to be inflicted (Fig. 14.2).
  - *Differential diagnosis of bruises*: Mongolian spots, erythema multiforme, coagulopathy (including leukemia), Henoch-Schonlein purpura, secondary syphilis, cultural rituals (coining, cupping), phytophotodermatitis (a cutaneous phototoxic reaction produced by contact with a variety of plant substances, followed by sunlight exposure).
  - It is important to look for specific shapes that suggest inflicted bruises, such as hand print, belt, or cords (see Figs. 14.3A and 14.3B).
- Burns:
  - Mechanisms include chemical, thermal, electrical, and radiation. Scald burns are the most common, accounting for 85% of burns.
  - Thermal burns:
    - *Forced immersion scalds* have uniform depth with sharp borders. Flexion creases are spared. Burns often are a result of the hands/feet or buttocks being held under hot water.

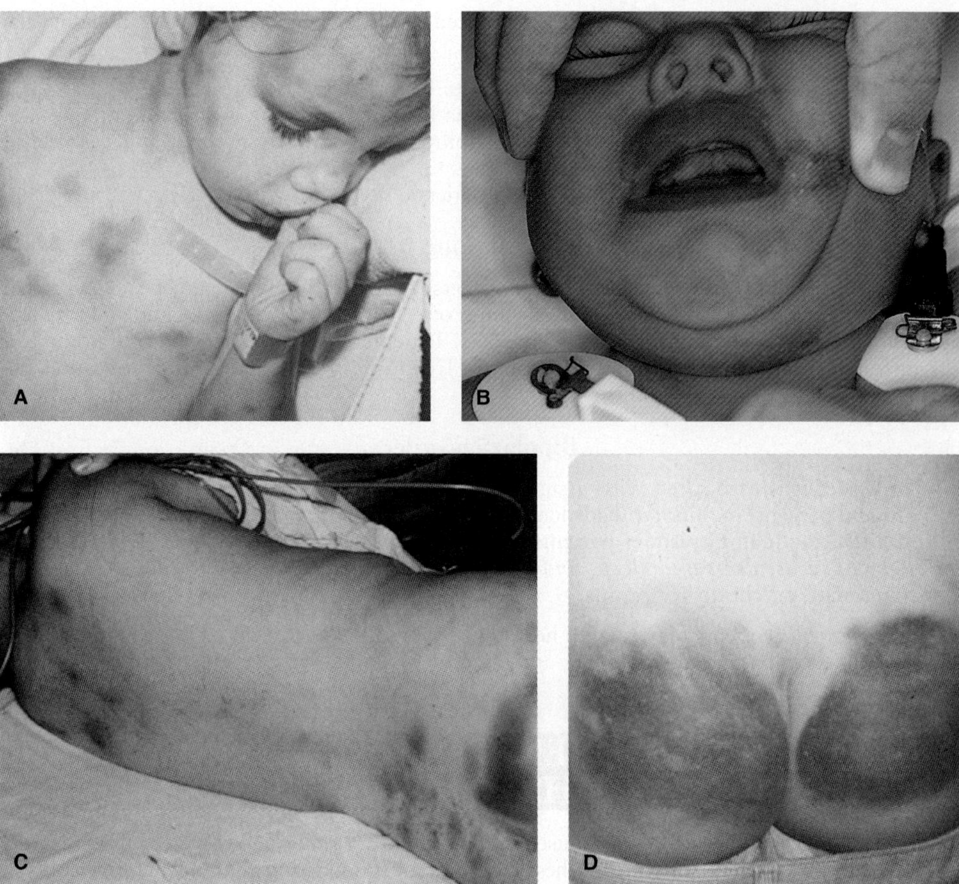

FIGURE 14.2. Cutaneous manifestations of child abuse. A: Multiple bruises in a central pattern. B: Bruises around the face. C: Bruises at various stages of healing. D: Buttocks bruises as a cause of myoglobinuria. (Used with permission from Fleisher GR, Ludwig S, Baskin MN. *Atlas of Pediatric Emergency Medicine*. Philadelphia, PA: Lippincott Williams & Wilkins, 2004.)

    - *Dry contact burns* are usually from irons, hair dryers, cigarette lighters, light bulbs, and cigarettes (Fig. 14.4).
- *Head injuries* are associated with more mortality and long-term morbidity than any other form of abuse. Signs and symptoms are often nonspecific, such as irritability, poor feeding, lethargy, and vomiting. Missing the diagnosis of inflicted head injury puts the child at risk for further trauma.
    - Types of head injuries include the following:
        - Scalp trauma, subgaleal bleed.
        - Skull fracture with or without associated epidural bleeding.
        - Subdural/subarachnoid bleeding.
        - Cerebral edema.

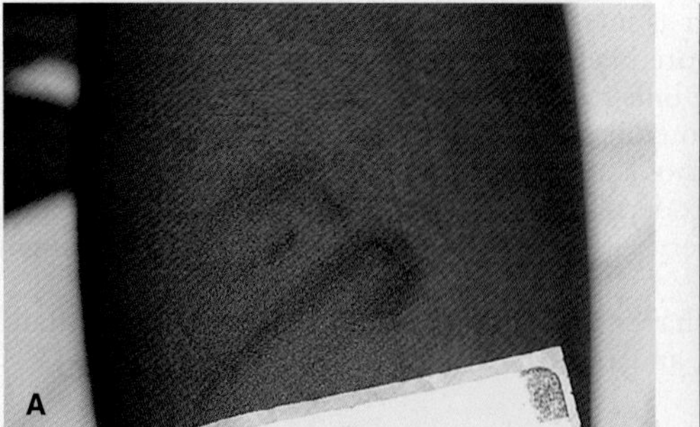

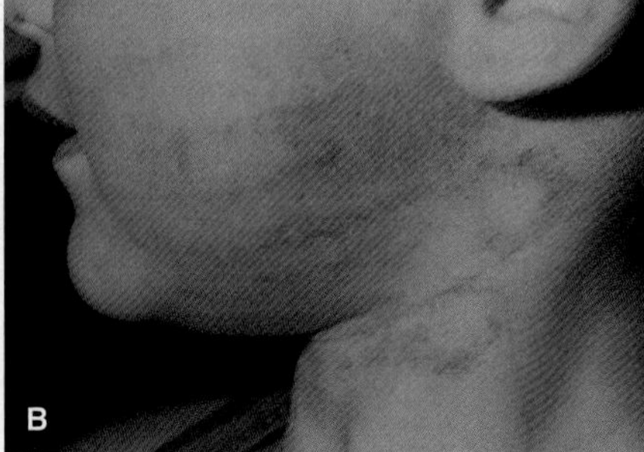

FIGURE 14.3. Curvilinear bruising from a looped cord. (Used with permission from Fleisher GR, Ludwig S, Baskin MN. *Atlas of Pediatric Emergency Medicine*. Philadelphia, PA: Lippincott Williams & Wilkins; 2004:425.) Inflicted handprint on the face of a child leaving an outline of the fingers. (From Reece RM, Ludwig S. *Child Abuse: Medical Diagnosis and Management*. 2nd ed. Philadelphia, PA: Lippincott Williams & Wilkins, 2001:28, 396, with permission.)

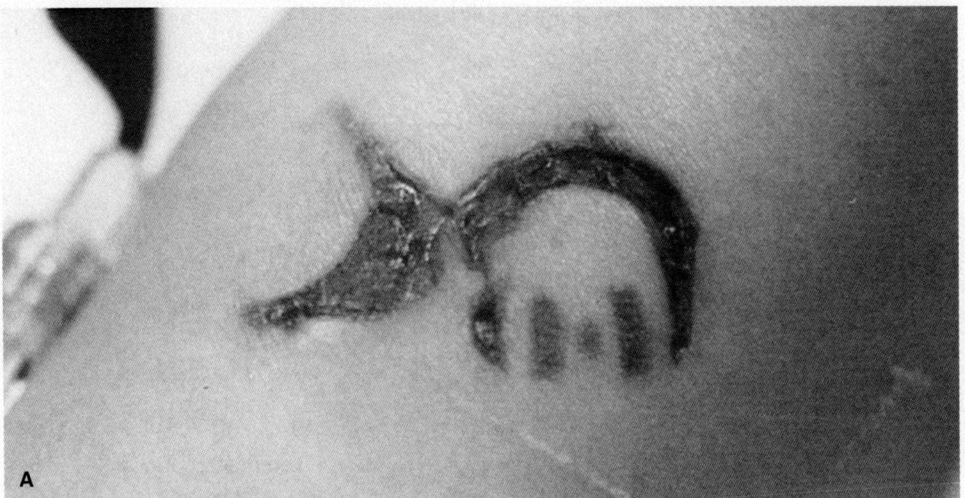

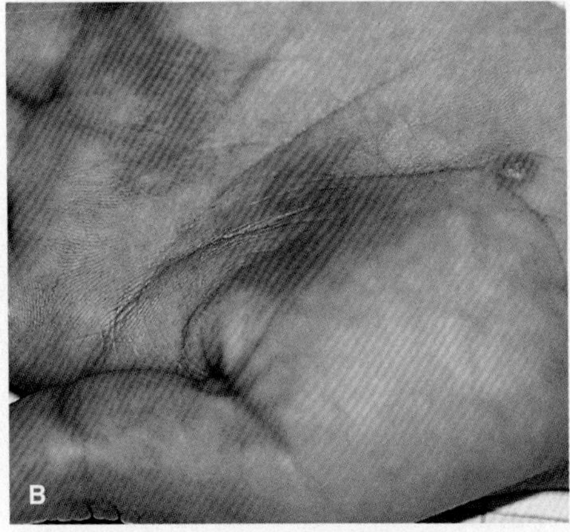

FIGURE 14.4. Hot solid burns. **A:** Pattern burn from cigarette lighter. **B:** Coin burn. From Reece RM, Ludwig S. *Child Abuse: Medical Diagnosis and Management*. 2nd ed. Philadelphia, PA: Lippincott Williams & Wilkins, 2001:455, with permission.)

    - Axonal injury.
    - Brain contusion or intraparenchymal bleeding.
  - In cases of suspected abusive head trauma, it is important to look for cutaneous injuries, intra-abdominal injuries, mucosal lesions such as torn frenulum, and retinal hemorrhages.
- *Shaken baby syndrome/Shaken impact syndrome* is often an attempt to stop uncontrollable crying. Shaking episodes are often followed by the impact of throwing the infant against a surface.
  - Shaking and sudden deceleration with impact can cause:
    - Rupture of bridging veins in the skull, leading to subdural hematoma and subarachnoid hemorrhage.
    - Direct trauma to brain itself.
    - Axonal shear injury and release of chemicals by injured neurons leading to vasospasm and oxygen deprivation.
  - The degree of symptoms and time to appearance of those symptoms is dependent on the length and force of shaking (Fig. 14.5).
  - Ophthalmologic evaluation is essential; *retinal hemorrhages are seen in 33% of children with nonaccidental head trauma* (vs. 2% of children with accidental trauma). Other possible injuries include retinal detachment, optic nerve injury (Fig. 14.6).
  - *Differential diagnosis* of retinal hemorrhages (note: all other causes are RARE or age-specific):
    - Vaginal deliveries—retinal hemorrhages occur in 40% of deliveries, but usually resolve by 10 to 14 days of age.
    - Bleeding disorders (should be associated with other sites of bleeding).
    - Arteriovenous malformation (rare in infants).
    - Increased ICP—usually from inflicted and accidental trauma.
    - Bacterial meningitis—retinal hemorrhages are only seen in approximately 1% of cases.
    - Accidental head trauma—rare cause of retinal hemorrhages.
- Skeletal injuries:
  - The majority of inflicted fractures (80%) are in children younger than 18 months. Only 2% of fractures in children within this age group are accidental.

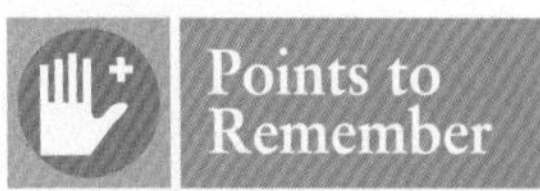

- **No type of fracture is pathognomonic or specific for abuse.**

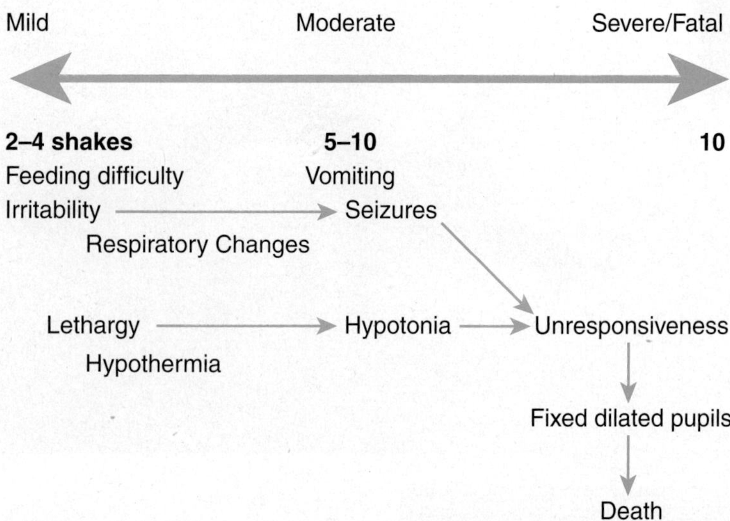

FIGURE 14.5. Conceptual model of the "dose-response" in shaken baby/shaken impact syndrome (SBS/SIS). (Reprinted with permission from McMillan JA, Feigin RD, DeAngelis C, et al. *Oski's Pediatrics: Principles and Practice*. 4th ed. Philadelphia, PA: Lippincott Williams & Wilkins, 2006.)

- A *toddler fracture* is a common *accidental* oblique fracture of the tibia in children aged 9 months to 3 years.
- *Metaphyseal fractures of long bones* are common fractures of abuse, and require significant torsional force. These are also known as "corner fractures" or "bucket handle fractures." The tibia is the most common site (Fig. 14.7).
- The humerus is the second most common long bone involved in fractures of abuse. These are often spiral and oblique fractures resulting from twisting.

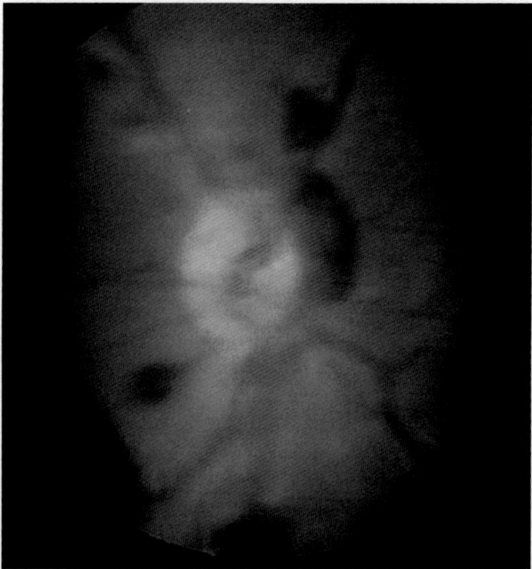

FIGURE 14.6. Retinal hemorrhage. (From Fleisher GR, Ludwig S, Baskin MN. *Atlas of Pediatric Emergency Medicine*. Philadelphia, PA: Lippincott Williams & Wilkins, 2004.

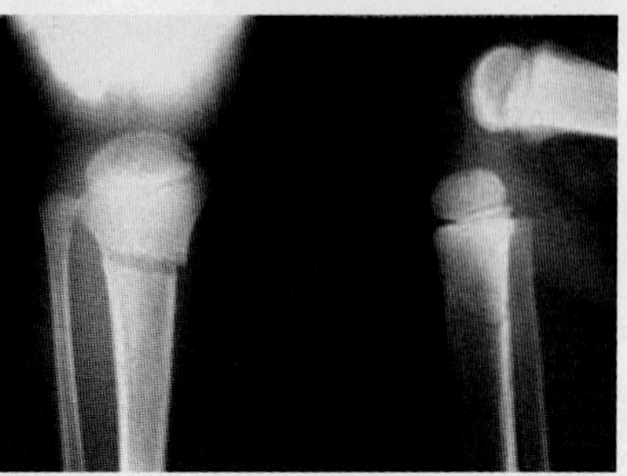

FIGURE 14.7. Anteroposterior (AP) and lateral radiographs of the proximal tibial metaphyseal fracture with an intact fibula in a 3-year-old child. (Reprinted with permission from Sharps CH, Cardea JA. Fractures of the shaft of the tibia and fibula. In: MacEwen GD, Kasser JR, Heinrich SD, eds. *Pediatric Fractures: A Practical Approach to Assessment and Treatment*. Baltimore, MD: Williams & Wilkins, 1993:321.)

TABLE 14.7

WHEN TO SUSPECT ABUSE

Metaphyseal fractures in children <2 y of age
Posterior rib fractures
Scapular fractures
Spine fractures
Sternal fractures
Multiple, especially bilateral, fractures
Fractures to hands or feet
Fractures in infants or very young children
Fractures seen in children in poverty
Fractures seen in former prematurely born children
Fractures seen in children with developmental handicaps
Fractures seen with associated other injuries not attributable to accidents

- Rib fractures are usually discovered on skeletal survey and not often suspected clinically. Posterior fractures are most common and are frequently multiple and bilateral.
- When to suspect abuse (see Table 14.7).
- *Differential diagnosis* of fractures in children:
    - Accidental trauma.
    - Obstetric trauma.
    - Prematurity (leads to osteopenia).
    - Nutritional deficiency (rickets).
    - Osteogenesis imperfecta (usually types I and IV confused with abuse).
    - Metabolic disorders.
    - Drug toxicity.
    - Infection.
    - Skeletal dysplasia.
    - Neoplasms.
- Human bites and intrathoracic and intra-abdominal injuries may also be manifestations of physical abuse.

Neglect

Definition

Caretaker fails to provide the child with the essentials for development and survival or causes the child to suffer either deliberately or through extreme inattentiveness. Neglect accounts for 60% of abuse in children, usually by the female parent.

Risk Factors

Risk factors for neglect are similar to those for physical abuse.

Types of Neglect

- *Physical neglect* can result in obesity or undernourishment, lack of appropriate shelter, or hygiene.
- *Medical neglect* includes refusal or delay of health care.
- *Supervisory neglect* results from failing to provide a safe environment, allowing the child to be exposed to domestic violence, abandonment, custody issues.
- *Emotional neglect* includes not providing adequate affection, permitting drug/alcohol abuse or delinquency, and having unrealistic expectations of child.
- *Educational neglect* is a failure to provide child with education according to the law.

Possible Indicators of Neglect

- *Behavioral indicators* in children include avoidance of eye contact, no smiling, lack of interest in the environment, difficult to console, negative response to cuddling, repetitive behaviors like head banging, and inappropriate seeking of affection from strangers.
- *Physical indicators* include severe diaper rash, impetigo, poor hygiene, protuberant abdomen (sign of malnutrition), flat occiput.

Points to Remember

- Socioeconomic status and race are NOT risk factors for sexual abuse.

Sexual Abuse

Epidemiology

Twenty percent of girls and 9% of boys have a history of sexual abuse. Boys are less likely to disclose abuse. The perpetrator is often someone known to the family.

Risk Factors

Risk factors include the presence of a male in the household that is not biologically related to child, and a poor parent-child relationship.

Diagnosis

- Disclosure by the victimized child. An attempt should be made to interview the child only once with proper documentation. Leading questions should be avoided. Interviews should ideally be performed by trained individuals.
- Observation by the parent or health care professional of sexual behaviors in the child. It is important to differentiate from developmentally appropriate behavior.
- When indicated, medical examination should include collection and documentation of forensic evidence and STD testing.
- *Physical examination*: An anogenital examination is essential, although a normal examination does not rule out abuse. Only approximately 10% of children will have evidence of injury on examination. Ideal positions for the examination are supine frog-leg and knee-chest (Fig. 14.8).

Points to Remember

- Vaginal bleeding and/or discharge is not always due to abuse. Look for urethral prolapse or evidence of foreign body such as toilet paper.

Munchausen-by-proxy (MBP)

Definition

In MBP, the child is a victim of the parent or guardian's mental illness. Illness in the child is simulated by a parent or guardian, usually the mother. The child comes for frequent medical evaluation and care, and undergoes many procedures.

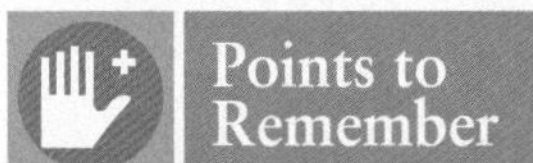

Points to Remember

- In cases of MBP, the child's symptoms improve when they are separated from the perpetrator.

Red Flags

- Recurrent serious illness with no obvious explanation and no response to the usual therapies.
- Reported symptoms are not observed by others and cannot be verified.
- A determination that any part of medical or family history has been fabricated.
- Unexplained illness or death in patient's siblings.
- Parent/guardian seems unusually calm when child is most ill.
- History of Munchausen syndrome in mother or guardian.

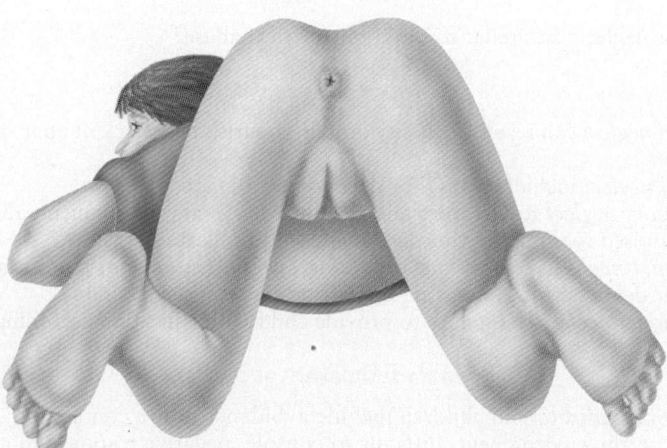

FIGURE 14.8. Knee-chest position used for conducting examination in cases of suspected sexual abuse. (Reprinted with permission from Bickley LS and Szilagyi P. *Bates' Guide to Physical Examination and History Taking*. 8th ed. Philadelphia: Lippincott Williams & Wilkins, 2003.)

Goal of Treatment

Goal of treatment is to prove that the condition is being produced or simulated, which can be difficult.

EXTERNAL INFLUENCES ON DEVELOPMENT/ BEHAVIOR: IMPACT OF FAMILY AND COMMUNITY

Many times children are faced with stressful situations and challenges that are outside of their control. These include a death in the family, being placed in foster care, and having a chronic illness. The final section in this chapter will provide a brief overview of these external events and circumstances that can affect a child's behavior and development.

Death and Bereavement

A child's response to death will depend on his or her age and level of cognitive development. Children younger than 5 years have a poor understanding of death and may feel guilty or responsible for the death in some way. An understanding of the finality of death develops around the age of 6 to 7 years. Responses may include the following:

- *Preschool*—sleep disturbance, anxiety, aggressive behavior, social withdrawal, regression of milestones, sadness.
- *School-age*—denial, may hide feelings of grief, poor school performance, somatic complaints.
- *Adolescents*—as above, also may act out or have increase in aggressive behavior.

Children may act resentful or angry either at the person who died or at surviving family members.

The opportunity for open grieving is important to ensure healthy emotional development with protection and support from remaining adults/family members. Honest and direct answers are best. It is also important to try and maintain a routine and keep the child's life as organized as possible.

Divorce

As with death and bereavement, a child's response to divorce is related to their age and cognitive development.

- *Preschool*—regression of milestones, feelings of guilt.
- *School-age*—guilt, feelings of sadness and rejection, fantasies about parents getting back together.
- *Older children/adolescents*—somatic symptoms, anger or acting out, aggression, mental health issues (depression, substance abuse).

The effect of the divorce itself on the child may be complicated by ongoing issues of discord between parents, including custody and visitation problems.

It is within the role of the pediatrician to ask about parental relationship, provide anticipatory guidance and advocate for the child in cases of separation/divorce, and involve mental health professionals if necessary.

Foster Care and Adoption

In the United States, children who end up in foster care or who are adopted are often those born to young, single parents from a low socioeconomic status, often with a history of psychiatric disease and/or drug/alcohol abuse. These children may have been victims of or exposed to violence. Older children who are adopted may have been in foster care prior to adoption, ~50% with more than one foster care placement. Prior to entrance into the foster care system, children often have poor access to health care and inadequate immunization and have incomplete or no screening for lead exposure, anemia, vision, or hearing.

In cases of international adoption, children often suffer from effects of institutionalization (see Table 14.8). Health care and screening vary widely from one country to another, so parents may have little, if any, medical information (past medical history, family history) about the child they are adopting, and the information available are not always accurate.

It is the role of the pediatrician to address concerns of adoptive parents, and perform careful evaluations of all adopted children.

TABLE 14.8

EFFECTS OF INSTITUTIONALIZATION ON CHILDREN

Exposure to infections
Lack of access to medical diagnosis and treatment
Lack of nurturing physical contact
Poor nutrition and growth
Delayed cognitive development
Physical neglect
Emotional neglect
Vulnerability to physical and sexual abuse
Exposure to poor hygiene

Medical Issues

Medical issues may include the following:

- Prenatal drug/alcohol exposure.
- History of neglect or abuse.
- Exposure to/infection with hepatitis, tuberculosis, HIV.
- Anemia, rickets, or other nutritional deficiencies.
- Metabolic or genetic disorders not picked up because of the lack of newborn screening (hypothyroidism, PKU).
- Lead poisoning.
- Growth delay and developmental delay are common.

Behavioral and Psychiatric Problems

These are common, including the following:

- Significant separation anxiety.
- Problems forming attachments.
- Sleep disturbance.
- ADHD, learning disabilities, other school-related problems.
- Depression, anxiety, PTSD.

Exposure to Violence

Exposure to violence affects emotional and moral development, the ability to learn, social interactions, and the development of relationships and intimacy. The true effect is dependent on nature of the violence, the child's relationship with the victim and/or perpetrator, and the length of exposure.

- *Toddlers*—sleep disturbance, irritability, increased separation anxiety, regression in language, or toilet training.
- *Preschool*—increased anxiety, sleep disturbance and night terrors, decreased verbalization, decreased motivation.
- *School-age*—increased anxiety, sleep disturbance, trouble paying attention, distraction, decreased motivation.
- *Adolescents*—learning problems and school difficulty, low self-esteem, aggressive behavior, substance abuse, psychiatric problems.

Children may exhibit signs of PTSD at any age and are at risk for development of other mental health disorders.

Effect of the Media

Studies show many potential harmful effects of increased exposure to television and other media including the following:

- Decreased active time/increased sedentary time leading to an increase in the number of children who are overweight/obese.
- Increased exposure to violence and sexual behavior.
- Increased aggressive behavior and an unrealistic/trivialized view of violence.
- Poor academic performance/achievement.
- A distorted view of beauty leading to a distorted body image and eating disordered behavior.
- Advertising influence on toys, clothes, food.

Television, internet, and video game time (i.e., sedentary time) should be limited to less than 2 hours per day and parents should control/limit what shows and Web sites can be accessed by their children. The AAP also recommends that parents have access to all sites visited by their children on the Internet (i.e., know their usernames and passwords).

Effects of Chronic Illness

Children with chronic illness often have tremendous fear and anxiety about the future but may not know how to express it, and frequently are confused about the nature of their illness. Younger children may deny their illness to try and fit in better with their peers. Older children and adolescents with chronic illness may be more at risk for body image problems, and may have trouble developing independence and forming lasting relationships. Children may maintain the "sick role" and be less motivated to participate in treatment if they feel that they are rewarded emotionally and otherwise by being "sick." Chronic illness affects the entire family. *Parents* may feel guilt and may blame themselves or one another for the illness and its effects. *Siblings* may feel neglected and resentful because of the amount of attention that the patient requires.

Vulnerable Child Syndrome

Definition

A vulnerable child is a physically healthy child whose parents feel is at greater risk for behavioral, developmental, or medical problems.

Risk Factors

Risk factors include the following:

- *Problems with the child* including prematurity, previous serious illness from which the child has recovered, previous injury or accident, congenital anomalies, feeding problems.
- *Problems with fertility, pregnancy or birth* including frequent miscarriages, or child born from an "at-risk" pregnancy.
- *Psychological problems in parents* including postpartum depression, unresolved grief reactions, emotional disturbances.

Diagnosis

Diagnosis is based on excessive use of health care services and unusually high parent anxiety.

Important Points

Parents tend to be overindulgent and have difficulty setting limits for these children. The child is at risk for sleep problems, hyperactivity, underachievement, and learning difficulties.

Treatment

- Address parental concerns including the true risks to the child and how long child will be at risk.
- Teach parents how to interpret signs and symptoms.
- Address behavioral issues in the child and reinforce discipline of the child.

SAMPLE BOARD REVIEW QUESTIONS

1. A 6-month-old boy presents to your office for well-child care. The mother tells you that he can roll front-to-back and back-to-front, and he can lift himself up onto his hands with his arms extended in the prone position. What other gross motor skill would you expect of an infant at this age?
    a. Crawling
    b. Cruising
    c. Sitting without support
    d. Sitting with support or propping
    e. Pulling to stand

    Answer: d. A 6-month-old boy should be expected to sit with support or propping but most children this age cannot yet sit unsupported. The other motor milestones reported by the mother are age-appropriate.

2. An 18-month-old girl presents to your office for well-child care. Her mother tells you that she has at least 15 to 20 words and is starting to put 2 words together. She can point

to and name some of her body parts. What other language skill is expected of an 18-month-old child?

a. Follow a one-step command with a gesture
b. Follow a two-step command
c. Follow a command with two actions and two objects
d. Follow a one-step command without a gesture
e. Follow a series of three simple instructions

Answer: b. An 18-month-old child should be able to follow a two-step command, such as "get your shoes and bring them to mommy."

3. A 10-month-old boy presents to your office for well-child care. He sits unsupported, pulls to stand but does not cruise, babbles using vowel sounds such as "oooh" and "aaah," is beginning to use a crude pincer grasp, and waves bye-bye. Which of these prompts further intervention?

a. Sits unsupported
b. Pulls to stand but does not cruise
c. Babbles using vowel sounds
d. Uses a crude pincer grasp
e. Waves bye-bye

Answer: c. A 10-month-old child should babble using consonant sounds and may even be starting to say "mama" and "dada" in a nonspecific way. This child should undergo a more thorough evaluation for language delay, which should include a detailed developmental assessment and hearing screen.

4. A 3-year-old child should be able to do which of the following?

a. Copy a cross
b. Copy a vertical line
c. Copy a circle
d. Copy a square
e. Copy a horizontal diamond

Answer: c. At 3 years a child should be able to copy a circle.

5. Glaucoma and cataracts can lead to which of the following if untreated?

a. Strabismus
b. Astigmatism
c. Amblyopia
d. Nystagmus
e. Diplopia

Answer: c. Amblyopia is a loss of visual acuity, usually in one eye, although it can affect vision in both eyes. This can be due to misalignment of the eyes (strabismus) or anything that interferes with clear vision from either eye (such as occurs with glaucoma or cataracts). The brain suppresses the image from the weaker eye, and without treatment the visual loss can be permanent.

6. A 6-week-old girl is transferred to your emergency department from a community hospital for further evaluation for suspected nonaccidental head trauma. The infant was brought to the hospital by her grandmother when she found her sleepy and difficult to arouse after her nap. At the outside hospital she was found to have a large boggy hematoma on the back of her skull concerning for a skull fracture. No history of a fall is reported. She is stabilized and undergoes a head CT. What is the next most important part of the evaluation of a suspected nonaccidental head trauma?

a. Abdominal CT to look for intra-abdominal injuries
b. Chest x-ray to evaluate for broken ribs
c. Ophthalmologic examination to evaluate for retinal hemorrhages
d. Screening labs such as CBC and chem 7
e. Social work consult

Answer: c. Retinal hemorrhages are seen in 33% of patients with abusive head trauma, and only 2% of patients with accidental head trauma. Given the patient's age, it is likely that her head injury is inflicted. Although all of these options may eventually be part of her evaluation, it is essential that she undergo a full ophthalmologic examination as soon as possible.

7. A 7-year-old boy presents to your office for well-child care. The mom is concerned because he does not seem to get along well with other children. She reports that he is very bright for his age, and tells you that he is "obsessed" with dinosaurs and knows

"absolutely everything about them." However, she has noticed that he tends to keep to himself at school and does not seem to enjoy playing with the other children. Other people have told her that he is just "shy," but she is concerned that there is something else wrong with him. Cognitive, language, and motor development have been normal to date. Which of the following disorders could this patient have?

a. Autistic disorder
b. Asperger syndrome
c. Rett syndrome
d. Separation anxiety disorder
e. Social phobia

Answer: b. Normal cognitive and language development with impaired social interactions and restricted interests are all characteristics of Asperger syndrome.

8. A mother brings her 2-year-old son into your office because he has recently started rocking his body back and forth in his crib before he goes to sleep at night. She has no other concerns about his behavior or development, and he has had no other medical problems. There have been no changes or new stresses at home. The most likely diagnosis is

a. Normal behavior
b. Autism
c. Childhood depression
d. Brain injury
e. Obsessive-compulsive disorder

Answer: a. Normal behavior. It is not unusual for toddlers to engage in repetitive, self-soothing behaviors such as head banging, rocking, thumb-sucking, or masturbation. These behaviors are more common in boys and usually resolve over time. Because the mother has no other concerns about his behavior and his history is otherwise unremarkable, the other options are all unlikely causes for his body rocking.

9. A mother calls your office because she is concerned about episodes that her 9-year-old daughter has been having at night. She reports that her daughter wakes up screaming but does not respond when her mother goes in to comfort her even though she is awake. She seems anxious and is breathing very quickly during these episodes. The child does not seem to remember these episodes, but the mother is worried. The episodes she is describing seem most consistent with

a. Seizures
b. Nightmares
c. Narcolepsy
d. Sleep apnea
e. Night terrors

Answer: e. Night terrors are characterized by abrupt awakening that often begins with a scream. In these episodes, the child sits up abruptly with signs of intense anxiety (dilated pupils, perspiration, tachycardia, tachypnea) but is unresponsive and difficult to arouse/awaken. The child often has no memory of these events, and they are far more disturbing to parents.

10. A 14-year-old girl presents to the emergency department with sudden onset weakness and numbness in her legs. She is anxious and concerned. She insists that she is unable to bear weight or walk and that she cannot feel anything below the waist. On examination, she withdraws to pain, has normal patellar and ankle reflexes, and appears to resist when you attempt to passively move her legs. The most likely diagnosis is:

a. Somatization disorder
b. Factitious disorder
c. Pain disorder
d. Conversion disorder
e. Hypochondriasis

Answer: d. In conversion disorder, patients truly believe that their symptoms are real. Often, patients will present with neurologic complaints that do not follow normal anatomic patterns on examination or will have complaints that are not corroborated on physical examination. In this case, the patient is complaining of numbness and weakness/paralysis but appears to have sensation and strength present in her legs on examination.

11. The most sensitive early marker for MR is

a. Learning disability
b. Hypotonia or motor delay
c. Language delay

d. Presence of dysmorphic features
e. Behavioral disturbance

Answer: c. Language delay. Although children with MR may have delays in all of the developmental streams, dysmorphic features in the case of certain genetic conditions, and behavioral disturbances, impaired language development is the most sensitive early marker of MR.

12. What is the most common form of child maltreatment in the United States?
a. Head injury (including shaken baby syndrome)
b. Fractures
c. Sexual abuse
d. Neglect
e. Burns

Answer: d. Neglect accounts for 60% of abuse cases, usually by the female parent/caretaker. Because of this, female perpetrators are more common than males in cases of abuse in this country.

SUGGESTED READINGS

GROWTH AND DEVELOPMENT

Johnson CP, Walker WO Jr. Mental retardation: management and prognosis. *Pediatr Rev.* 2006;27:249–256.

McMillan JA, DeAngelis CD, Feigin RD, et al. eds. *Oski's Pediatrics: Principles and Practice.* 4th ed. Philadelphia, PA: Lippincott Williams & Wilkins, 2006.

Rosenberg LE. Psychometrics. In: McMillan JA, DeAngelis CD, Feigin RD, et al. eds. *Oski's Pediatrics: Principles and Practice.* 3rd ed. Philadelphia, PA: Lippincott Williams & Wilkins, 1999:86.

Walker WO Jr, Johnson CP. Mental retardation: overview and diagnosis. *Pediatr Rev.* 2006;27:204–212.

BEHAVIOR

Berman BD. Foster care and adoption. In: Rudolph CD, Rudolph AM, Hostetter MK, et al. eds. *Rudolph's Pediatrics.* 21st ed. New York, NY: McGraw Hill, 2003.

Goldstein LH. Major family transitions: birth of a sibling and bereavement. In: Rudolph CD, Rudolph AM, Hostetter MK, et al. eds. *Rudolph's Pediatrics.* 21st ed. New York, NY: McGraw Hill, 2003.

Hanna GL, Fischer DJ, Fluent TE. Separation anxiety disorder and school refusal in children and adolescents. *Pediatr Rev.* 2006;27:56–63.

McMillan JA, DeAngelis CD, Feigin RD, et al. eds. *Oski's Pediatrics: Principles and Practice.* 4th ed. Philadelphia, PA: Lippincott Williams & Wilkins, 2006.

Johnson CF. Sexual abuse in children. *Pediatr Rev.* 2006;27:17–27.

Kass LJ. Sleep problems. *Pediatr Rev.* 2006;27:455–462.

Osofsky JD. Family and community violence. In: Rudolph CD, Rudolph AM, Hostetter MK, et al. eds. *Rudolph's Pediatrics.* 21st ed. New York, NY: McGraw Hill, 2003.

Pearson SR, Boyce WT. Consultation with the specialist: the vulnerable child syndrome. *Pediatr Rev.* 2004;25:345–349.

Schmidt ME, Rich M. Media and child health: pediatric care and anticipatory guidance for the information age. *Pediatr Rev.* 2006;27:289–298.

Sirotnak AP, Grigsby T, Krugman RD. Physical abuse of children. *Pediatr Rev.* 2004;25:264–277.

CHAPTER 15 ■ HEMATOLOGY

HEMA DAVE AND CALVIN K. LEE

ACS	Acute chest syndrome	HUS	Hemolytic uremic syndrome
AD	Autosomal dominant	INR	International normalized ratio
ALL	Acute lymphoid leukemia	ITP	Idiopathic (immune) thrombocytopenic purpura
AML	Acute myeloid leukemia	IVIG	Intravenous immunoglobulin
aPTTr	Activated partial thromboplastin time ratio	LDH	Lactate dehydrogenase
ANC	Absolute neutrophil count	MCHC	Mean corpuscular hemoglobin concentration
AR	Autosomal recessive	MCV	Mean corpuscular volume
ATP	Adenosine triphosphate	NO	Nitric oxide
BMT	Bone marrow transplant	NSAID	Nonsteroidal anti-inflammatory drug
CHF	Congestive heart failure	OSA	Obstructive sleep apnea
CML	Chronic myeloid leukemia	PAIgG	Platelet associated immunoglobulin G
CMV	Cytomegalovirus	PK	Pyruvate kinase
CXR	Chest x-ray	PMN	Polymorphonuclear leukocyte
DDAVP	Desmopressin acetate	PNH	Paroxysmal nocturnal hemoglobinuria
DIC	Disseminated intravascular coagulation	PRBC	Packed red blood cells
DNA	Deoxyribonucleic acid	PT	Prothrombin time
2,3-DPG	2,3-diphosphoglycerate	PTT	Partial thromboplastin time
DVT	Deep venous thrombosis	RBC	Red blood cells
EBV	Epstein–Barr virus	RDW	Red blood cell distribution width
Fe	Iron	RES	Reticuloendothelial system
FFP	Fresh frozen plasma	Retic	Reticulocyte count
FTT	Failure to thrive	RMSF	Rocky Mountain spotted fever
GBS	Group B streptococcus	RNA	Ribonucleic acid
G6PD	Glucose-6-phosphate dehydrogenase	RSV	Respiratory syncytial virus
GI	Gastrointestinal	SLE	Systemic lupus erythematosus
G-CSF	Granulocyte colony-stimulating factor	TAR	Thrombocytopenia absent radius
Hb	Hemoglobin	TCD	Transcranial doppler
Hb A	Adult hemoglobin	TIA	Transient ischemic attack
Hb A_2	Minor adult hemoglobin	TIBC	Total iron binding capacity
Hb F	Fetal hemoglobin	tPA	Tissue plasminogen activator
Hb S	Sickle hemoglobin	TTP	Thrombotic thrombocytopenic purpura
Hct	Hematocrit	vWF	von Willebrand factor
HIV	Human immunodeficiency virus	WBC	White blood cell
HLH	Hemophagocytic lymphohistiocytosis		
HSV	Herpes simplex virus		

CHAPTER OBJECTIVES

1. To understand and differentiate between important causes of anemia in infants and children
2. To understand the clinical manifestations, diagnosis, and treatment of sickle cell disease and the thalassemias
3. To review the causes, complications, and treatment of neutropenia
4. To review the function and importance of the spleen
5. To review the presentation, diagnosis, and management of congenital and acquired forms of thrombocytopenia

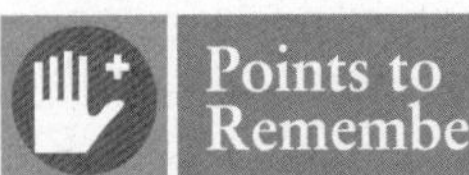

- The differential diagnosis for microcytic anemia includes iron deficiency, lead poisoning, and beta-thalassemia minor. The Mentzer index (MCV/RBC) helps differentiate between iron deficiency and thalassemia—a Mentzer index more than 13.5 suggests iron deficiency and less than 11.5 suggests thalassemia.
- The iron stores of a full-term infant are usually sufficient for the first 6 to 9 months of life, after which the infant's diet should be supplemented with Fe-fortified foods. Premature infants have lower iron stores and require supplementation as early as possible.
- Chronic GI blood loss is an important cause of Fe-deficient anemia worldwide and is often seen in patients with parasitic infections, Meckel's diverticulum, milk protein allergy, and/or peptic ulcer disease.
- Iron deficiency increases the rate of GI absorption of both iron and lead. Heavy metals such as lead decrease GI absorption of iron, thus potentiating the iron deficiency.

6. To understand the approach to and differential diagnosis of pancytopenia
7. To review the clotting cascade and understand the presentation, diagnosis, and treatment of important bleeding and clotting disorders.

ANEMIA

Normal hemoglobin levels vary according to age and gender. Hemoglobin is highest at birth and falls during the first 6 to 10 weeks of life to a physiologic nadir before increasing to childhood and adult levels.

Anemia is a common childhood condition characterized by a decrease in RBC mass or hemoglobin concentration. Anemia results from inadequate production or excessive destruction of RBCs.

- Inadequate RBC production can be due to **nutritional deficiencies** (e.g., iron deficiency, folate deficiency, Vitamin B12 deficiency) or a decrease in RBC precursors (e.g., Diamond–Blackfan anemia, transient erythroblastic anemia of childhood, parvovirus-associated aplastic crisis, acquired aplastic anemia, Fanconi syndrome).
- Excessive RBC destruction can be due to **cell membrane defects** (e.g., hereditary spherocytosis, hereditary elliptocytosis, paroxysmal nocturnal hematuria, hereditary stomatocytosis), enzyme deficiencies (e.g., PK deficiency, G6PD deficiency), or antibody-mediated destruction (e.g., autoimmune hemolytic anemia, Evans syndrome, cold antibodies).

Children with anemia can be asymptomatic or can present with signs and symptoms such as pallor, fatigue, tachycardia, and/or exercise intolerance.

RBC morphologic indices help categorize and differentiate types of anemia into microcytic, normocytic, and macrocytic anemias.

- **MCV**: describes the size of the RBCs and separates anemias into microcytic (low MCV), normocytic (normal MCV), and macrocytic (high MCV) anemias.
- **MCHC**: a marker of the Hb content in RBCs.
- **RDW**: describes the variability of RBC size.
- **Retic**: quantifies the percentage of immature RBCs in the circulation and is a marker of production of new RBCs.

Examples of anemias with different morphological features are shown in Figures 15.1 and 15.2.

Nutritional Anemias

Anemia can result from inadequate iron, folate, or vitamin B12. Iron-deficiency anemia is the single most common cause of childhood anemia. Nutritional anemias and their characteristics are shown in Table 15.1.

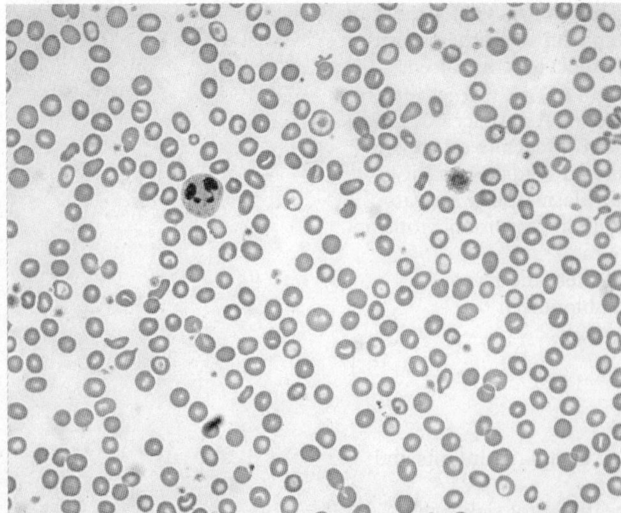

FIGURE 15.1. Microcytic hypochromic anemia (Fe deficiency, thalassemia, or lead poisoning). (Reprinted with permission from McMillan JA, Feigin RD, DeAngelis C, et al. *Oski's Pediatrics: Principles and Practice*. 4th ed. Philadelphia, PA: Lippincott Williams & Wilkins, 2006.)

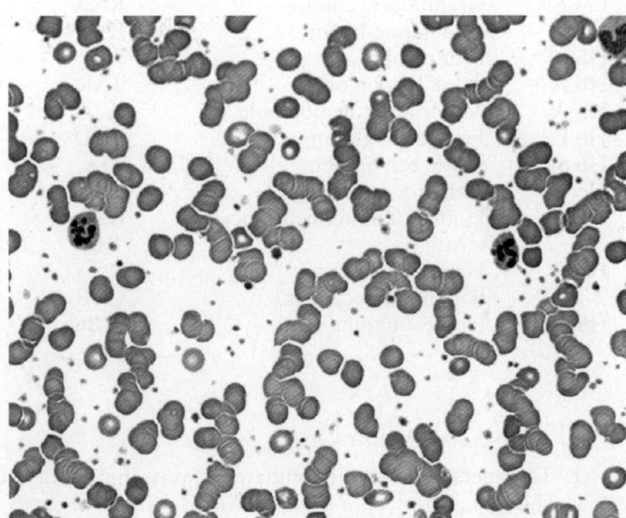

FIGURE 15.2. Macrocytic anemia with hypersegmentation of polymorphonuclear leukocytes (Vitamin B12 or folate deficiency). (Reprinted with permission from McMillan JA, Feigin RD, DeAngelis C, et al. *Oski's Pediatrics: Principles and Practice*. 4th ed. Philadelphia, PA: Lippincott Williams & Wilkins, 2006.)

TABLE 15.1

NUTRITIONAL ANEMIAS

Nutritional Deficiency	Prevalence and Causes	Morphology and Laboratory Findings	Treatment	Comments
Iron	Common High milk intake, prematurity, blood loss, vegetarian diet, elevated serum lead	Microcytic, hypochromic anemia (Fig. 15.1) with elevated RDW and low retic Fe studies demonstrate low iron, high TIBC, low ferritin, low transferrin	Iron (should see increase in retic in 2–3 d, increase in Hb in 1–4 wk, and increase in ferritin in 3 mo) Correction of underlying etiology when possible	Most common in children 9–24 mo of age Some children with Fe-deficiency have pica. Fe-deficiency anemia and even Fe-deficiency without anemia has adverse effects on attention span, behavior, and school performance
Folate	Rare Malabsorptive states, medications, defects in folate metabolism	Macrocytic anemia (Fig. 15.2) Low folate level, normal B12, low retic	Folate	Fruits and vegetables are the main dietary sources of folate
Vitamin B12	Rare Strict vegan diets, pernicious anemia, parasitic infections, diseases affecting terminal ileum	Macrocytic (Fig. 15.2) Low B12, normal folate, low retic	Vitamin B12	Intrinsic factor is needed for B12 absorption; the receptors for intrinsic factor are located in the terminal ileum. Thus, diseases affecting the terminal ileum (e.g., Crohn disease) can lead to B12 deficiency

RDW, red blood cell distribution width; TIBC, total iron binding capacity.

Anemia Due to Chronic Inflammation

Chronic inflammatory illnesses can lead to anemia. Increased cytokine production leads to increased amounts of hepcidin, a molecule that regulates the release of iron stores. Chronic illnesses commonly associated with anemia include HIV, rheumatoid arthritis, SLE, chronic renal disease, malignancies, and inflammatory bowel disease. Anemia of chronic disease is usually normocytic but can occasionally be microcytic. Other laboratory abnormalities include low serum iron, normal-to-high ferritin, and normal TIBC.

Points to Remember

- Patients receiving chronic blood transfusions are at risk for iron overload and hemosiderosis. Serum ferritin levels should be monitored closely and chelation therapy initiated if there is evidence of iron overload.

Pure Red Blood Cell Aplasias

Pure RBC aplasias are important but rare causes of severe anemia that result from inadequate production of erythroid precursors in the bone marrow. This is reflected by an inappropriately low serum retic. WBCs and platelets are normal. Pure RBC aplasias and their characteristics are shown in Table 15.2.

Points to Remember

- The normal life span of an RBC is 100 to 120 days.

Hemolytic Anemias

Hemolytic anemias result from increased destruction of RBCs and shortened life spans due to intrinsic RBC abnormalities or extrinsic factors. Most hemolytic anemias are due to one of three mechanisms:

1. Cell membrane defects leading to RBC instability and increased destruction in the spleen.
2. RBC enzyme abnormalities compromising ATP generation, leading to inability to meet metabolic demands of the cell and shortened RBC survival.
3. Immune-mediated destruction of RBCs via antibodies directed against RBCs leading to extrinsic hemolysis.

Clinical manifestations of hemolysis include signs and symptoms of anemia (e.g., pallor, fatigue, shortness of breath), jaundice, and/or splenomegaly. Patients with hemolytic anemia are also at increased risk of gallstones and parvovirus-related aplastic crisis.

Laboratory evidence of hemolysis includes a normocytic anemia, reticulocytosis, indirect hyperbilirubinemia, elevated LDH, and/or low haptoglobin.

The diagnosis, treatment, and characteristics of specific hemolytic anemias are shown in Table 15.3. Sickle cell disease and the thalassemias are also forms of hemolytic anemias and are discussed in the following section on hemoglobinopathies. ABO incompatibility in the newborn is also a type of immune-mediated hemolytic anemia and is discussed in Chapter 17.

Points to Remember

- Heinz bodies represent denatured and precipitated Hb within RBC secondary to oxidative stress. They damage the RBC membrane and cause acute hemolysis.
- Evan syndrome is concomitant autoimmune hemolytic anemia and ITP.
- The direct Coombs test detects autoantibodies or complement on a patient's RBCs. The indirect Coombs test detects autoantibodies in a patient's serum.

TABLE 15.2

PURE RED BLOOD CELL APLASIAS

Disease	Etiology	Clinical Manifestations	Findings	Treatment
Diamond–Blackfan anemia	Congenital No clear pattern of inheritance	Presents in infancy 25% of patients have associated abnormalities including short stature, facial dysmorphism, cardiac abnormalities, and/or renal abnormalities	Hb may be as low as 2.5 g/dL Macrocytic anemia with low Retic ↑ Hb F for age ↑ Erythropoietin, iron, and erythrocyte adenine deaminase Absent or markedly reduced erythroid precursors in bone marrow	Require continuous transfusions 2/3 respond to steroids BMT is curative for patients who do not respond to steroids
Transient erythroblastic anemia of childhood	Acquired Likely autoimmune; possibly postinfectious	Presents in children 1–5 y of age	Hb may be as low as 2.5 g/dL Normocytic anemia with low Retic Normal iron, HgF, and erythrocyte adenine deaminase Low erythrocyte precursors in bone marrow	Self-limited In severe cases, transfusions may be needed to support the patient until recovery occurs
Parvovirus-associated aplastic crisis	Parvovirus directly infects erythroid progenitor cells and inhibits erythrocyte production for 1–2 wk	Clinically insignificant in normal hosts but results in profound anemia (aplastic crisis) in patients with hemolytic anemias (e.g., sickle cell disease)	Drop in hemoglobin from baseline with severe reticulocytopenia and absence of erythrocyte precursors in bone marrow Positive antibody titers to parvovirus	Supportive care with blood transfusions as needed Does not recur in the same patient due to development of protective antibodies

BMT, bone marrow transplant; Hb F, fetal hemoglobin.

HEMOGLOBINOPATHIES

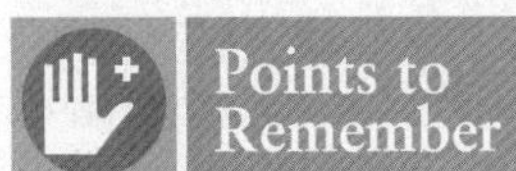

- **Hemoglobin electrophoresis results are not valid if a patient has recently been transfused; it must be repeated 3 to 4 months later.**

Hemoglobin is a tetramer of 2 alpha and 2 non-alpha polypeptide chains and an iron-containing heme group that binds oxygen. Normal hemoglobin types are shown in Table 15.4.

Hb F has a higher oxygen affinity than Hb A and is the primary form of hemoglobin until 3 to 6 months of age when Hb A predominates.

There are hundreds of known hemoglobin variants, but only a few of these (e.g., sickle cell disease, thalassemias) produce clinically significant disease. Electrophoresis is used to detect and characterize various hemoglobin variants and is part of newborn screening in most states.

Sickle Cell Disease

Hb S is a hemoglobin variant caused by a single amino acid substitution (glutamic acid → valine) in Hb A. In the deoxygenated form, Hb S polymerizes to form a spindle-shaped sickled erythrocyte. Sickled erythrocytes have markedly shortened survival and can obstruct small blood vessels and cause distal tissue ischemia and necrosis.

Individuals who are homozygous for Hb S (Hb SS) have sickle cell disease, a severe chronic hemolytic anemia. Individuals who are heterozygous for the gene have sickle cell trait and have a benign clinical course, as only 30% to 40% of their hemoglobin is Hb S, which is not enough to cause sickling.

Clinical Manifestations

Clinical manifestations of sickle cell disease usually do not appear until after 6 months of age, coincident with the postnatal decrease in Hb F and increase in Hb S. Acute and chronic complications of sickle cell disease are shown in Tables 15.5 and 15.6, respectively.

TABLE 15.3

HEMOLYTIC ANEMIAS

Disorder and Pathophysiology	Diagnosis	Therapy[a]	Comments
		Cell Membrane Defects	
Hereditary spherocytosis (Fig. 15.3) Spectrin defect results in accelerated loss of RBC membrane, membrane instability, and increased destruction in spleen	Hemolytic anemia with elevated MCHC Spherocytes on peripheral smear Abnormal osmotic fragility test	Splenectomy if severe disease	Mild cases can be asymptomatic 75% are AD, 25% are AR Increased incidence in people of Northern European descent
Hereditary elliptocytosis (Fig. 15.4) Structural abnormality of spectrin results in abnormally shaped fragile RBCs	Only 10% of patients have a hemolytic anemia Smear with elongated RBCs	Splenectomy for severe disease	AD inheritance Most cases are asymptomatic
Hereditary stomatocytosis Increased permeability of RBC membrane to cations	Hemolytic anemia Smear with swollen and cup-shaped RBCs with a mouth-like slit (stoma) instead of central pallor	Splenectomy for severe disease	Rare
Paroxysmal nocturnal hemoglobinuria (PNH) Clonal abnormality with *PIGA* gene mutation results in abnormal surface protein anchor and makes RBCs susceptible to complement-mediated destruction	Hemolytic anemia and hemoglobinuria Thrombocytopenia and leukopenia may also be present Flow cytometry shows absence of CD 59	Steroids limit the duration of hemolysis Bone marrow transplantation has been successful in some cases	Hemolysis is characteristically worse during sleep, and morning hemoglobinuria is typical Hemolysis is often precipitated by infection
		Enzyme Defects	
Pyruvate kinase deficiency PK-deficient RBCs are unable to produce ATP; increased 2,3-DPG leads to rightward shift of oxygen dissociation curve	Hemolytic anemia Increased levels of 2,3-DPG Smear with polychromatophilic RBCs	Splenectomy is not curative but may improve anemia in patients with severe disease	Most common of RBC glycolytic enzyme deficiencies AR inheritance
G6PD deficiency G6PD deficiency leads to decreased protection from oxidative stress	Hemolytic anemia precipitated by exposure to oxidative stress Decreased G6PD activity (G6PD may be normal during an acute crisis because of reticulocytosis)	Avoidance of oxidant substances (e.g., sulfonamides, naphthalene, antimalarials, fava beans)	X-linked Common in African Americans, Arabics, and Mediterraneans
		Autoimmune Hemolytic Anemias	
Autoimmune hemolytic anemia Patient produces antibodies directed against his or her own RBCs	Hemolytic anemia Smear with prominent spherocytosis and polychromasia Positive direct and indirect Coombs test	Acute cases respond to steroids and remit spontaneously within a few weeks or months Immunosuppressive agents and/or splenectomy for refractory disease Patients with underlying disease tend to have chronic anemia with prognosis determined by underlying disease	Two clinical patterns: fulminant acute disease and chronic prolonged course Antibody production can be idiopathic or secondary to an underlying disease (e.g., SLE, lymphoma, immunodeficiency), a viral or mycoplasma infection, or drug exposure

[a]Supportive care for all patients with hemolytic anemias includes folic acid supplementation and blood transfusions as needed.
AD, autosomal dominant; AR, autosomal recessive; ATP, adenosine triphosphate; MCHC, mean corpuscular hemoglobin concentration; RBC, red blood cell; SLE, systemic lupus erythematosus.

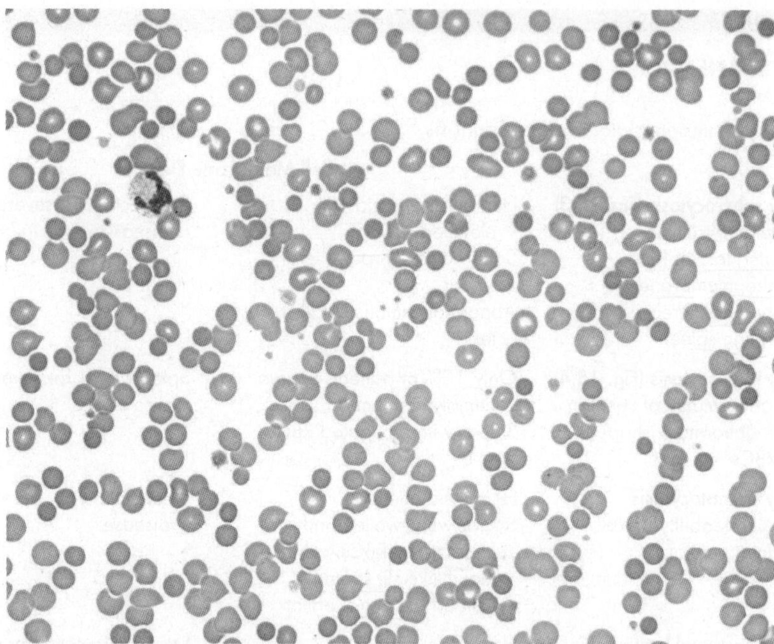

FIGURE 15.3. Spherocytosis. Small round red blood cells with less or absent central pallor. (Reprinted with permission from McMillan JA, Feigin RD, DeAngelis C, et al. *Oski's Pediatrics: Principles and Practice*. 4th ed. Philadelphia, PA: Lippincott Williams & Wilkins, 2006.)

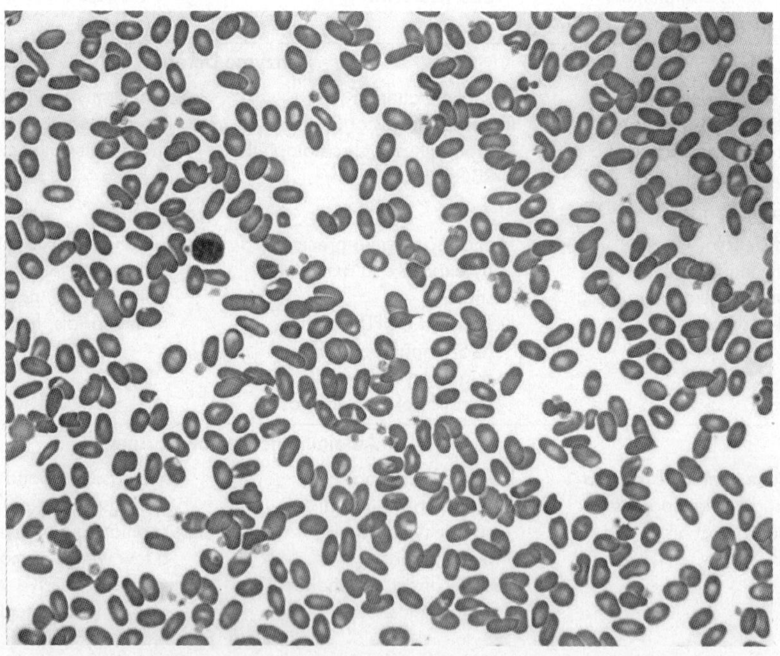

FIGURE 15.4. Elliptocytosis. Elongated red blood cells. (Reprinted with permission from McMillan JA, Feigin RD, DeAngelis C, et al. *Oski's Pediatrics: Principles and Practice*. 4th ed. Philadelphia, PA: Lippincott Williams & Wilkins, 2006.)

Points to Remember

- Sickle cell trait is present in 8% of African Americans. Having sickle cell trait confers partial resistance to falciparum malaria and so may provide a survival benefit in endemic parts of the world.
- Other sickle cell syndromes are as follows:
  - Hb SC patients: course is similar to but less severe than Hb SS
  - Hb S–β^0-thalassemia patients: course is similar to Hb SS in quality and severity
  - Hb S–β^+-thalassemia patients: course is similar to but less severe than Hb SS

TABLE 15.4

NORMAL HEMOGLOBIN TYPES

Type of Hb	Globin Chains	Adult Levels (%)
Adult Hb (Hb A)	$\alpha_2\ \beta_2$	>95
Minor Adult Hb (Hb A_2)	$\alpha_2\ \delta_2$	<3.5
Fetal Hb (Hb F)	$\alpha_2\ \gamma_2$	<2

TABLE 15.5

ACUTE COMPLICATIONS OF SICKLE CELL DISEASE

	Cause	Presentation	Treatment
Pain crisis	Vaso-occlusion of small vessels	Severe localized or diffuse pain triggered by dehydration, fever, cold, infection, etc.	Hydration, analgesia
Dactylitis	Infarcts of small bones in hands and feet	Painful swelling of hands and feet; usually seen in infancy	Hydration, narcotics
Sequestration crisis	Acute trapping of RBCs in spleen, causing an abrupt fall in Hb	Pallor, fatigue, splenomegaly	Transfusions, oxygen; splenectomy in severe refractory cases
Acute chest syndrome	Vaso-occlusion of pulmonary vessels leading to an often severe pulmonary process (e.g., infarct, fat emboli, infection)	Triad of fever, new infiltrate on CXR, and hypoxia	Hydration, oxygen, narcotics, antibiotics, positive-pressure ventilation, transfusions
Aplastic crisis	Infection with parvovirus B19 causing severe anemia with reticulocytopenia	Severe pallor, disappearance of baseline icterus	Transfusions
Stroke and TIAs	Exact etiology is unknown	Acute neurologic deficit 11%–20% of sickle cell patients have silent strokes that are not associated with acute neurologic deficits but cause long-term more subtle cognitive deficits	Supportive care for stroke, transfusions Early detection by routine annual transcranial doppler (TCD) Chronic transfusion therapy for patients with abnormal TCDs or history of stroke or TIA
Priapism	Vaso-occlusive obstruction of venous drainage of penis	Intermittent or painful, sustained erection >24 h	Hydration, narcotics, transfusion, epinephrine, penile aspiration, sildenafil
Infection	Splenic dysfunction leads to increased risk of infections; most common organisms include *Streptococcus pneumoniae, H. influenzae, Staphylococcus aureus*	Bacteremia, sepsis, pneumonia, meningitis, osteomyelitis	Antibiotics

CXR, chest x-ray; RBCs, red blood cells; TIA, transient ischemic attack.

TABLE 15.6

CHRONIC COMPLICATIONS OF SICKLE CELL DISEASE

	Cause	Presentation	Treatment
Gallstones	Biliary sludging	Asymptomatic, acute biliary colic, cholecystitis, cholangitis	Hydration, analgesia, elective cholecystectomy
Pulmonary hypertension	Intravascular sickling leads to reduced NO levels, causing endothelial dysfunction	Asymptomatic, right heart failure	Early detection with annual echo after 16 y of age; aggressive management of coexistent pulmonary disease (e.g., asthma)
Renal disease	Intramedullary sickling, papillary necrosis, renal tubular defect	Hyposthenuria, hematuria, microalbuminuria, proteinuria	ACE inhibitors effective for microalbuminuria, hydroxyurea
Ocular complications	Proliferative or nonproliferative retinopathy	Asymptomatic, decreased visual acuity	Early detection by annual eye exam starting at age 10 y
Avascular necrosis	Expansion of bone marrow and repeated bone infarction	Painful hip or knee	Analgesia, hip core decompression, physical therapy

ACE, angiotensin-converting enzyme.

Points to Remember

- Infection is the most common cause of death in sickle cell patients younger than 5 years.
- Blood cultures should be obtained and empiric antibiotic coverage should be provided in sickle cell patients with fever higher than 38.5°C without a source. In general, patients younger than 3 years and those with inadequate ability to follow-up should be hospitalized.
- The most common organisms implicated in ACS in patients older than 3 years are *Chlamydia pneumoniae* and mycoplasma. *Streptococcus pneumoniae* and other typical organisms are less common pathogens but are implicated in some cases. Antibiotic coverage, therefore, should include both ceftriaxone and a macrolide.
- Think about salmonella as a cause of osteomyelitis in sickle cell patients.
- Transfusions almost always consist of PRBC rather than whole blood and can be simple or exchange.
- Gallstones are common in patients with sickle cell disease and are present in 42% of patients 15 to 18 years of age.
- Because of the need for multiple transfusions, patients with sickle cell syndromes are at risk of iron overload.
- Retinopathy is more common in patients with Hb SC disease than in Hb SS disease.

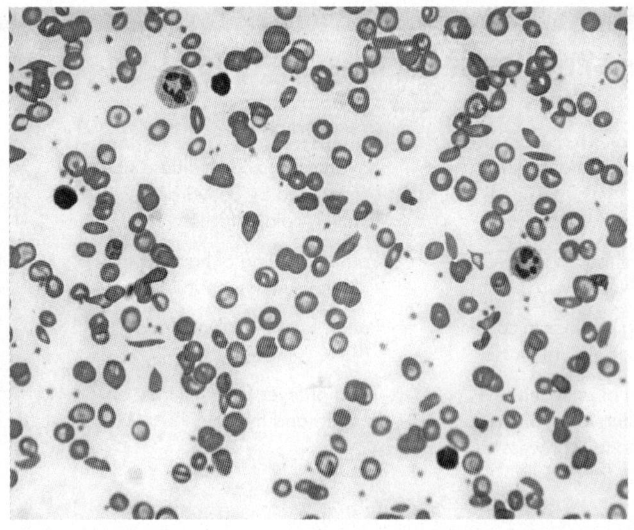

FIGURE 15.5. Peripheral blood smear in a patient with Hb SS disease showing sickled red blood cells, nucleated erythrocytes, and Howell–Jolly bodies. (Reprinted with permission from McMillan JA, Feigin RD, DeAngelis C, et al. *Oski's Pediatrics: Principles and Practice*. 4th ed. Philadelphia, PA: Lippincott Williams & Wilkins, 2006.)

Diagnosis

- Newborn screen with FSA hemoglobin.
- Lab abnormalities include anemia (Hb 5 to 9 g/dL) with reticulocytosis (retic 5% to 15%).
- Peripheral blood smear reveals sickled RBCs, nucleated erythrocytes, and Howell–Jolly bodies (nuclear remnants) (see Fig. 15.5).

Treatment

Treatment of sickle cell anemia is intended to minimize and treat complications.

- Treatment of associated complications is shown in Tables 15.5 and 15.6.
- Prevention of infection
  - Penicillin prophylaxis beginning at the age of 2 months and continuing until 5 years of age.
  - Routine childhood immunizations plus 23 valent pneumococcal vaccine at ages 2 and 5 years, meningococcal vaccine after 2 years, and yearly influenza vaccination.
- Hydroxyurea increases Hb F production and decreases pain crises, ACS, and need for transfusion.
- Chronic transfusion therapy to maintain Hb S less than 30% is indicated in patients with severe disease and helps prevent recurrent stroke, ACS, and recurrent pain crises.
- BMT is curative but is rarely done in the United States because of the associated risks.
- Routine surveillance with yearly TCD examination after the age of 2 years to assess stroke risk, yearly echocardiogram beginning at age 15 or 16 years to detect pulmonary hypertension, and yearly eye exam after the age of 10 years to evaluate for retinopathy.

Thalassemias

Thalassemias are a group of hereditary hypochromic microcytic anemias associated with defective synthesis of one of the polypeptide chains of hemoglobin. In the United States, thalassemias are most common in persons of Mediterranean and Southeast Asian ethnic backgrounds. In the heterozygous state, thalassemia genes produce mild anemia. In the homozygous form, however, they are associated with severe disease. Unbalanced polypeptide chain synthesis forms unstable hemoglobin complexes within the erythrocyte that cause early RBC death, mainly within the bone marrow. The result is ineffective erythropoiesis with severe hemolysis and compensatory hypertrophy of erythroid tissue in medullary and extramedullary sites.

Alpha Thalassemias

Alpha thalassemias are associated with defective alpha chain production and a relative excess of beta and gamma chains. Alpha chain production is determined by four identical genes on chromosome 16. Mutations in these genes result in different subtypes of alpha thalassemias as shown in Table 15.7.

Beta Thalassemias

Beta thalassemias are associated with defective beta chain production and a relative excess of alpha chains. Beta globin production is controlled by two genes on chromosome 11. There are two distinct gene mutations involved in beta thalassemias. The β^0 mutation results in the complete absence of beta chain production. The β^+ mutation results in variably decreased beta chain

TABLE 15.7

ALPHA THALASSEMIAS

Thalassemia	Globin Genotype	Subtype	Newborn Hb Electrophoresis	Clinical Manifestations	Treatment
1 gene deletion	$-, \alpha/\alpha, \alpha$	Silent carrier	1%–2% Bart's Hb	Asymptomatic Normal Hb	None
2 gene deletion	$-, \alpha/-, \alpha$ or $-, -/\alpha, \alpha$	Alpha-thalassemia trait	5%–10% Bart's Hb	Asymptomatic Mild anemia	None
3 gene deletion	$-, -/-, \alpha$	Hb H disease	20%–30% Bart's Hb, 5%–10% Hb H	Moderate-to-severe anemia	Periodic transfusions, folate, +/− splenectomy
4 gene deletion	$-, -/-, -$	Hydrops fetalis	89%–90% Bart's Hb No normal Hb	Severe anemia Hydrops fetalis	Fatal

Notes: Bart's Hb is made up of four gamma chains (γ_4); Hb H is made up of four beta chains (β_4).

production. Mutations in these genes result in different subtypes of beta thalassemias as shown in Table 15.8.

Clinical Manifestations in Children with Severe Thalassemias

- Signs and symptoms of anemia (e.g., pallor, fatigue, weakness, FTT, CHF).
- Abnormal facies due to extramedullary hematopoiesis and expansion of medullary spaces (e.g., maxillary hyperplasia, flat nasal bridge, frontal bossing).
- Pathologic bone fractures.
- Hepatosplenomegaly with hypersplenism.

Diagnosis

- Abnormal hemoglobin electrophoresis results as shown in Tables 15.7 and 15.8.
- Variable severity of hypochromic microcytic anemia with nucleated RBCs, poikilocytes, and target cells.

Treatment

Treatment of the thalassemias depends on the severity of the specific disease and is mainly supportive as shown in Tables 15.7 and 15.8.

- Transfusions may be required intermittently or regularly to maintain the hemoglobin level at 10 g/dL or more.
- Iron chelation with deferoxamine to prevent iron overload in patients requiring chronic transfusions.
- Splenectomy is indicated in severe cases with hypersplenism.
- BMT from HLA-identical and partly mismatched siblings can be curative.

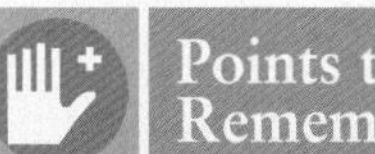

Points to Remember

- **Newborn screening in every state includes a hemoglobin electrophoresis that will detect sickle cell disease.**

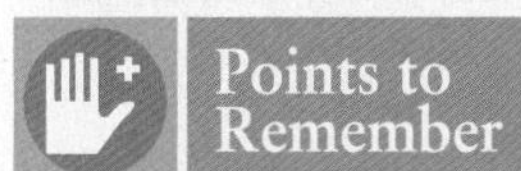

Points to Remember

- **In alpha thalassemia, a relative excess of beta and gamma chains leads to an increased amount of Bart's hemoglobin (γ_4) and Hb H (β_4).**
- **Hemoglobin electrophoresis is not helpful after the immediate postnatal period for diagnosing alpha thalassemias—it is only in the newborn period that electrophoresis shows 3% to 6% Bart's Hb instead of the normal Hb F.**

TABLE 15.8

BETA THALASSEMIAS

Thalassemia	Globin Genotype	Subtype	Hb Electrophoresis	Clinical Manifestations	Treatment
β^0 or β^+ heterozygote	β^0/A or β^+/A	Beta-thalassemia trait/minor	Elevated Hb A_2, variable elevation of Hb F	Mild anemia; usually asymptomatic	None
β^+-Thalassemia severe	β^+/β^+	Thalassemia intermedia	70%–95% Hb F, 2% Hb A_2, Trace Hb A	Moderate anemia presenting at 2 years of age	Periodic transfusions
β^0-Thalassemia homozygous or double heterozygotes	β^0/β^0 or β^+/β^0 or β^+/β^+	Beta-thalassemia major	98% Hb F, 2% Hb A_2	Severe anemia within first 6 mo of life; FTT and CHF within first year of life without treatment	Transfusion dependent

Note: β^+/β^+ can result in thalassemia intermedia or thalassemia major depending on the quantity of beta globin chain production by the abnormal β^+ genes.
CHF, congestive heart failure; FTT, failure to thrive.

Points to Remember

- In beta thalassemias, a relative excess of alpha chains and a normal amount of gamma and delta chains lead to an increased amount of Hb F ($\alpha_2\gamma_2$) and Hb A_2 ($\alpha_2\delta_2$).

HEMOSIDEROSIS

Hemosiderosis is the inevitable and fatal consequence of prolonged transfusion therapy. Every transfusion contains iron that cannot be physiologically excreted and builds up in vital organs.

- Elevated serum ferritin is an early marker of hemosiderosis.
- Noninvasive methods to aid in diagnosis include MRI ferrous scan and superconducting quantum interference device.
- Quantitative iron measurement by liver biopsy is the diagnostic gold standard.
- Chelation therapy (e.g., deferoxamine) is key for prevention and treatment.

POLYCYTHEMIA

Polycythemia is an excess of erythrocytes in relation to blood volume. It is defined as a Hb or Hct greater than two standard deviations above normal for age. Polycythemia can be primary or secondary.

Primary Polycythemia

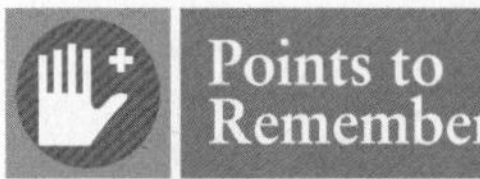

Points to Remember

- Erythropoietin levels are low in primary polycythemias and high in secondary polycythemias.

Primary polycythemia is rare in children. It results from mutations within the hematopoietic progenitor cells and can be acquired (polycythemia vera) or inherited (primary familial congenital polycythemia). It is characterized by low erythropoietin levels. Seventy-five percent of patients with polycythemia vera have a pan-myeloproliferative disorder and thus also have leukocytosis and thrombocytosis.

Secondary Polycythemia

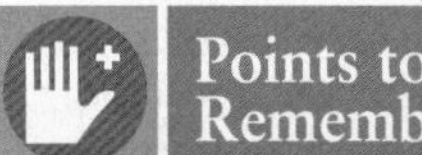

Points to Remember

- The normal number of neutrophils in the blood varies slightly according to age and race.
- All patients with neutropenia require early and aggressive treatment of suspected and confirmed infections. Gram-negative enterics are a particular concern.

Secondary polycythemia is caused by an increase in circulating erythropoietin. The increased erythropoietin may be physiologically appropriate or inappropriate.

- Appropriate increases in erythrocyte mass are seen in conditions that cause tissue hypoxia and are most often associated with cardiac or pulmonary abnormalities (e.g., OSA, chronic lung disease, cyanotic congenital heart disease).
- Inappropriate secretion of erythropoietin is associated with a variety of benign and malignant tumors, renal abnormalities (e.g., cysts, obstructive uropathy, posttransplantation), endocrine imbalances (e.g., Cushing syndrome, excess androgens, growth hormone therapy), and congenital abnormalities in the hypoxia-sensing pathway (e.g., Chuvash polycythemia).

Clinical Manifestations

- Can be asymptomatic.
- Patients may have a ruddy complexion.
- Hyperviscosity may cause headache, hypertension, and/or shortness of breath.
- Increased risk of thrombosis and/or hemorrhage.

Treatment

- **Primary polycythemia:** periodic phlebotomy, iron supplementation, antiplatelet agents, and/or hydroxyurea.
- **Secondary polycythemia:** periodic phlebotomy, treatment of underlying etiology.

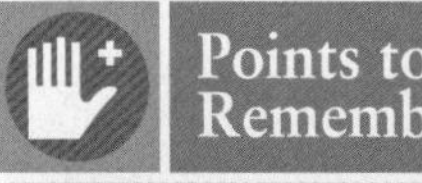

Points to Remember

- ANC = % (PMNs + bands) × total WBC

NEUTROPENIAS

Neutropenia is defined as an absolute decrease in the number of circulating neutrophils. Complications of neutropenia are related to the duration and severity and include bacterial and fungal infections such as sepsis, pneumonia, stomatitis, gingivitis, perirectal infections, and cellulitis.

The ANC is used to classify neutropenia according to severity as follows:

- ANC 1,000 to 1,500 = mild neutropenia.
- ANC 500 to 1,000 = moderate neutropenia.
- ANC less than 500 = severe neutropenia.

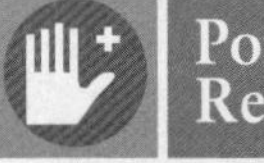

Points to Remember

- Congenital cyclic neutropenia is not benign—10% of patients with cyclic neutropenia die from infectious complications.

Chronic neutropenia is defined as neutropenia for 6 months or more.

Neutropenia exists in both congenital and acquired forms. Congenital forms of neutropenia are shown in Table 15.9.

TABLE 15.9

CONGENITAL FORMS OF NEUTROPENIA

Congenital Causes of Neutropenia				
	Inheritance	Clinical Features	Lab Findings	Treatment
Cyclic neutropenia	AD	During neutropenic phases, patients may suffer fever, malaise, oral ulcers, stomatitis, pharyngitis, lymphadenopathy, and/or serious bacterial and fungal infections. 10% of patients die from associated infections.	Regular, periodic episodes of severe neutropenia with ANC <200 occurring every 19–21 d and lasting 3–10 d ANC in between episodes may be normal or may not exceed 1,000. Bone marrow demonstrates granulocytic hypoplasia during episodes of neutropenia	G-CSF
Kostmann syndrome (severe congenital neutropenia)	AR	Presents in first few months of life with recurrent, unusual, and/or serious infections	Severe neutropenia with ANC <200 ± monocytosis, eosinophilia Bone marrow with arrest at promyelocyte and myelocyte stages	G-CSF BMT
Shwachman–Diamond–Oski syndrome	AR	Presents in infancy with failure to thrive, pancreatic insufficiency, metaphyseal dysostosis, eczema, neutropenia, anemia, thrombocytopenia, and infections Transformation to leukemia in 12%–25% of patients	Neutropenia, elevated stool fecal elastase, genetic testing	BMT
Dyskeratosis congenital	X-linked	Hyperpigmentation, leukoplakia, nail dystrophy 35% of patients have associated mild neutropenia and suffer increased infections	Mild neutropenia, decreased telomerase length	

AD, autosomal dominant; AR, autosomal recessive; ANC, absolute neutrophil count; BMT, bone marrow transplant; G-CSF, granulocyte colony-stimulating factor.

Acquired neutropenias can result from infections, autoimmune processes, drugs/toxins, and malignancies. Causes of acquired neutropenia are shown in Table 15.10.

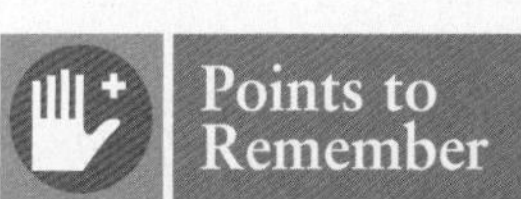

- Infectious diseases are the most common cause of acquired neutropenia in children.
- Autoimmune neutropenia is the most common cause of chronic neutropenia in young children. It typically presents between 6 and 26 months of age. Most children do not require intervention and recover without specific therapy. Steroids, IVIG, and/or G-CSF may be beneficial in select cases.

TABLE 15.10

ACQUIRED CAUSES OF NEUTROPENIA

	Specific Etiologies
Infection	*Viral*: hepatitis A/B, varicella, influenza, HSV, RSV, CMV, EBV, HIV, parvovirus *Bacterial*: overwhelming sepsis, tuberculosis *Misc*: rickettsial diseases (e.g., RMSF), malaria, toxoplasmosis
Drugs and toxins	*Antibiotics*: penicillins, aminoglycosides, sulfa drugs, cephalosporins *Anticonvulsants*: phenytoin, barbiturates, valproic acid *Antiinflammatory agents*: NSAIDs, aspirin *Misc*: chemotherapy agents, thiazides, quinidine, propranolol, antithyroid agents
Bone marrow infiltration	Leukemia, lymphoma, neuroblastoma, rhabdomyosarcoma, retinoblastoma, myelofibrosis, storage diseases
Autoimmune	Autoimmune neutropenia, SLE, rheumatic arthritis
Idiopathic	Chronic idiopathic neutropenia

CMV, cytomegalovirus; EBV, Epstein–Barr virus; HIV, human immunodeficiency virus; HSV, herpes simplex virus; NSAID, nonsteroidal anti-inflammatory drug; RMSF, Rocky Mountain spotted fever; RSV, respiratory syncytial virus; SLE, systemic lupus erythematosus.

SPLEEN

The spleen and lymph nodes are the two major components of the RES. Fixed phagocytic cells interact with circulating lymphocytes to filter and remove damaged cells and debris from the blood stream and also to deliver antigens to the immune system. By clearing circulating bacteria, the RES as a whole plays a critical role in the immune system. The spleen, however, is the only part of the RES that is able to effectively filter encapsulated bacteria.

Splenomegaly

Splenomegaly results from hyperplasia of the RES due to excessive antigenic stimulation, excessive destruction of cells, or passive congestion. Specific causes include viral infections (e.g., CMV, EBV), malignancies (e.g., lymphoma, HLH), portal venous congestion, and storage disorders.

Hypersplenism

An overactive spleen can lead to deficiencies in one or more peripheral cell lines, most commonly thrombocytopenia. Depending on the severity and underlying etiology, splenectomy may be indicated and is curative.

Hyposplenism

Hyposplenism may be anatomic or functional and congenital or acquired. An example of congenital anatomic hyposplenism is a patient who is born without a spleen. An example of congenital functional hyposplenism is a patient with congenital heart disease and polysplenia who has multiple spleens but none that function properly. An example of acquired functional asplenia is a sickle cell patient who becomes functionally asplenic as a result of splenic infarction.

- The presence or absence of a spleen can be documented via imaging techniques such as MRI or ultrasound. Functional assessment of a spleen is best studied via a technetium-99 radionuclide splenic scan. Howell-Jolly bodies may also be identified on peripheral blood smear.
- Patients who are functionally asplenic are at increased risk of serious infections with encapsulated organisms such as *S. pneumoniae*, *Haemophilus influenzae*, *and Neisseria meningitidis*.
- The most important aspect of treatment is prevention of infection via prophylactic penicillin, immunization against encapsulated organisms, and early treatment of suspected or confirmed infections.

DISORDERS OF PLATELETS

Abnormalities of platelets may be congenital or acquired and quantitative (i.e., abnormal number of platelets) or qualitative (i.e., platelets do not function normally).

Congenital Platelet Abnormalities

Important congenital platelet abnormalities are shown in Table 15.11.

Acquired Platelet Abnormalities

Idiopathic (Immune) Thrombocytopenic Purpura

ITP is the most common cause of acquired thrombocytopenia in childhood. The exact etiology is unknown, but it is thought to be an immune-mediated phenomenon likely in response to a viral infection. It is most common in children 1 to 4 years of age. A preceding viral illness 1 to 4 weeks before the onset of symptoms is described in more than half of patients.

Clinical Manifestations

- Acute onset of generalized petechiae, ecchymosis, and/or purpura in a well-appearing otherwise healthy child (see Fig. 15.6).
- Mucosal bleeding and/or submucosal hemorrhages are common (see Fig. 15.7).
- Physical examination is otherwise normal.
- CNS bleeding is the most feared complication but occurs in less than 1% of patients.

TABLE 15.11

CONGENITAL PLATELET ABNORMALITIES

	Inheritance and Defect	Clinical Manifestations	Lab Findings	Treatment
		Congenital Thrombocytopenias		
Thrombocytopenia absent radius (TAR)	AR	Presents in infancy with petechiae, purpura, limb deformities, and cardiac and/or renal anomalies	Peripheral thrombocytopenia Bone marrow with decreased megakaryocytes	Periodic platelet transfusions Thrombocytopenia typically resolves by age 2–3 y
Amegakaryocytic thrombocytopenia	AR Mutations in thrombopoietin receptor	Presents in infancy with petechiae and/or purpura Some patients develop neurologic deficits and generalized bone marrow dysfunction later in life	Peripheral thrombocytopenia	Bone marrow transplant
Wiskott–Aldrich syndrome	X-linked recessive	Presents with thrombocytopenia, eczema, and/or immunodeficiency	Peripheral thrombocytopenia Tiny platelets	IVIG, corticosteroids, bone marrow transplant
Other quantitative platelet disorders include Fanconi's anemia, Shwachman–Diamond syndrome, dyskeratosis congenita, trisomy 18 and 13, deletions of chromosome 22q11 (DiGeorge syndrome, velocardiofacial syndrome)				
		Congenital Qualitative Platelet Disorders		
Glanzmann thrombasthenia	AR Absence of glycoprotein IIb/IIIa from platelet membrane	Broad spectrum of bleeding severity ranging from mild to life threatening hemorrhage	Normal platelet number and morphology Abnormal in vitro platelet aggregation	Platelet transfusions, epsilon-aminocaproic acid for mucosal hemorrhage, recombinant factor VIIa
Bernard–Soulier syndrome	AR Absence of glycoproteins Ib, V, and IX from platelet surface	Severe hemorrhage	Abnormal in vitro platelet aggregation Large, bizarre platelets	Platelet transfusions, epsilon-aminocaproic acid for mucosal hemorrhage, recombinant factor VIIa
Gray platelet syndrome	AD >> AR Abnormalities of platelet granules	Bleeding diathesis usually apparent at birth	Washed-out or gray appearing platelets	
Qualitative platelet dysfunction can also occur in type I glycogen storage disease, cyanotic congenital heart disease, Epstein syndrome, TAR syndrome, Ehlers Danlos syndrome, Wiskott–Aldrich syndrome, and osteogenesis imperfecta				

AD, autosomal dominant; AR, autosomal recessive; IVIG, intravenous immunoglobulin.

Diagnosis

- CBC demonstrates isolated thrombocytopenia (platelet count often <20 K/μL).
- Blood smear shows a reduced number of platelets that are normal in morphology (normal WBC and RBC number and morphology).
- Bone marrow aspirate is not required for diagnosis but may be indicated if diagnosis is unclear and will reveal normal to increased number of megakaryocytes.

Treatment

- Treatment does not change the natural history of the disease but may be indicated in severe cases to decrease the risk of complications, primarily intracranial hemorrhage.
- Watchful waiting may be considered in mild cases with platelets greater than 20 K/μL.
- Treatment options for patients with platelets less than 20 K/μL, extensive bleeding, and/or who develop complications of ITP include IVIG, Anti-D immunoglobulin, and corticosteroids (see Table 15.12).

Prognosis

- More than 50% of children with ITP recover within 4 weeks without treatment and more than 80% recover spontaneously within 6 months.
- Chronic ITP is defined as symptoms lasting more than 6 months.
- Relapses are rare in acute ITP but common in chronic ITP.

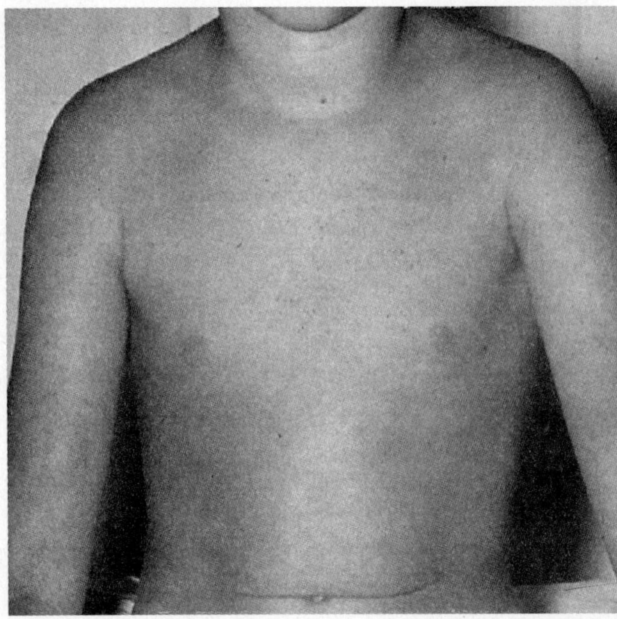

FIGURE 15.6. Petechiae in a patient with idiopathic (immune) thrombocytopenic purpura. (Reprinted with permission from McMillan JA, Feigin RD, DeAngelis C, et al. *Oski's Pediatrics: Principles and Practice*. 4th ed. Philadelphia, PA: Lippincott Williams & Wilkins, 2006.)

Drug-Induced Thrombocytopenia

A variety of drugs are known to cause thrombocytopenia in some patients. In some cases, the thrombocytopenia is due to the development of specific antibodies but nonimmune forms exist as well.

- Common offending drugs include penicillins, bactrim, digoxin, quinine, benzodiazepines, heparin, and valproic acid.
- Acute onset, typically within hours of drug administration.
- Thrombocytopenia is usually severe.
- Most cases resolve with withdrawal of offending agent.

Heparin-induced thrombocytopenia is a well-recognized phenomenon that deserves special mention. It occurs in two forms: (1) a non–immune-mediated form that occurs within 1 to 2 days of heparin administration and is mild and benign and (2) an immune-mediated form that occurs 4 to 10 days after heparin administration, is severe, and is associated with a paradoxical increased risk of arterial and venous thromboses.

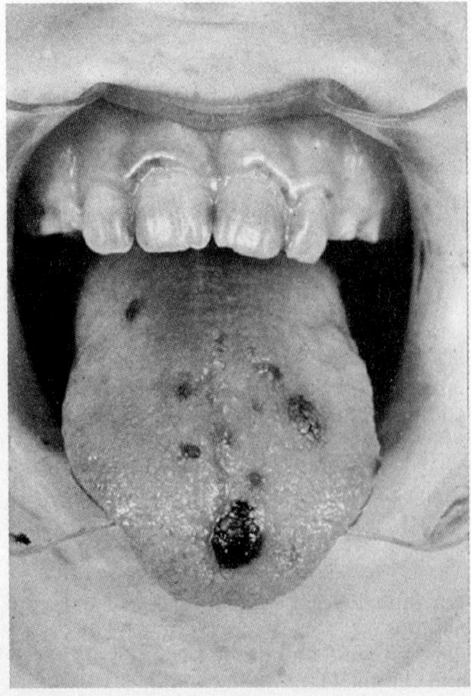

FIGURE 15.7. Submucosal hemorrhages in a patient with idiopathic (immune) thrombocytopenic purpura. (Reprinted with permission from McMillan JA, Feigin RD, DeAngelis C, et al. *Oski's Pediatrics: Principles and Practice*. 4th ed. Philadelphia, PA: Lippincott Williams & Wilkins, 2006.)

TABLE 15.12

TREATMENT OPTIONS FOR SEVERE AND/OR COMPLICATED ITP

Treatment	Mechanism	Comments
IVIG	Blocks RES and decreases splenic clearance of platelets, promotes clearance of antiplatelet antibodies, and inhibits phagocytosis of platelets	Response is rapid but short-lived Duration of treatment 1–5 d One-third of patients experience transient complications such as headache, nausea, and/or aseptic meningitis; allergic reactions can also occur
Anti–D immunoglobulin	Coats RBCs, and antibody-coated RBCs compete with antibody-coated platelets for uptake and clearance by the spleen	Only efficacious in Rh+ patients Response is rapid and more sustained than IVIG Duration of treatment 1–2 d Good safety profile; associated decrease in Hb of ~1.3 g/dL; severe anemia can occur but is rare
Corticosteroids	Decreases immune response	Response is slower and less robust Duration of treatment is several weeks Side effects include Cushing syndrome, hyperglycemia, hypertension

Notes:
Platelet transfusions are indicated only for severe acute bleeding in ITP because of shortened survival of the transfused platelets.
Splenectomy is curative for most patients but is indicated only for life-threatening emergencies and/or refractory disease because of the risks associated with asplenia.
Other immunosuppressive agents such as azathioprine and cyclosporine may be indicated in select cases.
IVIG, intravenous immunoglobulin; ITP, idiopathic (immune) thrombocytopenic purpura; RBCc, red blood cells; RES, reticuloendothelial system.

Neonatal Immune Thrombocytopenia

Two forms of neonatal immune thrombocytopenia exist: autoimmune and allo- or isoimmune.

Neonatal Autoimmune Thrombocytopenia

- Caused by passive transplacental transfer of antibodies from a mother with ITP.
- PAIgG detected on mother's platelets (direct platelet antibody test positive with mothers' platelets).
- Postnatal IVIG may be helpful.

Neonatal Alloimmune Thrombocytopenia

- Occurs in infants whose mothers have been sensitized to paternally inherited antigens present on the infant's platelets that belong to a different class than the mother's antigens (similar to Rh isoimmunization).
- Direct PAIgG test on mother is negative but mother's serum tested with infant's platelets is positive (indirect test).
- In severe cases, in utero platelet transfusions for infant and/or IVIG administered to mother decrease the risk of intracranial hemorrhage.

Microangiopathic Causes of Thrombocytopenia

Thrombocytopenia due to destruction of platelets within blood vessels occurs in HUS, TTP, and large hemangiomas.

Hemolytic Uremic Syndrome

- Typically presents with bloody diarrhea followed by renal failure, anemia, and thrombocytopenia.
- Most commonly implicated pathogen is *E. coli* O157:H7.
- Shortened platelet survival secondary to microangiopathic process involving fibrin deposition.
- Treatment is primarily supportive; dialysis is indicated in severe cases.
- Platelet transfusions should be given only for serious hemorrhage as the increase in the platelets will be very transient.

Thrombotic Thrombocytopenic Purpura

- Characterized by fever, neurological symptoms, microangiopathic hemolytic anemia, and thrombocytopenia.
- Less common in children than in adults.
- Thrombocytopenia results from platelet aggregation and clumping in vessels.
- Treatment is immunosuppression and plasma exchange.
- Platelet transfusions are contraindicated as they may exacerbate CNS and cardiac symptoms
- ADAMTS13 activity level is decreased.

Hemangiomas

- Platelets can be sequestered and subsequently destroyed in large hemangiomas, such as those found in patients with Kasabach–Merritt syndrome.
- Treatment is primarily supportive; for severe cases, treatment strategies include corticosteroids, platelets, cryoprecipitate, and interferon-alpha-2a.

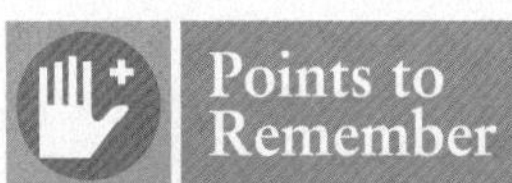

Points to Remember

- **Extreme thrombocytosis (often >1 million) is commonly seen in patients with Kawasaki disease and typically begins 7 to 14 days after the onset of the acute illness.**

Thrombocytosis

Thrombocytosis is most commonly secondary to an underlying cause, although rarely primary or familial thrombocytosis does occur.

- Common causes of secondary thrombocytosis include acute or chronic bleeding, inflammatory or infectious processes, and iron deficiency.
- Myeloproliferative syndromes such as polycythemia vera and CML are rare causes of thrombocytosis.
- Symptomatic thrombocytosis is rare; typically, no role for aspirin or other antiplatelet agents.

PANCYTOPENIA

Pancytopenia is defined as a decrease in two or more cell lines. Pancytopenia can result from a variety of causes, including both congenital and acquired etiologies. A thorough medical history and physical examination as well as examination of a peripheral blood smear is important in making the diagnosis and determining the etiology, but examination of the bone marrow is most important.

Table 15.13 lists causes of pancytopenia grouped based on the cellularity and status of the bone marrow. A more detailed discussion of aplastic anemia is presented in the following section. The other etiologies are discussed in more detail in other chapters.

Aplastic Anemia

Aplastic anemia is a clinical state characterized by varying degrees of peripheral pancytopenia resulting from reduced or absent production of blood cells in the bone marrow. Aplastic anemia may arise in the setting of inherited/congenital syndromes leading to marrow failure or may develop secondary to acquired abnormalities.

Aplastic anemia is classified as severe if two of the following peripheral blood abnormalities occur in combination with severe hypocellularity of the bone marrow: (a) ANC less than 500/μL, (b) platelets less than 20,000/μL, and (c) absolute retic less than 1%.

TABLE 15.13

CAUSES OF PANCYTOPENIA ACCORDING TO BONE MARROW FINDINGS

Hypocellular Marrow (Aplastic Anemias)	Cellular Bone Marrow	Replacement of Marrow by Infiltrative Process
Acquired aplastic anemia	**Primary bone marrow disease**	**Blood malignancies**
Drugs	Myelodysplastic syndrome (Monosomy 7)	AML
Chloramphenicol	Paroxysmal nocturnal hemoglobinuria	ALL
Antineoplastic agents		Hemophagocytic lymphohistiocytosis
Toxins	**Secondary to systemic disease**	**Metastatic solid tumors**
Ionizing radiation	SLE	Neuroblastoma
Infections	Sjogren syndrome	Rhabdomyosarcoma
EBV	Hypersplenism	Retinoblastoma, Osteopetrosis
CMV	Storage disorder	Myelofibrosis
Hepatitis B and C	Sarcoidosis	
Seronegative hepatitis		
HIV		
Parvovirus		
Inherited aplastic anemia		
Fanconi syndrome		
Diamond–Blackfan syndrome		
Shwachman–Diamond syndrome		
Dyskeratosis congenital		

ALL, acute lymphoid leukemia; AML, acute myeloid leukemia; CMV, cytomegalovirus; EBV, Epstein–Barr virus; HIV, human immunodeficiency virus; SLE, systemic lupus erythematosus.

Acquired Aplastic Anemia

Many drugs, infections, and environmental factors have been associated with the development of aplastic anemia as shown in Table 15.13.

Some agents are directly toxic to the bone marrow and regularly produce marrow hypoplasia in a dose-dependent manner (e.g., ionizing radiation, antineoplastic agents), whereas other agents only produce marrow hypoplasia in a small proportion of those exposed (e.g., chloramphenicol). Chloramphenicol is the drug most frequently associated with aplastic anemia, although only 1 in 20,000 to 50,000 persons taking chloramphenicol develop aplastic anemia.

Common viral causes of aplastic anemia include EBV, CMV, parvovirus, hepatitis B and C, and HIV. A particularly serious form of aplastic anemia occurs in the wake of viral hepatitis. In half of these patients, no causative factor for the hepatitis is found.

Clinical Manifestations

- Signs and symptoms of anemia (e.g., pallor, fatigue), leukopenia (e.g., infections), and/or thrombocytopenia (e.g., petechiae, easy bruising/bleeding).

Treatment

- Depends on the severity and specific etiology.
- Aplastic anemia secondary to a viral infection is often transient and self-limited.
- More severe forms of aplastic anemia require transfusions, immunosuppressive therapy (e.g., steroids, cyclosporine, cyclophosphamide), and/or BMT.

Congenital Aplastic Anemia

Congenital aplastic anemias are very rare. The most common congenital aplastic anemia is Fanconi anemia. Fanconi anemia is an AR disorder caused by a defect in DNA that renders the patient's cells susceptible to damage by environmental toxins, thus predisposing the patient to marrow failure. Diamond–Blackfan syndrome, Shwachman–Diamond syndrome, and dyskeratosis congenital are other inherited causes of aplastic anemia.

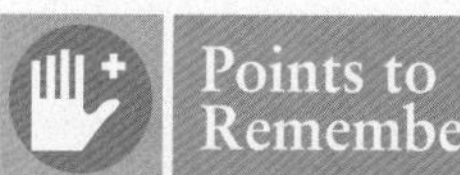

- The hematologic abnormalities associated with Fanconi syndrome are progressive and are usually not present during infancy and early childhood.

Clinical Manifestations of Fanconi Syndrome

- Progressive pancytopenia and hypoplasia of the bone marrow; thrombocytopenia usually develops prior to anemia and leucopenia; patients usually present with petechiae and bruising between the ages of 2 and 22 years (average is 7 years).
- Physical abnormalities are present in half of patients and may include short stature, generalized hyperpigmentation, thumb and/or radii abnormalities, and/or renal abnormalities.

Diagnosis of Fanconi Syndrome

- Should be suspected in patients with physical abnormalities described earlier.
- Macrocytosis and elevated levels of Hb F precede the onset of marrow failure.
- Severe pancytopenia and eventual bone marrow failure.
- Diepoxybutane test: peripheral lymphocytes exposed to diepoxybutane (an alkylating agent) show chromosomal abnormalities.

Treatment of Fanconi Syndrome

- Temporary relief via platelet and erythrocyte transfusions.
- Two-third of patients respond to androgenic hormone therapy but most eventually become refractory to androgens.
- BMT.

COAGULOPATHIES

The body's normal response to control bleeding includes vasoconstriction, platelet activation, and activation of the coagulation cascade. The coagulation cascade consists of the activation of several enzyme complexes that ultimately results in the activation of thrombin and the subsequent deposition of an insoluble fibrin clot (see Fig. 15.8).

Coagulation disorders can be divided into conditions with abnormal bleeding (i.e., hypocoagulable states) and those associated with the development of thrombosis (i.e., hypercoagulable states). Coagulopathies can be congenital or acquired and can be secondary to abnormalities of the blood vessels, platelets, and/or plasma clotting factors.

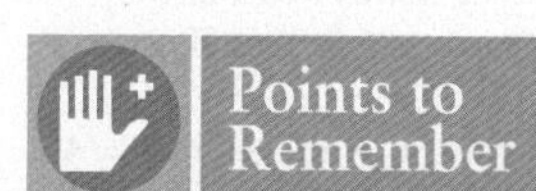

- Because spontaneous mutations are common, many patients with hemophilia A will not have a known family history of the disorder.

Congenital Coagulopathies

Factor VIII Deficiency (Hemophilia A) and Factor IX Deficiency (Hemophilia B)

Hemophilia A represents a defect in factor VIII procoagulant activity. It is one of the most common inherited bleeding disorders, affecting 1 in 5,000 male newborns. It is an X-linked disorder. Female

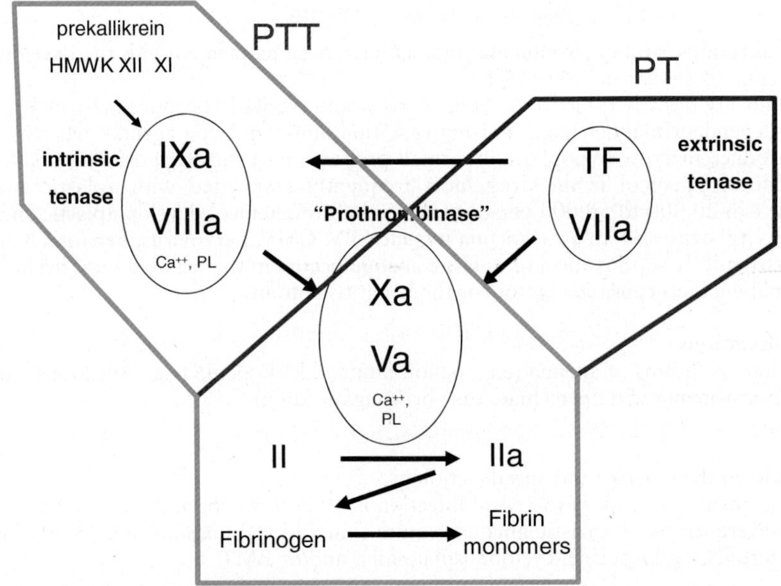

Note: Blue: Intrinsic pathway
Red: Extrinsic pathway
Points to remember: Deficiency of factors XII, XI, IX, VIII prolong PTT alone
Deficiency of factor VII prolongs PT

FIGURE 15.8. Coagulation cascade: physiology of clot formation and factors affecting partial thromboplastin time and prothrombin time.

carriers are asymptomatic. Spontaneous mutations are common. Hemophilia B is an X-linked defect in factor IX procoagulant activity. Hemophilia A and B are clinically indistinguishable.

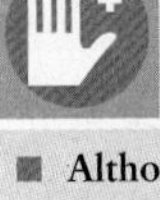

Points to Remember

- Although the severity of hemophilia is related to how much factor activity is present, life-threatening bleeding can occur even in patients with mild disease.
- Although bleeding may occur at virtually any anatomic site, the most common serious bleeding encountered in hemophiliacs is hemarthrosis.

Clinical Manifestations

- Severity is related to how much factor activity is present
  - Mild (5% to 25% of normal activity): usually bleed only after surgery or major trauma.
  - Moderate (1% to 5% of normal activity): usually develop significant bleeding only after some type of trauma.
- Severe (<1% of normal activity): subject to spontaneous bleeding.
- Lifelong tendency to bleed
  - Half of patients present with excessive bleeding after circumcision.
  - Mucosal bleeding and bruising.
  - Intracranial hemorrhage.
  - Hemarthrosis.
  - Excessive bleeding with dental procedures, sutures, surgeries, etc.

Diagnosis

- Screening testing: prolongation of aPTT with normal PT.
- Confirmatory testing:
  - Hemophilia A: low factor VIII activity with a normal vWF assay.
  - Hemophilia B: low factor IX activity.

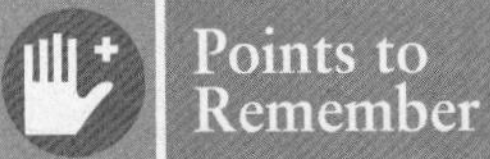

Points to Remember

- For acute bleeds, factor replacement should occur as soon as possible. For patients with hemophilia A, factor VIII levels will typically increase by 2% for every 1 unit/kg given. For patients with hemophilia B, factor IX levels will typically increase by 1% for every 1 unit/kg given.

Treatment

- Prevention of bleeding via avoidance of contact sports and similar activities.
- Replacement therapy with factor VIII for hemophilia A and factor IX for hemophilia B
  - Maintenance therapy to keep activity greater than 1%.
  - Prophylactically prior to procedures.
  - Acutely in response to acute bleeding episodes.
- Other supportive treatment measures that may provide some benefit include epsilon aminocaproic acid, tranexamic acid, FFP, and/or DDAVP.

Factor XI Deficiency

Factor XI deficiency is an AR disorder characterized by a mild bleeding tendency. It is a rare disorder with an incidence of 1 per 50,000. It is most common in Ashkenazi Jews. Symptoms include increased bruising, epistaxis, menorrhagia, and postoperative bleeding. Hemarthroses and deep soft tissue bleeding are rare.

TABLE 15.14

CLASSIFICATION OF VON WILLEBRAND DISEASE

	Type 1	Type 2	Type 3
Inheritance	Autosomal dominant	Autosomal dominant	Autosomal recessive
Ristocetin cofactor activity	Decreased	Decreased (except 2N)	Decreased
vWF antigen	Decreased	Normal to decreased	Severely decreased
Ristocetin induced platelet aggregation	Normal to decreased	Decreased	Severely decreased
Severity of bleeding	Mild to moderate	Severe	Severe
Treatment	DDAVP	vWF concentrates	vWF concentrates

DDAVP, desmopressin acetate; vWF, von Willebrand factor.

Factor VII Deficiency

Factor VII deficiency is a rare AR disorder that can present with symptomatic mucosal bleeding and/or intracranial hemorrhage. Diagnosis is made by finding isolated prolongation of PT with normal aPTT. Treatment is with recombinant factor VII and/or FFP.

Factor XIII Deficiency

Factor XIII deficiency classically presents with delayed bleeding from the umbilical stump. Coagulation studies are normal, but blood forms an unstable clot in urea. Treatment is with cryoprecipitate and/or plasma.

Von Willebrand Disease

Von Willebrand disease is the most common inherited coagulopathy, affecting 0.8% to 1.6% of the general population. It encompasses a heterogeneous group of disorders resulting from the deficiency or dysfunction of vWF. vWF mediates platelet adhesion at sites of tissue injury and also acts as a carrier for factor VIII. Thus, insufficient vWF activity results in decreased platelet adhesiveness, impaired agglutination of platelets, and prolonged bleeding time. The three major forms of von Willebrand disease are shown in Table 15.14.

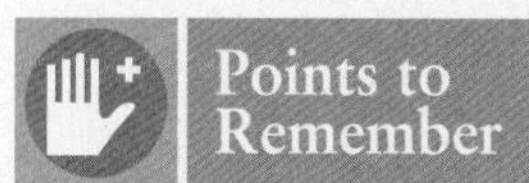
Points to Remember

- Type I von Willebrand disease is by far the most common form, accounting for 80% to 85% of cases.

Clinical Presentation

- Patients with type I disease have mild-to-moderate bleeding tendency
  - Epistaxis.
  - Menorrhagia.
  - Easy bruising.
  - Excessive bleeding after dental extractions.
- Patients with types II and III have more severe bleeding tendencies.

Diagnosis

- Screening labs demonstrate prolonged aPTT and prolonged bleeding time with a normal platelet count (except type IIa).
- Confirmatory testing reveals decreased activity of vWF measured by ristocetin activity and vWF antigen levels.

Treatment

- DDAVP
  - Useful for type 1 disease.
  - Given intranasally 20 to 30 minutes prior to minor procedures for prophylaxis and/or for minor bleeding.
- Aminocaproic acid
  - Useful for prophylaxis and/or for mucosal bleeding.
- vWF concentrates
  - Useful for severe bleeding in all types, not just 1 and 2.

Acquired Coagulopathies

Vitamin K Deficiency

Vitamin K is an important substrate for factors II, VII, IX, X, protein C, and protein S. Dietary vitamin K is found primarily in green, leafy vegetables. Causes of vitamin K deficiency include inadequate dietary intake, malabsorption (e.g., pancreatic insufficiency, biliary atresia, prolonged diarrhea), and drugs (e.g., phenytoin, rifampin, isoniazid).

Points to Remember

- Hemorrhagic disease of the newborn is rare now due to the routine practice of administering intramuscular vitamin K at birth. Be suspicious, however, in infants born at home or out of the traditional hospital setting who present with bruising and/or bleeding.

Hemorrhagic disease of the newborn is a special type of vitamin K deficiency. Newborns are particularly susceptible to vitamin K deficiency because of limited transplacental acquisition of vitamin K, limited ability to store vitamin K in the immature liver, and lack of gut flora to produce vitamin K.

Clinical Manifestations

- Bleeding tendency, easy bruising, oozing, visceral hemorrhage.

Diagnosis

- Disproportionate prolongation of PT in comparison with aPTT, normal fibrinogen.

Treatment

- Vitamin K (usually given PO or SQ, but can be given IV if life-threatening bleeding).

Liver Disease

Most of the clotting factors are synthesized in the liver. Factor VIII is the exception and has significant extrahepatic synthesis. Thus, any process that impairs liver synthetic function will result in coagulopathy with prolongation of both PT and aPTT.

Disseminated Intravascular Coagulation

DIC is characterized by a constellation of clinical and laboratory abnormalities associated with the activation of the coagulation system and subsequent deposition of fibrin in the microvasculature. Systemic causes of DIC include sepsis, shock, and exposure to certain snake venoms. Localized causes of DIC include hemangiomas and brain injury.

Points to Remember

- Purpura fulminans is a syndrome of DIC associated with hemorrhagic necrosis of the skin and widespread purpuric lesions.

Clinical Manifestations

- Excessive bruising and bleeding/oozing.
- Purpura and/or petechiae.
- Circulatory collapse.
- Increase risk of thrombosis.

Diagnosis

- No single test is diagnostic.
- Clinical findings as earlier plus lab abnormalities include thrombocytopenia, prolonged aPTT and PT, low fibrinogen, and/or increased D-dimer.
- Peripheral smear with microangiopathic changes in peripheral smear.

Treatment

- Treatment should be aimed at correcting the underlying cause.
- Supportive care for severe cases may include clotting factors and/or platelets (there is a theoretical risk of exacerbating the risk of thrombosis but benefits outweigh risks for severe disease).
- Heparin use in patients with thrombosis is controversial.

HYPERCOAGULABILITY

Points to Remember

- Many children with thromboses have multiple underlying risk factors rather than a single underlying predisposing factor.

Arterial and venous thromboses are relatively rare in infants and children, and when present, should prompt investigation for an underlying hypercoagulable condition. Thromboses can take the form of pulmonary emboli, DVT, renal artery or vein thromboses, stroke, catheter-related thrombosis, retinal artery occlusion, and/or peripheral artery or vein thromboses.

Inherited and acquired causes of hypercoagulability are shown in Tables 15.15 and 15.16, respectively.

Points to Remember

- Factor V Leiden is the most common inherited cause of hypercoagulability and is seen in 30% of children with DVTs.

Treatment

- Aggressiveness of treatment depends on severity of presentation and complications but may include anticoagulation and/or thrombolysis.
- Anticoagulation.
- Unfractionated heparin is the mainstay of treatment of acute thrombosis; typically given as a bolus followed by a continuous infusion; achieve and maintain therapeutic levels via monitoring of aPTTr and adjusting infusion appropriately (goal is 1.5 to 2.5 times the control).
- Long-term anticoagulation can be accomplished via warfarin or low-molecular-weight heparin.

TABLE 15.15

INHERITED CAUSES OF HYPERCOAGULABILITY

	Characteristics	Diagnosis
Protein C deficiency	■ AR and AD forms ■ Exists in heterozygous and homozygous states ■ Homozygous Protein C deficiency can present with purpura fulminans, and is often fatal without treatment	Low or absent protein C activity
Protein S deficiency	■ AD ■ Heterozygous form ■ Similar to heterozygous protein C deficiency	Low protein S activity
Factor V Leiden	■ AR ■ Single point mutation in factor V ■ Common; present in 2%–11% of the general population	Decreased activated protein C activity level, gene testing
Antithrombin III deficiency	■ AD ■ Can be associated with heparin resistance	Decreased antithrombin III activity
G20210A	■ AD ■ Single nucleotide mutation in prothrombin gene	Elevated PT levels, gene testing
Homocystinuria	■ AR ■ Deficiency of cystathionine beta-synthase	Low homocystine levels

AD, autosomal dominant; AR, autosomal recessive.

- Warfarin: administered orally; requires close monitoring of INR as levels are affected by different foods and various drugs; associated with increased risk of bleeding.
- Low-molecular-weight heparin: administered subcutaneously; more expensive than warfarin but less bleeding risk and decreased need for close monitoring (some people monitor antifactor Xa levels but the need to do so is controversial).
- Thrombolysis
  - Thrombolytic therapy with urokinase or t-PA if available should be strongly considered; catheter associated thrombolysis in an experienced setting allows smaller effective doses with potentially less bleeding.
- Disease-specific treatment.
- Protein C concentrate is useful for patients with protein C deficiency.
- Antithrombin III concentrates can be used for patients with antithrombin III deficiency
  - Folic acid supplementation is useful in the treatment of homocystinuria.

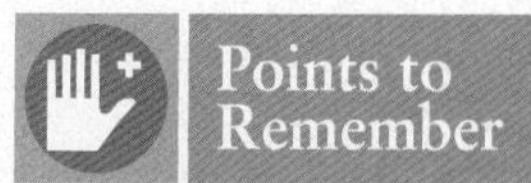

- When transitioning from heparin to warfarin, patients must receive heparin for a few days after initiating warfarin due to earlier fall in protein C and S levels than the other clotting factors and a paradoxical early hypercoagulability.

TABLE 15.16

ACQUIRED CAUSES OF HYPERCOAGULABILITY

	Specific Causes
Venous stasis	Immobilization, hyperviscosity, polycythemia, congestive heart failure, sickle cell disease
Intravasculature abnormality	Indwelling catheters, artificial heart valves, Kawasaki disease
Circulating anticoagulants	Lupus anticoagulant and anticardiolipin antibodies
Systemic diseases	Malignancy, liver disease, inflammatory bowel disease, PNH, nephrotic syndrome
Drugs	L-Asparaginase, warfarin, epsilon-aminocaproic acid, heparin

SAMPLE BOARD REVIEW QUESTIONS

1. An 18-month-old African American girl is noted to be anemic with a Hb of 10.1 gm/dL at a well child visit. MCV is low at 66 and RDW is elevated at 15.1. WBC and platelets are normal. The child appears to be asymptomatic and is growing and developing appropriately. Family history is significant for sickle cell trait in her mother. You suspect iron deficiency and start the patient on supplemental oral iron. Because of her family history, you send a hemoglobin electrophoresis that shows Hb A 65% and variant Hb 35%. You review the patient's newborn screen and find that it showed FAS. What is the most likely etiology of the patient's anemia?
   a. Sickle cell anemia
   b. Sickle cell trait
   c. Iron deficiency anemia
   d. Thalassemia

   Answer: c. Iron deficiency anemia. This patient has a microcytic anemia. The differential diagnosis for microcytic anemia includes iron deficiency, lead poisoning, and beta thalassemia. Iron deficiency anemia is by far the most common cause of anemia in young children and is further supported by this patient's elevated RDW. Iron deficiency is most common in children 9 to 24 months of age. Treatment is via supplemental oral iron. This patient also has sickle cell trait, but this is not the most likely cause of her anemia. This diagnosis is supported by the findings of FAS on her newborn screen and the hemoglobin electrophoresis showing 35% variant hemoglobin. Some labs are not able to detect sickled Hb and report it as variant hemoglobin. Individuals who are heterozygous for Hb S have sickle cell trait and have a benign course, as only 30% to 40% of their hemoglobin is Hb S. This is not enough to cause sickling or anemia.

2. You are evaluating a 15-month-old White female for short stature. Her past medical history is significant for eczema and three episodes of acute otitis media. She has never been hospitalized. She has never had any unusual or severe infections. Review of systems is significant for 6 to 8 stools per day and is otherwise negative. Physical examination shows a frail appearing toddler with a distended abdomen and bilateral clinodactyly. Weight is 25th% and height is 3rd%. CBC shows WBC of 3,200/mm^3, ANC 1,000, Hb 10.8 gm/dL, and platelets 130,000/mm^3. Which of the following is the most likely diagnosis in this patient?
   a. Cystic fibrosis
   b. Shwachman–Diamond syndrome
   c. Pearson syndrome
   d. Wiskott–Aldrich syndrome

   Answer: b. Shwachman–Diamond syndrome. Neutropenia in the setting of FTT and short stature should suggest Shwachman Diamond syndrome. This diagnosis is further supported by the patient's eczema, frequent stooling (likely secondary to pancreatic insufficiency), and clinodactyly. Shwachman–Diamond syndrome is an AR condition that typically presents in infancy or early toddlerhood with poor growth, pancreatic insufficiency, metaphyseal dysostosis, eczema, neutropenia, anemia, thrombocytopenia, and infections.

3. A 2-year-old female with Hb SS is brought to the ER with a 2-day history of decreased activity and pallor. Vital signs in triage are as follows: T 37.3, HR 174, bp 81/48, RR 24, and SaO_2 100% on RA. Initial labs reveal WBC 8,000/mm^3, Hb 3.5 gm/dL, platelets 100,000/mm^3, total bilirubin 4.5 mg/dL, and retic 10%. Which of the following physical examination findings supports the most likely etiology of this patient's acute deterioration?
   a. Grade 3/6 systolic ejection murmur
   b. Slapped cheek rash
   c. Scleral icterus
   d. Splenomegaly

   Answer: d. Splenomegaly. An acute drop in hemoglobin and reticulocytosis in a patient with Hb SS disease is concerning for splenic sequestration crisis. Vaso-occlusion within the spleen leads to trapping of RBCs in the spleen and an acute drop in hemoglobin. This life-threatening complication most commonly presents in infants and toddlers with Hb SS disease whose spleens have not yet undergone fibrosis from repeated infarcts. Patients with splenic sequestration crisis typically present with acute onset of fatigue and pallor. The anemia can be so severe that patients can develop hypovolemic shock if they do not receive adequate blood volume replacement via transfusions. Splenectomy is indicated in severe and/or refractory cases.

   A slapped cheek rash is suggestive of a parvovirus infection. Patients with sickle cell disease and other hemolytic anemias are at risk for parvovirus-related aplastic crisis, which is manifested by an acute drop in hemoglobin. Aplastic crisis, however, is associated with a reticulocytopenia rather than a reticulocytosis as is the case in this patient. A grade 3/6 SEM is consistent with the patient's anemia but does not provide any clue to the underlying etiology of the anemia. Scleral icterus is a sign of hyperbilirubinemia and is present at baseline in most patients with Hb SS disease. Thus, the presence of scleral icterus does not provide any clue to the underlying etiology of the anemia.

4. A 3-year-old female child is brought to the ER with a 3-day history of fever and progressive lethargy. Her physical examination in the ER is consistent with septic shock. She is given two 20 cm^3/kg normal saline boluses and started on broad-spectrum IV antibiotics. Initial labs are significant only for a leukocytosis and bandemia. CXR demonstrates dextrocardia but is otherwise normal without infiltrates. A head CT is normal. Lumber puncture is deferred because of the patient's instability. The patient's past medical history is significant for one hospitalization as an infant with *S. pneumoniae* bacteremia. Family history is noncontributory. Eight hours after being admitted to the intensive care unit, the laboratory reports that the patient's blood culture is positive for *Neisseria meningitidis*. Her peripheral smear is reviewed at that time and is shown in the accompanying image (insert peripheral smear with Howell–Jolly bodies). Which of the following is the most likely underlying disorder in this patient?
   a. Sickle cell disease
   b. Heterotaxy syndrome
   c. Complement deficiency
   d. Bruton's agammaglobulinemia

Answer: b. Heterotaxy syndrome. A second serious infection with an encapsulated bacterium should raise suspicion for splenic dysfunction. The presence of Howell–Jolly bodies (inclusion bodies in the RBCs from remnants of damaged DNA fragments) on her peripheral smear also raises concern for splenic dysfunction. Although there are many etiologies of splenic dysfunction, the finding of dextrocardia on her CXR makes heterotaxy syndrome the most likely etiology. The patient's normal hemoglobin and lack of sickled RBCs on peripheral smear is not consistent with a diagnosis of sickle cell disease. Furthermore, as long as the patient was born in the United States, sickle cell disease should have been detected on her newborn screen. Although patients with complement deficiencies can have increased risk for serious bacterial infections with encapsulated organisms, the findings of dextrocardia on CXR and Howell–Jolly bodies on peripheral smear make this diagnosis less likely than heterotaxy syndrome. Bruton's agammaglobulinemia is an X-linked disorder and does not affect females.

5. A 15-year-old White female with systemic lupus erythematosus presents with acute onset of low-grade fevers and altered mental status. Urine toxicology screen is negative. Head CT is normal. CBC is significant for anemia and thrombocytopenia. Her peripheral blood smear is shown in the accompanying image (insert peripheral smear showing hemolytic anemia with increased schistocytes). CMP is remarkable for an elevated creatinine, almost double that of her baseline. Which of the following interventions is most appropriate for this patient at this time?
   a. Platelet transfusion
   b. Plasmapheresis
   c. Broad spectrum IV antibiotics
   d. IVIG

Answer: b. Plasmapheresis. The constellation of altered mental status, microangiopathic hemolytic anemia, thrombocytopenia, and acute renal failure in this patient are consistent with TTP. TTP is rare in children and occurs at a higher incidence in children with underlying medical conditions such as this patient with SLE. TTP is a medical emergency. The most effective treatment is emergent plasma exchange. There is also a role for corticosteroids. Platelets are contraindicated as they may worsen CNS and cardiac symptoms. There is no role for antibiotics or IVIG in the treatment of patients with TTP.

6. A 9-year-old girl with Fanconi's anemia presents with a 3-week history of unexplained bruising. A bone marrow biopsy is performed and demonstrates severe myelosuppression and 10% blasts. Cytogenetic analysis reveals deletion of the short arm of chromosome 7. Of the following treatment strategies, which is the most curative?
   a. IV methylprednisolone
   b. IV Danazol
   c. Bone marrow transplant
   d. Platelet transfusion

Answer: c. Bone marrow transplant. Monosomy 7 is the most common chromosomal abnormality seen in the bone marrow of patients with inherited bone marrow failure syndromes such as Fanconi's anemia. The blasts in this patient's bone marrow suggest that she has progressed to AML. The only curative strategy in these patients is BMT. Androgen therapy and platelet transfusions can be supportive but are not curative. There is no role for IV methylprednisolone in the treatment of these patients.

7. A 16-year-old girl is admitted to your service with a DVT. You are treating her with IV heparin. Despite being on adequate therapy for a week, she continues to need higher doses of heparin to achieve therapeutic levels. Which of the following is the most appropriate next step in the management of this patient?
   a. Check antithrombin III levels
   b. Add vitamin K supplementation to her regimen
   c. Add high dose folic acid supplementation to her regimen
   d. Discontinue heparin therapy and initiate therapy with oral warfarin

Answer a: Check antithrombin III levels. This patient has heparin resistance. Because heparin needs antithrombin III to work, you should always think about antithrombin deficiency in patients with heparin resistance. If the patient is found to have antithrombin III deficiency, she should be treated with recombinant antithrombin III in addition to heparin during the acute phase of her treatment to ensure the efficacy of heparin.

8. A 4-month-old female infant with craniosynostosis is being evaluated by neurosurgery for surgical repair. Other than the craniosynostosis, the infant has no other known medical problems. She was born via uncomplicated SVD in a local hospital. She has been growing and developing appropriately while being fed formula. You are consulted by the neurosurgeons because the infant's preoperative labs show an isolated prolongation of PT. Her aPT and platelets are within normal limits. Her CBC and CMP are normal. Repeat labs demonstrate similar results. There is no history of easy bruising or bleeding in the infant. There is no history of bleeding disorders in the family but there is parental consanguinity. In terms of further diagnostic evaluation, which of the following is the most appropriate recommendation?
   a. Send factor VIII and IX levels
   b. Send vitamin K levels
   c. Send factor V and VII levels
   d. Send factor X levels

Answer c: Send factor V and VII levels. This patient has an isolated prolongation of PT. The differential diagnosis includes vitamin K deficiency (e.g., dietary, warfarin therapy), factor VII deficiency, and liver disease. The most likely etiology in this patient is factor VII deficiency, a rare AR bleeding disorder. Parental consanguinity makes offspring at an increased risk of all autosomal disorders. Factor VII deficiency can present clinically with symptomatic mucosal bleeding and/or intracranial hemorrhage or can be detected by an isolated prolongation of PT as is the case in this patient. Diagnosis is made by finding a low factor VII level. Replacement with recombinant factor VII product prior and during surgery will decrease the risk of extensive bleeding during surgery. FFP is also helpful to control bleeding in this patient. A low factor V level would suggest liver disease as it is synthesized by the liver. Liver disease, however, is unlikely in this patient who is growing and developing appropriately and has a normal CMP. Vitamin K deficiency is also very unlikely in this patient. Infants born in hospitals in the United States are given a dose of IM vitamin K at birth, and all infant formulas in the United States contain adequate amounts of vitamin K making insufficient dietary vitamin K unlikely in formula-fed infants. Hemorrhagic disease of the newborn is a special type of vitamin K deficiency due to limited transplacental acquisition of vitamin K, limited ability to store vitamin K in the immature liver, and lack of gut flora to produce vitamin K. Because infants born in hospital settings in the United States are routinely given an intramuscular dose of vitamin K at birth, however, this also is an unlikely cause of this patient's isolated prolongation of PT.

Factor VII and IX deficiency (Hemophilia A and B, respectively) are X-linked bleeding disorders and are not symptomatic in female carriers. Screening labs are significant for an isolated prolongation of aPTT with normal PT and platelets.

9. A previously healthy 3-year-old male presents to your primary care clinic with acute onset of generalized petechiae. He is otherwise well and review of symptoms is negative for weight loss, fatigue, recurrent fevers, and change in activity. On physical examination, the patient is a well-appearing toddler in no apparent distress with generalized petechiae. The remainder of his examination is normal. There is no history of a preceding viral illness. He does not take any medications. Family history of bleeding disorders is noncontributory. CBC is significant for severe thrombocytopenia with platelets of 12,000. WBC and hemoglobin are normal. Which of the following is the most likely diagnosis in this patient?

a. Leukemia
b. Idiapathic (immune) thrombocytopenic purpura (ITP)
c. Wiskott–Aldrich syndrome
d. Glanzmann thrombasthenia

Answer: b. Idiopathic (immune) thrombocytopenic purpura (ITP). ITP is the most common cause of isolated thrombocytopenia in childhood and is the most likely diagnosis in this otherwise healthy patient. ITP is most common in children 1 to 4 years of age and is thought to be an immune-mediated phenomenon in response to a viral infection. A history of a preceding viral illness 1 to 4 weeks before the onset of symptoms is elicited in more than half of patients but is not always present. The classic presentation is a well-appearing child with acute onset of generalized petechiae, ecchymosis, and/or purpura with an otherwise normal physical examination. CNS bleeding is the most feared complication but occurs in less than 1% of patients. Bone marrow aspirate is not required for diagnosis but may be indicated if diagnosis is unclear and will reveal normal to increased number of megakaryocytes. Treatment does not change the natural history of the disease but may be indicated in severe cases to decrease the risk of complications, primarily intracranial hemorrhage. Various treatment options include IVIG, anti–D immunoglobulin, corticosteroids, and immunosuppressive agents. Platelet transfusions are only indicated for severe acute bleeding in ITP because of shortened survival of the transfused platelets. Splenectomy is curative for most patients but is indicated only for life-threatening emergencies and/or refractory disease because of the risks associated with asplenia.

Watchful waiting may be considered in mild cases with platelets 20 K/μL. More than 50% of children with ITP recover within 4 weeks without treatment and more than 80% recover spontaneously within 6 months. Leukemia should be considered in any patient with thrombocytopenia but is more commonly associated with leucopenia and/or pancytopenia. Furthermore, review of systems and physical examination are often suggestive of an oncologic process. Wiskott–Aldrich syndrome is an X-linked recessive disorder associated with thrombocytopenia, eczema, and/or immunodeficiency. It is a much less common cause of thrombocytopenia than ITP. Glanzmann thromboasthenia is AR disorder of platelet aggregation due to the absence of glycoprotein IIb/IIIa from the platelet membrane. Platelets are present in normal number and morphology but are not able to form clots normally.

10. Which of the following RBC indices and laboratory markers are consistent with the diagnosis of iron-deficiency anemia?
   a. Low MCV, elevated RDW, elevated retic, low iron, low TIBC, low ferritin, low transferrin
   b. Low MCV, low RDW, low retic, low iron, low TIBC, low ferritin, low transferrin
   c. Low MCV, elevated RDW, low retic, low iron, elevated TIBC, low ferritin, low transferrin
   d. Elevated MCV, low RDW, elevated retic, low iron, elevated TIBC, low ferritin, low transferrin

Answer: c. Low MCV, elevated RDW, low retic, low iron, elevated TIBC, low ferritin, low transferrin. Iron-deficiency anemia is the most common cause of anemia in children 9 to 24 months of age. It is a microcytic (low MCV), hypochromic anemia. It is associated with an elevated RDW (reflecting a wide distribution of RBC sizes) and a low retic (reflecting lack of production of new RBCs). Fe studies demonstrate low iron, high TIBC, low ferritin, and low transferring. Risk factors for iron-deficiency anemia include high milk intake, prematurity, blood loss, vegetarian diet, and elevated serum lead. Fe-deficiency anemia and even Fe-deficiency without anemia has adverse effects on attention span, behavior, and school performance. Treatment is via correction of the underlying etiology when possible (e.g., decrease milk intake) and supplemental iron therapy.

SUGGESTED READINGS

ASH Image bank. American Society of Hematology. http://ashimagebank.hematologylibrary.org/

Buchanan GR. Thrombocytopenia during childhood: what a pediatrician needs to know. *Pediatr Rev*. 2005;26:401.

Bolton-Maggs PH, Paski KJ. Hemophilias A and B. *Lancet*. 2003;361:1801.

Custer JW, Rau RE, Lee CE. *The Harriet Lane Handbook*. 18th ed. Philadelphia, PA: Mosby, 2008.

Monagle P, Chalmers E, Chan A, et al. Antithrombotic therapy in neonates and children: American College of Chest Physicians Evidence-Based Clinical Practice Guidelines (8th Edition). *Chest*. 2008;133: 887S–968S.

McMillan JA, Feigin RD, DeAngelis C, et al. *Oski's Pediatrics: Principles and Practice*. 4th ed. Philadelphia, PA: Lippincott Williams & Wilkins, 2006.

Segel G et al. Managing anemia in pediatric office practice: Part 1 and 2. *Pediatr Rev*. 2002;23:75–84; 111–122.

CHAPTER 16 ■ INFECTIOUS DISEASES

PRANITA D. TAMMA

AAP	American Academy of Pediatrics
AIDS	Acquired immunodeficiency syndrome
AOM	Acute otitis media
BA	Bacillary angiomatosis
BCG	Bacille Calmette–Guérin
CDC	Centers for Disease Control
CHD	Congenital heart disease
CSD	Cat-scratch disease
CRP	C-reactive protein
CNS	Central nervous system
CSF	Cerebrospinal fluid
DIC	Disseminated intravascular coagulation
DFA	Direct fluorescent antibody
DT	Diphtheria and tetanus vaccine
DTaP	Diphteria, tetanus, and acellular pertussis
EBV	Epstein–Barr virus
ECM	Erythema chronicum migrans
EHEC	Enterohemorrhagic *Escherichia coli*
EIA	Enzyme immunoassay
ELISA	Enzyme-linked immunosorbent assay
EKG	Electrocardiogram
ESR	Erythrocyte sedimentation rate
GAS	Group A Streptococcus
GBS	Group B Streptococcus
GGT	Gamma-glutamyl transferase
HAART	Highly active antiretroviral therapy
HAV	Hepatitis A virus
H&E	Hematoxylin and Eosin stain
HiB	Haemophilus influenzae type B
HHV-6	Human herpes virus 6
HSV	Herpes simplex virus
HUS	Hemolytic uremic syndrome
IFA	Immunofluorescence assay
IgA	Immunoglobulin A
IgG	Immunoglobulin G
IgM	Immunoglobulin M
IVIG	Intravenous immunoglobulin
LAIV	Live, attenuated influenza vaccine
MCV4	Meningococcal quadrivalent conjugate vaccine
MMR	Measles, mumps, and rubella
MRI	Magnetic resonance imaging
NA	Neuraminidase
NNRTI	Nonnucleoside reverse transcriptase inhibitor
NRTI	Nucleoside reverse transcriptase inhibitor
NSAIDs	Nonsteroidal anti-inflammatory drugs
NTM	Nontuberculous mycobacterium
PCP	*Pneumocystis jiroveci*
PCR	Polymerase chain reaction
PCV7	Heptavalent pneumococcal conjugate vaccine
PMNs	Polymononuclear cells
PT	Prothrombin time
PTT	Partial thromboplastin time
RIG	Rabies immunoglobulin
RMSF	Rocky Mountain spotted fever
ROM	Rupture of membranes
RSV	Respiratory syncytial virus
SARS	Severe acute respiratory syndrome
Tdap	Tetanus, diphtheria, and acellular pertussis
TIG	Tetanus immunoglobulin
TIV	Trivalent inactivated influenza vaccine
TMP-SMX	Trimethoprim–sulfamethoxazole
TSS	Toxic shock syndrome
TST	Tuberculin skin test
UTI	Urinary tract infection
VATS	Video-assisted thoracoscopic surgery
VZIG	Varicella-zoster immunoglobulin
WBC	White blood cell

CHAPTER OBJECTIVES

1. To review the epidemiology of infectious processes that may be seen by the general pediatrician
2. To review the clinical manifestations associated with various infectious diseases
3. To review current diagnostic techniques used to identify infectious processes
4. To review therapeutic options available for the treatment of infectious diseases.

Infectious disease as a discipline is part of all pediatric subspecialties and its scope within pediatrics is broad. For the purposes of board review, this chapter will begin by highlighting immunity to infectious disease through immunization and specific infectious considerations among infants. This will be followed by a review of key infectious pathogens in alphabetical order and a summary by organ system to help solidify how infectious processes present clinically.

IMMUNITY THROUGH IMMUNIZATION

Immunity may be conferred either through passive or active immunization practices. Current immunization schedules as well as preadministration counseling basics are reviewed within the Preventive Pediatrics, Biostatistics, & Ethics chapter.

Passive Immunization

Administration of preformed antibodies to an infectious agent is termed "passive immunization." Passive immunization is indicated for patients with antibody deficiency states, as prophylaxis for those with exposure or a high likelihood of exposure to preventable infections and as treatment for certain diseases. Specific preparations of immunoglobulin with high levels of antibody to infectious agents such as hepatitis B, rabies, and tetanus are derived from humans or animals known to have high titers of the desired antibody. IVIG is derived from pooled human plasma and has a number of uses including pre-exposure prophylaxis (e.g., prevention of hepatitis A for children younger than 1 year traveling to endemic areas); postexposure prophylaxis against hepatitis A, measles, varicella, and other viral infections; and reduction of the consequences of immune-mediated conditions such as Kawasaki disease and immune-mediated thrombocytopenia.

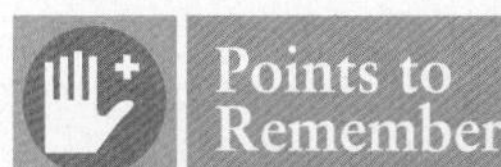

- IVIG recipients may have systemic reactions (fevers, chills, headaches, alterations in blood pressure, aseptic meningitis) and individuals with IgA deficiency may develop anti-IgA antibodies leading to serious allergic reactions.

Active Immunization

Administration of a vaccine or toxoid to stimulate humoral and/or cellular immunity results in active immunization. Vaccines can be attenuated forms of the live virus (weakened infectious agents), inactivated (killed agents), or subunit preparations (components, e.g., proteins or polysaccharides of infectious agents).

INFECTIOUS PROCESSES IN THE NEONATE

The neonate (infant <28 days of life) is uniquely susceptible to infection and therefore is considered in a category all its own. Although a neonate can be infected by any number of infections, those reviewed below are considered from an epidemiological standpoint to be the most important to treat, exclude, and diagnose as rapidly as possible. Further in-depth review is available within the "Neonatology" chapter.

Fever in the Neonate

Definition: Neonates are predisposed to infection as a result of immature neutrophil chemotaxis, phagocytosis and killing, as well as a lack of prior exposure to antigens. Factors that enhance the newborn's susceptibility to infection include prematurity, prolonged rupture of membranes, maternal fever, and chorioamnionitis. Infection should be suspected in any neonate with a temperature higher than 100.4°F, and a complete evaluation should be undertaken.

Epidemiology: Please see Table 16.1 for most likely pathogens involved.

1. *Group B Streptococcus* (Fig. 16.1)
   Protocol for prevention of early onset disease:
   a. Maternal screening for GBS colonization should be performed between 35 and 37 weeks' gestation.
   b. Prophylaxis should be given to mothers during delivery who meet the following criteria: A previous infant with invasive GBS disease, GBS bacteriuria, a positive GBS screen, an unknown GBS status and gestational age less than 37 weeks, ROM over 18 hours, or intrapartum temperature higher than 38.0°C.

TABLE 16.1

NEONATAL SEPSIS

	Early Onset	Late Onset
Timing	<7 d	7–30 d
Source of organism	Maternal genital tract	Maternal genital tract, community, nosocomial
Major pathogens involved	*Group B Streptococcus, Escherichia coli*, other enteric Gram-negative organisms, *Listeria monocytogenes*	*Group B streptococcus, Escherichia coli, Streptococcus pneumoniae, Staphylococcus aureus* (when considering nosocomial infections also consider *Candida* species, *Enterobacter, Serratia, Pseudomonas,* Coagulase-*negative staphylococcus,* and *Enterococcus* species

2. *Listeria monocytogenes*
   a. Consider in cases of preterm delivery to mother with a febrile, flu-like illness.
   b. Placenta often noted to have white nodules.
   c. Microabscesses may be seen on infant's organs.

Diagnosis: Any neonate with a temperature higher than 100.4°F requires a full sepsis evaluation: blood cultures, urine cultures, and lumbar puncture; if respiratory symptoms are present, obtain a chest x-ray. If gastrointestinal symptoms are present, a stool culture is indicated.

Treatment: Febrile neonates require admission while awaiting culture results and are generally treated empirically with IV ampicillin and IV gentamicin. Cefotaxime and gentamicin is often administered if neonatal meningitis is suspected, but Listeria has intrinsic resistance to this agent. Ampicillin should be administered if Listeria is a consideration.

Neonatal Herpes Simplex Virus Infection

Epidemiology: Neonatal HSV is most often caused by HSV-2 infection. An infant born via vaginal delivery to a mother with primary HSV genital infection has up to a 50% chance of acquisition of HSV infection due to a large quantity and prolonged duration of viral shedding. The risk of transmission with recurrent maternal genital herpes infection is 1% to 3%, reduced because a smaller quantity of virus is being shed and by the presence of maternal neutralizing antibody.

Clinical presentation: Neonatal herpes infection can manifest as disease localized to skin, eyes, and mouth (SEM disease); disseminated disease involving multiple organs; and localized CNS disease (Table 16.2; Figs. 16.2 to 16.4).

Other Viral Infections

Enteroviruses, influenza, and other respiratory tract viruses may also cause febrile infections in neonates. Respiratory tract symptoms may be minimal or undetected. Evaluation and treatment is dependent on the time of year, exposures, and results of bacterial studies.

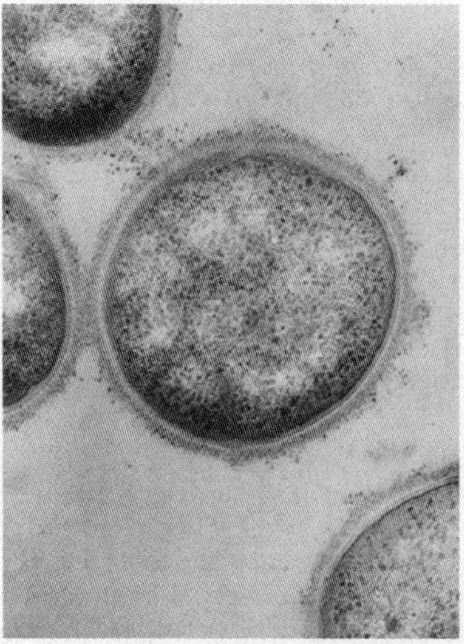

FIGURE 16.1. Transmission electron micrograph of group B Streptococcus. Organisms of group B Streptococcus were incubated with type-specific antiserum followed by ferritin-labeled anti-IgG. An irregular layer of capsular polysaccharide is visible exterior to the cell wall, decorated by ferritin particles (original magnification, 55,000×). (Reprinted with permission from Gorbach SL, Bartlett JG, et al. *Infectious Diseases.* Philadelphia, PA: Lippincott Williams & Wilkins, 2004.)

TABLE 16.2

NEONATAL HERPES SIMPLEX VIRUS INFECTIONS

	Skin, Eye, Mucous Membrane	Disseminated	Central Nervous System
Percentage of neonatal HSV infections	45	25	30
Peak age of presentation	7–14 d of life	5–10 d of life	14–21 d of life
Clinical manifestation	Discrete vesicular lesions	Fever, lethargy, irritability, respiratory distress, jaundice, seizures, shock with disseminated intravascular coagulation	Lethargy, seizures, fever, irritability
Diagnosis	Scraping base of vesicle may reveal multinucleated giant cells by Tzanck test, viral culture of skin lesions	CSF HSV PCR, mucous membrane swabs for viral culture, scrapings of vesicles (if present) for Tzanck test	CSF with positive HSV PCR, spinal fluid may reveal CSF pleocytosis with lymphocyte predominance, elevated protein, and significant red blood cells
Treatment	Intravenous acyclovir for at least 14 d	Intravenous acyclovir for 21 d	Intravenous acyclovir for 21 d
Prognosis	If untreated can lead to disseminated infection; prognosis with appropriate treatment very good	Mortality of 85% in untreated and 57% with treatment; morbidity in those who survive is significant	Mortality of 50% in untreated and 15% in treated with significant neurologic sequelae in survivors

CSF, cerebrospinal fluid; HSV, herpes simplex virus; PCR, polymerase chain reaction.

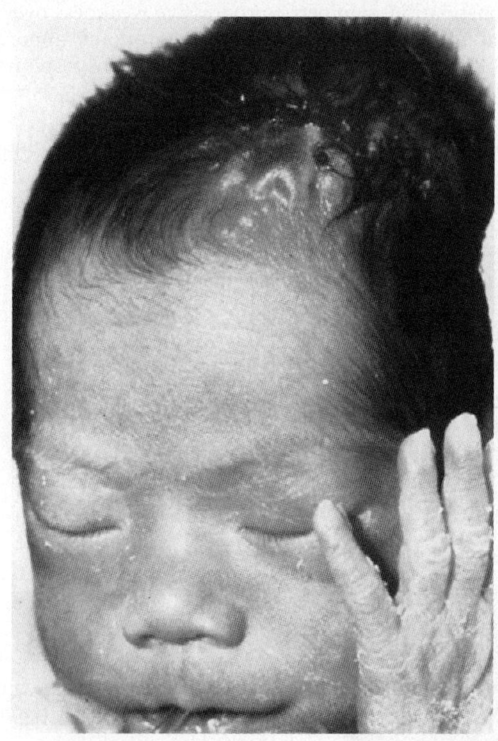

FIGURE 16.2. Clustered vesicles of neonatal herpes simplex virus infection that developed at the site of a scalp electrode. (Reprinted with permission from McMillan JA, Feigin RD, DeAngelis C, et al. *Oski's Pediatrics: Principles and Practice.* 4th ed. Philadelphia, PA: Lippincott Williams & Wilkins, 2006.)

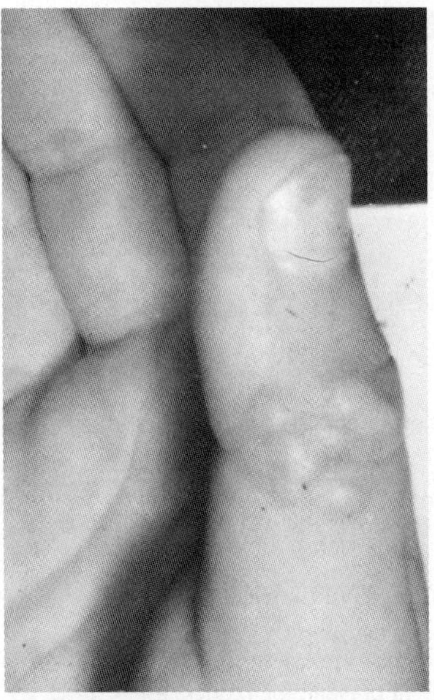

FIGURE 16.3. Herpes simplex infection should always be considered when grouped vesicles are present. (Reprinted with permission from McMillan JA, Feigin RD, DeAngelis C, et al. *Oski's Pediatrics: Principles and Practice*. 4th ed. Philadelphia, PA: Lippincott Williams & Wilkins, 2006.)

REVIEW OF SPECIFIC PATHOGENS

In the following section, we will review a number of common infections including vaccine-preventable diseases which may appear in populations where vaccines are not readily available or within a significant cohort of individuals who have refused vaccination. The review is generally organized so that infections defined by the organ system they most affect precede pathogen specific discussions.

Infantile Botulism

Epidemiology: Caused by *Clostridium botulinum*, intestinal colonization occurs from ingestion of spores from honey, dust, or soil. In infants, spores produce a neurotoxin in gastrointestinal tract, which binds to presynaptic nerve terminals and irreversibly prevents release of acetylcholine. Symptoms appear 12 to 36 hours after exposure. In older children, a preformed toxin must be ingested for disease to occur.

Clinical manifestations: Constipation, symmetric progressive weakness over days to weeks, decreased suck and cry, diplopia, ptosis, urinary retention, and autonomic abnormalities may be seen. Most untreated cases of infantile botulism progress to complete respiratory failure and require mechanical ventilation.

Diagnosis: Presence of botulinum toxin in stool.

Treatment: Supportive care and human-derived botulinum antitoxin. Aminoglycosides contraindicated because they may potentiate neuromuscular blockade.

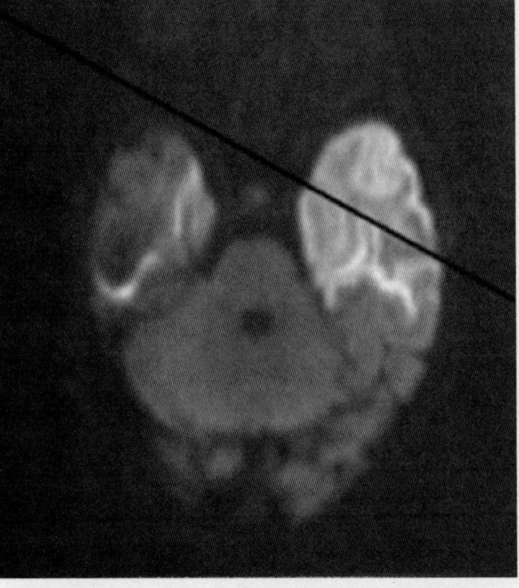

FIGURE 16.4. Diffusion weighted MRI. Both temporal lobes (left more than right) acute stroke in infant with HSV encephalitis.

EBV Infection

EBV infections can range from asymptomatic to severe lymphoproliferative disease with a wide range of presentations in between.

Epidemiology: A result of EBV infection which is transmitted via oropharyngeal secretions. The incubation period is 30 to 50 days.

Clinical manifestations: Infectious mononucleosis, the most recognizable syndrome associated with EBV infection, includes fever, exudative pharyngitis, tonsillar hypertrophy, malaise, lymphadenopathy, and hepatosplenomegaly. Complications include splenic rupture, hemolytic anemia/thrombocytopenia, encephalitis, and airway obstruction.

Diagnosis: In patients with infectious mononucleosis, CBC demonstrates leukocytosis—mostly atypical lymphocytes. Heterophile antibodies are present in more than 90% of children older than 4 years, but in younger children, specific serologic studies are preferred because of increased sensitivity.

Treatment: Supportive care is mainstay of therapy. Avoidance of contact sports until spleen size normalizes. Corticosteroids can be used when there is concern for airway obstruction. Rash is a frequent complication when ampicillin is given to patients with EBV infection.

Borrelia burgdorferi (Lyme Disease)

Infection with spirochete *Borrelia burgdorferi*. The deer tick (Ixodes species) is the vector.

Epidemiology: Infection requires more than 24 to 36 hours of attachment. Most cases occur in the summer. The deer tick vector is endemic in the United States, in southern New England, and in the eastern mid-Atlantic states.

Clinical manifestations:

- *Early localized phase* manifests 7 to 14 days after tick bite. ECM, a "bulls eye rash" or expanding annular erythematous lesion at the site of a recent tick bite, is seen, often accompanied by flu-like symptoms (Fig. 16.5).
- *Early disseminated phase* occurs days to weeks after the bite and manifests most commonly with multiple ECM lesions. Joints can be affected, a facial palsy (and other cranial nerve palsies) may appear, and aseptic meningitis and carditis (heart block) are other manifestations.
- *Late phase* occurs weeks to months after the bite and can present with arthritis in large joints, such as the knee, and polyneuritis.

Diagnosis: If ECM is present, no laboratory testing is needed. Diagnosis is generally clinical with serological confirmation (IgG or IgM by ELISA is positive; confirmed by Western blot). For Lyme meningitis, diagnosis is made by positive serology with CSF pleocytosis and clinical symptoms; CSF PCR has poor sensitivity. Of note, when typical symptoms are absent, a positive antibody test is likely to be a false positive. Lyme disease causes fever and arthritis that may be confused with juvenile rheumatoid (idiopathic) arthritis.

Treatment: For early localized and early disseminated disease, children younger than 8 years are treated with amoxicillin and older than 8 years are treated with doxycycline for 14 days. For Lyme meningitis and carditis (if severe), intravenous ceftriaxone for 21 to 28 days is generally recommended.

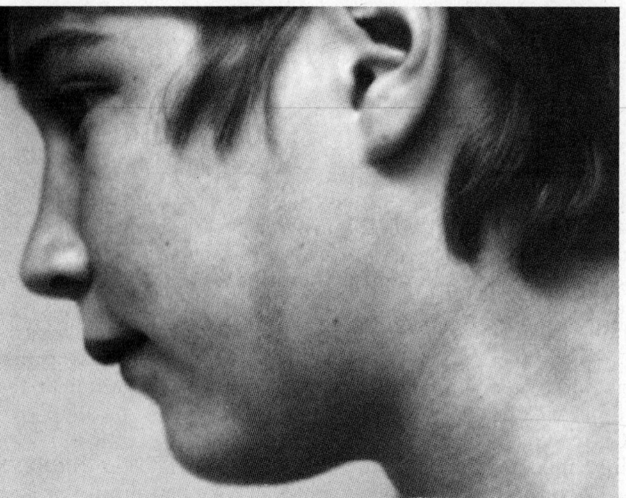

FIGURE 16.5. An enlarging lesion and multiple smaller annular lesions on the face of an 11-year-old boy diagnosed with Lyme disease who had been hiking in Westchester, NY. (Reprinted with permission from McMillan JA, Feigin RD, DeAngelis C, et al. *Oski's Pediatrics: Principles and Practice*. 4th ed. Philadelphia, PA: Lippincott Williams & Wilkins, 2006.)

Cat-Scratch Disease

An infection caused by *Bartonella henselae*—a fastidious, slow-growing, Gram-negative bacillus.

Epidemiology: Follows a scratch/bite of a cat by 1 to 8 weeks. Vast majority of patients have a recent history of contact with a cat, usually a kitten, as kittens can carry the organism without any clinical symptoms.

Clinical manifestations: Predominant feature is regional lymphadenopathy. May be associated with Parinaud oculoglandular syndrome (inoculation of eyelid conjunctiva results in conjunctivitis and ipsilateral preauricular lymphadenopathy), granulomas in the liver and spleen, and encephalitis. Immunocompromised patients may develop BA (proliferation of blood vessels, resulting in formation of tumor-like masses in the skin and other organs).

Diagnosis: Serology.

Treatment: Self-limited with resolution in 2 to 4 months. Antibiotics are not indicated in most cases, but they may be considered for severe or systemic disease. Reduction of lymph node size has been demonstrated with a 5-day course of azithromycin and may be considered in patients with severe, painful lymphadenopathy; however, no advantage is shown in the duration of symptoms. Treatment is mainly supportive; in cases of severe disease, intensive care unit admission may be necessary. It is unclear if there is a benefit of antimicrobials and corticosteroids for CSD encephalitis. Azithromycin, erythromycin, and doxycycline are effective in treating BA and bacillary peliosis.

Clostridium difficile

Epidemiology: Classically associated with clindamycin treatment but can occur after almost any antibiotic. Normal colonization in the gastrointestinal tract altered leading to overproduction of *C. difficile*, a spore-forming anaerobe that is toxin producing.

Clinical manifestations: *Pseudomembranous colitis* is characterized by diarrhea, abdominal cramps, fever, abdominal tenderness, and stools containing blood and mucus.

Diagnosis: Carriage without symptoms is common in younger than 1 year. Pathogen is diagnosed by presence of *C. difficile* toxin in the stool. Endoscopic findings demonstrate presence of pseudomembranes and hyperemic, friable mucosa.

Treatment: Discontinue any antibiotics if possible; oral metronidazole (first line) or *oral* vancomycin in those who do not respond to initial therapy.

Ehrlichiosis

Human ehrlichiosis is caused by Ehrlichia and Anaplasma species. They cause an acute, systemic, febrile illness.

Epidemiology: Generally presents in southeastern and mid-Atlantic United States in the spring and summer months.

Clinical manifestations: Clinically similar to RMSF as findings may also include leukopenia, anemia, and hepatitis. The absence of vasculitis and less common presence of a rash are distinguishing features. Complications can involve the liver, lung, and CNS and can be associated with renal failure and spontaneous hemorrhage.

Diagnosis: Serology or PCR. Pancytopenia, hyponatremia, and a transaminitis are frequently seen. Morulae may be seen on blood smear.

Treatment: Doxycycline is the treatment of choice even in children younger than 8 years and should continue for at least 3 days after patient defervesces for a minimum total course of 5 to 10 days.

Human Herpes Virus 6

Epidemiology: Primary infection peaks between 6 and 24 months of age. Transmission likely to occur from contact with infected respiratory secretions from asymptomatic adult caregivers. Once individuals have been infected, the virus persists in latent form throughout life.

Clinical manifestations: Roseola (exanthem subitum) is the most recognizable syndrome associated with this virus. Roseola can also be caused by human herpes virus 7. The illness typically presents with 3 to 5 days of high fever followed by a macular papular rash which appears on the trunk and spreads to the extremities, neck, and face as the fever resolves. It is associated with febrile seizures. Encephalitis and encephalopathy have been seen. Reactivation in the immunocompromised host may result in fever and, possibly, hepatitis (Fig. 16.6).

Diagnosis: Generally clinical, PCR when available.

Treatment: Supportive. For immunocompromised patients with serious HHV-6 disease, a few reports suggest the use of ganciclovir and other antiviral agents may be beneficial.

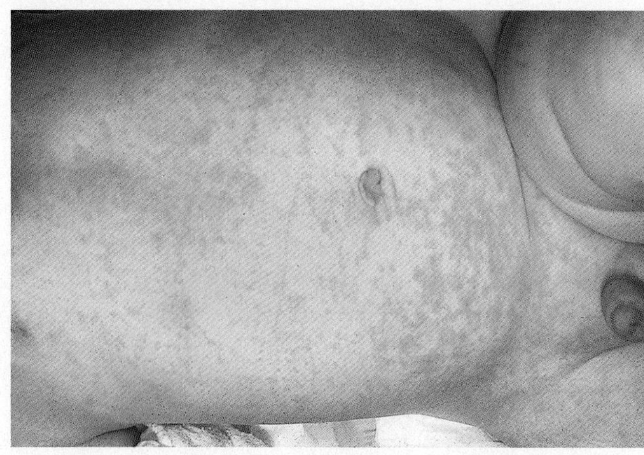

FIGURE 16.6. Roseola (courtesy of Bernard A. Cohen; http://www.dermatlas.org) (Reprinted with permission from Goodheart HP. *Goodheart's Photoguide of Common Skin Disorders: Diagnosis and Management*. Philadelphia, PA: Lippincott Williams & Wilkins, 2003:187.)

Points to Remember

- All infants born to HIV-positive mothers will be ELISA positive at birth because of passive transplacental transfer of antibodies persisting up to 18 months.

Human Immunodeficiency Virus

Infection occurs through exposure to infected human fluids including blood, breast milk, or during sexual intercourse. Tears and saliva are not significant modes of transmission. Vertical transmission may occur in utero, intrapartum, or postpartum (via breast feeding). Risk factors for transmission include high maternal viral load, low CD4 count, preterm delivery, chorioamnionitis, breast-feeding, prolonged rupture of membranes, and vaginal delivery.

Definition: HIV infection is caused by an enveloped RNA virus that causes CD4-lymphocyte depletion and dysgammaglobulinemia. Active viral replication slowly overwhelms the immune system causing severe immunodeficiency.

Clinical manifestations: Recurrent bacterial infections during the first year of life likely due to increased production of nonfunctional antibodies. Those who should be tested include all pregnant women, all sexually active adolescents, children with failure to thrive, generalized adenopathy, recurrent invasive bacterial disease, chronic parotitis, chronic diarrhea, unexplained hepatitis, loss of developmental milestones, and chronic/recurrent thrush after the age of 2 years.

Diagnosis: First screening test: ELISA (IgG-based antibody) if maternal HIV status unknown or was most recently negative.

The HIV Western blot is used as a confirmatory test for patients older than 2 years with two positive ELISA tests. HIV RNA PCR is a quantitative test for detecting viral load. In general, the higher the viral load, the greater the risk of progression to AIDS. AIDS is defined as the presence of a CD4 count of 200/mm^3 or less in a patient with HIV or the presence of an opportunistic infection in such a patient.

Treatment: Zidovudine is given to the mother prenatally and during labor and delivery and to the infant for the first 6 weeks of life. TMP—SMX is given twice a day three times a week beginning at 4 to 6 weeks of life for prophylaxis against PCP; discontinue if HIV-negative status is confirmed. In the absence of marked immunosuppression, children should receive MMR and varicella vaccines. All HIV-infected children require care of HIV treatment specialist to aid in the management of resistance profiles, side effects, drug interactions, etc.

Points to Remember

- Measurement of CD4 count and percentage allows for staging of immunodeficiency (use age-adjusted norms).
- *Evaluation of the HIV-exposed infants*: Diagnostic testing with HIV-1 DNA or RNA assays recommended at 14 to 21 days of age and, if results are negative, repeated at 1 to 2 months of age and again at 4 to 6 months of age. Viral diagnostic testing in the first few days of life recommended by some experts to allow for the early identification of infants with infection acquired in utero. For children with negative virologic tests, many experts confirm absence of HIV-1 infection with HIV-1 antibody assay testing at 12 to 18 months of age.

Influenza

Epidemiology: Spread by direct contact or respiratory droplets. Incubation period of 24 to 72 hours.

Clinical manifestations: Includes chills, fevers, malaise, myalgias, and respiratory symptoms. Complications include secondary bacterial infections with *Streptococcus pneumoniae*, *Streptococcus pyogenes*, or *Staphylococcus aureus*; pneumonia; otitis media; myocarditis; myositis; encephalitis; and Guillain—Barre syndrome.

Diagnosis: Rapid diagnostic tests for identification of influenza A and B antigens in the respiratory tract are available. Viral culture or PCR confirms diagnosis.

Treatment: Appropriate use of NA inhibitors requires prompt and accurate diagnosis of influenza infection, because early initiation of treatment appears to be the most important determinant of treatment efficacy. Zanamivir (older than 7 years) and Oseltamivir (older than 1 year) are NA inhibitors available for treatment of influenza A and B. Therapy with NA inhibitors is not indicated for minor nonfebrile illnesses or when symptoms are of greater than 2 days duration in immunocompetent individuals. Amantadine and rimantadine have been used for treatment and prophylaxis for influenza A. Some circulating influenza A and B strains have developed resistance to both NA inhibitors and the adamantanes (amantadine and rimantadine). Public health authorities make annual recommendations regarding antiviral therapy for circulating strains.

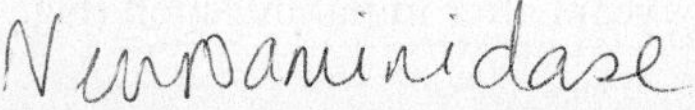

Points to Remember

- Antiretroviral agents include NRTI, NNRTI, protease inhibitors, and fusion inhibitors. When initiating therapy, use combinations of 3 or 4 agents, from at least two classes.

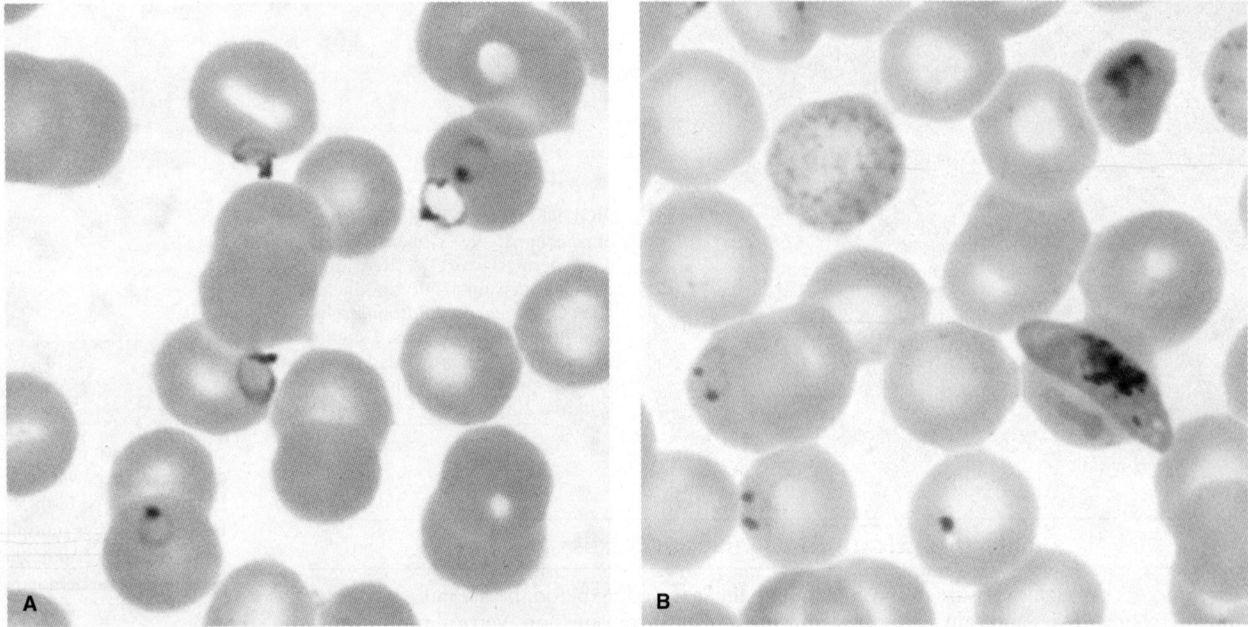

FIGURE 16.7. Microscopic image of *Plasmodium falciparum*. **A:** ring stage and **B:** gametocyte. (Reprinted with permission from McMillan JA, Feigin RD, DeAngelis C, et al. *Oski's Pediatrics: Principles and Practice*. 4th ed. Philadelphia, PA: Lippincott Williams & Wilkins, 2006.)

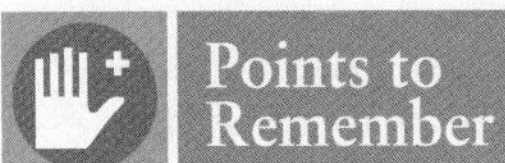
Points to Remember

- Public health authorities make annual recommendations regarding antiviral therapy for circulating strains. For emerging strains, such as Novel H1N1 influenza virus, vaccination and antiviral treatment recommendations evolve as the nature and burden of disease is understood. For current information, refer to the CDC Web site (www.cdc.gov).
- H5N1 [Avian Flu]. This influenza strain is so named as it is endemic among bird and poultry populations in Asian countries. The first transmission of this strain to humans was noted in 1997 in Hong Kong when 18 people were infected during a poultry outbreak in a live-bird market.
- TIV is inactivated or killed virus administered by intramuscular injection, which is approved for use beginning at 6 months of age in healthy and at-risk persons.
- Live, attenuated influenza vaccine is an intranasal spray, approved for use between 2 and 49 years of age in healthy, nonpregnant persons.

Malaria

Epidemiology: Endemic in tropical areas; infection acquired by the saliva from a female *Anopheles* mosquito.

Clinical manifestations: Classic symptoms are high fever with chills and other constitutional symptoms. *Plasmodium falciparum* can cause CNS disease. Anemia and hyperbilirubinemia can be seen as a result of hemolysis. Cerebral malaria presents with increased intracranial pressure, seizures, and progression to coma and death.

Diagnosis: Identification of parasitic organism on thick and thin blood smears. Rapid antigen test available for detection of *P. falciparum* (Fig. 16.7).

Treatment: Treatment should be guided by three main factors: the infecting plasmodium species, clinical status of the patient, and the drug susceptibility of the infecting parasites as determined by the geographic area where the infection was acquired. Patients diagnosed with uncomplicated malaria can be effectively treated with oral antimalarials. However, patients who have one or more of the following should be treated aggressively with parenteral antimalarial therapy: impaired consciousness, severe normocytic anemia, renal failure, pulmonary edema, acute respiratory distress syndrome, circulatory shock, DIC, spontaneous bleeding, acidosis, hemoglobinuria, jaundice, repeated generalized convulsions, and/or parasitemia of more than 5%. Please see the CDC website for more information on therapy. (http://www.cdc.gov/malaria/diagnosis_treatment/index.html)

Prevention: In malaria endemic areas, reducing exposure to infective mosquito bites by the use of personal protection measures (long-sleeve clothing and bed nets) has been successful in preventing disease. In addition, for travelers, routine antimalarial prophylaxis is an essential preventive measure.

Measles

Measles is a highly contagious disease spread by airborne means or by contact with respiratory droplets.

Epidemiology: Outbreaks are rare in the United States because of herd immunity resulting from near universal immunization. Isolated cases in the United States occur within communities with low immunization rates. Patients are generally contagious about 5 days before to 4 days after the appearance of the pathognomonic rash.

Clinical manifestations: Prodrome of fever, cough, coryza, conjunctivitis, and cough followed by the development of the pathognomonic morbilliform rash which appears approximately day 5 of illness in a cephalocaudad progression fading in the order that it appeared; skin may desquamate. Koplik's spots are pathognomonic gray/white spots on buccal mucosa. Complications of the disease include otitis media, pneumonia, croup, and subacute sclerosing panencephalitis which is a rare degenerative encephalitis characterized by dementia and intellectual deterioration and seizures occurring many years after initial infection (Fig. 16.8).

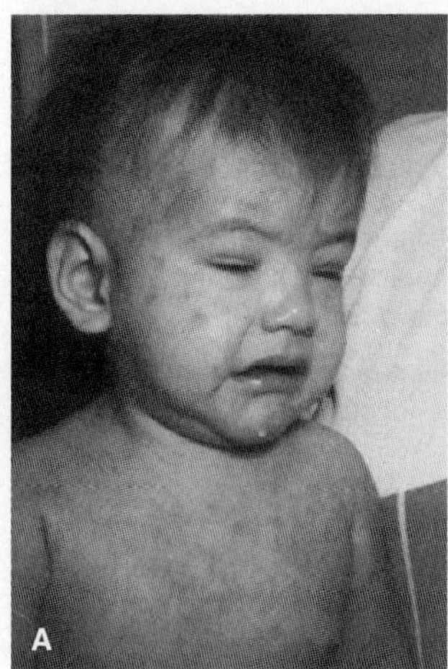
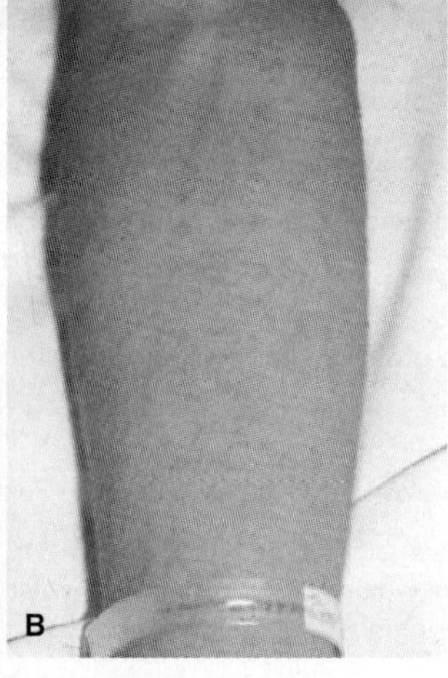

FIGURE 16.8. Maculopapular rash. **A:** Typical measles. (Courtesy of Dr. Gail J. Demmler.) **B:** Atypical measles. (Reprinted with permission from McMillan JA, Feigin RD, DeAngelis C, et al. *Oski's Pediatrics: Principles and Practice*. 4th ed. Philadelphia, PA: Lippincott Williams & Wilkins, 2006.)

Diagnosis: Clinical diagnosis can be verified with serology.

Treatment: Generally supportive. IVIG indicated intramuscularly within 6 days of exposure regardless of previous immunization status for immunocompromised patients, pregnant women, and infants younger than 1 year.

Meningococcal Infections

Epidemiology: *Neisseria meningitidis* is a Gram-negative diplococcus. Transmission occurs from person to person via respiratory droplets. Disease primarily affects children younger than 5 years and adolescents. Serogroups A, C, Y, and W-135 are contained in a tetravalent meningococcal polysaccharide—protein conjugate vaccine. There is no vaccine available in the United States to prevent serogroup B which causes most disease in infant.

Clinical manifestations: Meningococcal sepsis results in a febrile illness and an associated toxic appearance, often with a petechial rash. Begins with influenza-like symptoms (fever, upper respiratory symptoms, lethargy) that may last hours to days and in this time period, a nonspecific maculopapular rash evolves to a petechial or purpuric rash. Invasive infection results in meningococcemia, meningitis, or both. In fulminant disease, the patient is toxic and ill-appearing, and clinical deterioration can occur within minutes to hours, leading to shock, DIC, coma, and death (Fig. 16.9).

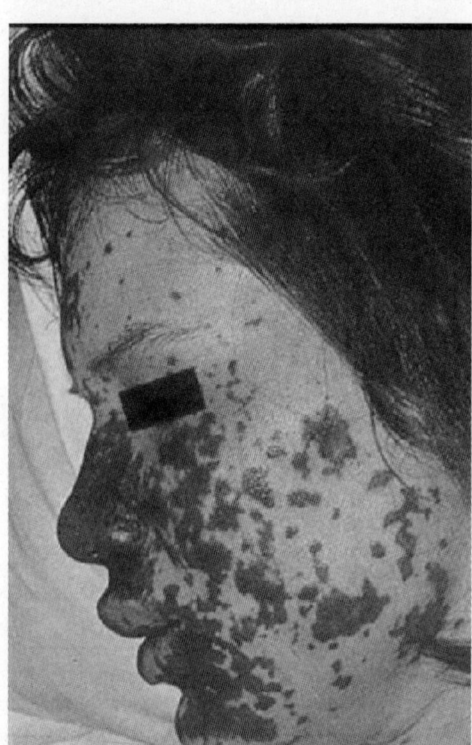

FIGURE 16.9. Purpura fulminans in a child with fulminant meningococcal sepsis. Purpura may evolve rapidly even in an initially nontoxic appearing child. (Reprinted with permission from McMillan JA, Feigin RD, DeAngelis C, et al. *Oski's Pediatrics: Principles and Practice*. 4th ed. Philadelphia, PA: Lippincott Williams & Wilkins, 2006.)

Points to Remember

- *Plasmodium vivax* and *ovale* can result in relapse due to their latent hepatic stages, whereas *Plasmodium malariae* can cause chronic asymptomatic parasitemia that can persist for several years.

Points to Remember

- Patients with mild HIV should be given MMR vaccine.
- During an outbreak of measles infant older than 6 months may receive one dose of a measles-containing vaccine, preferably monovalent if available. Children receiving measles-containing vaccine before 12 months of age require two additional doses of a measles-containing vaccine separated by at least 1 month starting at 12 to 15 months of age. IVIG administration is another option for preventing measles in infants younger than 12 months following household exposure. Measles-containing vaccine should be deferred if IVIG is administered for at least 5 months (after administration of 0.25 mL/kg) or 6 months (after administration of 0.5 mL/kg.

TABLE 16.3

CHEMOPROPHYLAXIS

Pathogen	Special Conditions	Prophylaxis
Pneumocystis jiroveci	HIV, leukemia	Trimethoprim–sulfamethoxazole, aerosolized pentamidine, dapsone, or atovaquone
Catalase-producing bacteria	Chronic granulomatous disease	Trimethoprim–sulfamethoxazole, fluconazole if history of fungal infections
Streptococcus pneumoniae	Functional or anatomic asplenia	Penicillin
Group B streptococcus	Pregnant women colonized in recto-vaginal region in labor	Penicillin to mother
Candidiasis	Steroids, recurrent infections	Nystatin, fluconazole
Mycobacterium avium complex	HIV	Azithromycin, clarithromycin, rifabutin (if tuberculosis excluded)
Bordetella pertussis	Contacts	Erythromycin
Neisseria meningitidis	Household contacts and those with exposure to patient's oral secretions (includes daycare)	Rifampin, ceftriaxone, ciprofloxacin
Mycobacterium tuberculosis	Children living with known infected adults	Isoniazid
Haemophilus influenzae	Close contacts of HiB should receive chemoprophylaxis despite prior vaccination if there is an unvaccinated child younger than 4 years in the home	Rifampin
HIV	Exposed neonates	Zidovudine

Diagnosis: Blood and CSF cultures are diagnostic. Gram stain and PCR can also be of benefit until cultures confirm diagnosis.

Treatment: Penicillin G for 5 to 7 days.

Postexposure chemoprophylaxis: Antibiotics are indicated for all individuals with potential contact to oral secretions of an infected patient; therefore, all household, classroom, and child care contacts are recommended to receive antibiotics (Table 16.3).

Prevention: Routine vaccination with tetravalent meningococcal protein conjugate vaccine recommended at ages 11 to 12 years. Routine vaccination also is recommended for college freshmen living in dormitories and for other populations at increased risk (i.e., military recruits, travelers to areas in which meningococcal disease is hyperendemic, patients with anatomic or functional asplenia, and patients with terminal complement deficiency).

Mumps

Epidemiology: Transmitted by respiratory droplets.

Clinical manifestations: General symptoms of fever, headache, malaise, and muscle aches with swelling of one or more salivary gland (usually parotid gland). Complications include meningoencephalitis, orchitis in pubescent males, arthritis, myocarditis, and pancreatitis. Note that orchitis causes infertility infrequently.

Diagnosis: Clinical diagnosis supported with serology.

Treatment: Supportive.

Points to Remember

- **Do not confuse mumps with bacterial parotitis which generally presents with a higher fever and more toxic appearance.**

Parvovirus B19

Epidemiology: Transmitted by respiratory route, exposure to blood products, and vertical transmission. Recognized as the etiologic agent of **erythema infectiosum** (**fifth disease**). This virus is also the cause of at least 90% of the episodes of aplastic crisis in children with sickle cell disease.

Children with erythema infectiosum are no longer contagious once the rash has developed. Children with aplastic crisis remain contagious for weeks and should be isolated if hospitalized.

Clinical manifestations: Primarily causes infection in school-aged children. Most infections are asymptomatic. Erythema infectiosum is manifested by a "slapped cheek" facial rash followed by a lacy, reticular rash on the trunk and extremities. The rash may be preceded by about 10 days of fever, headaches, and myalgias.

Complications:

- A symmetrical, self-limited polyarticular arthritis can occur, more commonly in adolescents.
- Transient aplastic crisis can occur and is of clinical significance in those with hemoglobinopathies. Severe anemia can also occur in those with HIV/AIDS.
- Primary maternal infection is associated with a congenital infection syndrome that can result in **fetal hydrops** (see "Neonatology" chapter).

Diagnosis: Detection of serum parvovirus B19 specific IgM antibody is preferred diagnostic test.

Treatment: Generally only requires supportive care. Patients with aplastic crises may require transfusions.

Pertussis

Epidemiology: Respiratory infection caused by *Bordetella pertussis*, a Gram-negative aerobic coccobacillus. Adolescents and adults often serve as a source of infection for infants and young children as their symptoms are not recognized as pertussis.

Clinical manifestations: Begins with a mild upper respiratory prodrome for a week (catarrhal stage), followed by severe cough for 1 to 3 months (paroxysmal stage) that may be associated with a classic inspiratory whoop; during convalescent stage, symptoms resolve gradually. Patients are usually afebrile throughout the illness. Older children and adults usually have milder URI symptoms.

Diagnosis: PCR, DFA, or culture. Peripheral blood leukocytosis with lymphocytosis.

Treatment: Infants younger than 6 months commonly require hospitalization for supportive care.

After paroxysmal phase begins, treatment does not lessen severity of disease but may limit spread. Treat with erythromycin for 14 days or azithromycin for 5 days.

Prevention: Infants are routinely immunized with the DTaP vaccine at several intervals within the first 2 years of life (2, 4, 6, and 15 months) as well as at 4 years of age. Adolescents aged 11 to 18 years should receive a single dose of Tdap instead of Td for booster immunization against Tetanus, Diphtheria, and Pertussis. Those exposed to Pertussis, regardless of immunization status, should be treated prophylactically with a macrolide to prevent spread.

Rabies

The vehicle of rabies virus transmission is infected animal saliva, which can be inoculated by a bite or scratch. After local tissue replication over weeks to months, the virus moves along peripheral nerves at the rate of 100 mm/day or higher. Once in the spinal cord, the virus spreads rapidly to the brain.

Epidemiology: Consider after bite or scratch of skunks, raccoons, foxes, coyotes, woodchucks, or any exposure to a bat—including being asleep in the same room as a bat. Rabies infection is considered low risk from rabbits, squirrels, guinea pigs, hamsters, mice, or rats.

Clinical manifestations: Weeks to months following the bite, infection produces a rapidly progressive encephalopathy with manifestations such as seizures, delirium, dysphagia, and hydrophobia. Once symptoms have developed, prognosis is very poor.

Treatment: Postexposure prophylaxis entails washing of the wound with soap and water and administration of human RIG along with administration of the rabies vaccine at a different site from RIG. Following bites from dogs, cats, and ferrets with unknown vaccination status, the animal should be held for 10 days and observed for signs of rabies. If observation cannot occur, prophylaxis is indicated.

Rocky Mountain Spotted Fever

Definition: A systemic, febrile illness cause by *Rickettsia rickettsii*. The dog tick (Ixodes species) is the vector.

Epidemiology: Generally presents in southeastern and mid-Atlantic United States in the spring and summer months.

Clinical manifestations: Presents with fever, headache, arthralgias/myalgias, mental status changes, anorexia, photophobia, nausea, and vomiting. An erythematous rash that can become maculopapular or petechial may first appear on the distal extremities 2 to 3 days after onset of

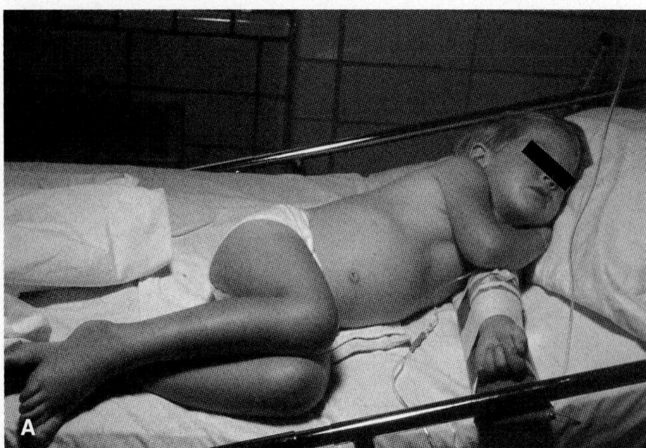

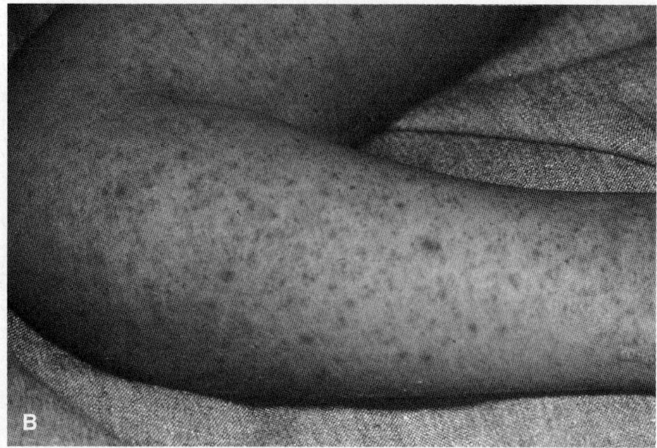

FIGURE 16.10. **A:** Patient with Rocky Mountain spotted fever. Rash is most extensive on extremities, with lesser intensity on trunk. Lesions are maculopapular, petechial, and purpuric. Facial edema and swelling of feet are evident. The protuberant abdomen is related to enlargement of the liver and spleen in this patient. **B:** Close-up picture of extremity showing intense rash with many maculopapular, petechial, and purpuric lesions. (Reprinted with permission from McMillan JA, Feigin RD, DeAngelis C, et al. *Oski's Pediatrics: Principles and Practice*. 4th ed. Philadelphia, PA: Lippincott Williams & Wilkins, 2006.)

Points to Remember

- **If RMSF is suspected, treatment should be initiated immediately while awaiting serology results.**

illness. The rash spreads proximally to the trunk. Complications can include involvement of virtually every organ system, the development of DIC, and death (Fig. 16.10).

Diagnosis: Laboratory studies may demonstrate thrombocytopenia and hyponatremia. Detection of serum antibodies reactive with *R. rickettsii* by indirect IFA can be used for confirmation. A fourfold increase in titers take about a month apart or a single titer 1:64 is diagnostic.

Treatment: Doxycycline is the drug of choice—even for children younger than 8 years because of the significant morbidity and mortality of this disease. Therapy should be continued for at least 3 days after unequivocal evidence of clinical improvement is seen. The minimum duration of treatment is 5 to 7 days; longer courses may be warranted in more severe disease.

Rubella

Epidemiology: Virus is transmitted by droplets or direct contact. Infected individuals are contagious from a few days before to 7 days after the onset of rash. Because of comprehensive vaccination and routine antibody screening by obstetricians, congenital rubella syndrome has nearly been eliminated in the United States.

Clinical manifestations: Asymptomatic infections are common. Rubella infection can produce mild erythematous maculopapular rash, fever, and lymphadenopathy. Transient polyarthralgias and polyarthritis are common in adolescent females. The disease is of major medical importance because of congenital rubella syndrome (see "Neonatology" chapter)

Diagnosis: IgM serology.

Treatment: Supportive.

Points to Remember

- **Spores are highly resistant to disinfection by chemicals or heat, but vegetative forms are susceptible to the bactericidal effect of heat, chemical disinfectants, and a number of antibiotics.**

Tetanus

Clostridium tetani is a gram-positive bacillus that exists in vegetative and sporulated forms.

Definition: Tetanus toxin primarily gains access to nervous system via neuromuscular junction, where it migrates retrograde transsynaptically, protected from neutralizing antitoxin, predominantly to inhibitory synapses to prevent release of acetylcholine.

Epidemiology: Wounds contaminated by soil or excreta present a risk for tetanus. Neonatal tetanus is seen in developing countries where women are unimmunized and nonsterile umbilical clamps are used.

Clinical manifestations: *C. tetani* exotoxin causes severe neurologic disease including trismus and severe muscular spasms. Weakness and inability to suck are most common manifestations of neonatal tetanus, often appearing between 7 and 14 days of age. Later, generalized tetanic spasms, rigidity, and opisthotonos occur.

Diagnosis: Clinical.

Treatment: See Table 16.4.

Points to Remember

- **When injury involves, a nail puncture wound through a shoe also consider pseudomonas infection (this can cause osteomyelitis/ osteochondritis).**

Tuberculosis

Epidemiology: Result of infection with acid-fast bacillus which is transmitted by airborne droplets. Risk factors include travel to or residence in endemic countries, close contact with an

TABLE 16.4

TETANUS PROPHYLAXIS

Number of Doses of Tetanus Toxoid Vaccine	Clean Wounds—Td or TdaP	Contaminated Wounds—Td or TdaP[a]	Clean Wounds—TIG	Contaminated Wounds—TIG
<3 or unknown	Yes	Yes	No	Yes
3 or more	No unless >10 y since last dose	No unless >5 y since last dose	No	No

[a]For children younger than 7 years, DTaP for wound prophylaxis Td, tetanus, diphtheria; Tdap, tetanus, diphtheria, and acellular pertussis vaccine; TIG, tetanus immunoglobulin.

individual with a positive TST, and exposure to individuals with HIV, who are homeless, or in prison.

Clinical manifestations: Cough, weight loss, night sweats/fevers, meningitis, bone lesions.

Diagnosis: Place TST (see Table 16.5).

A positive TST indicates possible infection with *Mycobacterium tuberculosis*. Negative TST may occur in presence of overwhelming tuberculosis, neonates, and the immunosuppressed. False-positive TSTs may result from cross-reaction with other Mycobacterium species and prior BCG vaccine.

The diagnosis is established by isolation of organism from gastric aspirates, sputum, pleural fluid, CSF, bronchial washings, or any biopsy specimens. Obtain chest radiography for all with positive TST. A chest x-ray may demonstrate lymphadenopathy of the hilar, mediastinal, or cervical nodes; atelectasis, cavitary lesions, or pleural effusions may also be seen (Fig. 16.11).

Treatment: Latent TB is treated with 9 months of isoniazid. Pulmonary TB is treated with 2 months of isoniazid, rifampin, and pyrazinamide followed by 4 months of isoniazid and rifampin. Treatment is extended to 9 months for coinfection with HIV and 12 months for TB meningitis. Consult infectious diseases specialist for multidrug-resistant TB. Affected patients can return to work/school after receiving antituberculous therapy and three consecutive negative sputum/gastric lavage smears for acid-fast bacillus. Children younger than 10 years with pulmonary tuberculosis are generally not considered to be contagious unless they have cavitary lesions or extensive disease.

Varicella-Zoster Infection

Primary infection or "chickenpox" manifests as a generalized, pruritic vesicular rash with mild fever and other systemic symptoms. Reactivation of varicella-zoster virus causes localized, usually painful vesicular rash referred to as zoster or shingles.

Epidemiology: Children are contagious 1 to 2 days before the varicella rash until the lesions are crusted over. Incubation period is about 10 to 21 days. Person-to-person transmission occurs by direct contact with patients with varicella or airborne spread from respiratory secretions. The incidence has declined dramatically in the United States, but it may still be seen in unimmunized US children and immigrants.

Clinical presentation: The rash begins as papules, progresses to vesicles which occur in crops, followed by pustules, and crusting. All four stages of the lesions exist simultaneously. Complications include bacterial superinfection of skin lesions (especially GAS), pneumonia, encephalitis, osteomyelitis, hepatitis, glomerulonephritis, and arthritis. Reye syndrome can follow chickenpox, but the incidence of Reye syndrome has dramatically declined since salicylates

TABLE 16.5

CRITERIA FOR POSITIVE TUBERCULIN SKIN TESTS IN CHILDREN

>5 mm	■ Contact of a known or suspected case ■ Clinical or chest x-ray evidence of active disease ■ Immunosuppressed patients
>10 mm	■ Age younger than 4 years ■ Children from endemic areas or who have traveled to endemic areas ■ Children exposed to high-risk adults ■ Children with chronic medical conditions
>15 mm	■ Children older than 4 years without risk factors

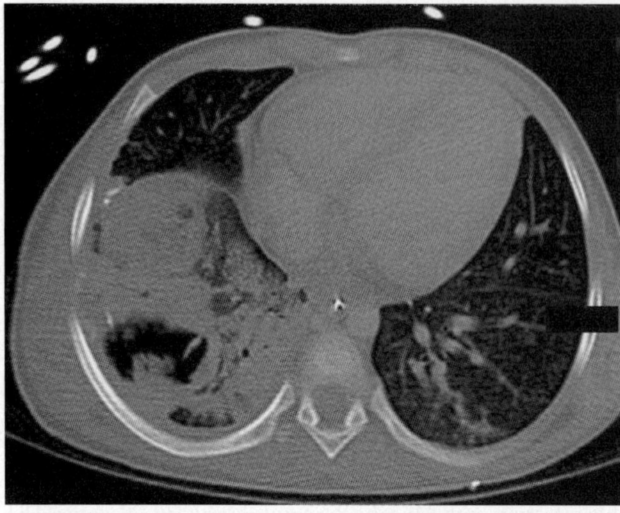

FIGURE 16.11. Cavitary lesion in a patient with *Mycobacterium tuberculosis*.

are no longer used in children. In the immunocompromised, the lesions are often deep-seated, larger, and umbilicated and disseminated disease is more likely. Infections in infants of a nonimmune mother may be severe or fatal (see "Neonatology" chapter) (Figs. 16.12 and 16.13). Reactivation (zoster) usually occurs many years after primary (varicella) infection. Lesions erupt in a dermatomal pattern and may be preceded by sensitivity or pain in the same dermatomal region. Disseminated zoster may occur in immunocompromised patients.

Diagnosis: PCR of fluid, serology, or Tzanck smear.

Treatment: The AAP does not recommend antiviral treatment for uncomplicated varicella in healthy children. Oral acyclovir or valacyclovir (three to five times improved bioavailability) should be considered for otherwise healthy people at increased risk of moderate-to-severe varicella. This includes people older than 12 years, people with chronic cutaneous or pulmonary disorders, and people receiving long-term steroids. Intravenous acyclovir is recommended for the severely immunocompromised and those with severe disease (encephalitis, pneumonia, and hepatitis). For immunocompromised patients, pregnant women, and newborns whose mothers had an onset of chickenpox 5 days before or 2 days after delivery, VariZIG, or, if not available, IVIG, given within 96 hours of exposure can prevent or modify the course of disease. Varicella vaccine administered within 3 days of exposure may provide some protection for nonimmune individuals.

INFECTION REVIEW BY ORGAN SYSTEM

Infections: Ear, Nose, and Throat

The following groups of diseases are caused by infections localized to the head, neck, and upper airways. Most of these are extremely common to pediatric practice both in the outpatient and

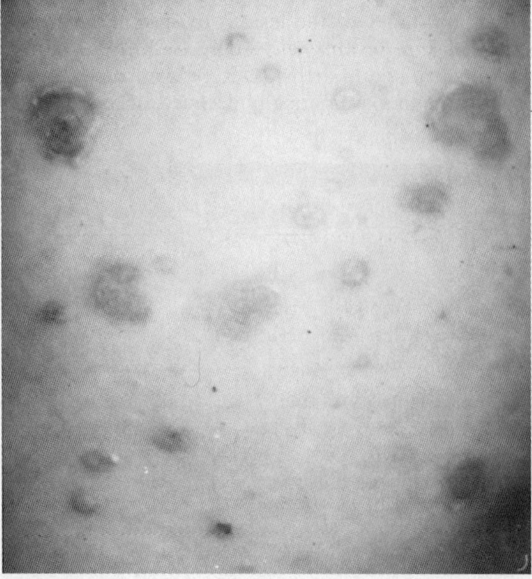

FIGURE 16.12. Bullae and round erosions of bullous impetigo complicating varicella. (Reprinted with permission from McMillan JA, Feigin RD, DeAngelis C, et al. *Oski's Pediatrics: Principles and Practice*. 4th ed. Philadelphia, PA: Lippincott Williams & Wilkins, 2006.)

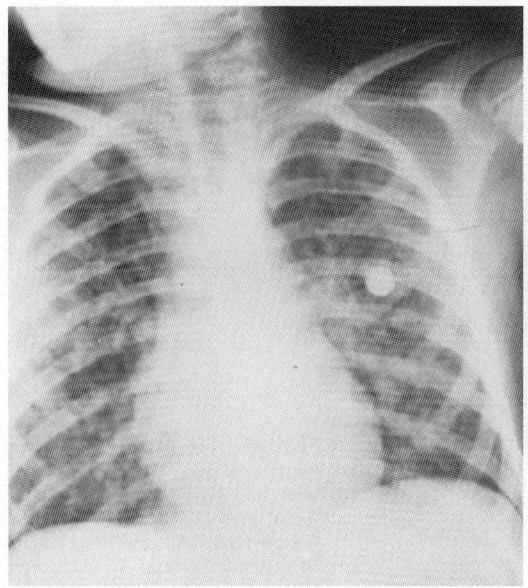

FIGURE 16.13. Varicella pneumonitis in a boy with leukemia and chickenpox. Symptoms include cough, dyspnea, tachypnea, and chest pain. Initial roentgenographic findings include peribronchial nodular infiltrates that may extend throughout the lung. Because varicella pneumonitis is a medical emergency, the patient should be admitted for intensive respiratory care as well as administration of antiviral chemotherapy. (Reprinted with permission from McMillan JA, Feigin RD, DeAngelis C, et al. *Oski's Pediatrics: Principles and Practice.* 4th ed. Philadelphia, PA: Lippincott Williams & Wilkins, 2006.)

inpatient clinical settings; therefore, questions pertaining to these diseases are likely to appear both on the Boards and in your practices. For further review, please see the "Ear, Nose, and Throat" chapter.

Acute Otitis Media

Inflammation of the mucosa lining the middle ear. Most episodes of otitis media with effusion are a result of viral infections, which are self-limited; the most common bacterial causes of otitis media include *S. pneumoniae*, *Haemophilus influenzae*, and *Moraxella catarrhalis*. This is true for infants younger than 6 weeks as well as for older infants and children. Complications of otitis media include conductive hearing loss, cholesteatoma, tympanic membrane perforation, intracranial abscess, lateral sinus thrombosis, and meningitis. Chronic suppurative otitis media is defined as purulent drainage from a perforated tympanic membrane for more than 6 weeks.

Epidemiology: Ninety percent of children have at least one episode by 2 years of age. Peak incidence usually occurs within the fall and winter months. Risk factors include craniofacial anomalies, immunodeficiencies, bottle-feeding, day-care attendance, and tobacco smoke exposure. Breast-feeding is protective.

Diagnosis: Usually visual. Tympanocentesis indicated for the relief of severe pain, to confirm diagnosis in the very young and immunocompromised, or for failed antibiotic therapy and for the treatment of mastoiditis.

Treatment: Optimize pain control. Use of antihistamines and decongestants has no proven value. For children younger than 2 years, antibiotics are recommended, but for all others if illness is not severe, initial observation without antibiotics should be considered with plan to treat if no improvement within 48 to 72 hours. High-dose amoxicillin (80 mg/kg/day divided BID) is first-line treatment. When there is absence of response to therapy in 48 to 72 hours, or if a resistant organism is cultured, amoxicillin–clavulanate or ceftriaxone (for 3 days) can be used. For non–type 1 penicillin-allergic patients, cefdinir can be used; in type 1 penicillin-allergic patients, use azithromycin, clarithromycin, or clindamycin. Tympanostomy tubes are recommended for chronic otitis media, failed antibiotics for recurrent AOM, and tympanic membrane retraction with ossicular erosion or cholesteatoma formation.

Bacterial Tracheitis

Most commonly caused by *S. aureus*, *S. pyogenes*, *S. pneumoniae*, *M. catarrhalis*, and anaerobes—usually following viral upper respiratory infection.

Epidemiology: Greatest incidence in children aged 3 months to 3 years.

Clinical presentation: Toxic appearance, high fever, stridor, and copious secretions.

A chest x-ray demonstrates a "ragged" tracheal air column.

Treatment: Parenteral antibiotics, humidification of entrained air, and oxygen. Severe disease requires intubation or tracheostomy until secretions have decreased or resolved.

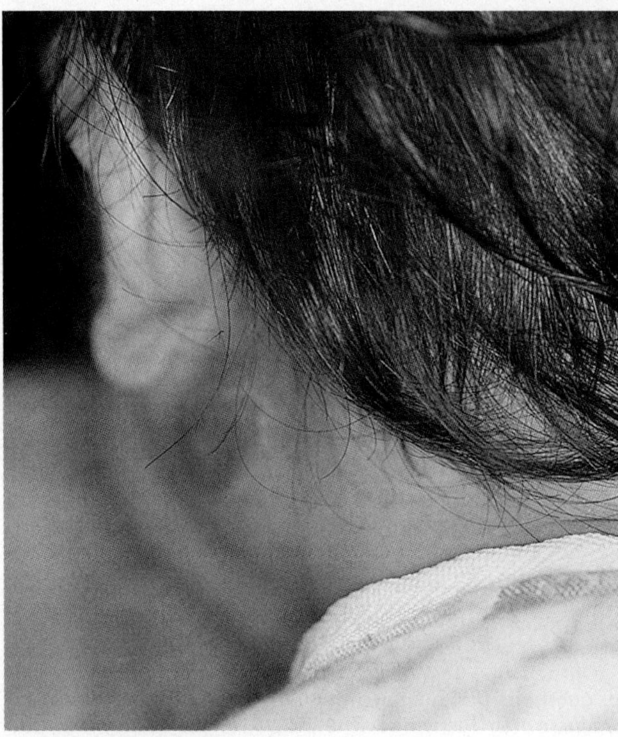

FIGURE 16.14. Mycobacterial lymphadenitis. This young girl, who had recently returned from India, presented with an inflamed lymph node and additional signs of systemic disease. An excisional biopsy showed caseating granulomas. (Reprinted from Fleisher GR, Ludwig W, Baskin MN. *Atlas of Pediatric Emergency Medicine*. Philadelphia, PA: Lippincott, Williams & Wilkins, 2004.)

Cervical Lymphadenitis

Typically occurs between ages 1 and 4 years. For bilateral disease, consider viral etiologies. For acute, unilateral disease, consider *S. aureus* and *S. pyogenes*. For subacute and more chronic cervical lymphadenitis, consider *B. henselae*, NTM.

Diagnosis: When nonviral causes suspected, fluid or pathology is diagnostic. For NTM, a TST is usually 5 to 9 mm (Fig. 16.14).

Treatment: Empiric therapy (depending on local epidemiology) with cephalexin, dicloxacillin, or clindamycin. NTM requires surgical resection of affected nodes. *B. henselae* infection resolves without therapy, though azithromycin may hasten resolution.

Croup (Laryngotracheitis)

Most common etiologies are parainfluenza types 1, 2, and 3; influenza; RSV; and adenovirus. It is the result of inflammation of the trachea and larynx, particularly the subglottic area.

Epidemiology: Tends to occur in the late fall and winter. Peak incidence is at 18 months.

Clinical manifestations: Presents as a dry, barking cough that worsens at night; hoarse voice; inspiratory stridor; and use of accessory muscles of respiration. Bacterial superinfection (*S. aureus*, *S. pyogenes*, *S. pneumoniae*, and *H. influenzae*) is the most common complication. Neck radiographs may reveal a tapered subglottic narrowing (steeple sign) (Fig. 16.15).

Treatment: Cool misted air may soothe inflamed mucosa and decrease the viscosity of tracheal secretions. Corticosteroid (dexamethasone oral or intramuscular) decreases laryngeal mucosal edema. Nebulized epinephrine is used to reduce laryngeal swelling in severe croup. Endotracheal intubation may be required.

Epiglottitis

Clinical manifestations: Consider in an unimmunized patient (pathogenesis: *H. influenzae* type b). Children will have a toxic appearance, high fever, drooling, dysphagia, and neck hyperextension with "tripoding" (sitting and leaning forward with hands on the knees).

Diagnosis: Clinical diagnosis; on neck radiograph, a "thumb sign" (swollen epiglottis) may be seen; definitive diagnosis obtained by visualization of the epiglottis. Blood culture or swab of the epiglottis yields pathogenic bacteria.

Treatment: Because rapid progressive respiratory demise may occur, urgent endotracheal intubation by an experienced anesthesiologist/otolaryngologist is recommended. Treat with beta-lactamase resistant antibiotics.

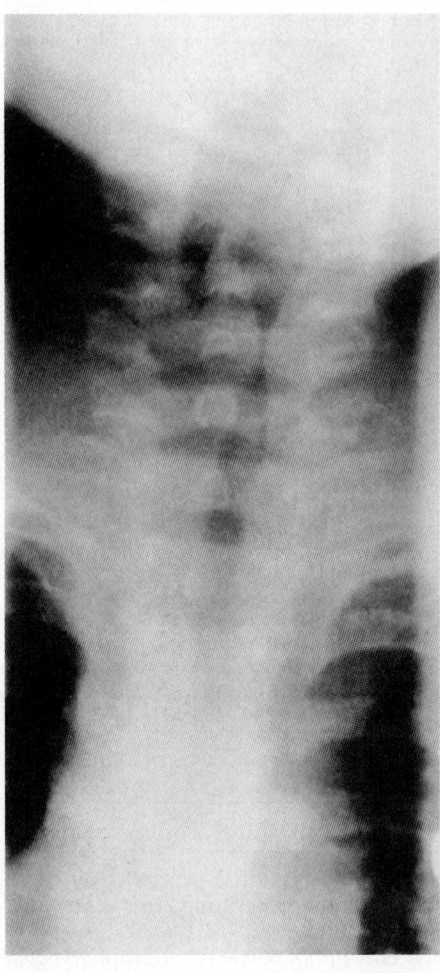

FIGURE 16.15. Steeple sign. This radiograph shows the characteristic narrowing of the subglottis indicative of acute laryngotracheobronchitis. (Reproduced with permission from Cotton RT, Myer CM. *Practical Pediatric Otolaryngology*. Philadelphia, PA: Lippincott Williams & Wilkins, 1999.)

Mastoiditis

An infection of the middle-air cell system with or without bone destruction caused by spread of middle-ear infection to mastoid. Similar bacterial pathogens to AOM but when result of chronic infection, also consider *S. aureus*, *P. aeruginosa*, and *S. pyogenes*.

Diagnosis: On physical examination, the mastoid is swollen, causing the ear to protrude; tenderness and erythema are present. A contrast-enhanced head CT scan defines the extent of disease (Fig. 16.16).

Treatment: Parenteral antibiotics (ampicillin–sulbactam or third-generation cephalosporin) and myringotomy to drain the middle ear and to obtain culture. If fever and otalgia persist for more than 48 hours, or if infection is progressing, a mastoidectomy is recommended.

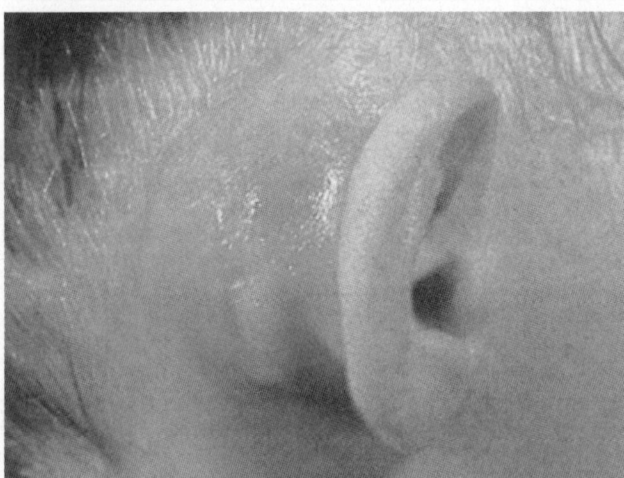

FIGURE 16.16. Mastoiditis. (Reprinted with permission from McMillan JA, Feigin RD, DeAngelis C, et al. *Oski's Pediatrics: Principles and Practice*. 4th ed. Philadelphia, PA: Lippincott Williams & Wilkins, 2006.)

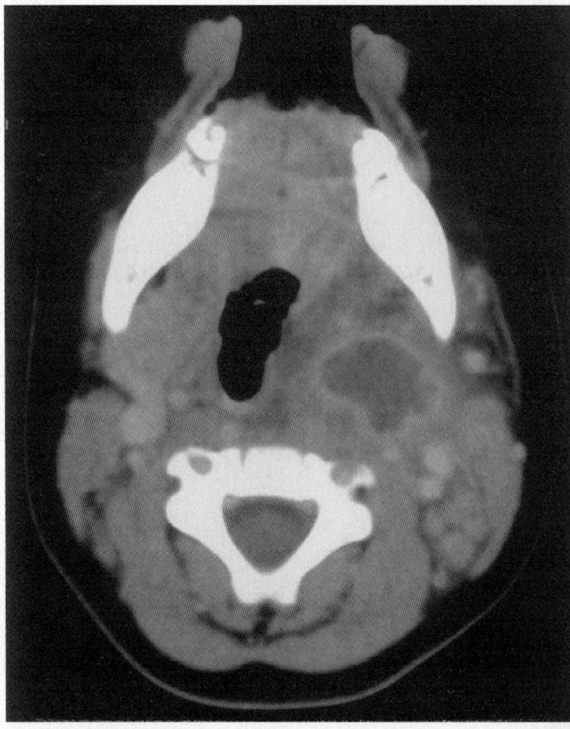

FIGURE 16.17. Appearance on a computed tomography scan of a focal, ring-enhancing retropharyngeal abscess with a scalloped contour to the abscess wall. (Reprinted from Kirse DJ, Robersin DW. Surgical management of retropharyngeal space infections in children. *Laryngoscope.* 2001;111:1413.)

Peritonsillar and Retropharyngeal Abscesses

Peritonsillar abscesses consist of purulent collections in the tonsillar fossa generally caused by oral flora. A retropharyngeal abscess is an infection of the lymph nodes found in the potential space between the posterior pharyngeal wall and the prevertebral fascia.

Epidemiology: Peritonsillar abscesses usually occur in adolescents. Retropharyngeal abscesses generally occur in children younger than 5 years.

Clinical manifestations: Peritonsillar abscesses presents with trismus, drooling, and a "hot potato voice." On examination of a peritonsillar abscess, unilateral tonsillar swelling with a deviated uvula is seen. Retropharyngeal abscesses are usually complications of bacterial pharyngitis and present with high fever, difficulty swallowing, a hyperextended neck, and drooling and may also result in neck pain or stiffness (Fig. 16.17).

Diagnosis: A lateral neck x-ray is the initial diagnostic study of choice for diagnosis of retropharyngeal abscess. CT scan confirms the diagnosis of a retropharyngeal abscess, delineates the extent, and distinguishes abscess from cellulitis.

Treatment: Peritonsillar abscesses require drainage and 10 to 14 days of antibiotics; intravenous penicillin is the first-line antibiotic therapy. Retropharyngeal abscesses are treated with intravenous antibiotics including treatment for *S. aureus*. Drainage of the abscess should be undertaken as soon as possible.

Pharyngitis

Most cases are viral (adenovirus, EBV, influenza, parainfluenza). Bacterial causes include *S. pyogenes*, *Arcanobacterium haemolyticum*, *Mycoplasma pneumoniae*, and *Neisseria gonorrhea*. Most infections causing pharyngitis are spread by contact with respiratory secretions (or, in the case of *N. gonorrhea*, by contact with genital secretions). *A. haemolyticum* can cause an acute pharyngitis, primarily in young adults and adolescents, which on some occasions can lead to invasive disease such as peritonsillar abscesses, pneumonias, and septicemia.

Epidemiology: Peaks in late winter and early spring. Risk factors include day care attendance and crowded living conditions.

Diagnosis: GAS rapid antigen detection studies have sensitivities of greater than 80% and specificities greater than 95%; GAS culture is the gold standard and recommended if there is a high clinical suspicion with a negative rapid test.

Treatment: Penicillin V is the first-line oral agent for GAS; macrolides or clindamycin can be used for penicillin-allergic patients. Treatment for GAS reduces symptoms rapidly and prevents rheumatic fever; it does not prevent poststreptococcal glomerulonephritis. Diphtheria is prevented by immunization; when infection with this organism is suspected, administer diphtheria antitoxin in addition to penicillin. Treat *A. haemolyticum* with macrolides.

Sinusitis

Maxillary and ethmoid sinuses are present at birth, sphenoid sinuses pneumatize by the age of 5 years, and frontal sinuses develop in preadolescence. Classification depends on the duration of symptoms—acute (<30 days), subacute (1 to 4 months), and chronic (>4 months). Organisms involved in acute and subacute infections are similar to AOM, while chronic infections may also be caused by anaerobes and *S. aureus*.

Complications: Intracranial spread of infection can lead to significant morbidity and mortality, especially in adolescent males. Complications include periorbital and orbital cellulitis, cerebral abscesses, cavernous or sagittal sinus thrombosis, and frontal (Pott's puffy tumor), and maxillary osteomyelitis.

Diagnosis: CT imaging is recommended for suspected complications of sinusitis, persistent or recurrent symptoms, and anticipated surgical interventions. Nasal swab and throat cultures may not produce the same results as sinus aspirates.

Treatment: For acute and subacute infections, 10 to 14 days of high-dose amoxicillin is recommended. Surgery recommended for chronic sinusitis not responsive to maximal medical therapy. Patients with orbital or CNS infections should be hospitalized and treated with ampicillin–sulbactam or third-generation cephalosporins. Antistaphylococcal antibiotic should be used in cases of chronic infection.

INFECTIONS: PULMONARY

In the following pages, diseases of the lower airway will be reviewed. For full detail, please refer to the "Pulmonary" chapter.

Bronchiolitis

Epidemiology: Most common cause is RSV, other causes include parainfluenza, adenovirus, human metapneumovirus, and influenza. Risk for severe disease is increased for premature infants, those with chronic lung or CHD, neuromuscular conditions, and children exposed to environmental smoke; breast-feeding is protective. Bronchiolitis is the most common hospital admission diagnosis in the United States for children. Reduction of nosocomial transmission is achieved by use of contact precautions and good hand hygiene.

Clinical manifestations: Often presents with 2 to 3 days of history of low-grade fever, cough, and rhinorrhea progressing to expiratory wheeze, retractions, tachypnea, and cyanosis. Apnea can occur in infants younger than 6 months.

Diagnosis: RSV can be diagnosed by rapid EIA, fluorescent antibody test, PCR, or viral culture of nasopharyngeal aspirate. Chest x-ray may demonstrate diffuse infiltrates and hyperinflation.

Treatment: Supportive therapies, including fluid administration and supplemental oxygen, are mainstays. Inhaled short-term beta-agonists (albuterol) may show modest short-term improvement in clinical features, but their use has not been shown to impact the rate or duration of hospitalization. Systemic steroids may be beneficial for patients with previous wheezing or severe illness. Monthly palivizumab prophylaxis reduces RSV hospitalization for at-risk infants. Prophylaxis is recommended for children younger than 2 years born less than 32 weeks' gestation or with significant risk factors for severe disease such as chronic lung disease and/or CHD.

Lymphocytic Interstitial Pneumonitis

Second only to PCP pneumonia among pediatric AIDs-defining conditions.

Clinical manifestations: Clinically differs from PCP in that onset is insidious. Cough and tachypnea are usually present. Examination of chest usually reveals few auscultatory abnormalities. Marked generalized lymphadenopathy, hepatosplenomegaly, and salivary gland enlargement may be noted.

Diagnosis: Chest radiography typically reveals symmetrical, bilateral reticulonodular and interstitial infiltrates, sometimes in association with hilar adenopathy. No typical lab abnormality; marked increase in serum immunoglobulin concentrations may be seen. Definitive diagnosis by open-lung biopsy.

Treatment: Largely supportive. Spontaneous clinical remission sometimes observed. Progressive hypoxemia may respond to corticosteroid therapy.

Pleural Effusion

Clinical manifestations: Suspect if pleuritic chest pain present, fever 48 hours or more after starting treatment for pneumonia, or clinical deterioration during treatment of pneumonia. *S. pneumoniae*,

TABLE 16.6

EVALUATION OF PLEURAL FLUID

Laboratory Value	Transudate	Exudate
pH	>7.2	<7.1
Glucose	>40 mg/dL	<40 mg/dL
Lactate dehydrogenase	<1,000 IU/mL	>1,000 IU/mL
Pleural protein/serum protein	<0.5	>0.5

S. aureus, and *S. pyogenes* are the most common etiologies. Mycoplasma has also been shown to cause parapneumonic effusions (inflammatory fluid collections adjacent to a pneumonia).

Diagnosis: Chest ultrasound and lateral decubitus films are helpful in differentiating free flowing versus loculated fluid. Send plural fluid for studies (see Table 16.6). Exudates are likely to be caused by bacterial infection, and transudates may be caused by viruses or bacteria.

Treatment: Empiric antibiotic therapy should treat *S. pneumoniae*, community-acquired methicillin-resistant *S. aureus*, and *S. pyogenes*. The traditional approach is to obtain fluid by needle aspiration, followed by administration of antibiotics. A chest tube may need to be placed when there is re-accumulation of the pleural effusion and resulting respiratory compromise. In severely affected individuals, more aggressive approaches may be needed such as VATS or lysis of adhesions.

Pneumonia

Epidemiology: *S. pneumoniae* remains most common bacterial cause. See Table 16.7.

Clinical manifestations/diagnosis: Atypical bacteria (*M. pneumoniae*, Chlamydia) (Fig. 16.18) and viruses generally cause a diffuse or bilateral interstitial pattern on chest x-ray. The onset of Mycoplasma pneumonia is not well defined. It begins with a constellation of malaise, headache, sore throat, fever; cough is usually nonproductive. *Chlamydia trachomatis* pneumonia presents during the 4th to 12th weeks of life with a staccato cough, tachypnea, and without a fever; chest x-ray reveals an interstitial pneumonia. Blood cultures are positive in less than 10% of patients with presumed bacterial pneumonia. Diagnosis is based on typical clinical findings (cough, tachypnea, fever, and rales) and chest x-ray demonstrating focal infiltrates (Fig. 16.19).

Treatment: For first month of life, treat with ampicillin and gentamicin. If more than 28 days of life, use high-dose amoxicillin for outpatient therapy and second-generation cephalosporins/ampicillin for inpatient treatment. Add a macrolide if considering *M. pneumoniae*, *Chlamydia pneumoniae*, or *B. pertussis*. The typical duration of treatment is 10 to 14 days.

Pneumocystis jirovecii (PCP Pneumonia)

PCP is one of the most severe complication for HIV-infected infants in the first year of life. PCP pneumonia also occurs in oncology/bone marrow transplant patients and others with severe compromise of T cell immunity.

Clinical manifestations: Consider in infant with tachypnea, rales, hypoxemia, and fever.

Diagnosis: Diagnose with histologic smear of lung fluid or DFA for PCP. Chest radiography typically has a "ground-glass" appearance; elevated serum LDH reflects lung injury. HIV RNA

TABLE 16.7

ETIOLOGY OF PNEUMONIA BY AGE

Age	Organisms
Birth–3 wk	Group B streptococcus, Gram-negative enteric bacteria
3 wk–3 mo	*Chlamydia trachomatis, respiratory syncytial virus* (RSV), *Streptococcus pneumoniae, Bordetella pertussis*
3 m–5 y	Viral pneumonia (*RSV, parainfluenza, influenza, human metapneumovirus, adenovirus, rhinovirus*); *Streptococcus pneumoniae, non-typeable Haemophilus influenzae, Staphylococcus aureus*
5–15 y	*Mycoplasma pneumoniae, Streptococcus pneumoniae, Streptococcus pyogenes, Staphylococcus aureus*

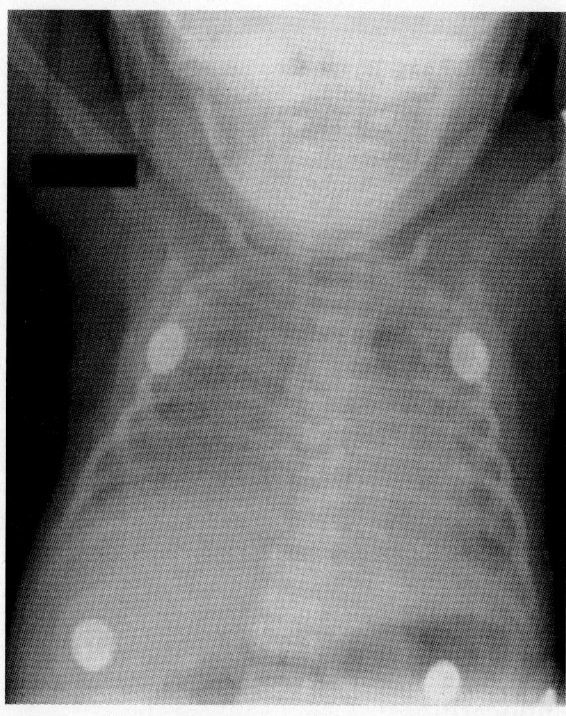

FIGURE 16.18. *Chlamydia Pneumonia* in an infant.

(viral load) is also helpful if HIV exposure/diagnosis has not already been determined. Suspect congenital immunodeficiency in non–HIV-infected infants with PCP pneumonia.

Treatment: Treat with high-dose IV TMP–SMX with or without steroids (depending on severity of hypoxemia). Prophylaxis for PCP is TMP–SMX; alternatives for allergic patients include aerosolized pentamidine, oral dapsone, and oral atovaquone.

INFECTIONS: CARDIOLOGY

Infections involving the heart—endocarditis, myocarditis, and pericarditis—are reviewed in the following section. Please refer to the chapter dedicated to "Cardiology" for more complete review.

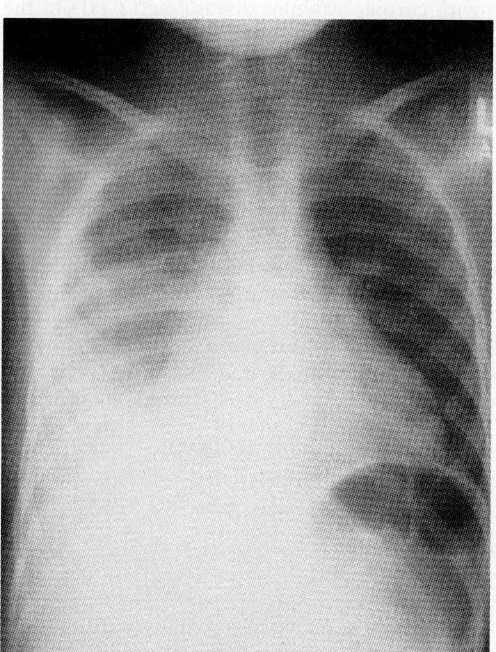

FIGURE 16.19. A child with bacterial pneumonia. This radiograph of the chest shows lobar consolidation and a pleural effusion on the right. Note the meniscus indicating the presence of fluid in the pleural cavity. (Reprinted from Fleisher GR, Ludwig S, Baskin MN, eds. *Atlas of Pediatric Emergency Medicine*. Philadelphia, PA: Lippincott Williams & Wilkins, 2004:196.)

TABLE 16.8

DIAGNOSIS OF INFECTIVE ENDOCARDITIS

Symptom/Finding	Incidence (%)
Fever	56–100
Anorexia/weight loss	8–83
Malaise	40–79
Arthralgias	16–38
Gastrointestinal problems	9–36
Chest pain	5–20
Heart failure	9–47
Splenomegaly	36–67
Petechiae	10–50
Embolic events	14–50
New/changing murmur	9–44
Clubbing	2–42
Osler nodes	7–8
Roth spots	0–6
Janeway lesions	0–10
Splinter hemorrhages	0–10

Reprinted with permission from McMillan JA, Feigin RD, DeAngelis C, et al. *Oski's Pediatrics: Principles and Practice.* 4th ed. Philadelphia, PA: Lippincott Williams & Wilkins, 2006.

Endocarditis

Infection of the endocardial surface of the heart including the valves. In children, it is usually associated with congenital heart defect and rheumatic heart disease but can also occur in children with normal hearts with bacteremia due to poor dental care, indwelling central venous catheters, or intravenous drug use.

Epidemiology: *Viridans streptococci* is the most common organism. *Enterococci*, *S. aureus*, *S. epidermidis*, and HACEK organisms (fastidious oropharyngeal organisms, including Haemophilus, Actinobacillus, Cardiobacterium, Eikenella, and Kingella) are other possible pathogens. Culture negative endocarditis can result from Q fever, brucellosis, *Bartonella*, and fungi.

Clinical manifestations: Key findings include fever, malaise, change in an existing murmur or a new murmur, worsening cardiac function, peripheral septic emboli, or new neurological findings.

Diagnosis: Diagnose with Duke criteria, which is a combination of blood culture and clinical, laboratory, and echocardiography findings. Vegetations can be visualized with echocardiography—transesophageal echocardiography is more sensitive (see Table 16.8).

Treatment: Treat with bactericidal antibiotics; length of therapy depends on etiology.

Prophylaxis: Cardiac conditions associated with the highest risk of endocarditis for which prophylaxis with dental procedures is recommended include prosthetic cardiac valve, previous endocarditis, cardiac transplantation recipients with cardiac valvular disease, and CHD in the following categories: (a) unrepaired cyanotic CHD, including those with palliative shunts and conduits; (b) completely repaired CHD with prosthetic material or device, whether placed by surgery or catheter intervention, during the first 6 months after the procedures; (c) Repaired CHD with residual defects at the site or adjacent to the site of a prosthetic patch or prosthetic device (which inhibit endothelialization).

Myocarditis

Myocardium damaged by direct infection of myocytes followed by immune-mediated inflammation. Commonly caused by infection with enteroviruses (particularly Coxsackie A and B), adenoviruses, influenza, and parvovirus.

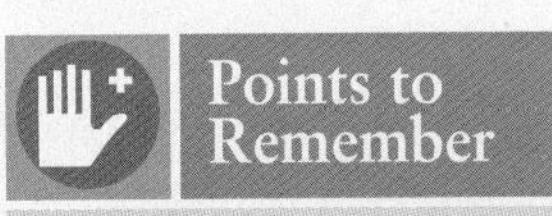

- Consider Chagas disease in a child with myocarditis from South America.

Clinical manifestations: Presentation includes palpitations, fatigue, tachypnea, cyanosis, and exercise intolerance. Chest x-ray may demonstrate cardiomegaly, and EKG may show low-voltage and may demonstrate arrhythmias. Troponin I typically elevated. Chronic myocarditis can result in dilated cardiomyopathy.

Diagnosis: Clinical. Definitive diagnosis achieved with endomyocardial biopsy (Fig. 16.20).

Treatment: Supportive care (inotropes, antiarrhythmics). Progressive disease may require heart transplantation.

Pericarditis

May result from viral or bacterial bloodstream infections or as an extension of myocarditis, lung infection, or a postsurgical chest infection. In summer months, pericarditis is most likely caused

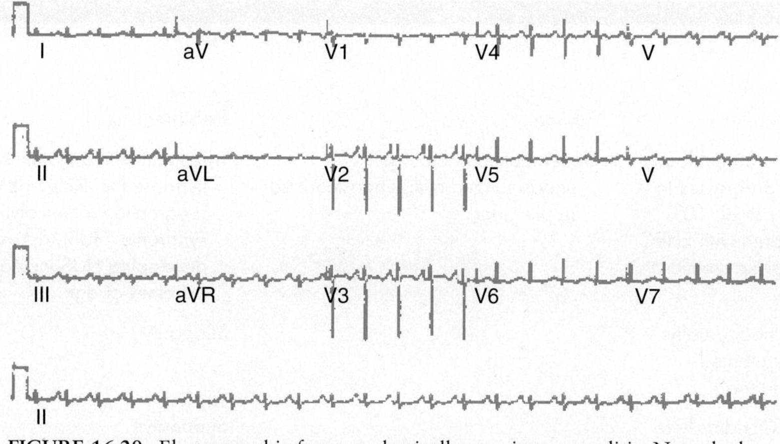

FIGURE 16.20. Electrographic features classically seen in myocarditis. Note the low-voltage QRS complexes. (Reprinted with permission from McMillan JA, Feigin RD, DeAngelis C, et al. *Oski's Pediatrics: Principles and Practice*. 4th ed. Philadelphia, PA: Lippincott Williams & Wilkins, 2006.)

by enteroviruses, and in winter months, it is most likely caused by influenza. Noninfectious causes include collagen vascular disease, rheumatic fever, sarcoidosis, drugs (phenytoin, hydralazine), neoplasms, trauma, and Kawasaki disease.

Clinical Presentation: More common in children younger than 2 years. Typical presentations include fever, tachypnea, tachycardia, and precordial pain associated with muffled heart sounds, friction rub, and signs of right-heart failure (if constrictive physiology is present). A pulsus paradoxus of more than 10 mm Hg suggests cardiac tamponade.

Diagnosis: Chest-x-ray may show enlarged cardiac silhouette. Send pericardial fluid for Gram stain/bacterial cultures, acid-fast stain/mycobacterial culture, viral cultures, and KOH/fungal cultures.

EKG shows nonspecific ST-T wave changes and low-voltage QRS complexes.

Treatment: Manage with bed rest, NSAIDs, and cardiac monitoring; drain pericardial fluid urgently if tamponade develops. Specific treatment is directed at the underlying pathogen, when antimicrobial therapy is available.

INFECTIOUS DIARRHEA

Campylobacter Infections

Epidemiology: Vehicles of transmission include improperly cooked meat, particularly chicken; untreated/unchlorinated water; unpasteurized milk; and direct contact with an infected pet (puppy or kitten).

Clinical manifestations: Predominant symptoms include diarrhea, abdominal pain, malaise, and fever; abdominal pain can be severe. May cause immunoreactive complications such as Guillain–Barre syndrome.

Diagnosis: Organism grows in stool culture; stools may contain visible or occult blood.

Treatment: Macrolides can shorten duration of illness and prevent relapse.

Cryptosporidium

Parasitic pathogen that spreads via person to person, from environmentally contaminated water, or from contaminated food. Zoonotic transmission from calves well documented.

Clinical manifestations: In immunocompetent hosts, causes a self-limiting profuse watery diarrhea that can contain mucus but rarely contains white or red blood cells and resolves in about 10 to 14 days. Half of patients have crampy abdominal pain, nausea, and emesis. Immunocompromised patients have prolonged, debilitating disease. Biliary tract disease is well documented in immunocompromised hosts.

Diagnosis: Usually by EIAs or IFAs of stool. Definitive diagnosis relies on identifying oocysts in stool or biopsy.

Treatment: Immunocompetent hosts require supportive therapy only. Nitazoxanide is the only approved therapy for cryptosporidiosis and is approved for this condition in children.

TABLE 16.9

ESCHERICHIA COLI DIARRHEA

	Clinical Manifestations	Source	Treatment
Enterohemorrhagic *E. coli* 0157:H7 (EHEC)	Usually begins as a nonbloody diarrhea and progresses to grossly bloody stool; 10% of young children with EHEC develop hemolytic uremic syndrome	Undercooked hamburgers, unpasteurized milk, unpasteurized apple cider	Treatment with antibiotics may increase the likelihood of progression to hemolytic-uremic syndrome (HUS); risks of developing HUS increased with extremes of age
Enterotoxigenic *E. coli*	Self-limited diarrhea, usually nonbloody nicknamed "traveler's diarrhea"		Supportive
Enteroinvasive *E. coli* (EIEC)	EIEC causes bloody diarrhea and fever similar to shigella		Supportive
Enteropathogenic *E. coli*	Mostly found in developing countries and causes nonbloody acute or chronic diarrhea in neonates and young children		Supportive

Escherichia coli Diarrhea

See Table 16.9.

Gastroenteritis with Non-Bloody Stool

Children with significant dehydration or protracted diarrhea and those with the appearance of serious infection warrant diagnostic evaluation including stool microscopy, fecal lactoferrin, stool guaiac test, and stool culture (see Table 16.10 for bacterial causes and treatment).

TABLE 16.10

BLOODY DIARRHEA

Bacteria	Notes	Treatment
Campylobacter		Erythromycin
Clostridium difficile		Discontinue current antibiotics Oral metronidazole or vancomycin
Salmonella	Treatment indicated for those at risk for invasive disease (malignancies, severe colitis, or immunocompromised, or infants younger than 3 mo)	Ampicillin/amoxicillin, trimethoprim/sulfamethoxazole, ceftriaxone (if treatment needed, antibiotic susceptibility testing is recommended)
Shigella	Most clinical infections are self-limited (48–72 h) and do not require antimicrobial therapy unless patients have severe disease or underlying immunosuppression	Trimethoprim/sulfamethoxazole, ceftriaxone, azithromycin (antimicrobial susceptibility testing of clinical isolates is indicated)
Vibrio cholera		Trimethoprim/sulfamethoxazole, doxycycline, tetracycline
Yersinia enterocolitica bacteremia	Gastroenteritis does not generally require antimicrobial treatment; treat septicemia or focal infections (osteomyelitis, peritonitis, abscesses)	Trimethoprim/sulfamethoxazole, aminoglycosides, cefotaxime

Viral causes include rotavirus, caliciviruses, astroviruses, enteric adenoviruses (types 40 and 41). If the incubation period is less than 6 hours, consider pre-formed toxins (*S. aureus*, *B. cereus*). Positive fecal leukocyte examination indicates presence of an invasive or cytotoxin-producing organism. If erythema nodosum is present, consider *C. jejuni*, *Salmonella* spp., or *Y. enterocolitica*. If reactive arthritis is present, consider *C. dificile*, *C. jejuni*, *Shigella* spp., *Salmonella* spp., and *Y. enterocolitica*.

Salmonella

Epidemiology: Gram-negative bacillus that can be acquired from food (chickens, eggs, contaminated vegetables) and may be transmitted from reptiles, chickens.

Clinical manifestations: Nontyphoidal salmonella organisms can cause asymptomatic carriage, gastroenteritis, bacteremia, and focal infections—which include osteomyelitis and meningitis. Nontyphoidal strains cause diarrhea, abdominal pain, and fever. *Salmonella typhi* can cause typhoid fever—fever, constitutional symptoms, abdominal tenderness, hepatosplenomegaly, rose spots, and mental status changes.

Diagnosis: Organism grows in stool culture; neutrophils present in stool.

Treatment: Healthy children with nontyphoid salmonella are not treated. Treatment does not shorten duration of illness and can prolong excretion of bacteria; however, antibiotics (ampicillin, TMP–SMX, third-generation cephalosporin) are indicated for infants younger than 3 months, typhoid fever or enteric fever, invasive disease such as osteomyelitis or meningitis, immunosuppressed patients and patients with hemoglobinopathies.

Shigella

Clinical manifestations: Gram-negative bacillus that causes watery/bloody diarrhea, fever, and abdominal pain. Associated with Reiter syndrome, hemolytic-uremic syndrome, and new-onset seizures (produces neurotoxin).

Diagnosis: Organism isolated in stool culture; neutrophils present in stool; peripheral leukocytosis with bandemia may be seen.

Treatment: Treat with antibiotics (ampicillin, TMP–SMX, azithromycin). Affected patients to be excluded from daycare until symptoms have resolved and stool cultures are negative.

Yersinia Infections

Epidemiology: Gram-negative rod. Principle reservoir of *Yersinia enterocolitica* is swine.

Clinical manifestations: Typically manifests as fever and diarrhea in young children. In older children, a "pseudoappendicitis syndrome" can occur with fever, tenderness in the right lower quadrant, and leukocytosis. Bacteremia most often occurs in children younger than 1 year and in older children who are immunocompromised. Postinfectious sequelae include erythema nodosum, glomerulonephritis, and reactive arthritis which occur in older children and adults.

Diagnosis: Stool often contains blood, mucus, and leukocytes; grows in stool culture.

Treatment: Antibiotic therapy not beneficial in most healthy patients. Patients with bacteremia or infection other than gastroenteritis should receive antimicrobial therapy; generally susceptible to TMP–SMX, aminoglycosides, or cefotaxime.

INFECTIONS: ABDOMINAL DISEASE PRESENTATIONS

Cholangitis

Epidemiology: Pathologic biliary system inflammation usually caused by enteric Gram negatives, enterococcus spp., and anaerobes. Patients who have undergone Kasai procedure, liver transplantation, or with Alagille syndrome are at increased risk.

Clinical manifestations: Classic triad consists of fevers/chills, right upper quadrant pain, and jaundice.

Treatment: Treat empirically with ampicillin–sulbactam, if more resistant enteric flora is suspected, consider piperacillin-tazobactam, carbapenems, or third-generation cephalosporins + metronidazole.

Hepatitis

Definition: Acute hepatitis is defined as less than 6 months of liver inflammation, and chronic hepatitis indicates an inflammatory process which has been present for 6 or more months. The most common cause of hepatitis outside of the United States is schistosomiasis.

TABLE 16.11

VIRAL HEPATITIS

	Epidemiology	Transmission	Presentation	Diagnosis	Therapy
Hepatitis A (RNA virus)	Epidemics in child care facilities	Fecal-oral	May be asymptomatic or may present with diarrhea, fever, malaise, jaundice, anorexia	Anti-Hep A IgM ab	No specific therapy, vaccine-preventable, postexposure prophylaxis available with vaccine or immunoglobulin for <1 year of age
Hepatitis B (DNA virus)		Parenteral, sexual, and perinatal transmission	Varies from asymptomatic to fulminant fatal hepatitis, may be associated with hepatoma and extraintestinal manifestations (serum sickness, polyarteritis nodosa, glomerulonephritis) Chronic infection associated with hepatocellular carcinoma	Hepatitis B surface antigen, hepatitis B core antibody (Fig. 16.21)	Vaccine-preventable, no specific therapy for acute infection, interferon alpha or lamivudine for chronic infection
Hepatitis C (RNA virus)		Parenteral, sexual, and perinatal transmission	Presents with fever, jaundice, malaise, and anorexia High risk to develop chronic infection (and subsequently cirrhosis and hepatocellular carcinoma)	HCV-RNA by PCR, serum antibody to HCV >3 mo after infection	Interferon alpha plus ribavirin; pegylated interferon plus ribavirin (not approved by the Federal Drug Administration)

Anti-Hep A IgM ab, anti-hepatitis A immunoglobulin M antibodies; HCV, hepatitis C virus; PCR, polymerase chain reaction.

Clinical manifestation: Presentation of hepatitis generally consists of fever, fatigue, and anorexia. Physical examination demonstrates jaundice, scleral icterus, abdominal pain, pruritus, and dark urine.

Diagnosis: Laboratory findings include transaminitis sometimes in combination with elevations in bilirubin, alkaline phosphatase, and/or GGT (signs of cholestasis). Markers of synthetic liver function (albumin, PT, and PTT) are often abnormal. Serologic tests for hepatitis viruses aid in diagnosis. Abdominal ultrasound of the liver, biliary tree, and spleen assists with diagnosis (Table 16.11).

Peritonitis

Definition: Primary spontaneous bacterial peritonitis is diagnosed by the identification of pathogenic bacteria in peritoneal fluid without an identified intra-abdominal source. It can occur in conditions such as nephrotic syndrome or cirrhosis of the liver. Secondary bacterial peritonitis is a peritoneal infection secondary to an abdominal source, such as perforation of an abdominal viscus (ruptured appendicitis, necrotizing enterocolitis).

Epidemiology: *S. pneumoniae* is the most common pathogen in previously healthy children and children with nephrotic syndrome. *S. epidermidis* followed by *S. aureus* are the most common pathogens in children with dialysis catheters and ventriculoperitoneal shunts. Gram-negative bacteria are found in children with cirrhosis.

Clinical manifestations: Defined by its clinical presentation of ascites, fever, and generalized abdominal pain.

Diagnosis: Fluid in bacterial peritonitis generally demonstrates low pH and glucose as well as elevated protein and LDH levels. WBC count of more than 250 cells/μL with more than 50% neutrophils increases likelihood of bacterial cause; peritoneal fluid should be evaluated with Gram stain and culture.

Treatment: Empirically treat with third-generation cephalosporin and an aminoglycoside until pathogens are identified. Add vancomycin for life-threatening, catheter-related infections. With persistence of the infection (tertiary peritonitis), therapy may need to be broadened to treat resistant organisms: vancomycin-resistant *Enterococcus*, methicillin-resistant *Staphylococcus aureus*, *Pseudomonas* spp, resistant *Bacteroides*, and *Candida* species.

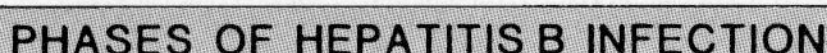

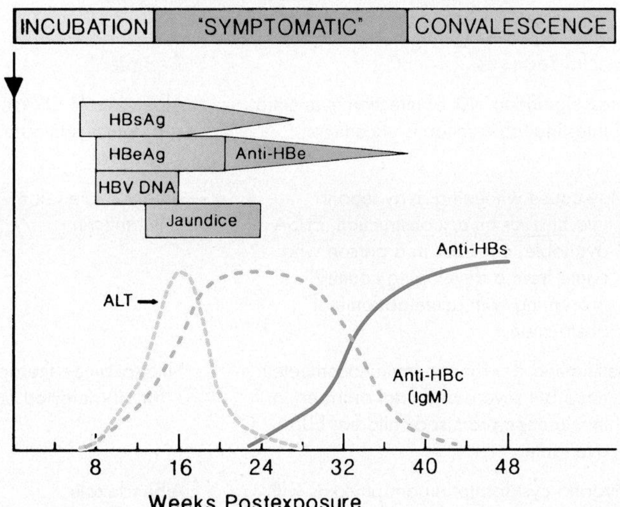

FIGURE 16.21. Typical course of hepatitis B infection. After exposure to hepatitis B virus (HBV; *arrow*), the earliest detectable serum marker is a rise in HBsAg, which may appear at any time (weeks 1 to 10) postexposure; HBV DNA and HBAg follow closely. HBeAg is detectable 2 to 8 weeks before the onset of the symptomatic phase, which is heralded by an increase in alanine aminotransferase (ALT) levels, serum bilirubin concentrations, and constitutional signs. Clearance of HBsAg by immune aggregation with anti–hepatitis B core antigen (HBc) occurs by 6 to 8 months postinfection; those who fail to clear are termed HBsAg carriers. Anti-HBc, which appears just before the symptomatic phase, is the first detectable, host-induced immunologic marker of hepatitis B infection. Anti-HBc of the IgM class may be the only marker of HBV infection in serum after clearance of HBsAg and before a rise in anti-HBs. Anti-HBc is not a neutralizing antibody and therefore, in contrast to anti-HB, is not protective. (Reprinted with permission from McMillan JA, Feigin RD, DeAngelis C, et al. *Oski's Pediatrics: Principles and Practice*. 4th ed. Philadelphia, PA: Lippincott Williams & Wilkins, 2006.)

Intestinal Helminthic Infections

See Table 16.12.

Proceeding from the GI tract, infections of the genitourinary system, skin/soft tissue, and joints are reviewed in brief. All sexually transmitted infections are covered within the "Adolescent Health" chapter.

INFECTIONS: RENAL AND GENITOURINARY

Renal Abscesses

Epidemiology: Caused by an ascending UTI (Gram-negative enteric) of hematogenous spread.

Clinical manifestations: Consider renal abscess when a patient has failed UTI treatment, there is fever without a source after urinary or abdominal surgery, or fever with urinary tract obstruction.

Diagnosis: Blood cultures positive in about 33% of patients; urine cultures positive in 50% of patients. Renal ultrasound is helpful in defining presence of renal abscess.

Treatment: Intravenous antibiotics to treat both Enterobacteriaceae and *S. aureus*. If no response after 2 to 3 days of antibiotic therapy, consider surgical drainage.

Urinary Tract Infections/Pyelonephritis

Epidemiology: Risk factors include presence of foreskin, poor genital hygiene, sexual intercourse, constipation, urinary obstruction, neurogenic bladder. *E. coli* is the most common cause followed by *Klebsiella* spp., *Proteus* spp., *Pseudomonas* spp., and *Enterobacter* spp.; *Staphylococcal saprophyticus* is a common Gram-positive pathogen in adolescents.

Clinical manifestation: Frequency, urgency, and dysuria are frequent presenting complaints in older children and adolescents but complaints are less specific in children and infants where clues to infection include emesis, fever, flank pain, abdominal pain.

TABLE 16.12

HELMINTHS

Protozoa/Helminth	Common Name	Special Features	Treatment
Ankylostoma duodenale	Hookworm (Fig. 16.22)	Most significant risk of infection is anemia; intestinal obstruction is uncommon	Albendazole OR mebendazole OR pyrantel pamoate OR endoscopic removal
Ascaris lumbricoides	Roundworm (Fig. 16.23)	May cause wheezing, may lead to intestinal or biliary obstruction, ELISA available, consider in a person who came from a developing country presenting with acute abdominal obstruction	Albendazole OR mebendazole OR ivermectin
Cryptosporidium		Self-limited diarrhea in immunocompetent hosts but severe and fatal diarrhea in immunocompromised children; ELISA available	Nitazoxanide therapy only necessary for HIV infected patients
Echinococcus		Hydatid cyst formation anaphylaxis with cyst rupture (Fig 16.24)	Albendazole
Entamoeba histolytica		Clinical course ranges from asymptomatic to minor or severe; Amebiasis presents with 1–2 wk of abdominal pain, diarrhea, and tenesmus with stools containing blood and mucus; may lead to hepatic and brain abscesses as well as lung disease, ELISA available, stool cultures generally positive	Metronidazole
Enterobius vermicularis	(Fig. 16.25)	Nocturnal anal pruritus, Tape test	Mebendazole OR pyrantel pamoate OR albendazole
Giardia		Found in school children, ELISA available for diagnosis	Metronidazole OR tinidazole OR nitazoxanide (no treatment indicated for asymptomatically infected children)
Necator americanus	Hookworm	Infections can lead to iron-deficiency anemia	Mebendazole OR albendazole OR pyrantel pamoate
Schistosoma species			Praziquantel
Strongyloides stercoralis		May cause wheezing	Ivermectin OR albendazole
Trichinella spiralis		Found worldwide where pork is consumed, may lead to pneumonitis, myocarditis, and encephalitis	Mebendazole OR albendazole PLUS corticosteroids
Taenia solium	Cysticercosis	Brain is most common site for cysticercosis and also is site that most commonly results in symptomatic disease (Neurocysticercosis); presents with seizures, headache, altered mental status; highest prevalence is Latin America, India, sub-Saharan Africa (Fig. 16.26)	Treatment depends on number and location of cyst, their viability, and inflammatory response. Niclosamide or praziquantel with corticosteroids are generally used with treatment indicated
Toxocara canis		Ingestion of dog or cat roundworm eggs; eggs hatch in gut and larvae migrate to various organs (visceral larva migrans); can cause ocular larva involvement; presents with fever, cough, wheezing, urticaria, and hepatosplenomegaly; can be diagnosed with ELISA; associated with significant eosinophilia and hypergammaglobulinemia	Albendazole or mebendazole

ELISA, enzyme-linked immunosorbent assay.

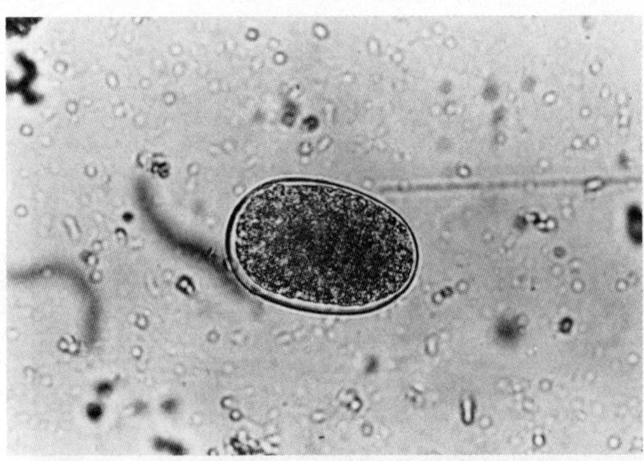

FIGURE 16.22. Hookworm ova (×396) in stool. (Reprinted with permission from McMillan JA, Feigin RD, DeAngelis C, et al. *Oski's Pediatrics: Principles and Practice*. 4th ed. Philadelphia, PA: Lippincott Williams & Wilkins, 2006.)

Diagnosis: In children who are not toilet trained, urine should be collected for culture by catheterization or suprapubic aspiration. A clean catch specimen is not appropriate for collection of urine in non–toilet-trained children (see Table 16.13).

Imaging: Renal ultrasound (demonstrates hydronephrosis), VCUG (demonstrates active reflux and grades it), and radionuclide scan (can demonstrate active infection and presence of scarring).

Treatment: If the child is toxic appearing, severely dehydrated, or unable to tolerate oral antimicrobials, initial antibiotics should be parenteral and hospitalization should be considered. Recommended oral agents for uncomplicated UTIs include TMP–SMX, amoxicillin, and cephalosporins.

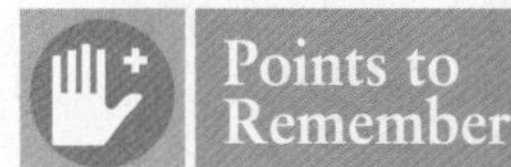

Points to Remember

- **Who should be imaged at first UTI? All children younger than 2 years and all boys and febrile girls younger than 5 years with their first UTI.**

Sexually Transmitted Infections

Please see "Adolescent Health" chapter for full discussion.

INFECTIONS: SKIN

Cellulitis

Definition: Infection of skin with varying extension into subcutaneous tissues.

Epidemiology: Most common pathogens are *S. aureus* and *S. pyogenes*. In an unvaccinated child with facial cellulitis, think about *H. influenzae* type b.

Diagnosis: Culture pus from site if possible; blood culture rarely positive.

Treatment: Drain when possible. If antibiotics deemed necessary, empiric antibiotic therapy should include activity against beta-hemolytic streptococci and *S. aureus* (empirically treat for MRSA in areas of high prevalence).

Impetigo

Definition: Superficial skin infection generally caused by *S. pyogenes* and *S. aureus* (*S. aureus* more likely to cause bullous impetigo).

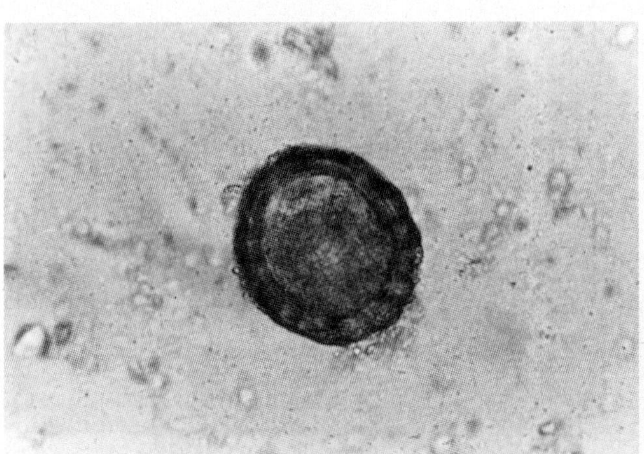

FIGURE 16.23. Eggs of *Ascaris lumbricoides* (×396) in freshly passed stool. (Reprinted with permission from McMillan JA, Feigin RD, DeAngelis C, et al. *Oski's Pediatrics: Principles and Practice*. 4th ed. Philadelphia, PA: Lippincott Williams & Wilkins, 2006.)

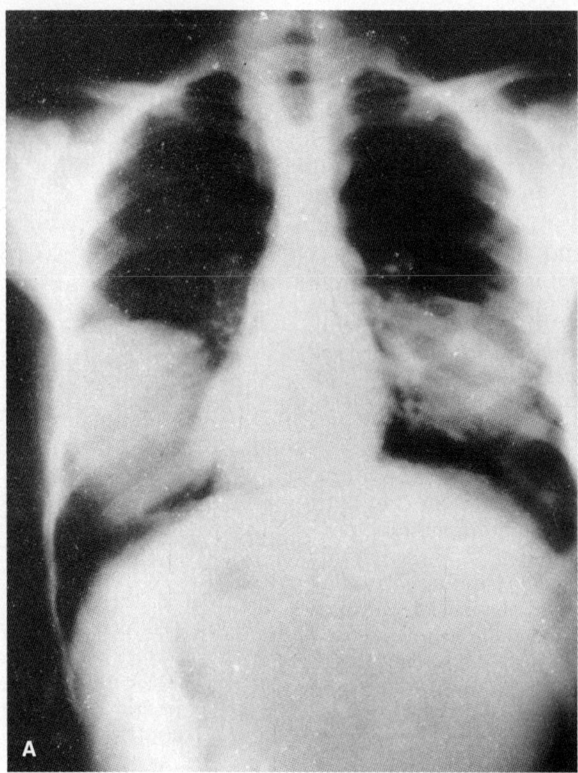

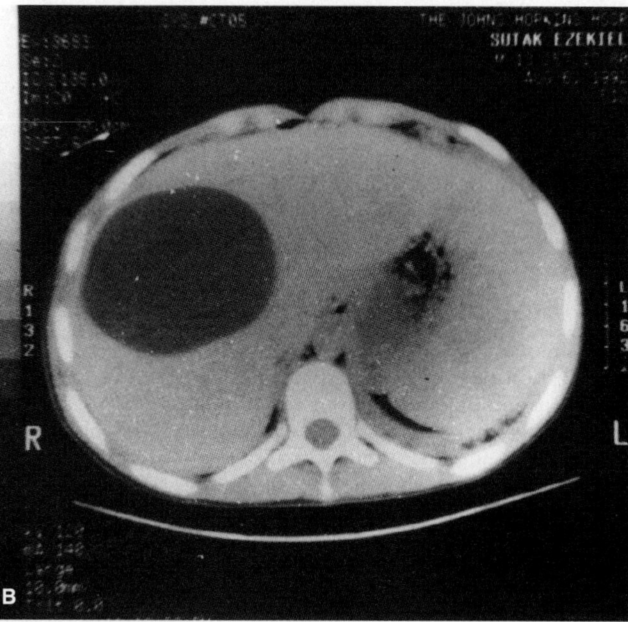

FIGURE 16.24. **A:** Chest roentgenogram showing bilateral pulmonary echinococcal cysts. **B:** Computed tomographic scan of the abdomen showing a solitary cyst in the liver of an 11-year-old boy. (Reprinted with permission from McMillan JA, Feigin RD, DeAngelis C, et al. *Oski's Pediatrics: Principles and Practice*. 4th ed. Philadelphia, PA: Lippincott Williams & Wilkins, 2006.)

Clinical manifestations: Characterized by pruritic, honey-crusted exudates on face and extremities; bullous form characterized by single or clustered bullae on face, perineum, extremities, and periumbilical area. Most bullous lesions resolve spontaneously (Fig. 16.27).

Treatment: For localized nonbullous lesions, use topical mupirocin. Oral anti-staphylococcal agents recommended for bullous impetigo and for widespread impetigo.

Necrotizing Fasciitis

Definition: Extensive cellulitis with severe involvement of subcutaneous tissue including fascia, muscle, or both, resulting in tissue necrosis. Pyogenic exotoxins lead to cytokine production and tissue damage; infection spreads along fascial plans, eventually producing myonecrosis and gangrene (Fig. 16.28).

Epidemiology: Patients may report a history of recent surgery, trauma, omphalitis, or varicella infection. Often polymicrobial; organisms include *S. aureus*, *S. pyogenes*, Gram-negative enterics, *P. aeruginosa*, and anaerobes (*Peptostreptococcus* spp., *Clostridium* spp., and *Bacteroides* spp.).

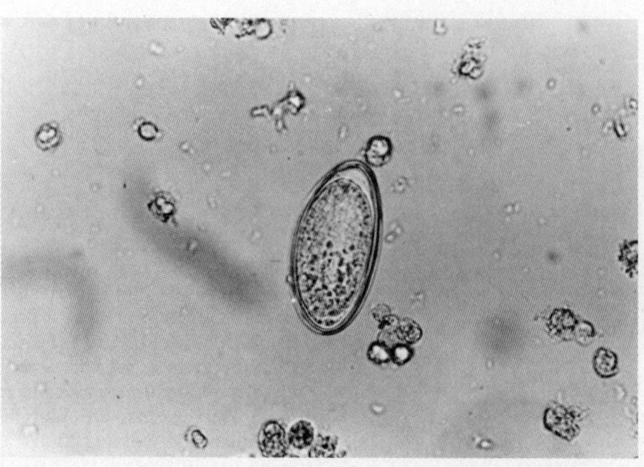

FIGURE 16.25. *Enterobius vermicularis* ova (×396) collected from the perianal skin. (Reprinted with permission from McMillan JA, Feigin RD, DeAngelis C, et al. *Oski's Pediatrics: Principles and Practice*. 4th ed. Philadelphia, PA: Lippincott Williams & Wilkins, 2006.)

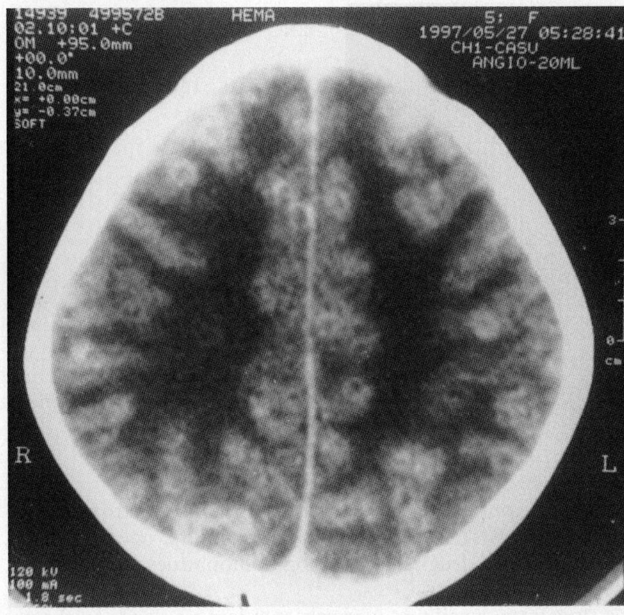

FIGURE 16.26. Computed tomographic scan of the brain showing multiple parenchymal neurocysticerci. (Reprinted with permission from McMillan JA, Feigin RD, DeAngelis C, et al. *Oski's Pediatrics: Principles and Practice*. 4th ed. Philadelphia, PA: Lippincott Williams & Wilkins, 2006.)

Clinical manifestations: Erythema, edema, and tenderness with pain out of proportion to the physical findings, progressing to the development of ischemia and tissue necrosis. Systemic signs will be present (fever, myalgias, anorexia, malaise).

Diagnosis: Supported by CT or MRI findings and confirmed by biopsy. Direct surgical exploration allows definitive diagnosis and cultures.

Treatment: Emergent, wide surgical debridement is critical and may need to be repeated. Antibiotic therapy in the absence of surgical debridement is ineffective. Initial antibiotics should treat both aerobic and anaerobic Gram-positive and -negative organisms.

INFECTIONS: SKELETAL

Diskitis

Clinical manifestations: Presents with refusal to walk, backache, and irritability in ambulatory children. Refusal to sit in preambulatory children. Palpation of the spine reveals localized tenderness. May have fever, leukocytosis, and elevation of ESR. *S. aureus* is the most common culprit. Other organisms that may be involved include *S. epidermidis* and *Kingella kingae*, anaerobes, Gram-negative enterics, and *S. pneumoniae*.

Diagnosis: Findings on plain film are normal early in the course. Bone scan may demonstrate increased uptake of technetium 99 m at the level of disk space involvement. CT scan can demonstrate narrowing of disk space and vertebral body involvement early in the course. MRI can confirm diagnosis. Place TST if tuberculosis is a consideration.

Treatment: Most children respond promptly with bed rest. Immobilization of spine sometimes required. Failure to respond to immobilization suggests diagnosis is incorrect. Empirical use of antistaphylococcal agent is appropriate.

Osteomyelitis

Epidemiology: Acute hematogenous osteomyelitis generally occurs in younger than 5 years.

TABLE 16.13

DIAGNOSIS OF URINARY TRACT INFECTION

Method of Collection	Diagnosis of UTI (CFU/mL)
Supra-pubic analysis	>1,000
Bladder catheterization	>10,000
Clean catch (mid-stream)	>100,000

CFU, colony forming units.

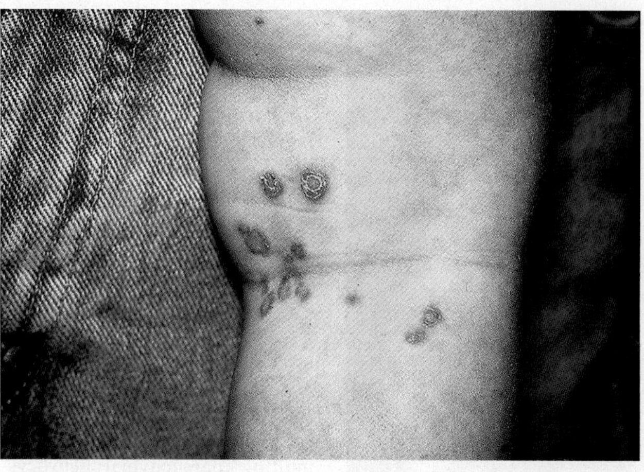

FIGURE 16.27. Impetigo. This photo does not show intact blisters, only the flaccid remains of the lesions. (From Goodheart HP. *Goodheart's Photoguide of Common Skin Disorders*. 2nd ed. Philadelphia, PA: Lippincott Williams & Wilkins, 2003.)

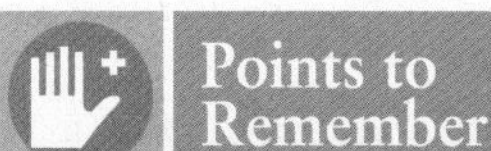

- Consider salmonella infection as a cause for osteomyelitis in patients with sickle cell disease (functional asplenia).

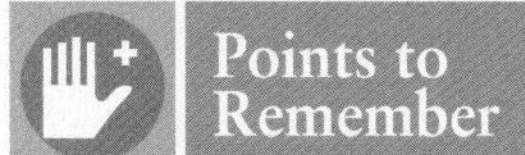

- Pelvic osteomyelitis may present with abdominal pain and difficulty walking.
- Consider vertebral osteomyelitis when back pain and fever are present.
- Foot puncture wounds through the sole of a shoe are associated with *Pseudomonas osteochondritis*.

In infants, infection may spread from contiguous septic arthritis because of transphyseal vessels (which recede in the first year of life). Risk factors include minor injury, open fractures, orthopedic surgery, decubitus ulcers, intravenous drug abuse, hemoglobinopathies, and diabetes. Caused by the same pathogens as septic arthritis.

Clinical manifestations: Fever, localized swelling, warmth, tenderness, and erythema. Refusal to walk in ambulatory children.

Diagnosis: If multiple sources are cultured (blood, bone, and joint fluid), a bacterial cause can be found in about 50% to 80% of cases. ESR and CRP are generally elevated. MRI with contrast is generally considered most useful modality to delineate affected area. Technetium bone scan is especially useful for detecting multifocal disease. X-ray findings of periosteal bone formation are usually not present until 2 weeks after onset of symptoms.

Treatment: Antimicrobial therapy should be tailored to cultured organism and generally continued for 4 to 6 weeks.

Septic Arthritis (Pyogenic Arthritis)

Epidemiology: Most commonly affects children younger than 3 years. A result of hematogenous spread, direct inoculation, or contiguous extension from an adjacent osteomyelitis. Common pathogens include *S. aureus*, *S. pyogenes*, *S. pneumoniae*, *K. kingae*, and *H. influenzae*; in neonates, consider GBS.

Clinical manifestation: Presents with acute onset of fever, refusal to use a limb, and localized joint swelling, tenderness, or erythema. Generally monoarticular, involving large joints (hip joint in infants and knee in older children). Lyme arthritis most commonly affects the knee. *N. gonorrhea* frequently affects the knee, hand, or wrist and may present with fevers, chills, polyarthralgia, and hemorrhagic pustules on the extensor surfaces of affected joints.

Diagnosis: Aspirate joint fluid and send culture, Gram stain, and cell count—usually more than 50,000 WBCs/mm^3. Specifically request Lyme PCR and cultures for *N. gonorrhea* if appropriate history raises suspicion for these infections.

Treatment: Drainage is both diagnostic and therapeutic. In cases of septic arthritis of the hip, emergent drainage is critical because blood supply to the acetabulum is compromised by

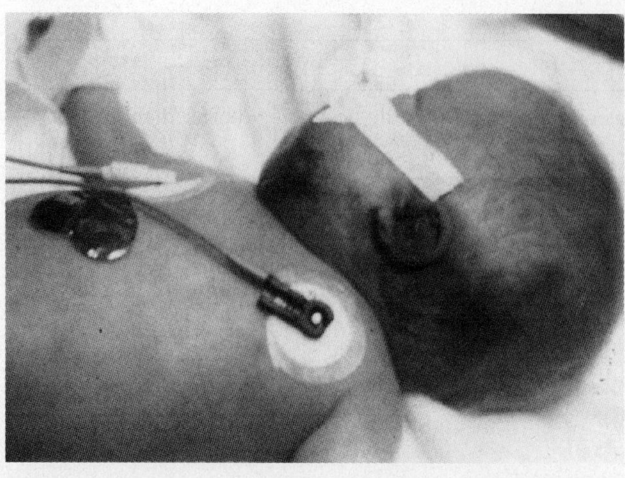

FIGURE 16.28. Necrotizing fasciitis of the submandibular area and pinna in a 3-month-old premature infant with late-onset group B streptococcal sepsis. (Reprinted with permission from McMillan JA, Feigin RD, DeAngelis C, et al. *Oski's Pediatrics: Principles and Practice*. 4th ed. Philadelphia, PA: Lippincott Williams & Wilkins, 2006.)

synovial fluid. Initiate empiric intravenous antibiotics with antistaphylococcal coverage. In younger children, where *Kingella kingae* and *H. influenzae* (especially if unvaccinated) are concerns, consider addition of a third-generation cephalosporin. Treat Lyme arthritis with amoxicillin (younger than 8 years) or doxycycline (8 years or older).

Toxic Synovitis (Transient Synovitis)

Clinical manifestations: Usually a painful limp or hip pain of acute origin; often unilateral; commonly presents between 2 and 6 years.

Diagnosis: Diagnosis of exclusion. Temperature, WBC, ESR are normal or slightly elevated, and these values plus clinical status can help decide if needle aspiration of joint is warranted to exclude septic arthritis.

Treatment: Bed rest and analgesics.

INFECTIONS: NERVOUS SYSTEM

Neurological and ophthalmic infections usually require prompt action to avoid disastrous results. This review should help solidify key facts often tested.

Cerebral Abscesses

Epidemiology: Etiology includes viridans streptococci, anaerobes, *S. aureus*, and occasionally gram negatives; in immunocompromised patients, consider fungi—especially aspergillus. Risk factors include cyanotic heart disease, neonatal meningitis (especially *Citrobacter*), chronic sinusitis, chronic otitis, dental and lung abscesses, and penetrating trauma.

Clinical manifestations: Fever, headaches, and focal neurologic signs are common.

Diagnosis: Risk of herniation is a concern if intracranial pressure is increased; therefore, head CT should be performed before a lumbar puncture is attempted and LP deferred if CT reveals evidence of increased ICP.

Treatment: Empiric antibiotics similar to those for epidural abscesses and subdural empyemas.

Encephalitis

Inflammation of the brain parenchyma, often accompanied by meningeal involvement. Can be infectious (caused by various viruses) or postinfectious (believed to be immune mediated). Viral infections of the brain cause cellular damage and provoke inflammatory responses. Most affected children have no predisposing illnesses.

Clinical manifestations: Characterized by the acute onset of a febrile illness and headache associated with altered consciousness and behavioral disturbances. When a cause is identified, enteroviral infections are most frequently identified; however, the list of possible causes is extensive as detailed in brief below.

- Enterovirus infections, including echovirus and coxsackie—generally present in the summer and fall but can occur year-round.
- Arboviruses most likely to cause encephalitis in the United States include the following: Eastern equine encephalitis, Western equine virus, St. Louis encephalitis, California encephalitis, and West Nile virus.
- Cat-scratch encephalitis, infection with *B. henselae*, occurs after scratches or bites from cats (especially kittens); usually has a good prognosis.
- Mycoplasma encephalitis may be seen after respiratory infection, as encephalitis may be postinfectious; however, it is unclear if treatment for this organism changes prognosis.
- HSV encephalitis beyond the neonatal period is uncommon; in older children, presents with fevers, headaches, personality changes, focal seizures, and coma.

Diagnosis: For *B. henselae* and Mycoplasma encephalitis, send serology. For HSV encephalitis, CSF HSV PCR is the preferred test (see Table 16.14).

For herpes encephalitis, electroencephalogram may demonstrate periodic lateralized epileptiform discharges in the temporal lobes and an MRI may demonstrate increased temporal lobe signal.

Treatment: Supportive care. Acyclovir should be given for possible HSV encephalitis, but specific therapies for other viruses are not available.

Meningitis

Infection and inflammation of the meninges surrounding the brain by direct inoculation or hematogenous spread across venules/lymphatics which drain portions of the face.

TABLE 16.14

CEREBROSPINAL FLUID EVALUATION

	Normal	Bacterial	Viral	Lyme Meningitis	Tuberculosis
WBC per mL	0–5 (allow up to 30 in neonates)	100–100,000	50–1,000	50–1,000	100 s
Glucose (mg/dL)	45–65	Low	Normal	Normal	Low
Protein (mg/dL)	20–45	High	Slightly increased	Slightly increased to high	High
Gram stain	Negative	Positive	Negative	Negative	Negative

Epidemiology: See Table 16.13 for epidemiology. "There has been a shift in the relative frequency of pathogens causing bacterial meningitis in children since the introduction of Hib and PCV-7 vaccines." In a retrospective review of 231 cases of bacterial meningitis in children (1 month through 18 years of age) who presented to 20 pediatric emergency departments in the United States between 2001 and 2004, the most frequent pathogens varied according to age as follows:

- ≥1 month and <3 months—GBS (39%), Gram-negative bacilli (32%), *S. pneumoniae* (14%), *N. meningitidis* (12%).
- ≥3 months and <3 years—*S. pneumoniae* (45%), *N. meningitidis* (34%), GBS (11%), Gram-negative bacilli (9%).
- ≥3 years and <10 years—*S. pneumoniae* (47%), *N. meningitidis* (32%).
- ≥10 years and <19 years—*N. meningitidis* (55%).

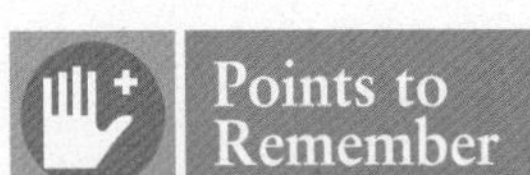

Points to Remember

- Incidence of *H. influenzae* type b meningitis has decreased dramatically as a result of immunization.

Most serogroups of meningococcal disease can be prevented by immunization; vaccination does not protect against serogroup B, which causes majority of meningococcal disease in infants.

S. pneumoniae is the most common cause of bacterial meningitis in children in the United States, but its incidence has fallen significantly since the availability of conjugated, 7-valent *S. pneumoniae* vaccine. There has been an increase in certain Pneumococcal serotypes, especially 19a, which are not present in the 7-valent vaccine because of a phenomenon known as serotype replacement but some of these, including serotype 19a, are found in the 13-valent Pneumococcal vaccine.

Clinical manifestations: Fever, headache, photophobia, vomiting, seizures, altered mental status, and nuchal rigidity. Infants may show nonspecific signs such as poor feeding, irritability, abnormal cry, and somnolence. Neurologic sequelae include focal deficits, seizures, hearing loss, and vision impairment. The most common permanent neurologic sequel is hearing loss. Complications include subdural effusion, intracranial infection (subdural empyema, brain abscess), cerebral infarction, hydrocephalus, diabetes insipidus, and disseminated infection (arthritis, pneumonia).

Diagnosis: See Table 16.14.

Treatment: In neonates, initiate ampicillin plus cefotaxime. Cefotaxime will treat GBS and Gram-negative enterics and penetrates the CSF. Ampicillin is mainly used for its effectiveness against *Listeria monocytogenes*. In infants and children outside of the neonatal age group, a third-generation cephalosporin is generally used empirically, as it treats pathogens most likely recovered at this age, including *S. pneumoniae*, *N. meningitidis*, and GBS. Vancomycin is added for resistant *S. pneumoniae*. Dexamethasone shown to decrease hearing loss in those with meningitis due to *H. influenzae* type b (given before or concurrently with first dose of antibiotics).

Antibiotic prophylaxis of close contacts to those with meningococcal meningitis and *H. influenzae* type b meningitis is indicated.

Subdural Empyemas and Epidural Abscesses

Definition: Intracranial infection may be confined to the spaces between the dura and the inner table of the skull or spinal column (epidural abscess), or between the meninges and dura (subdural empyema).

Epidemiology: Risk factors include bacterial meningitis (subdural), otitis, or sinusitis (subdural or epidural) (Fig. 16.29).

A spinal epidural abscess may develop as a complication of vertebral osteomyelitis or as a consequence of bacteremia. As a complication of bacterial meningitis, subdural empyemas may be caused by *S. pneumoniae* or *H. influenzae*; however, most subdural effusions complicating bacterial meningitis are sterile. If extension of sinusitis or otitis, also consider anaerobes, gram-negative aerobes, and *S. aureus*. Complications include cerebral herniation and thrombosis of the vertebral or venous sinuses.

Diagnosis: CT with contrast/MRI is essential. LP often shows pleocytosis with negative cultures.

Treatment: Surgical drainage and antibiotics (vancomycin plus a third-generation cephalosporin empirically). If associated with chronic sinusitis or chronic otitis media, consider ceftazidime and metronidazole.

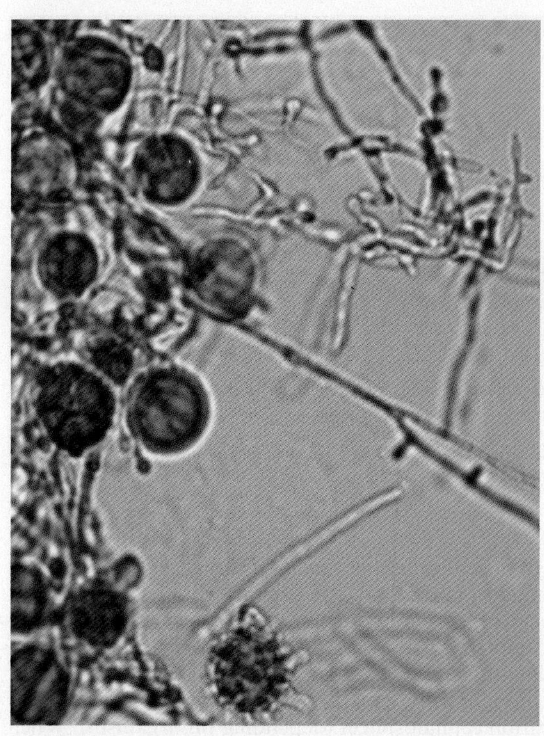

FIGURE 16.29. Macroconidia of the mold form of *Histoplasma capsulatum*.

Ventriculoperitoneal Shunt Infections

Epidemiology: Shunts usually become infected as a result of contamination during surgery, shunt aspiration, or by ascending infection from the gastrointestinal tract.

Most commonly caused by coagulase-negative Staphylococcus. For indolent infections, consider coagulase-negative staphylococcus and *Propionibacterium acnes*.

Clinical manifestations: Often presents with nonspecific fever, vomiting, and irritability with specific meningeal signs being less common. On exam, assess for signs of increased intracranial pressure, meningeal inflammation, erythema along path of catheter, and abdominal ecchymosis or tenderness.

Diagnosis: Culture and Gram stain and culture of CSF obtained from the shunt. Consider imaging to look for a fluid collection at ventricular or peritoneal tip.

Treatment: Removal of shunt with interim use of extraventricular drainage. Initial antibiotic treatment with vancomycin and a third-generation cephalosporin is recommended pending culture and susceptibility testing.

INFECTIONS: OPHTHALMIC

Neonatal Conjunctivitis

Epidemiology: Prophylaxis includes 1% tetracycline, 0.5% erythromycin, or 1% silver nitrate. Prophylaxis significantly decreases incidence of gonococcal conjunctivitis in the newborn. There are conflicting studies regarding reduction in incidence of chlamydial conjunctivitis in the newborn; it does not prevent *C. trachomatis* pneumonia acquired from exposure to maternal genital flora. Chlamydia conjunctivitis is the most common cause of conjunctivitis in the United States. Silver nitrate application can cause chemical conjunctivitis, which occurs on the first day of life—resolves spontaneously without treatment.

Clinical manifestations, Diagnosis, and **Treatment:** See Table 16.15 (Fig. 16.30).

Orbital and Periorbital Cellulitis

Definition: Periorbital (preseptal) cellulitis is an infection of the skin and soft tissue anterior to the orbital septum. Orbital cellulitis is an infection of the tissues posterior to the orbital septum.

Clinical manifestations: Differentiate periorbital from orbital cellulitis. Limitations of extraocular eye movements or proptosis are suggestive of orbital cellulitis.

Diagnosis: If suspicious of orbital cellulitis, obtain an orbital CT scan.

TABLE 16.15

NEONATAL CONJUNCTIVITIS

	Chlamydia trachomatis	*Neisseria gonorrhea*	HSV Conjunctivitis
Age of presentation	Second week of life	First week of life	Second to fourth week of life
Clinical presentation	Varies from mild conjunctival injection with scant mucoid discharge to severe mucopurulent conjunctivitis with chemosis and pseudomembrane formation; can result in corneal scarring without treatment	Copious purulent discharge; can result in corneal ulceration or perforation, endophthalmitis, arthritis, sepsis, and meningitis	Erythema of conjunctivae, possibly with vesicular rash of surrounding area. Chorioretinitis, cataracts, and corneal scarring
Diagnosis	Identification of the organism by culture, PCR, or nucleic acid amplification	Gram stain and culture of pus	Viral culture of conjunctival swab
Treatment	14 d of oral erythromycin	One dose of ceftriaxone	10 d of acyclovir

Treatment: Hospitalize all children with orbital cellulitis, consult ophthalmology, and treat with intravenous antibiotics. Empiric antimicrobial therapy for orbital cellulitis should treat *S. aureus*, *S. pyogenes*, anaerobic bacteria of the upper respiratory tract, and the usual pathogens of sinusitis (*S. pneumoniae*, *H. influenzae*, and *M. catarrhalis*). For periorbital cellulitis, if etiology is trauma, manage with an antistaphylococcal antibiotic for 10 to 14 days of oral therapy. When periorbital cellulitis is thought to be caused by hematogenous spread, treat with penicillin, ampicillin, or a third-generation cephalosporin (depending on organism). When the etiology is thought to be due to inflammatory edema of sinusitis, a second-generation cephalosporin which treats *S. pneumoniae*, *H. influenzae*, and anaerobes can be used—as can amoxicillin/clavulanate.

INFECTIONS: OTHER SPECIAL CONDITIONS

Treatment for bites and toxin-producing organisms are commonly tested subjects. Review appears here as well as within the "Critical Care and Emergency Medicine" chapter.

Cat and Dog Bites

Epidemiology: Cat bites are responsible for only about 5% of bites but more likely to cause infection than dog bites. Dog bites are responsible for about 80% to 90% of bites. Bite wounds are generally polymicrobial; pathogens include *Staphylococcus spp., Pasturella multocida, Bacteroides spp., Prevotella, Streptococcus spp., Eikenella corrodens, and Capnocytophaga canimorus.*

Clinical manifestations: Pain, erythema, swelling, and purulent drainage of the bite wound site, usually developing 1 to 2 days after the bite. Pasteurella infections cause pain and swelling within 12 to 24 hours.

Treatment: Irrigation and debridement of devitalized tissues. Assess tetanus and rabies immunization status (see later). Antibiotics (amoxicillin–clavulanate) are indicated prophylactically for puncture wounds; bites on the hands, face, or genitals; when devitalized tissue or a crush injury is present; and in immunocompromised/asplenic patients. For penicillin-allergic

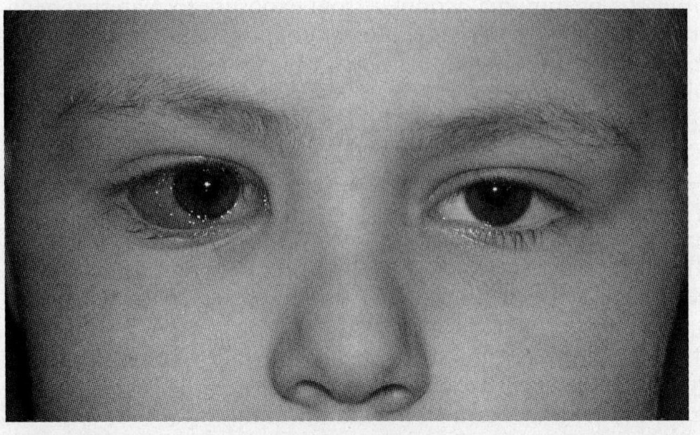

FIGURE 16.30. Right conjunctivitis. Note conjunctival chemosis, redness, and discharge. (Reprinted with permission from McMillan JA, Feigin RD, DeAngelis C, et al. *Oski's Pediatrics: Principles and Practice*. 4th ed. Philadelphia, PA: Lippincott Williams & Wilkins, 2006.)

patients, TMP–SMX and clindamycin can be used. A 7- to 10-day antibiotic course is usually sufficient for soft tissue infections; duration of treatment for bite-associated bone infections is at least 4 weeks.

Human Bites

Epidemiology: Responsible for about 5% of bite wounds. Causative organisms include *Staphylococcal* spp., *Streptococcal* spp., *Haemophilus* spp., anaerobes, and *Eikenella corrodens*.

Treatment: Same treatment as for cat/dog bites.

Toxic Shock Syndrome

Clinical manifestations: An acute febrile illness caused by bacterial exotoxins from *S. aureus* or *S. pyogenes*. *S. aureus* more associated with profuse diarrhea and foreign body at site of infection (e.g., tampon); *S. pyogenes* more commonly associated with localized soft-tissue infection.

Diagnosis: *Major criteria (all required)*: (a) fever, (b) diffuse erythrodermatous rash that desquamates 1 to 2 weeks after disease onset, and (c) hypotension. *Minor criteria (any three)*: vomiting, diarrhea, liver dysfunction, renal dysfunction, respiratory dysfunction, mental status changes, mucous membrane inflammation, and muscle abnormalities.

Blood cultures are rarely positive in *S. aureus* TSS but often positive in *S. pyogenes* disease.

Treatment: Removal of foreign body (e.g., tampon) if one exists, fluid replacement, and management of cardiac or respiratory failure. Antibiotics: beta-lactam plus clindamycin (mostly to decrease toxin production).

Fungal Infections

Although all children can develop fungal infections, invasive fungal disease is often a signal of an immunocompromised state. See Table 16.16.

Fever and Neutropenia

Definition: Neutropenia is an absolute neutrophil count less than 500/mm^3 or less than 1,000 mm^3 and falling.

Treatment: Prompt empiric broad-spectrum antimicrobials are vital, as there is a broad differential of possible pathogens. Potential regimens include B-lactams with anti-Pseudomonal coverage including piperacillin-tazobactam, ceftazidime, cefepime, or carbapenems. Vancomycin may need to be added when central lines are in place. If fever lasts for more than 5 days, consider fungal etiology and start presumptive antifungal therapy (amphotericin B) and consider viral etiology (CMV, HHV-6, adenovirus, etc.).

EMERGING INFECTIONS

Severe Acute Respiratory Syndrome

Definition: SARS was so named by the World Health Organization (WHO) in March 2003 when this acute respiratory illness appeared in the Guangdong province of China. It is suspected to be a new viral strain from the coronavirus family.

Epidemiology: At the time of writing this book, the most recent outbreak was reported in China, April 2004. For more information, please see the CDC Web site: www.cdc.gov/ncidod/sars/.

Clinical manifestations: A suspected case is defined by the WHO as an individual presenting with

- Fever higher than 38°C (≥100.5°F) plus.
- Cough or difficulty breathing plus.
- Close contact with a person who has been diagnosed with SARS and/or history of travel or residence in an area with recent local transmission of SARS within 10 days of symptom onset.

Diagnosis: ELISA testing for IgG antibody to the SARS virus.

Treatment: Supportive. Although antivirals have been used, there is no clearly established therapy currently available.

TABLE 16.16

FUNGAL INFECTIONS

	Etiology	Clinical Symptoms	Treatment
Candida spp.	Mucocutaneous candida may be caused by antibiotic use; invasive candidiasis most commonly seen in malignancies, bone marrow transplant recipients, prolonged corticosteroid use, parenteral nutrition use, extensive burns	Mucocutaneous candidiasis includes oral-pharyngeal infections "thrush" or vaginal candidiasis; invasive candidiasis can involve virtually any organ and can be rapidly fatal	Topical nystatin for mucocutaneous candidiasis or if severe fluconazole or amphotericin B
Aspergillus spp.	Ubiquitous in environment, causes invasive disease in the immunocompromised	Most often causes sinopulmonary disease; aspergillomas (fungal balls) grows in preexisting cavities in patient with cystic fibrosis or tuberculosis; consider allergic bronchopulmonary aspergillosis in asthmatics with worsening symptoms despite treatment	Treat invasive aspergillosis with voriconazole or amphotericin B; surgical excision of a localized aspergilloma is often warranted
Cryptococcus neoformans	An encapsulated yeast generally acquired by inhalation; isolated primarily from soil (Fig. 16.31)	Primary infection often asymptomatic; can cause pulmonary disease (cough and constitutional symptoms); meningitis and dissemination to other organs occurs in children with defects in cell-mediated immunity	Treat with amphotericin + flucytosine for serious infections
Coccidioidomycosis	Consider in people with recent travel to southwestern United States; found in soil	Flu-like symptoms generally develop within a month of exposure; can be asymptomatic	Antifungal therapy is not indicated for uncomplicated infection (self-limited). Treat with amphotericin B, fluconazole, or ketoconazole if treatment is indicated.
Histoplasma capsulatum	Found throughout Ohio, Missouri, Mississippi river valleys from bird droppings	Most people asymptomatic; patients who become ill are generally immunocompromised (may present with flu-like symptoms with pulmonary infiltrates); progressive disseminated histoplasmosis can develop in otherwise healthy infants (prolonged fever, hepatosplenomegaly, failure to thrive) (Fig. 16.29)	Treatment is usually not necessary (self-limited), but if disease is disseminated or host is immunocompromised, use amphotericin, fluconazole, or itraconazole
Blastomyces dermatitidis	Generally found in southeastern United States; acquired from inhalation; found in soil	Clinical manifestations include pulmonary (flu-like symptoms with infiltrates on chest x-ray), cutaneous (often subcutaneous abscesses), and disseminated	Amphotericin B for severe infections, itraconazole or fluconazole for mild infections
Sporotrichosis schenckii	Often caused by traumatic inoculation by rose thorns	Chronic subcutaneous fungal infection that invades regional lymphatics; inoculation occurs at a site of minor trauma and lesions proceed to develop along the lymph nodes proximal to the lesion; disseminated disease can occur in immunocompromised hosts (Figs. 16.32 and 16.33)	Amphotericin B for pulmonary or disseminated sporotrichosis; itraconazole for cutaneous disease

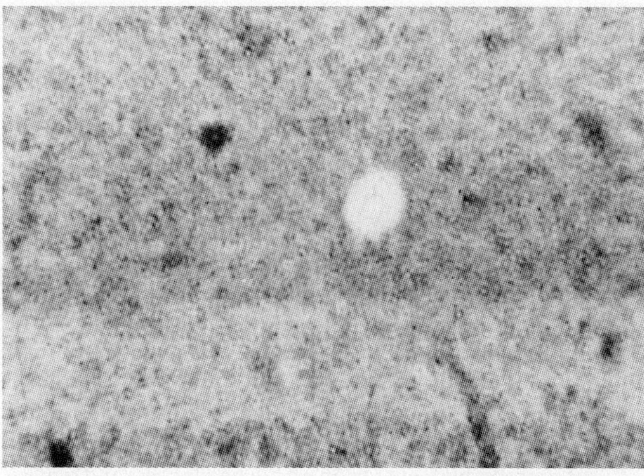

FIGURE 16.31. India ink preparation of cerebrospinal fluid showing budding yeast with prominent capsule. (Reprinted with permission from McMillan JA, Feigin RD, DeAngelis C, et al. *Oski's Pediatrics: Principles and Practice.* 4th ed. Philadelphia, PA: Lippincott Williams & Wilkins, 2006.)

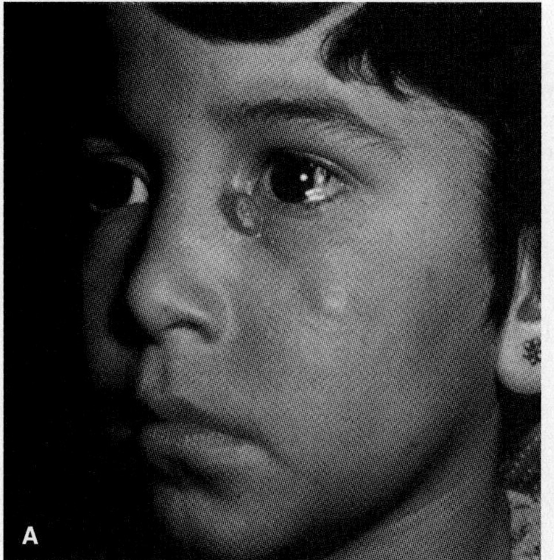

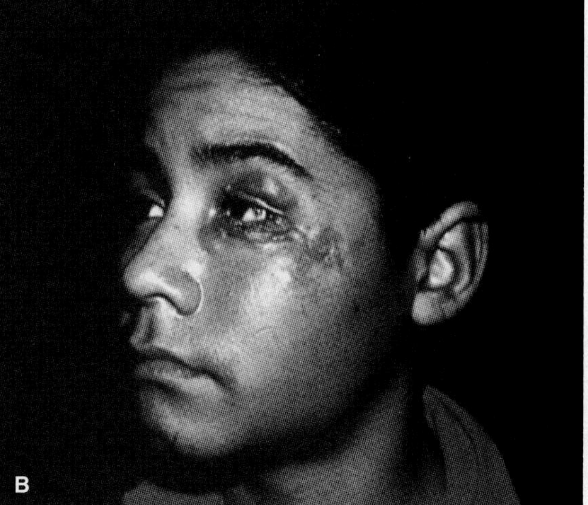

FIGURE 16.32. **A:** Sporotrichosis in its classic appearance as a solitary lesion on the face of a child. **B:** Sporotrichosis spread. (Reprinted with permission from McMillan JA, Feigin RD, DeAngelis C, et al. *Oski's Pediatrics: Principles and Practice.* 4th ed. Philadelphia, PA: Lippincott Williams & Wilkins, 2006.)

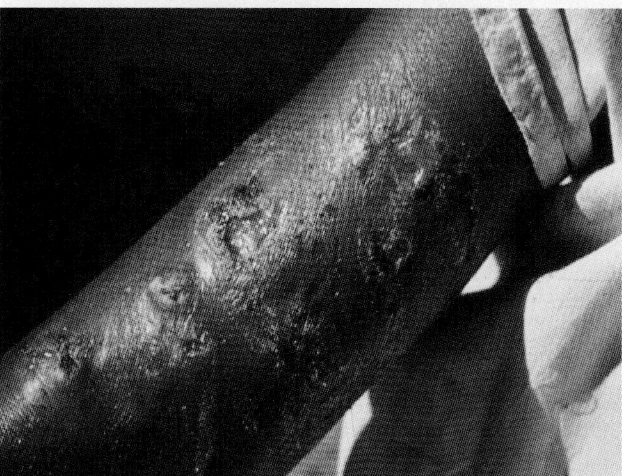

FIGURE 16.33. Sporotrichosis presenting on an arm. (Reprinted with permission from McMillan JA, Feigin RD, DeAngelis C, et al. *Oski's Pediatrics: Principles and Practice.* 4th ed. Philadelphia, PA: Lippincott Williams & Wilkins, 2006.)

SAMPLE BOARD REVIEW QUESTIONS

1. A 13-year-old boy presents to the emergency room with puffiness around his left eye. On further questioning, he has had severe frontal headaches for the past week and has been having nasal drainage for 2 weeks. He has had about 2 days of fevers and has had some emesis over the past 24 hours. On examination, he is febrile to 101.7°F and slightly tachycardic but with otherwise normal vital signs. He is slow to respond to questions and is not oriented to time and date. His pupils are equally reactive and he has full range of eye movements. He complains of facial tenderness over his left frontal, maxillary, and ethmoid sinuses. Of the following, the best diagnostic procedure would be
   a. Urine toxicology screen
   b. Nasal swab for diagnosis of sinusitis
   c. Lumbar puncture to rule out meningitis
   d. No further diagnostic procedure is necessary, as this patient has periorbital cellulitis
   e. Computerized tomography scan of the head with intravenous contrast

   Answer: e. The presence of mental status changes in the setting of sinusitis is suggestive of intracranial extension. The headaches and emesis are concerning for increased intracranial pressure. Serious complications of sinusitis include orbital cellulitis, cerebral abscess, cavernous or sagittal sinus thrombosis, and frontal (Pott's puffy tumor) or maxillary osteomyelitis. Head computerized tomography scan is preferred for this patient because of the constellation of pain, confusion, and morning emesis which makes a focal intracranial mass a possibility. Contrast with the CT scan improves visualization of a fluid collection.

2. All of the following statements regarding comparisons between TIV and LAIV are **correct, except which of the following?**
   a. TIV uses noninfectious viruses; LAIV uses live attenuated viruses that can only replicate efficiently at temperatures present in the nasal mucosa
   b. TIV is administered intramuscularly via injection; LAIV is administered intranasally
   c. TIV is licensed for use among persons as young as 6 months; LAIV is licensed for use among nonpregnant persons aged 2 to 49 years
   d. Both TIV and LAIV can be safely administered to persons with medical risk factors for influenza-related complications
   e. All of these answers are correct

   Answer: d. LAIV is not approved for administration to persons with medical risk factors for influenza-related complications. High-risk groups include chronic pulmonary (including asthma), cardiovascular, metabolic, renal disorders, and hemoglobinopathies; those receiving immunosuppressive therapy or salicylates; and any condition that can cause respiratory distress. TIV is recommended for children with these conditions.

3. The following groups of people are eligible to routinely receive the tetravalent meningococcal conjugate vaccine (MCV4) **except?**
   a. Children aged 11 to 12 years with no underlying medical issues
   b. College freshman living in dormitories
   c. HIV-infected individuals aged 11 to 55 years
   d. Children aged 2 to 10 years with no underlying medical issues
   e. The vaccine is licensed for all of the above groups

   Answer: d. Routine vaccination of young adolescents with a single dose of MCV4 intramuscularly is recommended at the preadolescent health-care visit. For adolescents that have not previously received MCV4, vaccination can be given before high-school entry. A single dose of MCV4 is recommended for groups at high risk of infection with *N. meningitidis* aged 11 to 55 years: college freshman living in dormitories, persons traveling to areas where *N. meningitidis* is hyperendemic or epidemic, microbiologists routinely exposed to *N. meningitidis*, military recruits, people with terminal complement deficiencies and persons with anatomic or functional asplenia, and persons with HIV infection.

4. You are seeing a 17-year-old adolescent male who received the tetanus and diphtheria toxoid (Td) vaccine at the age of 11 years. Which of the following statements is the recommendation with regard to the tetanus toxoid, reduced diphtheria toxoid, and acellular pertussis vaccine (Tdap)?
   a. Administer a second dose of Td now, as there is no benefit of administering Tdap at this time
   b. Administer a single dose of Tdap to provide protection against pertussis as well as diphtheria and tetanus

c. No further vaccination with regard to tetanus toxoid, diphtheria toxoid, and pertussis is needed at this time
d. Consider administration of Tdap only if a traumatic injury occurs
e. Consider administration of Tdap only if an infant lives in the household

Answer: b. Adolescents aged 11 to 18 years should receive a single dose of Tdap. An interval of at least 5 years between Td and Tdap is encouraged to reduce risk of any reactions after Tdap vaccination (interval as little as 2 years can be used if necessary—health care worker, new mother in postpartum period). There is currently a recommendation for only one booster of Tdap in a lifetime. For future protection against tetanus, one can revert back to Td.

5. Which of the following statements most accurately describes the changing epidemiology of pneumococcal disease since the introduction of the 7-valent pneumococcal conjugate (PCV7) vaccine from 1998–1999 to 2003?
   a. The incidence of vaccine-type invasive pneumococcal disease among children younger than 5 years has decreased by approximately 94% without a significant effect on herd immunity
   b. The incidence of vaccine-type invasive pneumococcal disease among children younger than 5 years has decreased by approximately 94% with a significant effect on herd immunity
   c. The incidence of vaccine-type invasive pneumococcal disease among children younger than 5 years has decreased by approximately 54% without a significant effect on herd immunity
   d. The incidence of vaccine-type invasive pneumococcal disease among children younger than 5 years has decreased by approximately 54% with a significant effect on herd immunity.
   e. Because of an increase in replacement serotypes (serotypes not found in the PCV7 vaccine), there has been no significant change in the prevalence of pneumococcal disease

Answer: b. From 1998–1999 to 2003, the incidence of vaccine type invasive pneumococcal disease among children younger than 5 years has decreased by 94%. Indirect effects of PCV7 are believed to be caused by decreased nasopharyngeal carriage of vaccine-type strains among immunized children, which results in decreased transmission to nonimmunized children and adults (i.e., herd immunity).

6. Which of the following is a true statement regarding *B. henselae* infection?
   a. Fleas are responsible for cat-to-cat transmission of *B. henselae*
   b. Corticosteroids are the mainstay of therapy for patients with CSD encephalitis
   c. Older cats are the main mode of transmission of *B. henselae* to humans
   d. Cats with *B. henselae* bacteremia tend to be ill appearing
   e. The majority of patients with CSD encephalitis have significant long-term neurological sequelae

Answer: a. *B. henselae* is a fastidious, slow-growing, Gram-negative bacillus and is the organism that causes the clinical syndrome of CSD. CSD results from scratch, lick, or bite of cat, and usually a kitten. Fleas transmit *B henselae* between cats. There has been no documented person-to-person transmission.

7. An 18-month-old female presents with low-grade fevers and the inability to walk. Imaging demonstrates a right hip septic arthritis with involvement of her right proximal femur. Fluid from her joint is aspirated and the bacterial culture reveals *Kingella kingae*. Which of the following is true regarding this organism?
   a. It mainly causes invasive disease in immunocompromised patients
   b. It tends to cause invasive disease mainly in teenagers
   c. It is a gram-negative coccobacillus which usually grows in less than 24 hours
   d. It is an organism which can colonize the respiratory and oropharyngeal tract of healthy children
   e. It is highly resistant to beta-lactams

Answer: d. *Kingella kingae* is a fastidious, Gram-negative coccobacillus. It has been shown to cause osteomyelitis/septic arthritis in young children, bacteremia in infants, and endocarditis in school-aged children and adults. It is a member of the HACEK group of organisms (*Haemophilus* spp., *Actinobacillus* spp., *Cardiobacterium* spp., *Eikenella* spp., and *Kingella* spp.). The majority of children with invasive disease due to this organism are not immunosuppressed. It is known to colonize the respiratory and oropharyngeal tract of children. The Gram stain of synovial fluid shows WBCs but frequently is negative for organisms due to the fastidious nature of the bacteria, and culture often take several days to grow. It is recommended that laboratories hold the culture for 7 days when there is a suspicion for this organism. *K. kingae* is highly susceptible to many antimicrobials including penicillin.

8. A 5-year-old female who recently emigrated from Honduras presents to your clinic. Her father describes her as complaining of colicky abdominal pain for the past 3 weeks. He does not report a change in her stooling habits. She has bowel sounds on examination and appears to have diffused mild abdominal tenderness. She has no rebound or guarding. After deep palpation of her abdomen, she has an episode of emesis. The emesis contains a long, slim, roundworm that measures approximately 20 cm in length. Of the following, the best treatment choice is
   a. Iodoquinol
   b. Albendazole
   c. Praziquantel
   d. Metronidazole
   e. Immediate surgical intervention

   Answer: b. Ascariasis is an infection caused by the roundworm *Ascaris lumbricoides*. It is seen most frequently in tropical climates where there are poor sanitation systems. Adult worms live in the small intestines and produce eggs which are excreted in the stool. Occasionally, larvae pass from the small intestine into the bloodstream and travel to the lungs and liver. Treatment of ascariasis that is not associated with intestinal obstruction consists of a single dose of albendazole, pyrantel pamoate, or mebendazole.

9. A 19-year-old female who returned from a trip to Eastern Europe 4 months ago presents in the summer time in Texas with a 2-day history of fever, chills, confusion, and weakness in her arms and legs. On exam, she has asymmetric weakness in both of her arms and legs. She has hyporeflexia and her sensation is intact. She has a normal peripheral WBC count. Her CSF demonstrates 15 WBCs/mm^3, 90% lymphocytes, protein of 230 mg/dL, glucose of 43 mg/dL. An MRI of her brain and spine demonstrate no abnormalities. Electromyogram and nerve conduction studies reveal severe asymmetric peripheral neuropathy. She has no travel history other than her recent trip to Eastern Europe and has received all her childhood vaccinations. The most likely cause for this syndrome is which of the following?
   a. Epidural abscess
   b. Japanese encephalitis
   c. Guillain–Barre syndrome
   d. Botulism
   e. West Nile virus

   Answer: e. West Nile virus can present as an acute flaccid paralysis. Patients present with a syndrome similar to polio and involvement of the anterior horn cells of the spinal cord and motor axons is seen. Weakness is generally asymmetric and there is no pain or sensory loss seen. Guillain–Barre syndrome does not typically present with fever and is a symmetric process that may involve both sensory and motor function. There is no epidemiologic risk of Japanese encephalitis, as this occurs only in Asia. The distribution of weakness is not plausible with an epidural abscess. Botulism is a serious paralytic disease caused by the botulinum toxin. All forms lead to paralysis that typically starts with the muscles of the face and then spreads toward the limbs.

10. A 15-year-old boy living in Maryland was bitten on the hand by a feral cat. The bite occurred 9 hours ago after the boy tried to feed the cat. Examination of the hand reveals several puncture wounds and some edema and tenderness. No exudates are seen. The two younger sisters of the boy also petted the cat but were not licked, scratched, or bitten. In addition to review of his tetanus immunization status and immunization if necessary, which of the following is recommended?
   a. If the cat has escaped, RIG is not necessary, but rabies vaccine should be administered to the 15-year-old boy
   b. If the cat has escaped, rabies vaccine should be administered in one thigh and RIG in the other thigh to the 15-year-old boy and his sisters
   c. If the cat has escaped, RIG should be administered in one thigh and the rabies vaccine in the other thigh to the 15-year-old boy only
   d. If the cat has escaped, rabies prophylaxis is unnecessary as a cat is an unlikely host
   e. If the cat can be monitored for 10 days and demonstrates no signs of illness, rabies prophylaxis is unnecessary for anyone

   Answer: e. Rabies is a rapidly progressive disease in dogs and cats after they become infectious, so observation for 10 days is sufficient to exclude this disease. This appears to be a provoked bite, so the likelihood of the cat being infected with rabies is low. If the cat cannot be observed, the best option would be to administer immune globulin into the bitten hand and to administer the reminder in another site. A course of rabies vaccination should also be begun, giving the initial injection into a site other than the site the immune globulin was administered. Cats are not generally infected in the United States, but this does not mean that they cannot be infected. Since the younger children were not exposed to the cat's saliva, they do not need prophylaxis.

11. A 19-year-old male who has been noncompliant with HAART presents with 8 days of fevers and chills. On exam, his only finding is a 1-cm purple nodule on his forearm. This was noticed by the patient to have developed on the first day of his fever. He has a peripheral WBC count of 31,000 cells/mm^3. He has recently been cleaning out an old attic and has developed some scratches from cats and mice. The patient is hospitalized. Parenteral antibiotics are started and a biopsy is performed. An hematoxylin and eosin stain demonstrates "lobular collections of endothelial cells with vascular infiltrates composed mostly of neutrophils." Numerous bacilli are seen on Warthin–Starry stain. The organism causing disease in this patient was most likely transmitted by which of the following?

a. Ticks
b. Mosquitos
c. Cats
d. Cockroaches
e. Rats

Answer: c. This patient has BA likely due to *B. henselae*. BA is characterized by the proliferation of blood vessels, resulting in the formation of tumor-like masses in the skin and other organs. The vector appears to be cats which are bacteremic with this organism. If a cat is carrying *B. henselae*, it may not exhibit any symptoms. Transmission to humans is thought to occur via flea feces inoculated into a cat scratch or bite, and transmission between cats occurs only in the presence of fleas. Although most patients with this disease have AIDS, other immunosuppressed patients have been reported to develop the disease.

12. A 5-year-old girl presents approximately 100 hours after being bitten by a dog in her left arm. Her mother states that she developed fever and swelling of the affected arm over the past 12 hours. Physical examination reveals a nontoxic, febrile female. Her wound site has visible purulence and surrounding erythema. The most likely pathogen that would be cultured from this wound is which of the following?

a. *Streptococcus pyogenes*
b. *Staphylococcus aureus*
c. *Pasturella multocida*
d. *Escherichia coli*
e. *Kingella kingae*

Answer: b. The patient described in this vignette developed an infection 4 days after sustaining a bite wound. Late infections that produce purulence are usually due to *Staphylococcus aureus* or *Eikenella*, or *both*. Infections with *Pasturella multocida* can occur after an animal bite but usually develop within 24 hours. Although dogs may be colonized with *Streptococcus pyogenes*, wound infections with this organism after a bite are uncommon. *Kingella* is not a usual cause of bite wound infection.

13. You are taking care of a 4-year-old previously healthy male who has never been vaccinated against varicella. He presents with a rash consistent with chickenpox. On examination, he is generally well appearing and his rash is present in various stages. You advise the mother to do which of the following?

a. Initiate therapy with oral acyclovir
b. Initiate therapy with intravenous acyclovir
c. Because oral absorption is improved with valacyclovir, initiate therapy with valacyclovir
d. Administer varicella-zoster immune globulin and antiviral therapy
e. None of the above

Answer: e. Antiviral therapy is not recommended for routine use in otherwise healthy children with varicella. Antiviral therapy should be considered for children at risk of moderate-to-severe varicella, such as people older than 12 years, people with chronic cutaneous or pulmonary disorders, people receiving long-term salicylate therapy, and people receiving corticosteroids. Some experts also recommend use of oral acyclovir for secondary household contact cases in which the disease is usually more severe than the primary case.

14. A 4-year-old child recently diagnosed with acute myelogenous leukemia has received induction chemotherapy. She is admitted for fever and found to have an absolute neutrophil count of 300 cells/mm^3. Her blood pressure is 64/46. Of the following, the best empiric antimicrobial therapy would be

a. Piperacillin–tazobactam and gentamicin
b. Ceftriaxone
c. Ceftriaxone and clindamycin
d. Vancomycin
e. Vancomycin and ceftriaxone

Answer: a. When considering causes for fever and neutropenia, *Pseudomonas aeruginosa* is a major concern. Piperacillin–tazobactam is an extended spectrum penicillin that has the most activity against *P. aeruginosa* of the antimicrobial agents listed.

15. Which of the following persons is at increased risk for HAV infection should be routinely vaccinated?

a. A 4-year-old child traveling to India for a vacation
b. A 17-year-old male who has sex with other males
c. A 16-year-old female who admits to injection drug use
d. A 7-year-old boy with factor VIII deficiency
e. A 3-year-old child with Alagille syndrome
f. All of the above

Answer: f. The Advisory Committee on Immunization Practices recommends the routine vaccination of children older than 1 year in the United States with the hepatitis A vaccine. Persons from developed countries who travel to developing countries are at substantial risk for acquiring hepatitis A. Hepatitis A outbreaks among males who have sexual intercourse with males have been reported frequently. Outbreaks have been reported with increasing frequency among users of injection and noninjection drugs. In the United States, data suggests that persons with hemophilia might be at increased risk for HAV infection. Although not at increased risk for HAV infection, persons with chronic liver disease are at increased risk for fulminant hepatitis A.

16. A mother brings her twin 5-year-old daughters in because of the sudden onset of a fever. After taking a history from the mother and completing your physical examination, you discover that they also have headaches, pharyngitis, bilateral conjunctivitis, and nasal conjunctivitis. They recently attended a classmate's birthday pool party and several other children from the party have had similar symptoms. You give the mother reassurance and inform her that the organism that is likely responsible for their symptoms is which of the following?

a. Epstein–Barr virus
b. Cytomegalovirus
c. Adenovirus
d. Parvovirus
e. Coxsackie B virus

Answer: c. Adenovirus most commonly infects the respiratory tract. It frequently causes rhinorrhea, cough, fever, sore throat, pharyngitis, conjunctivitis. Community outbreaks of pharyngoconjunctival fever have been attributed to exposure to water from contaminated swimming pools. The onset of symptoms is acute and fever and associated symptoms usually last 3 to 5 days.

17. A 19-year-old college student returned 5 days ago from Greece where he had contact with raw animal herds. He had initially experienced only mild upper respiratory tract symptoms, but 3 days later was brought to the emergency room with fever, severe dyspnea, cyanosis, and tachycardia. You receive a call from the microbiology technician because the Gram stain reveals large, gram-positive rods with subterminal spores. What is the most likely identity of this organism?

a. *Clostridium botulinum*
b. *Bacillus anthracis*
c. *Clostridium perfringens*
d. *Leptospira interrogans*
e. *Bacillus subtilis*

Answer: b. Anthrax is a zoonotic disease that occurs in many rural areas of the world. Depending on the route of infection, anthrax can occur in three forms: cutaneous, inhalation, and gastrointestinal. Inhalation anthrax is a cause of serious morbidity and mortality. A nonspecific prodrome of fever, sweats, headache, myalgia, and malaise generally occur initially. Over the next few days, it progresses to a fulminant phase which can present with hypotension, dyspnea, cyanosis, hypoxia, and shock. A high index of clinical suspicion and rapid administration of appropriate antibiotics is essential. Naturally occurring disease can be treated with penicillins and tetracyclines. For bioterrorism-associated disease, fluoroquinolones are generally recommended.

18. A previously healthy, 16-year-old Ecuadorian immigrant is brought to an emergency room in Houston because of seizures. A head CT reveals a solitary calcified lesion, 2 cm in diameter, in the right cerebral hemisphere. Which of the following is the most likely diagnosis?
    a. Extraintestinal amebiasis
    b. CNS coccidioidomycosis
    c. Cerebral cysticercosis
    d. Cerebral echinococcosis
    e. Progressive multifocal leukoencephalopathy

Answer: c. Cysticercosis is a parasitic infection that results from ingestion of eggs from the adult tapeworm, *Taenia solium*. When cysticercosis involves the CNS, it is called neurocysticercosis. Neurocysticercosis is the most common parasitic infection of the brain and a leading cause of epilepsy in the developing world, especially Latin America, India, Africa, and China. Neurocysticercosis is acquired through consumption of food contaminated with feces of a *T. solium* tapeworm carrier (i.e., through fecal–oral contract). Neurocysticercosis typically presents with seizures (70% to 90% of acutely symptomatic patients) or headache. Headache usually indicates the presence of hydrocephalus, meningitis, or increased intracranial pressure. Brain imaging can demonstrate the stages of neurocysticercosis: vesicular (viable larval cyst), colloidal (enhancing cyst, without a well-defined scolex), and calcified granulomas.

19. A previously normal, full-term infant developed bilateral conjunctivitis at 2 weeks of age. The conjunctivitis was followed by severe coughing, but the infant remained afebrile. When the infant was 8 weeks old, a chest x-ray showed bilateral symmetrical interstitial infiltrates. The WBC count was 14,000/mm^3 with 29% segmented neutrophils, 58% lymphocytes, and 9% eosinophils. Which of the following is the most likely infectious agent?
    a. *Chlamydia trachomatis*
    b. *Streptococcus agalactiae*
    c. *Haemophilus influenzae*
    d. *Pneumocystis jiroveci* pneumonia
    e. Cytomegalovirus

Answer: a. Infants who become infected with chlamydia during birth frequently develop a type of neonatal conjunctivitis of the eyes, sometimes referred to as ophthalmia neonatorum. *C. trachomatis* infection is the most common cause of neonatal conjunctivitis in industrially developed countries. Conjunctivitis develops between 5 and 14 days after delivery, usually in one eye but affecting the other after 2 to 7 days. Edema and erythema of the eyelids is common, along with eye discharge that may be watery initially but becoming purulent later. Infants can also develop pneumonia caused by nasopharyngeal *C. trachomatis* infection or aspiration of infected genital secretions during delivery. Pneumonia typically occurs at around 6 weeks of age. These babies generally have a low-grade fever with an increased respiratory rate. Often a persistent cough interferes with feeding. A chest x-ray generally demonstrates hyperinflation and diffused infiltrates.

SUGGESTED READINGS

Durbin WJ, Stille C. Pneumonia. *Pediatr Rev.* 2008;29:147–160.
Lewis P, Glaser CA. Encephalitis. *Pediatr Rev.* 2005;26:353–363.
Powell KR. Orbital and periorbital cellulitis. *Pediatr Rev.* 1995;16:163–167.
Woodin KA, Morrison SH. Back to basics: antibiotics: mechanisms of action. *Pediatr Rev.* 1994;15:440–447.
Report of the Committee on Infectious Diseases. *Red Book. Passive Immunization.* 28th ed. 2009:55–61.
Report of the Committee on Infectious Diseases. *Red Book. Antimicrobial Prophylaxis.* 28th ed. 2009: 819–827.

CHAPTER 17 ■ NEONATOLOGY

SHAZIA BHOMBAL AND EVA GRANZOW

ABR	Auditory brainstem response
AFP	Alpha-fetoprotein
AGA	Average for gestational age
BIND	Bilirubin-induced neurologic dysfunction
BP	Blood pressure
bpm	Beats per minute
CAH	Congenital adrenal hypoplasia
CBC	Complete blood count
CCAM	Congenital cystic adenomatoid malformation
CNS	Central nervous system
CPAP	Continuous positive airway pressure
CRP	C reactive protein
CSF	Cerebrospinal fluid
CT	Computed tomography
CVS	Chorionic villus sampling
CXR	Chest x-ray
CMV	Cytomegalovirus
DIC	Disseminated intravascular coagulation
DR	Delivery room
ECF	Extracellular fluid
ECMO	Extracorporeal membrane oxygenation
EDD	Expected date of delivery
ex	prior
GA	Gestational age
GBS	Group B *Streptococcus*
HCG	Human chorionic gonadotropin
HDN	Hemorrhagic disease of the newborn
HIE	Hypoxic-ischemic encephalopathy
HR	Heart rate
HSV	Herpes simplex virus
HTN	Hypertension
IDM	Insulin-dependent diabetes mellitus
IM	Intramuscular
IUGR	Intrauterine growth restriction
IVH	Intraventricular hemorrhage
LGA	Large for gestational age
LMP	Last menstrual period
MAS	Meconium aspiration syndrome
MEN2	Multiple endocrine neoplasia type 2
NEC	Necrotizing enterocolitis
NICU	Neonatal intensive care unit
NSVD	Normal spontaneous vaginal delivery
PDA	Patent ductus arteriosus
PG	Phosphatidylglycerol
PKU	Phenylketonuria
PTU	Propylthiouracil
RBC	Red blood cell
RDS	Respiratory distress syndrome
ROP	Retinopathy of prematurity
RSV	Respiratory syncytial virus
SGA	Small for gestational age (<10th percentile)
SIDS	Sudden infant death syndrome
SLE	Systemic lupus erythematosus
TBW	Total body water
TEF	Tracheoesophageal fistula
TSH	Thyroid stimulating hormone
TTN	Transient tachypnea of the newborn
TTTS	Twin-to-twin transfusion syndrome
VP	Ventriculoperitoneal
VZIG	Varicella-zoster immune globulin

CHAPTER OBJECTIVES

1. To learn methods for evaluation of the fetus as well as DR management
2. To be familiar with normal newborn management and recognize normal physical examination findings
3. To be aware of the fetal implications of maternal conditions, such as lupus and HTN
4. To be familiar with neonatal congenital anomalies and recognize signs and symptoms relating to the diseases/malformations
5. To be aware of the causes of neonatal sepsis and properly evaluate and treat the various disease processes.

TABLE 17.1

PERINATAL LAB PATTERNS

Downs Syndrome	Trisomy 18, Turners	Neural Tube, Abdominal Wall Defects
AFP decreased (↓)	decreased (↓)	increased (↑)
HCG increased (↑)	decreased (↓)	normal
Estriol (uE3) decreased (↓)	decreased (↓)	normal
Inhibin A increased (↑)	normal (trisomy 18)	

Smith-Lemli-Opitz—very low uE3, slightly low AFP/HCG.
AFP, alpha-fetoprotein; HCG, human chorionic gonadotropin.

PERINATAL ASSESSMENT

There are many tools to evaluate the status of the fetus, as well as identifying a pregnancy with an increased chance of diagnosable fetal disorder. Many of these methods are noninvasive to the fetus, such as ultrasound or testing maternal serum for the quadruple screen. However, some are invasive, such as amniocentesis or percutaneous umbilical blood sampling and can provide necessary information about the fetal status.

Noninvasive Prenatal Testing

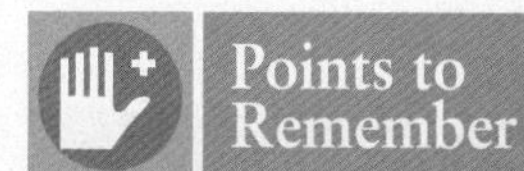

■ Quadruple screen does not detect closed spina bifida.

The Quadruple Screen is done in the second trimester (ideally between 15 to 18 weeks gestation); it tests AFP, HCG, inhibin A, and unconjugated estriol (uE3) levels. These data are interpreted as follows (see Table 17.1).

Prenatal Ultrasound

Used to determine EDD as these results are typically more accurate than LMP or physical examination, even when menstrual dates are certain. Interpretation in cases of date discrepancy is as follows:

- First trimester ultrasound: use LMP dates unless ultrasound EDD is more than 7 days off.
- Second trimester ultrasound: change EDD to ultrasound estimate if dates differ by more than 2 weeks. If dates are changed, a follow-up ultrasound in 2 weeks is indicated to confirm whether the dating is correct.
- Third trimester ultrasound: a 3-week discrepancy between LMP dates and ultrasound dates is accepted.
- Prenatal ultrasound is also used along with the triple/quadruple screen to detect congenital anomalies. Optimal timing for this screening is between 16 and 20 weeks gestation.

Amniocentesis

Has multiple indications, including assessment of fetal lung maturity (ideal sampling after 32 weeks), obtaining samples for prenatal genetic studies, and as a therapeutic measure to remove excess amniotic fluid.

- It is technically possible to perform after 11 weeks GA. For prenatal diagnoses is performed between 15 and 17 weeks GA, with results available in 7 days.
- This procedure is performed transabdominally under ultrasound guidance. The complication rate is less than 1 in 1,000 and includes direct/indirect fetal injury, membrane rupture, infection, and fetal loss.

Chorionic Villus Sampling

Involves obtaining a small sample of placenta for chromosomal or DNA analysis. This procedure can be performed transcervically or transabdominally.

- As it can be performed after 10 weeks of GA, this is the earliest detection option available for diagnosis of fetal anomalies. Note: knowledge of the chorionicity of multiple gestations is essential prior to CVS, as this gives information on the number of samples to be taken.
- Results of DNA analysis can be available within hours or days of testing.

Percutaneous Umbilical Blood Sampling (Cordocentesis)

Technique used to sample blood from near umbilical cord insertion into the placenta.

- The sample is at risk for contamination with maternal blood and usually amniocentesis, which is safer, can provide the same diagnostic results.
- If used, fetal blood sampling is most useful for rapid karyotype analysis in the second and third trimesters and for diagnosis of fetal hyper/hypothyroidism and thrombocytopenia.

FETAL ASSESSMENT

The *Nonstress Test*

Points to Remember

- **Less than 32 weeks gestation—two accelerations of at least 10 bpm, lasting for 10 seconds or more, over a 20-minute interval is reassuring for fetal wellbeing.**

The *Nonstress Test* is the most common technique used to evaluate the fetus during the antepartum period.

- This test can be performed when fetal neurological maturation allows for accelerations in the fetal HR, typically between 26 and 28 weeks, and is most commonly used to screen for fetal hypoxemia in high-risk pregnancies. Results are valid only for the actual time of testing; a reassuring pattern indicates that there is no fetal hypoxemia.
- Interpretation is as follows:
  - Reactive Test (if >32 weeks gestation): presence of two or more fetal HR accelerations of 15 bpm above baseline rate, lasting for 15 seconds, over a 20-minute period. A reactive test is reassuring for fetal well being.

Points to Remember

- **Obstetricians may warn you of these decelerations on rhythm strips during labor:**
  - **Early decelerations: due to head compression, not concerning**
  - **Variable decelerations: Most common, due to cord compression, may be concerning**
  - **Late decelerations: Uteroplacental insufficiency, concerning!!**

The *Contraction Stress Test*

The *Contraction Stress Test* is performed using an infusion of oxytocin and a fetal HR tracing is observed until three contractions occur in 5 to 10 minutes.

- Nonreassuring test (positive test): late fetal HR decelerations following 50% or more of contractions.
- Reassuring test (negative test): no late or significant variable decelerations.

Biophysical Profile

- An assessment tool based on five parameters, each of which is scored from 0 to 2 points (akin to APGARS).
- If these five parameters are present, it is unlikely that there is fetal CNS hypoxemia or acidosis at the time of testing (Table 17.2).

Assessment of Fetal Lung Maturity

The fetal lung is one of the last organ systems to fully mature; therefore, determination of lung maturity is important when deciding on iatrogenic preterm delivery.

The most common time to perform testing is after 32 weeks in pregnancies complicated by preterm labor where accurate dates are not available.

TABLE 17.2

BIOPHYSICAL PROFILE COMPONENTS AND SCORING

Parameter	Points
Fetal movement	Two points if two discrete body parts move within 30 minutes of observation
Fetal tone	Two points if extension and return to flexion of spine or extremity
Fetal breathing	Two points if rhythmic breathing for more than 20 seconds within 30 minutes
Amniotic fluid volume	Two points if adequate (at least >1 cm in two perpendicular planes) (e.g., amniotic fluid index more than 5 cm)
Nonstress test	Two points if reactive

Score <8 is concerning.

TABLE 17.3

APGAR SCORE

	0	1	2
Skin color	Blue all over	Acrocyanosis	Pink all over
Heart rate	Absent	>60	>100
Reflex irritability	No response to stimulation	Grimace, feeble cry	Sneeze, cough, pulls away
Muscle tone	None	Some flexion	Active movement
Breathing	Absent	Weak or irregular	Strong

Scores <6 are indication of neonatal distress.

The following tests are those most commonly used:

- *Lecithin to sphingomyelin ratio (L:S)*: These two pulmonary substances can be found in the amniotic fluid. Until 32 to 33 weeks, the concentrations of lecithin and sphingomyelin remain the same, but after this time production of lecithin increases more than that of sphingomyelin.
- *PG* is a minor component of surfactant and increases in amniotic fluid after the rise in lecithin. The advantage of this test is that it is not affected by contaminants such as blood or meconium.
  - A value of more than 3.0 of PG predicts minimal risk of RDS.

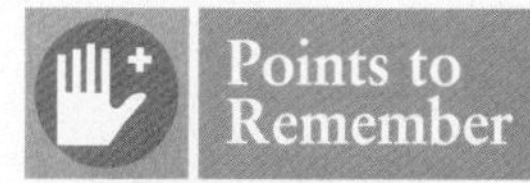

- **Risk for RDS is lowest when the L:S is 2.0 or more (reaches 2 around 35 weeks GA.)**

DELIVERY ROOM MANAGEMENT

The *Apgar* score evaluates a newborn's wellbeing on the basis of five criteria, each assigned a score of 0 to 2. The score typically is assigned at 1 and 5 minutes and gives an indication of fetal well-being as well as any response to resuscitation. The criteria are outlined in Table 17.3.

Traumatic Delivery

1. Forceps Delivery

Possible Complications

- Facial marks, bruising, lacerations, hematomas, facial nerve injury, skull fractures, intracranial bleeding, subgaleal hematomas.

2. Vacuum Delivery

Possible Complications

- Bruising, lacerations, hematomas, skull fractures, intracranial bleeding, subgaleal hematomas. Risks are somewhat lower than that with forceps delivery.

Brachial Plexus Injuries

- Erb-Duchenne palsy (most common)—injury to C5–7 resulting in an arm rotated internally, extended at the elbow, and flexed at the fingers—"waiter's tip".
- Klumpke palsy—injury to C7-T1 resulting in wrist and fingers extended, digits neutral—"claw hand"
  - Involvement of T1 can result in Horner syndrome (ptosis, meiosis, and anhydrosis).

MATURATIONAL ASSESSMENT

This section will discuss intrauterine growth and multiple gestation and their potential complications.

Weight

AGA—between 10th to 90th percentile
LGA—above 90th percentile
SGA—below 10th percentile
IUGR

- Deviation and reduction in expected fetal growth pattern.
- Occurs in 5% to 8% of all pregnancies.
- Associated with higher perinatal morbidity and mortality rates.
- Please see Table 17.4 for comparison between symmetric and asymmetric IUGR.

TABLE 17.4

SYMMETRIC VS. ASYMMETRIC IUGR/ SMALL FOR GESTATIONAL AGE (<10%)

Symmetric	Asymmetric
Early onset prior to third trimester	Late onset in third trimester
Catch up growth longer than 6 months	Catch up growth usually by 6 months
Head circumference proportional to body	Head circumference% > weight%
Etiology: Usually intrinsic—chromosomal abnormalities, congenital infection, maternal drugs, inborn errors of metabolism	Etiology: Usually extrinsic—for example, due to uteroplacental insufficiency—maternal vascular disease, often due to preeclampsia, chronic hypertension, or severe diabetes

IUGR, intrauterine growth restriction.

Gestational Age

Preterm—less than 37 weeks
Term—37 to 41 weeks
Postterm—more than 42 weeks

Multiple Gestation

Frequency = $80^{(n-1)}$, where n = number of fetuses (e.g., triplet frequency = $80^{(3-1)}$ = 1/6,400 (Table 17.5)

Dizygotic Twins (Two-Thirds of Twins)

Definition: Fertilization of two eggs, result of ovulation of multiple follicles, dichorionic (two placentas)

Epidemiology: Traditionally incidence varies geographically; rates are highest in West Africa and lowest in Southeast Asia; however, because of the increased use of fertility augmentation, there has been a notable rise in the overall rate of multiple gestations.

Monozygotic Twins (One-Third of Twins)

Definition: Genetically identical twins as a result of one fertilized egg splitting into two embryos within the first 2 weeks of development.

Epidemiology: Incidence of approximately 1:3.5/1,000 constant worldwide.

Twin-to-Twin Transfusion Syndrome (TTTS)

- Complication for approximately 5% to 15% of monochorionic-diamniotic twins.

TABLE 17.5

TYPES OF GESTATIONAL VARIANTS FOR MONOZYGOTIC TWINS

Type	Description
Dichorionic, diamniotic	Early division
Monochorionic, diamniotic	Division > 3 d after fertilization **Most common type (95%)** Increased risk of twin-twin transfusion
Monochorionic, monoamniotic	Division after amnion formed **Rarest type (<1%)** Greater risk of cord problems High mortality rate

- Caused by intertwin vascular anastomoses (usually artery-to-vein) in the monochorionic placentas.
- May be acute or chronic transfer of blood from one twin to the other.
- Donor twin complications
  - Anemia, oligohydramnios, decrease birth weight, growth restriction.
- Recipient twin complications
  - Polyhydramnios, polycythemia, cardiac hypertrophy, hydrops, increased birth weight.
- Prognosis if untreated is poor.
- Possible treatments include amniocentesis for polyhydramnios, laser ablation of vascular anastomoses, septostomy between the two amnions, selective reduction of donor twin.

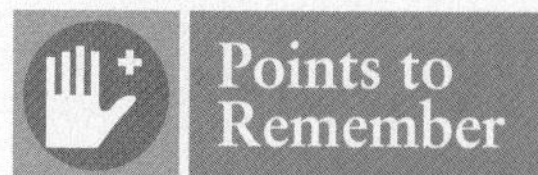

Points to Remember

- Conjoined twins occur from cleaving of embryonic plate 13 to 15 days after conception (1% monozygotic twins, more common in female twins).

ROUTINE CARE OF THE NEWBORN

For a majority of newborn infants, transition to extrauterine life occurs without significant intervention. However, as research continues to find ways to improve neonatal outcomes, various interventions have become norms. This section will discuss routine care of the newborn, as well as screening tests and normal physical examination findings.

Vitamin K

- Given at birth to prevent HDN.
- Protective during the first week after birth (classic/early HDN).
- IM use is preferred over PO administration because of variable compliance with oral vitamin K and potential inadequate absorption.
- Administer 1 mg IM × 1 to term neonates; 0.5 mg for infants weighing less than 1,000 g.

Note: see discussion at the end of the chapter.

Eye Prophylaxis

- Given within the first hour of life with 0.5% erythromycin, 1% silver nitrate, or 1% tetracycline ophthalmic preparations.
- Prevents ocular *Neisseria gonorrhoeae;* Reduces the incidence of Chlamydia trachomatis ophthalmia and pneumonia but does not prevent them (Table 17.6).

Newborn Feeding and Fluid Requirements

- A term newborn has a TBW content of 75% and an ECF fraction of 45%.
- Term infants usually lose 5% of their body weight in the first week of life.
- Preterm infants lose 10% to 15% of their body weight in the first week of life.
- Caloric requirements are approximately 120 to 150 kcal/kg/day for preterm neonates and 100 kcal/kg/day for term neonates.
- Weight gain is more than 15 g/kg/day for infants weighing less than 2 kg and more than 20 g/day for infants weighing more than 2 kg.

TABLE 17.6

CONJUNCTIVITIS

Type	Onset	Treatment
Chemical (i.e., silver nitrate)	First 24 h	None—resolution
Bacterial (i.e., Staph)	Commonly 24–48 h, can be anytime	Topical—erythromycin for Gram positive, gentamicin or tobramycin for Gram negative
Gonococcal	2–4 d of life	Topical erythromycin and systemic third-generation cephalosporin
Viral	4–5 d or later if HSV	Herpes—systemic acyclovir
Chlamydia	5–12 d of life	Oral erythromycin

HSV, herpes simplex virus.

Points to Remember

- In the United States, all 50 states and all territories perform universal screening for PKU and congenital hypothyroidism. Additional screening protocols vary widely among states/ territories.

Newborn Screen

- Detects endocrinopathies, hemoglobinopathies, infectious diseases, and inborn errors of metabolism.
- Identifies patients who need further testing, and abnormal results should be evaluated emergently.
- Asymptomatic siblings of an identified case should also be tested.
- The incidence of false negatives is increased in premature infants, infants who have received blood transfusions (obscures diagnosis of galactosemia), patients who have undergone dialysis, and patients tested at less than 24 hours of age (obscures diagnosis of PKU). Infants in these categories should have follow-up testing.

Points to Remember

- Any cord that persists beyond 3 weeks is considered delayed and infants should be evaluated for leukocyte adhesion defects and neutrophil function. Delayed separation can also represent an urachal abnormality.

Umbilical Cord Care

- Needs depend on the sanitary conditions at delivery and postnatally.
- Antiseptic cord care reduces the risk of omphalitis. The cord itself should separate by 1 to 2 weeks of life but may take longer if topical antiseptic treatments are used, as phagocytes mediate tissue breakdown and epithelialization of the stump.

Newborn Rashes

Please see Table 17.7 and Dermatology chapter for information on newborn rashes.

Newborn Reflexes

Please see Table 17.8 for information on newborn reflexes.

TABLE 17.7

NEWBORN RASHES

	Timing	Location	Appearance	Cell Types	Treatment
Erythema toxicum (Fig. 17.1)	Not present at birth, appear at 24–48 h of life. Resolves in 5–7 d. May wax and wane	Trunk and proximal extremities	Multiple erythematous macules and papules that progress to pustules	Eosinophils on Wright stain of pustule contents	None needed
Transient neonatal pustular melanosis	May be present at birth, lesions may exist in different stages at the same time	Variable	Lesions progress through three stages: (1) pustules on an erythematous base. (2) Erythematous macule with collarette of scale (3) hyperpigmented macule	Neutrophils on Wright stain	No treatment needed
Neonatal Acne (Fig. 17.2)	Onset at around 3 weeks of life. Males > females	Mostly on face and scalp (sebaceous glad stimulation by maternal androgens)	Papules, pustules and comedones		Usually resolves by 4 months of age, no treatment needed
Miliaria (Fig. 17.3)	Not usually present at birth, develops in the first week of life	Face, scalp, intertriginous areas	Thin-walled papules filled with white-colored keratin, formed over blocked sweat glands.		Usually resolve when infant is in a cooler environment, no treatment is needed

TABLE 17.8

COMMON NEWBORN REFLEXES

Reflex	Age
Moro reflex	Present in normal newborns and disappears by 3–6 months of age
Grasp reflexes (palmar and plantar)	Present in normal newborns and disappears by 3 months of age
Lower extremity crossed extension reflex	Present at birth and disappears by 1 month of age
Extensor plantar response	Variably present in normal newborns and disappears by 8–12 months of age
Placing reflex	Present at birth and disappears by 1–2 months of age
Stepping reflex	Present at birth and disappears by 1–2 months of age
Asymmetric tonic neck reflex	Variably present in normal newborns and disappears by 3–6 months of age

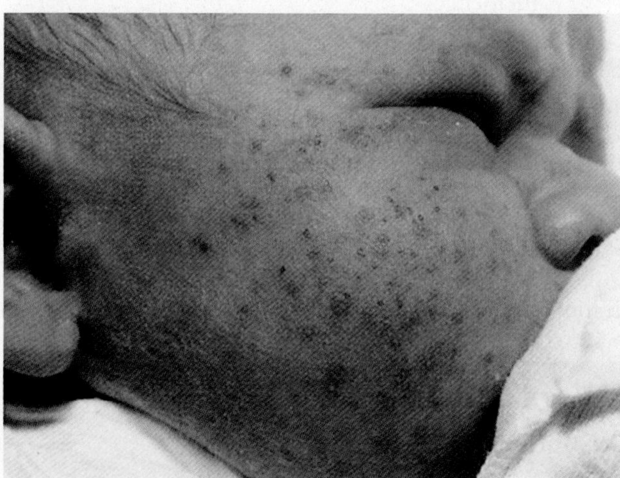

FIGURE 17.1. Erythema toxicum. These yellow or white pustules are surrounded by a red base and are commonly noted in normal newborns. (Reprinted with permission from Fletcher MA. *Physical Diagnosis in Neonatology*. Philadelphia, PA: Lippincott Williams & Wilkins, 1998.)

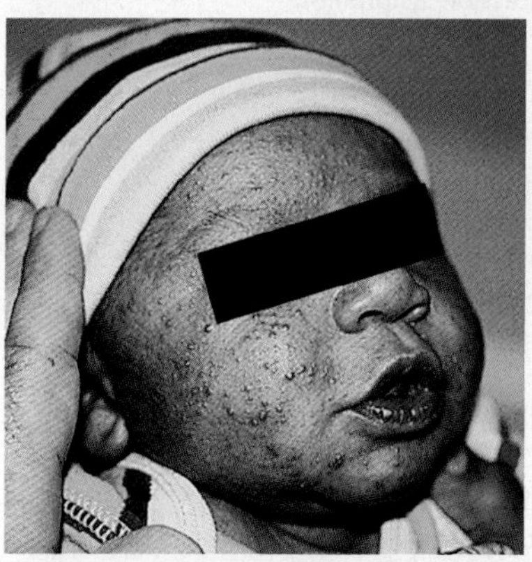

FIGURE 17.2. Neonatal acne. Erythematous pustular rash on cheeks of a 3-week-old neonate. (Courtesy of George A. Datto, III, MD.)

MATERNAL DISORDERS, MEDICATIONS, AND SUBSTANCE USE AFFECTING THE NEWBORN

Infant of a Diabetic Mother

Diabetes is a complicating factor in many pregnancies, with gestational diabetes comprising a larger number of patients than diabetes acquired prior to pregnancy. Infants of diabetic mothers have an increased rate of anomalies, as well as increased problems during pregnancy including a two-fold increase in preeclampsia.

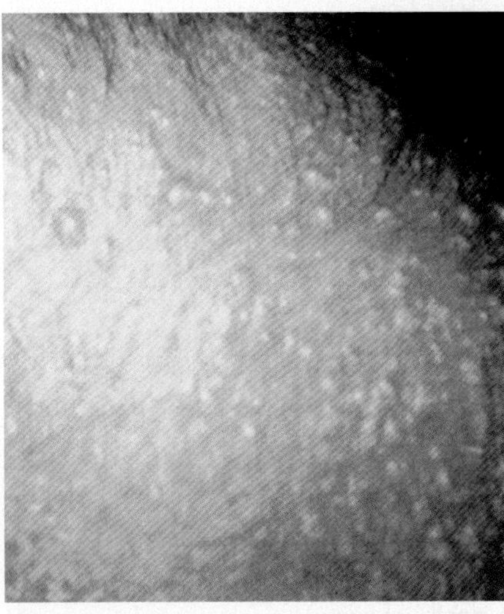

FIGURE 17.3. Miliaria crystallina alba. (Reprinted with permission from Fletcher MA. *Physical Diagnosis in Neonatology*. Philadelphia, PA: Lippincott Williams & Wilkins, 1998.)

Incidence

Gestational diabetes develops in approximately 2.5% of mothers. Most screening occurs between 24 and 28 weeks but can be done earlier if risk factors are identified (i.e., obese, history of abnormal glucose tolerance test, family history of diabetes).

- There is an increased risk of congenital malformations in infants of insulin-dependent diabetic mothers as the critical period for teratogenesis is within the first 3 to 6 weeks gestation; thus, prevention of complications depends on achieving good glycemic control prior to pregnancy.
- Premature births are more common due to increased incidence of preeclampsia (2 times) in mothers with diabetes.

Points to Remember

- The risk of having an infant with macrosomia increases when the maternal glucose level is greater than 130 mg/dL; however, an infant may be SGA if a mother has uteroplacental insufficiency due to severe vascular effects of diabetes.

See Table 17.9 for neonatal complications associated with maternal diabetes.

TABLE 17.9

NEONATAL COMPLICATIONS ASSOCIATED WITH GESTATIONAL AND INSULIN-DEPENDENT MATERNAL DIABETES

Neurological	Anencephaly, caudal regression syndrome, spina bifida
Respiratory	Respiratory distress syndrome—surfactant deficiency
Cardiac	Hypertrophic cardiomyopathy—present ~30% patients, usually resolves by 1 yr Congestive cardiomyopathy Incidence of congenital heart disease
Abdomen	Hypoplastic left colon
Metabolic	Hypoglycemia—due to hyperinsulinism, hypocalcemia
Hematology	Hyperbilirubinemia (due to polycythemia), polycythemia (fetal hypoxia stimulates fetal erythropoietin production)
Musculoskeletal	Shoulder dystocia (2–4 higher in IDM), brachial plexus trauma

IDM, insulin-dependent diabetes mellitus.

Maternal Systemic Lupus Erythematosus

Neonatal lupus erythematosus is a rare disorder acquired by only approximately 1% of infants who are positive for antibodies from maternal SLE. It is acquired by transfer of anti-Ro and anti-La antibodies across placenta.

TABLE 17.10

MANIFESTATIONS OF NEONATAL LUPUS ERYTHEMATOUS

System	Incidence	Clinical Findings	Treatment/Outcome
Cardiac	2% Infants with anti-Ro antibodies	Congenital heart block—usually third degree Occurs during 18–30 wk gestation Complete heart block can lead to hydrops fetalis	~24% mortality 50% of surviving infants require pacemaker
Skin	50% of affected infants	Usually annular erythematous scaling plaques on sun exposed areas in first 2 wk of life. (Fig. 17.4)	Spontaneously disappears by 6 months (once maternal antibodies are depleted) May use corticosteroids
Heme	~10%	Thrombocytopenia	Transient
Liver		Hepatitis	Resolve by 1 yr of age

Diagnosis

Pre/postnatal maternal screening or neonatal screening for anti-Ro(SSA)and anti-La(SSB) antibodies

- Usually presents within first 2 months of life.
- See Table 17.10 for manifestations of neonatal lupus.

Maternal Thyroid Disorder

Hypothyroidism occurs in approximately 0.2% to 3% of pregnancies.

- Endemic iodine deficiency is the most common cause worldwide; main cause in iodine-repleted countries is chronic autoimmune thyroiditis.
- Other causes: maternal Graves disease and excessive PTU therapy, Hashimoto thyroiditis, familial genetic defect in thyroxine synthesis, treatment with iodides or lithium, exposure to radioactive iodine during pregnancy.
- Three-fold risk of placental abruption and two-fold risk of premature delivery.

Hyperthyroidism occurs in approximately 0.2% of pregnancies.

- Graves disease is the cause in 85% of cases.
  - Graves disease—maternal IgG crosses placenta.
    - Newborn symptoms include irritability, tachycardia, HTN, poor weight gain, and exophthalmos.
    - Mortality rate may be 25% in severe disease.
    - Diagnosis may be delayed 8 to 9 days as maternal medication depletes in infant and conversion of T4 to active T3 occurs shortly after birth.
    - Usual clinical course is 3 to 12 weeks as maternal antibodies degrade.
    - Treatment includes PTU and propranolol.
  - Other causes include maternal thyroiditis, Hashimoto thyroiditis.

If concerned for hypo- or hyperthyroidism, check TSH, free T4, thyroid antibody at 2 to 7 days.

- If hypothyroid, treat with levothyroxine (Synthroid).
- If hyperthyroid, treat with PTU and propranolol.

Maternal Myasthenia Gravis

Neonatal myasthenia gravis manifests in neonates because of maternal antibody transfer and antiacetylcholine receptor antibodies.

Incidence/Clinical Presentation

Approximately 10% to 20% of infants of mothers with myasthenia gravis develop symptoms including respiratory distress, weak suck and cry, and generalized hypotonia.

- Usually presents approximately 12 to 48 hours after birth; persists for 3 weeks on average but can last up to 15 weeks.

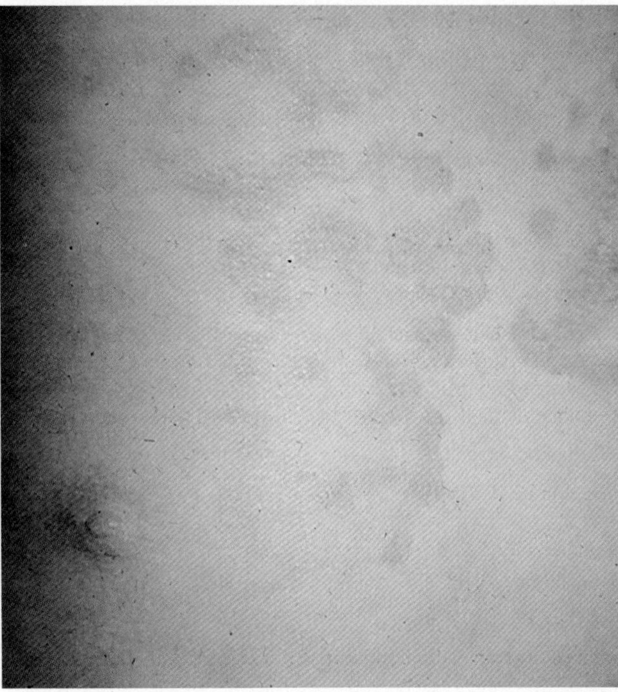

FIGURE 17.4. Neonatal lupus rash (Courtesy of the teaching files of Dr. Joan Hodgman and Dr. Lorayne Barton).

Suspect disease in infants of an affected mother; diagnosis is made by administration of a rapid-acting anticholinesterase inhibitor (edrophonium—Tensilon test).

Note: This test should only be done in a setting where resuscitation is available.

Treatment/Complications

Treat with anticholinesterases if severe; 90% of infants recover by 2 months of age. May lead to fetal arthrogryposis (rare)

Maternal Hypertension

Maternal HTN occurs in approximately 6% to 8% of pregnancies and can lead to a myriad of complications for the neonate and mother.

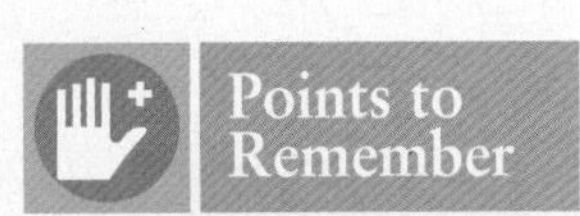

- If preeclampsia is severe, it can lead to HELLP syndrome (hemolysis, elevated liver enzymes, low platelets)

Diagnosis

Preeclampsia is defined as HTN documented more than twice and proteinuria.

- Diastolic BP above 90 mmHg or systolic BP above 140 mmHg after 20 weeks gestation in a woman who was normotensive prior to pregnancy.

Complications

Fetal risks include IUGR, possiblee premature delivery, thrombocytopenia, and neutropenia.

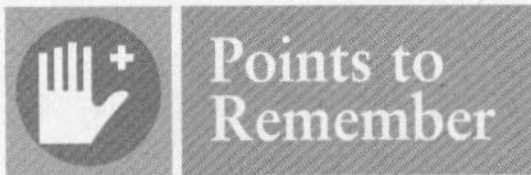

- Accelerated lung maturity can be seen in infants of mothers with HTN.

Advanced Maternal Age

Although there is no universal definition for advanced reproductive age in women, a commonly used number is >35 years of age.

- Advanced maternal age increases risk of miscarriage, chromosomal abnormalities, premature delivery, pregnancy-induced HTN, gestational diabetes, and maternal mortality.
- Increased risk of trisomy 21, 13, and 18.
- Trisomy 21 risk increases with age (Table 17.11).

TABLE 17.11

MATERNAL AGE AND TRISOMY RISK AT TIME OF EXPECTED LIVE BIRTH

Age	Risk of Down Syndrome	Total Risk for Chromosomal Abnormalities
20	1/1,667	1/526
25	1/1,250	1/476
30	1/952	1/385
35	1/385	1/202
40	1/106	1/65
49	1/11	1/7

Reprinted with permission from McMillan JA, DeAngelis C, Feigin RD, et al. *Oski's Pediatrics: Principles and Practice.* 3rd ed. Philadelphia, PA: Lippincott Williams & Wilkins, 1999.

Neonatal Withdrawal Syndrome

Affects 16% to 90% of infants whose mothers use opiates (heroin or methadone); symptoms usually appear within 48 hours of birth.

Clinical Presentation

Neonatal abstinence syndrome is characterized by a constellation of signs and symptoms including the following:

- Neurologic excitability (jitteriness, irritability, increased tone/moro reflex, seizures).
- Gastrointestinal manifestations (diarrhea, difficulty feeding, poor weight gain, poor suck).
- Autonomic instability (fever, sweating, mottling, temperature control).

Treatment

Medical treatment mainstay for opiate withdrawal is opiates—e.g., methadone and morphine for controlled and graduated weaning.

Please see Table 17.12 for complications associated with maternal medication/drug use.

TABLE 17.12

MATERNAL MEDICATIONS/DRUG USE

ACE inhibitor	Greatest risk in third trimester (category D in second and third trimesters), risks include renal tubular dysplasia
Alcohol	Most common teratogenic exposure to fetus; earlier exposure worsens outcome Fetal alcohol syndrome: Long, smooth philtrum, thin upper lip, short palpebral fissures, lower IQ, hyperactivity, cardiac anomalies (septal defects, PDA)
Amphetamines	Prematurity, IUGR
Carbamazepine	Neural tube defects
Cigarette smoking	IUGR/SGA, SIDS, spontaneous abortion
Cocaine	Placental abruption, premature delivery
Phenytoin	Digit and nail hypoplasia IUGR
Retinoic acid	Hydrocephalus, cardiac defects, microtia (pregnancy category D) (isotretinoin)
Lithium	Ebstein anomaly—displacement of tricuspid valve into body of right ventricle
Salicylates	Risk of fetal closure of PDA, bleeding; note- low doses are used to treat some medical conditions without fetal harm
Tetracycline	Yellow-brown discoloration of teeth
Valproic acid	Neural tube defects (1% infants exposed in first trimester category D)

ACE, angiotensin converting enzyme; IUGR, intrauterine growth restriction; PDA, patent ductus arteriosus; SGA, small for gestational age ($<10^{th}$ percentile); SIDS, sudden infant death syndrome.

RESPIRATORY DISORDERS

Respiratory distress is a common presentation of disease in the newborn infant. Physical signs include tachypnea (>60 breaths per minute), retractions, cyanosis, nasal flaring, and grunting on expiration (indication of neonate attempting to autopeep to keep alveoli open). This section will explore the multiple causes of respiratory distress in the neonate.

Respiratory Distress Syndrome

RDS occurs because of insufficiency of pulmonary surfactant and is a major cause of morbidity and mortality in the premature infants. It usually occurs in premature infants (incidence of 60% at 29 weeks GA). Surfactant administration to at risk neonates decreases RDS by approximately 50%.

Epidemiology

- More common in males than in females.
- Predisposing factors include prematurity, perinatal asphyxia, maternal diabetes, maternal hemorrhage, C-section without labor.
- Protective factors include premature rupture of membranes, intrauterine growth retardation, maternal stress.

Diagnosis/Evaluation

Lecithin to sphingomyelin ratio of greater than 2 in amniotic fluid indicates fetal lungs likely mature; immature if the ratio is less than 1.5.

CXR: ground glass appearing lung fields, diffuse atelectasis, loss of lung volume (Fig. 17.5)

Clinical Presentation

Peak severity usually at 1 to 3 days—if uncomplicated, recovery can start after 48 hours.

Symptoms include grunting (closure of glottis—maintains lung volume and gas exchange during exhalation), tachypnea, retractions, and cyanosis.

Treatment/Prevention

Surfactant replacement after birth

Prevention: delivery at term or administration of prenatal glucocorticoids (usually betamethasone—two doses 24 hours apart with delivery 24 hours after last dose or dexamethasone—four doses, each 12 hours apart)

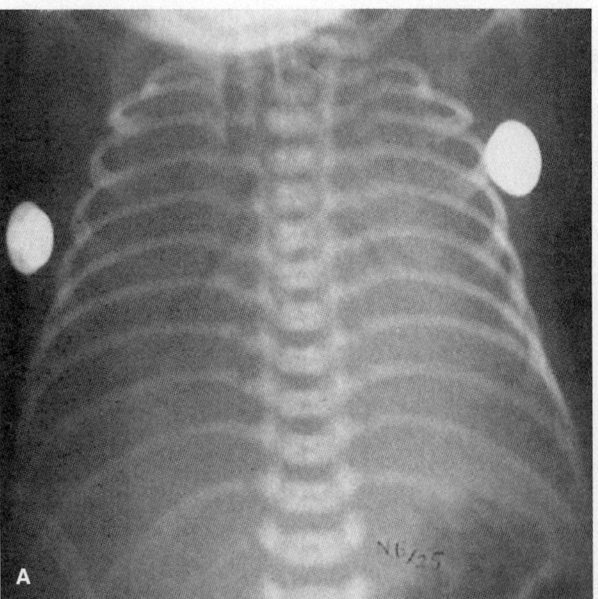

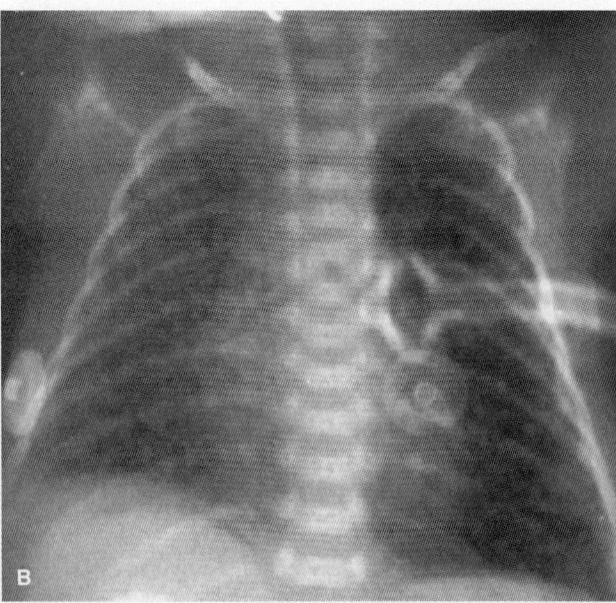

FIGURE 17.5. (A) This premature infant presented with grunting, retractions, and cyanosis after delivery. The diffuse reticular–granular opacification, air bronchograms, and decreased lung volumes in the chest radiograph film indicate respiratory distress syndrome. (B) Chest x-ray film of pulmonary interstitial emphysema (PIE). A premature infant with severe respiratory distress syndrome requiring mechanical ventilation developed worsening respiratory acidosis and hypoxia refractory to increased ventilatory support. An anteroposterior chest x-ray film demonstrates a salt-and-pepper pattern resulting from radiolucent interstitial air surrounding compressed lung tissue. A left chest tube was placed to treat pneumothorax, a common complication of pulmonary interstitial emphysema. (Reprinted with permission from MacDonald MG, Seshia MMK, Mullett MD, et al. *Avery's Neonatology: Pathophysiology & Management of the Newborn.* 6th ed. Philadelphia, PA: Lippincott Williams & Wilkins, 2005.)

Transient Tachypnea of the Newborn

TTN is a benign, self-limited condition, usually due to delayed clearance of fetal lung fluid. It is seen primarily in full-term infants, more commonly in those born by C-section without labor.

Risk Factors

C-section, maternal diabetes, maternal sedation, precipitous delivery, perinatal depression, delayed cord clamping

Clinical Presentation

Tachypnea, grunting, retractions, nasal flaring
CXR—Hyperaeration, fluid in the fissures, especially right middle fissure

Treatment

Supportive, CPAP/O_2
Usually resolves by 24 to 48 hours

Pneumonia

Pneumonia in the neonate can occur shortly after birth (early onset—first 2 to 3 days), or after the first week (late onset). The most common pathogens are GBS and Gram-negative rods such as *Escherichia coli* and *Klebsiella*

- Early onset (within first few days)—GBS, *E. coli*, *Klebsiella*, *Listeria*.
- Late onset (after first week)—as above, also *Staphylococcus aureus*, *Pseudomonas*, *Chlamydia*, fungi (especially *Candida*).
- Other—syphilis, viruses (CMV, herpes, RSV, enterovirus), ureaplasma, mycoplasma.

Clinical Presentation

Symptoms include signs of respiratory distress—grunting, tachypnea, nasal flaring, retractions
History of maternal chorioamnionitis, prolonged rupture of membranes, signs of shock, and poor perfusion in the neonate indicate that respiratory distress is more likely to be caused by pneumonia CXR can be similar to RDS initially, especially if caused by GBS.

Note: For further review of Pneumonia please see the Infectious Disease chapter

Meconium Aspiration Syndrome

Infants with MAS can present with mild symptoms of respiratory distress or can be extremely sick to the point of requiring ECMO.

Incidence

Meconium staining occurs in approximately 10% to 26% of all deliveries; however, almost all infants with meconium staining do not develop MAS.
Risk factors include postdates, sepsis.

Pathogenesis

Aspirated meconium produces mechanical obstruction that leads to atelectasis with hyperinflation.

- After approximately 24 to 48 hours, chemical pneumonitis develops—infiltration of alveolar septa by neutrophils, small airway obstruction—necrosis of alveolar and airway epithelia, accumulation of proteinaceous debris within the alveoli.
- A neonate with MAS is at risk for developing persistent pulmonary HTN, bacterial pneumonia, and pneumothorax.

Clinical Presentation

History of Meconium-stained amniotic fluid
Worsening respiratory distress, coarse rales
CXR: hyperinflation of lung with patchy infiltrates (Fig. 17.6)

Treatment

Tracheal suctioning at delivery if patient is not vigorous/crying; ventilator management, surfactant and antibiotic administration may be beneficial.

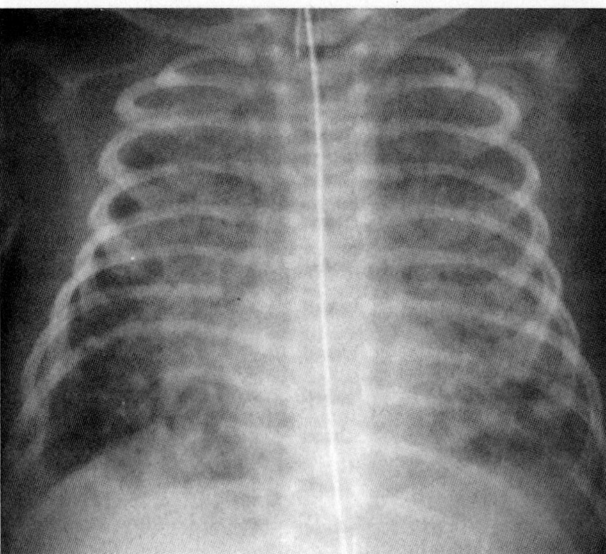

FIGURE 17.6. This full-term infant was born with fetal bradycardia and thick meconium in the amniotic fluid. Cyanosis and respiratory distress were evident within minutes of delivery. The chest radiograph film demonstrates coarse, irregular infiltrates, hyperinflation (left and right diaphragms at ribs 10 to 11) and right pleural effusion indicative of meconium aspiration syndrome. Endotracheal and nasogastric tubes are in position. (Reprinted with permission from MacDonald MG, Seshia MMK, Mullett MD, et al. *Avery's Neonatology: Pathophysiology & Management of the Newborn.* 6th ed. Philadelphia, PA: Lippincott Williams & Wilkins, 2005.)

Apnea

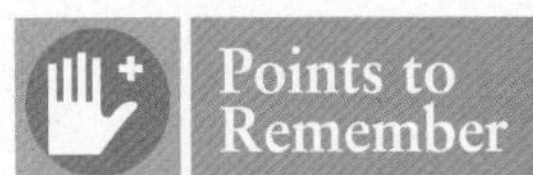

Points to Remember

- Apnea of Prematurity is the most common cause of apnea in the neonate

Definition

Apnea in the neonate is defined as the cessation of breathing for more than 20 seconds.

- *Primary apnea*: Post delivery, recover with O_2 and stimulation.
- *Secondary apnea*: Central (10% to 25%), obstructive (10% to 20%), mixed (50% to 70%).
  - Positive pressure ventilation needed for secondary apnea event.

Etiology

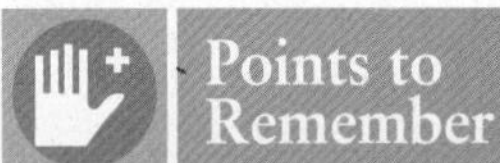

Points to Remember

- *Periodic breathing:* a normal manifestation of immature ventilatory control—regular cycles interrupted by pauses of 5 to 10 seconds.

- Prematurity (usually less than 35 weeks GA).
- Sepsis.
- Maternal medications (including magnesium, narcotics).
- Neonatal medication (including prostaglandins).
- Gastroesophageal reflux.
- CNS disorder (e.g., seizure, intracranial hemorrhage).

Treatment

Caffeine, aminophylline, CPAP, treating underlying etiology, intubation, and mechanical ventilation if needed.

Pneumothorax

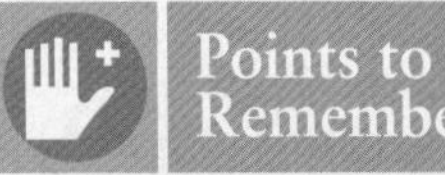

Points to Remember

- Tension pneumothorax (shift of cardiac apex, decreased breath sounds, asymmetric chest) requires urgent treatment—needle aspiration, chest tube.

Spontaneous pneumothorax occurs in 1% to 3% of all live births.

Clinical Presentation

Many neonates are asymptomatic, however, some present with signs of respiratory distress severe enough to require intubation. May have cardiovascular compromise if tension pneumothorax occurs.

Pneumothorax can be detected by transillumination of chest (part of chest with air leak may be more translucent than normal lung).

Sites of air leak: Pleural cavities (pneumothorax; Fig. 17.7), mediastinum (pneumomediastinum), lung interstitial tissue (interstitial emphysema), pericardial sac (pneumopericardium), and peritoneal cavity (pneumoperitoneum).

Treatment

Administration of 100% O_2 may be sufficient for resolution if minimal distress and no tension.

May require needle aspiration and/or chest tube placement if unstable or if pneumothorax large or under tension.

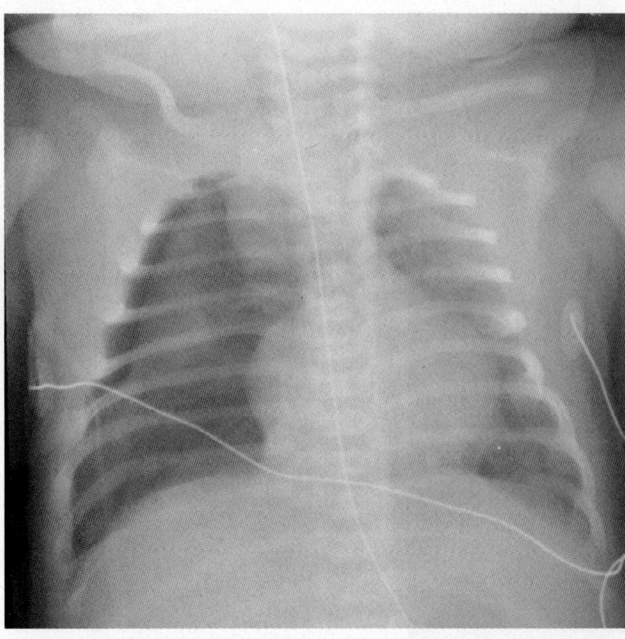

FIGURE 17.7. Right side pneumothorax (Courtesy of the teaching files of Dr. Joan Hodgman and Dr. Lorayne Barton).

Congenital Abnormalities of the Lung

- *Congenital lobar emphysema*—most common neonatal cystic lung malformation.
- *CCAM*—numerous cysts of lung tissue that communicates with tracheobronchial tree (Fig. 17.8).
- *Pulmonary hypoplasia*—Etiology: in utero compression (e.g., by congenital diaphragmatic hernia), neuromuscular disease.
- *Bronchogenic cyst*—cystic mass that may or may not communicate with airways.
- *Bronchopulmonary sequestration*—nonfunctioning lung tissue that receives blood supply from systemic vessels
  - Can present in childhood with history of recurrent pneumonias.
  - Associated with Potter syndrome.
- *Congenital diaphragmatic hernia* (Fig. 17.9)
  - *Incidence*: 1 in 3,000 live births, left-sided abnormal development of the diaphragm in 85% to 90% of cases.
  - *Mortality*: 40% to 62%.

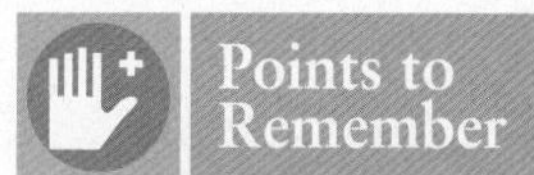

Points to Remember

- **Combination of scaphoid abdomen and respiratory distress—think CDH!**

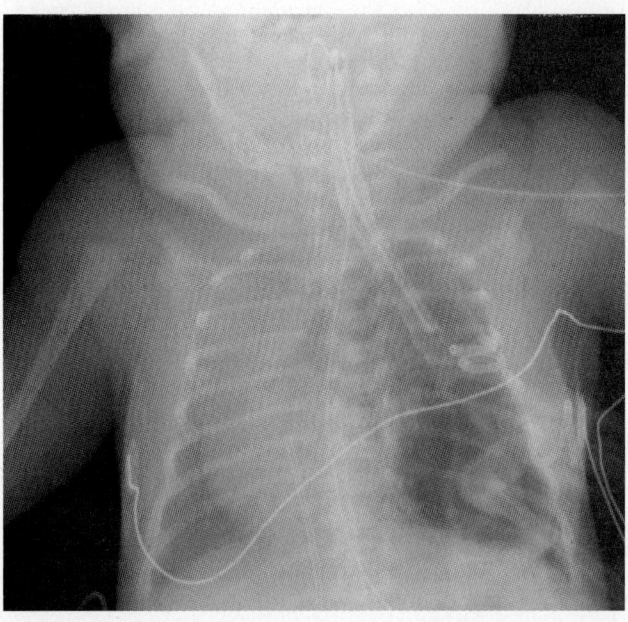

FIGURE 17.8. Left side congenital cystic adenomatoid malformation (Courtesy of the teaching files of Dr. Joan Hodgman and Dr. Lorayne Barton).

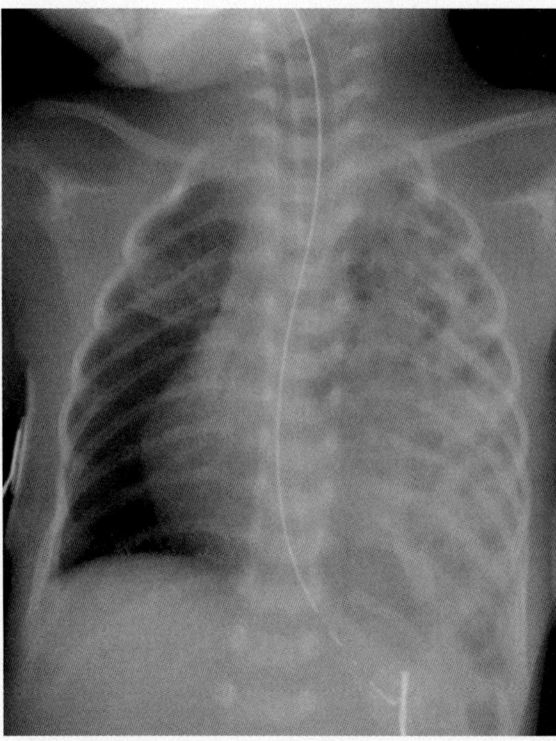

FIGURE 17.9. Congenital diaphragmatic hernia (Courtesy of the teaching files of Dr. Joan Hodgman and Dr. Lorayne Barton).

CARDIOLOGY

For full discussion please see the Cardiology chapter.

Transitional Circulation

- Blood enters fetus from placenta through one umbilical vein -> ductus venosus -> inferior vena cava; leaves fetus from descending aorta -> internal iliac artery -> two umbilical arteries -> placenta.
- Studies have shown that neonatal pulmonary artery pressure falls significantly within approximately 2 weeks after delivery.

Patent Ductus Arteriosus

- Connects left pulmonary artery near origin to the descending aortic distal to the left subclavian artery (isthmus).
- Usually closes in first few days in full-term infants—patent in approximately 1 in 2,000 births (5% to 10% of all congenital heart disease).
- Initially, right-to-left shunting due to increased pulmonary vascular resistance.
  - As resistance decreases, left-to-right shunting develops.
    - Can result in pulmonary overcirculation and eventually to Eisenmenger syndrome.
- Increase in pulmonary vascular resistance and right heart failure.
- Increased incidence in premature infants.
- *Treatment*: Ibuprofen, indomethacin, surgical ligation.

Congenital Heart Disease

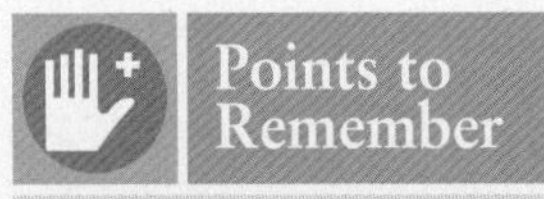

- **Think about hypoplastic left heart syndrome in infants 1 to 2 weeks of life that present to the ER in shock!!**

- Incidence of congenital heart disease is approximately 8 to 10 in 1,000.
- Life-threatening cardiac disease in newborns occurs in approximately 3 in 1,000 live births.
- Cyanotic heart disease—4 Ts
  - Transposition of great arteries.
  - Tetralogy of Fallot.
  - Tricuspid atresia.
  - Total anomalous pulmonary venous return.
  - Also consider coarctation once PDA closes
- For cyanotic heart disease, use prostaglandin to keep PDA open—beware of side effect of apnea and hypotension!

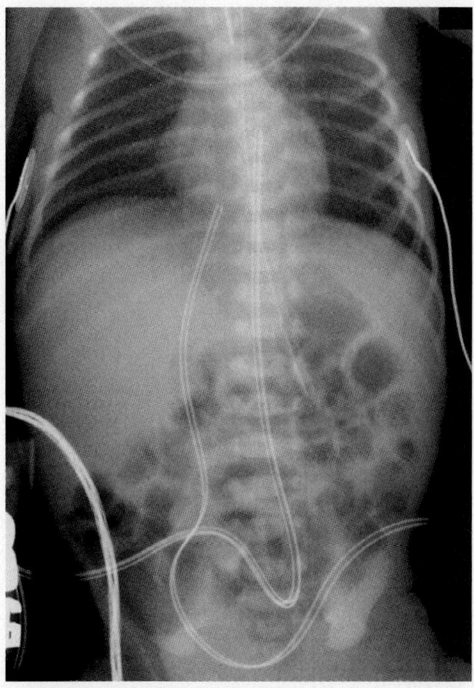

FIGURE 17.10. Umbilical lines.

- Hyperoxia test—Measure arterial PaO_2 on room air and 100% FiO_2—PaO_2 more than 150 mmHg on 100% FiO_2 indicates a decreased likelihood of congenital heart disease.

Arrhythmias

- HR less than 50 bpm most commonly associated with complete heart block and presence of anti-Ro or anti-La immune responses.
- HR 250 bpm most commonly associated with supraventricular tachycardia
  - Treatment of choice is adenosine.

Umbilical Lines

- Umbilical venous catheter—Placed for nutrition, medication administration (Fig. 17.10)
  - Location: Umbilical vein.
  - Duration of line usually 7 to 14 days.
    - Complications: thrombosis
- Umbilical arterial catheter—blood draws, BP assessment
  - Location: Umbilical artery -> hypogastric artery -> internal iliac artery -> descending aorta.
  - Placement acceptable between T6 and T10 or low-lying between L3-4.
  - Duration of line usually maximum 7 days.
    - Complications: thromboembolic complications in 1% to 9% (aortic or renal artery thrombosis).
- Consider thrombosis if infant develops HTN, intraventricular hemorrhage, NEC.

NEUROLOGICAL DISORDERS

Intraventricular Hemorrhage

Intracranial bleeding, which occurs in the periventricular germinal matrix, primarily in infants born before 32 weeks (germinal matrix begins to involute at 34 weeks) (Fig. 17.11).

Incidence

Occurs in approximately 15% to 30% of infants weighing less than 1,500 g

Post hemorrhagic hydrocephalus is a known consequence, as is poor myelination, brain growth, and abnormal cortical development.

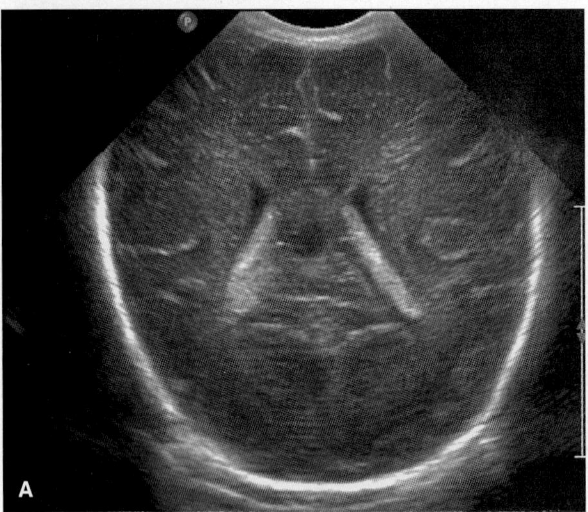

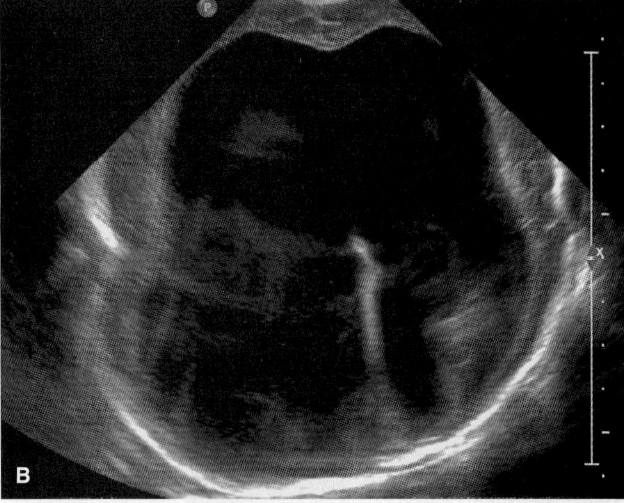

FIGURE 17.11. (A) Grade I intraventricular hemorrhage. (B) Grade IV intraventricular hemorrhage.

Treatment

Supportive, including maintaining stable BP and treating seizures.
Please see Table 17.13 for IVH grading.
Neonatal seizures can have multiple causes—please see Table 17.14 for details.

Hypoxic-Ischemic Encephalopathy

Usually occurs in infants born at or near term. Incidence is approximately 6 in 1,000 live births at term. The initial hypoxic injury results in anaerobic glycolysis in the tissue of the heart, brain, and muscles.

Prepartum risks: IUGR severe preeclampsia, postdates pregnancy, placental abnormalities, and maternal thyroid disease.

Intrapartum risks: persistent posterior position of the occiput, maternal fever, emergency cesarean section, operative vaginal delivery, and placental abruption or uterine rupture.

- The severity of HIE correlates with the length and degree of asphyxia.
- Constellation of symptoms develops over the first 72 hours of life.

Clinical Presentation

Infants demonstrate abnormal tone, abnormal reflexes, altered level of consciousness, apnea, and seizures.

Treatment and Prognosis

Supportive, studies demonstrate that head/body cooling improves outcomes, especially if initiated less than 6 hours after delivery (however, has not been demonstrated to help infants with severe encephalopathy).

TABLE 17.13

INTRAVENTRICULAR HEMORRHAGE GRADE AND IMAGING FINDINGS

Grade	Findings
Grade I	Germinal matrix hemorrhage only
Grade II	Intraventricular hemorrhage without ventricular dilation
Grade III	Intraventricular hemorrhage with ventricular dilation
Grade IV	Germinal matrix hemorrhage or intraventricular hemorrhage with parenchymal involvement

TABLE 17.14

NEONATAL SEIZURES—1% TO 20% OF NEWBORNS

Cause	Onset and Description
Perinatal asphyxia	First 24 h of life
Neonatal stroke	1:4,000 term births; usually term or late preterm infants; left MCA most common; 25%–40% have seizures (generally focal); risk factors include cyanotic heart disease (embolism), meningitis, DIC, polycythemia, severe fetomaternal hemorrhage
Subarachnoid hemorrhage	Second day of life. Infants are well between seizures
IVH	Premature infants <34 wk, usually within first 72 h of life and are usually subtle, decerebrate seizures
Subdural hemorrhage	After injury/trauma. Focal seizures
Metabolic disturbance	May be early if due to hypocalcemia in a premature infant can be anytime electrolytes are abnormal
Infections	GBS meningitis, HSV encephalitis
Drug withdrawal	Opiates: onset 48–72 h after birth Barbiturates: first 24 h, up to 14 d of age

DIC, disseminated intravascular coagulation; GBS, group B *Streptococcus*; HSV, herpes simplex virus; IVH, intraventricular hemorrhage; MCA, middle cerebral artery.

Neural Tube Defects

- Malformations of the brain and spinal cord.
- Lesions differ depending on when and where the neural tube closure was disrupted.

Anencephaly: *Incidence 1 in 1,000*, defective closure of the upper anterior neural tube. The brain and the calvarium are absent above the orbits. The tissue that remains is generally destroyed by exposure to the intrauterine environment. Polyhydramnios is often present; approximately 15% stillborn, the rest die shortly after birth (Fig. 17.12).

Encephalocele: *Incidence 1 in 5,000*, more commonly associated with other birth defects or occurs as part of genetic syndrome; usually closed, usually occipital herniation of brain and/or meninges through a skull defect.

Myelomeningocele (most common form of spina bifida): *Incidence 1 in 2,000 live births*, failure of the posterior neural tube to close. There are malformations of the brain and spinal cord, usually associated with Chiari II malformations and hydrocephalus (in 75%).

Spina bifida occulta: *Incidence approximately 15% of general population*; vertebral defects herniation of contents of spinal canal, most commonly lumbosacral region.

Holoprosencephaly: *Incidence 1 in 13,000*; cerebral hemispheres are a single, sphered structure with large central ventricle; majority die shortly after birth

Points to Remember

- Folic acid supplementation of 0.4 mg/day (or up to 3 mg/day if there is a family history of neural tube defects), prior to conception and during early gestation, can decrease the incidence of neural tube defects by 70%.

Points to Remember

- Spina bifida: a protrusion of an uncovered neural plate. 80% are in the lumbar area.

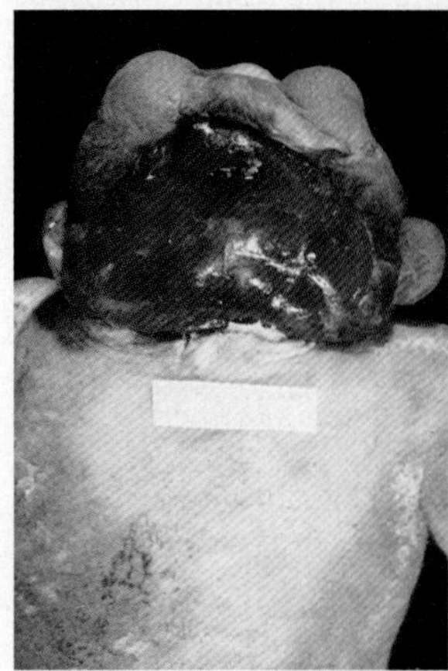

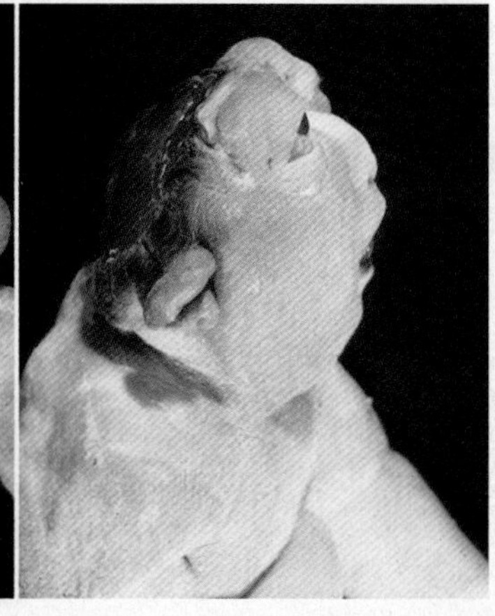

FIGURE 17.12. Anencephaly is the most severe neural tube defect. (Reprinted with permission from McConnell TH. *The Nature of Disease Pathology for the Health Professions*. Philadelphia, PA: Lippincott Williams & Wilkins, 2007.)

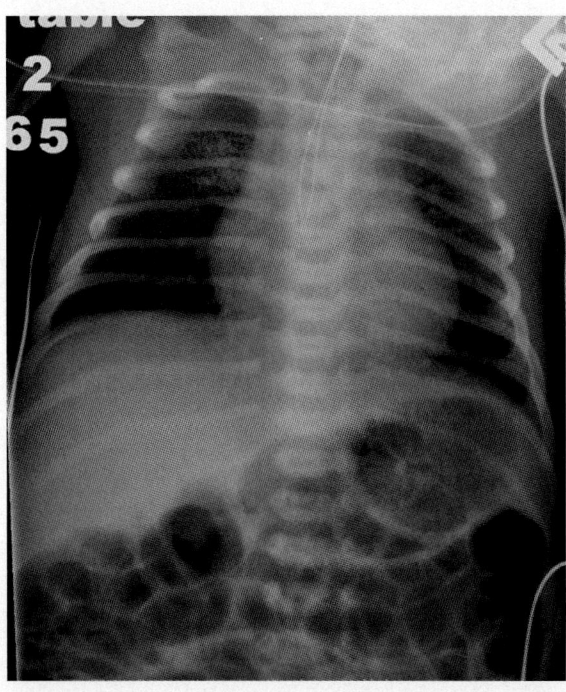

FIGURE 17.13. Transesophageal fistula.

GASTROINTESTINAL DISORDERS

Tracheoesophageal Fistula

TEF occurs in approximately 1:3,500 live births and is caused by failed separation of the foregut to form into the trachea and esophagus. It can be associated with VACTERL syndrome (vertebral anomalies, anorectal malformations, cardiac defects, TEF, renal or radial anomalies, and limb malformations) (Fig. 17.13).

Clinical Presentation

Usually present at birth with respiratory distress, considerable amount of oral secretions, and aspiration. Failure to pass an orogastric/nasogastric tube into stomach is diagnostic. Gas in the abdomen indicates presence of a TEF.

Treatment

Primary anastomosis if possible, with ligation of fistula if present. If gap is too large, surgery may be delayed and/or undergo colonic interposition can be performed.

- Please see Table 17.15 for further information on TEF.

Points to Remember

- Esophageal atresia is the most common esophageal malformation—1 in 2,000 to 5,000 live births

Intestinal Obstruction

Duodenal atresia is more common than more distal atresias and is thought to have different etiology than jejunal or ileal atresia. Jejunal and ileal atresia are thought to be the result of ischemic events in utero (i.e., volvulus, internal hernias), whereas duodenal atresia is likely caused by abnormal recanalization of the intestinal lumen. Can be associated with polyhydramnios in utero.

TABLE 17.15

MOST COMMON AND LEAST COMMON TYPES OF TRACHEOESOPHAGEAL FISTULA

Type	Frequency	Location	Symptoms	Treatment
A-type	85% of cases	Proximal esophageal pouch with distal TEF	Immediately symptomatic: drooling, respiratory distress, unable to feed	Surgical
H-Type	0.5% of cases	No esophageal atresia	Small defects may present late, with frequent pneumonia due to aspiration	Surgical

TEF, tracheoesophageal fistula.

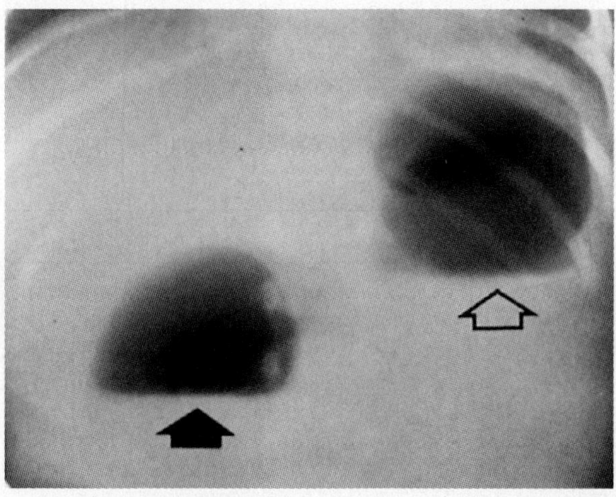

FIGURE 17.14. Duodenal atresia with double-bubble sign. The left bubble (*open arrow*) represents air in the stomach; the right bubble (*solid arrow*) reflects duodenal gas. There is no gas in the small or large bowel distal to the level of the complete obstruction. (Reprinted with permission from Eisenberg RL. *An Atlas of Differential Diagnosis*. 4th ed. Philadelphia, PA: Lippincott Williams & Wilkins, 2003.)

Incidence

Duodenal atresia incidence approximately 0.5 to 1 in 10,000; distal atresias (i.e., jejunal and ileal) 1 in 20,000 live births. Duodenal atresia may be associated with Down syndrome, congenital heart disease, TEF, malrotation, and renal anomalies.

Clinical Presentation

Usually present in neonatal period with bilious emesis, abdominal distention.

Diagnosis

Usually seen on abdominal x-ray as multiple dilated loops of bowel with air fluid levels (Fig. 17.14). Contrast enema can be diagnostic and often therapeutic if the obstruction is moveable.

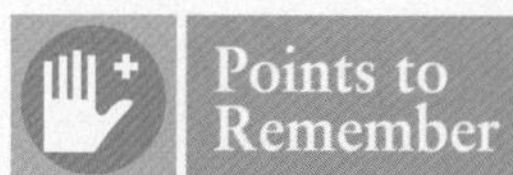

- **Duodenal atresia is classically associated with the "double-bubble" sign on abdominal x-ray.**

Treatment

Supportive: NG tube to suction and IV fluids and nutrition. Surgical repair/management.

Malrotation and Volvulus

Arrest of the normal embryonic rotation of the developing gut. Most common developmental abnormality of the intestine. Malrotation on its own may not be symptomatic, but the resulting volvulus of the mesentery can cause ischemia and is a MEDICAL EMERGENCY!!

Clinical Presentation

Can occur at any age, but usually present in early infancy with bilious vomiting (90% of infants with volvulus), abdominal distension, pain, passage of blood via rectum. May have less severe symptoms if volvulus is intermittent including episodic vomiting, failure to thrive, and anorexia.

Diagnosis

Upper GI tract with small bowel follow through is diagnostic. Malrotation appears as an abnormal position of the ligament of Treitz (usually left side of abdomen) and proximal jejunum on right of abdomen. Volvulus is demonstrated by "corkscrew" appearance of the distal duodenum.

Treatment

Surgical, including Ladd's procedure wherein abnormally fixed duodenum, jejunum, and colon are freed.

Meconium Ileus

Meconium ileus may be separated into two types, uncomplicated and complicated. Uncomplicated is defined as obstruction of the distal ileum with meconium pellets; compromise of intestinal viability defines complicated meconium ileus.

Incidence

10%–15% of infants with cystic fibrosis present with meconium ileus. At least one-third to one-half of cases were complicated by volvulus, atresia, pseudocyst, or meconium peritonitis.

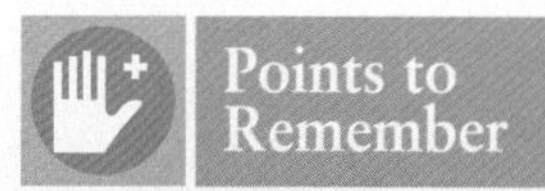

- **Majority of neonates with meconium ileus have cystic fibrosis.**

Clinical Presentation

Abdominal distention, emesis, no passage of meconium; "doughy abdomen"—firm movable, palpable masses in abdomen. Radiologic examination demonstrates dilated loops of bowel, calcification indicative of meconium peritonitis. Contrast enema demonstrates proximal bowel dilation and microcolon.

Treatment

Sixty percentage improve with diagnostic gastrografin (used because it is hypertonic, water-soluble) enema; otherwise surgical intervention is required.

Hirschsprung Disease

Motor disorder of the gut due to failed migration of neural crest cells. The affected bowel fails to relax and the functional obstruction is visible on contrast enema as a dilated proximal colon, which then narrows into a distal small caliber lumen.

Incidence, Types and Treatment

1 in 5,000, male to female ratio of 3.8:1. Hirschsprung disease is associated with trisomy 21, ventricular septal defects, congenital central hypoventilation syndrome, Waardenburg syndrome, MEN2, and Smith-Lemli-Opitz syndrome.

Clinical Presentation

Infants present with signs of distal obstruction (bilious emesis, failure to pass stool after first 48 hours of life). The gold standard diagnostic study is a rectal biopsy. Complication includes enterocolitis, caused by exposure of a dilated bowel to increased bacteria and toxins. Enterocolitis can be a significant cause of morbidity and mortality with foul-smelling bloody diarrhea, abdominal distention, and systemic illness.

Treatment

Surgical intervention with colostomy, myotomy, and/or pull-through.

Imperforate Anus

Occurs because of abnormal division of the cloaca into urogenital and rectal portions. Describes the lack of an anal opening of proper location or size, usually with a fistula from the distal rectum to the perineum or urogenital tract.

Incidence, Types and Treatment

1 in 5000 live births, with approximately one-half associated with other anomalies (e.g., VACTERL) Two types:

- High imperforate anus: the rectum ends above the puborectalis sling. Treatment is surgical colostomy.
- Low imperforate anus: rectum has traversed the puborectalis sling, and there may be a perineal fistula. Treatment is surgical anaplasty or dilation.

Imaging

All infants with imperforate anus should receive radiographs of the lumbosacral spine and urinary tract to detect associated anomalies, also ultrasound or CT to identify level of lesion (important to determine surgical intervention).

Abdominal Wall Defects

Please see Table 17.16 for comparison of gastroschisis and omphalocele.

TABLE 17.16

ABDOMINAL WALL DEFECTS

Gastroschisis	Omphalocele
Deformation	Malformation
Full thickness abdominal wall defect	Anterior abdominal wall defect causing the abdominal contents to protrude into the umbilical cord base
Defect is due to a vascular accident, which alters abdominal wall development	**Usually covered** by a membrane
Not covered by a membrane	Incidence can be sporadic
Increased risk in children born of women <20 years old	Often associated with trisomy 13, trisomy 15, trisomy 16, trisomy 18, Beckwith-Wiedemann
Treatment: surgery	Treatment: surgery

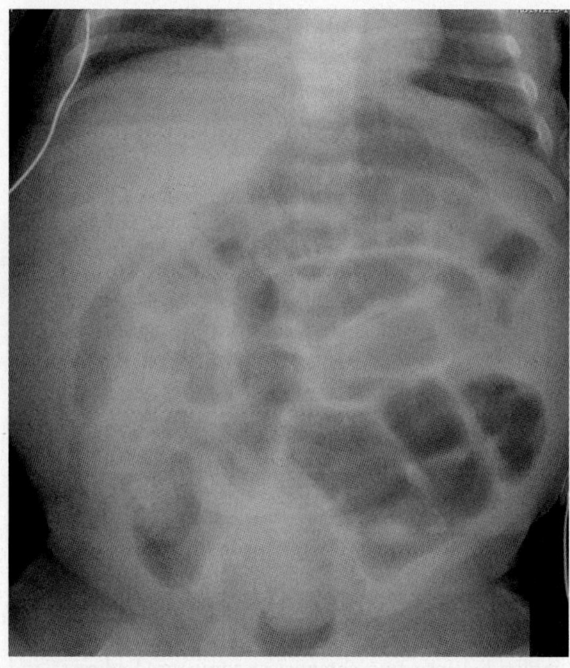

FIGURE 17.15. Pneumatosis.

Necrotizing Enterocolitis

NEC is the most common GI emergency of the newborn infant. The incidence decreases with increasing GA, and affected infants may be previously healthy, feeding, and growing.

Incidence

2.4 in 1,000 live births; 1% to 5% of all infants requiring NICU care; nearly 90% of cases occur in preterm infants.

Clinical Presentation

Initial signs can be nonspecific, including apnea, lethargy, poor feeding, and hypotension. Signs specific to the abdomen include abdominal distention, gastric retention, abdominal tenderness, vomiting, diarrhea, and bloody stools.

NEC is staged as follows:

Stage IA: "Suspected NEC." Nonspecific general and abdominal signs, may have mild ileus or distention on abdominal x-ray. May also have a normal x-ray.

Stage IIA: "Proven NEC." Includes the above signs and also absent bowel sounds and possible abdominal tenderness. Abdominal x-ray shows pneumatosis intestinalis and/or ileus and/or dilatation (Fig. 17.15). Infant is mildly ill.

Stage IIB: Same as IIA plus metabolic acidosis, thrombocytopenia, ascites on x-ray, and a moderately ill infant.

Stage IIIA or B: "Advanced NEC." Infant is critically ill, IIIA with intact bowel, IIIB with perforated bowel. Both include signs as in II but with additional hypotension, bradycardia, severe apnea, and possibly DIC.

Treatment

Supportive Care

- Bowel rest and GI decompression with intermittent NG suction.
- Total Parental Nutrition.
- Fluid replacement.

Antibiotics - various empiric broad spectrum regimes.
Lab and radiographic monitoring for progression of disease
Surgical management for those with evidence of necrosis, suspected necrosis, or perforation.

HEMATOLOGY

- Jaundice and hyperbilirubinemia can be physiologic or pathologic (Table 17.17).
- The danger of elevated bilirubin from any cause is that bilirubin that is not bound to albumin can cross the blood-brain barrier and is toxic to the CNS.

TABLE 17.17

PHYSIOLOGY VERSUS NONPHYSIOLOGIC HYPERBILIRUBINEMIA

Type	Bilirubin Level/ Timing	Rate of Rise	Conjugated Bilirubin	Duration	Etiology
Physiologic hyperbilirubinemia	First week of life	Slow	Low	First week of life	Increase bilirubin load due to high RBC mass and shorter RBC lifespan, defective uptake of bilirubin by immature liver, defective hepatic conjugation of bilirubin due to decreased activity of glucuronyl transferase in the newborn liver
Nonphysiologic hyperbilirubinemia	Bilirubin >13 in a term infant, elevated bilirubin in first 24 h of life	>5 mg/dL/d	>2 mg/dL	Persisting longer than 1 wk in a full-term infant	See below for table

- Total serum bilirubin level of more than 25 to 35 mg/dL is associated with an increased risk for bilirubin-induced neurologic dysfunction (BIND).
- Kernicterus is the chronic and permanent sequelae of BIND and can develop even if infants are adequately treated.

Nonphysiologic hyperbilirubinemia is divided into two categories: conjugated (direct) and unconjugated (Indirect) hyperbilirubinemia. Differential diagnosis of each outlined in Table 17.18.

Polycythemia

Refers to a hematocrit level greater than 2 standard deviations above the FA mean (hematocrit level of more than 65 in a full-term infant).

- Risks of polycythemia include hyperviscosity and its sequelae such as stroke, and hyperbilirubinemia from increased red cell mass.
- The most common causes include delayed umbilical cord clamping and increased fetal RBC production due to placental insufficiency.

Clinical Presentation

Many infants are asymptomatic, but some exhibit symptoms, which usually occur in the 2 hours following birth. These include acrocyanosis, heart failure, sluggish pulses, hypoglycemia, neurologic signs consistent with stroke, hyperbilirubinemia, and thrombocytopenia.

TABLE 17.18

CAUSES OF UNCONJUGATED VERSUS CONJUGATED HYPERBILIRUBINEMIA

Unconjugated (Indirect) Hyperbilirubinemia	Conjugated (Direct) Hyperbilirubinemia
Hemolytic anemia (ABO or Rh incompatibility, red cell structural defects)	*Extrahepatic:*
Polycythemia	Biliary atresia
Crigler-Najjar I and II	Choledochal cyst
Gilbert syndrome	Bile duct stasis
Hypothyroidism	*Intrahepatic*:
Glucuronyl transferase inhibition	Inspissated bile
Breast feeding failure jaundice	Paucity of intrahepatic bile ducts
Breast milk jaundice	*Hepatocellular disease:*
Galactosemia (usually conjugated)	Alpha-1 antitrypsin deficiency
Gastric obstruction	Cystic fibrosis
	Zellweger syndrome
	Dubin-Johnson syndrome
	Rotors syndrome
	Galactosemia
	TPN cholestasis
	Infections
	Idiopathic neonatal hepatitis
	Neonatal hemochromatosis

Management/Treatment

Infants can be managed with observation if they are asymptomatic and the hematocrit level is less than 70. If there are symptoms or the hematocrit level is above 70, partial volume exchange transfusion is performed.

Neonatal Immune-Mediated Thrombocytopenia

Neonatal immune-mediated thrombocytopenia an be divided into the following two types:

- *Alloimmune*: Maternal antiplatelet antibodies against a platelet antigen that the infant has inherited from the father. In this case, maternal IgG crosses the placenta and attacks the fetus' platelets. The most serious complication is intraventricular hemorrhage, which may occur in utero.
- *Autoimmune*: Maternal conditions such as SLE and ITP cause the formation of maternal antibodies that react with the infant's platelets. Infants are generally healthy at birth but may have bruising and petechiae.
- Grading: Mild (100 to 150 $\times$ 10^9 platelets/L), moderate (50 to 100 $\times$ 10^9), severe (<50 $\times$ 10^9).

Hemorrhagic Disease of the Newborn/ Vitamin K Deficient Bleeding (VKDB)

Direct result of failure to administer vitamin K in the immediate newborn period; incidence is 0.25% to 1.7% of neonates without vitamin K administration.

Clinical Presentation

Presents as oozing from the umbilical stump and any puncture sites as well as petechiae. PT and PTT are prolonged. There are two types:

- Early onset (classical) occurs from 24 hours to 7 days, and usually presents on the first day of life. It may occur when the mother is receiving medications that impair vitamin K uptake, such as some anticonvulsants and warfarin or in the setting of a home birth where vitamin K was not administered.
- Late onset (starting beyond the first 2 weeks of life) is associated with intestinal malabsorption of vitamin K.

Prevention

Routine intramuscular administration of Vitamin K at delivery. See Routine Care of the Newborn earlier in this chapter.

OPHTHALMOLOGY

Retinopathy of Prematurity

ROP is a neovascular disease affecting premature infants. Blood vessels in the retina fail to grow and develop normally. Poor vision and blindness can result. Etiology includes hypoxemia and hyperoxic damage.

Incidence

Approximately 50% in infants weighing less than 1,200 g

Diagnosis

Retinal examination by an ophthalmologist is recommended for all neonates born <30 weeks gestation or weighing less than 1,500 g at birth. Neonates >1,500 g with an unstable clinical course also require an evaluation. Follow up examinations are recommended between 4–6 weeks of life.

Please see Ophthalmology chapter for further information.

INFECTIOUS DISEASES

Sepsis

Neonatal sepsis affects approximately 2 in 1,000 live births. Etiologies for neonatal sepsis include the following:

TABLE 17.19

EARLY VERSUS LATE NEONATAL SEPSIS

	Risk Factors	Pathogens	Symptoms	Treatment
Early onset (first 72 h of life)	Prematurity #1 Chorioamnionitis Prolonged rupture of membranes (>18 h) Maternal colonization with known pathogens (e.g., GBS)	Most commonly: *Escherichia coli* and GBS Also, *Streptococcus* sp., *Listeria monocytogenes*, and nontypeable *Haemophilus influenzae*	95% show symptoms within first 72 h of life Bacteremia in 80% Pneumonia in 7%–10% If bacteremia, meningitis in 5%–15% Nonspecific symptoms most common—in severe cases, apnea, hypotension, DIC	Ampicillin and gentamicin × 48–72 h for rule out, 7–10 d if positive cultures or high degree of suspicion Treat meningitis × 14–21 d Mortality 5%–20%
Late onset (Usually 8–30 d of life)	Prematurity Invasive procedures and devices (e.g. catheters, ventilators, VP shunts)	Coagulase negative *Staphylococcus aureus* most common (CONS) Others: *S. aureus*, GBS, *Enterococcus*, *Candida*, *E. Coli*	Onset more insidious, fever frequent 66% have bacteremia, 20%–30% have meningitis	Treatment based on culture-proven or suspected pathogen Handwashing most effective intervention to decrease nosocomial infection rate

DIC, disseminated intravascular coagulation; GBS, group B *Streptococcus*; VP, ventriculoperitoneal.

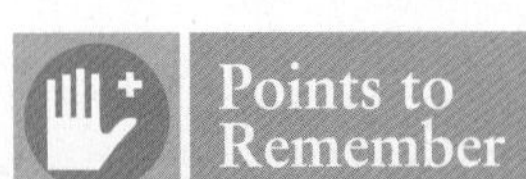

Points to Remember

- **Chorioamnionitis: Cause of 30% to 40% of premature deliveries (see Table 17.20)**

1. Congenital infection (see discussion below)—major risk factor is maternal infection.
2. Early onset infection—transplacental, ascending, or intrapartum.
3. Late onset infection—acquired in hospital, home, or community
   - *Evaluation*: CBC with differential, CRP (in some institutions), blood culture, urine culture (if >48 to 72 hours of life), CXR in patient with clinical signs of sepsis, lumbar puncture (especially if patient symptomatic).
   - Suspect sepsis if total WBC count is less than 5,000 or more than 30,000, I to T ratio grater than 0.2 (immature WBCs including bands, divided by total neutrophils).
   - 25% of septic infants have thrombocytopenia at diagnosis.
   - Please see Table 17.19 for early versus late neonatal sepsis.
     - ➢Most result from ascending bacterial or mycoplasma infection.
     - ➢Bacteria causes includes *E. coli*, *Mycoplasma hominis*, *Ureaplasma urealyticum*, GBS, *Staphylococcus*, *Pseudomonas*, *Proteus*, *Klebsiella*, and *Fusobacterium* sp.
     - ➢Ureaplasma/Mycoplasma infection linked to increased risk of bronchopulmonary dysplasia in preterm infants.
4. GBS
   - GBS colonizes genital tract in 5% to 40% of pregnant women.
   - More than 98% of neonatal infections are due to vertical transmission from genital tract of mother to infant.
   - *Early onset*: Defined as onset within the first week of life; 75% symptomatic in first 24 hours, 80% to 90% by 48 hours of life, usually respiratory distress (60%); CXR indistinguishable from hyaline membrane disease.
   - *Late onset*: May occur as late as 12 to 16 weeks, usually in infants 8 to 30 days old; most characteristic finding is meningitis, but other focal infection occurs (e.g., osteomyelitis, cellulitis, lymphadenitis), most often insidious onset.
   - Please see Tables 17.21 and 17.22 for discussion of risk factors for GBS and management of neonates born to group B *streptococcus* screening culture positive women.

TABLE 17.20

CHORIOAMNIONITIS SIGNS AND SYMPTOMS

Fever (an intrapartum temperature >100.4°F or 37.8°C)
Significant maternal tachycardia (>120 bpm)
Fetal tachycardia (>160 bpm)
Purulent or foul-smelling amniotic fluid
Uterine tenderness
Maternal leukocytosis (total blood leukocyte count >15,000 cells/μL)

TABLE 17.21

RISK FACTORS FOR GBS

Preterm labor at less than 37 wk
Rupture of membranes for more than 18 h
Intrapartum fever of 100.4°F or higher
GBS bacteriuria
Prior delivery of an infant with GBS disease

GBS, group B *Streptococcus*.

Meningitis

GBS and *E. coli* most commonly (combined accounts for 70% of cases); *Listeria monocytogenes* found in 5% of cases in first week of life, other pathogens include *Haemophilus influenzae* and *Streptococcus pneumoniae*; if hospitalized more than 1 week, *S. epidermidis* most common.

Incidence

0.2 to 0.5 in 1,000 live births

Clinical Presentation

Lethargy, feeding difficulties, altered temperature, respiratory distress, emesis, apnea, diarrhea, jaundice, abdominal distention, **seizures in 40%**. Positive CSF culture provides proof of infection; suspicious CSF results include the following:

- Elevated WBC count in CSF (by 1 month of age, >5 cells/mL concerning) with neutrophils predominating (except in *L. monocytogenes*).
- CSF to blood glucose ratio of more than 0.6.
- Protein may be normal (in newborns, up to 170 mg/dL normal).
- Blood culture positive in 50% to 85% of patients with positive CSF culture.

Treatment

Prolonged antibiotic course, including ampicillin and gentamicin

- GBS and *L. monocytogenes* treat with penicillin or ampicillin × 14 days.
- Gram-negative bacteria treat for at least 14 to 21 days.
- If catheter or VP shunt is present, may consider vancomycin.
- Repeat lumbar puncture 24 to 72 hours after initiation of therapy to assess sterilization in cases of Gram-negative meningitis.
- Consider imaging in patients with meningitis, especially with Gram-negative pathogens to exclude parameningeal foci and abscess.

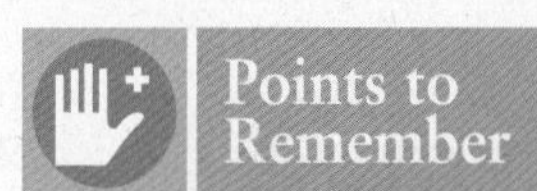

- *Citrobacter koseri* and *Enterobacter sakazakii* are frequently associated with the development of brain abscesses.

Prognosis

20% mortality, 50% morbidity (neurologic damage including deafness, blindness, hydrocephalus, and brain abscess)

TABLE 17.22

MANAGEMENT OF NEONATES BORN TO GROUP B *STREPTOCOCCUS* SCREENING CULTURE POSITIVE WOMEN[a]

IAP Indicated
- Previous infant with invasive GBS disease (early or late onset)
- GBS bacteriuria during current pregnancy
- Positive GBS screening culture during current pregnancy (unless cesarean section scheduled)
- Unknown GBS status and any of the following:
  - Delivery at <37 wk of gestation
  - Membrane rupture ≥18 h
  - Intrapartum fever ≥100.4°F (≥38.0°C)

IAP Not Indicated
- Previous pregnancy with positive GBS culture (unless culture is positive during current pregnancy)
- Scheduled cesarean section delivery in the absence of labor or membrane rupture
- Negative vaginal and rectal GBS screening culture, regardless of intrapartum risk factors

[a]Vaginal and rectal GBS cultures at 35 to 37 weeks gestation for all pregnant women.
GBS, group B *Streptococcus*; IAP, intrapartum antibiotic prophylaxis.
Adapted from Pickering LK, ed. *Red Book*. Elk Grove Village, IL: American Academy of Pediatrics, 2003.

TABLE 17.23

TORCH INFECTIONS

	Clinical Findings	Diagnosis	Treatment
T = toxoplasmosis (1–8/10,000)	Increased severity when acquired early in pregnancy, but higher transmission rates when acquired later in pregnancy *90% infected infants asymptomatic at birth CNS involvement is hallmark—chorioretinitis, diffuse intracranial calcifications, and hydrocephalus	Serologic assays for measurement of antibodies to *T. gondii* in serum and body fluids—gold standard is Sabin-Feldman dye test	Combined: Pyrimethamine, sulfadiazine, leucovorin (folinic acid)
O = other (e.g., syphilis, parvovirus B19, HIV, varicella)	**Syphilis**—Most infants born to women with syphilis have infection, though 50% have clinical symptoms Premature delivery, stillbirth, nonimmune hydrops Early congenital syphilis (symptoms present within 2 yr of age) Late congenital syphilis (symptoms >2 yr) Snuffles (nasal discharge), rash (maculopapular bullae on extremities), osteochondritis and periostitis in 80%–90%, frontal bossing, saber shins, Hutchinson teeth (upper central incisors wide, short, wide gap) hepatosplenomegaly (50%–90%); neurosyphilis (40%–60%)—acute syphilitic leptomeningitis, chronic meningovascular syphilis **Parvovirus B19**—10%–27% of cases of nonimmune hydrops fetalis; risk highest during second trimester **HIV**—Perinatal transmission if mother untreated—20%–30% worldwide average; if treated with AZT, ~8% transmission **Congenital varicella syndrome**—syndrome occurs in neonate in 2% of maternal infections in first trimester—skin scarring, limb deformities, eye involvement; may develop zoster during first few years of life	**Syphilis** Nontreponemal: RPR and VDRL—congenital syphilis if neonate nontreponemal antibody level four times higher than maternal Treponemal: FTA-ABS—confirm after diagnosis with nontreponemal test Dark field microscopy of Treponema **Parvovirus**—Maternal antibodies or PCR in neonate/fetus **HIV**—HIV PCR-DNA at birth, 1 mo, and 3–4 mo **Varicella**—VZV IgG, IgM, scraping of skin lesions (large multinucleated giant cells with Tzanck smear)	**Syphilis**—Penicillin **Parvovirus**—Spontaneous resolution in one-third of pregnancies; early fetal transfusion **HIV**—AZT × 6 wk for all HIV-exposed neonates **Varicella**—acyclovir for severe infections. Give VZIG to newborns when mother develops varicella 5 days before or 2 days after delivery.
R = rubella (<0.5/100,000)	Maternal infection during first trimester most damaging Up to 20% of fetuses aborted if maternal primary infection within first 8 wk of pregnancy Classic triad: sensorineural hearing loss, cataracts, and congenital heart disease (PDA, pulmonary stenosis, valve abnormalities in 45%–70%) *Blueberry muffin babies—extramedullary hematopoiesis	Maternal antibodies Neonate—IgM, rise in rubella IgG titer, culture, PCR Laboratory tests—thrombocytopenia, leucopenia, hyperbilirubinemia	Supportive *Immunization against rubella contraindicated during pregnancy
C = cytomegalovirus (1% of live births)	Most infected infants are asymptomatic; small percentage have hearing loss only *Leading infectious cause of brain damage and hearing loss Primary infection in third trimester worst outcome Classic presentation: petechiae, ecchymoses, jaundiced, hepatosplenomegaly	PCR or culture within first 2 wk of life (urine or blood) 70%–80% of symptomatic infants have abnormal CT findings. *Classic periventricular calcifications	Controversial—ganciclovir may decrease viral shedding while on medication, though studies unclear whether decreases sequelae including hearing loss
H = herpes simplex virus (1–3/20,000 births) (HSV-2 = 70%–85% of neonatal HSV infections)	*Very rarely a congenital infection—85% transmitted at delivery Usually not symptomatic at birth Disseminated disease begins toward end of first week (skin vesicles in 50%, poor feeding, lethargy, hypertension, fever, DIC) Localized disease appears second to third week of life (keratoconjunctivitis, chorioretinitis, pneumonitis, if CNS—seizures, irritable)	Culture Tzanck smear on skin scrapings HSV PCR CSF (lymphocytosis noted) Disseminated disease—LFT elevation EEG abnormal in 80% of patients with disseminated disease	Acyclovir × 14 d in localized disease, × 21 d in disseminated or CNS disease Overall mortality = 20% *C-section recommended if active lesions

CNS, central nervous system; CSF, cerebrospinal fluid; DIC, disseminated intravascular coagulation; HSV, herpes simplex virus; LFT, liver function test; PCR, polymerase chain reaction; PDA, patent ductus arteriosus; RPR, rapid plasma regain; VDRL, venereal disease research laboratory.

Congenital Infections and TORCH

Congenital infections are defined as those transmitted anytime during gestation except the last 5 to 7 days. The most commonly acquired include CMV, HIV, and parvovirus B19.

Please see Table 17.23 for further details on congenital/TORCH infections.

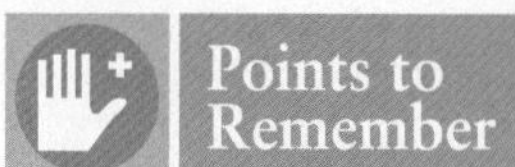

- Give VZIG to newborns when mother develops varicella 5 days before or 2 days after delivery.

ENDOCRINE

See Endocrine chapter for full discussions.

Congenital Hypothyroidism

1 in 4,000 neonates have congenital hypothyroidism.

5% to 10% have transiently abnormal thyroid function tests because of maternal antibodies against thyrotropin receptors of thyroid gland.

These antibodies decline in the first 3 months of birth. Congenital hypothyroidism benefits from rapid early detection and treatment to decrease the incidence of intellectual impairment and poor growth. See Box 10.1 for signs and symptoms of congenital hypothyroidism.

Congenital Adrenal Hyperplasia

- Most commonly 21-hydroxylase deficiency—incidence approximately 1 in 15,000 worldwide.
- Results in impaired production of cortisol and excess androgen production.

Clinical Presentation

- Females with CAH demonstrate ambiguous genitalia (see Figure 10.1)
- Neonates can present in adrenal crisis with hyponatremia, hyperkalemia, and dehydration.

Treatment

Hydrocortisone [glucocorticoid] and fludrocortisone [mineralocortocoid] replacement are the mainstay of therapy Sick patients may require aggressive fluid and electrolyte management in addition to stress dose hydrocortisone. Adequacy of glucocorticoid dosing can be assessed via 17-OHP level. Stress dose steroids are needed during illness or other times of stress. Surgery may be required on the female genitalia depending on the degree of virilization

NEONATAL EMERGENCIES

- **Bilious emesis;** for NEC see above discussion—always be concerned if called about bilious emesis—an emergency upper GI is needed to rule out malrotation.
- **Abdominal distention/bloody stools**—concern for NEC, enterocolitis due to Hirschsprung disease.
- **Sudden respiratory decompensation**—remember ABC's—airway management with bag and mask ventilation and intubation as needed; if intubated, assess tube position, if asymmetric chest movement, CXR or illumination of chest may demonstrate pneumothorax requiring needle aspiration and/or chest tube.
- **Anuria**—fluid bolus, assess renal function, place Foley catheter, consider surgical consultation if abdominal distension and concern for compartment syndrome (increased abdominal pressure possibly leading to decreased perfusion of kidneys).
- **Fetal hydrops**—can lead to neonatal compromise in the DR, increased fluid in at least two compartments (e.g., abdominal ascites, pleural effusion), may require aspiration in the DR.

SAMPLE BOARD REVIEW QUESTIONS

1. You are called to the newborn nursery to examine a 41-week-old boy of an insulin-dependent gestational diabetic mother. The nurse noted that the baby is pale and capillary refill is greater than 3 seconds. What is the next course of action?
   a. Give the infant a formula feed
   b. Check the calcium level
   c. Obtain an echocardiogram
   d. Administer an NS bolus with added dextrose
   e. Obtain a cranial ultrasound

Answer: d. Approximately 30% of neonates born to diabetic mothers have some degree of hypertrophic cardiomyopathy. Infants with inadequate circulation may be pale, limp, poor cap refill, have low BP, which may indicate hypertrophic cardiomyopathy with outflow tract obstruction. Inotropic agents such as dopamine should be avoided in these infants because of the potential worsening of the outflow tract obstruction. This infant could be hypoglycemic requiring dextrose, but feeding an unstable infant would not be optimal—a dextrose infusion would be more appropriate. Checking calcium levels is important, as hypocalcemia can be seen in infants of diabetic mothers; however, this would not be the immediate intervention. An echocardiogram of this neonate should be obtained to assess for hypertrophic cardiomyopathy and congenital heart disease, but again, this would not be the immediate intervention, nor is obtaining a cranial ultrasound.

2. You are called to the bedside of a 31-week infant who the nurse frantically reports oxygen saturations in the sixties, seconds, decreased BP, and increased work of breathing. They are bagging the infant without improvement. On examination, you note decreased breath sounds on the left side and an asymmetric chest. What is the immediate management?
   a. Obtain a chest x-ray
   b. Needle aspiration of the left side
   c. Administer a normal saline bolus
   d. Intubate with low pressures
   e. Position the infant right side up and place on 100% oxyhood

Answer: b. This infant has evidence of a tension pneumothorax with evidence of cardiovascular compromise. The immediate management is needle aspiration with possible need for chest tube. If this patient had a pneumothorax with mild respiratory symptoms without evidence of a tension pneumothorax, he could have been placed on 100% oxyhood for nitrogen washout.

3. Administration of this supplement can decrease the rate of neural tube defects by 70%.
   a. Calcium
   b. Vitamin B_{12}
   c. Folate
   d. Iron
   e. Vitamin A

Answer: c. Folate. The optimal time of starting folate is 3 to 4 months prior to fertilization.

4. The NICU recently had a recent outbreak of *E. coli* infection in the unit. The infection control team visited the NICU and made several recommendations. Which recommendation is the most effective intervention to decrease nosocomial infection rate?
   a. Negative pressure rooms
   b. Sterilizing all ventilator equipment
   c. Wearing masks prior to examining the neonates
   d. Handwashing
   e. Deep cleaning the unit once per month

Answer: d. Nosocomial infections cause a number of cases of morbidity and mortality in the hospital setting. The most effective way to decrease nosocomial infection rates is to promote handwashing.

5. An SGA, ex 34-week-old infant failed the hearing screen in the NICU. On an outpatient ABR at 2 months of age, the infant passed her hearing on the right side but failed on the left. What is the most likely infectious cause of her hearing loss?
   a. Syphilis
   b. Rubella
   c. Cytomegalovirus
   d. Parvovirus
   e. Herpes simplex virus

Answer: c. CMV affects approximately 1 in 40,000 live births. CMV is the leading infectious cause of brain damage and hearing loss. Primary infection in the third trimester has the worst outcome. Classic signs include petechiae, ecchymoses, hepatosplenomegaly. 70% to 80% of symptomatic infants have abnormal CT finding, classically periventricular calcifications. Rubella can also cause hearing loss (sensorineural), part of the classic triad of hearing loss, cataracts, and congenital heart disease. Both syphilis and HSV can have neuro involvement but not necessarily hearing loss.

6. On examination of a 2-day-old full-term infant, the mother is concerned about red spots on the trunk and arms. On examination, you note multiple erythematous macules and papules (1 to 3 mm in diameter) with occasional pustules on an erythematous base. You reassure

the mother that the lesions are benign and should resolve in 5 to 7 days. If you were to take a sample of the pustules contents, what would you expect to see on microscopy?

a. Eosinophils on Wright stain
b. Neutrophils on Wright stain
c. Keratin
d. Gram-positive cocci in clusters
e. B and D

Answer: a. This neonate has erythema toxicum, a benign newborn rash that typically can appear at 24 to 48 hours of life and resolves in 5 to 7 days. No treatment is necessary. It is usually found on the trunk and proximal extremities. The lesions of transient neonatal pustular melanosis contain neutrophils on Wright stain. Keratin can be seen in miliaria, papules formed over blocked sweat glands that can develop in the first day of life. These lesions are not typical for *Staphylococcus* infection.

7. You have been called to counsel a 32-year-old woman with type 1 diabetes. She is poorly controlled, with a hemoglobin A1c of 12. You discuss with her the potential complications of a baby born to a mother with poorly controlled diabetes. Of the following, which is NOT associated with infants of diabetic mothers?

a. Shoulder dystocia
b. Caudal regression syndrome
c. Polycythemia
d. Hypoplastic left colon
e. Improved lung maturity

Answer: e. Gestational diabetes develops in approximately 2.5% of pregnancies. Prolonged exposure to maternal hyperglycemia and poorly controlled diabetes can lead to multiple congenital anomalies. Infants of diabetic mothers have a two to three times greater risk of major malformations than that of the general population. These infants have a higher incidence of respiratory distress due to decreased lung maturity.

8. A 1-week-old neonate is brought to the emergency department by the paramedics limp and pale. His parents report that he had been doing well until the past day when he started feeding poorly. His breathing became more labored per parents. In the emergency department, the patient is intubated and given multiple normal saline boluses because of poor perfusion. Of the following, which medication should be added?

a. Adenosine
b. Prostaglandin E2
c. Indomethacin
d. Caffeine
e. Dexamethasone

Answer: b. Ductal-dependent cyanotic heart disease, such as hypoplastic left heart syndrome and coarctation of the aorta, can present within the first few weeks of life as the duct closes. These infants can present pale, have poor perfusion, and have a similar presentation to an infant with septic shock. While it would be important to work this patient up for septic shock and start antibiotics, congenital heart disease should be considered, in which case starting PGE to reopen a closed duct could be lifesaving.

9. The lecithin to sphingomyelin (L:S) ratio is used prenatally to assess lung maturity in pregnancies complicated by preterm labor. The test is performed on amniotic fluid, which is partly composed of fetal lung fluids. As the fetus matures, the L:S ratio changes. Which numerical value for the L:S ratio indicates lung maturity?

a. 0.25
b. 1.5
c. 0.15
d. 2.5

Answer: d. The L:S ratio indicates lung maturity when it is more than 2. The L:S ratio reaches 2 at approximately 35 weeks of gestation.

10. Vitamin K is administered orally to a newborn after parents refuse "a shot." You counsel the parents about the risk of late HDN and include the following fact about this disorder:

a. It starts in week one of life
b. It is caused by intestinal malabsorption of vitamin K
c. It can be caused by maternal medications such as warfarin
d. Signs include joint swelling and hemarthroses

Answer: b. Late HDN has an onset of approximately 2 weeks of life and is caused by poor absorption of vitamin K in the newborn gut. It is preventable with parenteral administration of vitamin K in the immediate newborn period. Oral vitamin K does not protect against late HDN.

11. Newborn eye prophylaxis with 0.5% erythromycin, 1% silver nitrate, or 1% tetracycline ophthalmic preparations is given to prevent:
    a. *C. trachomatis*
    b. *N. gonorrhea.*
    c. *L. monocytogenes*
    d. *E. coli*

Answer: b. Given to prevent ocular *N. gonorrhea*. These agents also reduce the incidence of *C. trachomatis* ophthalmia disorders but do NOT prevent them.

12. A 19-year-old primigravid woman enters prenatal care in her second trimester. She thinks her LMP was about 5 months ago, but her periods have never been regular. An ultrasound is performed for dating the pregnancy. Which of the following statements is true?
    a. Ultrasound dating at this GA is equally as accurate as LMP
    b. LMP dating is preferred at this GA
    c. A 2-week difference in LMP and ultrasound dating is grounds to use LMP dating and rescan in 2 weeks
    d. A 2-week difference in LMP and ultrasound dating and LMP is grounds to use ultrasound dating and rescan in 2 weeks

Answer: d. This patient is in her second trimester. Guidelines are as follows: in the first trimester, if date difference between LMP and ultrasound is less than 7 days, use LMP for due date. In the second trimester, if ultrasound is more than 2 weeks different from LMP dates, use ultrasound dates, and rescan in 2 weeks to confirm. In the third trimester, if ultrasound dates are within 3 weeks of LMP dates, use LMP dates.

13. A full-term infant is born via NSVD with a true umbilical cord knot. During delivery, some late decelerations were noted and the infant is blue and with no cry when you receive her. After stimulation and oxygen administration, at 1 minute, her HR is 72, she has a feeble cry, her extremities have no active movement, she has weak breathing, and is blue. What is the significance of her Apgar score?
    a. It indicates she has recovered from her initial insult
    b. It indicates she will have lifelong neurological sequelae from birth events
    c. It indicates she needs further resuscitation
    d. It indicates she is ready to be wrapped and placed on her mother's abdomen

Answer: c. Her Apgar score is 5, indicating continued neonatal distress. The Apgar score is an assessment of a neonate's response to birth and to resuscitation efforts, not an indication of future outcomes. An indication of a successful resuscitation is an increasing Apgar score at each interval.

14. An obese but otherwise previously healthy pregnant 24-year-old woman has an abnormally high glucose tolerance test at 28 weeks and is diagnosed with gestational diabetes. Which of the following complications is most likely?
    a. Congenital cardiac defect
    b. Caudal regression syndrome
    c. Shoulder dystocia
    d. Hypoplastic left colon

Answer: c. This previously healthy woman likely had normal blood sugar during the first, organogenic, trimester of pregnancy, as gestational diabetes is a condition which typically develops in the late second/early third trimester. Therefore, it is unlikely that her infant will suffer from congenital structural abnormalities related to high blood sugar, such as caudal regression syndrome or congenital cardiac abnormalities. More likely is that the infant will be large at birth, especially if her gestational diabetesis poorly controlled. This can lead to shoulder dystocia at delivery, among other complications.

SUGGESTED READINGS

Gotoff SP. Group B streptococcal infections. *Pediatr Rev*. 2002;23:381–386.

Luo G, Norwitz E. Revisiting amniocentesis for fetal lung maturity after 36 weeks' gestation. *Rev Obstet Gynecol*. 2008;1(2):61–68.

Onyebuchi O, Marx H, Lazarus J. Medical management of thyroid dysfunction in pregnancy and the postpartum. *Expert Opin Pharmacother.* 2008;9(13):2281–2293.

Revello MG, Gerna G. Diagnosis and management of human cytomegalovirus infection in the mother, fetus, and newborn infant. *Clin Microbiol Rev*. 2002;15(4):680–715.

Schneider D, Moore J. Patent ductus arteriosus. *Circulation*. 2006;114:1873–1882.

CHAPTER 18 ■ NEUROLOGY

KRISTIN W. BARANANO

ACC	Agenesis of the corpus callosum	GI	Gastrointestinal
AD	Autosomal dominant	HGPRT	Hypoxanthine-guanine phosphoribosyltransferase
ADEM	Acute disseminated encephalomyelitis	HSV	Herpes simplex virus
ADHD	Attention-deficit/hyperactivity disorder	ICP	Intracranial pressure
ADOS	Autism Diagnostic Observation Schedule	IIH	Idiopathic intracranial hypertension
AED	Antiepileptic drug	JME	Juvenile myoclonic epilepsy
AIDP	Acute inflammatory demyelinating polyneuropathy	MLD	Metachromatic leukodystrophy
ALD	Adrenoleukodystrophy	MRA	Magnetic resonance angiography
ALT	Alanine aminotransferase	MRI	Magnetic resonance imaging
AR	Autosomal recessive	MRV	Magnetic resonance venography
AST	Aspartate aminotransferase	MS	Multiple sclerosis
AVM	Arteriovenous malformation	MSLT	Multiple sleep latency test
BECTS	Benign epilepsy with centrotemporal spikes	NF	Neurofibromatosis
CBC	Complete blood count	NMO	Neuromyelitis optica
CCM	Cerebral cavernous malformation	NSAID	Nonsteroidal anti-inflammatory drug
CIDP	Chronic inflammatory demyelinating polyneuropathy	NREM	Nonrapid eye movement
CIS	Clinically isolated syndrome	OT	Occupational therapy
CK	Creatinine kinase	PML	Progressive multifocal leukoencephalopathy
CMP	Comprehensive metabolic panel	PT	Physical therapy
CMV	Cytomegalovirus	PVS	Persistent vegetative state
CN	Cranial nerve	REM	Rapid eye movement
CNS	Central nervous system	SIDS	Sudden infant death syndrome
CP	Cerebral palsy	SSRI	Selective serotonin reuptake inhibitor
CSF	Cerebrospinal fluid	TBI	Traumatic brain injury
CT	Computed tomography	tPA	Tissue plasminogen activator
CTA	CT angiogram	TIA	Transient ischemic attack
DMD	Duchenne muscular dystrophy	TSC	Tuberous sclerosis complex
EMG	Electromyogram	UBO	Unidentified bright object
GBS	Guillain-Barre syndrome	VLCFA	Very-long-chain fatty acid
GCL	Globoid cell leukodystrophy	VST	Venous sinus thrombosis
		VZV	Varicella zoster virus

CHAPTER OBJECTIVES

1. To be familiar with the presentation of specific neurologic disorders, including stroke, myasthenia gravis, brachial plexus injuries, GBS, ADEM, muscular dystrophies, and the neurophakomatoses
2. To understand the role of lumbar puncture in the diagnosis of various infections of the CNS
3. To be aware of the various neurodegenerative disorders, which are a consideration when a child presents with loss of milestones
4. To be familiar with the normal development of the CNS and how perturbations can result in various CNS malformations

5. To be aware of guidelines regarding the evaluation of first time seizures, common epilepsy syndromes, and principles of selection of AED therapy.

SIGNS AND SYMPTOMS OF NEUROLOGIC ABNORMALITY

Headache

Resource: The International Headache Society has published diagnostic criteria (http://ihs-classification.org/en/).

Overview: Headaches are a common childhood issue and can be divided into three broad categories.

1. **Primary headaches:** migraine, tension-type, cluster.
2. **Secondary headaches:** those caused by medication overuse or intracranial pathology, such as IIH, or pseudotumor cerebri (see section on increased ICP, below), Chiari malformation type I, and meningitis.
3. **Central neuralgias and central and primary facial pain** includes diagnoses uncommon in children, such as trigeminal neuralgia.

Clinical Manifestations

History: focus on whether the pain is acute or chronic, recurrent or progressive.

- **Acute headaches** involve a single episode and can be associated with a variety of systemic illnesses. Although rare, subarachnoid hemorrhage due to aneurysm rupture can occur in children. Adults often describe this as "the worst headache of my life."
- **Acute recurrent headaches** are headaches separated by pain-free intervals. When associated with nausea and vomiting and photophobia or phonophobia, the diagnosis is often migraine headaches. Compared with adults, migraines in children can be shorter in duration and the pain is less likely to be unilateral.
- **Chronic progressive headaches** may indicate increased ICP. Red flags on history include a new headache or change in prior pattern, extremely severe headache, headache that wakes the child from sleep or is worse in the morning, or headache that is worse with coughing or straining. Increased ICP can cause nausea or vomiting. Funduscopic examination to evaluate for papilledema should always be performed with a complaint of headaches.
- **Chronic nonprogressive headaches** can include chronic tension-type headaches or chronic daily migraine (transformed migraine). Stress and medication overuse frequently play a role. There can also be overlay of acute recurrent headaches (migraines) onto chronic nonprogressive headaches.

Key elements of a history: number and types of headaches, location, character, duration, frequency, warning signs (aura), presence of photophobia or phonophobia, nausea or vomiting, alleviating factors (ex: sleep), exacerbating factors (dehydration, skipping meals), caffeine intake, exercise frequency, sleep schedule, frequency of medication use, relationship to menses, and family history.

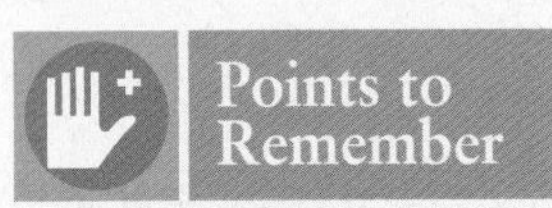

Points to Remember

- Red flags suggesting imaging is indicated: new headache or changing headache, a headache that awakens a child from sleep, or a headache that worsens with straining or coughing.

Diagnosis

In general, a greater than 6-month history of headaches with a normal neurologic examination (including funduscopic examination and blood pressure measurements) and a positive family history of migraines = no indication to image.

Migraine variants in children include cyclical vomiting, abdominal migraine, and benign paroxysmal vertigo.

Treatment of migraines starts with addressing lifestyle factors elicited in history (see above). Headache diaries are helpful.

Abortive therapies: *NSAIDs* (ibuprofen at 10 mg/kg/dose or naproxen) or a triptan (such as *sumatriptan*; the nasal preparation is especially effective if nausea is present). Triptans are not approved for children younger than 17 years, and there is a theoretical interaction with SSRIs.

Prophylactic treatment: When headaches are frequent and/or disruptive (not easily treated with ibuprofen and/or patient is missing school), consider the following options: *cyproheptadine* (good choice for young children), *amitriptyline* (often a first choice for teenagers), *topiramate* (good choice if patient is overweight), *valproic acid* (at bedtime, especially for boys without without weight issues or with mood problems). Beta blockers and calcium channel blockers can also be used in children.

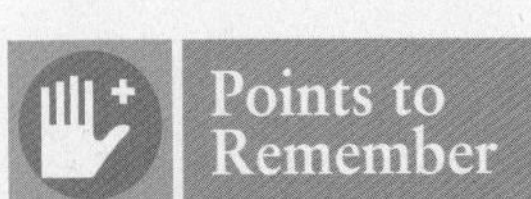

Points to Remember

- In general, positive family history for migraine with a greater than 6-month history of headaches and a normal neurological examination = no indication to image.

TABLE 18.1

CAUSE OF ALTERED LEVEL OF CONSCIOUSNESS

Category	Etiologies to Consider
Metabolic	Hypoglycemia Diabetic ketoacidosis Hypo- or hypernatremia Hypo- or hypercalcemia Hyperammonemia Hypercapnia Hypothyroidism Uremia Adrenal crisis Hypo- or hyperthermia
Infectious	Sepsis Focal infection (abscess, subdural empyema) Encephalitis
Vascular	Ischemic stroke Hemorrhage Venous sinus thrombosis Hypertensive encephalopathy
Inflammatory	Acute disseminated encephalomyelitis (ADEM)
Toxins	Carbon monoxide Alcohol Methanol Ethylene glycol Lead Organophosphates Ingestions of medications
Other	Trauma Hypoxia Hypotension Hydrocephalus Neoplasm Status epilepticus or postictal state
Mimics	Conversion reaction Catatonia Locked-in syndrome Neuromuscular weakness

Altered Level of Consciousness

See Table 18.1 for details on potential causes of altered level of consciousness.

Ataxia

Introduction: Ataxia is a sign of cerebellar dysfunction.

Clinical Signs

Clinical signs of cerebellar involvement include the following:

- Truncal ataxia (wide-based gait, "drunken sailor"), which when severe can include head bobbing (titubation).
- Dysmetria (difficulty performing finger-nose-finger test).
- Nystagmus.
- Vertigo.
- Scanning speech.

Also assess for signs of CN involvement, which could be a sign of ischemia in the posterior circulation of the brain (off the vertebral arteries).

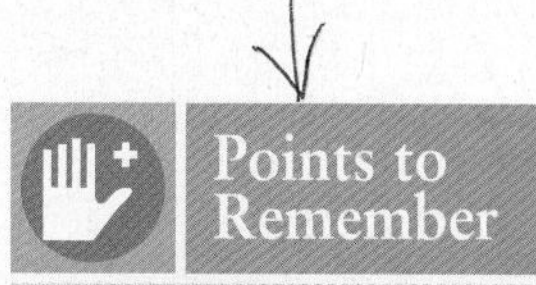

- truncal ataxia = lesion of midline cerebellar vermis; appendicular ataxia = lesions of cerebellar hemispheres.

History: Focus on time course, for example, sudden versus gradual onset, episodic versus continuous.

Differential Diagnosis

- **Acute onset ataxia**: intoxication (i.e., phenytoin overdose), infection (such as *Bartonella*), postinfectious (classic scenario: toddler with recent viral illness, previously often seen after VZV infection), postvaccination, demyelinating events (ADEM, childhood MS, Miller Fisher variant of GBS [Look for associated eye movement abnormalities and areflexia]), migraine (vestibular migraine can present with ataxia and vertigo, not always associated with headache).
- **Subacute onset ataxia**: cerebellar hemorrhage or ischemic stroke, encephalitis, acute labyrinthitis (vestibular neuronitis), tumors of posterior fossa, paraneoplastic (opsoclonus-myoclonus, with multidirectional chaotic eye movements, evaluate for neuroblastoma).
- **Chronic or progressive ataxia**: developmental defects, tumors, paraneoplastic, genetic etiologies (spinocerebellar ataxias, Friedreich ataxia, ataxia telangiectasia).
- **Recurrent ataxia**: episodic ataxias (EA1 and EA2, with AD inheritance), metabolic disorders (various mitochondrial disorders, Hartnup disease, urea cycle defects, intermittent forms of maple syrup urine disease).

Diagnosis: based on

1. **Careful history**, especially related to time course and antecedent events.
2. **Physical examination**, with special attention to eye movements, CN function, and reflexes.
3. **Other tests and imaging studies**: such as a toxicology screen, imaging (a head CT scan is a good primary study to rule out hemorrhage whereas MRIs are preferred to look for posterior fossa lesions or demyelination), and lumbar puncture when infectious etiologies are considered.

Movement Disorders

Tics

Clinical Manifestations. Tics are sudden, involuntary movements. Distinguish motor tics (blinking, shoulder shrugs) from vocal tics (grunting, coughing). Typical age of onset of tics is around 7 years. There is often a family history. Tics typically wax and wane in severity and can be exacerbated by stress and fatigue; new types of tics may develop. Some children will have premonitory sensation (i.e., the sense of an "itch" that is relieved by producing a tic). Tics often coexist with obsessive-compulsive features and attention-deficit disorder.

Diagnosis. Tics are often a transient phenomenon. A chronic motor or vocal tic disorder is present when it persists for more than 1 year. Tourette syndrome is defined by the combination of motor and vocal tics with onset before the age of 18 years, at least 1 year in duration, causing distress or impairment in daily functioning.

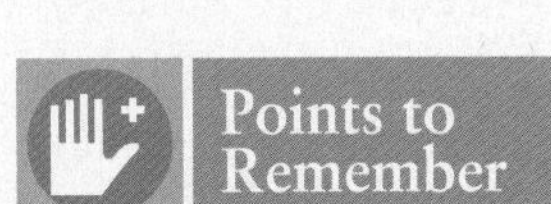

- Tourette syndrome is a combination motor and vocal tic disorder with more than 1 year of duration with onset before the age of 18 years, causing distress or impairment in daily functioning.

Treatment. Consider treatment if tics are causing physical discomfort or injury or psychosocial distress. First-line agents are *clonidine* or *guanfacine*. Second tier agents modulate the dopaminergic system (*haloperidol*, *pimozide*).

Prognosis: Two-thirds of cases will remit or be substantially better by adulthood, one-third will persist into adulthood.

Stereotypes: Stereotyped, complex movements (i.e., hand flapping). Stereotypes usually have an earlier age of onset than tics. Often more pronounced when the child is relaxed or engrossed. Associated with autism, but also seen in normal children. Parental reassurance is the treatment of choice.

Spasmus nutans is a benign, self-limited condition during infancy. It is characterized by odd head positions, head bobbing, and nystagmus. Brain imaging should be performed to rule out optic pathway and thalamic gliomas.

Tremors are oscillating, rhythmic movements about a fixed point. Distinguish between tremor at rest (rare in children) and action tremor (including postural tremors, when holding a limb in a position, against gravity). Enhanced physiologic tremor occurs in normal individuals. Often related to medication effects (e.g., valproic acid, lithium). Classic: *familial essential tremor*, inherited in AD fashion, worsens with age. For some, alcohol improves. Usually defer treatment (beta-blocker such as propranolol) until adulthood, so long as able to write and feed self.

Chorea is part of the group of disorders called *dyskinesias* and is characterized by random movements that flow into one another. Chorea may occur with *athetosis*, which refers to twisting or writhing movements, typically of the distal extremities. Causes of chorea include kernicterus, juvenile Huntington disease, choreoathetoid CP, and Wilson disease. Chorea is treated by modulating basal ganglia function (increasing GABAergic or blocking dopaminergic signaling) with agents such as valproic acid, carbamazepine, diazepam, and haloperidol.

Iatrogenic movement disorders: With increasing use of newer generation atypical neuroleptics in pediatric patients, it is important to be aware of potential side effects. *Tardive dyskinesias* (more common with older agents such as haloperidol) can present after prolonged use as involuntary movements of mouth, including tongue. Abrupt withdrawal of agents can cause *withdrawal dyskinesias*. Neuroleptics can cause *akathisia*, the urge to move constantly.

Points to Remember

- *Sydenham chorea* is an immune-mediated response following group A streptococcal infection and is one of the major criteria of acute rheumatic fever. It is often accompanied by associated emotional volatility. If suspected, send ASO titer (but titer is often waning by the time chorea develops) and DNase B. Treatment is penicillin VK. Steroids may hasten recovery.

Increased Intracranial Pressure

Introduction: CSF is produced by the choroid plexus in the lateral ventricles. It flows through the interventricular foramina (**foramen of Monro**) into the third ventricle, then through the cerebral aqueduct (**aqueduct of Sylvius**) into the fourth ventricle. It exits through two lateral apical roof apertures (**foramina of Luschka**) and one median posterior roof aperture (**foramen of Magendie**) into the pontine cistern and cisterna magna. CSF then flows down the spinal cord and over the cerebral hemispheres.

Obstruction in CSF flow at any point along with path can result in a *noncommunicating hydrocephalus*. Common causes include congenital aqueductal stenosis, Chiari II malformation (typically associated with myelomeningocele), Dandy-Walker malformation, and obstructing cysts. A *communicating hydrocephalus* can be caused by failure of CSF to be appropriately reabsorbed by the *arachnoid granulations*. Common causes include intraventricular hemorrhage (as may be seen with a germinal matrix bleed associated with prematurity), increased CSF protein following meningitis, or due to overproduction of CSF, such as from a choroids plexus tumor.

Points to Remember

- Dyskinesias and akathisia can be a result of medication use or withdrawal.

For acute management of elevated ICP: see chapter on Critical Care.

IIH, or pseudotumor cerebri, is a diagnosis of exclusion. The pathophysiology is thought to involve excess production of CSF, impaired absorption of CSF, and/or stenosis of the venous sinuses. When it presents in younger children, there is no association with obesity or gender. After puberty, obesity and female gender are major risk factors. IIH can be associated with the use of certain medications, including growth hormone, tetracyclines such as minocycline, vitamin A derivatives, and steroids.

Clinical Manifestations

Patients present with headaches and papilledema. There can be associated CN palsies (especially CN VI).

Diagnosis

IIH is a diagnosis of exclusion. Head CT scan should be performed prior to lumbar puncture to rule out a mass and/or noncommunicating hydrocephalus (which could cause herniation during lumbar puncture). Lumbar puncture with opening and closing pressures should be performed, and CSF sent for routine studies (results should be normal in IIH). MRI of the brain, including MRV, should be performed to exclude sinus venous thrombosis (prior to the era of antibiotics, *otitic hydrocephalus* was common).

Treatment

Risk of vision loss should prompt urgent treatment, which can include serial large-volume lumbar punctures to lower ICP. Patients should be closely followed by ophthalmology to monitor color vision and visual fields. Potentially offending medications should be withdrawn and patients counseled regarding weight loss (even a 10% weight loss can result in significant clinical improvement). Pharmacologically, *acetazolamide*, and in some cases, *topiramate*, are used. Rarely, shunting or optic nerve fenestration is required to preserve vision.

Benign external hydrocephalus is a cause of macrocephaly in the first year of life. On imaging, there is extra-axial fluid, but no concern for obstruction. As the arachnoid granulations mature, the excess fluid is absorbed and head size normalizes.

Weakness

Overview: The motor examination includes assessment of muscle tone, bulk, and power.

Key Questions

1. Evidence of asymmetry?
2. Are proximal or distal muscles more involved?

TABLE 18.2

UPPER MOTOR NEURON VERSUS LOWER MOTOR NEURON SIGNS

Upper Motor Neuron Signs (Involvement of Cortical Motor Neurons)	Lower Motor Neuron Signs (Damage to Spinal Cord Motor Neurons)
Spasticity	Weakness
Brisk reflexes	Muscle atrophy
Upgoing toes (positive Babinski sign, but toes are normally upgoing until about 18 months of age).	Fasciculations

3. Where does the lesion localize? (brain, spinal cord, peripheral nerve, neuromuscular junction, muscle)?

See Table 18.2 for more information on upper motor neuron versus lower motor neuron signs.

Case Example: Evaluation of the floppy infant. Hypotonia (low tone) can be caused by lesions in the central or peripheral nervous system. It is important to assess if muscle strength or reflexes are affected.

The localized causes of hypotonia are outlined in Table 18.3.

CNS Infections

Bacterial Infections

Refer to the chapter on Infectious Diseases for further review.

Overview. Meningitis refers to inflammation of the leptomeninges.

Clinical Manifestations. Classic presentation includes fever, nuchal rigidity, photophobia, and headache. Meningeal signs are unreliable in infants.

TABLE 18.3

LOCALIZATION OF HYPOTONIA

Location of Defect	Some Possible Causes	Diagnostic Testing
Brain	Structural brain abnormalities, static encephalopathy (such as caused by anoxia), Prader-Willi, Tay-Sachs	MRI, genetic testing
Spinal cord	Trauma, such as transection during delivery	MRI
Anterior horn cell	Spinal muscular atrophy	EMG, gene testing
Neuromuscular junction (NMJ)	Botulism (presents with weakness of bulbar and extraocular muscles, constipation, dilated and sluggishly responsive pupils)	EMG, stool culture for *Clostridium botulinum*
	Hypermagnesemia (due to maternal treatment with magnesium for pre-eclampsia)	Electrolyte levels
	Neonatal myasthenia gravis	Repetitive nerve stimulation, test dose of acetylcholinesterase inhibitor
Muscle	Neonatal myotonic dystrophy, congenital myopathies, muscular dystrophies, Pompe disease (acid maltase deficiency).	Muscle biopsy, genetic testing.
Systemic causes	Down syndrome, hypothyroidism	Karyotype, thyroid studies

EMG, electromyogram.

TABLE 18.4

CAUSES AND EMPIRIC ANTIBIOTIC TREATMENT OF BACTERIAL MENINGITIS

Neonates (0–3 months)	Empiric Antibiotic Therapy	Older Infants and Children	Empiric Antibiotic Therapy
Group B *Streptococcus* *Escherichia coli* *Listeria monocytogenes*	Ampicillin + cefotaxime	*Streptococcus pneumoniae* Neisseria meningitidis Haemophilus influenzae type b (if unvaccinated)	Cefotaxime (or ceftriaxone) + vancomycin

Diagnosis/Treatment. Early recognition and initiation of antibiotic therapy is essential, even if the situation necessitates administration prior to obtaining lumbar puncture. Corticosteroid treatment is recommended for patients with *Haemophilus influenzae* meningitis by some experts and if administered it should be given along with or within 30 minutes of the first dose of antibiotic. Corticosteroid treatment is recommended for adults with *Streptococcus pneumoniae* meningitis, but its value for children is uncertain. For recommendations regarding empiric antibiotic treatment, refer to Table 18.4.

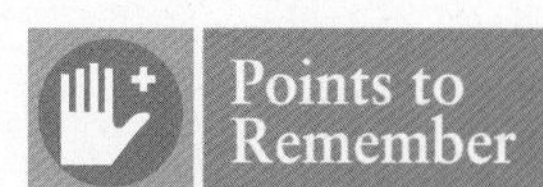

- Findings in CSF in bacterial meningitis:
  - a predominantly polymorphonuclear pleocytosis
  - elevated protein
  - low glucose.

Potential Sequelae

Acute: seizures, ventriculitis, hyponatremia, increased ICP.

Long term: sensorineural hearing loss, hydrocephalus, blindness, paralysis, developmental delay.

Tuberculous meningitis follows a subacute course. Spinal fluid may relatively unremarkable, with low glucose as the only clue. Yield of AFB culture increases with a large volume of CSF (>5 cc fluid). Tuberculomas may be seen on imaging.

Brain abscesses: relatively uncommon in children, classically associated with emboli related to cyanotic congenital heart disease and bacterial endocarditis.

Diagnosis: neuroimaging, either CT or MRI.

Viral Infections—Meningitis and Encephalitis

Viruses can cause both meningitis and encephalitis (inflammation of the brain). *Viral meningitis* is often benign and self-limited. CSF shows fewer white blood cells than seen in bacterial meningitis, usually a mononuclear predominance (although may initially be polymorphonuclear), mildly elevated protein, and normal or slightly decreased glucose. Signs of *viral encephalitis* include fever, altered mental status, and seizures. History should include questions about travel, recent sick contacts, exposure to animals (such as horses, birds, and rodents), mosquitoes, and ticks. Even with a thorough investigation, etiology of viral CNS infections is determined only about half the time.

Enterovirus infections include *Coxsackie*, *echovirus*, numbered enterovirus strains, and *poliomyelitis*. They are transmitted primarily through infected fecal material. Poliomyelitis remains a problem in some developing countries. The virus can infect motor neurons and cause an asymmetrical flaccid paralysis.

Arboviruses are transmitted via blood sucking arthropods. Well-known agents include *La Crosse encephalitis*, *St. Louis encephalitis*, and *western and eastern equine encephalitis*. *West Nile Virus* can cause a flaccid paralysis similar to poliomyelitis.

HSV type 1 is associated with orofacial infections, while type 2 is associated with genital infections. CNS disease can be caused either by primary infection or reactivation of a latent infection. Neonates exposed to HSV during birth may present within 3 weeks of life with encephalitis or disseminated disease. In older patients, HSV can be associated with meningitis or encephalitis. HSV has a predilection for infection of the temporal lobes and can cause hemorrhagic encephalitis. Acyclovir should be started as soon as possible if HSV CNS infection is suspected.

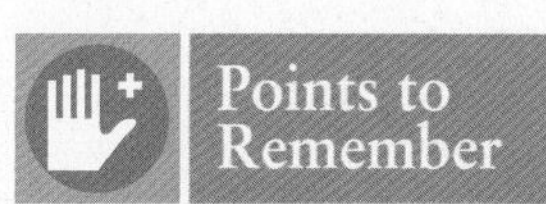

- Infection of the temporal lobes—suspect HSV.

VZV: Primary VZV infection results in chickenpox; reactivation causes herpes zoster, or shingles. Immunocompromised patients may develop encephalitis, meningitis, or disseminated VZV infection.

Congenital CNS Infections

Please refer the chapter on Neonatology.

Special Topics in Neuro-ID

HIV Infection and AIDS

Children and adolescents may present either with congenital infection or primary HIV infection. Neurologic manifestations of HIV infection include those associated with both the initial infection (an aseptic meningoencephalitis or cranial neuropathies) and sequelae of immune compromise. In patients with a low CD4 count, neurologic symptoms, and lesions on brain imaging, consider the following:

- Vasculitis (either due to the HIV infection itself or in association with VZV infection).
- Opportunistic infections (especially when affecting the basal ganglia), including toxoplasmosis (should demonstrate calcification and ring-enhancement after contrast administration) or a cryptococcoma; tuberculosis.
- Primary CNS lymphoma (also ring-enhancing).
- CMV encephalitis.
- PML—demyelination caused by reactivation of JC virus.

Lyme Disease

Lyme disease (also refer to the chapter on Infectious Diseases) in the United States is caused by *Borrelia burgdorferi*, and transmitted by infected deer ticks. Initial symptoms include the erythema chronicum migrans rash and constitutional symptoms. Subsequent infection of the CNS (neuroborreliosis) can have diverse manifestations, including facial palsy, aseptic meningitis, radiculitis, nonspecific white matter changes on MRI, other cranial neuropathies, and a pseudotumor cerebri-like presentation.

Treatment. In the United States, Lyme meningitis or any neurologic symptoms plus CSF pleocytosis is treated with an appropriate parenteral antibiotic. Studies involving the European varieties of *Borrelia* have shown that oral doxycycline is equivalent to treatment with IV ceftriaxone. Recommended duration is 14 days, although it is commonly extended to 28 days. Facial palsy alone can probably be adequately treated with oral doxycycline. There has been controversy over a possible post-Lyme syndrome (residual chronic symptoms following appropriate antibiotic treatment). Several Class I trials have demonstrated in adults that the symptoms of post-Lyme syndrome do not respond to prolonged treatment with antibiotics.

*Worldwide, **neurocysticercosis** is the leading cause of epilepsy.* Because of immigration from Latin America, it is being seen with increasing frequency in the United States. It is caused by the pork tapeworm, *Taenia solium*, and transmitted via ingestion of the eggs, often on food irrigated with water contaminated with human fecal material. After the eggs hatch, the embryos invade the bowel wall, travel hematogenously, and develop as cysticerci in the brain parenchyma. This infection is often asymptomatic. Eventually, the cysticerci die and the cysts become calcified, creating a seizure focus (Fig. 18.1)

Degenerating or dying cysticerci can provoke an inflammatory response and seizures. Cysts in the CSF can cause obstruction of CSF flow and increased ICP. *Treatment*, if necessary, is with albendazole and anticonvulsants.

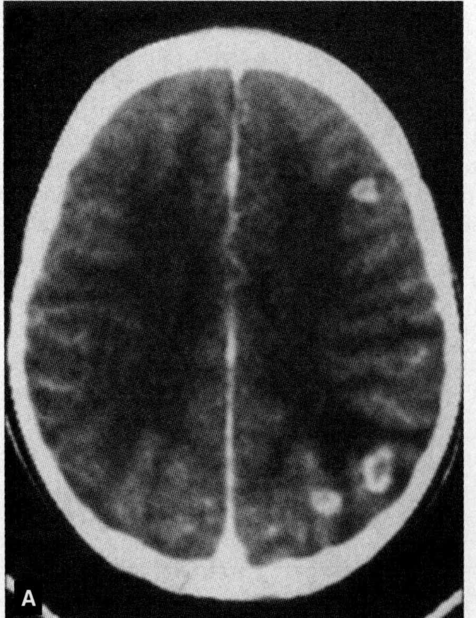

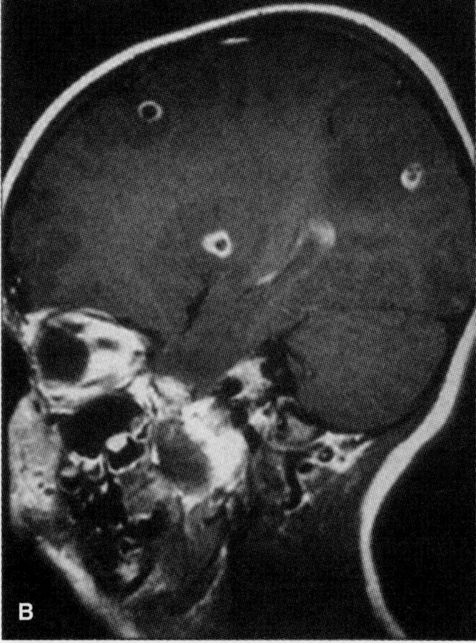

FIGURE 18.1. Neurocysticercosis. (**A**) Cysticercosis. Appearance of head (CT scan). (**B**) Cysticercosis. Appearance of head (MRI). (Reprinted with permission from Ludwig S. *Visual Handbook of Pediatrics and Child Health: The Core*. Philadelphia, PA: Lippincott Williams & Wilkins, 2008.)

Degenerative Conditions

Leukodystrophies

Overview: The leukodystrophies are degenerative conditions affecting primarily the white matter. Suspicion should be raised with a history of loss of milestones or intellectual decline and a gait disorder or signs of spasticity. Seizures can be variably present, sometimes later in the disease course. Most leukodystrophies have subtypes categorized by age of onset (infantile, juvenile, adult), with infantile onset being most common.

Adrenoleukodystrophy (ALD) is the most common, affecting 1 in 10,000 males (X-linked). The most common subtype is the cerebral form, which presents in boys aged 5 to 8 years with cognitive impairment, spasticity, and seizures. The gene mutated in ALD controls the transport of very long chain fatty acids (VLCFA) into the peroxisome, where they normally undergo beta oxidation. Thus, VLCFA accumulate, and ALD can be diagnosed by detection of elevated VLCFA. The characteristic MRI shows demyelination first in occipital regions, progressing anteriorly. Potential therapies include dietary therapy (Lorenzo's oil) and bone marrow transplantation.

There are two leukodystrophies caused by lysosomal storage disorders. **MLD** is caused by a defect in glycolipid metabolism. The enzyme *arylsulfatase A* is required to convert sulfatides to ceramides, so sulfatides accumulate in lysosomes. **GCL, or Krabbe disease,** is caused by a deficiency in *galactocerebrosidase* (GALC), leading to accumulation of galactosylsphingosine in lysosomes. Diagnosis is made by assaying GALC enzyme activity in leukocytes.

Two leukodystrophies that can present with macrocephaly are **Canavan disease** (spongy degeneration of the cerebral white matter). Inheritance is AR, and there is a high carrier rate in the Ashkenazi Jewish population. Diagnosis: elevated urinary N-acetylaspartic acid. **Alexander disease** is caused by mutation in *GFAP*. Inheritance is AD, but most mutations are de novo. MRI changes are seen, predominantly in frontal regions.

Pelizaeus-Merzbacher disease is an X-linked disorder of myelin formation. It is caused by deletion or duplication in the *PLP* gene and presents with nystagmus and spasticity.

Lysosomal storage disorders, peroxisomal diseases, and **neuronal ceroid lipofuscinoses** can have marked neurologic sequelae. See the chapter "Genetics and Metabolism" for further discussion.

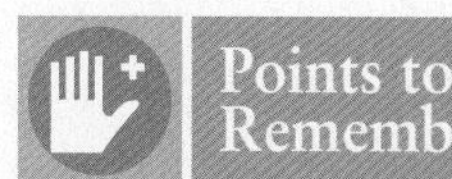

- Canavan disease and Alexander disease are the two leukodystrophies that present with macrocephaly. Tay-Sachs disease (a lysosomal storage disorder in which lack of the enzyme hexosaminidase A causes the accumulation of GM2 gangliosides in neurons) can also present with loss of milestones and macrocephaly.

Mitochondrial Cytopathies

Overview

Mitochondria provide energy for the production of ATP through oxidative phosphorylation. There are five respiratory chains of enzymes (complexes I to V), with subunits encoded either by mitochondrial or nuclear DNA. Inheritance of mitochondrial defects may be either AR (nDNA) or maternal (mtDNA).

Clinical Presentation

Multiple systems are affected, usually those requiring high levels of energy. Some examples of these diseases include skeletal or cardiac myopathies, diabetes mellitus, hearing loss, and retinitis pigmentosa.

Diagnosis

Evaluation of serum lactate, serum pyruvate, CSF lactate, and urine organic acids are useful initial studies. Muscle biopsy to quantify activity of the different complexes or the presence of ragged red fibers may be required. Sequencing of the mitochondrial genome is now available.

- **MELAS** (mitochondrial encephalopathy with lactic acidosis and stroke-like episodes) is caused by mutations in the leucine tRNA.
- **MERRF** (myoclonic epilepsy with ragged-red fibers) is caused by mutations in the lysine tRNA.
- **Kearns-Sayre syndrome** consists of external ophthalmoplegia, retinitis pigmentosa, and myopathy, and or/ataxia and is caused by large-scale deletions of mDNA.
- **Leigh encephalopathy** presents in infancy and can be caused by a number of different mutations causing deficiency in pyruvate dehydrogenase or the various complexes.
- **NARP** (neuropathy, ataxia, retinitis pigmentosa) is caused by the same mutation in the mitochondrial ATPase-6 gene that if present in a higher percentage will cause Leigh encephalopathy.
- **Alpers syndrome,** one of the mitochondrial depletion syndromes, presents with gray matter degeneration and liver failure and is caused by mutations in the mitochondrial DNA polymerase (*POLG*) gene.

Treatment

Largely supportive, including avoidance of metabolic stressors. Supplementation with various vitamins and cofactors ("mitochondrial cocktail") may be of some benefit.

Miscellaneous Mutations

In typical cases of **Rett syndrome**, girls initially develop normally until 6 to 12 months of age, and then developmental regression occurs and microcephaly develops. Typical features include hang wringing, intermittent hyperventilation, and autistic behavior. Most cases are caused by mutations in *MeCP2*, involved in transcriptional repression.

Wilson disease (hepatolenticular degeneration) is caused by a defect in a copper transporting protein causing liver cirrhosis and deposition of copper in the basal ganglia. Degeneration of the basal ganglia causes extrapyramidal symptoms (dystonia, chorea). Inheritance is AR. *Diagnosis* can be made by finding Kayser-Fleischer rings around the iris, low levels of serum ceruloplasmin, or large quantities of copper in a liver biopsy. *Treatment* is copper chelation or liver transplant.

Menkes disease (kinky hair disease) is also caused by a defect in a copper transporting protein, causing deficiencies in copper-containing enzymes. This results in gray matter degeneration, seizures, and the pathognomic kinky hair. Patients have both low serum copper and ceruloplasmin levels; treatment is parenteral copper.

Lesch-Nyhan syndrome is caused by a disorder of purine metabolism. It is characterized by hyperuricemia, spasticity, choreoathetosis, and self-injurious behavior. It is an X-linked disorder caused by mutations in the enzyme HGPRT.

Developmental Malformations and Static Neurologic Deficits

Neural Tube Defects

Closure of the neural tube occurs during the fourth gestational week. The incidence of **neural tube defects** has declined with maternal folic acid supplementation.

- **Anencephaly** results from disruption or failure of rostral neuropore closure.
- **Spina bifida** refers to failure of fusion of the caudal vertebral column, allowing herniation of meninges (**meningocele**) or meninges plus spinal cord tissue or roots (**meningomyelocele**).
- **Spina bifida occulta** occurs when the posterior vertebral arches fail to fuse, without herniation of meninges or tissue.
- A **tethered cord** occurs when a defect causes restricted movement of the spinal cord roots. Initial symptoms may be subtle, including bowel and bladder dysfunction.
- **Sacral agenesis** (absence of the coccyx and lower sacral vertebrae) is associated poor maternal glucose control during pregnancy complicated by diabetes.

Most children with lumbar or lumbosacral meningomyelocele also have **Chiari II** malformations. This hindbrain malformation is characterized by downward displacement of the medulla and fourth ventricle, kinking of the medulla, and protrusion of the cerebellar tonsils through the foramen magnum. This can result in impaired outflow of CSF and hydrocephalus. A **syrinx**, or enlargement of the central canal, is often present. In contrast, a **Chiari I** malformation refers to downward displacement of the cerebellar tonsils alone. A **Dandy-Walker** malformation is characterized by agenesis of the cerebellar vermis and cystic dilation of the fourth ventricle (Fig. 18.2).

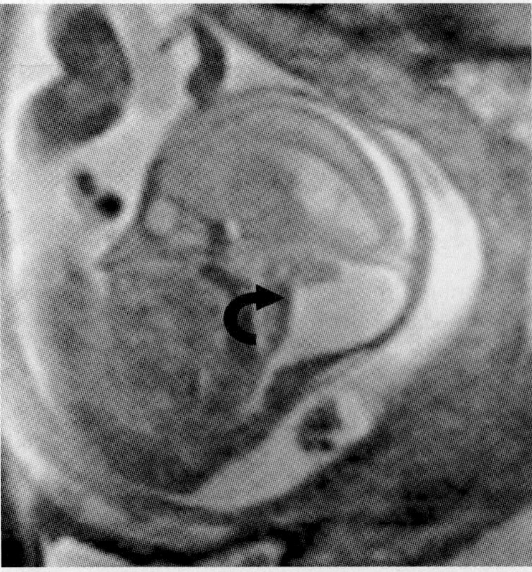

FIGURE 18.2. Sagittal T2 weighted image of a 22-week gestation demonstrates a Dandy-Walker cyst with absent inferior vermis. (Reprinted with permission from MacDonald MG, Seshia MMK, Mullett MD, et al. *Avery's Neonatology Pathophysiology & Management of the Newborn*. 6th ed. Philadelphia, PA: Lippincott Williams & Wilkins, 2005.)

Midline Defects

Holoprosencephaly is a disorder of the cleavage of the forebrain. In order of increasing severity, holoprosencephaly may be lobar, semilobar, or alobar. It can be associated with trisomy 13, 18, and defects in the sonic hedgehog signaling pathway. Children are at high risk for associated hypothalamic-pituitary dysfunction.

Septo-optic dysplasia is also a defect in midline cleavage, with agenesis of the septum pellucidum and hypoplasia of the optic nerves, and often agenesis or hypoplasia of the corpus callosum.

ACC can be found in isolation, or in conjunction with other structural anomalies or genetic syndromes. There is an extremely high risk of developmental delay associated with ACC, but individuals can also be completely normal, with this noted as an incidental finding.

Neurogenesis occurs in the walls of the lateral ventricles and then neurons migrate to their final location in the cortical plate.

- **Lissencephaly** refers to smooth brain, reflecting lack of successful neuronal migration. **Pachygyria** is a less severe form, with broad, simplified gyri.
- **Polymicrogyria** consists of small and excessive gyri. It occurs because of some sort of insult prior to the fifth month of gestation.
- **Heterotopias** are islands of abnormally placed neurons. There maybe complete arrest of migration (as seen in **bilateral periventricular nodular heterotopia**, which may be associated with filamin mutations), or an abnormal layer of cells (as seen in **subcortical laminar heterotopia**, or band heterotopia, which is related to mutations in the doublecortin gene).
- **Schizencephaly**, or cleft brain, is characterized by a cleft extending from the cortical surface to the ventricular system. It is frequently accompanied by heterotopias.
  - In contrast, porencephaly, or **porencephalic cysts**, arise as sequelae of intrauterine stroke or infection, as necrotic tissue reorganizes. **Arachnoid cysts** are fluid filled cavities within the arachnoid space, often incidentally noted. Infrequently they cause compression.
  - In contrast to schizencephalic clefts, neither porencephalic nor arachnoid cysts are associated with migrational defects.

Points to Remember

- Asymmetric crying facies, a relatively common finding in the newborn nursery, is caused by hypoplasia of the depressor anguli oris. It is considered a minor congenital anomaly and has only cosmetic consequences. This is in contrast to a congenital facial nerve paralysis, which can be associated with trauma or developmental causes (and potentially associated with a number of syndromes), which can lead to difficulty with eyelid closure (leaving the cornea susceptible to damage) and to feeding difficulties.

Craniosynostosis refers to premature fusion of one or more of the cranial sutures. It may be associated with various genetic conditions, such as Apert, Crouzon, and Pfeiffer syndromes.

With the successful institution of the "Back to Sleep" campaign, which has reduced the incidence of SIDS, there has been an increase in **positional plagiocephaly** associated with decreased tummy time. This needs to be differentiated from lambdoidal craniosynostosis and can often be treated conservatively, such as with a positioning pillow.

CP is by definition a static, nonprogressive defect in the motor system. For unknown reasons, cortical motor neurons are particularly susceptible to injury associated with extreme prematurity. CP may be classified as spastic, dyskinetic (dystonic or choreoathetoid) or ataxic-hypotonic. *Treatment* may include addressing increased tone through aggressive PT and OT, bracing to prevent flexion contractures and maximize function, pharmacotherapy with lorazepam and/or baclofen, injection of muscles with botulinum toxin, and orthopedic surgery.

CN defects: There are several noteworthy congenital defects in CNs. **Duane syndrome** is caused by failure of normal development of the abducens nerve (CNVI), resulting in miswiring of the lateral rectus muscle and impaired abduction of the eye. **Moebius syndrome** is characterized by bifacial weakness and abnormal eye movements, relating to abnormal development of CN nuclei (usually CNVI and VII).

SEIZURES

General Approach to Seizures

Seizures are abnormal electrical discharges in the brain. To be diagnosed with epilepsy, a child must have two or more unprovoked seizures. When eliciting a history, ask what the seizure looked like and encourage imitation. Was the child responsive during the seizure? Did the head turn or the eyes deviate? How long did the seizure last? Was there loss of bladder or bowel continence or tongue biting?

Points to Remember

- To be diagnosed with epilepsy, a child must have two or more unprovoked seizures.

Seizures are classified on the basis of two features:

1. Simple versus complex and partial versus generalized.
   - Simple seizure: no alteration of consciousness.
   - Complex seizure: with alteration of consciousness.
   - Partial seizure: seizure arises in a part of the brain, giving rise to focal findings such as head turning and eye deviation.
   - Generalized seizure: entire brain involved.

   Seizure types include tonic, tonic-clonic, atonic (drops), absence (petit mal), myoclonic (jerks).

Points to Remember

- By definition, if clonic activity is present on both sides, the seizure is generalized, but it may have started with a partial seizure that then secondarily generalized.

2. Diagnostic evaluation of **first-time nonfebrile seizure**.

Points to Remember

- **A first seizure includes all occurrences within a 24-hour period with recovery of consciousness between seizures. An EEG is recommended.**

Points to Remember

- **Following a first-time seizure, the risk of seizure recurrence with a normal EEG is about 25%; with an abnormal EEG it is about 50%.**

Points to Remember

- **Always consider cytochrome P450 interactions when prescribing AEDs.**

A practice parameter has been published by the American Academy of Neurology, and applies to children older than 1 month (excluding neonatal seizures) (see Suggested Readings). It applies to seizures with no immediately provoking cause (febrile seizures, seizures due to trauma, infection, electrolyte abnormalities, etc.). It does not apply to status epilepticus (a seizure lasting more than 30 minutes). Definition of a first seizure includes those with multiple recurrences within a 24-hour period with recovery of consciousness between seizures.

Laboratory tests should be ordered on the basis of clinical history or findings, and toxicology screening should be strongly considered. Routine lumbar puncture is not recommended but should be strongly considered for young children (<6 months), patients with persistently altered mental status or failure to return to baseline, or meningeal signs. In the acute setting, with a nonfocal neurologic examination, the likelihood that a head CT scan would reveal an abnormality that would warrant a therapeutic intervention is quite low. Emergency imaging should be considered if the child does not return to baseline or has a focal deficit. MRI is the nonurgent imaging modality of choice, and the most likely to find subtle causes of seizures such as heterotopias or hippocampal sclerosis.

EEG is recommended. An EEG done within 24 hours is most likely to show abnormalities, either epileptiform activity or slowing. However, as some abnormalities, such as slowing, may be transient, it is reasonable to delay performing an EEG until 24 to 48 hours after the seizure. EEG should be performed with the child both awake and asleep, as well as with hyperventilation (if not contraindicated, such as with structural heart disease or asthma) and intermittent photic stimulation.

In general, in counseling parents in the acute setting following a first-time seizure in a developmentally normal child, there is a **one in three risk of recurrence.**

Treatment

AEDs are generally not started after a first unprovoked seizure in a child or adolescent, given the risk of side effects and the low likelihood of recurrence. Starting treatment after the first seizure does not affect the ultimate rate of remission.

Initiation and choice of AED therapy should be based on seizure description, EEG results, clinical setting, and compliance. For example, carbamazepine and oxcarbazepine are good choices for seizures with a partial onset. For JME, a medication like zonisamide with once daily dosing may promote compliance in adolescents. Topiramate may be a better choice than valproic acid in an overweight child with generalized epilepsy. Always consider cytochrome P450 interactions when prescribing AEDs. For example, lamotrigine can be a good choice for adolescent girls, especially given its lower risk of teratogenicity, but it will lower levels of oral contraceptives.

Specific Antiepileptics

Phenobarbital is usually the first medication of choice in the neonatal period. It is easily dosed, with an initial 20 mg/kg load leading to a blood level of 20 (with usual goal of 20 to 40). It must slowly be weaned because of the risk of irritability and withdrawal seizures. If a child continues to require AED therapy, transition to another agent should be accomplished by the age of 1 year due to possible cognitive effects of phenobarbital.

Phenytoin is one of the oldest AEDs (first used in 1938). It is inexpensive and can be dosed once a day in adults, but requires more frequent dosing in children. Long-term use can cause cerebellar atrophy and gingival hyperplasia. It has a relatively narrow therapeutic window, as its metabolism transitions abruptly from first-order to zero-order kinetics. There is a risk of fetal hydantoin syndrome for infants born to mothers taking phenytoin.

Carbamazepine is an excellent choice for seizures with a partial onset. However, it can worsen generalized epilepsy syndromes. It autoinduces its own metabolism, so levels will drift down with time. Blood counts and liver enzymes should be monitored. It can interfere with thyroid function.

Oxcarbazepine is a cousin of carbamazepine and also works best for seizures with a partial onset. Patients should be monitored for hyponatremia. In contrast to carbamazepine, there is no reported leukopenia or aplastic anemia.

Valproic acid is particularly effective for generalized seizures with a spike-wave appearance on EEG. It also has mood-stabilizing properties. Significant side effects include weight gain, hair loss, and pancreatitis. CBC and CMP should be monitored. Avoid in adolescent girls because of the risk of teratogenicity.

Lamotrigine is a good choice for generalized seizures, including absence seizures. It may exacerbate myoclonic jerks. It is necessary to increase the dose very slowly initially to lessen the risk of an idiosyncratic Stevens-Johnson rash, so it is not a good choice when immediate onset of action is required. Because of drug interactions, it must be started at a lower dose with concomitant valproic acid use.

Ethosuximide is the first-line agent for childhood absence epilepsy, but it may not be adequate therapy in cases of juvenile absence epilepsy. Its major side effect is GI upset.

Topiramate can be effective in both generalized and partial onset seizures. It can cause acute angle-closure glaucoma and decreased sweating. It may cause glaucoma and decreased sweating. Some patients experience cognitive dulling. It may promote weight loss.

Zonisamide is similar to topiramate. Because of a very long half-life, it can be dosed daily. Side effects include kidney stones, decreased sweating, and weight loss (less than with topiramate).

Levetiracetam works for many seizure types, is excreted by the kidneys, and it reaches therapeutic levels quickly. However, there is a high risk of irritability in children, which may limit its use.

Ketogenic diet is a high-fat diet, which simulates a fasting state, forcing the brain to use ketone bodies for fuel. Its anticonvulsant properties are the subject of ongoing studies but are currently poorly understood.

Vagus nerve stimulator can be used as an adjunct in cases of intractable epilepsy.

Selected Seizures and Epilepsy Syndromes

Neonatal seizures: see the chapter on Neonatology

Febrile seizures typically occur between 6 months and 6 years of age. There is often a family history of febrile seizures. Circulating cytokines associated with illness may trigger the seizure, rather than the fever itself. Parents should be reassured that they do not need to administer around the clock antipyretics when children are ill in an attempt to prevent a febrile seizure. The American Academy of Pediatrics has published a management algorithm (see Suggested Readings). Simple febrile seizures are defined as seizures that last less than 15 minutes and do not recur within 24 hours. Management includes addressing the source of fever and consideration of lumbar puncture for younger infants. Routine head imaging or EEG is NOT recommended.

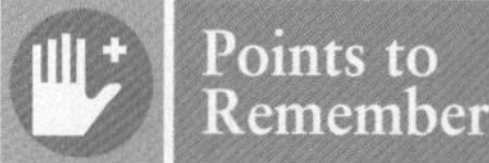

Points to Remember

- For febrile seizures, routine head imaging or EEG is NOT recommended. Circulating cytokines are thought to trigger the seizure event rather than fever itself.

Infantile spasms typically have onset around 6 months. The seizures consist of clusters of arm flexion with head bobs. Infantile spasms are most common just after awakening and rarely occur during sleep. The pathognomonic EEG finding is *hypsarrhythmia*, a high voltage, chaotic pattern, which is present interictally. The initial evaluation is aimed at identifying an underlying etiology. There is a long list of disorders associated with infantile spasms, including tuberous sclerosis, Down syndrome, and congenital brain malformations. Approximately 25% to 33% of cases are classified as cryptogenic, with no underlying etiology determined after a comprehensive evaluation. These infants have the best prognosis for ultimate developmental outcome if their preceding development was normal. Infantile spasms can eventually evolve into **Lennox-Gastaut syndrome**, with a disorganized EEG and multiple seizure types. The gold standard treatment of infantile spasms is ACTH, although there is credible data supporting the use of prednisolone, the ketogenic diet, and topiramate. Vigabatrin is the first choice for infants with tuberous sclerosis, although it can cause a permanent visual field defect.

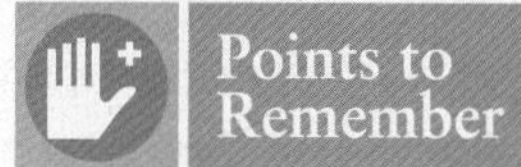

Points to Remember

- The gold standard treatment for infantile spasms is ACTH. The pathognomonic EEG finding is *hypsarrhythmia*.

Absence seizures can occur in multiple forms of epilepsy; however, absence epilepsy refers to epilepsy defined solely by absence seizures. Absence epilepsy is typically defined by age of onset (see Table 18.5 below). Both forms of absence epilepsy have a characteristic three cycles per second spike and wave on EEG and can be provoked by hyperventilation.

JME consists of a combination of absence seizures, generalized seizures, and myoclonic jerks (typically most noticeable in the morning). First-time generalized tonic-clonic seizures may be provoked by sleep deprivation (going off to college for the first time). JME is not outgrown. Treatment is with valproic acid, topiramate, lamotrigine, or levetiracetam and tailored on the basis of which seizure types are most prominent.

TABLE 18.5

CHILDHOOD VERSUS JUVENILE ABSENCE EPILEPSY

Absence Seizure Type	Childhood Absence Epilepsy (CAE)	Juvenile Absence Epilepsy (JAE)
Age	Between ages 5 to 10 years	Onset between 7 and 16 years
Distinguishing feature	Usually outgrown by puberty	Can be associated with generalized tonic-clonic seizures, less benign course
First-line treatment	Ethosuximide	Valproic acid or lamotrigine

BECTS, or benign rolandic epilepsy, is the most common epilepsy syndrome in children. There are characteristic centrotemporal spikes, especially with sleep, on EEG. A typical seizure occurs shortly after falling asleep, with twitching on one side of the face that may spread to an arm. These seizures may rarely generalize or occur during the day. If treatment is indicated (which it may not be, if seizures are infrequent and only at night), carbamazepine and levetiracetam are the usual choices. BECTS has its onset between ages 4 to 12 years and is outgrown in puberty.

Myoclonic epilepsies are often catastrophic and associated with degenerative syndromes with poor prognoses.

Mimickers of Seizure

Breathholding spells can be pallid or cyanotic. There is frequently a family history, and there may be an association with iron deficiency anemia. A small convulsion can be witnessed at the end of the spell.

- **Syncope:** a postsyncopal convulsion can often be seen.
- **Pseudoseizures,** or psychogenic nonepileptic seizures can coexist in patients with true seizures.
- **Sandifer syndrome:** arching associated with severe gastroesophageal reflux.
- **Infantile self-gratification:** typically seen in young girls.

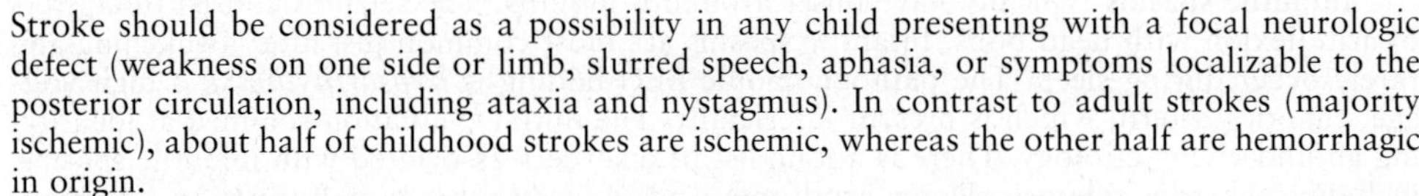

CEREBROVASCULAR DISEASE

Stroke

Overview/Clinical Manifestations

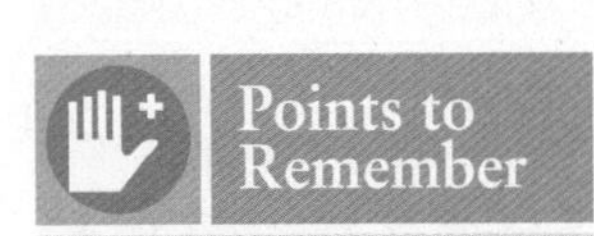

Points to Remember

- In contrast to adult strokes (majority ischemic), about half of childhood strokes are ischemic, whereas the other half are hemorrhagic in origin.

Stroke should be considered as a possibility in any child presenting with a focal neurologic defect (weakness on one side or limb, slurred speech, aphasia, or symptoms localizable to the posterior circulation, including ataxia and nystagmus). In contrast to adult strokes (majority ischemic), about half of childhood strokes are ischemic, whereas the other half are hemorrhagic in origin.

Particularly at-risk populations include children with **sickle cell disease** and **congenital heart disease** with a right-to-left shunt. A thorough history should be undertaken, which may reveal **VZV or HIV** infection (causing a vasculopathy), recurrent episodes with illness or hyperventilation, or a history of cognitive decline or regression (**MELAS, moyamoya disease**), or symptoms suggestive of a deep vein thrombosis or a family history of **thrombophilia** or early stroke. A history of **trauma**, especially to the head and neck, may suggest dissection as a cause. Even a relatively minor trauma can cause a tear in the intimal layer of an artery, with subsequent formation of clot at the site of the tear, which can then embolize.

Diagnosis

- Evaluation of a child with suspected stroke should begin with an MRI of the brain and an MRA (or CTA) of the intracranial vessels. Stroke in a nonvascular distribution raises concern for MELAS or for a VST, and thus an MR venogram would be indicated.
- In suspected dissection, MRA of the neck (fat saturated T1 sequence is particularly helpful and must be specifically requested) and/or CTA of the neck from the aortic arch to the circle of Willis should be performed. Conventional angiography may be required to make a firm diagnosis of dissection.
- EKG (to evaluate for supraventricular tachycardia) and echocardiogram should be performed, including testing for a patent foramen ovale.
- Laboratory evaluation should be directed toward screening for hypercoagulability.

In children, the etiology of stroke is often multifactorial; therefore, thorough investigation is warranted.

Treatment

- tPA is not FDA approved for the treatment of ischemic stroke in patients younger than 18 years. However, its use may be considered in exceptional cases, especially when less than 3 hours from onset of symptoms. For hemorrhagic stroke, consider administration of fresh frozen plasma and platelets.
- For dissections, anticoagulation is generally appropriate to prevent the formation of further clot while the tear heals.

VST may occur in infants, typically after an inciting factor, such as dehydration or sepsis. Hypercoagulability evaluation should be performed. In teenage girls, oral contraceptives can predispose to the formation of blood clots. VST should be considered in cases of new headache, especially with evidence of increased ICP. Otitic hydrocephalus, caused by thrombosis of a transverse sinus as a complication of untreated otitis media, was seen more frequently prior to the era of antibiotics.

Vascular malformations are being diagnosed with increased frequency, in particular as incidental findings in scans performed for other reasons. Vascular malformations are characterized by the component elements and their connections; for example, in an AVM, the artery and vein are directly connected, without an intervening capillary bed. A CCM represents a cluster of abnormally dilated vessels. *Vein of Galen malformations* are due to the failure of this midline vein to regress during fetal development. Infants may present with increasing head circumference, a bruit audible at the fontanelle, and congestive heart failure. *Aneurysms* are abnormal dilations of arteries, and can be saccular or fusiform. The risks of intervention versus the risk of rupture, bleeding, or rebleeding of vascular anomalies such as these must be carefully weighed. Options may include observation, surgery, irradiation, or neurointerventional techniques such as glue embolization or coiling.

Moyamoya ("puff of smoke") disease is caused by progressive stenosis of intracranial vessels, causing formation of abnormal collaterals that appear on imaging as a puff of smoke. Children can present with recurrent TIAs or stroke.

PERIPHERAL NERVE AND NEUROMUSCULAR JUNCTION

Brachial Plexus

Erb's palsy ("waiter's tip") is caused by injury to the upper trunk of the brachial plexus, often due to stretching related to shoulder dystocia during delivery. Clinically, the shoulder is slumped and internally rotated, the elbow extended, and the forearm flexed. The biceps reflex on the affected side is diminished, and there will be an asymmetric Moro reflex.

A **Klumpke palsy** is caused by an injury to the lower trunk of the brachial plexus, primarily affecting the flexors of the wrist and fingers. Grasp reflex will be lost, and a *Horner's syndrome* (ptosis, miosis, anhydrosis) may be present because of injury to the cervical sympathetic fibers.

A **radial nerve palsy** ("Saturday night palsy") is caused by compression of the radial nerve as it spirals around the humerus, for example, by falling asleep with an arm draped over the edge of a chair or by improper use of crutches. There will be a wrist drop and inability to extend the fingers.

An idiopathic brachial plexitis (**Parsonage-Turner syndrome**) can occur, with variable pain and weakness.

Peripheral Nerve

Bell's palsy refers to an acute paralysis of the face, specifically related to those muscles innervated by CNVII (the facial nerve). A facial paralysis due to a peripheral cause should also have associated weakness of the forehead (in contrast to facial droop caused by a cortical stroke) and alteration of taste in the anterior two-thirds of the tongue. There may be hyperacusis, due to paralysis of the stapedius muscle. Bell's palsy may be due to an antecedent viral infection, but other causes should be considered, including herpes infection (**Ramsay Hunt syndrome**, examine ear canal for evidence of vesicles), Lyme disease, or otitis media. Initial treatment is typically with oral corticosteroids and lubrication of the cornea, which is at risk for ulceration due to incomplete eye closure. There is less support for empiric use of acyclovir.

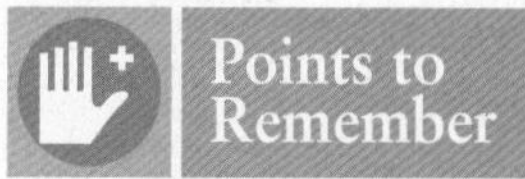

- Ramsay Hunt syndrome is a result of a VZV infection of the CNS. Facial weakness, hearing loss, and vertigo are examples of symptoms that may be associated with this syndrome.

GBS, or AIDP is caused by autoimmune-mediated demyelination of peripheral nerves and spinal nerve roots. An illness such as an upper respiratory tract infection or gastroenteritis often precedes the development of symptoms. The weakness may be subtle at first, and there are often complaints of pain. Classically, the weakness is symmetric and ascending, with loss of tendon reflexes. The hallmark finding on CSF is *cytoalbuminologic dissociation* (elevated protein without pleocytosis). Early in the course of the disease, CSF may be normal. Paralysis of respiratory muscles and autonomic dysfunction may occur; therefore, careful monitoring is required until the trajectory of decline is determined. Patients usually reach the nadir after about 3 weeks. Treatment is plasmapheresis or infusion of IVIg; there is no role for steroids.

- In the **Miller Fisher** variant, there is a triad of ophthalmoplegia, ataxia, and areflexia.
- In CIDP, the onset of weakness is usually slower, and symptoms progress over at least 2 months. Attacks often recur, and immune modulatory therapy may be required.

Neuromuscular Junction

Myasthenia gravis should be suspected with symptoms such as fatigable weakness, especially of proximal muscles, ptosis, diplopia (with variable involvement of eye muscles), difficulty chewing or swallowing, or dysphonia. Autoantibodies are often detected, either directed against the acetylcholine receptor or the MuSK tyrosine kinase receptor.

Diagnosis is classically made via the *Tensilon test* (edrophonium, an acetylcholinesterase inhibitor, will cause a brief improvement in symptoms).

Treatment is symptomatic, with the administration of an oral anticholinesterase inhibitor (Mestinon or pyridostigmine) and then immunomodulatory therapy (steroids, IVIg, plasmapheresis, or steroid-sparing agents). Thymectomy is generally performed after symptoms have stabilized. Certain medications should be avoided, as they may worsen symptoms and precipitate a myasthenic crisis (e.g., aminoglycoside antibiotics, penicillamine).

Neonatal myasthenia gravis is seen when infants are born to affected mothers. Affected infants may be hypotonic and have difficulty sucking and crying. The illness is transient. This is in contrast to **congenital myasthenic syndromes**, caused by mutations in components of the acetylcholine synapse components; these variably respond to anticholinesterase treatment.

In cases of flaccid paralysis, the possibility of **tick paralysis** should be entertained. This is caused by a neurotoxin produced by a tick, which may be well-hidden in the patient's hair. Recovery promptly ensues following removal of the tick.

Muscle Disease

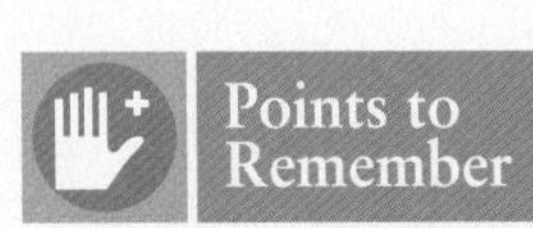

- Gowers' sign indicates weakness of the proximal muscles, primarily of the lower limbs. Patients use their hands to "walk" up their lower limbs to get from a squatting to a standing position.

Muscular dystrophies are diseases with progressive myofiber degeneration caused by specific genetic mutations, often in cytoskeletal elements important in the structural integrity of these contracting cells, or in extracellular matrix molecules. The most common muscular dystrophy is **DMD**, caused by a deletion in the *dystrophin* gene. This is an X-linked disorder. Boys may have elevations in CK levels even before they become symptomatic. The classic finding is *pseudohypertrophy* of the calves as fatty infiltration occurs and a *Gowers' sign*. **Becker muscular dystrophy** is also due to a mutation in dystrophin, but boys are less severely affected. Corticosteroid treatment in DMD prolongs function. Patients are now surviving beyond teenage years and should be followed by a multidisciplinary team, including a neurologist, a cardiologist (to follow for development of a cardiomyopathy) and a pulmonologist (to address issues of pulmonary toilet and respiratory support).

When liver enzymes are elevated (especially when AST > ALT), a muscle source should be suspected and the CK checked. However, not all muscular dystrophies are associated with elevations in CK.

The typical appearance of an adult male patient with **myotonic dystrophy** is frontal balding, atrophy of facial muscles and bifacial weakness, and inability to release a handshake (due to myotonia, or inability of the muscles to relax). Classical myotonic dystrophy is due to an expansion of a triplet repeat in the *DMPK* gene. This disorder displays anticipation, such that offspring of an affected mother are more severely affected, resulting in **congenital myotonic dystrophy**. These children are hypotonic and weak, with facial diplegia. Myotonia appears later, as do cardiac conduction defects, cataracts, and diabetes.

Congenital myopathies, in contrast to the muscular dystrophies, do not show progressive degeneration of the myofibers. Diagnosis often requires muscle biopsy.

Dermatomyositis is an idiopathic inflammatory myopathy. It is a systemic illness and may be accompanied by a low-grade fever and elevated inflammatory markers. Weakness is proximal, and bulbar muscles may be affected. There is a skin rash, which may include a violaceous discoloration of the eyelids (*heliotrope rash*) and *Gottron papules* on the knuckles. **Polymyositis** is rare in children.

Central Nervous System Trauma

Overview: According to the *Monro-Kelly doctrine*, the cranial vault is a fixed volume, with three components: blood, CSF, and brain. Should the volume of one component increase, another must decrease to compensate. For example, if a TBI causes intraparenchymal bleeding, ICP will increase. This will displace CSF and reduce the flow of arterial blood into the brain. If there is not sufficient compensation, brain tissue will herniate to relieve pressure. Management of increased ICP is discussed in the chapter "Critical Care and Emergency Medicine."

Typical patterns of injury are seen following trauma. *Contrecoup injury*, contralateral to the point of impact, occurs especially in cases of acceleration injury. On MRI, *diffuse axonal injury* can be appreciated, referring to the result of shear injury. *Cerebral contusions* result in *cytotoxic edema*, which is increased water content caused by cellular injury. In contrast to *vasogenic edema* (due to breakdown of the blood-brain barrier, such as that seen with brain tumors), cytotoxic edema is not responsive to steroid treatment. *Epidural hematomas* occur when blood accumulates between the skull and the dura, such as following a skull fracture. There is typically a lucid interval between the time of the injury and the rapid accumulation of blood from damaged arterioles. Radiographically, epidural hematomas have a lentiform appearance. In contrast, *subdural hematomas* are collections of blood between the dura and the arachnoid, but also cause compression of the underlying parenchyma. Trauma can also cause *subarachnoid hemorrhages* and *intraventricular hemorrhages*.

Coma is a disorder of level of arousal, in which a person is unable to respond to external stimuli. In cases of severe brain injury, coma may evolve into a PVS. In PVS, there can be spontaneous eye opening, reflexive responses, and sleep-wake cycles, but no evidence of awareness of self or the environment.

Concussion: According to the American Academy of Neurology (see Suggested Readings), **concussion** is a trauma-induced alteration in mental status that may or may not involve loss of consciousness.

- *Grade 1 concussions* involve only transient confusion, no loss of consciousness, and resolution of symptoms within 15 minutes.
- *Grade 2 concussions*, symptoms last for more than 15 minutes.
- Any concussion involving loss of consciousness is a *grade 3*.

Regarding athletic activities, children and adolescents who experience multiple grade 1, a grade 2, or a brief grade 3 concussion should wait 1 week to return to play, assuming complete resolution of symptoms (see Table 22.7). Those who suffer multiple grade 2 or a prolonged grade 3 should wait 2 weeks. Individuals who experience multiple grade 3 concussions should wait 1 month or longer. See the chapter "Orthopedics and Sports Medicine" and http://www.cdc.gov/concussion/clinician.html for more information.

INFLAMMATORY/AUTOIMMUNE DISORDERS

Acute Disseminated Encephalomyelitis

Overview

ADEM typically occurs in younger children, often following a viral infection. *Clinical manifestations*: Patients may present with focal neurologic deficits and alteration of consciousness. Both brain and spinal cord may be involved. Seizures do occur on occasion.

Diagnosis

MRI typically demonstrates fluffy patches that are bright on T2/FLAIR and may enhance with contrast. Spinal fluid examination may demonstrate a monocytic pleocytosis. In suspected demyelinating disease, CSF should also be examined for protein, glucose, oligoclonal bands, IgG index, and possibly myelin basic protein, in addition to testing for possible infectious causes.

Treatment

Children with ADEM and substantial neurologic deficits will benefit from a course of steroids, followed by an oral taper.

Prognosis/Natural History

In general, one-third return to baseline, one-third have some sort of residual deficit, and one-third may not have substantial recovery. ADEM may rarely recur.

Pediatric Multiple Sclerosis

In children, the distinction between recurrent ADEM and MS may initially be difficult to establish. Demyelinating attacks in MS tend to have a different radiographic appearance, including lesions perpendicular to the lateral ventricles (*Dawson's fingers*). Either disorder may demonstrate contrast enhancement on MRI.

When a child has a first demyelinating attack, with brain lesions suspicious for MS, the initial diagnosis is a **CIS**. For a diagnosis of MS, there must be **two or more attacks separated in time and space**, or radiographic evidence of disease progression. Some data support the initiation of immune-modifying therapy after a CIS, to delay subsequent attacks and improve outcome. Options include *glatiramer acetate* or *interferon beta*.

Transverse Myelitis, Optic Neuritis, and Neuromyelitis Optica

Transverse myelitis is demyelination of the spinal cord. It can be a CIS, but can also be associated with MS (usually a small patch of spinal cord involved) or NMO (with three or more segments of the cord involved). In NMO, which is also called *Devic's disease*, patients typically have recurrent attacks of transverse myelitis and/or **optic neuritis**, and a more aggressive course than MS. About half of the cases are associated with a positive NMO antibody, which reacts against the aquaporin-4 channel.

Sleep

Overview: The American Academy of Sleep Medicine divides sleep into two types, NREM and REM sleep. NREM is further subdivided into stage 1, stage 2, and slow wave (previously stages 3 and 4) sleep, each of which is defined by characteristic EEG patterns. NREM and REM sleep cycle multiple times in the course of the night.

The amount of sleep needed changes dramatically with age.

- Infants (3 to 11 months): 14 to 15 hours.
- Toddlers: 12 to 14 hours.
- Preschoolers: 11 to 13 hours.
- School-aged children: 10 to 11 hours.
- Teenagers: 9 to 10 hours.

Sleep Disorders

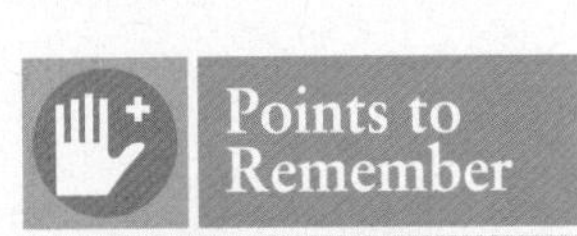

- Both sleep terrors and somnambulism arise from NREM sleep usually without memory of the occurrence. Nightmares arise from REM sleep.

Parasomnias frequently occur in childhood. *Sleep terrors* (pavor nocturnus) present with abrupt arousal from slow wave (NREM) sleep, with signs of intense fear and inconsolable crying. The child is difficult to awaken and has no memory of the event. *Somnambulism* (sleep walking) also arises from NREM sleep. *Nightmares* occur out of REM sleep. Generally, the diagnosis is clear and parasomnias can be managed with reassurance and, if necessary, securing the sleep environment. Rarely, bedtime doses of a medication such as *clonazepam* are employed.

With nocturnal sleep disturbances, seizures are also a possibility, so if there is any question about the diagnosis, a sleep study with extra EEG electrodes is warranted. *Restless leg syndrome* is being increasingly recognized in children. It involves the sensation of needing to move the legs while awake, worse in the evenings, and periodic leg movements during sleep. Sleep studies are also useful to evaluate for *obstructive sleep apnea*, which may contribute to attentional problems and headaches. *Narcolepsy* is a sleep disorder characterized by excessive daytime sleepiness, cataplexy (sudden loss of muscle tone), sleep paralysis, and hypnagogic or hypnopompic hallucinations.

In narcolepsy, an MSLT (nap study) will reveal inappropriate intrusion of REM sleep into wakefulness.

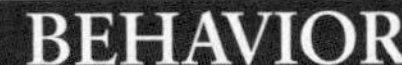

BEHAVIOR

Autism

For further discussion, please refer the Growth and Development chapter.

Overview/Clinical Manifestations

Autism is a disorder of communication. It is characterized by three elements: (1) impaired language, (2) impaired interpersonal interactions, and (3) repetitive behaviors. Signs of autism are generally present by 18 to 24 months of age. Classical autism affects 1:500 children; autism spectrum disorders (including Asperger syndrome) are diagnosed in 1:150. Autism is more common in boys (5:1) and in children with disorders such as Fragile X syndrome, Down syndrome, and NF. Despite popular press, scientific data do not support the idea of an "autism epidemic" or any link to vaccinations.

Diagnosis

Autism is a clinical diagnosis. Recognition begins with routine developmental surveillance as part of well child care. If a child fails to babble or gesture by the age of 12 months, have single words by 16 months, two-word spontaneous speech (not just echolalia) by 24 months, or loss of language or social skills at any age, they should undergo further developmental evaluation. Any child with developmental delay and/or concern for autism should undergo audiologic assessment. Lead screening should be considered. A rigorous diagnosis of autism requires use of one of the standardized interviews or observational rating scales (e.g., the ADOS). Children with a diagnosis of autism should undergo a medical and neurologic evaluation to consider the need for genetic and metabolic testing.

Treatment/Prognosis

Early recognition of children with autism allows for intensive early intervention during the toddler and preschool years, which improves the outcome for most young children with autism.

Attention-Deficit/Hyperactivity Disorder

Overview/Clinical Manifestations

ADHD is one of the most common childhood psychiatric disorders. Symptoms cluster around the domains of inattention, impulsivity, and hyperactivity. Children are commonly referred around the age of 7 years for evaluation of the possibility of ADHD (starting elementary school, with increased academic and social demands).

Differential diagnosis: learning disabilities, absence epilepsy (especially for ADHD, inattentive subtype).

Diagnosis

ADHD is diagnosed on the basis of fulfilling the diagnostic criteria set forth in the *DSM-IV*. A number of standardized questionnaires (e.g., Connors, Vanderbilt) incorporate these criteria and should be completed by both parents and teachers to confirm that impairment occurs in multiple settings. The possibility of comorbid symptoms (learning disorders, oppositional defiant disorder, anxiety, depression, tics) should be explored.

Treatment

Behavioral therapy can play a role, but stimulant medications are the mainstay of therapy. There are a number of *methylphenidate* and *amphetamine* preparations, which vary in their onset and duration of action, as well as delivery systems. *Atomoxetine*, a selective norepinephrine reuptake inhibitor, is also FDA approved for the treatment of ADHD. Alpha2-adrenergic agonists (*clonidine*, *guanfacine*) may also be beneficial.

Children or adolescents with pre-existing heart disease or symptoms suggestive of cardiovascular disease (palpitations, chest pain, syncope, exercise intolerance, family history of sudden death) should be evaluated by a cardiologist prior to considering stimulant therapy. In otherwise healthy individuals, there is no evidence currently supporting the need for routine cardiac evaluation (e.g., EKG, ECHO) prior to starting ADHD medication. Height and weight should be monitored on a regular basis, as well as re-evaluating the efficacy of medication and need for continuation.

PHAKOMATOSES

Neurofibromatosis

Overview

The most common form of NF is **NF1** (1:3,000 vs. 1:40,000 for NF2). NF1 is caused by mutation in the neurofibromin gene on chromosome 17.

Clinical Manifestations/Diagnosis

NF1 is a clinical diagnosis, based on fulfilling two or more of the following NIH criteria:

- Six or more café au lait macules (>5 mm in children, >15 mm after puberty).
- Two or more neurofibromas or one plexiform neurofibroma (Fig. 18.3).
- Axillary or inguinal freckling.
- Optic glioma.
- Two or more Lisch nodules (iris hamartomas).
- Distinctive bone lesion (sphenoid dysplasia or tibial pseudoarthrosis).
- First-degree relative with NF1.

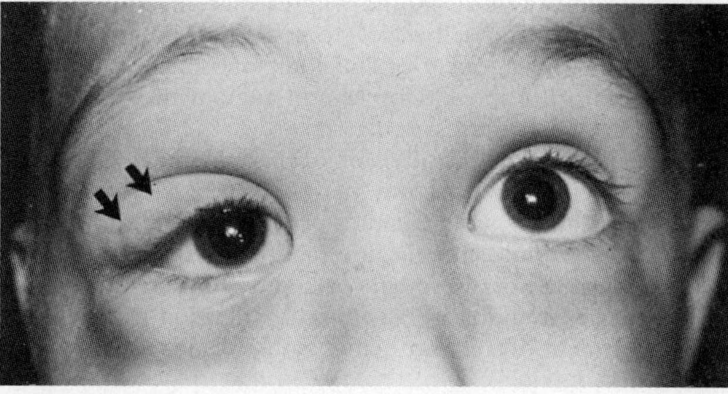

FIGURE 18.3. Plexiform neurofibroma of the lid (*arrows*) in a child with neurofibromatosis. (Reprinted with permission from McMillan JA, Feigin RD, DeAngelis C, et al. *Oski's Pediatrics: Principles and Practice*. 4th ed. Philadelphia, PA: Lippincott Williams & Wilkins, 2006.)

Prognosis/Natural History

NF1 is an AD genetic disorder with 100% penetrance, but expression is variable. Dermal manifestations increase with age. MRI of the brain commonly finds UBOs (T2/FLAIR bright signals of no clinical significance). Children should have yearly ophthalmologic examinations to monitor for the possibility of optic pathway gliomas. Because these tumors tend to be indolent, routine MRI of the brain is not recommended. Blood pressure should be monitored because of the risk of hypertension and vasculopathy. Malignant peripheral nerve sheath tumors can occur.

NF2 is caused by mutation in the Merlin gene on chromosome 22; it is also an AD genetic disorder. In comparison to NF1, the pathologic features of NF2 primarily involve the development of tumors and their complications (bilateral vestibular schwannomas, schwannomas along other CNs, spinal roots, and peripheral nerves, meningiomas, gliomas). Lens opacities may initially develop in childhood, but rarely progress to cataracts.

Tuberous Sclerosis Complex

Overview

TSC is caused by mutations in the *TS1* and *TS2* genes, encoding the proteins hamartin and tuberin. Clinically, *TS1* and *TS2* are indistinguishable. Incidence is 1:5,000 to 10,000. This is an AD genetic disorder with 100% penetrance but variable expression.

Clinical Manifestations/Diagnosis

Diagnostic criteria include the following:

- Definite TSC: two major features or one major feature and two minor features.
- Probable TSC: one major feature and one minor feature.
- Possible TSC: one major feature or two or more minor features.

TSC major features are the following:

- Facial angiofibromas (adenoma sebaceum) or forehead plaque.
- Ungual or periungual fibromas.
- Three or more hypomelanotic macules (ash leaf spots).
- Shagreen patch.
- Retinal nodular hamartomas.
- Cortical tuber.
- Subependymal nodule.
- Subependymal giant cell astrocytoma.
- Cardiac rhabdomyoma.
- Lymphangiomyomatosis.
- Renal angiomyolipoma.

TSC minor features are the following:

- "Confetti" skin lesions (multiple 1 to 2 mm hypomelanotic macules).
- Multiple renal cysts.
- Retinal achromic patch.
- Nonrenal hamartomas.
- Gingival fibromas.
- Cerebral white matter radial migration lines.
- Bone cysts.
- Hamartomatous rectal polyps.
- Randomly distributed dental enamel pits.

Prognosis/Natural History

About 80% of children with TSC will develop seizures. Infantile spasms are common. Cognitive deficits and autistic features are common. Children with TSC should be followed on a regular basis by a number of subspecialists, including cardiology (if diagnosed with cardiac rhabdomyomas), neurology (periodic MRIs to monitor for risk of giant cell astrocytomas, seizure management), ophthalmology, and dermatology (for cosmetic management of facial angiofibromas). They also should have regular renal ultrasounds to monitor for the development of angiomyolipomas.

Sturge-Weber syndrome (SWS) is a rare congenital vascular disorder characterized by a facial port wine stain (usually in the distribution of the first division of the trigeminal nerve) and a leptomeningeal angioma. Glaucoma is common. It is not heritable and the etiology is unknown. Calcified vessels are apparent on head CT scan. Seizures occur in 80%.

Von Hippel-Lindau syndrome (VHL) is an autosomally dominant inherited cancer syndrome, characterized by hemangioblastomas of the brain, spinal cord, and retina; renal cell carcinomas; and pheochromocytomas. Retinal hemangioblastomas typically develop in childhood and can cause hemorrhage and visual impairment. Cerebellar hemangioblastomas usually occur in adult and can present with headaches and ataxia.

SAMPLE BOARD REVIEW QUESTIONS

1. A 15-year-old adolescent girl presents to your office, complaining of a 1-year history of headaches. They occur twice a month, are throbbing in character, and have associated photophobia and nausea. Her mother suffers from similar headaches. Her examination, including funduscopic examination, is normal. You
   a. Elicit further history regarding her sleep, caffeine, eating, and exercise habits
   b. Recommend over-the-counter ibuprofen or naproxen
   c. Prescribe sumatriptan
   d. Prescribe topiramate
   e. Order an MRI

   Answer: a. You elicit additional information regarding possible provoking factors that may be triggering her headaches. It would also be reasonable to recommend over-the-counter NSAIDs, while cautioning against medication overuse and the risk of rebound headaches. In the setting of a greater than 6-month history, reassuring examination, and a family history, the most likely diagnosis here is migraine headaches.

2. Which of the following is a serious and potentially permanent sequelae of untreated IIH (pseudotumor cerebri)?
   a. Chronic daily headaches
   b. Vision loss
   c. Venous thrombosis
   d. Stroke

   Answer: b. Permanent vision loss is the most feared complication of untreated or inadequately treated IIH.

3. A 7-year-old boy is brought to your office because of concern for frequent eye blinking and throat clearing for the past 2 months. His diagnosis is:
   a. Acute tic disorder
   b. Chronic tic disorder
   c. Tourette syndrome

   Answer: a. The boy is exhibiting motor and vocal tics, less than 1 year in duration.

4. Regarding the patient in the preceding question, you recommend the following:
   a. Reassurance
   b. Behavioral therapy
   c. Initiation of clonidine therapy

   Answer: a. Acute tic disorders in this age group are often transient. Indications for treatment are physical discomfort or psychosocial distress.

5. A 4-year-old boy frequently engages in hand flapping when he is excited or engrossed. This behavior is:
   a. A tic
   b. A stereotypy
   c. Worrisome for autism
   d. A seizure
   e. Evidence of developmental delay

   Answer: b. Stereotypies are generally seen earlier in life than tics. Although associated with autism and mental retardation, they are frequently seen in normal children, and may persist into adulthood.

6. A 2-month-old infant presents with several days of lethargy, poor feeding, and constipation. You note that he has ptosis and poorly reactive pupils. You are most concerned about:
   a. Spinal muscular atrophy
   b. Congenital myopathy
   c. Infantile myasthenia gravis
   d. Botulism
   e. Sepsis

   Answer: d. Bulbar and eye involvement are the hallmark of infantile botulism.

7. A 15-month old child presents to the emergency department with a fever to 41 degrees, is difficult to arouse, and has a stiff neck. Initial appropriate antibiotic therapy would be:
   a. Vancomycin alone
   b. Ceftriaxone alone

c. Ampicillin and ceftriaxone
d. Ampicillin and vancomycin
e. Ampicillin and gentamicin

Answer: d. Ceftriaxone at meningitic dosing, plus vancomycin to cover for possibly resistant *S. pneumoniae.*

8. A 15-year-old adolescent girl wakes one morning in June and notices that she is drooling from the right side of her mouth and her right eyelid will not close completely. She has no fever, rash, meningismus, headache, or photophobia. She does not recall any tick bites, but she does live in an area where Lyme disease is endemic. She does not have any other neurologic symptoms. You elect to:
   a. Treat presumptively with oral steroids after sending serum for Lyme antibody testing
   b. Reassure the patient that she likely has sequelae from a viral infection
   c. Treat presumptively with oral doxycycline
   d. Perform a lumbar puncture to test CSF for Lyme antibody
   e. Obtain a CT scan

   Answer: a. The girl has symptoms of a peripheral facial nerve palsy, which could be due to the sequelae of a viral infection or to Lyme disease. It would be reasonable to treat with oral corticosteroids (plus or minus acyclovir), which has been demonstrated to improve recovery, and then treat for Lyme disease only if titers are positive. She should also be prescribed lubrication for her eye to protect the cornea.

9. A 10-year-old girl, a recent immigrant from Central America, presents to the emergency department with a first-time seizure. A head CT scan reveals several areas of calcification. Highest on your differential is:
   a. CNS lymphoma
   b. Toxoplasmosis
   c. HIV
   d. Neurocysticercosis
   e. Herpes simplex encephalitis

   Answer: d. Worldwide, neurocysticercosis is the leading cause of epilepsy.

10. Although normal at birth, a 12-month-old boy has begun to have regression of milestones and develop spasticity in his extremities. His head circumference has notably increased. You are concerned about which of the following disorders?
   a. Adrenoleukodystrophy
   b. Canavan disease
   c. Krabbe disease
   d. Pelizaeus-Merzbacher disease

   Answer: b. Canavan and Alexander disease are the two leukodystrophies associated with the development of macrocephaly. Tay-Sachs disease (a lysosomal storage disorder) can also include macrocephaly in the presentation.

11. A 2-year-old girl was developing normally for the first year of life. She then began to display developmental regression and microcephaly became apparent. She is nonverbal and has frequent hand wringing and seizures. She most likely has a mutation in which of the following genes?
   a. *POLG*
   b. *FMR1*
   c. *MECP2*
   d. *DMPK*

   Answer: c. Mutations in *MECP2* are associated with Rett syndrome. More recently, mutations in the gene *CDKL5* have also been demonstrated to be responsible for some cases.

12. A 7-year-old girl has been performing poorly in school and her teacher has noted spells of "day dreaming." An EEG demonstrates three per second spike and wave discharges during hyperventilation. Which medication should be started?
   a. Methylphenidate
   b. Valproic acid
   c. Lamotrigine
   d. Ethosuximide

   Answer: d. Ethosuximide is generally the first-line agent for treating childhood absence epilepsy, but valproic acid or lamotrigine would also be effective.

13. Which of the following is NOT a potential side effect of topiramate?
   a. Weight loss
   b. Kidney stones
   c. Cognitive slowing
   d. Hair loss

Answer: d. Hair loss is a potential side effect of valproic acid.

14. The most common epilepsy syndrome in childhood is:
   a. Childhood absence epilepsy
   b. Benign epilepsy with centrotemporal spikes
   c. Juvenile myoclonic epilepsy
   d. Lennox-Gastaut syndrome

Answer: b.

15. A 6-month-old infant with known tuberous sclerosis develops clusters of head bobs with arm extensions. EEG is most likely to reveal:
   a. Three per second spike and wave
   b. Hypsarrhythmia
   c. Periodic spikes
   d. Focal atrophy
   e. Periventricular hemorrhage

Answer: b. Hypsarrhythmia is the EEG finding associated with infantile spasms.

16. A 5-year-old boy falls from the monkey bars on the playground and hits his head on the ground. He resumes play. A few hours later, he becomes progressively sleepy and confused. A head CT scan is likely to reveal:
   a. Subdural hematoma
   b. Epidural hematoma
   c. Subarachnoid hemorrhage
   d. Intraparenchymal hemorrhage

Answer: b. A lucid interval is characteristic of an epidural hematoma.

17. A 17-year-old football player is tackled during a game and briefly loses consciousness. He quickly returns to baseline and wishes to return to the game. He may return to play in:
   a. Immediately
   b. 1 week
   c. 1 month
   d. He should remain on the sidelines for the season

Answer: b. Assuming no residual neurologic symptoms and no prior concussions.

18. A 16-year-old girl is in your office for a well-child check. Her mother complains that she is difficult to arouse in the mornings for school and sleeps until noon on the weekends. You counsel the family that teenagers require how much sleep each night?
   a. 13 to 14 hours
   b. 11 to 12 hours
   c. 9 to 10 hours
   d. 7 to 8 hours

Answer: c.

19. An 18-month-old boy babbles but does not have any recognizable words at his well-child check. At this point, the most appropriate management is:
   a. Parental reassurance
   b. Referral to a geneticist
   c. Referral for further developmental assessment, including audiologic assessment
   d. MRI of the brain
   e. Social services assessment of the family

Answer: c. Failure to babble or gesture by 12 months, have single words by 16 months, or two-word spontaneous speech by 24 months should prompt further evaluation.

20. Which of the following is NOT a feature of tuberous sclerosis?
   a. Facial angiofibromas
   b. Cardiac rhabdomyomas
   c. Lisch nodules
   d. Renal angiomyolipomas

Answer: c. Lisch nodules are associated with NF type 1.

SUGGESTED READINGS

Hirtz D, Ashwal S, Berg A, et al. Practice parameter: evaluating a first nonfebrile seizure in children: report of the quality standards subcommittee of the American Academy of Neurology, The Child Neurology Society, and The American Epilepsy Society. *Neurology*. 2000;55:616–623.

Jordan LC. Stroke in childhood. *Neurologist.* 2006;12:94–102.

Krupp LB, Banwell B, Tenembaum S, et al. Consensus definitions proposed for pediatric multiple sclerosis and related disorders. *Neurology*. 2007;68:S7–S12.

McCrory P, Meeuwisse W, Johnston K, et al. Consensus statement on Concussion in Sport 3rd International Conference on Concussion in Sport. *Clin J Sport Med.* 2009;19:185–200.

O'Shea M. Cerebral palsy. *Semin Perinatol.* 2008;32:35–41.

Practice parameter: the management of concussion in sports. *Neurology.* 1997;48:581–585.

Practice parameter: the neurodiagnostic evaluation of the child with a first simple febrile seizure. American Academy of Pediatrics. Provisional Committee on Quality Improvement, Subcommittee on Febrile Seizures. *Pediatrics* 1996;97:769–72.

CHAPTER 19 ■ NUTRITION

LAURA L. STEINBERG

ARA	Arachidonic acid	LDL	Low-density lipoprotein
BMI	Body mass index	MCT	Medium chain triglyceride
DHA	Docosahexaenoic acid	MRI	Magnetic resonance imaging
HDL	High-density lipoprotein	RDI	Recommended daily intake
HIV	Human immunodeficiency virus		

CHAPTER OBJECTIVES

1. Review the nutritional requirements of children, including the daily recommended intakes for children of all ages
2. Review the risks and consequences of improper nutrition, including the symptoms of macronutrient, micronutrient, and vitamin deficiency and excess
3. Compare the contents of and indications for breast milk and infant formula
4. Review alternative methods of providing nutrition to children with chronic disease.

Proper nutrition is the cornerstone to the expression of normal growth and development in children. Nutritional deficiencies, whether organic or environmental, often start a cascade of developmental problems. Understanding the basic needs and requirements in pediatric nutrition is fundamental to the pediatric discipline.

MACRONUTRIENTS

We will begin with a review of the macronutrients: carbohydrates, protein, and fat.

Carbohydrates serve as the major source of fuel for metabolism, whereas protein and fat serve as the building blocks for tissues and cells. Carbohydrates are not essential nutrients in humans as protein and fat can be used for energy as well. The brain, however, prefers glucose as its energy substrate. Although glucose can be metabolized from protein and fat, it is more efficiently obtained from carbohydrates. There are simple and complex carbohydrates. Simple carbohydrates are the monosaccharides and disaccharides that are found in highly processed foods, such as juice, soda, candy, chips, and pastries. Simple carbohydrates cause rapid, large spikes in blood glucose. The resulting vigorous insulin response can cause the blood glucose level to drop excessively, resulting in hunger and excess caloric intake when simple carbohydrates are consumed throughout the day. Complex carbohydrates are the polysaccharides found in whole grains, fruits, and vegetables. Complex carbohydrates are more difficult to break down resulting in slower release of glucose and insulin into the blood stream allowing for a sustained sensation of fullness and lower caloric intake.

Protein consists of amino acids. Out of the 20 different amino acids, there are 8 that must be consumed in the diet as our bodies cannot synthesize them in sufficient quantity. These are termed essential amino acids. Animal products, such as meat, eggs, and milk, generally have higher bioavailability of essential amino acids than plant products, such as nuts and legumes.

Fat consists of fatty acids. Fatty acids may be saturated, wherein all carbon atoms contain as many hydrogens as possible without formation of double bonds, or unsaturated, in which carbon atoms do not contain as many hydrogens as possible and some form double bonds. Saturated fatty acids form straight chains that can be packed together very tightly, allowing for dense chemical energy storage. This can be problematic when saturated fats are consumed in excess. Unsaturated fatty acids may form straight chains when they are in trans configuration (hydrogen atoms are bound to opposite sides of the double bond) or bent chains when they are in cis configuration (hydrogen atoms are bound to the same side of the double bond). Fatty acids in trans configuration, or trans fats, are not found in nature and are produced by industrial hydrogenation of plant oils. By unclear mechanisms, trans fats have been shown to raise serum triglycerides and LDL and lower HDL. Consumption of trans fats correlates more closely with atherosclerosis and coronary artery disease than consumption of non-trans fats.

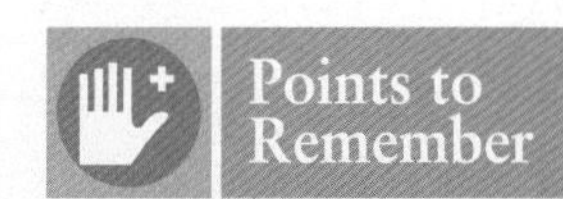

- **Essential fatty acids are linoleic and alpha-linoleic acid.**

Points to Remember

- Phototherapy in newborns increases the risk for B_2 deficiency.
- B_6 supplementation is indicated for those taking isoniazid.
- B_{12} absorption relies upon gastric intrinsic factor and terminal ileum receptors.
- Vitamin C deficiency can trigger a hemolytic crisis in those with G6PD deficiency.
- Anticonvulsants interfere with vitamin D metabolism.
- Vitamin K deficiency occurs in newborns, malabsorption syndromes, and chronic antibiotic use.
- Deficiencies of vitamin C, iron, and copper all cause microcytic anemia.

There are two unsaturated cis fatty acids, linoleic and alpha-linoleic acid, that we cannot produce and are therefore essential fatty acids that should be consumed in our diet. These fatty acids are needed for prostaglandin and cell membrane synthesis and can be found in plant oils. Deficiency of either may result in poor hair growth, flaky dermatitis, diarrhea, thrombocytopenia, and increased risk of infection. Consumption of essential fatty acid supplements in the setting of dietary imbalance has been associated with reduction in violent behavior and increased attention span in school-aged children. The mechanism of these effects and the association with vision and IQ are still unclear. DHA and ARA are unsaturated fatty acids found in fish oil. While we can make DHA and ARA, these unsaturated fatty acids can help fulfill our essential fatty acid requirement and should be consumed in our diet.

Carbohydrates, protein, and fat make up the calories we consume throughout the course of a day. Tables 19.1 and 19.2 quantify the RDIs for calories, macronutrients, vitamins, and micronutrients according to age. Side effects may result when we consume too little or too much of a given macronutrient, vitamin, or micronutrient. The next sections will further discuss undernutrition and overweight. Please see Tables 19.3 to 19.5 for a review of the deficiencies and toxicities that may result from improper vitamin and mineral consumption. Please also see Table 19.6 for a listing of unique diets that may result in specific vitamin and micronutrient deficiencies.

Undernutrition

Failure to thrive is defined as weight less than 2 standard deviations below the mean for sex and age or weight that has fallen more than 2 percentile lines on the growth chart after having achieved a previously stable pattern. There are many possible etiologies for failure to thrive. The etiologies can be separated into four categories:

- Inadequate intake secondary to swallow dysfunction, anorexia, or altered mental status.
- Increased metabolic rate secondary to fever, infection, or chronic disease.
- Insufficient utilization of ingested calories secondary to maldigestion or malabsorption.
- Psychosocial factors include poverty, unusual health beliefs, inadequate parenting/feeding skills, stress, violence, social isolation, and substance abuse.

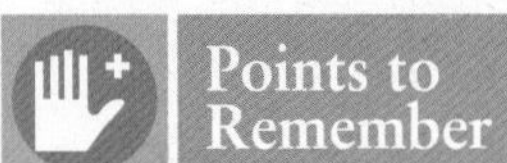

Points to Remember

- Failure to thrive is further discussed in the chapter "Growth and Development."

The evaluation of failure to thrive involves a thorough history and physical examination as well as laboratory evaluation. If the history and physical examination are not suggestive of a specific organic etiology, then a basic laboratory assessment can be done first with further diagnostic assessment as indicated. The initial basic laboratory assessment often includes the following:

- Complete blood cell count.
- Electrolytes, protein, albumin, and renal and hepatic panels.
- Urinalysis.

Other laboratory evaluation to consider, if the history and physical examination are suggestive, includes the following:

- HIV testing.

TABLE 19.1

AVERAGE RECOMMENDED CALORIC INTAKE FOR INDIVIDUALS ACCORDING TO AGE, ADAPTED FROM *AAP PEDIATRIC NUTRITION HANDBOOK*, 6TH EDITION

Age	Estimated Energy Requirement (kcal/day)
0–3 mo	89 × Weight (kg) + 75
4–6 mo	89 × Weight (kg) − 44
7–12 mo	89 × Weight (kg) − 78
13–36 mo	89 × Weight (kg) − 80
3–8 yr (boys)	108.5 − (62 × Age [yr]) + PA × (26.7 × Weight [kg] + 903 × Height [m])
3–8 yr (girls)	155 − (31 × Age [yr]) + PA × (10 × Weight [kg] + 934 × Height [m])
9–18 yr (boys)	113.5 − (62 × Age [yr]) + PA × (26.7 × Weight [kg] + 903 × Height [m])
9–18 yr (girls)	160 − (31 × Age [yr]) + PA × (10 × Weight [kg] + 934 × Height [m])

PA, Physical Activity Coefficient; m, meter; yr, year.
PA for boys: sedentary = 1, low active = 1.13, active = 1.26, very active = 1.42.
PA for girls: sedentary = 1, low active = 1.16, active = 1.31, very active = 1.56.

TABLE 19.2

AVERAGE RECOMMENDED MACRONUTRIENT, MICRONUTRIENT, AND VITAMIN INTAKES FOR INDIVIDUALS ACCORDING TO AGE, ADAPTED FROM *AAP PEDIATRIC NUTRITION HANDBOOK*, 6TH EDITION

	0–6 mo	7–12 mo	1–3 yr	4–8 yr	9–13 yr (boys)	9–13 yr (girls)	14–18 yr (boys)	14–18 yr (girls)	Pregnancy ≤18 yr	Lactation ≤18 yr
Carbohydrates (g/d)	60	95	130	130	130	130	130	130	175	210
Fiber (g/d)[a]			19	24	31	26	38	26	28	29
Protein (g/kg/d)	1.5	1	1	1	1	1	0.9	0.9	1	1.3
Fat (g/d)[a]	31	30								
Vitamin A (μg/d)	400	500	300	400	600	600	900	700	750	1200
Vitamin B_1 (mg/d)	0.2	0.3	0.5	0.6	0.9	0.9	1.2	1	1.4	1.4
Vitamin B_2 (mg/d)	0.3	0.4	0.5	0.6	0.9	0.9	1.3	1	1.4	1.6
Vitamin B_3 (mg/d)	2	4	6	8	12	12	16	14	18	17
Vitamin B_5 or Pantothenic Acid (mg/d)	1.7	1.8	2	3	4	4	5	5	6	7
Vitamin B_6 (mg/d)	0.1	0.3	0.5	0.6	1	1	1.3	1.2	1.9	2
Vitamin B_{12} (μg/d)	0.4	0.5	0.9	1.2	1.8	1.8	2.4	2.4	2.6	2.8
Folate (μg/d)	65	80	150	200	300	300	400	400	600	500
Biotin (μg/d)	5	6	8	12	20	20	25	25	30	35
Vitamin C (mg/d)	40	50	15	25	45	45	75	65	80	115
Vitamin D (μg/d)	5	5	5	5	5	5	5	5	5	5
Vitamin E (mg/d)	4	5	6	7	11	11	15	15	15	19
Vitamin K (μg/d)	2	2.5	30	55	60	60	75	75	75	75
Calcium (mg/d)	210	270	500	800	1300	1300	1300	1300	1300	1300
Copper (μg/d)	200	220	340	440	700	700	890	890	1000	1300
Fluoride (mg/d)	0.01	0.5	0.7	1	2	2	3	2	3	3
Iron (mg/d)	0.27	11	7	10	8	8	11	15	27	10
Magnesium (mg/d)	30	75	80	130	240	240	410	360	400	360
Phosphorus (mg/d)	100	275	460	500	1250	1250	1250	1250	1250	1250
Selenium (μg/d)	15	20	20	30	40	40	55	55	60	70
Zinc (mg/d)	2	3	3	5	8	8	11	9	13	14

[a]Normal values are not available for recommended fat intake for older children and fiber intake for infants. Fat intake should represent 20% to 30% of total caloric intake for older children.

- Tuberculosis skin testing.
- Sweat test for cystic fibrosis.
- Thyroid function tests.
- Stool elastase, alpha 1 antitrypsin, and reducing substances for malabsorption.
- Genetic testing.

The management of failure to thrive includes the treatment of underlying medical illnesses as well as enhancing the nutritional status of the child (Table 19.7). Some patients can be managed as an outpatient, whereas others require inpatient admission. Factors that might lead a provider to consider admitting a patient for failure to thrive include severe acute malnutrition, severe dehydration, concern for child abuse or neglect, parental substance abuse, or failure of outpatient management. Whether or not the child who is failing to thrive is admitted to the hospital, the tenets of care remain the same:

- Supplement the diet with high-calorie foods to allow for weight gain. One can calculate the necessary caloric requirement for weight gain using the following equation: kcal/kg/d = (RDI for age [kcal/kg] × ideal weight for height [kg])/actual weight (kg).

TABLE 19.3

THE FUNCTION OF THE WATER-SOLUBLE VITAMINS AND THEIR ASSOCIATED DEFICIENCY AND TOXICITY STATES

Vitamin	Function	Signs of Deficiency	Toxic Effects
Vitamin B_1 (thiamin)	Carbohydrate metabolism	Wet beriberi (heart failure) Dry beriberi (polyneuritis)	Unknown
Vitamin B_2 (riboflavin)	Enzyme cofactor	Photophobia, glossitis, cheilosis (Fig. 19.1), seborrheic dermatitis	Unknown
Vitamin B_3 (niacin)	Enzyme cofactor	Pellagra with diarrhea, dermatitis, dementia	Flushing/vasodilation, pruritus
Vitamin "B_5" (pantothenic acid)	Enzyme cofactor	Depression, hypotension, weakness	Unknown
Vitamin B_6 (pyridoxine)	Enzyme cofactor	Microcytic anemia, glossitis, cheilosis, peripheral neuritis In infants: irritability and seizure	Unknown
Vitamin B_{12} (cyanocobalamin)	Enzyme cofactor, red blood cell maturation, CNS metabolism	Pernicious anemia, neuropathy, demyelination	Unknown
Biotin	Enzyme cofactor	Seborrheic dermatitis, alopecia, muscle pain, anorexia	Unknown
Folate	Nucleoprotein synthesis	Megaloblastic anemia, impaired cellular immunity, neural tube defects (Fig. 19.2)	Masks vitamin B_{12} deficiency
Vitamin C (ascorbic acid)	Collagen synthesis, folic acid metabolism, iron absorption/transport	Scurvy (Fig. 19.3) with hemorrhage, hysteria, depression, poor wound healing	Oxalate/cysteine kidney stones

- Multivitamin.
- Ferrous sulfate if the child has a microcytic anemia.
- Education regarding childhood nutrition.
- Behavior modification to improve feeding techniques.
- Weekly to monthly outpatient or home visits to document weight and monitor compliance.

When a child who is undernourished is placed on a high-calorie diet to promote weight gain, fluid and electrolyte abnormalities may develop, which is otherwise referred to as *refeeding syndrome*. Patients at risk for refeeding syndrome include those who have experienced prolonged periods of starvation, vomiting, diarrhea, or nasogastric suction and those with anorexia nervosa, recent major surgery, cancer, or alcoholism. Refeeding syndrome develops when starvation results

TABLE 19.4

THE FUNCTION OF THE FAT-SOLUBLE VITAMINS AND THEIR ASSOCIATED DEFICIENCY AND TOXICITY STATES

Vitamin	Function	Signs of Deficiency	Toxic Effects
Vitamin A (retinol)	Vision epithelial integrity, bone cell function	Night blindness, Bitot's spots Hyperkeratosis, pruritus Decreased antibody production Poor bone growth	Acute: pseudotumor cerebri Chronic: alopecia, scaly skin, hepatic fibrosis, hyperostosis
Vitamin D (calciferol)	Bone resorption	Rickets (Fig. 19.4) Osteomalacia (See Endocrine chapter for full discussion)	Hypercalcemia Hyperphosphatemia Azotemia Nephrocalcinosis
Vitamin E (alpha-tocopherol)	Stabilizes membranes Antioxidant	Hemolytic anemia Peripheral neuropathy leading to ataxia Obstructive jaundice	Unknown
Vitamin K (phylloquinone)	Blood clotting via factors II, VII, IX, and X	Hemorrhage	Hyperbilirubinemia

TABLE 19.5

THE FUNCTION OF THE MINERALS AND THEIR ASSOCIATED DEFICIENCY AND TOXICITY STATES

Mineral	Function	Signs of Deficiency	Toxic Effects
Calcium	Bone/tooth mineralization Muscle contraction Nerve function Blood clotting Blood pressure	Rickets Osteomalacia Tetany Seizures	Confusion Muscle pain Calcium kidney stones Constipation
Copper	Red blood cell production Connective tissue synthesis Nerve function	Sideroblastic anemia Osteoporosis Neutropenia	Wilson's disease Liver dysfunction
Fluoride	Tooth remineralization Disrupts bacterial metabolism to reduce caries	Dental caries	Fluorosis (Fig. 19.5)
Iodine	Component of thyroid hormone	Goiter Hypothyroidism Cretinism	Hyper or hypothyroidism
Iron	Forms hemoglobin and myoglobin	Microcytic anemia Pica Impaired wound healing Impaired growth Developmental delay	Diabetes Liver disease Arrhythmia
Magnesium	Bone mineralization	Weakness, cramps Arrhythmias	Weakness Hypotension Nausea
Phosphorus	Bone/tooth mineralization Energy transfer	Rickets Neuropathy	Low calcium
Selenium	Antioxidant	Cardiomyopathy Anemia	Mucous membrane irritation Pallor
Zinc	Component of enzymes Taste Wound healing Immunity	Anorexia Acrodermatitis enteropathica (Fig. 19.6) Growth and puberty delay Slow wound healing	Aggravates copper deficiency

in loss of lean mass, minerals, and water. When enteral or parenteral refeeding is initiated, the carbohydrate load induces insulin secretion and cellular uptake of electrolytes (potassium, phosphorus, magnesium, calcium). Tissue anabolism further increases cellular demand for phosphorus in the form of ATP, potassium, glucose, and water. The carbohydrate load also leads to avid sodium and water retention and edema. These electrolyte and fluid shifts may result in rhabdomyolysis, respiratory failure, cardiac failure, arrhythmia, seizure, delirium, coma, or sudden death. The following interventions are recommended for the prevention of refeeding syndrome:

- Start feeding at 25% estimated caloric requirements.
- Increase calories slowly over several days.

TABLE 19.6

UNIQUE DIETS AND THEIR ASSOCIATED VITAMIN AND MICRONUTRIENT DEFICIENCIES

Diet	Definition	Deficiency
Goat milk	Avoidance of cow milk	Folate
Semi-vegetarian	Limited to no red meat consumption	Iron
Lacto-ovo vegetarian	Avoid flesh foods, but eat dairy and eggs	Iron
Vegan	Avoid all meats and animal products	Vitamin B_{12}, vitamin D, calcium, iron

TABLE 19.7

COMPONENTS OF HISTORY AND PHYSICAL EXAMINATION TO INCLUDE IN FAILURE TO THRIVE ASSESSMENT

History	Physical Examination
Maternal assessment (drug use, congenital infections, health during pregnancy)	Anthropometric data (weight, height, weight for height, head circumference)
Birth history (labor, delivery, neonatal events)	Observe parent-child interaction
Child's past medical history (medical illnesses, surgeries, infections, medications, immunizations, development)	Comprehensive physical examination (general appearance, head, neck, lungs, heart, abdomen, genitals, extremities, skin, neurologic system)
Growth history of patient and family members	
Nutrition history (feeding behavior, food sensitivities/allergies, quantitative assessment of intake)	
Current symptoms (dysphagia, emesis, bowel movements, dysuria, fever, activity level)	
Social history (life stresses, social and economic supports)	

- Check and correct electrolytes initially and then daily for at least 4 days after feeding is initiated or until electrolytes are stabilized.
- When serum phosphorus falls below 1 mg/dL, infuse intravenous phosphate to prevent or treat symptoms.

There are two categories of undernutrition: overall calorie deficiency, called marasmus (Fig. 19.7), or more specific protein deficiency, called kwashiorkor (Fig. 19.8).

Marasmus, also termed infantile atrophy, generally occurs in infants and may result from increased caloric needs secondary to acute or chronic infection, impaired absorption with chronic diarrhea or other malabsorptive states, or inadequate caloric intake secondary to transition from breast feeding to nutrient poor foods.

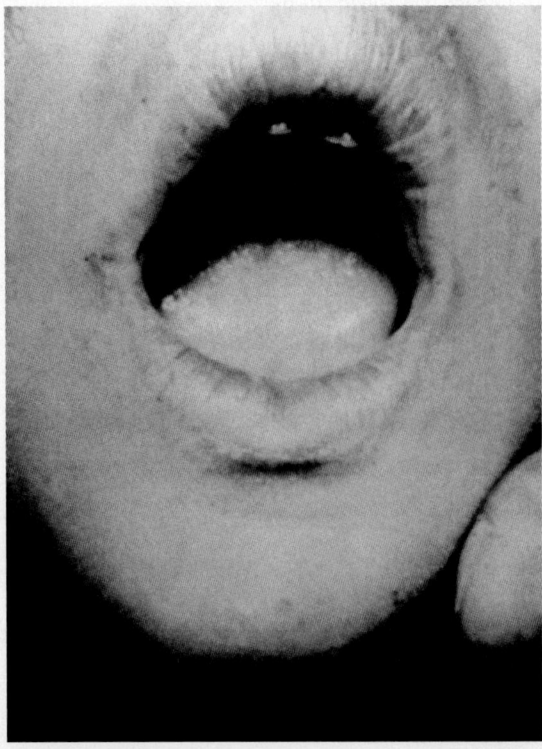

FIGURE 19.1. This patient presented with angular lesions of the lips, or cheilosis due to a vitamin B_2 deficiency. With a vitamin B_2 deficiency, the lips become dry, scaly, and swollen, and lesions develop at the corners of the mouth known as cheilosis. The gums or gingivae become inflamed and have a tendency to bleed easily. (Reprinted from CDC/Nutrition Program.)

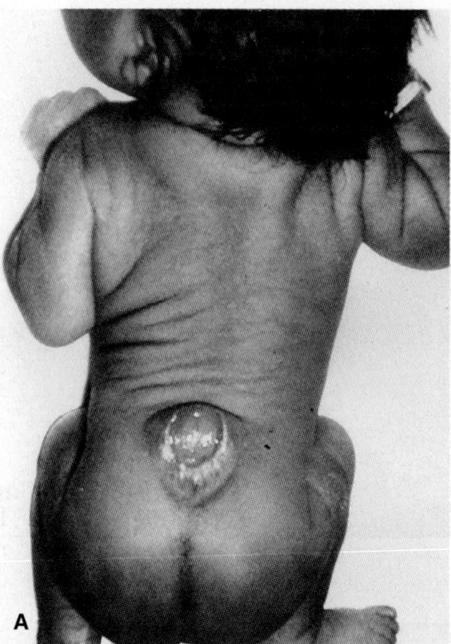

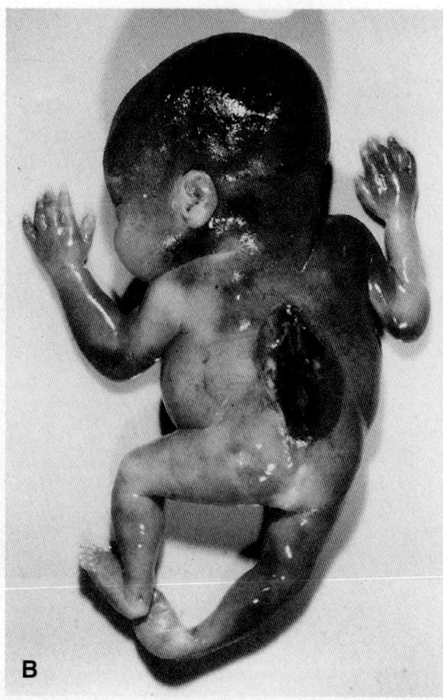

FIGURE 19.2. Lumbosacral region of patients with neural tube defects. (**A**) Patient with a large meningomyelocele. (**B**) Patient with a severe defect in which the neural folds failed to elevate throughout the lower thoracic and lumbosacral regions, resulting in rachischisis. (Courtesy of Dr. MJ Sellers, Division of Medical and Molecular Genetics, Guys Hospital, London.)

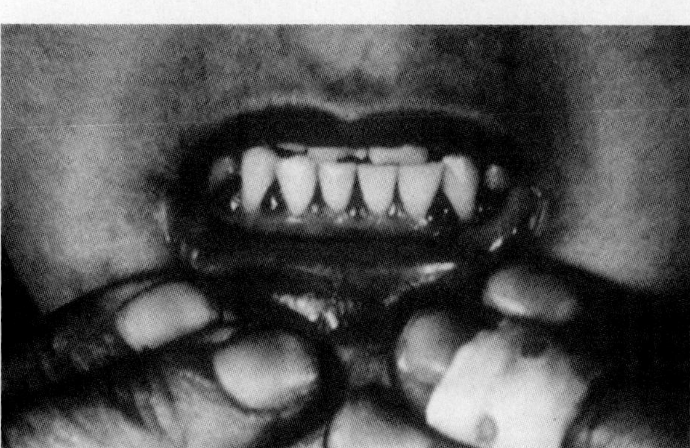

FIGURE 19.3. This patient presented with scorbutic gums due to a vitamin C deficiency, a symptom of scurvy. The condition referred to as scorbutic gums involves inflammation of the gums or gingivitis, as well as gingival hemorrhages due to the breakdown of capillary components of the gingival vascular system. (Reprinted from CDC.)

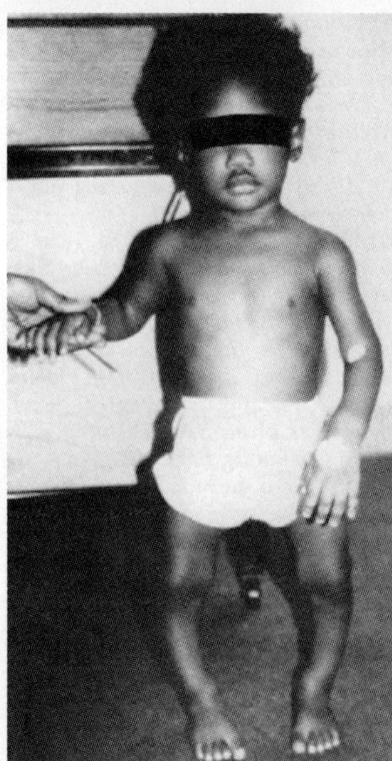

FIGURE 19.4. Nutritional rickets (vitamin D deficiency) in a 3-year-old boy. Note the severe bowing of the lower extremities and the wider wrists and ankles. (Reprinted with permission from Becker KL, Bilezikian JP, Brenner WJ, et al. *Principles and Practice of Endocrinology and Metabolism.* 3rd ed. Philadelphia, PA: Lippincott Williams & Wilkins, 2001.)

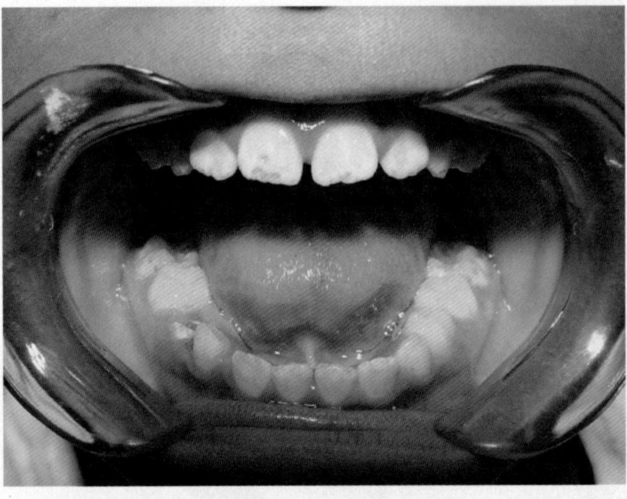

FIGURE 19.5. Fluorosis. (Courtesy of Michael Lemper, DDS.)

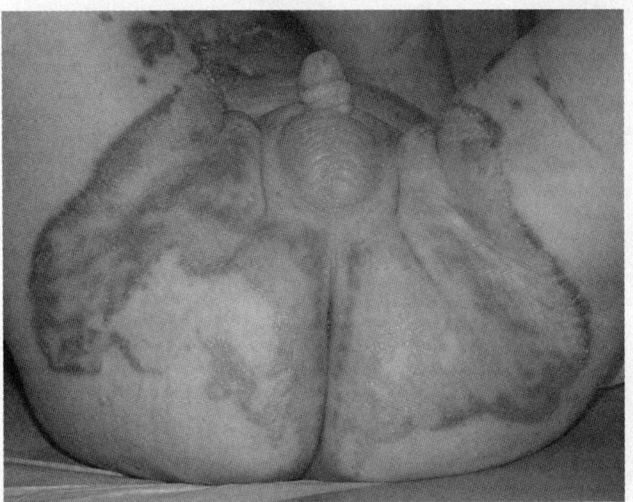

FIGURE 19.6. Acrodermatitis enteropathica. (Reprinted with permission from MacDonald MG, Seshia MMK, Mullett MD, et al. *Avery's Neonatology Pathophysiology & Management of the Newborn*. 6th ed. Philadelphia, PA: Lippincott Williams & Wilkins, 2005.)

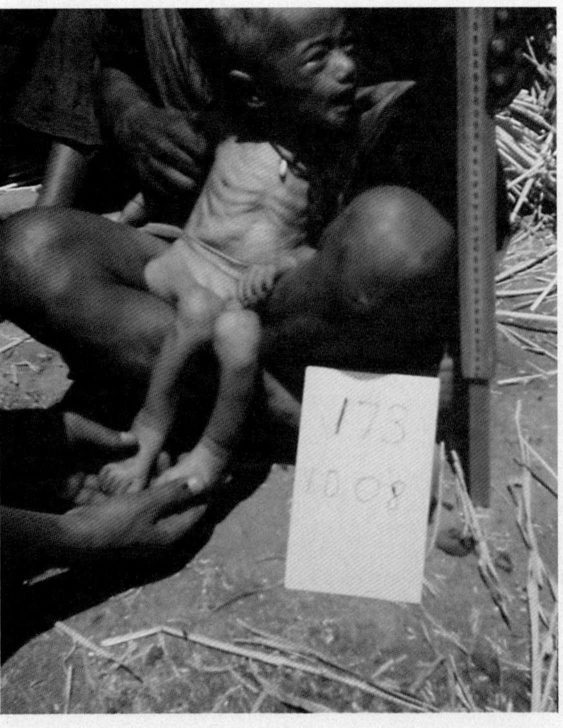

FIGURE 19.7. The signs of marasmus are loose, folded skin, and a protruding rib cage with the manifestation of such symptoms in a developing child, whose body is in need of vast quantities of nutrients, being quite rapid and producing profound consequences. (Reprinted from CDC/Dr. Edward Brink.)

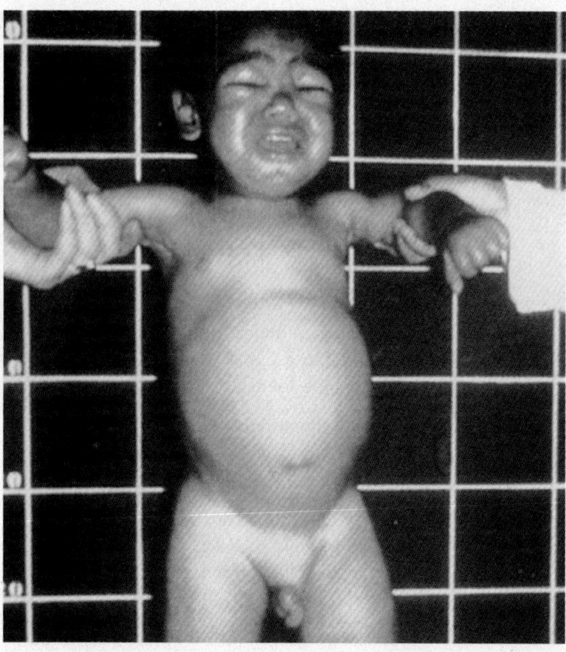

FIGURE 19.8. A child with kwashiorkor often has been abruptly weaned and may have a distended abdomen and muscle wasting. (Reprinted with permission from Klossner NJ, Hatfield NT. *Introductory Maternity & Pediatric Nursing: Basis of Human Movement in Health and Disease.* 4th ed. Philadelphia, PA: Lippincott Williams & Wilkins, 2005.)

Kwashiorkor on the other hand, generally occurs in children between 1 and 4 years of age and may result from abnormal losses of protein with burns or nephrotic syndrome, inadequate production of protein with chronic liver disease, impaired absorption of protein with chronic diarrhea, or inadequate protein intake secondary to inadequate food supply with drought or famine. Table 19.8 provides a comparison of the features seen in each form of malnutrition. Management of both marasmus and kwashiorkor includes oral rehydration, slow increase in caloric intake, and close monitoring for refeeding syndrome. Children with marasmus may require up to 150 kcal/kg/day to achieve catch-up growth.

Not all children with chronic disease are undernourished, but it is important to be aware of the nutrition-related challenges posed by certain types of chronic disease as reviewed in Table 19.9.

Nutritional Support

Enteral supplemental nutrition includes those feeds that are given via nasogastric, gastrostomy, and duodenal tubes. There are various indications for enteral feeds including conditions leading to oromotor dysfunction and increased caloric requirement.

TABLE 19.8

FEATURES OF CHILDREN WITH MARASMUS AND KWASHIORKOR

Marasmus	Kwashiorkor
Significant weight loss	Minimal weight loss
Slowed vertical growth	Slowed vertical growth
Emaciated and weak appearing with striking loss of subcutaneous fat	Muscle wasting masked by generalized edema
Thin skin and hair	Hyperkeratotic, depigmented, peeling skin Red, straight, thin hair
Constipation	Diarrhea
Ravenous hunger	Irritability
Low prealbumin, but albumin may be normal	Elevated sodium and chloride Low potassium, protein, albumin, and blood urea nitrogen

TABLE 19.9

CHRONIC DISEASE-SPECIFIC NUTRITION PROBLEMS AND SOLUTIONS

Disease	Problem	Solution
Neurologic impairment	Oromotor dysfunction Gastroesophageal reflux	Occupational therapy Prokinetics and/or H_2 blockers Enteral tube feeding
Cardiac disease	Hypermetabolism Fatigue with feeding	Calorie-dense diet Enteral tube feeds
Cystic fibrosis	Malabsorption Hypermetabolism	Fat-soluble vitamins, pancreatic enzymes Calorie-dense diet Enteral tube feeds
Short bowel syndrome	Malabsorption	Parenteral nutrition Amino acid formula with medium chain fatty acids
Liver disease	Encephalopathy	Low-protein diet, branch-chain amino acid formula Increased soluble fiber to reduce ammonia absorption
Renal disease	Hyperkalemia Hyperphosphatemia Hypertension/edema Malnutrition with excess restriction	Restrict potassium (orange, banana, dried fruit, potato, tomato) Restrict phosphorus (milk, meat, nuts) Restrict sodium (packaged or canned foods, cured/smoked meats, salty chips or crackers) Follow-up to ensure that restriction decisions are appropriate
Sickle cell disease	Increased energy requirement Folate deficiency	Hydration Calorie-dense diet Folate supplementation
Cancer	Hypermetabolism Anorexia Chemotherapy toxicity (nausea, vomiting, altered taste, pain, diarrhea, etc.)	Calorie-dense diet Enteral tube feeding Parenteral nutrition
HIV	Anorexia Malabsorption Hypermetabolism	Occupational/behavioral therapy Appetite stimulants Enteral tube feeding Highly active antiretroviral therapy (HAART)

The advantages of enteral nutrition over parenteral nutrition include the following:

- Supports the integrity of the gastrointestinal tract.
- More complete range of nutrients including glutamine, long-chain polyunsaturated fatty acids, short-chain fatty acids, and fiber.
- Less expensive.
- Fewer infectious risks.

Parenteral nutrition is given via peripheral or central access. Indications for parenteral nutrition are similar to those for enteral nutrition and include gastrointestinal disease contraindicating use of the gastrointestinal tract and severe malnutrition. Side effects of parenteral nutrition include hepatic disease with cholestasis in infants and steatohepatitis in older children and reversible intestinal mucosal atrophy. Blood stream infection is an additional risk.

Overweight

A child with a healthy weight has a BMI (weight in kg/height in m^2) between the 5th and the 84th percentiles. Overweight is defined as a BMI between the 85th and 94th percentiles, and obesity is defined as a BMI greater than the 95th percentile. Overweight and obesity develop as a result of caloric intake being greater than energy expenditure. Most commonly, children

TABLE 19.10

THE SYMPTOMS AND SIGNS OF THE COMPLICATIONS OF OBESITY

Complication	Symptom	Sign
Pseudotumor cerebri	Headache, blurry vision, nausea, vomiting	Papilledema
Sleep apnea	Snoring, night waking, enuresis, daytime inattention or somnolence	Tonsillar hypertrophy
Hypertension	Asymptomatic or headache	Persistently elevated blood pressure
Hypercholesterolemia	Asymptomatic	
Nonalcoholic fatty liver disease	Asymptomatic or right upper quadrant pain	Hepatomegaly
Constipation	Abdominal pain, enuresis	Abdominal mass
Polycystic ovarian syndrome	Amenorrhea	Acne, hirsutism
Type 2 diabetes mellitus	Polyuria, polydipsia	Acanthosis nigricans
Slipped capital femoral epiphysis	Hip or knee pain	Limp, leg rests in abduction, decreased flexion and adduction

develop overweight or obesity as a result of being fed more calories than their daily activities require, but there are genetic (e.g., Prader-Willi) and endocrine (e.g., hypothyroidism, Cushing's) syndromes that may contribute as well.

The assessment of a child who is overweight or obese should include a thorough history of the child's diet (types and amounts of foods and drinks consumed daily and willingness to change), activity (types and frequency of physical and sedentary activities and barriers to increasing physical activity), and family history of cardiovascular disease and associated risk factors including hypertension, diabetes, and hypercholesterolemia. The review of systems and physical examination should give particular attention to complications of obesity as seen in Table 19.10. Laboratory evaluation should be done on every child who is overweight or obese at least every 2 years. Table 19.11 lists the laboratory tests that should be obtained on the basis of the child's BMI and risk factors, which include family history of obesity and/or obesity-related diseases, personal history of smoking or of obesity-related diseases, or history or physical examination suggestive of comorbidities. Additional targeted tests may also be obtained as suggested by the history or physical examination.

The management of overweight and obesity involves alterations of both diet and activity. The following dietary suggestions might be made to a parent of an overweight or obese child:

- Eat three meals daily with additional small, healthy snacks as needed.
- Minimize sweetened beverage consumption to 6 ounces daily.
- Decrease fast food.
- Eat five servings of fruits and vegetables daily.
- Small steps will be much more successful and long-lasting than radical change.

TABLE 19.11

LABORATORY TESTS TO BE OBTAINED ON THE BASIS OF A CHILD'S BMI AND RISK FACTORS

BMI ± Risk Factors	Recommended Laboratory Testing
85th–94th, No risk factors	Fasting lipid levels
85th–94th, Has risk factors	Fasting lipid levels, fasting glucose, transaminases
≥95th	Fasting lipid levels, fasting glucose, transaminases

BMI, body mass index.

The following activity suggestions might be made to a parent of an overweight or obese child:

- Limit sedentary activities and/or screen time to 2 hours daily.
- Engage in moderate physical activity for at least 60 minutes daily.

Breast Feeding

According to the American Academy of Pediatrics, breast feeding should be the exclusive source of nutrition for children during the first 6 months of life and it should be continued, regardless of the timing of introduction of complementary foods, for 12 months or longer if mutually desired by the parent and child. There are many benefits of breast feeding, including nutritional and maternal, as listed below:

- Human milk has a dynamic nutrient composition that differs throughout lactation, over the course of a day, within a feeding, and among women.
  - Colostrum is the milk produced during the first 3 to 5 days. Its protein content is higher, including immunoglobulins and carotene, and it contains enzymes to stimulate gut maturation.
  - Mature milk is present after 10 days of breast feeding. Mature human milk has less protein and more fat and lactose than colostrum and cow milk.
- Human milk has unique protein content as shown in Table 19.12. There is more whey, which is more easily digested and promotes more rapid gastric emptying, as well as lactoferrin and immunoglobulin (specifically secretory IgA), which are proteins involved in host defense. Infants who are breast fed have been shown to have fewer cases of otitis media, lower respiratory tract infections, and gastroenteritis.
- Human milk has unique pattern of fatty acids including very-long-chain polyunsaturated fatty acids, ARA, and DHA associated with visual function and neurodevelopment.
- Human milk has more lipase than formula allowing for superior fat absorption.
- Human milk contains unabsorbed lactose, which contributes to softer stool, more non-pathogenic fecal flora, and improved absorption of minerals.
- Human milk contains oligosaccharides that mimic bacterial antigen ligands, preventing bacterial attachment to host mucosa.
- Human milk contains minerals that are more bioavailable than those in formula as they are bound to digestible proteins.
- Mothers who breast feed have enhanced bonding with their infant.
- Mothers who breast feeds lose weight postpartum more rapidly.
- Mothers who breast feed have delayed resumption of normal ovarian cycles allowing for natural contraception.
- Mothers who breast feed have decreased incidence of breast and ovarian cancer.

There are few instances in which breast feeding is contraindicated. These include the following:

- Infant has galactosemia.
- Maternal HIV (in the United States).
- Herpes, chicken pox, or syphilis of the maternal breast.
- Maternal tuberculosis prior to receiving at least 2 weeks of therapy.
- Maternal cancer requiring chemotherapy.
- Maternal drug abuse.

TABLE 19.12

COMPARISON OF THE PERCENT PROTEIN CONTENT OF HUMAN AND COW MILK

Protein	Components	Human Milk (%)	Cow Milk (%)
Casein		**40**	**82**
	Alpha-casein		39
	Beta-casein	35	29
	Gamma-casein		3
	Kappa-casein		10
Whey		**60**	**18**
	Beta-lactoglobulin		10
	Alpha-lactalbumin	28	4
	Serum albumin	3	1
	Immunoglobulin	8	3
	Lactoferrin	21	

Although mothers of premature infants can and are encouraged to breast feed, these infants often require additional caloric supplementation.

Infants who are breast fed are at risk for vitamin K, vitamin D, iron, and fluoride deficiencies as breast milk does not contain sufficient amounts of these vitamins and minerals. All infants receive an intramuscular dose of vitamin K at birth to prevent bleeding associated with vitamin K deficiency that results from breast feeding alone. In November 2008, the American Academy of Pediatrics published a new statement to replace their 2003 vitamin D supplementation guidelines. The 2008 report recommends that all infants and children receive vitamin D supplementation beginning in the first few days of life. Infants who are breast fed and infants and children who consume less than 1,000 mL of vitamin D fortified formula or breast milk should be prescribed 400 IU/day vitamin D. Human milk contains less iron than cow milk, but the iron in human milk is more bioavailable. Infants who do not consume sufficient iron-containing foods by 6 months of age require iron supplementation. Two servings of meat (half ounce per serving) or iron-fortified dry cereal (15 g per serving) are needed to meet the daily iron requirement. Those who do not meet the daily iron requirement should be prescribed 1 mg/kg/day elemental iron. Infants who do not take in sufficient fluoride supplemented water are at higher risk of developing dental caries. Infants who are exclusively breastfed or who take in ready-to-feed formula should receive 0.25 mg fluoride daily starting at 6 months of age.

Infant Formulas

Term infants require 100 to 120 kcal/kg/day or 150 to 180 mL/kg/day. When the recommended volume is provided, all the formulas listed in Table 19.13 contain adequate macronutrients, vitamins, and minerals to serve as the sole source of nutrition for an infant. An ounce of

TABLE 19.13

INFANT FORMULA CONTENTS AND INDICATIONS

Type	Examples	Contents	Indications
Preterm	Preemie Enfamil Similac Special Care Enfacare Neosure	22–24 kcal/ounce Higher vitamin and mineral content Protein: nonfat cow milk, whey Carbohydrate: lactose, corn syrup Fat: soy, coconut, MCT	Preterm infants until they reach 44 wk postconceptive age
Term	Enfamil Lipil Similac Advance Nestle Good Start	Protein: nonfat cow milk, whey Carbohydrate: lactose Fat: soy, coconut, safflower, or sunflower oil	Term infant
Soy	Prosobee Isomil Good Start Soy	Protein: soy, methionine Carbohydrate: corn syrup Fat: soy, coconut, safflower, or sunflower oil	IgE-mediated cow milk protein allergy Galactosemia Hereditary lactase deficiency Vegetarian preference **Not recommended for preterm infants, prevention of colic or allergy, or non—IgE-associated cow milk protein allergy
Lactose free	Lactofree Similac Sensitive	Protein: nonfat cow milk Carbohydrate: corn syrup Fat: soy, coconut, sunflower	Lactose intolerance Secondary lactase deficiency Galactosemia
Hydrolyzed	Nutramigen Alimentum Pregestimil	Protein: casein hydrolysate Carbohydrate: corn syrup or sucrose Fat: soy, MCT, safflower, sunflower, coconut, or corn	Cow milk protein allergy Cystic fibrosis Malabsorption
Amino acid	Elecare Neocate	Protein: free amino acids Carbohydrate: corn syrup Fat: soy, safflower, MCT	Multiple allergies Severe malabsorption Short gut Intestinal transplant
Fat modified	Tolerex Portagen	Protein: free amino acids Carbohydrate: modified corn starch or corn syrup Fat: MCTs, corn, or safflower oil	Chylothorax Severe steatorrhea

MCT, medium chain triglyceride.

TABLE 19.14

MECHANISMS FOR COW MILK PROTEIN ALLERGY AND THE ASSOCIATED PRESENTATIONS

IgE-Mediated	IgE- or Non–IgE-Mediated	Non–IgE-Mediated
Urticaria	Atopic dermatitis	Contact dermatitis
Angioedema	Asthma	Food-induced pulmonary hemosiderosis
Rhinoconjunctivitis	Eosinophilic esophagitis	Food-induced enterocolitis
Acute bronchospasm	Eosinophilic gastritis	Food-induced proctocolitis
Oral allergy syndrome	Eosinophilic gastroenteritis	Food-induced enteropathy
Gastrointestinal anaphylaxis		Gastroesophageal reflux disease

formula generally contains 20 kcal unless otherwise indicated. Unprocessed cow milk is not recommended for infants as it contains inadequate iron, excess protein, and electrolytes leading to excess renal load, a higher phosphorus content that can lead to hypocalcemia, and it can also lead to gastrointestinal bleeding.

Milk Protein Allergy

Milk protein allergy can occur in infants. Table 19.14 lists the characteristics of food hypersensitivity according to mechanism for the allergy. Infants with IgE-associated symptoms should not be given cow milk protein but may receive soy. If the child is breast feeding, his/her mother should eliminate cow milk protein from her diet, but may consume soy. The child may also transition to a soy formula until 1 year of age. Infants with non–IgE-associated symptoms should not be given cow milk protein or soy as there is significant crossover between allergens in this group. If the child is breast feeding, his/her mother should eliminate cow milk protein and soy from her diet. Alternatively, the child may transition to a hydrolyzed or an amino acid–based formula until 1 year of age.

SAMPLE BOARD REVIEW QUESTIONS

1. A 1-year-old child presents to your office for a well-child visit. The parents are strict vegetarians and would like their child to consume a vegetarian diet that excludes all meat, fish, and animal products. They inquire whether there are any risks associated with children adhering to strict vegetarian or vegan diets.
   You inform them that they should be worried about development of which of the following deficiencies?
   a. Caloric
   b. Protein
   c. Vitamin B_{12}
   d. Vitamin K
   e. Fluoride

   Answer: c. Children who adhere to strict vegetarian or vegan diets are at risk for vitamin B_{12}, vitamin D, calcium, and iron deficiency. Parents should be educated about providing calorie-dense foods to ensure that the child receives sufficient calories for growth, although calorie and protein malnutrition rarely, if ever, result from vegetarian diets. Similarly, vitamin K and fluoride deficiency are not the consequence of a vegetarian diet.

2. Breast milk and infant formula have many differences. Regarding macronutrients, formula has more of which of the following?
   a. Carbohydrate
   b. Fat
   c. Protein

   Answer: c. Formula has more protein as compared with breast milk. The protein in formula consists primarily of casein whereas breast milk has a greater percentage of whey. Breast milk has more fat as compared with formula. There are comparable amounts of carbohydrate in breast milk and formula.

3. Which of the following is a contraindication to breast feeding for mothers living in the United States?
   a. Maternal hepatitis B
   b. Maternal CMV

c. Maternal tuberculosis that has been fully treated
d. Mastitis
e. Maternal HIV

Answer: e. There is a short list of contraindications to breast feeding that can be found in the text. Maternal HIV is a contraindication in countries where malnutrition is not a major concern. CMV, hepatitis B, and tuberculosis treated for more that 2 weeks are all compatible with breast feeding. Breast feeding with mastitis helps promotes maternal healing and is not dangerous for the child.

4. A 4-month-old boy presents to your office for well-child care. At the end of the visit, you provide anticipatory guidance on the initiation of solid foods. You describe that the infant can begin with cereals over the next 2 months and then expand to pureed fruits and vegetables after 6 months of age. The infant's mother states that she is a fruitarian and would like to give her infant fruits and vegetables but is not interested in introducing cereal. Which of the following should you consider supplementing at this time if the infant if not going to receive cereal?
a. Vitamin K
b. Vitamin D
c. Iron
d. Fluoride

Answer: c. Although the iron in breast milk is more bioavailable than the iron in formula, the iron content of breast milk is insufficient to maintain normal body stores alone. Most infants begin taking iron fortified cereal between 4 and 6 months of age, which in combination with breast milk can provide sufficient iron for an infant. Breast fed infants who do not take cereal should receive iron supplements to prevent iron deficiency and anemia. The recommended dose is 1 mg/kg daily of elemental iron.

5. A 6-month-old infant presents to your office for well-child care. The child has been breast fed since birth. Over the course of the visit, you determine that the parents have introduced cereal and a few pureed fruits and vegetables over the course of the last month. The infant's mother also incidentally comments that they try to use bottled water for the preparation of all the foods they provide for the baby. Which of the following supplements should be initiated at this visit?
a. Vitamin K
b. Vitamin A
c. Iron
d. Fluoride

Answer: d. Most city water is supplemented with fluoride, but well water and bottled water are not. Infants who take powdered or concentrated formula or foods prepared with city water generally receive sufficient fluoride to help prevent dental caries. Infants who take ready to feed formula, who breast feed, or whose families only use well water or bottled water are not exposed to sufficient amounts of fluoride and should be supplemented. The recommended dose is 0.25 mg daily.

6. A mother brings her 2-week-old full-term girl to your office with concern for blood in her stools. The infant is formula fed and has become increasingly fussy with feeds. The infant has otherwise been without fever, vomiting, change in appetite. You consider the differential diagnosis for neonatal hematochezia, which includes swallowed maternal blood, anal fissure, necrotizing enterocolitis, and milk protein allergy. After initial evaluation, you decide that milk protein allergy is most likely cause for the hematochezia and recommend that they switch to which of the following formulas?
a. Soy
b. Lactose free
c. Hydrolyzed
d. Amino acid
e. Fat modified

Answer: c. Hematochezia as a result of milk protein is a non–IgE-mediated allergy. About 30% to 50% of children with non–IgE-mediated allergy to milk protein have continued symptoms when transitioned to soy. A hydrolyzed formula is indicated for this infant. Lactose-free and fat-modified formulas still contain milk protein. Although amino acid formulas could also be used, they are more expensive and thus only indicated when multiple allergies are present.

7. A previously healthy 12-month-old boy presents to your office for well-child care. You briefly glance at the growth parameters that the nurse obtained at the beginning of the

visit. You notice that his weight has fallen from the 50th to just below the 10th percentile since 6 months of age. You obtain a thorough history looking for any explanation for the inadequate weight gain. You discover that he takes formula as well as a variety of solid foods, but it is difficult to get a specific dietary history as he spends 60 hours each week in daycare. His examination is unremarkable with the exception of the aforementioned change in weight. His height and head circumference are stable at the 50th percentile. You suspect a psychosocial etiology for failure to thrive but decide to request some laboratory studies. Which of the following studies are appropriate at this point?

a. Complete blood cell count, electrolytes, protein, albumin, renal and hepatic panel, and urinalysis
b. Complete blood cell count, HIV, tuberculosis skin testing
c. Sweat test for cystic fibrosis
d. Stool elastase and reducing substances
e. MRI and chromosomal analysis

Answer: a. You might have decided to contact the daycare provider to obtain more diet history before obtaining laboratory tests, but it is not in appropriate to send to screening laboratories at this point. Laboratory screening consists of complete blood cell count, electrolytes, protein, albumin, renal and hepatic panel, and urinalysis. The remainder of the laboratory tests and diagnostics are indicated if the history and physical examination are suggestive of risk for HIV or tuberculosis, cystic fibrosis, malabsorption, or a genetic syndrome.

8. An 11-year-old girl presents to your office for well-child care. You calculate her BMI at the 90th percentile. Her personal and family histories are otherwise unremarkable. Her blood pressure is normal for her gender and height. On examination, you notice that she has acanthosis nigricans over the posterior aspect of her neck. Which of the following laboratory evaluations are appropriate at this time?

a. Fasting lipid levels
b. Fasting lipid levels, fasting glucose, transaminases
c. Fasting lipid levels, fasting glucose
d. Fasting glucose

Answer: b. This patient is overweight with acanthosis nigricans, which is suggestive of insulin resistance. Given the possible comorbidity of type 2 diabetes mellitus, she should undergo laboratory screening with fasting lipid levels, fasting glucose, and transaminases.

9. A 4-year-old boy presents to the emergency department for significant burns over the trunk and lower extremities sustained during a house fire. After debridement, he is admitted for skin care and fluid management. Given the severity of his burn, he is at risk for which of the following deficiencies:

a. Zinc
b. Vitamin C
c. Iron
d. Copper
e. Protein

Answer: e. Children with severe burns have significant protein losses. If their nutrition is not carefully managed as they heal, they may develop protein deficiency or Kwashiorkor.

10. Which of the following deficiencies results in anemia?

a. Vitamin B_6, vitamin B_{12}, folate, vitamin C, vitamin E, copper, iron, selenium
b. Vitamin K, vitamin C, vitamin B_{12}, folate, iron
c. Magnesium, zinc, iron, vitamin A
d. Vitamin D, calcium, phosphorus

Answer: a. All of the vitamins and minerals listed in choice A can cause anemia. Vitamin B_{12} and folate cause megaloblastic anemia. Vitamin B_6, vitamin C, copper, and iron all cause microcytic anemia.

11. A 6-month-old infant presents with a severe diaper rash over the labia and surrounding the anus. It appears eczematous with overlying bullae. Parents report that they have tried over-the-counter diaper creams, antifungal creams, and steroids without improvement. You suspect the following deficiency:

a. Vitamin B_2
b. Vitamin B_3
c. Biotin
d. Zinc

Answer: d. Acrodermatitis enteropathica is a rash that results from zinc deficiency. It appears as an eczematous rash with overlying vesicles, bullae, or pustules. It typically surrounds body orifices (mouth, anus) but can also be found on the scalp, hands, and feet. The rash is generally unresponsive to the aforementioned topical therapy and resolves with zinc supplementation.

12. A 24-month-old boy presents to the emergency department with refusal to bear weight. There is no known history of trauma. His parents report that he has always been bow legged, but that he has never had difficulty walking or refusal to bear weight until today. You decide to obtain radiographs of the lower extremities, which demonstrate cortical thinning and genu varum bilaterally and a greenstick fracture of the right femur. You suspect the following deficiency:

a. Vitamin A
b. Vitamin D
c. Pantothenic acid
d. Copper
e. Zinc

Answer: b. Vitamin D deficiency manifests with genu varum (bow legs) in toddlers and genu valgum (knock knees) in older children. Bones tend to be very weak and are prone to greenstick fractures. Other distinct bony changes include a square skull and costochondral swelling appearing as a rachitic rosary.

13. A 4-year-old boy presents to the emergency department with bleeding gums and a rash. His past medical history is significant for evaluation in feeding clinic at 2 years of age. His parents report that he is a very picky eater, but that he is no longer followed in feeding clinic because he is growing well. They report that his diet mostly consists of milk, cereal, pop tarts, and cheese pizza. You suspect the following deficiency:

a. Vitamin C
b. Vitamin A
c. Vitamin D
d. Vitamin B_3

Answer: a. Hemorrhage can result from vitamin C or vitamin K deficiency. Vitamin C deficiency results in scurvy, which manifests initially as bleeding from mucous membranes and dark purple macules primarily over the legs. Advanced vitamin C deficiency is associated with dental decay, open nonhealing wounds, and chronic diarrhea.

14. A 15-year-old boy with history of acne presents with progressively worsening headache and blurry vision. He reports he started taking a natural supplement to treat his acne a few weeks ago. He cannot remember the name, but he reports that he has started taking more because it really seems to be helping his acne. You suspect that he may be taking excess amounts of which of the following vitamin:

a. Biotin
b. Vitamin B_{12}
c. Vitamin A
d. Vitamin B2
e. Vitamin E

Answer: c. Hypervitaminosis A in the acute phase can result in pseudotumor cerebri, which manifests as headache and blurry vision. Tretinoin is the acid form of vitamin A that is prescribed by dermatologists for management of severe acne. Patients who are taking tretinoin are very closely monitored for side effects. Some health food stores advertise vitamin A supplements as treatment for acne. As in the case of this patient, unsupervised administration of vitamin A supplements for management of acne can be very dangerous. Long-term complications of vitamin A excess include hepatic fibrosis, osteoporosis, desquamation, and hair loss.

SUGGESTED READINGS

Finberg L. Feeding the healthy child. In: McMillan JA, DeAngelis CD, Feigin RD, et al. eds. *Oski's Pediatrics: Principles and Practice.* 4th ed. Philadelphia, PA: Lippincott Williams & Wilkins, 2006:109–118.

Kirkland RT. Failure to thrive. In: McMillan JA, DeAngelis CD, Feigin RD, et al. eds. *Oski's Pediatrics: Principles and Practice.* 4th ed. Philadelphia, PA: Lippincott Williams & Wilkins, 2006:900–906.

Kleinman RE, ed. *Pediatric Nutrition Handbook.* 5th ed. Elk Grove Village, IL: American Academy of Pediatrics, 2004.

Marinella MA. The refeeding syndrome and hypophosphatemia. *Nutr Rev.* 2003;61:9.

Schulman AJ. An obesity action plan. *Contemp Pediatr.* 2008;25:4.

Stein F. Continuous drip feeding. In: McMillan JA, DeAngelis CD, Feigin RD, et al. eds. *Oski's Pediatrics: Principles and Practice.* 4th ed. Philadelphia, PA: Lippincott Williams & Wilkins, 2006:2582.

Story RE. Manifestations of food allergy in infants and children. *Pediatr Ann.* 2008;37:8.

CHAPTER 20 ■ ONCOLOGY

RACHEL E. RAU

AFP	Alpha fetal protein	IVC	Inferior vena cava
AML	Acute myelogenous leukemia	IVIG	Intravenous immunoglobulin
ANC	Absolute neutrophil count	JRA	Juvenile rheumatoid arthritis
ALL	Acute lymphoblastic leukemia	FISH	Fluorescent in situ hybridization
APL	Acute promyelocytic leukemia	LCH	Langerhans' cell histiocytosis
BM	Bone marrow	LDH	Lactate dehydrogenase
BMT	Bone marrow transplantation	MIBG	Meta-iodobenzylguanidine
CBC	Complete blood cell count	MRI	Magnetic resonance imaging
cHL	Classical Hodgkin lymphoma	NB	Neuroblastoma
CML	Chronic myeloid leukemia	NHL	Non-Hodgkin lymphoma
CSF	Cerebral spinal fluid	NLP	Nodular lymphocyte predominant
CXR	Chest x-ray	NSAIDs	Nonsteroidal anti-inflammatory drugs
DIC	Disseminated intravascular coagulation	OM	Opsoclonus-myoclonus
EFS	Event-free survival	PB	Peripheral blood
FAB	French–American–British	RBC	Red blood cell
FCD	Fibrous cortical defect	RFA	Radiofrequency ablation
FEL	Familial erythrophagocytic lymphohistiocytosis	SMS	Superior mediastinal syndrome
GCTs	Germ cell tumors	SVC	Superior vena cava
HLH	Hemophagocytic lymphohistiocytosis	SVCS	Superior vena cava syndrome
HSCT	Hematopoietic stem cell transplantation	TLS	Tumor lysis syndrome
ICP	Intracranial pressure	WBC	White blood cell
ITP	Idiopathic thrombocytopenic purpura	WT	Wilms' Tumor

CHAPTER OBJECTIVES

1. To be familiar with the epidemiology of the most common childhood malignancies
2. To recognize the typical presenting signs and symptoms of malignancy in children
3. To understand the appropriate evaluation for children with suspected malignancy
4. To become familiar with the management of common childhood malignancies
5. To recognize and be able to manage common complications of malignancies and their treatments.

EPIDEMIOLOGY OF CHILDHOOD CANCER

From 2001 to 2005, the incidence of cancer in children was 16.7 cases per 100,000 for children aged 0 to 19 years. Cancer mortality in children is 2.7 per 100,000. The overall incidence is slightly higher in Whites (17.7 per 100,000) compared with Blacks (12 per 100,000). The most common childhood cancer is acute leukemia with 4.5 cases per 100,000 each year.

ONCOLOGIC EMERGENCIES

Fever In the Neutropenic Patient

Patients with neutropenia secondary to cancer and chemotherapy are at high risk for serious infections. Patients can quickly decompensate if not managed aggressively with antibiotics and supportive care.

Evaluation

In addition to a typical history and physical examination, febrile neutropenic patients require a thorough evaluation including several key assessments looking for specific sources of infection.

Important historical questions:
- Symptoms (chills, diaphoresis, pallor) with central line flushes—possible bacteria in the line.
- Pain with bowel movements—indicating possible perirectal cellulitis.
- Abdominal pain—possible typhlitis.

Physical examinations:
- Vital signs—first sign of shock is often an increased heart rate.
- Exam of vascular access sites—cellulitis.
- Assessment of perirectal area (NO digital rectal exam!)—perirectal cellulitis.

Important laboratory studies:
- CBC with differential and calculation of ANC.
- Blood cultures (all lumens of central lines).
- Urine culture (no catheterization).
- Comprehensive metabolic panel.

Typical ANC nadir occurs 10 to 14 days after the initiation of myelosupressive chemotherapy.

Consider other studies based on symptoms including CXR, sinus CT, abdominal CT. Some authors suggest a CXR in all febrile neutropenic patients regardless of symptoms.

Points to Remember

- *Typhlitis*: Inflammation of the small bowel wall in neutropenic patients. Predilection for the cecum. Classic presentation: RLQ pain and fever. Imaging: CT scan/ultrasound—bowel wall thickening, pneumatosis (air in the wall of the bowel), and free air if perforated. Management: NPO, broad-spectrum antibiotics including anaerobic coverage, serial exams, and early surgical consultation.

Management

In general, patients with an ANC of less than 500/μL (or <1,000 and falling) and fever require hospitalization and broad-spectrum antibiotics including adequate coverage for pseudomonas species. Single agents that are acceptable include third- and fourth-generation cephalosporins (ceftazidime and cefepime) and carbapenems (imipenem and meropenem).

Points to Remember

- ANC = WBC × (% bands + % neutrophils)
  For example, WBC = 2,300/μL, 40% neutrophils, 2% bands
  ANC = 2,300 × (0.4 + 0.02) = 966.

Tumor Lysis Syndrome

Leukemia and lymphoma cells turn over rapidly and are broken down quickly, especially after initiation of chemotherapy. When broken down, these cells release their contents into the circulation, which can result in TLS. TLS occurs most commonly with Burkitt's lymphoma and ALL, especially T-cell ALL.

Classic laboratory findings are hyperuricemia, hyperkalemia, and hyperphosphatemia with secondary hypocalcemia.

TLS can lead to acute renal failure secondary to uric acid and calcium phosphate crystal precipitation in the microvasculature of the kidneys. This can exacerbate hyperkalemia, which, if untreated, can lead to fatal arrhythmias.

Management

Prevention:
- Allopurinol (250 to 500 mg/m^2/day, max: 800 mg daily) to prevent the formation of uric acid.
- Aggressive hydration (usually at two times maintenance rate) to adequately flush the kidneys (fluids should not contain potassium).
- Alkalinization to increase the excretion of uric acid.
  - Monitor urine pH with a goal of 7.0 to 7.5: less than 7.0 can lead to uric acid precipitation; more than 7.5 can lead to calcium phosphate crystal formation.
- Frequent monitoring of serum electrolytes is essential.

Treatment:
- When metabolic abnormalities occur, treatment should be initiated immediately (e.g., Kayexalate for hyperkalemia).
- If renal failure occurs, dialysis is required.

Hyperleukocytosis

Hyperleukocytosis is defined as a WBC greater than 100,000/μL. Patients most at risk for complications are those with AML, those with ALL and other hematologic malignancies typically do not experience complications unless WBC is greater than 200,000/μL. Hyperleukocytosis can lead to sludging of viscose blood in small vessels. Three organ systems are predominantly affected: pulmonary, central nervous system, and renal (see Table 20.1). These patients are also at high risk for TLS.

TABLE 20.1

COMPLICATIONS OF HYPERLEUKOCYTOSIS

System	Complication	Signs/Symptoms
Pulmonary	Pulmonary leukostasis and secondary pulmonary hemorrhage	Dyspnea, hypoxia, cyanosis, acidosis
Central nervous system	Leukostasis in cerebral vasculature Hemorrhagic stroke (more commonly) Ischemic stroke (rare)	Mental status changes, headache, blurry vision, seizure, coma, focal neurologic deficits, papilledema
Renal	Leukostasis in microvasculature Renal failure	Oliguria, anuria, hyperkalemia
Other	Leukostasis in small vessels Hemorrhage	Priapism, dactylitis, GI bleeding, pericardial tamponade

Management

- Initiate the usual preventative regimen for TLS with aggressive hydration, alkalinization, and allopurinol.
- Keep platelet count at least more than 20,000/μL to prevent hemorrhage.
- Avoid RBC transfusions as they increase viscosity. If RBC transfusion is necessary, consider exchange transfusion.
- If symptoms of leukostasis are present, consider leukapheresis to quickly decrease WBC. *Note*: exchange transfusion and leukapheresis are only temporizing measures. The definitive treatment is initiation of chemotherapy as quickly as is safely possible.

Spinal Cord Compression

- Masses compressing the spinal cord, conus medullaris, or cauda equina constitute medical emergencies.
- Should be suspected in any child with cancer and back pain.
- If cord compression remains undiagnosed, progressive neurologic symptoms are usually present, including weakness, paresis, and sensory deficits and may be irreversible; therefore, immediate diagnosis and appropriate management is vital.

Evaluation

- A thorough neurologic examination including strength, sensory, deep tendon reflex exam, and rectal sphincter tone. Absence of neurologic symptoms does not rule out cord compression.
- MRI is the radiographic study of choice to diagnose spinal cord compression.
- Spine radiographs are abnormal in less than 50% of patients with spinal cord compression, but, given their ease of availability, may be useful in the early evaluation of a child with suspected cord compression while awaiting MRI.

Management

- If history and physical exam suggest **cord dysfunction,** the patient should receive 1 to 2 mg/kg of dexamethasone and then undergo MRI.
- If cord compression is suspected but there is **no neurologic dysfunction,** the patient should be given dexamethasone at a lower dose of 0.25 to 0.5 mg/kg orally every 6 hours and an MRI should be scheduled within 24 hours.
- Occasionally emergent radiation therapy is necessary and rarely surgical decompression is required to relieve the compression.

Mediastinal Masses

Tumors in the anterior mediastinum can lead to compression of the trachea resulting in SMS. They can also cause compression or obstruction of the SVC resulting in SVCS. Both of these conditions constitute medical emergencies. (See Box 20.1 for mediastinal masses that most commonly cause SMS/SVCS.)

Evaluation

Use the least invasive method possible to obtain diagnosis.

Box 20.1 Common Causes of Mediastinal Masses

Hodgkin disease	Teratoma
Non-Hodgkin lymphoma	Acute lymphoblastic leukemia (most commonly T cell)
Germ cell tumor	Sarcomas
Neuroblastoma	

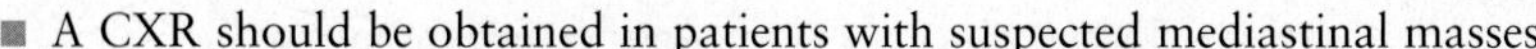

- A CXR should be obtained in patients with suspected mediastinal masses.
- CT scan delineates the extent of tracheal compression (perform in prone position if the supine position aggravates respiratory symptoms).
- Echocardiogram to investigate possible thromboembolism.

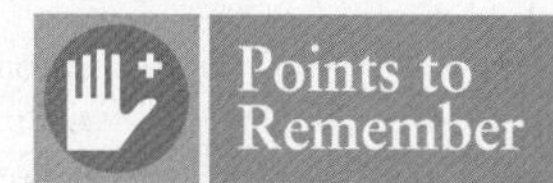

Points to Remember

- **In patients with mediastinal mass, conscious sedation and anxiolytics are contraindicated!**

Caution: General anesthesia can lead to relaxation of airway smooth muscles and worsening of airway obstruction, and tracheal intubation can be extremely difficult. If sedation or anesthesia is necessary, it should be performed in the operating room with fibroscopic equipment available should intubation prove difficult.

Management

- **Emergent initiation of steroids** and/or chemotherapy for presumed leukemia/lymphoma can be instituted.
- Emergent **radiation therapy** can also be used but may be less readily available and younger children often require sedation.
- **Surgery** may be required for tumors such as teratomas, which are less likely to respond to radiation and chemotherapy.

Initiation of emergent treatment may lessen the chance of making a tissue diagnosis, but institution of therapy may be necessary to prevent mortality or severe morbidity.

LEUKEMIA

Acute Lymphoblastic Leukemia

ALL is a hematologic malignancy that arises in the lymphoid cell lineage and can be either B cell or T cell derived. No underlying predisposing condition exists in most cases; however, known risk factors include Down syndrome, ataxia-telangiectasia, and prior exposure to ionizing radiation.

Epidemiology

- Accounts for approximately one-third of all childhood cancer.
- Approximately 80% to 85% of all childhood acute leukemia is ALL.
- Approximately 5,000 new cases in the United States each year.
- Disease of young children, with a peak age at diagnosis of 2 to 3 years.

Presentation

Signs and symptoms that bring a child with ALL to medical attention are secondary to infiltration of normal organs by leukemic blasts (see Table 20.2 for presenting signs and symptoms). Patients can also present with oncologic emergencies including TLS, hyperleukocytosis, SVC and/or airway compression syndrome secondary to a mediastinal mass, and fever in the face of neutropenia (see "Oncologic Emergencies" section)

Differential Diagnosis

A child presenting with ALL can have features that overlap with a number of different childhood illnesses. In general, a careful physical exam, blood smear evaluation, and BM aspirate will help establish the correct diagnosis.

- JRA can present with fever, pallor, joint pain, and hepatosplenomegaly. Perform a BM aspiration before initiating steroids.
- ITP is common in childhood, but only the platelet count should be affected.
- Infectious mononucleosis can also present much like acute leukemia with hepatosplenomegaly, lymphadenopathy, and mild cytopenias. On PB smear, it can be difficult to distinguish atypical lymphocytes (characteristic of infectious mononucleosis) and leukemic blasts (see Fig. 20.1).

TABLE 20.2

ORGAN INVOLVEMENT AND RESULTING SIGNS/SYMPTOMS IN ACUTE LEUKEMIA

Involved Organ	Signs/Symptoms	Involved Organ	Signs/Symptoms
Bone marrow	Anemia ■ Fatigue ■ Pallor ■ Dyspnea ■ Tachycardia ■ Lightheadedness ■ Congestive heart failure (rarely) Thrombocytopenia ■ Bruising ■ Bleeding ■ Petechiae Neutropenia ■ Fever and infection Pain secondary to marrow crowding ■ Limp ■ Refusal to bear weight	Lymph nodes Kidneys Gums Testis Thymus Skin Other	Lymphadenopathy Renal insufficiency Gingival hypertrophy ■ Most common in infants Testicular enlargement Anterior mediastinal mass ■ Most common with T-cell ALL ■ Can cause SVC syndrome and airway compression Leukemia cutis ■ Most common in infants Chloromas ■ Tumors of leukemia cells ■ Occur most commonly in the orbits resulting in proptosis
Liver/spleen	Hepatosplenomegaly		

SVC, superior vena cava.

- Aplastic anemia can present with cytopenias and related symptoms but should not have an increased blast count.
- Other malignancies can metastasize to the BM including NB, sarcomas, and retinoblastoma. If the BM involvement is extensive, patients can have a clinical picture like ALL.

Evaluation

- Thorough physical examination—lymphadenopathy, hepatosplenomegaly, pallor, bruising, signs of infection.
- Evaluation of the PB, BM, and CSF.
- Special testing of the PB and BM, including flow cytometry to establish cell type and FISH to look for recurrent chromosomal abnormalities.
- Labs to assess for TLS.

Management

At diagnosis, manage symptoms, treat infection, and initiate chemotherapy as soon as is medically feasible. There are multiple phases of chemotherapy including remission induction, consolidation with non–cross-resistant drugs to eradicate any remaining disease, and maintenance therapy to ensure complete elimination of disease and minimize the risk of relapse. All patients

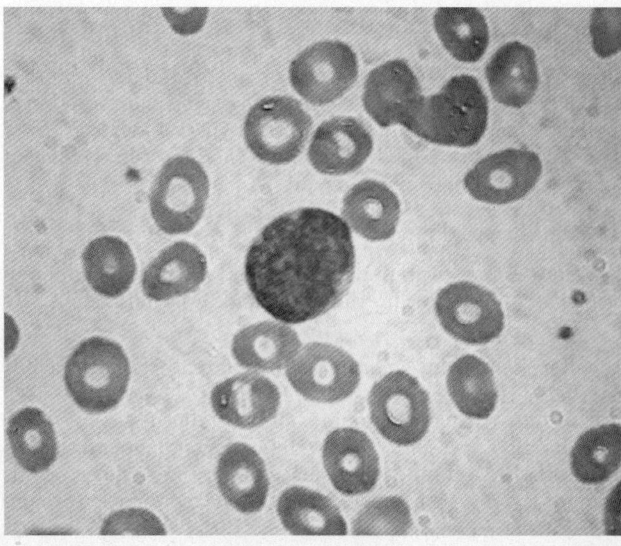

FIGURE 20.1. Lymphoblast. (Courtesy of Clifford Takemoto, MD.)

are given intrathecal chemotherapy to treat or prevent CNS involvement. Currently, boys are treated 1 year longer than girls to minimize testicular relapse risk.

Prognosis

The overall EFS for children with ALL is 85% to 90%. Patients with a WBC count more than 50,000/μL at diagnosis and those less than 1 year or more than 10 years at diagnosis are deemed high risk with EFS in the 60% to 70% range. These patients receive more intensive chemotherapy compared with patients with standard-risk ALL.

Acute Myelogenous Leukemia

AML represents a group of hematologic malignancies that arise within myeloid, monocyte, erythroid, or megakaryocytic cell lineages.

Epidemiology

- Approximately 15% to 20% of all childhood acute leukemia is AML, equaling roughly 1,000 new cases of AML annually in the United States.
- Prevalence Male = Female, Hispanics > Blacks and Whites.
- Most do not have a predisposing exposure or condition; however, ionizing radiation, benzenes, and prior chemotherapy increase the risk of AML.
- Inherited risk factors: Down syndrome, Li–Fraumeni syndrome, Neurofibromatosis type I, Klinefelter syndrome, and BM failure syndromes such as Fanconi's anemia, Shwachman–Diamond syndrome, and Ataxia telangiectasia.

Traditionally, AML is characterized based on morphology according to the FAB classification (see Table 20.3). Currently, immunophenotyping and cytogenetic analysis are also used to characterize AML blasts and help direct therapy.

Presentation

Typical presenting signs and symptoms are, like ALL, secondary to infiltration of the BM and other organs with leukemic blasts, anemia, thrombocytopenia, neutropenia, bone pain, hepatosplenomegaly, and lymphadenopathy. Extramedullary involvement can result in gingival hypertrophy and leukemia cutis (palpable raised plaques). These are more common in the

TABLE 20.3

FRENCH–AMERICAN–BRITISH (FAB) CLASSIFICATION OF AML

FAB Class	Name	Frequency	Special Features	Genetic Associations
M0	Undifferentiated	Rare		
M1	Acute myeloblastic—no maturation	~20% pediatric AML		
M2	Acute myeloblastic—with maturation	~30% pediatric AML		t(8;21)
M3	Acute promyelocytic	~5%–10% pediatric AML	High risk of DIC Treated with ATRA	t(15;17)
M4	Acute myelomonocytic	~25%–30% pediatric AML	Extramedullary involvement common M4Eo—variant in which cells are abnormal eosinophil precursors	Inv (16)
M5	Acute monocytic	~15% pediatric AML (~50% AML in children <2y)	Extramedullary involvement common	t(9;11)
M6	Acute erythroleukemia	Rare		
M7	Acute megakaryocytic	~5%–10% pediatric AML Most common subtype in DS	Associated with myelofibrosis and hepatic fibrosis	

AML, acute myelogenous leukemia; ATRA, all-trans retinoic acid; DIC, disseminated intravascular coagulation; DS, Down syndrome.

M4 and M5 subtypes (see Table 20.2 for other subtype-specific presenting signs/symptoms). Chloromas can be present throughout the body and are commonly found in the orbits and occasionally in the spinal cord.

Evaluation

- Thorough physical examination—lymphadenopathy, hepatosplenomegaly, pallor, bruising, signs of infection.
- Evaluation of the PB, BM, and CSF.
- Special testing of the PB and BM, including flow cytometry to establish cell type and FISH to look for recurrent chromosomal abnormalities.
- Coagulation studies should be obtained to evaluate for DIC.
- Labs to assess for TLS.

Treatment and Prognosis

Intensive chemotherapy with remission induction and postremission consolidation with either BM transplant or further chemotherapy. All current AML treatment protocols include prophylaxis against CNS disease, with intrathecal chemotherapy.

Long-term survival of children with AML is currently 40% to 60% with the exception of patients with M3 AML and patients with Down syndrome who do significantly better.

Chronic Leukemias

Chronic leukemias, unlike acute leukemias, have a predominance of mature cells and an indolent course. These diseases are extremely rare in childhood. Chronic lymphocytic leukemia essentially never occurs in children and therefore is beyond the scope of this review. CML is more common in children but makes up less than 5% of all childhood leukemias.

Chronic Myeloid Leukemia

The chronic phase of CML results in hyperproliferation of mostly mature BM cells.

Presentation

Fever, night sweats, fatigue, hepatomegaly and splenomegaly. CML can evolve into a myeloproliferative disease or a blast phase, which is essentially an acute leukemia with blasts in the PB and BM. Patients in blast phase present like patients with de novo acute leukemias.

Lab findings: Leukocytosis (rarely hyperleukocytosis) with a left shift, elevated levels of eosinophils and basophils, anemia, and often thrombocytosis.

Characterized by a genetic **translocation t(9;22)(q34;q11), known as the Philadelphia chromosome.** This translocation results in a **fusion protein, bcr/abl,** which appears to be important in the pathogenesis of CML.

Treatment

Historically, chemotherapy and stem cell transplant has been used to treat CML; however, imatinib mesylate (Gleevec), a small molecule inhibitor of bcr/abl, has revolutionized the treatment of CML. Imatinib is now first-line therapy for chronic phase CML. Blast phase CML is generally treated like acute leukemia with dismal response rates.

LYMPHOMA

Hodgkin Lymphoma

Hodgkin lymphoma is a B-cell–derived neoplasm. There are two main subtypes of Hodgkin lymphoma: NLP and cHL (see Table 20.4).

Presentation

- Painless lymphadenopathy.
- Approximately two-third also have a mediastinal mass; therefore, may have signs and symptoms of SMS/SVCS (see "Mediastinal Masses" section).
- Systemic symptoms can include fever, weight loss, and drenching night sweats ("B" symptoms).

Differential Diagnosis

Consider other causes of lymphadenopathy: infectious mononucleosis, atypical mycobacterium and toxoplasmosis, NHL, and metastatic adenopathy of other primary sites. See Box 1 for other causes of mediastinal masses.

TABLE 20.4

SUBTYPES OF HODGKIN LYMPHOMA

Subtype	Histology
Nodular lymphocyte predominant	Nodular architecture Lymphocytic and histiocytic cells surrounded by inflammatory cells
Classic Hodgkin lymphoma ■ Nodular sclerosis ■ Mixed cellularity ■ Lymphocyte rich ■ Lymphocyte depleted	Reed–Sternberg cells ■ Characterized by two large eosinophilic nuclei Subtypes classified based on presence of fibrosis and the features of the associated inflammatory infiltrate

Evaluation

- **Labs:** CBC with differential, ESR or CRP, renal, and hepatic function tests, alkaline phosphatase level.
- **Imaging studies:** To evaluate for a mediastinal mass—CXR/chest CT. To evaluate the extent of disease—CT of the neck, chest abdomen, and pelvis. Those with bone pain and/or elevated alkaline phosphatase should have a bone scan.
- **Biopsies:** Biopsy of enlarged lymph nodes and BM biopsies.

Treatment and Prognosis

Combination of surgery, chemotherapy, and radiation therapy is the mainstay of treatment for Hodgkin lymphoma. With multimodal therapy, the prognosis for patients is overall favorable. Patients with localized disease have an EFS of more than 90%. Patients with high-stage disease have an EFS of 60% to 80%. Some risk factors associated with inferior outcome include male gender, high WBC count, bulky mediastinal disease, and low hemoglobin.

Non-Hodgkin Lymphoma

NHLs are a group of malignancies arising from cells and organs of the immune system and are essentially any malignant lymphoma not classified as Hodgkin lymphoma. With common cells of origin, there is significant overlap between NHL and ALL. Disease is designated ALL if the BM has more than 25% lymphoblasts and NHL if there is less than 25%.

There are many variants of NHL; however, there are essentially three main types that occur in childhood, Burkitt's/B-large cell lymphoma, lymphoblastic lymphoma, and large cell lymphoma (most commonly anaplastic large cell lymphoma). See Table 20.5 for cell of origin, presentations, and outcomes.

Epidemiology

- More common in children younger than 10 years, whereas Hodgkin lymphoma is two times more common in children aged 15 to 19 years.
- Male predominance.
- Whites > Blacks.

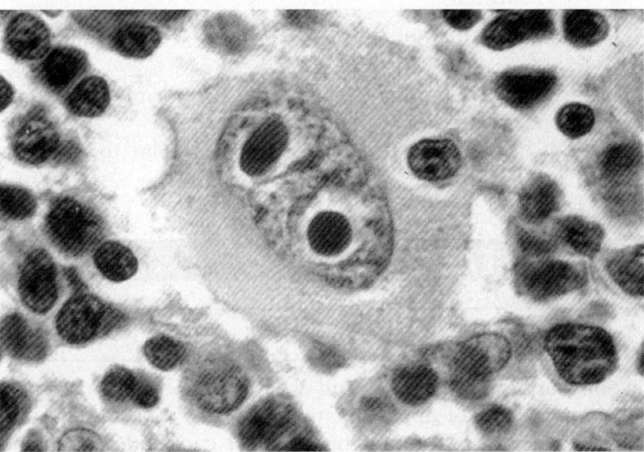

FIGURE 20.2. Reed–Sternberg cells typical of Hodgkin lymphoma. (Reprinted with permission from Rubin R, Strayer DS. *Rubin's Pathology: Clinicopathologic Foundations of Medicine.* 5th ed. Philadelphia, PA: Lippincott Williams & Wilkins, 2008.)

TABLE 20.5

NHL BY SUBTYPE

Subtype	Cell of Origin	Presentation	Outcome (EFS)
Burkitt's/B-large cell	B lymphocyte	Rapidly growing abdominal mass **Intussusception** **Massive TLS** LAD—mesentery, retroperitoneum Head and neck—jaw and orbit Spinal cord compression BM involvement CNS involvement	80%–90%
Lymphoblastic	T lymphocyte	LAD—cervical, SC, axillary Mediastinal mass Effusions HSM Cytopenias secondary to BM involvement CNS involvement	80%–90%
Large cell	■ B lymphocyte ■ Anaplastic	Head and neck masses LAD Mediastinal masses Soft tissue involvement—skin, bone, GI	90% for low-stage disease 60%–70% for high-stage disease

BM, bone marrow; CNS, central nervous system; EFS, event-free survival; GI, gastrointestinal tract; HSM, hepatosplenomegaly; LAD, lymphadenopathy; SC, supraclavicular; TLS, tumor lysis syndrome.

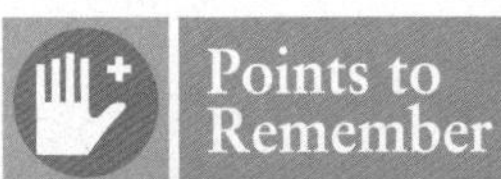

Points to Remember

- **Burkitt's lymphoma can present as intussusception secondary to masses originating from the Peyer's patches in the terminal ileum. Endemic Burkitt's lymphoma occurs in regions in Africa and is characterized by involvement of the maxilla, orbit, and other facial bones.**

Etiology

NHL arises in lymphoid cells after genetic alterations that affect cell proliferation and differentiation. For example, the most common genetic aberration is t(8;14) which results in the fusion of cMyc with a gene for an immunoglobulin chain and occurs in most Burkitt's lymphomas.

Endemic Burkitt's lymphoma, which occurs in areas of equatorial Africa and is characterized by involvement of the head and neck, appears to be caused by EBV, perhaps in the setting of chronic malaria. The role of EBV in nonendemic Burkitt's lymphoma, characterized by primarily abdominal involvement, is less clear.

Children with underlying congenital immune deficiency and those post–solid organ transplant are also at high risk for developing NHL in response to EBV. Also, patients with HIV are at risk for the development of NHL, predominantly Burkitt's lymphoma.

Evaluation

- Tissue resection or biopsy as well as BM, CSF, PB (CBC, morphology), and labs to assess for TLS.
- Imaging studies:
  - CT or MRI of the primary site.
  - Neck and chest CT should be obtained before any sedation given the risk of SMS.
  - Abdominal CT scan to rule out metastatic disease.

Treatment

- Burkitt's lymphoma: short intensive chemotherapy and CNS prophylaxis with intrathecal chemotherapy.
- Lymphoblastic lymphomas are treated essentially like ALL with multiple phases of chemotherapy including a maintenance phase lasting many months.
- Anaplastic large cell lymphoma can be treated with chemotherapy similar to Burkitt's lymphoma or lymphoblastic with similar results.

SOLID TUMORS

Brain Tumors

Brain tumors are the most common solid tumors in children and are the second most common cancer in childhood after acute leukemia. There are approximately 2,500 to 3,000 new cases diagnosed per year in the United States. They also **account for the most cancer deaths in the**

TABLE 20.6

HISTOLOGIC CLASSIFICATION OF BRAIN TUMORS

Cell Type	Cells	Tumor
Neuroglial cells	Astrocytes	Astrocytic tumors (gliomas) Pilocytic (low grade) Fibrillary Diffuse fibrillary (low grade) Anaplastic astrocytoma (high grade) GBM (high grade)
	Oligodendrocytes Ependyma Choroids plexus	Oligodendroma Ependymoma Choroid plexus papilloma Choroid plexus carcinoma
Neuronal/embryonal	Neurons/embryonal cells	Medulloblastoma Pineoblastoma Supratentorial PNET Atypical teratoid/rhabdoid tumor
Other		CNS lymphoma Germ cell tumor Craniopharyngioma

GBM, glioblastoma multiforme; PNET, primitive neuroectodermal tumor.

pediatric population. Several classifications of brain tumors exist. One useful way to classify brain tumors is by histology (see Table 20.6).

Presentation

Brain tumors can present in a variety of ways. They can have general and nonlocalizing symptoms, signs/symptoms of increased ICP if the tumor is in a location that obstructs the flow of CSF or is large enough to increase ICP, and localizing signs that are dependent upon the location of the tumor (see Table 20.7).

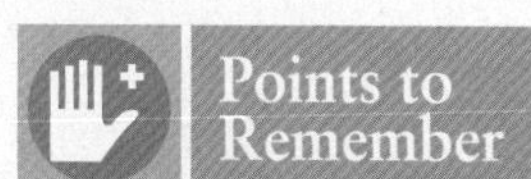

- **The majority of pediatric brain tumors are located in the infratentorial region (70%), whereas the vast majority of adult brain tumors are supratentorial.**
- **Parinaud syndrome: paralysis of conjugate upward gaze without paralysis of convergence, associated with tumors of the midbrain.**

Diagnosis

The initial study typically obtained in patients suspected of having a brain tumor is a CT scan. However, **MRI is the preferred study** because

- Visualization of the posterior fossa is superior to that of CT scans.
- Improved MRI techniques often delineate the appearance and location well enough to, in certain circumstances, eliminate the need for biopsy.

Given the risk of "drop metastasis" to the spine, all patients with brain tumors should undergo MRI of the spine and evaluation of the CSF (preferably prior to surgical resection of the primary mass).

Treatment

Combination of surgery, radiation therapy and chemotherapy.

For most brain tumors, patients have a higher chance of cure if a complete resection is possible; however, many are not amenable to complete surgical resection, and therefore radiation therapy and chemotherapy play a more central role.

Prognosis

Although overall survival for all CNS malignancies is approximately 70%, prognosis depends upon the type of tumor, the biologic features of the tumor, its location, and whether or not it can be completely resected. For example, medulloblastoma, the most common pediatric CNS malignancy, has a survival of approximately 80% when localized, whereas brain stem gliomas carry a dismal prognosis with a survival of less than 10% at 2 years. In addition to potential mortality, patients with CNS tumors often suffer significant morbidity from their disease and its treatment. These sequelae can include seizures, focal neurologic deficits, headaches, cognitive deficits, and behavioral abnormalities. Endocrinologic dysfunction, including growth failure, thyroid deficiency, and gonadotropin deficiency, can also occur as a result of radiation to the hypothalamus. With cranial radiation therapy, neurocognitive deficits can be particularly pronounced, especially if the patient was younger than 8 years at the time of treatment.

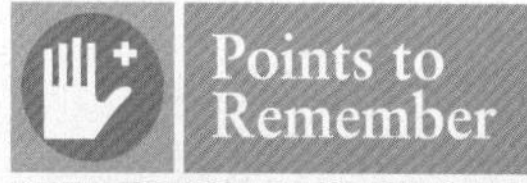

- **Currently, CNS malignancy accounts for more pediatric cancer deaths than any other malignancy.**

TABLE 20.7

SIGNS AND SYMPTOMS OF BRAIN TUMORS

Location and Common Tumors	Signs and Symptoms
Infratentorial: Cerebellar MB Cerebellar astrocytoma Ependymoma Brainstem Pontine glioma Exophytic brainstem glioma	Cranial neuropathies: visual loss, head tilt, diplopia, gaze palsy, hearing loss, facial weakness, etc. Drooling/swallow dysfunction Partial Horner syndrome Ataxia Nystagmus Dysmetria Slow or halting speech
Supratentorial: PNET GBM LGA GCTs Choroid plexus tumors	Hemiparesis/hemisensory loss Hyperreflexia Early handedness/change in handedness Seizures—exceedingly rare even with supratentorial tumors Visual complaints secondary to tumors along the optic path
Suprasellar/sellar region craniopharyngioma	Visual field defects Endocrinopathies: short stature, DI
Hypothalamus: Most often GTCs	Endocrinopathies: growth failure and DI, can be present years prior to diagnosis Behavioral and emotional changes
Pineal region tumors: GCTs Pineoblastoma	Parinaud syndrome Focal motor deficits
General, non-localizing	Headaches Vomiting Behavioral changes Developmental delay Weight loss/gain Failure to thrive Endocrine dysfunction Autonomic dysfunction
Increased ICP	Headache Irritability Lethargy Nausea/vomiting Bulging fontanelle Papilledema Anisocoria Ataxia Parinaud syndrome

MB, medulloblastoma; PNET, primitive neuroectodermal tumor; GBM, glioblastoma multiforme; LGA, low-grade astrocytoma; GCTs, germ cell tumors; DI, diabetes insipidus; ICP, intracranial pressure.

Neuroblastoma

NB cells arise from neural crest cells that were destined to differentiate into sympathetic neurons. See Figure 20.2 for catecholamine metabolism pathway.

Histologically, NB is a small round blue cell tumor. **A classic finding is Homer-Wright pseudorosettes; however, this is in actuality an infrequent finding.** There are many associated genetic abnormalities in tumor cells. The most common and prognostically significant is **amplification of the N-Myc gene** on chromosome 2p24.

Epidemiology

- Most common extracranial solid tumor of childhood.
- Approximately 8% of all childhood cancer.
- Male > Female.
- Median age at diagnosis = 22 months; 90% <5 years at diagnosis.

TABLE 20.8

PRESENTING SYMPTOMS OF NEUROBLASTOMA BASED ON SITE OF INVOLVEMENT

Site of Involvement	Symptoms
Abdominal	Abdominal pain Palpable mass Constipation Respiratory compromise in infants with massive liver infiltrate Lower extremity and/or scrotal edema secondary to occlusion of venous and lymphatic drainage Hypertension secondary to occlusion of renal vessels
Paraspinal	Radicular pain Paraplegia Bowel/bladder dysfunction
Thoracic/cervical	SVC syndrome Horner syndrome (ptosis, myosis, anhydrosis)
Orbital	Ptosis and periorbital ecchymosis (Raccoon eyes)
Skin	"Blueberry-muffin" nodules of tumor cells
Bone marrow	Cytopenias
Any site—symptoms from catecholamine overproduction	Hypertension Flushing Tachycardia Diaphoresis
Paraneoplastic	Opsoclonus-myoclonus (Dancing eyes, dancing feet) Secretory diarrhea

SVC, superior vena cava.

Clinical Presentation

The presenting features at the time of diagnosis vary depending upon the site of involvement. At diagnosis, the adrenal medulla is the most common primary site followed by paraspinal regions (35% and 30%, respectively). Twenty percent of patients present with thoracic primary tumors. Rarely, primary tumors will be found in the pelvis or cervical area. See Table 20.8 for presenting symptoms based on site of involvement.

Opsoclonus Myoclonus is a paraneoplastic syndrome occuring in 2% to 3% of patients with NB. Symptoms include myoclonic jerks of limbs and trunk, random eye movements, ataxia. Patients with OM have improved outcome with respect to their NB, but are at high risk for long-term cognitive, motor, language deficits, and behavioral problems. Treatment: steroids, high-dose IVIG, and gabapentin with variable success.

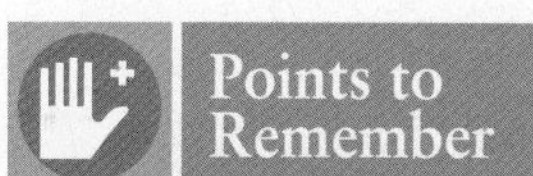

- **Opsoclonus-myoclonus (dancing eyes, dancing feet).**

Evaluation

- Imaging:
  - **CT scan or MRI** of the primary tumor.
  - **MIBG** scintiscan. MIBG is an analogue of catecholamine precursors and concentrates in NB cells and localizes to tumor cells in 90% to 95% of patients. Can be useful to follow for response to therapy, minimal residual disease, and recurrence. Caution: MIBG can damage the thyroid. To protect it, super-saturated potassium iodine is given prior to MIBG.
  - Evaluate for metastasis to the cortical bone via plain films or bone scan.
- Biopsy or resection of the primary tumor for histology and molecular studies. BM aspirate and biopsies from at least two sites.
- Labs: CBC, LDH, ferritin, and urine HVA and VMA.

Treatment

- Low-stage disease: surgery alone. Of note, many young patients with localized disease have spontaneous resolution of their tumor; however, when identified, the standard of care is still resection.
- Intermediate risk: combination of surgery, chemotherapy, and often radiation therapy.
- High risk: surgery, chemotherapy, radiation therapy. Autologous stem cell transplant is becoming a mainstay of therapy. Retinoic acid is also used as this medication can lead NB cells into differentiation.

Points to Remember

- Stage IV-S disease is a unique group of patients: infants younger than 1 year with a localized tumor with metastatic disease limited to the liver, skin, and/or BM. If they do not have N-Myc amplification or unfavorable histology, they typically regress spontaneously and do not require treatment unless they have symptoms secondary to mass effect.

- Patients with stage IV-S disease represent a unique subset of patients.
  - With favorable biologic features (i.e., favorable histology and lack of N-Myc amplification), the typical natural history is complete resolution of disease. Thus, observation alone is often sufficient.
  - If there is unfavorable tumor biology or if the patient is symptomatic, that is, respiratory symptoms secondary to an enlarged liver chemotherapy is given.

Prognosis

Localized NB: EFS of more than 95% even if ipsilateral lymph nodes are involved.

If the tumor has N-Myc amplification and/or unfavorable histology or distant metastasis at diagnosis, their prognosis is unfavorable (EFS, 30% to 50%).

Exception: Stage IV-S disease, though by definition have metastatic disease, do very well. If these patients have favorable biological features, they have an EFS of more than 95%.

Wilms' Tumor

- WT accounts for approximately 6% of all childhood cancer in the United States.
- Blacks > whites >> Asians.
- Unilateral disease: mean age at presentation is ~3.5 years for boys, ~4 years for girls.
- Bilateral disease: mean age at presentation is ~2.5 years for both sexes.
- Few congenital syndromes with well-established association with WT (Table 20.9).

Presentation

- Often parent notices abdominal fullness/mass while changing or bathing the child.
- Abdominal pain.
- Gross hematuria.
- 25% will also have hypertension at the time of diagnosis.

Evaluation

- Labs: renal and liver function tests, calcium, CBC, urinalysis, urine catecholamines to help differentiate from NB, and coagulation assays to examine for acquired von Willebrand disease, as this occurs in approximately 8% of patients at diagnosis.
- Imaging:
  - Initial study—ultrasound with Doppler to differentiate a solid from cystic mass and can identify the organ of origin.
  - Doppler study including the IVC is useful, as the tumor can extend into the IVC reaching as far as the right atrium.
  - CT scan of the chest, abdomen, and pelvis.
  - Baseline CXR.
- Prior to initiating therapy, a surgical specimen helps ensure the correct diagnosis has been established.

TABLE 20.9

CONGENITAL ANOMALIES AND SYNDROMES ASSOCIATED WITH WILMS' TUMOR

Syndrome	Features	Associated Genetic Mutations
WAGR syndrome	**W**ilms tumor (>30% of patients with WAGR will develop WT) **A**niridia **G**enitourinary malformations **R**etardation of mentation and growth	Germline mutation at chromosome 11p13 including *WT1* gene
Denys–Drash syndrome	Pseudohermaphroditism, degenerative renal disease (nephrotic syndrome or glomerulonephritis), Wilms' tumor	Associated with mutations in chromosome 11p
Beckwith–Wiedemann syndrome	Overgrowth syndrome with gigantism or regional hyperplasia, visceromegaly, macroglossia, hyperinsulinemic hypoglycemia, predisposition to embryonal tumors	Familial form maps to chromosome 11p15, same region as *WT2* gene and *IGFII* gene
Sporadic hemihyperplasia	Seen in ~ 25% of patients with WT	
Other	Cryptorchidism: in 46.6% of males with WT Hypospadias: in 20% of males with WT	

IGFII, insulin-like growth factor II.

Treatment

Treatment of WT consists of a multimodality approach. All patients undergo surgery. If resection is possible (typically a nephrectomy), this is the preferred initial therapy. If resection is not possible because of bilateral disease or bulky disease that would require extensive surgery, biopsy should be performed. All patients with WT are treated with chemotherapy. Patients with higher staged disease also receive radiation therapy.

Prognosis

Patients with WT overall do quite well. Patients with low-stage disease and favorable histology have an EFS of 90%. Patients with distant metastases at diagnosis and those with unfavorable histology have an EFS of 66%.

Bone Tumors

Ewing Sarcoma

Ewing sarcoma is an aggressive, small round blue cell tumor. Eighty-five percent of Ewing sarcomas have a reciprocal translocation between chromosomes 11 and 22, t(11;22)(q24;q12). In the majority of tumors without this translocation, there are other structural rearrangements of the same region of chromosome 22.

Epidemiology

- Second most common malignant bone cancer in patients younger than 20 years with an incidence of 2.9 per million.
- Male > Female.
- Caucasians > Asians and African Americans.
- By far more common in adolescents with a median age of 15 years.

Presentation. Localized pain is the most common presentation of Ewing sarcoma. Given many of these patients are in the peak of growth acceleration, this pain is often mistaken for "growing pains" or injury. "Red flags":

- Localized pain lasting longer than 1 month.
- A palpable mass at the site of pain.
- Pain without adequate trauma to explain the pain.
- Pain continuing at night.

Other symptoms may be present including fever and malaise, which occur in about one-third of patients.

Most Ewing sarcomas occur in bones, more commonly in the axial skeleton. The most common sites are the pelvis, chest wall, and long bones of the legs. Ewing sarcomas in long bones tend to occur in the diaphyseal region, whereas osteosarcoma tends to occur in the metaphyseal region. One-third of patients will present with metastasis, most commonly to the lungs.

Evaluation

- Imaging: plain films of the site of pain/mass and an MRI of the primary site. Plain films classically show a **diaphyseal lesion** that is predominantly radiolucent (see Fig. 20.3). There is typically associated periosteal reaction seen as **Codman's triangle** (see Fig. 20.4) or **onion-skinning** on plain film.
- Search for metastasis: chest CT, BM biopsies, a bone scan, or a FDG-PET scan.
- Labs: studies are typically normal but elevated LDH has been correlated with poor outcomes.
- Surgical biopsy.

Treatment. A multimodal treatment approach is utilized including systemic treatment with chemotherapy and local control with surgical resection and/or radiation.

Prognosis. The overall prognosis is relatively poor. With nonmetastatic disease, approximately two-thirds of patients can be cured. In patients with metastatic disease, only about one-third will survive their disease.

Osteosarcoma

- Osteosarcoma is the **most common malignant neoplasm of bone in patients younger than 20 years.**
- Peak incidence is in the second decade during the adolescent growth spurt suggesting that the pathogenesis of osteosarcoma is related to rapid bone growth.
- Children with osteosarcoma are taller on average than other children.

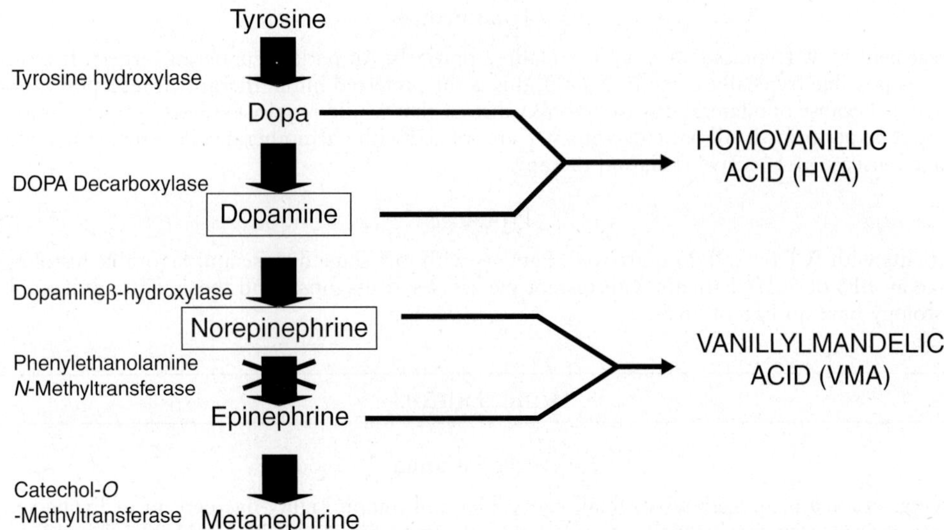

FIGURE 20.3. Catecholamine metabolism in NB cells. Unlike normal sympathetic neurons, NB cells lack phenylethanolamine *N*-methyltransferase, causing the buildup of dopamine, norepinephrine, and their metabolites HVA and VMA. HVA and VMA are excreted in the urine and are useful diagnostic markers. (Adapted from Pizzo and Poplack: *Principles and Practice of Pediatric Oncology.* 5th ed. Philadelphia, PA: Lippincott Williams and Wilkins, 2006.)

- Girl's peak age of diagnosis is earlier than boys corresponding to their earlier growth spurt.
- Patients with a history of bilateral retinoblastoma (with mutation in the tumor suppressor Rb gene) are at a significantly higher risk.

Presentation

- Most patients present with pain at the involved site ± a palpable mass.
- Usually affects the **metaphyseal portion of long bones.**
- **Most common sites are the distal femur, proximal tibia, and proximal humerus.**
- Approximately 15% to 20% of patients will have visible metastatic disease at diagnosis, most commonly in the lungs.

Evaluation

- Laboratory studies: typically unremarkable at diagnosis; however, 40% of patients have elevation of alkaline phosphatase and 30% have elevation of LDH at diagnosis.

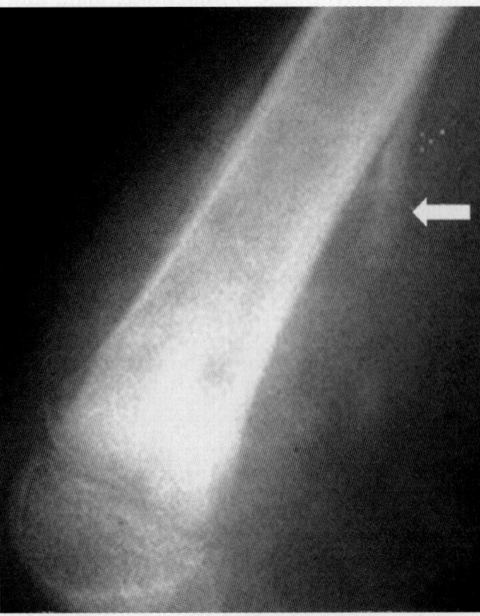

FIGURE 20.4. Codman's triangle (*arrow*). (Reprinted with permission from the Department of Pathology, New Jersey Medical School, University of Medicine & Dentistry of New Jersey [http://njms2.umdnj.edu/tutorweb/].)

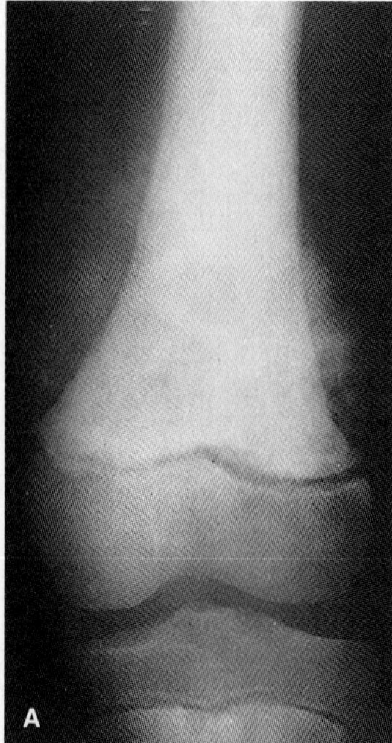

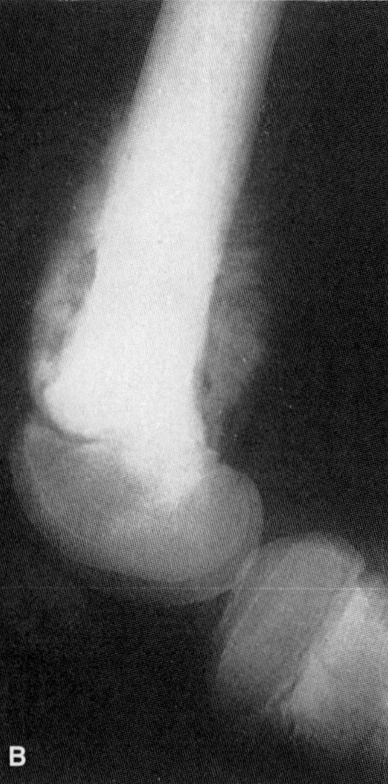

FIGURE 20.5. Osteosarcoma. Note the soft tissue mass with a "sunburst" pattern (*arrow*). (Reprinted with permission from Yochum TR, Rowe LJ. *Yochum And Rowe's Essentials of Skeletal Radiology*. 3rd ed. Philadelphia, PA: Lippincott Williams & Wilkins, 2004.)

- Radiographic studies:
  - Plain radiograph—a destruction of normal bone with indistinct margins, periosteal reaction (Codman's triangle) typically at the metaphyseal region of a long bone. A soft tissue mass is also often present with osteoid production that results in the classic finding of a **"sunburst" pattern** (see Fig. 20.5).
  - MRI for surgical planning.
  - Radionuclide bone scan to define the extent of the primary tumor and evaluate for bony metastasis.
  - Chest CT to evaluate for pulmonary metastasis.
- Definitive diagnosis: biopsy of the primary mass.

Treatment. Requires both local control with surgical resection and systemic treatment for micrometastatic disease. Typically, patients receive a few cycles of chemotherapy (termed neoadjuvant chemotherapy) and then undergo surgical resection of the primary mass. Given that most of these tumors are located at the ends of long bones, they are usually amenable to surgical resection. Amputation or limb-salvage surgery can be performed for most patients. After surgery, another several cycles of chemotherapy are given to prevent the spread of disease.

Prognosis. The prognosis of patients with nonmetastatic distal extremity tumors has been greatly improved by the combination of chemotherapy and surgical resection with an EFS of 60% to 70%. Patients with tumors that are not easily resectable, that is, those in the axial skeleton, and patients with metastatic disease do far worse.

Benign Bone Tumors

It is important and sometimes difficult to distinguish benign bone tumors from malignant ones. Some of the most common benign bone tumors in children include osteoid osteoma, cortical fibroma, and bone cysts.

Osteoid Osteoma

- 90% of patients are between 5 and 25 years of age.
- Uncommon in Blacks.
- *Typical clinical presentation is bone pain, usually worse at night, greatly relieved by NSAIDs.*
- Osteoid osteoma of the spine may result in scoliosis.

On plain x-ray: Radiolucent lesion in cortical bone associated with variable degrees of cortical and endosteal sclerosis (see Fig. 20.6). These lesions do not grow and often regress spontaneously.

Treatment: CT-guided RFA, ethanol, laser, or thermocoagulation therapy.

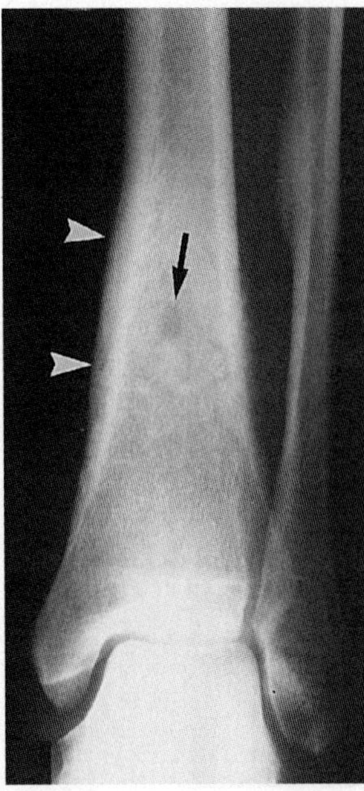

FIGURE 20.6. Osteoid osteoma. (Reprinted with permission from Yochum TR, Rowe LJ. *Yochum and Rowe's Essentials of Skeletal Radiology*. 3rd ed. Philadelphia, PA: Lippincott Williams & Wilkins, 2004.)

Fibromas. Fibromas (FCD, nonossifying fibroma) are benign tumors composed of spindle-shaped fibroblasts.

- Lesions occur most commonly in the metaphyseal region of tubular long bones.
- ***Usually found incidentally on plain film obtained for unrelated reasons.***
- 30% to 40% of children will have one or more FCDs.
- Rarely, pathologic fractures can occur in large lesions.

Radiographs reveal a sharply marginated eccentric lucency in the cortex, which may be multilocular and expansile (see Fig. 20.7). Most spontaneously regress. Lesions occupying more than 50% of bone diameter should undergo curettage and bone grafting to prevent pathologic fracture.

Unicameral Bone Cyst. Unicameral bone cysts (simple bone cysts) are fluid-filled lesions which occur in children 3 years to skeletal maturity (Fig. 20.8). They usually occur in the medullary portion of long bones, often extending to the physis. Patients are *usually only diagnosed incidentally* or after pathologic fracture, often after minor trauma. On x-ray, they appear as a solitary, centrally located lesion. Lesions can be treated with injection of methylprednisolone or BM, curettage, and bone grafting.

Aneurysmal Bone Cyst. Aneurysmal bone cysts are rapidly expanding lesions filled with blood and aggregates of tissue. They most commonly occur in the metaphyseal portion of the femur, tibia, and spine. *Patients present with pain and swelling.* Lesions in the spine may lead to

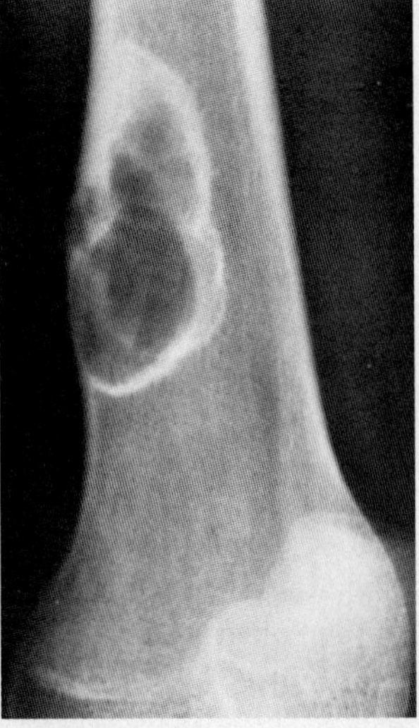

FIGURE 20.7. Fibroma. (Reprinted with permission from Eisenberg RL. *An Atlas of Differential Diagnosis*. 4th ed. Philadelphia, PA: Lippincott Williams & Wilkins, 2003.)

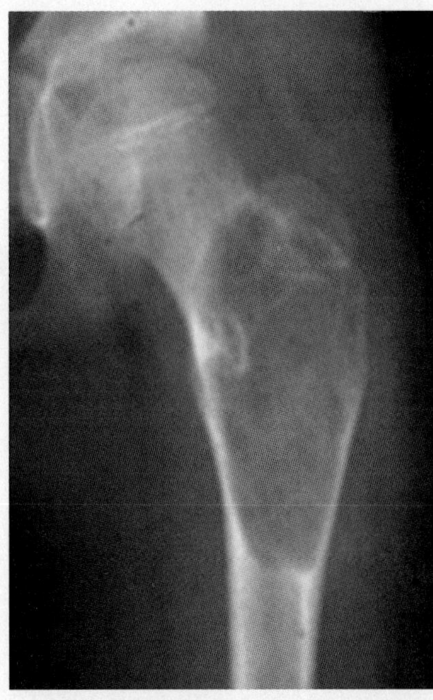

FIGURE 20.8. Unicameral bone cyst. (Reprinted with permission from the Department of Pathology, New Jersey Medical School, University of Medicine & Dentistry of New Jersey [http://njms2.umdnj.edu/tutorweb/].)

neurologic symptoms secondary to nerve root compression. Plain films reveal a lytic lesion surrounded by sclerotic rim (see Fig. 20.9). Treatment involves curettage and bone grafting or excision.

Histiocytosis Syndromes

Histiocytes are cells of the monocyte-macrophage series. They arise from precursors in the BM and mature into PB monocytes. Monocytes undergo terminal differentiation in tissues throughout the body. Histiocytosis syndromes are disorders in which there is an abnormal accumulation and infiltration of these cells in the involved tissues. They are classified into one of three categories; see Table 20.10 for presentation, laboratory findings, and treatment of these diseases.

Class I: LCH is a proliferative disorder of Langerhans' cells most commonly found in **bone** (lytic lesions) and the **skin** (lesions that can be confused with other dermatitis such as seborrhea, eczema, and candida) (see Fig. 20.10). Other at-risk organs include lymph nodes, lungs, the spleen, liver, and BM. Histologically, the lesions are characterized by **Birbeck granules** (see Fig. 20.11).

Class II: HLHs are histiocytosis of monocyte-macrophage cells. In HLH, monocyte-macrophages become overactive and phagocytose normal blood cells (see Fig. 20.12). HLH is subdivided into FEL and reactive HLH.

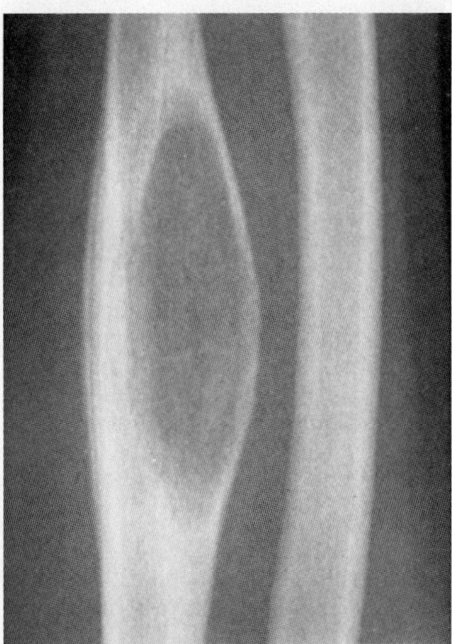

FIGURE 20.9. Aneurysmal bone cyst. (Reprinted with permission from Eisenberg RL. *An Atlas of Differential Diagnosis*. 4th ed. Philadelphia, PA: Lippincott Williams & Wilkins, 2003.)

TABLE 20.10

HISTIOCYTIC DISORDERS

Disease		Presentation	Laboratory Findings	Treatment
Class I: LCH	Bone: most commonly **skull,** femur, ribs, vertebra, humerus	Pain Palpable lesion	Cytopenias Hypoalbuminemia Elevated IL2 Hypernatremia	Infants with only skin involvement—observation only Combination chemotherapy for all others including corticosteroids and Velban with or without other agents Curettage of bone lesions may be beneficial
	Skin	Papular rash Seborrheic rash Other: pustular, petechial, vesicular, purpuric		
	Lymph nodes	Matted soft cervical nodes Mediastinal nodes mimicking lymphoma		
	Liver	Hepatomegaly Hypoalbuminemia without elevation of liver enzymes		
	Spleen	Splenomegaly		
	Lungs	Cystic/nodular disease Spontaneous pneumothorax		
	BM	Cytopenias		
	Pituitary	**DI** Growth hormone deficiency		
Class II: HLH	Fever[a] Hepatomegaly Splenomegaly[a] Neurologic symptoms Rash Lymphadenopathy Jaundice Respiratory distress Coagulopathy		Cytopenias (at least two cell lines)[a] Hypertriglyceridemia[a] Hypofibrinogenemia[a] Hemophagocytic cells seen in BM[a] Elevated ferritin levels Low NK cell number and activity Elevation of liver enzymes Hyperbilirubinemia Hypoalbuminemia Pleocytosis in CSF	Chemotherapy including dexamethasone etoposide, CSA, and IT MTX Patients with familial HLH and those with relapsed or refractory disease undergo Patients with familial HLH and those with relapsed or refractory disease undergo HSCT
Class III: Malignant histiocytic disorders	Histiocytic leukemia: like other acute leukemias (see "Leukemia" section) Histiocytic lymphoma: like other lymphomas (see "Lymphoma" section)		Cytopenias Elevation of LFTs Metabolic abnormalities if TLS is present	Chemotherapy

[a]Diagnostic criteria.
LCH, Langerhans' cell histiocytosis; IL2, interleukin 2; HLH, hemophagocytic lymphohistiocytosis; DI, diabetes insipidus; BM, bone marrow; NK, natural killer; CSF, cerebrospinal fluid; CSA, cyclosporine; IT, intrathecal; MTX, methotrexate; HSCT, hematopoietic stem cell transplant.

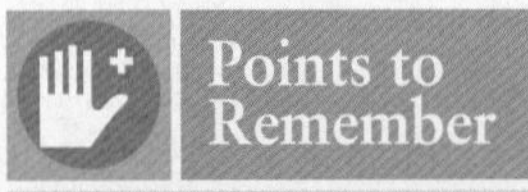

- HLH that is secondary to JRA or lupus is also termed "macrophage activation syndrome." Clinical and laboratory features are essentially the same as other forms of HLH. Treatment consists of cyclosporine and steroids.

- In FEL, there are three known and well-described genetic mutations, mutations of the perforin gene, Munc 13–4 mutations, and syntaxin 11 mutations.
- Reactive HLH includes
  - Infection-associated hemophagocytic syndrome.
    - **EBV (most commonly)**, CMV, parvovirus, herpes simples, varicella-zoster, measles, HHV-8, and HIV. Rarely bacterial and fungal infections.
  - HLH secondary to autoimmune disease such as JRA and lupus.
  - HLH secondary to leukemias/lymphomas.

Class III: Malignant forms, including acute monocytic leukemia (discussed in "Acute Myelogenous Leukemia" section), malignant histiocytosis, and true histiocytic lymphoma. These are exceedingly rare diagnoses in children. See section "Acute Myelogenous Leukemia" for further discussion of acute monocytic leukemia.

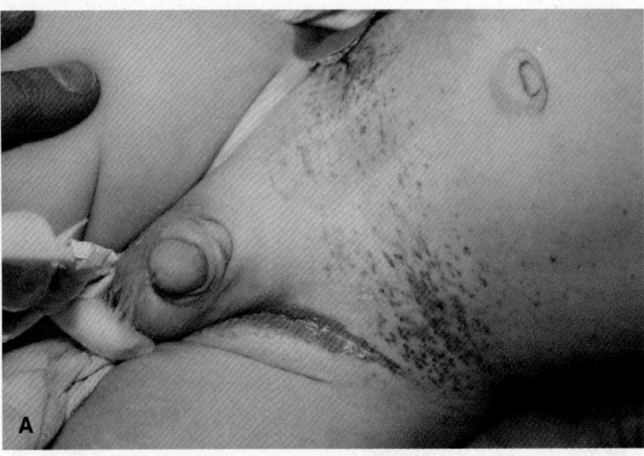

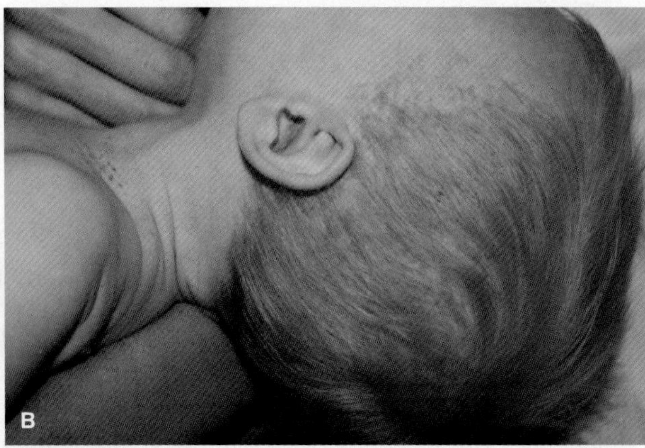

FIGURE 20.10. A: LCH skin lesion in the diaper region. **B:** LCH skin lesions of the neck and scalp. (Reprinted with permission from Cohen B. DermAtlas; http://www.dermatlas.org.)

Germ Cell Tumors

GCTs are a group of tumors that arise from primordial germ cells. These cells tend to persist in the midline, which is, therefore, where the vast majority of these tumors arise (see Table 20.11). **Approximately 90% of GCTs arise in the testes or ovaries.** In contrast to adults, **most tumors that arise in the testes and ovaries of children and adolescents are GCTs.** GCTs are relatively rare, accounting for only 3% of all childhood cancer. There are two peaks in incidence: 2 years of age and 20 years of age. Whites >> Blacks.

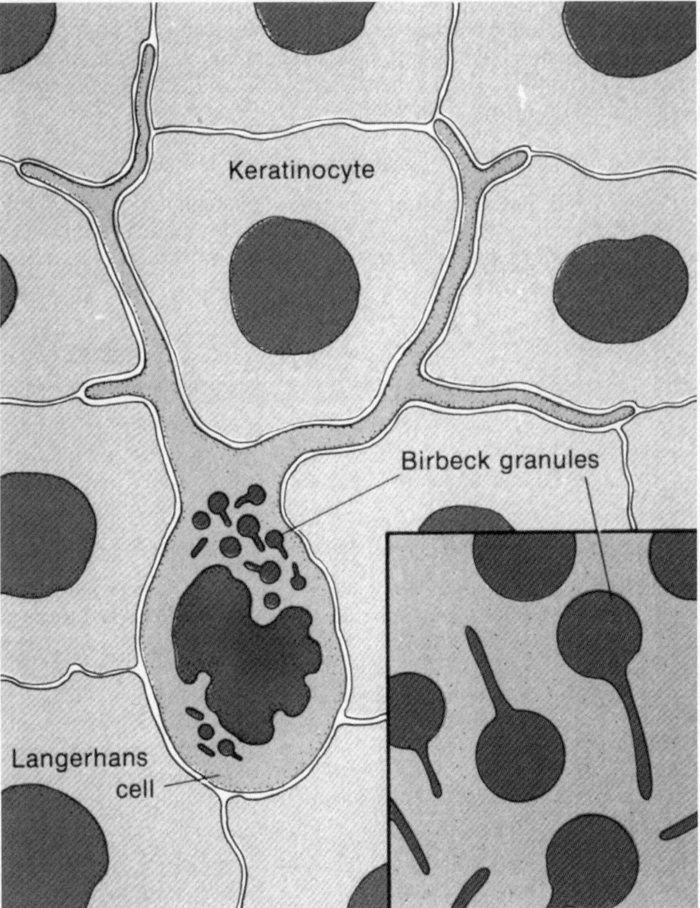

FIGURE 20.11. Tennis racket-shaped Birbeck granules which are found in Langerhans' cells. (Reprinted with permission from Rubin E, Farber JL. *Pathology*. 3rd ed. Philadelphia, PA: Lippincott Williams & Wilkins, 1999.)

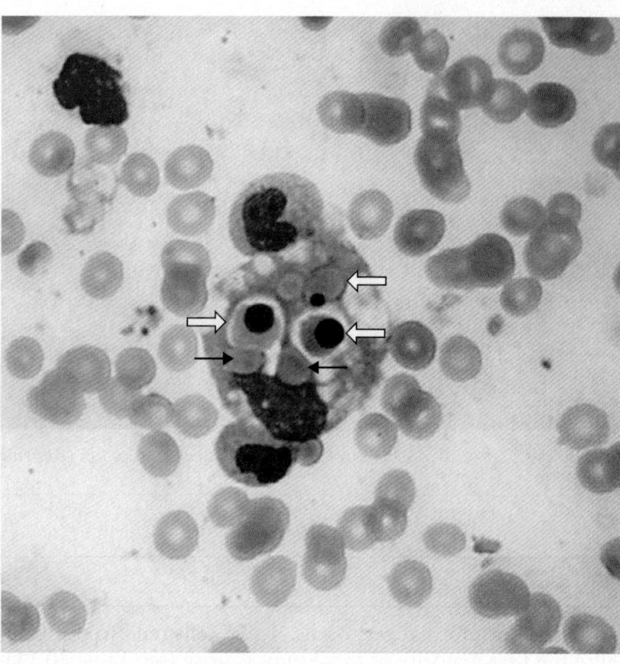

FIGURE 20.12. Hemophagocytosis of immature red blood cells (*arrows*) and a white blood cell (*arrow head*). (Courtesy of Clifford Takemoto, MD.)

Presentation

Typical presentation depends upon the location of the mass.

- Testicular GCTs: enlargement of a testis.
- Ovarian masses: abdominal pain and a palpable mass in the lower abdomen.
- Pineal tumors: Parinaud syndrome and focal motor deficits.
- Mediastinum: respiratory symptoms such as coughing, wheezing, and SVC syndrome.
- Teratomas in infants often are in the sacral region and occasionally the cervical region, typically first seen on neonatal ultrasound.

Treatment

Treatment for benign teratomas is surgical resection. For malignant GCTs, multimodal treatment is utilized with surgical resection and chemotherapy. Seminomas are very radiation sensitive, so they are treated with radiation therapy as well. GCTs in the CNS are also treated with radiation therapy.

TABLE 20.11

GERM CELL TUMORS (GCTs)

GCT (Normal Developmental Counterpart)	Percentage of GCTs	Associated Laboratory Finding	Most Common Location	Comments
Endodermal sinus tumor/yolk sac tumor (yolk sac)	44	**High AFP**	Sacrum/testes of infants Ovary/testes of adolescents	**Most common malignant GCT in testes of infants and young boys**
Choriocarcinoma (chorion)	4	**High βHCG**	Testes/ovary	Usually occurs as part of a mixed GCT
Germinoma/seminoma/dysgerminoma (ovum/sperm)	15	None	Ovary/testes (undescended), dysgenetic gonads	Most common malignant GTC in the ovary and CNS in children **Most common malignant testicular tumor in men >20 y,** rare <20 y
Embryonal carcinoma (gastrula)	10	**± AFP**	Testes	Usually occurs as part of a mixed GCT
Teratoma (embryo)	24	None	Ovary Sacrum of infants Anywhere in midline, commonly anterior mediastinum	**Most common GCT in ovary** Consist of three germ cell layers (ectoderm, mesoderm, endoderm) 65% benign, 5% immature, 30% malignant

TABLE 20.12

COMMONLY USED CHEMOTHERAPEUTIC AGENTS

Class of Drug	Mechanism of Action	Drugs	Specific Toxicities
Tubulin binders	Inhibits tubulin polymerization	Vincristine	**Constipation** **Peripheral neuropathy—foot drop and loss of DTRs** Jaw pain Shin pain Hepatotoxicity
		Vinblastine	Mild neurotoxicity Mucositis
Anthracyclines	Intercalate into DNA. Also induce Topoisomerase II–mediated DNA strand breaks	Doxorubicin	Severe tissue damage with extravasation Worsens the effects of XRT Acute cardiac toxicity—arrhythmias, acute drop in LV function, pericarditis **Chronic cardiomyopathy**
		Daunomycin	Severe tissue damage with extravasation Worsens the effects of XRT Acute cardiac toxicity—arrhythmias, acute drop in LV function, pericarditis **Chronic cardiomyopathy**
Alkylating agents	Lead to DNA damage by DNA–DNA and DNA–protein crosslinks	Cisplatin	Highly emetogenic Renal toxicity—Mg wasting, azotemia **Permanent hearing loss** Sensory peripheral neuropathy
		Carboplatin	Permanent hearing loss Delayed myelosuppression Hypersensitivity reactions
		Ifosfamide	**Hemorrhagic cystitis** SIADH Proximal tubular damage Neurotoxicity—somnolence disorientation, lethargy
		Cyclophosphamide	**Hemorrhagic cystitis** SIADH Cardiac toxicity with high doses
Topoisomerase inhibitors	Interfere with topoisomerase II leading to DNA strand breaks	Etoposide	Hepatotoxicity Hypersensitivity reactions **Secondary acute leukemia**
Antimetabolites	Structural analogs of cofactors or intermediates in the biosynthetic pathways of DNA and RNA Inhibit synthesis of nucleic acids or are incorporated into DNA/RNA resulting in defective production	Cytarabine	**"Ara-C" syndrome:** **High fever, malaise, rash, conjunctivitis, myalgias** Relieved by coadministration of corticosteroids Mucositis Neurotoxicity
		Mercaptopurine	Hepatotoxicity Mucositis
		Thioguanine	Hepatotoxicity Mucositis
		Methotrexate	Mucositis Rash Hepatotoxicity Nephrotoxicity—avoid by using hydration, alkalinization, and leucovorin Neurotoxicity—acute stroke-like encephalopathy and seizures
Molecularly targeted	Target abnormalities specific to cancer cells	Imatinib	Nausea Transient elevation of LFTs Fatigue Diarrhea

(continued)

TABLE 20.12
CONTINUED

Class of Drug	Mechanism of Action	Drugs	Specific Toxicities
		Tretinoin (ATRA)	**Teratogenicity** **Pseudotumor cerebri** Cheilitis Conjunctivitis Headache Xerosis ATRA syndrome: Weight gain Respiratory distress Serous effusions Cardiac and renal failure
Miscellaneous	Intercalates between DNA base pairs leading to DNA strand breaks	Dactinomycin	Severe tissue damage with extravasation Hepatic VOD Mucositis Can worsen effects of XRT
	Forms complex with iron which intercalates between DNA base pairs leading to strand breaks	Bleomycin	**Interstitial pneumonitis that can lead to pulmonary fibrosis** Dermatologic toxicity Mucositis Fever Hypersensitivity Raynaud's phenomenon
	Depletes asparagine, which cannot be synthesized by sensitive leukemia and lymphoma cells. Without asparagine, protein synthesis is inhibited	Asparaginase	Allergic reactions **Coagulopathy** Hepatotoxicity **Pancreatitis**
	Binds glucocorticoid receptors on cancer cells, translocate to the nucleus, bind DNA response elements, and lead to apoptosis	Corticosteroids	Weight gain Mood changes Hypertension Myopathy **Avascular necrosis of hips** Osteopenia Hyperglycemia Coagulopathy Peptic ulcer

DTRs, deep tendon reflexes; XRT, radiation therapy; LV, left ventricular; Mg, magnesium; SIADH, syndrome of inappropriate antidiuretic hormone; LFTs, liver function test; ATRA, all-trans-retinoic acid; VOD, veno-occlusive disease of the liver.

THERAPEUTIC CONSIDERATIONS

Chemotherapy

Chemotherapy is the mainstay of treatment for many oncologic diagnoses in children. There are numerous chemotherapeutic agents with varying mechanisms of action, pharmacokinetics, and side effect profiles. Typically, combinations of drugs with differing mechanisms of action and resistance patterns are utilized to maximize effectiveness. Myelosuppression, alopecia, and nausea/vomiting are frequent early side effects of many chemotherapeutic agents. Long-term sequelae common to many chemotherapeutic agents include infertility and neurocognitive deficits. See Table 20.12 for some of the most commonly used chemotherapeutic medications and their mechanisms of action and unique toxicities.

Bone Marrow Transplantation

BMT offers a potential cure for many malignant and nonmalignant conditions. The most common indication is to enable the delivery of otherwise lethal doses of chemotherapy for diseases incurable by conventional therapy such as cancers with poor prognosis or relapsed/refractory

TABLE 20.13

ADVANTAGES AND DISADVANTAGES OF STEM CELL SOURCES

Source of Stem Cells	Advantages	Disadvantages
Bone marrow	Less risk of GVHD compared with PBSCT Shorter engraftment time (average 14 d) than cord blood	Painful procedure for donor
Peripheral blood	Shortest time to engraft (average 10 d)	Higher risk of GVHD Need to give mobilizing agents to donor (GCSF)
Cord blood	Lowest risk of GVHD given immunologic immaturity of graft Can accept some mismatch of HLA type	Longest time to engraftment with average of 21 d May not contain enough cells for adult size recipients

GVHD, graft-versus-host disease; PBSCT, peripheral blood stem cell transplant; GCSF, granulocyte colony stimulating factor.

malignancies. Also, BMT provides immunotherapy for some malignant disease such as leukemia (graft-versus-tumor effect). Some nonmalignant diseases are also potentially curable with BMT including metabolic disease such as Hurlers, hematologic disorders such as sickle cell disease, and immune diseases such as severe combined immunodeficiency.

BMT is probably more accurately termed "HSCT," as it is stem cells that are actually transplanted from donor to recipient. HSCTs are either autologous, meaning the stem cells are obtained from the patient and stored for later use, or allogeneic, meaning the stem cells come from another person who has been HLA matched. There are three sources of stem cells that can be used for HSCT: BM, PB into which stem cells have been mobilized from the BM, and cord blood. See Table 20.13 for advantages and disadvantages of each type.

Typically, patients receive intense chemotherapy plus or minus radiation therapy prior to receiving the stem cell transplant. This chemoradiotherapy serves to eliminate malignant cells and to prevent graft rejection. Many complications can arise during this intense time of treatment, including infection secondary to extreme and prolonged neutropenia, significant nausea and vomiting with electrolyte disturbance, and toxicities specific to the type of chemotherapy the patient is receiving (see Table 20.12 for common side effects of chemotherapeutic agents). After BMT, patients can have a number of complications (see Table 20.14).

TABLE 20.14

COMPLICATIONS AFTER HEMATOPOIETIC STEM CELL TRANSPLANT

Complication	Timing	Signs/Symptoms	Treatment
Infection	During prep After transplant while awaiting engraftment After engraftment—still innately immunodeficient	Fever Vital sign instability Malaise Localizing signs/symptoms of infection	Hospitalization and broad-spectrum antibiotics with any fever or illness up to 6–12 mo posttransplant (or as long as patient is on immunosuppressive therapy)
Veno-occlusive disease of the liver—From damage to the sinusoidal endothelial cells of hepatic venules. Leads to obstruction of these vessels	Day 0–day 28	**Weight gain** Increased abdominal girth **RUQ pain** Hepatomegaly Hyperbilirubinemia Elevated LFTs **Reversal of portal blood flow** on Doppler U/S Can be fatal	Supportive care Fluid and sodium restriction Anticoagulants have not proven useful
Acute GVHD Secondary to the immune cells of the donor recognizing the recipient tissues as foreign and mounting an immune response	After engraftment Up to 100+ d after transplant	Skin: Erythematous rash Liver: Elevated LFTs Elevated bilirubin GI tract: Profuse diarrhea Abdominal pain	Immunosuppressants: Corticosteroids Tacrolimus Cyclosporin Others

RUQ, right upper quadrant; LFTs, liver function tests; U/S, ultrasound; GVHD, graft-versus-host disease; GI, gastrointestinal.

SAMPLE BOARD REVIEW QUESTIONS

1. A 15-year-old male with Ewing sarcoma is on day 10 of his fifth cycle of chemotherapy. He presents to the emergency department with fever of 39.4°C. He reports no other symptoms.
   Physical exam: temperature (T) 39.4°C, heart rate (HR) 122 beats/minute, respiratory rate (R) 24 breaths/minute, blood pressure (BP) 112/60.
   Lungs are clear to auscultation; there is a soft II/VI systolic murmur loudest at the left upper sternal border. His abdomen is soft, non-tender with normal bowel sounds, and no organomegaly. He has no skin lesions. Neurologic exam is normal. Laboratory studies reveal a WBC count of 500 with an ANC of 0, Hgb 7.9, platelet count 18,000.
   The patient in the scenario above is given a dose of cefotaxime in the emergency department. During the infusion, he becomes diaphoretic and pale. His blood pressure is now 70/30.
   What is the most likely etiology of his fever?
   a. Tumor fever
   b. Gram-negative bacteremia
   c. Aspergillus pneumonia
   d. Bacteremia with coagulase negative staphylococcus
   e. Viral infection

   Answer: b. The patient has recently received chemotherapy and is neutropenic. Therefore, he is at high risk for serious bacterial infections. Gram-negative organisms when exposed to cytotoxic antibiotics release endotoxins which can cause shock with hypotension and poor perfusion.

2. A 14-year-old male presents to his pediatrician with persistent cough of 3 weeks duration. On exam, the patient is afebrile and has decreased breath sounds on the right with tracheal deviation to the left. A CXR is obtained and reveals a large mediastinal mass. The patient is sent to the emergency room.
   What is the appropriate next study to evaluation of this patient?
   a. Sedated bronchoscopy
   b. Airway fluoroscopy
   c. Surgical resection of the mass
   d. Chest CT scan
   e. Chest MRI

   Answer: d. Conscious sedation and anxiolytics are contraindicated in patients with mediastinal masses, as this can lead to relaxation of the airway resulting in airway compression. Once a mass is detected on CXR, if the patient is stable, a chest CT should be performed to delineate the mass and the extent to which it compresses the airway. Always use the least invasive method possible to obtain a diagnosis in patients with mediastinal masses.

3. Children with this genetic syndrome are at high risk to develop acute leukemia, but, if diagnosed at 4 years of age or younger, have a much better prognosis compared with children who develop leukemia who do not have this syndrome.
   a. Down syndrome
   b. Prader–Willi syndrome
   c. Treacher Collins syndrome
   d. Ataxia telangiectasia
   e. Klinefelter syndrome

   Answer: a. Children with Down syndrome are at increased risk to develop both ALL and AML, typically M7 AML. However, when children with DS develop acute leukemia at an early age (which is typical), their prognosis is excellent. Children with ataxia telangiectasia and Klinefelter are also at increased risk to develop AML; however, they do not have a more favorable prognosis than other children with AML.

4. A 4-year-old girl presents to the emergency room with intermittent abdominal pain. Ultrasound reveals intussusception, which cannot be relieved by air enema. An abdominal CT scan is performed and demonstrates a large abdominal mass. Which of the following complications is this patient at highest risk for at the time of presentation?
   a. Gastrointestinal bleeding
   b. Sepsis
   c. TLS

d. Respiratory failure
e. DIC

Answer: c. This girl has Burkitt's lymphoma, which can often present as nonreducible intussusception when it originates from a Peyer's patch in the GI tract. Burkitt's lymphoma cells are rapidly dividing, with a high turnover rate. Therefore, many of these cells are dying and releasing their intracellular contents even before the initiation of chemotherapy rendering these patients at high risk for TLS. Therefore, it is imperative to initiate aggressive hydration and allopurinol as soon as the diagnosis is suspected.

5. A 10-month-old male is diagnosed with NB. Evaluation for metastasis finds disease in the liver, skin, and BM. His tumor was found to have favorable histology and was not N-myc amplified.

The appropriate treatment for this patient is

a. Chemotherapy alone
b. High-dose chemotherapy with autologous stem cell transplant
c. Chemotherapy plus radiation therapy
d. Radiation therapy alone
e. Observation only

Answer: e. This patient has stage IV-S NB defined as a child 1 year of age or younger with a localized mass and metastasis limited to the skin, liver, and/or BM. These patients in general have an excellent outcome without any therapy, as the natural course of the disease is spontaneous resolution. The only exceptions are those patients with stage IV-S who also have N-myc amplification or unfavorable histology, in which case aggressive therapy is required.

6. A 12-year-old girl presents to the office complaining of pain in her right leg just distal to the knee. The pain is worse at night. She reports that occasionally, it is severe enough to prevent sleep. She often takes ibuprofen for the pain with great relief. An x-ray is obtained that reveals a radiolucent lesion in the cortical bone of the right proximal tibia. There is no periosteal reaction.

What is the most likely diagnosis?

a. Osteoid osteoma
b. Osteosarcoma
c. Ewing sarcoma
d. Histiocytosis
e. Osteomyelitis

Answer: a. This is the classic presentation of osteoid osteoma, a benign bone tumor frequently occurring in young people. The typical presentation is bone pain that is worse at night and readily relieved by NSAIDs. The x-ray findings are also classic of osteoid osteoma, a radiolucent cortical lesion with variable degrees of cortical and endosteal sclerosis. Most lesions resolve on their own; occasionally, they will require treatment with RFA, thermocoagulation, or instillation of ethanol. Lesions in the spine can cause scoliosis.

7. A 5-year-old female presents to the emergency room with a chief complaint of difficulty walking. Her parents report that over the past week, the girl's gait has been becoming increasingly unstable such that now she is unable to walk without assistance. She is also having difficulty in sitting upright without support. Her parents also report that over the past 2 weeks, she intermittently has unusual jerking movements of her arms. On examination, you note significant ataxia, but no obvious weakness and sensation is in tact. You also note that intermittently her eyes dart back and forth.

A brain MRI is performed which is normal.

The following test is likely to reveal her underlying diagnosis:

a. An EMG
b. A psychological evaluation
c. CT scan of the neck, chest, and abdomen/pelvis
d. CSF evaluation for West Nile virus
e. A hearing test

Answer: c. This patient has opsoclonus-myoclonus, "dancing eyes, dancing feet." OM is a syndrome in which patients have ataxia, myoclonic jerks of the arms and legs, and abnormal random eye movements. The most frequent cause of OM in childhood is NB. OM occurs in 2% to 3% of patients with NB and is a paraneoplastic syndrome. In children with OM, NB must be ruled out. As NB typically occurs in the abdomen or paraspinal regions and less commonly in the thorax, neck, and pelvis, CT scans of these regions should be obtained.

8. A 19-year-old female who was treated for Ewing sarcoma at the age of 12 years now presents with progressive shortness of breath, exercise intolerance, and peripheral edema. A transthoracic echocardiogram is performed and reveals severe cardiomyopathy with an ejection fraction of 15%.

   What chemotherapy likely resulted in her cardiomyopathy?
   a. Vincristine
   b. Doxorubicin
   c. Etoposide
   d. Bleomycin
   e. Carboplatin

   Answer: b. One of the most severe potential long-term side effects of the anthracycline chemotherapeutic agents (doxorubicin and daunorubicin) is cardiomyopathy. Patients at highest risk for cardiomyopathy secondary to anthracyclines include those who received high cumulative doses of anthracyclines, those who received radiation therapy that involved the heart, young age (<5 years) at the time of treatment, female gender, and Black/African descent. Patients who have received anthracyclines should be followed with regular echocardiograms.

9. A 13-year-old girl presents to the emergency room with severe bleeding from a wisdom tooth extraction site several hours after the procedure was completed. She reports otherwise feeling well and has had no fevers or other symptoms. On further physical examination, she is found to have splenomegaly and hepatomegaly. She is mildly tachycardic and has numerous ecchymoses over the leading edges of her lower extremities.

   Laboratory evaluation reveals a WBC count of 34,000/μL with a differential remarkable for 80% blasts, a hemoglobin of 7.4 g/dL, and a platelet count of 80,000/μL. She also has a D-dimer of 18, a fibrinogen of 82, a PT of 23 seconds, and a PTT of 89 seconds.

   The most likely cause for this patient's DIC is
   a. ALL
   b. Severe factor VIII deficiency
   c. Sepsis
   d. APL or M3 AML
   e. ITP

   Answer: d. DIC has been observed in patients with all types of AML; however, by far it most commonly occurs in patients with APL. APL cells abnormally express high levels of annexin II, which increases the production of plasmin, a fibrinolytic protein, leading to DIC in these patients. Patients with APL overall have a more favorable prognosis in terms of their leukemia compared with other AML variants; however, there is a high rate of mortality around the time of diagnosis secondary to severe DIC-related hemorrhage. Therefore, any patient suspected of having leukemia should have a DIC panel sent and any patient with DIC of uncertain etiology should be evaluated for APL. The most effective therapy for APL-induced DIC is the early institution of therapy including ATRA.

10. A 3-year-old girl presents to the emergency room with difficulty walking that has worsened over the previous several weeks, headaches beginning 2 days ago, and a several hour history of persistent vomiting. On physical exam, she is noted to have ataxia, nystagmus, and dysmetria.

    The diagnostic study of choice for her suspected diagnosis is
    a. EEG
    b. Brain MRI
    c. Lumbar puncture
    d. Ophthalmologic exam under anesthesia
    e. Head CT

    Answer: b. This patient has presenting symptoms suggestive of an intracranial mass, and this diagnosis must be ruled out. Although a CT scan may reveal a mass, it does not adequately image the posterior fossa, the most common site for pediatric brain tumors. This patient does have signs suggestive of a cerebellar lesion; nystagmus, ataxia, and dysmetria; therefore, imaging to adequately visualize this area, brain MRI is imperative.

11. A 22-month-old male child with a history of severe diaper dermatitis unresponsive to multiple topical antifungal therapies undergoes CXR for possible pneumonia and is incidentally found to have multiple discrete lytic lesions in the ribs and vertebrae. Biopsy of the diaper lesion and a lytic rib lesion are obtained.

The most likely finding on pathological examination of the specimens is

a. Reed–Sternberg cells
b. Small round blue cells
c. Homer-Wright pseudorosettes
d. Birbeck granules
e. Inclusion bodies

Answer: d. This child has LCH which is a proliferative disorder of Langerhans' cells. The disease typically causes skin lesions that can be easily confused with diaper dermatitis of other etiologies and lytic lesions in the bones. Histologically, the lesions are characterized by Birbeck granules which have a classic tennis racket appearance.

12. A 13-year-old girl presents with pain just distal to her left knee. An x-ray is performed that reveals a mass with destruction of normal bone and periosteal reaction as well as a soft tissue mass described as a sunburst pattern by the radiologist.

The most likely site of metastasis of this disease is

a. Brain
b. Liver
c. Bone marrow
d. Lungs
e. Skin

Answer: d. Osteosarcoma is the most likely diagnosis. Osteosarcoma typically occurs in young people in the second decade of life, around the time of the adolescent growth spurt. Further, osteosarcoma typically occurs in the metaphyseal portion of long bones, most commonly the distal femur and proximal tibia. The x-ray finding is classic of osteosarcoma as the soft tissue mass seen on plain film represents osteoid production by the tumor creating the "sunburst pattern." The most common site of metastasis of osteosarcoma is the lung; therefore, a chest CT at diagnosis is necessary.

13. A 3-year-old female presents with pallor, fatigue, bruising, and fever. A CBC is performed which is significant for a WBC of 345,000/mm^3, a hemoglobin of 4.5 g/dL, and platelet count of 8,000/mm^3. Differential is significant for 82% blasts, 2% neutrophils, 12% lymphocytes, and 4% monocytes. Flow cytometry confirms the diagnosis of pre–B-cell ALL.

Which of the following laboratory abnormalities is the patient most likely to experience?

a. Hypokalemia
b. Hypercalcemia
c. Hyperphosphatemia
d. Hyponatremia
e. Hyperglycemia

Answer: c. Patients with acute leukemia, particularly Burkitt's leukemia/lymphoma and ALL (especially T-cell ALL), are at risk for TLS. This patient is particularly at risk given the high WBC at presentation. Patients can already have TLS at presentation given the rapid turnover of cells. The risk further increases when chemotherapy is begun, causing an even more brisk breakdown of cells which release their contents into circulation. These cells contain high levels of uric acid, potassium, and phosphate leading to the classic laboratory finding: hyperuricemia, hyperkalemia, and hyperphosphatemia with secondary hypocalcemia. Management consists of vigorous hydration, alkalinization, and allopurinol.

14. A 14-year-old male was recently diagnosed with ALL. He is currently on day 12 of induction. He is noted to have significant pain and swelling on his left upper extremity. Doppler ultrasound reveals an occlusive venous thrombus extending into the subclavian vein. A heparin drip is initiated and catheter-directed thrombolysis is performed.

The induction chemotherapeutic agent that has likely predisposed the patient to the development of this thrombus is

a. Vincristine
b. Asparaginase
c. Cyclophosphamide
d. Daunorubicin
e. Methotrexate

Answer: b. The mechanism of action of asparaginase is to inhibit protein production. In addition to inhibiting protein production in cancer cells, it also inhibits the production of many normally produced proteins including several proteins in the coagulation cascade leading to increased risk of bleeding, but more commonly thrombosis secondary to decreased production of antithrombin III, protein C, and protein S.

15. A 4-year-old boy presents to the emergency department with a 3-week history of constipation. On exam, a large right upper abdominal mass is palpated. On further physical examination, it is noted that the boy is less than the 5th percentile for height and weight. He is also noted to lack both irises. His past medical history is significant for repaired hypospadias.

The mass is most likely
a. WT
b. NB
c. Hepatoblastoma
d. GCT
e. Rhabdomyosarcoma

Answer: a. This child has WAGR syndrome, which includes aniridia, genitourinary anomalies, retardation of growth/mentation, and a high risk of Wilms' tumor (>30% of patients with WAGR will develop WT). Children with aniridia and no other anomalies are also at higher risk than the average child, so the index of suspicion for WT should be high in any child with aniridia and an abdominal mass.

SUGGESTED READINGS

Adelman WP, Joffe A. Consultation with the specialist: testicular masses/cancer. *Pediatr Rev.* 2005;26: 341–344.
Aune G, Serwint JR. Brief reports: Wilms tumor. *Pediatr Rev.* 2008;29:142–143.
Brown P. Answers to key questions about childhood leukemia–for the generalist. *Contemp Pediatr.* 2006;23(3):81–84.
Kelly CS, Kelly RE Jr. Lymphadenopathy in children. *Pediatr Clin North Am.* 1998;45:875–888.
Meck MM, Leary M, Sills RH. Late effects in survivors of childhood cancer. *Pediatr Rev.* 2006;27:257–263.
Park JR, Eggert A, Caron H. Neuroblastoma: biology, prognosis, and treatment. *Pediatr Clin North Am.* 2008;55:97–120.
Pui C, Evans WE. Acute lymphoblastic leukemia. *N Engl J Med.* 1998;339:605–615.

CHAPTER 21 ■ PEDIATRIC OPHTHALMOLOGY

JADE MARIE TAN

CSF	cerebrospinal fluid	PCR	polymerase chain reaction
HSV	herpes simplex virus	ROP	Retinopathy of prematurity

CHAPTER OBJECTIVES

1. To recognize ophthalmic disorders occurring during infancy
2. To formulate a differential diagnosis of the red eye in children
3. To understand obstructive ophthalmic disorders
4. To understand alignment and movement disorders
5. To understand trauma, masses, and swelling of the eye

OPHTHALMOLOGIC DISORDERS OF INFANCY

Retinopathy of Prematurity (ROP)

Definition

ROP results from an interruption in the vascularization and growth of new vessels within the retina. The greater the severity of ROP, the greater the risk of retinal detachment.

The *greatest* risk factor for development of ROP is *low birth weight*. Infants whose birth weight is less than 1,500 g or whose gestational age is less than 28 weeks are at a risk for ROP. Infants weighing less than 1,200 g are considered at high risk; incidence of ROP is approximately 50%.

Other risk factors for ROP include:

- Early gestational age
- Oxygen concentration and duration
- Shift of oxygen dissociation curve by transfused adult hemoglobin
- Sepsis
- Hypothermia
- High light intensity
- Hypoxia
- Occurrence of apnea

Diagnosis

Ophthalmic assessment should begin when the infant is clinically stable and is 4 to 6 weeks of age, or between 31 and 33 weeks postconceptional age, whichever occurs earlier. ROP is classified by both stage and zone.

- **Stage:** defines extent or severity of disease (Table 21.1)
- **Zone:** defines location of disease (Fig. 21.1). The various stages can be localized to one of the three zones of posteroanterior involvement. The more posterior the separation between vascularized and nonvascularized retina, the lower the zone. The lower (or more posterior) the zone of disease process, the more likely is the progression to a poor visual outcome
- **Plus disease:** dilated and tortuous posterior pole retinal vessels close to the optic disc place the disease level at the "plus" level, and the disease becomes more likely to progress to more advanced stages

Treatment

Cryotherapy or laser surgery to the avascular retina to arrest progression of the disease is generally performed. Surgery (vitrectomy and scleral buckling) is performed in stages IV and V of

TABLE 21.1

INTERNATIONAL STAGING OF ROP

Stage 1	Demarcation line dividing vascular from avascular retina
Stage 2	Ridge. Line of Stage 1 acquires volume and rises above surface retina to become a ridge
Stage 3	Ridge with extraretinal fibrovascular proliferation
Stage 4	Subtotal retinal detachment
Stage 5	Total retinal detachment

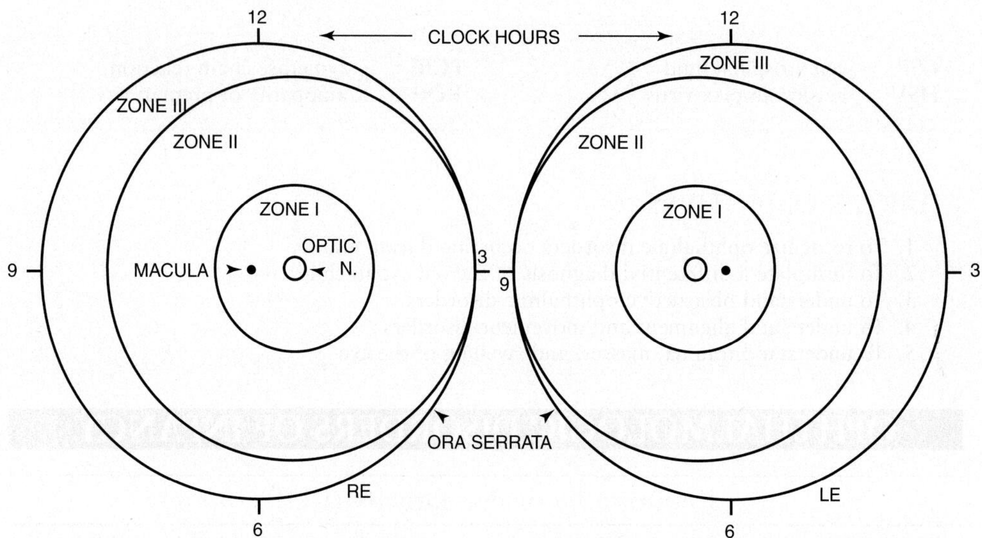

FIGURE 21.1. Schematic of the left and right eyes showing the clock hours and the states and zones of retinopathy of prematurity (ROP). (*Reprinted with permission from* The Committee for the Classification of Retinopathy of Prematurity. An International Classification of Retinopathy of Prematurity. *Arch Ophthalmol* 1984;102(8):1130–1134.)

the disease. In stages IV and V, visual results are generally poor, with patients only occasionally achieving ambulatory vision. Long-term complications are myopia and angle-closure glaucoma.

Congenital/Infantile Glaucoma

Definition

Primary infantile glaucoma refers to increased intraocular pressure occurring from birth to age 3. It occurs in 1/100,000 live births. Inheritance is autosomal recessive. Clinical presentation can vary.

Case Example (Seidman et al)

An infant was born by normal spontaneous vaginal delivery at 40 weeks of gestation. The mother noted her infant's eye to be "pink" at 3 months of age, at which point her pediatrician prescribed eye drops for "pink eye." Two weeks later, the infant's eye was pink and tearing constantly. The infant became increasingly irritable, crying frequently, and hiding her head when exposed to sunlight. At 4.5 months of age, an eye examination was requested by the mother. Profuse tearing, photophobia, blepharospasm, and enlarged hazy corneas were noted bilaterally. Examination by ophthalmology under anesthesia revealed bilateral elevated intraocular pressures, and glaucoma surgery was performed. Subsequently, the corneas cleared, intraocular pressure was controlled, and the optic nerves appeared healthy with good vision in each eye.

Clinical Presentation

Signs of glaucoma presenting within the first year of life include:

- Tearing
- Buphthalmos—large, prominent eye due to stretching of all ocular layers

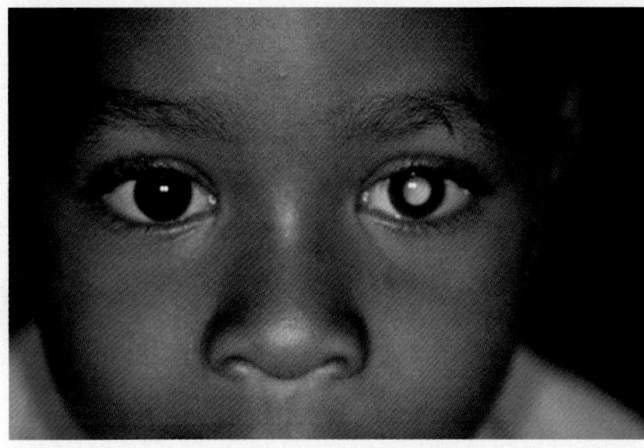

FIGURE 21.2. Leukocoria. (*Reprinted with permission from* Chung EK, Boom JA, Datto GA. *Visual Diagnosis in Pediatrics.* Philadelphia: Lippincott Williams & Wilkins, 2006.)

- Photophobia
- Blepharospasm (eyelid squeezing)
- Corneal clouding due to edema and optic nerve cupping
- Elevation of intraocular pressure is the hallmark of congenital glaucoma. After 3 years, usually only optic nerve changes occur

Treatment

Initially, infantile glaucoma requires immediate medical management (acetazolamide) to reduce intraocular pressure. Surgical treatment is also generally required.

Leukocoria (Fig. 21.2)

Definition

Leukocoria (white pupil) is a white or tan reflex in the normally black pupillary area. The reflex may result from opacification of any structure behind the iris (e.g., lens, vitreous, retina, choroid).

This subject is also reviewed in Preventive Medicine chapter.

Causes of Leukocoria (Table 21.3)

Cataracts (Fig. 21.3)

Definition. Cataracts are opacities of the crystalline lens. They may be unilateral or bilateral, may exist as isolated defects, or may be accompanied by other ocular disorders or systemic disease.

Clinical Presentation. Leukocoria, poor fixation, strabismus, or nystagmus (or both) may be the presenting complaints. In the newborn, absence of a red reflex should suggest the possibility of a cataract (Table 21.2).

Diagnosis. Unilateral cataracts: conduct TORCH diagnostic evaluation.

- Toxoplasmosis IgM antibody titers
- Rubella IgM antibody titers

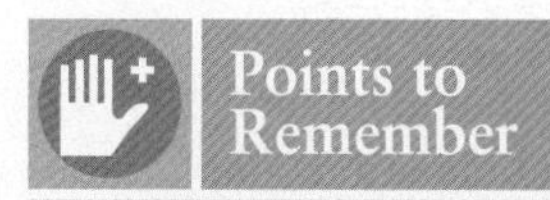

- **Infectious etiologies: Think rubella, HSV, varicella. Metabolic etiologies: Think galactosemia.**

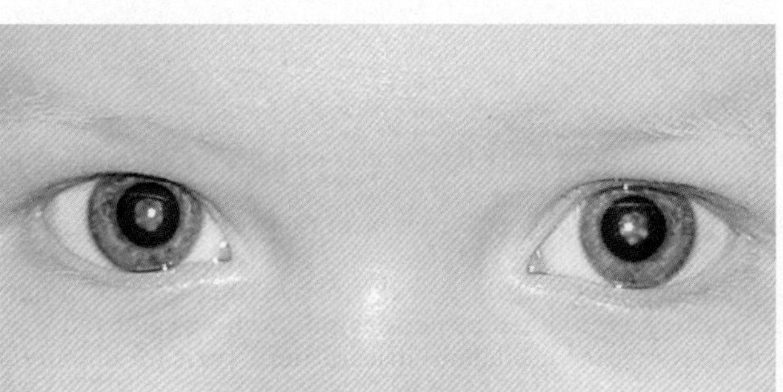

FIGURE 21.3. Bilateral central cataracts. (*Reprinted with permission from* Chung EK, Boom JA, Datto GA. *Visual Diagnosis in Pediatrics.* Philadelphia: Lippincott Williams & Wilkins, 2006.)

TABLE 21.2

CHROMOSOMAL AND HEREDITARY CONDITIONS ASSOCIATED WITH CATARACTS

Chromosomal disorders
- Trisomy 13
- Trisomy 18
- Trisomy 21

Metabolic disorders
- Galactosemia
- Galactokinase deficiency
- Albright pseudohypoparathyroidism
- Wilson's disease
- Fabry's disease
- Refsum's disease
- Homocystinuria
- Myotonic dystrophy

Skin diseases
- Incontinentia pigmenti
- Ectodermal dysplasia
- Rothmund–Thompson syndrome
- Werner syndrome
- Mandibulofacial syndromes
- Hallermann–Streiff syndrome
- Stickler syndrome with Pierre–Robin sequence
- Rubinstein–Taybi syndrome

Connective tissue and skeletal syndromes
- Conradi syndrome
- Marfan syndrome
- All syndromes involving dislocated lenses

Other bone dysplasias

Renal diseases
- Lowe oculocerebrorenal syndrome
- Alport syndrome

Central nervous system diseases
- Marinesco–Sjögren syndrome
- Sjögren syndrome

Reprinted with permission from McMillan JA, Feigin RD, DeAngelis C, et al. *Oski's Pediatrics: Principles and Practice*, 4th ed. Philadelphia: Lippincott Williams & Wilkins, 2006.

- Cytomegalovirus (CMV) traditional culture or shell viral culture of urine; PCR of urine or serum; IgM antibody titers
- Herpes simplex virus (HSV) cultures of skin, mouth/nasopharynx, eyes, urine, blood, rectum/stool, and CSF. PCR assay is useful for identifying HSV DNA in cerebrospinal fluid
- Inquire about history of maternal varicella infection during pregnancy

Bilateral cataracts: Viral diagnostics and history as above. Obtain urine for reducing substances and check newborn metabolic screen.

Treatment. Bilateral complete cataracts should be extracted early. In the case of congenital cataracts, surgery is done as early as 2 weeks to 1 month of age to avoid severe sensory amblyopia. The infant is fitted with a contact lens soon after the surgery. In the case of a unilateral cataract, the normal eye is patched for an increasing number of hours each day through middle childhood to treat amblyopia. Conservative management of partial cataracts includes the use of mydriatics if the opacity is central and patching of the uninvolved eye for treatment and prevention of amblyopia.

Retinoblastoma

Definition. Retinoblastoma is the most common primary intraocular malignancy of childhood.

Epidemiology. Annual incidence is 11 per million children from birth to 4 years.

Clinical Presentation. The most common manifestation is leukocoria. Other manifestations include: convergent or divergent strabismus, hyphema, periorbital swelling, and red eye. Average age at diagnosis is approximately 1 year for bilateral disease and 2 years for unilateral disease.

TABLE 21.3

DIFFERENTIAL DIAGNOSIS OF A WHITE PUPILLARY REFLEX (LEUKOCORIA)

- Hereditary conditions
- Norrie's disease
- Congenital cataract
- Coloboma
- Congenital retinoschisis
- Incontinentia pigmenti
- Familial exudative vitreoretinopathy
- Developmental anomalies
- Posterior hyperplastic primary vitreous
- Cataract
- Coloboma
- Retinal dysplasia
- Congenital retinal fold
- Myelinated nerve fibers
- Morning glory disc anomaly
- Congenital corneal opacities
- Inflammatory conditions
- Nematode endophthalmitis (toxocariasis)
- Congenital toxoplasmosis
- Congenital cytomegalovirus retinitis
- Herpes simplex retinitis
- Peripheral uveoretinitis
- Metastatic endophthalmitis
- Orbital cellulitis
- Tumors
- Retinoblastoma
- Retinal astrocytoma
- Medulloepithelioma
- Glioneuroma
- Choroidal hemangioma
- Retinal capillary hemangioma
- Combined retinal hamartoma
- Miscellaneous conditions
- Retinal telangiectasia with exudation (Coats disease)
- Retinopathy of prematurity
- Rhegmatogenous retinal detachment
- Vitreous hemorrhage
- Perforating ocular injuries
- Battered child syndrome

Modified from Shields JA, Augsburger JJ. Current approaches to the diagnosis and management of retinoblastoma. *Surv Ophthalmol* 1981;25:347

The genetics of retinoblastoma includes the 2 hit hypothesis, which states that retinoblastoma can be inherited or secondary to a sporadic mutation.

First hit: mutation of one allele inherited as autosomal dominant.

Second hit: second allele mutation, which is somatic. Both alleles must be affected to express the disease.

Treatment. Large tumors are generally treated by enucleation. Smaller tumors can be treated with external beam radiation or chemotherapy reduction. If the tumor is bilateral, every attempt should be made to save at least one eye. The use of chemotherapy to decrease tumor size, followed by laser or cryotherapy, has been effective in eyes with salvageable vision.

The Red Eye

Conjunctivitis

It is important to differentiate simple conjunctivitis from iritis, acute glaucoma, traumatic corneal abrasions, and infectious corneal ulceration. In conjunctivitis, vision, pupillary reflexes, intraocular pressure, and corneal clarity should be *normal* and pain should be mild, if present at all (Tables 21.4 and 21.5).

TABLE 21.4

CHARACTERISTICS OF NEONATAL CONJUNCTIVITIS

Etiology	Onset/Presentation	Conjunctival Scraping	Treatment
Silver nitrate	Within 24 h; Watery discharge	Negative Gram stain, few PMN	None
Neiserria gonorrhea	2–4 d; purulent discharge, lid swelling	Gram negative intracellular diplococci and culture +	Ophthalmic irrigation IV cefotaxime
Chlamydia	4–10 d; variable severity of lid swelling and serous or purulent discharge	Giemsa stain basophilic cytoplasmic inclusion bodies, positive direct immunofluorescence assay, culture +	Po erythromycin for 14 d
HSV	6 d to 2 wks; usually unilateral, serous discharge with keratitis, positive corneal staining	Gram stain multinucleated giant cells, Papanicolaou stain with intranuclear inclusion bodies, and herpes culture +	IV acyclovir

PMN, polymorphonuclear leukocytes; IV, intravenous; PO, per os (oral); d, days; wks, weeks; h, hours; HSV, herpes simplex virus.

TABLE 21.5

DIFFERENTIAL DIAGNOSIS OF CONJUNCTIVITIS

Finding	Acute Conjunctivitis	Allergy	Iritis	Acute Glaucoma	Corneal Abrasion/Ulcer
Pain	Mild	None	Moderate	Moderate	Severe
Tearing	Mild to moderate	Moderate	Moderate	None	Severe
Discharge	Moderate to copious	Moderate	None	None	Watery/purulent
Incidence	Very common	Very common	Uncommon	Uncommon	Common/uncommon
Vision	Normal	Normal	Mildly decreased	Decreased	Decreased
Injection	Diffuse	Diffuse	Perilimbal	Perilimbal	Diffuse
Cornea	Clear	Clear	Clear	Clear to cloudy	Clear/hazy
Intraocular pressure	Normal	Normal	Normal	Increased	Normal
Pupil size	Normal	Normal	Small	Mid-dilated	Normal
Pupillary reaction	Normal	Normal	Poor	Very poor	Normal
Culture	Causative organism	Normal	Normal	Normal	Normal/causative agent

Modified from DeAngelis C. The eye. In: DeAngelis C, ed. *Pediatric Primary Care*, 3rd ed. Boston: Little, Brown, 1984:221. (*Reprinted with permission from* McMillan JA, Feigin RD, DeAngelis C, et al. *Oski's Pediatrics: Principles and Practice*, 4th ed. Philadelphia: Lippincott Williams & Wilkins, 2006.)

Viral Conjunctivitis

Clinical Presentation

- Conjunctival erythema
- Discharge is generally watery but may appear purulent
- Tearing, lid swelling, with or without preauricular lymphadenopathy are prominent features
- All age groups

Treatment. Treatment is symptomatic and includes applying warm compresses and practicing appropriate hand hygiene (except HSV that requires acyclovir).

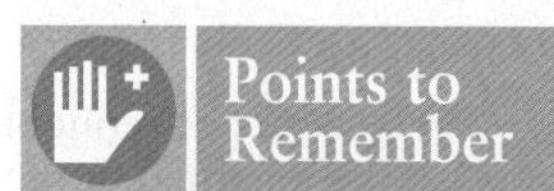

- **Most likely viral etiology is adenovirus. One should also think of HSV and enteroviruses.**

Bacterial Conjunctivitis (Fig. 21.4)

Clinical Presentation

- Conjunctival hyperemia is marked
- Moderate-to-copious *purulent discharge* occurs
- Regional lymphadenopathy is not a common finding
- Staphylococcal blepharitis or chronic inflammation at lid margins are common associated findings
- All age groups

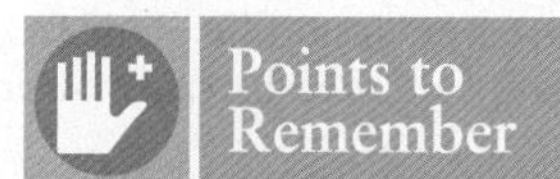

- **Common etiologies include: *S. pneumoniae*, nontypeable *Haemophilus* species, *M. catarrhalis*, *S. aureus*.**

Treatment. Ophthalmic antibiotics may prevent recurrences and shorten the disease course, but the infection usually resolves within 4 to 5 days without treatment. Empiric antibiotics include: erythromycin ophthalmic ointment, polymyxin B sulfate/trimethoprim ophthalmic drops, and fluoroquinolone ophthalmic drops.

Allergic Conjunctivitis

Clinical Presentation

- Hallmark is *itching*
- Usually associated with a stringy mucoid discharge
- Occurrence may be seasonal or associated with hay fever
- The patient frequently has a history of allergic disorders

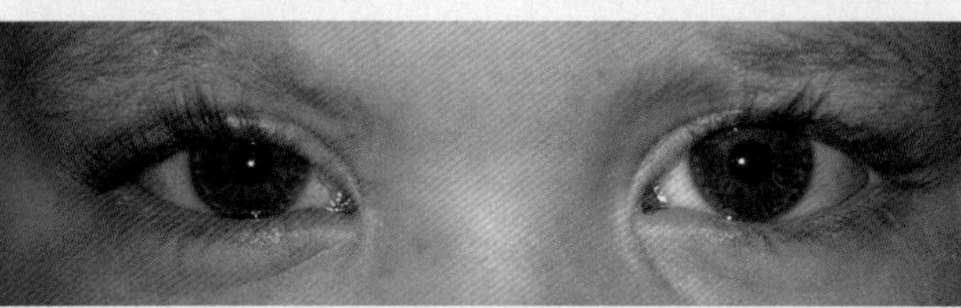

FIGURE 21.4. Bacterial conjunctivitis. (*Reprinted with permission from* Chung EK, Boom JA, Datto GA. *Visual Diagnosis in Pediatrics*. Philadelphia: Lippincott Williams & Wilkins, 2006.)

Treatment. Symptomatic treatment of eye complaints includes using warm compresses, topical antihistamines such as olopatadine (Patanol) and levocabastine (Livostin), and topical mast cell stabilizers such as cromolyn sodium, lodoxamide (Alomide), and pemirolast. Topical corticosteroids should be used only for short periods of time and only after consultation with an ophthalmologist.

Chemical Conjunctivitis

Clinical Presentation. Any chemical that reaches the ocular surface is potentially toxic. The classic example is the one induced by silver nitrate prophylaxis in newborns. The most serious of the chemical conjunctivitis are those caused by alkali (common household detergents).

Treatment. An ophthalmologist should be consulted immediately in the case of suspected ocular alkali burns. Pending ophthalmologist's examination, topical anesthetic drops should be instilled and the eye irrigated copiously with at least 2-L normal saline or until litmus paper test reveals a normal pH. Any debris or foreign bodies should be washed out of the conjunctival fornices.

Kawasaki Disease

For full discussion, please refer to Rheumatology chapter.

One of the five criteria for diagnosis of Kawasaki Disease includes a nonpurulent conjunctivitis that spares the limbic area.

Periorbital (Preseptal) and Orbital Cellulitis

For full discussion, please refer to Infectious Disease (ID) Chapter.

Periorbital Cellulitis

Infection remains anterior to the orbital septum, a fibrous structure located in the lids and separating the orbit proper from subcutaneous lid structures.

Orbital Cellulitis

Infection involves the orbit proper and may affect all orbital structures, including extraocular muscles, sensory and motor nerves, and optic nerve.

If orbital cellulitis is suspected, immediate ophthalmology consultation and CT scan of the orbits are advised.

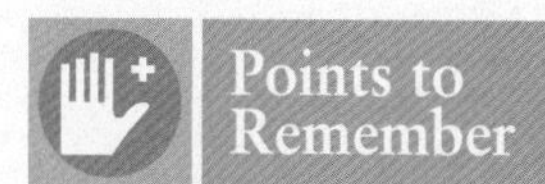

- Proptosis and pain or limitation of ocular motility aid in differentiating orbital from periorbital cellulitis. Fever, lid swelling, redness, and warmth occur in both.

Subconjunctival Hemorrhage and Hyphema

Subconjunctival Hemorrhage

Etiology can be traumatic or spontaneous. Clinical history is important as it may indicate the presence of significant ocular trauma.

Treatment. Reassurance that it will resolve spontaneously in 2 weeks. If recurrent, a systemic evaluation is indicated for diseases such as systemic hypertension, bleeding diathesis, or diabetes mellitus.

Hyphema (Fig. 21.5)

Definition. Blood in the anterior chamber from a ruptured vessel located near the root of the iris or in the anterior chamber angle. Most frequently caused by blunt ocular trauma.

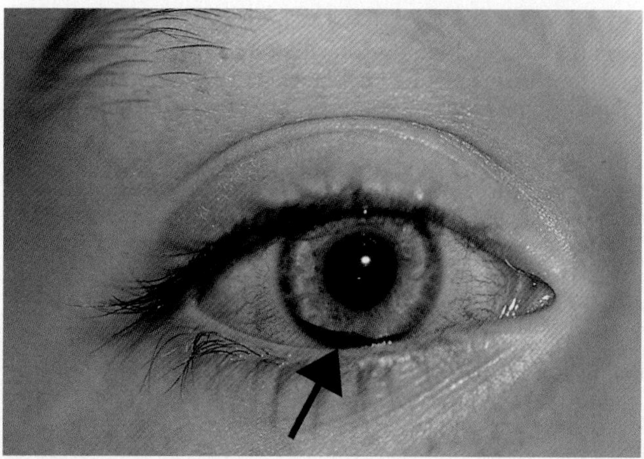

FIGURE 21.5. Hyphemas. This 7-year-old girl was struck by a hard rubber ball and presented with blurred vision. The 1-mm hyphema (**arrow**) was only visible when she was upright. (Courtesy of Dr. Andrew Capraro.) (*Reprinted with permission from* Fleisher GR, Ludwig S, Baskin MN. *Atlas of Pediatric Emergency Medicine.* Philadelphia: Lippincott Williams & Wilkins, 2004.)

Complications include the following:

- Late rebleeding into the anterior chamber
- Increased intraocular pressure
- Corneal blood staining

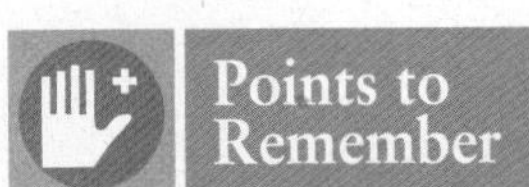

- All African Americans whose sickle cell status is unknown should be tested if hyphema is observed because those with sickle cell disease are at a risk for acute loss of vision.

Diagnosis. Ophthalmology consultation is required since it indicates severe ocular trauma and possible concurrent injuries to the retina or other ocular tissues.

Treatment. Treatment is bed rest, elevation of the head to a 45-degree angle, and use of an eyeshield. There is mixed evidence regarding the benefit of systemic antifibrinolytic agents, such as aminocaproic acid, which stabilize blood clots and reduce the risk of rebleeding. Given the close balance between the risk of thrombotic and other adverse events with the benefit, aminocaproic acid is not a first-line therapy and is usually reserved for patients who have rebled once or more.

Glaucoma (For Infantile Glaucoma See Previous Section)

Definition

Glaucoma is increased intraocular pressure that causes damage to ocular structures and loss of vision. Pediatric glaucoma can be congenital/infantile (0–3 years) or acquired/juvenile (3–30 years) and unilateral or bilateral. It is also classified on an anatomic basis into two types: open angle and closed angle.

Glaucoma occurs with *ocular syndromes* (aniridia, anterior segment disorders, e.g., Peters and Rieger anomaly) and *systemic syndromes* (Sturge–Weber syndrome, Klippel–Trenaunay–Weber syndrome, Pierre Robin syndrome, Neurofibromatosis 1).

Clinical Presentation

The age of onset of juvenile glaucoma is after 3 years. Unilateral glaucoma is more easily recognized as the difference in ocular size becomes apparent; bilateral disease is more difficult to diagnose as the increased ocular size is often considered attractive.

Treatment

Treatment is medication to reduce intraocular pressure and/or surgery.

Blepharitis

Definition

Blepharitis is inflammation of the eyelid margin. It is characterized by crusty debris at the base of the lashes, varying degrees of erythema at the lid margins, and in severe cases, secondary corneal changes such as punctuate erosions, vascularization, and ulcers.

Clinical Presentation

The two most common types of blepharitis are Staphylococcal blepharitis and meibomian gland dysfunction.

- Staphylococcal: Children complain of itching and burning and often awaken with their eyelids stuck together with crusting. Other signs include crusting and scales at the base of the eyelashes. When conjunctivitis accompanies it, the condition is known as blepharoconjunctivitis.
- Meibomian gland dysfunction: Meibomian glands are sebaceous glands with orifices at the eyelid margins. Their secretions provide a covering to the tear film. Dysfunction of the gland orifice by desquamated epithelial cells results in local inflammation and formation of hordeola. Clinical symptoms include irritation, burning, and redness of the lid margins and conjunctiva.

Treatment

Treatment of Staphylococcal blepharitis includes eyelid hygiene and topical antibiotic ointment, usually erythromycin. The treatment of meibomian gland dysfunction is eyelid hygiene with baby shampoo lid washes and eyelid massage to express the meibomian glands.

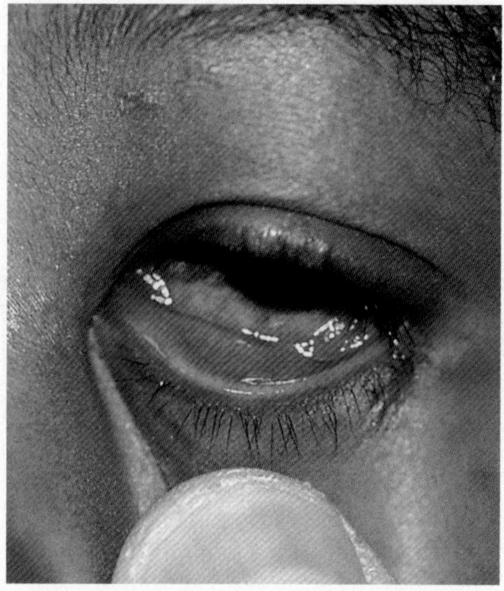

FIGURE 21.6. Uveitis. (*Reprinted with permission from* Chung EK, Boom JA, Datto GA. *Visual Diagnosis in Pediatrics.* Philadelphia: Lippincott Williams & Wilkins, 2006.)

Uveitis (Fig. 21.6)

Definition

Intraocular inflammation involving the uveal tract (iris, ciliary body, and choroid).

Anterior uveitis affects the anterior chamber and iris. Common causes include: juvenile idiopathic arthritis (formerly juvenile rheumatoid arthritis), HSV, and sarcoidosis.

Posterior uveitis affects the choroid and retina. The most common cause is toxoplasmosis.

Clinical Presentation

Uveitis may present with pain, photophobia, lacrimation, and blepharospasm, with or without the complaint of disturbance of vision. Ciliary injection is usually present, distinguishing uveitis from conjunctivitis. Other children may be completely asymptomatic. As with adults, boys are affected twice as frequently as girls are.

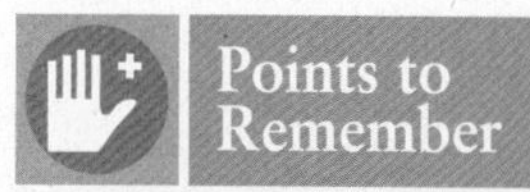

Points to Remember

- **Children with juvenile idiopathic arthritis, especially the pauciarticular type, should have periodic screening examinations for uveitis every 6 months since it may be present without signs or symptoms.**

Treatment

Treatment generally consists of administration of topical corticosteroids and topical mydriatics to keep the pupil mobile and to avoid papillary scarring.

Episcleritis

Definition

Inflammatory condition of the connective tissue between the sclera and conjunctiva. It occurs in adolescents and young adults as a unilateral or, more often, bilateral conjunctivitis.

Clinical Presentation

Patients present with localized injection of the conjunctiva and deeper episcleral tissue. There is often pain on eye movement, distinguishing episcleritis from allergic or infectious conjunctivitis.

Points to Remember

- **Pain with eye movement helps distinguish episcleritis from conjunctivitis.**

Treatment

Treatment is usually topical nonsteroidal anti-inflammatory agents or topical corticosteroids. Systemic anti-inflammatory agents such as ibuprofen may be required.

OBSTRUCTIVE DISORDERS

Nasolacrimal Duct Obstruction (Dacryostenosis)

Definition

Obstruction most commonly caused by a failure of the distal membranous end of the nasolacrimal duct to open during fetal development.

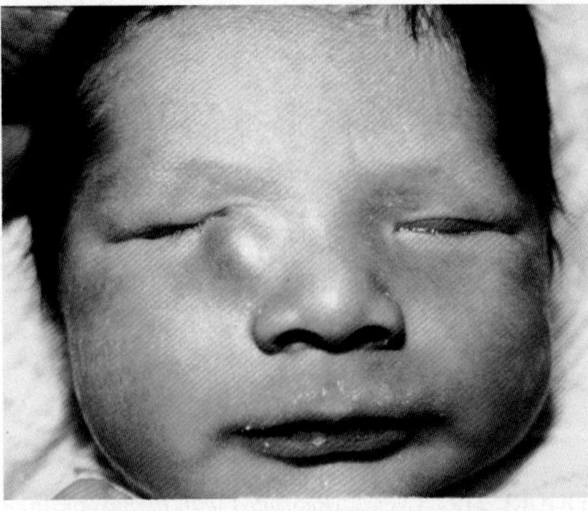

FIGURE 21.7. Dacrocystocele. (*Reprinted with permission from* Chung EK, Boom JA, Datto GA. *Visual Diagnosis in Pediatrics*. Philadelphia: Lippincott Williams & Wilkins, 2006.)

Clinical Presentation

Infants present with a wet-eye appearance, persistent or intermittent tearing, and various degrees of mucopurulent discharge over the medial canthal area and lids. Pressure over the lacrimal sac area expresses yellow/white material. Obstruction is bilateral in up to one-third of cases.

Treatment

Most (90%) resolve spontaneously by 18 months of age, and lid hygiene alone is the indicated treatment. Fingertip or cotton-tip applicator massage over the lacrimal sac area, with massage directed inferiorly while the upper end of the lacrimal system is blocked, may be tried for a short period of time. Superimposed dacrocystitis, dacrocystoceles, or fistulas may develop. The patient should be referred for nasolacrimal duct probing if it does not spontaneously resolve.

Dacrocystocele (Fig. 21.7)

Definition

Swelling of the nasolacrimal sac, caused by accumulation of fluid within the sac, as a result of nasolacrimal duct obstruction.

Clinical Presentation

A few days after birth, a bluish swelling appears in the medial canthal area, representing fluid that is sequestered within a distended nasolacrimal sac.

Treatment

For a noninfected dacrocystocele, treatment is local massage. If decompression does not occur within a few days, infection or dacrocystitis is almost certain. Once infected, treatment consists of IV antibiotics and urgent nasolacrimal duct probing to relieve obstruction and to drain the abscess.

Ptosis

Definition

Congenital ptosis is upper-lid drooping in children and young adults caused by faulty development of the levator palpebrae muscle.

- Usually unilateral with varying degrees of severity
- Infants with vision-threatening ptosis, in which the eyelid obstructs a portion of the pupil, usually assume a chin-up head posture and look with both eyes in downward gaze

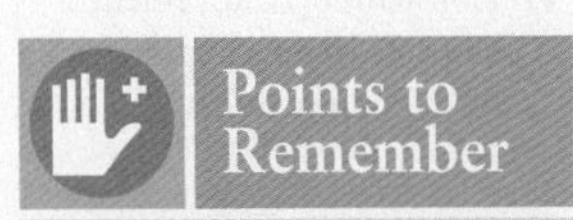

Points to Remember

- Horner syndrome: sympathetic denervation from compression or lesion of one side of the cervical or thoracic sympathetic chain leads to mild ptosis, miosis (constricted pupil), and anhidrosis of the ipsilateral face

Treatment

If ptosis threatens vision, there is a high risk of permanent vision impairment of the affected eye; therefore, surgical correction is often done early in infancy. Otherwise, cosmetic surgery is usually delayed until the child attends school.

Acquired ptosis demands special attention because it usually indicates potentially serious neurological disease.

ALIGNMENT AND MOVEMENT DISORDERS

Strabismus

Definition

Strabismus is a condition of ocular misalignment of one eye in relation to the other including:

- **Horizontal deviation:** eye turned in (esotropia) or turned out (exotropia)
- **Vertical deviation:** eye turned up or down

If strabismus occurs early, before 4 to 6 years of age, the child's brain/cortex will suppress the image from the deviated eye to prevent double vision. This mechanism of vision loss, **amblyopia**, is thought to be of central nervous system origin and is reversible in children if treated early. If untreated by age 6, strabismus will result in loss of binocular vision, and amblyopia of the nonpreferred, deviated eye may be irreversible.

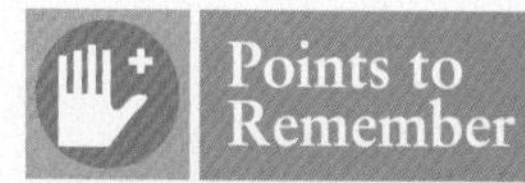

- **Amblyopia is vision loss caused by disuse of one eye and predominant use of the other. There is no organic or visual pathway lesion.**

Treatment

A major aim of strabismus treatment is prevention or reversal of amblyopia, in addition to the restoration of good ocular alignment and of binocular vision. Therapy of amblyopia consists of patching the better eye to allow stimulation of the central visual centers from the deviated eye. Atropine cycloplegia of the better functioning eye may be used as an alternative to part-time occlusion. Treatment of strabismus itself is the use of corrective glasses and/or surgery.

Please see Preventive Medicine chapter for further discussion.

Pseudostrabismus

Definition

This is a false impression of ocular misalignment as a result of a prominence of epicanthal folds, closely placed eyes, flat nasal bridges, or variations in orbital alignment in a young child.

Diagnosis

Distinguishing between pseudostrabismus and strabismus can be done with the following tests:

- **The cover test:** The child "fixes" on a distant object while the other eye is covered. The process is repeated with the other eye covered. The eye with strabismus "deviates" instead of fixating on the object.
- **Corneal light reflexes:** Well-centered corneal light reflexes in both eyes, and normal fixation patterns are usually sufficient to rule out true strabismus.

Nystagmus

Definition

Nystagmus is involuntary, rhythmic oscillations of the eyes that occur independently of normal movements. Nystagmus can be horizontal, vertical, or rotary (twisting of the eye). Nystagmus can be congenital or acquired. There are two types:

- **Pendular:** movements have equal velocity in each direction
- **Jerk:** fast eye movement in one direction and a slow eye movement in the opposite direction.

Congenital nystagmus: typical onset by 6 to 8 weeks of age. Visual acuity usually is decreased. Patients often adopt a compensatory facial turn to place the eyes at the null point (position of gaze where nystagmus diminishes) to enhance visual acuity. Albinism is often associated with nystagmus in childhood.

Treatment

Any child with abnormal eye movements should be promptly referred to an ophthalmologist for full ocular evaluation.

Third-, Fourth-, and Sixth-Nerve Palsies

Third-nerve palsy involves all the extraocular muscles except the lateral rectus (sixth) and superior oblique (fourth). The levator muscle of the upper eyelid is also innervated by the third cranial nerve, and ptosis is usually present. The pupil is large and nonreactive in complete third-nerve palsy. It is most commonly caused by trauma or increased intracranial pressure, and it may be complete or incomplete.

Fourth-nerve palsy: the superior oblique muscle is a depressor and intortor (twists eye nasally). Fourth-nerve palsy causes vertical strabismus. It is commonly caused by trauma or tumor, but many are idiopathic and present at birth. The patient tilts his or her head to the opposite side of the palsy to keep eyes aligned.

Sixth-nerve palsy is the most common ocular palsy in children. It results in limited abduction and an esotropia that is worse on the side of the palsy. It may indicate neurologic disease but is often transitory and benign following a viral infection. Benign sixth-nerve palsy in children develops 1 to 3 weeks after a febrile illness and usually subsides within 6 months. Other causes include head trauma, intracranial tumors, mastoiditis, Lyme disease, and meningitis.

TRAUMA, MASSES, AND SWELLING

For full discussions, please see Oncology chapter.

Neuroblastoma

Definition

Neuroblastoma is a tumor of embryonic sympathetic neuroblasts. Metastatic neuroblastoma accounts for approximately 3% of orbital tumors in children. Orbital metastases indicate stage 4 neuroblastoma and are associated with a poor prognosis. Patients most commonly present with proptosis and may have periorbital swelling and lid ecchymosis.

Retinoblastoma

Reviewed previously in this chapter under the section on Leukocoria.

Dermoid Cyst

Definition

These are benign tumors that arise from retained ectodermal tissue along the lines of closure of fetal bone fissures. Dermoid cysts can be present in the lid, brow, or orbit. Typically they are nontender and doughy or rubbery in consistency. Dermoid cysts account for 40% of orbital tumors of childhood.

Diagnosis is made on clinical grounds and with the assistance of ultrasonography and computed tomography.

Treatment is excision.

Corneal Abrasion

Definition

Corneal abrasion occurs when the corneal epithelium is removed. Clinical presentation is generally severe pain, tearing, and photophobia. Patients usually have the sensation that there is something in the affected eye, even in the absence of a foreign body. Differential diagnosis includes HSV keratitis, bacterial ulcer, or retained corneal foreign body.

Diagnosis

Fluorescein staining and examination with Wood's lamp show fluorescein uptake at the site of an abrasion.

Treatment

After ruling out corneal foreign body or infiltrate, an antibiotic ointment is applied. In most cases, a corneal abrasion will heal after 24 to 48 hours. Patching is no longer recommended.

Trauma to the Eye and Foreign Bodies

- Serious ocular injury must be presumed even if only minimal external signs exist
- Patients who have sustained blunt orbital trauma should be evaluated for a fracture of the orbital floor or the medial orbital wall
- In cases of penetrating injury, the key to examination is to be brief and gentle so as not to complicate the injury. Immediately after identifying an ocular injury as penetrating, further examination should be conducted in the operating room under general anesthesia
- In general, refer to an ophthalmologist for any penetrating injury, hyphema, pupil irregularity, or significantly reduced visual acuity

Foreign Bodies

Common conjunctival and corneal foreign bodies include:

- Dust
- Dirt
- Cosmetic eyelashes

Often the patient will continue to feel a foreign body sensation even after the foreign body is removed because of an associated abrasion.

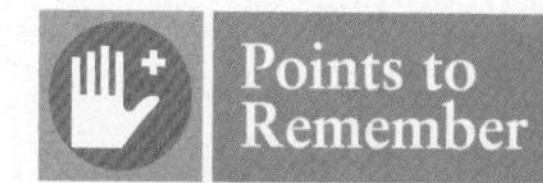

- **Retinal hemorrhages in infants are highly suggestive of battered child syndrome.**

HORDEOLUM AND CHALAZION

Hordeolum (Stye)

Definition

A hordeolum is an *acute infection* of the meibomian glands. It is characterized by warmth, swelling, erythema, and pain near the lid margin. The inflammatory process leads to the formation of a small abscess that points and ruptures to the outside within a few days.

Treatment

The main treatment consists of frequent application of warm compresses. Antibiotic ophthalmic ointment may be used, though there is mixed evidence to support its benefit in hastening resolution.

Chalazion (Fig. 21.8)

Definition

A chalazion is a *granulomatous inflammation* of the meibomian glands, not due to infection. It appears as a small bump within the lid tissues over the tarsal plates. A chalazion is usually painless and develops more chronically.

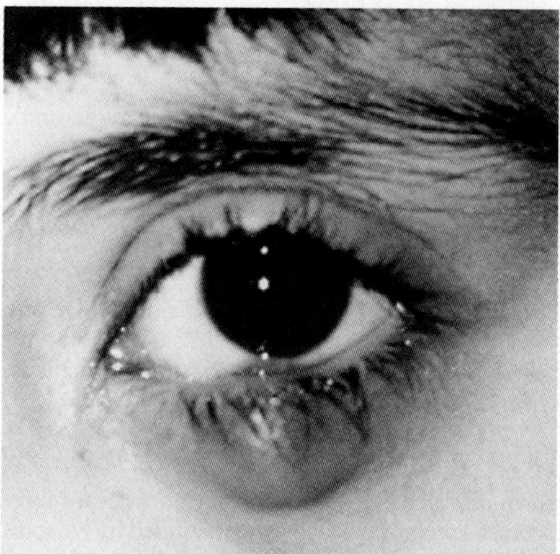

FIGURE 21.8. Chalazion. (*Reprinted with permission from* McMillan JA, Feigin RD, DeAngelis C, et al. *Oski's Pediatrics: Principles and Practice*, 4th ed. Philadelphia: Lippincott Williams & Wilkins, 2006.)

Treatment

Consists of warm compresses and antibiotic ointment for 2 to 4 weeks. If a chalazion fails to resolve and is cosmetically blemishing, it can be excised by an ophthalmologist.

MISCELLANEOUS MASSES

Capillary Hemangioma

Definition

This is a vascular tumor composed of proliferating capillaries that can arise in the periorbital area. A bluish discoloration of overlying skin, a tangled vascular mass, or the classic strawberry mark may be seen. One-third are present at birth, and 95% are diagnosed by the age of 6 months. Lesions continue to grow after birth but eventually regress spontaneously. Regression is complete in approximately 75% of patients by the age of 7 to 8 years.

Local complications include: ptosis, occlusion of the visual axis, ulceration and bleeding from the tumor surface, and infection.

Treatment

Treatment consists of observation if the visual axis is clear and there is no astigmatism. Systemic corticosteroids and intralesional injections of Celestone are the mainstay of therapy in vision-threatening capillary hemangioma. In vision-threatening cases, prompt referral to an ophthalmologist is recommended.

Lymphangioma

Definition

Lymphangiomas are benign, vascular hamartomas that usually appear in childhood. They tend to increase in size when a child has a viral illness. These tumors have a tendency to spontaneously hemorrhage and develop hematomas.

Clinical Presentation

Often the first sign of a lymphangioma is the rapid onset of proptosis secondary to acute bleeding within the tumor, which may necessitate urgent surgical decompression.

Treatment

Conservative management consists of preventing trauma and limiting the child's activity.

Xanthogranuloma

Definition

Patients with juvenile xanthogranuloma, usually younger than 1 year of age, may develop unilateral, asymptomatic, fleshy, yellow-brown tumors on the surface of the iris. If extensive and untreated, they may permanently affect vision from complications of glaucoma and recurrent intraocular hemorrhage.

Treatment

Treatment is surgical excision, systemic and topical steroids, and acetazolamide (for glaucoma).

Other Important Diagnostic Findings

Coloboma

A coloboma results from failed fusion of the embryonic fissure of the optic cup. It can involve any ocular structure, most commonly the iris. It can occur as an isolated defect or in association with systemic syndromes such as the CHARGE association (coloboma of retina or iris, heart abnormalities, atresia of the choanae, retarded growth, genital hypoplasia in males, ear anomalies).

Kayser–Fleischer Rings

Kayser–Fleischer rings appear as brown to gray-green discolorations in the posterior cornea, representing copper deposits on the inner surface of Descemet's membrane. They are identified in Wilson's disease if neurologic disease exists but may be absent in younger patients with liver disease only.

Aniridia

Aniridia is a feature in WAGR (Wilms' tumor, aniridia, genital abnormalities, retardation). Iris structures are present only as rudimentary findings.

Brushfield Spots

Brushfield spots, found in patients with Down syndrome, are tiny areas of normal iris stroma that are surrounded by rings of mild iris hypoplasia.

Anisocoria

Anisocoria refers to pupils that are unequal in size (impaired dilation or constriction of one pupil). It signifies a lesion of the parasympathetic or sympathetic pathways.

Port Wine (around the Eye)

A port wine stain of the face is a pink-to-red, macular lesion comprising mature capillaries. The characteristic features of Sturge–Weber syndrome are a port wine stain of the face and ipsilateral angiomatosis of the leptomeninges, which commonly leads to seizures and mental retardation. Typically, distribution of the stain is over the first or second division of the trigeminal nerve.

Papilledema

Papilledema, or optic disc swelling, signifies increased intracranial pressure transmitted to the optic nerve sheath.

Pterygia

Pterygia are elevated conjunctival lesions near the nasal or temporal corneoscleral limbus that enlarge and impinge on the cornea. Ultraviolet radiation is thought to play a role in the pathogenesis. Lesions consist of degenerated collagen.

Conjunctival Phlyctenule

Conjunctival phlyctenule is the result of a cell-mediated hypersensitivity reaction, and it can be associated with tuberculosis infection. Phlyctenular lesions are small, pink-white vesicles or pustules in the center of hyperemic areas of the conjunctiva.

SAMPLE BOARD REVIEW QUESTIONS

1. A 12-year-old male presents to his pediatrician's office with 1 day of worsening left eye swelling. During the preceding several days, he has had symptoms of purulent rhinorrhea, cough, and headache. Initially, there was mild redness around the skin of his left eye, but over the last day, the redness and swelling have greatly increased. On examination, there is marked swelling and erythema periorbitally with difficulty retracting the eyelid open secondary to swelling. The periorbital area is tender to palpation. Pupils are equally round and reactive to light. Extraocular muscles are intact, but the patient complains of pain in his left eye when asked to gaze upward and medially. There is no proptosis. There is no change in vision. The patient denies fever, trauma, or insect bites. He does relay that he has a tendency to get recurrent "colds" that last for several weeks at a time. The most appropriate course of action for the pediatrician is:
   - **a.** Prescribe oral clindamycin for 10 days with follow-up in 1 day
   - **b.** Prescribe oral amoxicillin/clavulanate for 10 days with follow-up in 1 day
   - **c.** Recommend admission for IV antibiotics with cefotaxime and clindamycin
   - **d.** Recommend admission for CT imaging of the orbits and sinuses, IV antibiotics with cefotaxime and clindamycin, and otolaryngology consultation
   - **e.** Place a referral to otolaryngology clinic for evaluation of the possibility of sinus surgery

   Answer: d. The patient has signs concerning for orbital cellulitis in the setting of chronic sinusitis. Signs include marked swelling causing inability to retract the eyelid and, more importantly, pain with extraocular movement in the affected eye. Appropriate diagnostic work-up for orbital cellulitis is CT scan to image the orbits. Empiric IV antibiotics should be started while awaiting imaging and otolaryngology should be subsequently consulted. Oral antibiotics without imaging would be an appropriate therapy for suspected periorbital cellulitis.

2. During a routine newborn visit, a healthy 1-week-old female is noted by the pediatrician to have only a very small amount of iris tissue bilaterally. Which of the following should be included in the evaluation for this infant?

a. MRI of the brain and spinal cord
b. Renal ultrasound
c. Echocardiogram
d. Plasma amino acids and urine organic acids
e. Plain radiographs of bilateral forearms

Answer: b. This patient has aniridia, which is congenital hypoplasia of the iris. Aniridia can occur alone, with other ocular defects, or in association with systemic defects, such as Wilms' tumor, genitourinary abnormalities, or mental retardation. Evaluation in a patient with aniridia for Wilms' tumor would include a renal ultrasound.

3. The parents of a healthy 10-month-old female bring their daughter to the pediatrician's office stating that their daughter's "eyes are crossed." On examination, the patient is a well-developed, well-appearing female infant. Pupils are equally round and constrict normally. Red reflexes are symmetric. She has closely placed eyes and a flat nasal bridge. On inspection, the patient's right eye appears to deviate nasally. The cover test reveals no shift. Both corneal light reflexes are well centered bilaterally. The best advice to her parents is:
   a. Reassurance that their daughter's eyes and vision are normal and the apparent "cross-eyes" will likely resolve with growth
   b. Reassurance that their daughter's eyes and vision are normal but she will require a more formal ophthalmology examination in 6 months
   c. Their daughter should be referred for an immediate ophthalmology appointment to evaluate for possible surgery
   d. Prescribe corrective lenses to prevent visual acuity loss
   e. Prescribe an eye patch to the right eye to be worn at all times until her next visit at the age of 24 months

Answer: a. This question requires knowledge of the differences between strabismus and pseudostrabismus. In strabismus, there is true eye misalignment and the affected eye is deviated medially (esotropia) or laterally (exotropia). In strabismus, the cover test will reveal an eye shift in the alternate eye when the affected eye is covered. Pseudostrabismus is the false impression of misalignment. Closely spaced eyes, flat nasal bridges, and epicanthal folds contribute to pseudostrabismus. In pseudostrabismus, both the cover test and corneal light reflex tests are normal. Only reassurance is necessary.

4. A 1-month-old male infant is noted to have a flat, pink-red discoloration overlying the left forehead and left upper eyelid. The remainder of the physical examination is normal. During this male's lifetime, he is most at risk for which of the following ophthalmic disease?
   a. Cataracts
   b. Retinoblastoma
   c. Amblyopia
   d. Glaucoma
   e. Uveitis

Answer: d. The skin lesion described here is a port wine stain or cutaneous angioma. These macular lesions are usually light pink in color initially and may progress to a dark red or purple nodular lesion. Roughly one-third of patients with a port wine stain have Sturge–Weber syndrome. This syndrome is a neurocutaneous disorder, consisting of leptomeningeal and cutaneous angiomas typically involving the ophthalmic and maxillary divisions of the trigeminal nerve. Patients, especially those with port wine stains involving the eyelid, are at risk for glaucoma in the ipsilateral eye. Glaucoma can present at birth or develop at any age.

5. A 10-day-old male was seen by his pediatrician for "red eyes" and discharge from the right eye for 2 days. There is mild periorbital swelling on examination and the palpebral conjunctiva is erythematous with a moderate amount of serous discharge from the right eye. After testing, the most appropriate treatment will likely be:
   a. IV cefotaxime
   b. IV ampicillin
   c. PO acyclovir
   d. PO erythromycin
   e. Topical erythromycin ointment

Answer: d. Neonatal conjunctivitis can be distinguished, in part, by the timing of clinical symptoms. Chemical or irritant conjunctivitis typically occurs within 12 to 24 hours from birth, though the incidence has decreased with the use of ophthalmic erythromycin instead of silver nitrate. Gonococcal conjunctivitis typically presents between days 2 and 5 of life and is characterized by thick, purulent discharge, marked lid swelling, and conjunctivitis. Chlamydial conjunctivitis typically occurs later, between 1 and 2 weeks of life. Both lid swelling and eye discharge can be variable, ranging from serous to purulent. Though testing is important to confirm, this infant presenting at day 10 of life with conjunctivitis, serous discharge, and mild periorbital swelling most likely has chlamydial conjunctivitis. First-line treatment is oral erythromycin.

6. A 3-week-old infant presents with 1 week of discharge from both eyes. The discharge is described as watery. At times, there is also a stringy, mucoid discharge. There is no scleral injection. The infant is otherwise thriving. The most appropriate management is:
   a. Administration of topical erythromycin ointment twice daily for 7 days
   b. Instructions for nasolacrimal massage, eyelid hygiene, and reassurance
   c. Fluorescein staining of the corneas
   d. Referral to ophthalmology for nasolacrimal duct probing
   e. Instillation of atropine drops twice daily

Answer: b. This infant's examination is consistent with congenital nasolacrimal duct obstruction, or blocked tear ducts. This is a common condition in infants, presenting from birth to several months of age. Infants usually present with watery-to-mucoid discharge, either unilateral or bilateral. There is no evidence of conjunctivitis. Treatment is generally supportive, including good eyelid hygiene and massage over the nasolacrimal sac, which may rupture the membrane and enhance drainage. If still present past 12 months of age, ophthalmology referral should be done for consideration of nasolacrimal duct probing.

7. A 14-year-old boy is struck in the right eye by a golf ball. He complains of double vision. On physical examination, there is edema, marked ecchymosis, and tenderness of the periorbital area. Pupillary reflexes are normal. There is no blood in the anterior chamber, and optic disc margins are sharp. Vision is 20/20 in the left eye and 20/30 in the right eye. Which of the following diagnoses is most likely?
   a. Orbital floor or "blow out" fracture
   b. Hyphema
   c. Corneal abrasion
   d. Retinal detachment
   e. Traumatic iritis

Answer: a. This patient likely has an orbital floor fracture. Orbital floor fractures are common when the eye is struck with a blunt object (ball, baseball bat, fist) that is equal to or greater than the orbital aperture. Symptoms and signs vary but can include: edema, ecchymosis, diplopia, often vertical, and decreased visual acuity.

8. Which of the following is the *most* important risk factor for the development of ROP?
   a. Gestational age of 32 weeks
   b. Gram negative sepsis at 2 weeks of age
   c. Oxygen therapy for the first 21 days of life
   d. Birth weight of 900 g
   e. History of three red blood cell transfusions in the neonatal period

Answer: d. While all of the answers are risk factors for development of ROP, the greatest risk factor is low birth weight (<1,500 g).

9. A newborn infant is noted to be small for gestational age. He is afebrile and otherwise appears well. A detailed examination is conducted, including an ophthalmology evaluation, which reveals bilateral cataracts. Which of the following diagnostic studies should be conducted to help determine the etiology of the baby's small size?
   a. Urine test for reducing substances and evaluation for congenitally acquired infections (toxoplasmosis, rubella, CMV, HIV)
   b. Bacterial cultures of blood, urine, and cerebrospinal fluid
   c. CT brain
   d. Viral culture of the eyes
   e. Culture of the eyes for chlamydia

Answer: a. The differential diagnosis of bilateral cataracts includes congenitally acquired infections (rubella, CMV, and toxoplasma infections), galactosemia, and other metabolic and genetic disorders. Please see Table 21.2 of this chapter for differential diagnosis. Appropriate initial diagnostic work-up for bilateral cataracts would include urine test for reducing substances to evaluate for galactosemia and evaluation for congenital infection.

10. A 15-month-old male presents to his pediatrician for a routine visit. His parents are concerned that his left eye appears "different" than his right eye in recent pictures compared

to pictures taken when he was younger. On examination, a white pupillary reflex is seen in the left eye. The infant should be evaluated for which of the following diagnoses?

a. Esotropia
b. Retinoblastoma
c. Keratitis
d. Papilledema
e. Hordeolum

Answer: b. The white reflex in the normally black pupillary area seen in this patient's left eye seen is suggestive of leukocoria, which is opacification of any structure behind the iris. This infant should be evaluated for retinoblastoma, an important cause of leukocoria. Other etiologies include: cataracts, ROP, coloboma, and uveitis.

11. Children with juvenile idiopathic arthritis should be screened for anterior uveitis, an important potential complication, every 6 months. Anterior uveitis is most commonly observed in this type of juvenile idiopathic arthritis:

a. Systemic onset juvenile idiopathic arthritis
b. Pauciarticular onset juvenile idiopathic arthritis, ANA positive
c. Pauciarticular onset juvenile idiopathic arthritis, ANA negative
d. Polyarticular onset juvenile idiopathic arthritis, ANA positive
e. Polyarticular onset juvenile idiopathic arthritis, ANA negative

Answer: b. The risk of developing anterior uveitis is highest in the pauciarticular form of juvenile idiopathic arthritis, ANA positive. Patients should be screened by ophthalmology every 4 to 6 months. Risk is intermediate in polyarticular onset juvenile idiopathic arthritis, ANA positive. Risk is lowest is systemic onset juvenile idiopathic arthritis.

12. A 4-year-old female had the acute onset of a tender, erythematous "pimple" on the edge of her left outer eyelid. It grew initially after presentation for the first 3 days but afterwards spontaneously resolved over the next several days. The diagnosis was most likely:

a. Chalazion
b. Hordeolum
c. Blepharitis
d. Seborrheic keratitis
e. Molluscum contagiosum

Answer: b. A hordeolum is an acute, focal infection involving either the glands of Zeis (internal hordeolum) or the meibomian glands (external hordeolum). A hordeolum generally presents with signs of acute inflammation: a tender, warm, erythematous, swollen lump on the eyelid. *Staphylococcus aureus* is the most common organism. In contrast, a chalazion is a chronic, granulomatous inflammation of the meibomian gland. It is usually nontender and firm.

13. Objective visual acuity screening with standard eye charts should begin at what age?

a. 1 year
b. 3 years
c. 5 years
d. 6 years
e. 7 years

Answer: b. The American Academy of Pediatrics and the American Academy of Ophthalmology recommend routine objective vision screening beginning at 3 years of age. Assessment can be done with a picture, tumbling "E," or alphabet chart.

14. During a 6-month-old health maintenance visit, you note bilateral key-shaped pupils. Which is the appropriate next step?

a. Immediate MRI of the brain and orbits
b. Immediate CT scan of the brain and orbits
c. Urgent ophthalmology referral for examination and genetics consultation
d. Immediate eye pressure lowering medications for presumed glaucoma
e. No intervention at this time and close follow-up at 9 months of age

Answer: c. An iris coloboma is a congenital defect or cleft of the iris, resulting from failure to fuse during embryonic development. A full ophthalmologic examination should be conducted to evaluate for other eye abnormalities that may involve the lens, retina, optic nerve, and choroid. While a coloboma may occur in isolation, genetics consultation is recommended to evaluate for congenital syndromes, such as Aniridia–Wilms' tumor association or cat's eye syndrome, which may occur in association.

15. It is important to diagnose and treat strabismus to prevent which of the following sequelae?

a. Nystagmus
b. Ptosis
c. Amblyopia
d. Refractive error
e. Third-nerve palsy

Answer: c. The feared sequelae of undetected and untreated strabismus is amblyopia. Amblyopia is decreased visual acuity that is caused by decreased inputs to the central visual pathways of the affected eye. It is not caused by any optic nerve or anatomic eye pathology.

SUGGESTED READINGS

Diamant JI. Ocular infections: update on therapy. *Ophthalmol Clin North Am* 1999;12:15–20.
Hay WW. *Current Diagnosis and Treatment in Pediatrics*, 18th ed. Columbus: McGraw-Hill Companies, 2006.
Leibowitz HM. The red eye. *N Engl J Med* 2000;343:345–351.
Magramm I. Amblyopia: etiology, detection, and treatment. *Pediatr Rev* 1992;13:7–14.
McMillan JA. *Oski's Pediatrics: Principles and Practice*, 4th ed. Philadelphia: Lippincott Williams and Wilkins, 2006.
Morrow GL, Abbott RL. Conjunctivitis. *Am Fam Physician.* 1998;57(4).
Sankar PS, Chen TC, Grosskreutz CL, et al. Traumatic Hyphema. *Int Ophthalmol Clin.* 2002;42(3):57–68.
Seidman DJ, et al. Signs and symptoms in the presentation of primary infantile glaucoma. *Pediatrics* 1986;77:399–404.
Tingley D. Vision screening essentials: screening today for eye disorders in the pediatric patient. *Pediatr Rev* 2007;28:54–61.
Wagner RS. The differential diagnosis of the red eye. *Contemp Pediatr* 1991;8:26–48.
Wright KW. *Pediatric Ophthalmology for Primary Care*, 3rd ed. American Academy of Pediatrics, 2007.
Zitelli BJ. *Atlas of Pediatric Physical Diagnosis: Text with Online Access*, 5th ed. St. Louis: Mosby, 2007.

CHAPTER 22 ■ ORTHOPEDICS

AMY E. VALASEK

CHAPTER OBJECTIVES

1. To review musculoskeletal disturbances of prenatal origin
2. To review disorders of skeletal tissue, connective tissue, and growth
3. To review common osteochondroses and overuse injuries in the pediatric athlete
4. To review common pediatric fractures, dislocations, and subluxations
5. To review preparticipation examination and concussion management

COMMON DEFINITIONS

Abduction: movement away from midline
Adduction: movement toward midline
Apophysis: cartilaginous structure at the insertion of muscle groups into bone that is susceptible to over use or acute fracture in children
Apophysitis: inflammation of apophysis due to repetitive traction
Cartilage: cellular tissue that forms a template for bone formation and growth
Cavus: excessive height of the longitudinal foot arch
Condyle: rounded process at the end of long bones
Diaphysis: shaft of long bone
Epiphyseal line: part of the long bone that produces growth
Epiphysis: part of long bone, which develops from center of ossification
Equinus: plantar flexed position of ankle
Heterotopic ossification: formation of bone in nonosseous tissue usually after trauma
Kyphosis: curvature of the spine that is convex posteriorly
Lordosis: curvature of the spine that is convex anteriorly
Mesomelia: disproportional length of the forearms and lower legs
Metaphysis: broad portion of the long bone adjacent to the joint
Myositis ossificans: abnormal bone production in muscle
Osteonecrosis: death of bone from obstruction of blood supply
Phocomelia: absent long bones with flipper like appearance of hands/feet
Physis: specialized cartilage between the epiphysis and metaphysis, which serves as growth plate
Planus: flattening of the arch of the foot
Rhizomelia: disproportional length of the proximal limb (e.g., achondroplasia)
Spondylolisthesis: forward slippage of one vertebral body in relation to the vertebral body below
Spondylolysis: stress fracture in the pars interarticularis of vertebrae

MUSCULOSKELETAL DISTURBANCES OF PRENATAL ORIGIN

Metatarsus Varus

- Definition: deformity of forefoot with medial deviation of all metatarsals secondary to intrauterine molding.
- Epidemiology: more common in females and left foot.
- Associated syndromes: 10% of affected newborns also have DDH.
- Treatment: resolves spontaneously and if fails to correct, casting may be necessary in addition to active stretching.

Metatarsus Primus Varus

- Definition: often hereditary deformity with broad forefoot and medial deviation of first metatarsal only.
- Epidemiology: more in females than in males.
- Treatment: surgical osteotomy is reserved for severe cases.

Talipes Calcaneovalgus

- Definition: intrauterine position causes excessive dorsiflexion of ankle and eversion of foot.
- Treatment: stretching exercises are recommended for rigid deformities. If the deformity fails to correct, casting may be necessary.

Talipes Equinovarus (Clubfoot)

- Definition: foot deformity that can be idiopathic, neurogenic, or indicative of syndrome.
- Epidemiology: 1/1,000 births; 50% of cases are bilateral; more in males than females.
- Three features required for diagnosis are as follows:
  - Ankle equinus.
  - Heel varus.
  - Metatarsus adductus.
- Treatment: serial castings (Ponseti management), percutaneous heel-cord lengthening, and splinting to prevent recurrence. After correction, a nighttime brace is required for maintenance. Surgical treatment is required in 15% to 50% of cases to release contractures that are resistant to casting.

Points to Remember

- Even with successful treatment, the affected foot and ipsilateral calf will show residual stiffness and hypoplasia.

Developmental Dysplasia of Hip (DDH)

- Definition: spectrum of conditions with an abnormal relationship between proximal femur and acetabulum, which is divided in two types: idiopathic and teratogenic. Different types of dysplasias are outlined in Table 22.1.

TABLE 22.1

TYPES OF DEVELOPMENTAL DYSPLASIA OF HIP

	Idiopathic	Teratogenic
Associations	Family history	Club feet Torticollis Metatarsus adductus Infantile scoliosis
Range of presentation	Laxity Dislocations	Dislocation
Intrauterine position	Yes	No

- Epidemiology: peak incidence: infancy to early childhood
  - 1/1,000 live births.
  - More in females than males.
  - Unilateral more than bilateral.
- Risk factors: first born Caucasian females in breech position.
- Clinical manifestations are as follows:
  - Asymmetric thigh and buttock folds.
  - Shorted limb length is noted on examination when it is unilateral.
  - Positive Galeazzi sign (Fig. 22.1).
  - Positive Barlow's sign: clunk (posterior dislocation) w/adduction.
  - Positive Ortolani's sign: click (relocation) w/abduction and internal rotation.
- Diagnosis: physical examination and signs of instability are most accurate. Ultrasound is best modality prior to 6 months to evaluate femoral head and acetabulum. After 6 months of age, radiographs are the modality of choice.
- Treatment: aim of therapy is to restore contact between the femoral head and acetabulum. Dislocated hips should be treated at the time of diagnosis. In early infancy, unstable hips can be treated with a splint (Pavlik harness) where the hip is maintained in flexion

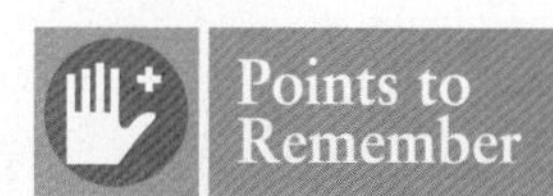

- Ortolani and Barlow have limited usefulness outside the neonatal period due to decreased mobility.

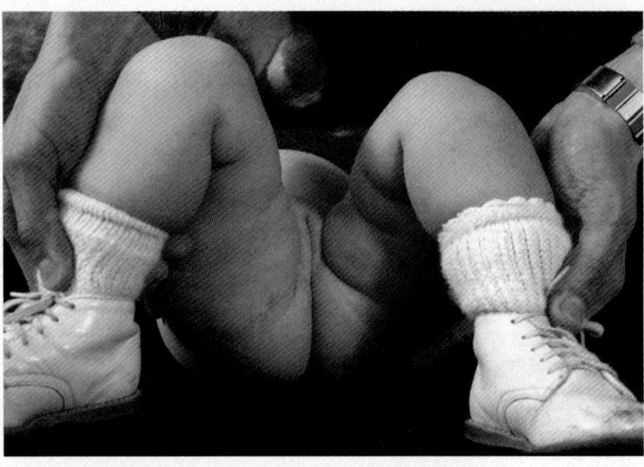

FIGURE 22.1. Positive Galeazzi sign. Note asymmetry in femoral heights. (Courtesy of Douglas A. Barnes, MD.)

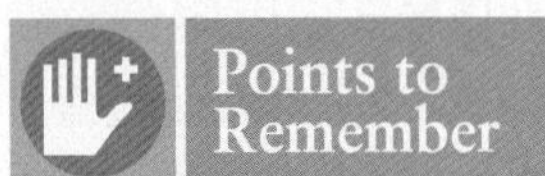

Points to Remember

- Use of double or triple diapers is not recommended for treatment.

and abduction. If noted 6 to 18 months, preoperative traction for 2 to 3 weeks brings the femur in contact with acetabulum. After closed reduction, a hip spica is needed for 6 months.

Congenital Torticollis (Wryneck)

- Definition: positional abnormality secondary to fibrosis and contraction of sternocleidomastoid muscle. The head is tilted toward the affected side.
- Epidemiology: 20% also have developmental dysplasia of hip.
- Risk factors: Breech position and forceps delivery.
- Clinical manifestation: palpable swelling or "tumor" in the muscle.
- Diagnosis: clinical examination and ultrasound of the hips to r/o DDH.
- Treatment: passive stretching during the first year of life or surgical release if condition persists after first year of life.

Phocomelia (Fig. 22.2)

- Definition: congenital disorder characterized by very short or absent long bones and flipper-like appearance of hands; the feet may also be involved.

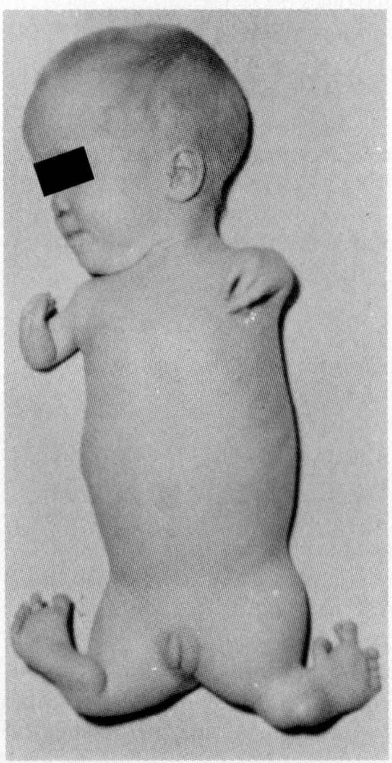

FIGURE 22.2. Patient with a form of meromelia called phocomelia. The hands and feet are attached to the trunk by irregularly shaped bones. (*Reprinted with permission from* Sadler T. *Langman's Medical Embryology*, 9th ed. Baltimore: Lippincott Williams & Wilkins, 2003.)

- Epidemiology: may be inherited or sporadic due to teratogen exposure such as thalidomide.
- Risk factors: associated finding in Holt–Oram syndrome and fusion of the carpal bones is found in almost every affected individual.

GENERALIZED DISORDERS OF THE SKELETAL AND CONNECTIVE TISSUES

Arthrogryposis Multiplex Congenita (Amyoplasia Congenita)

- Definition: nonprogressive muscle disorder of unknown etiology possibly due to failed muscle development or muscle degeneration that leads to decreased mobility, joint contractures, and degeneration of motor neurons.
- Epidemiology:
  - Neurological causes: Trisomy 13.
  - Trisomy 18.
  - Smith-Lemli-Opitz syndrome.
  - Zellweger syndrome.
  - Walker–Warburg syndrome.
  - Marden-Walker syndrome.
  - Spinal cord injury.
  - Amyoplasia congenital.
  - Infantile spinal muscular atrophy.
  - Infantile neuronal degeneration.
  - Non-neurological causes: cartilaginous abnormalities.
  - Physical constraint to movement *in utero*.
- Treatment: passive mobilization with removable splints and physical therapy.

Marfan Syndrome (Please see the Connective Tissue Diseases Chapter for Further Details)

- Definition: connective tissue disorder characterized by a constellation of findings: reduced upper-to-lower segment ratio, arachnodactyly, pectus carinatum or excavatum, scoliosis greater than 20 degrees, dilatation or dissection of the ascending aorta, mitral valve prolapse or regurgitation, and ectopia lentis.
- Athletic precaution: All athletes should be screened during preparticipation examination for Marfan syndrome. Athletes with this syndrome may need restriction from all contact sports based on degree of aortic dilatation.

Klippel–Feil Syndrome

- Definition: congenital malformation from failed segmentation of some or all cervical vertebrae, which is highly variable in presentation.
- Associated defects are as follows:
  - Congenital scoliosis.
  - Rib deformities.
  - Spina bifida.
  - Torticollis.
  - Deafness.
  - Sprengel deformity.
  - Renal/cardiac/pulmonary anomalies.
- Clinical manifestations: short broad stiff neck, low set hairline, possible webbed appearance (Fig. 22.3).
- Treatment: stretching exercises of neck musculature.
- Athletic precaution: contact sports to be avoided because of the risk for severe neck injury due to the limited mobility of the cervical area.

Sprengel Deformity

- Definition: congenital malformation in which one or both scapulas are abnormally small and limit ROM of upper extremity.
- Associated defects: Klippel–Feil syndrome, torticollis, scoliosis.
- Epidemiology: familial predisposition and most cases are unilateral.

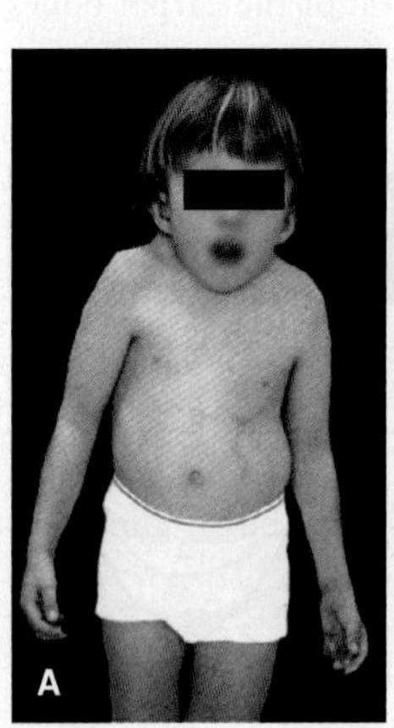

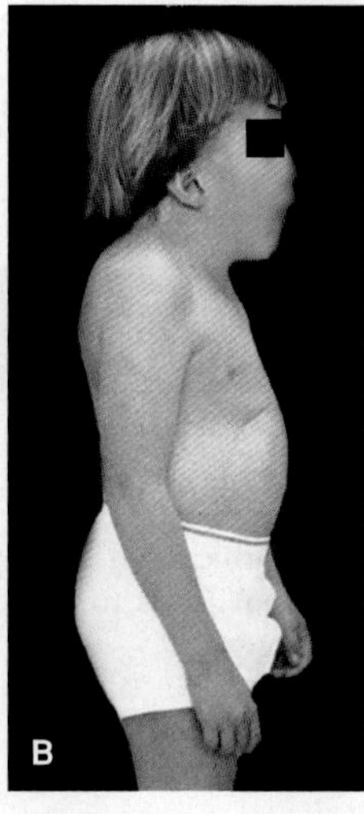

FIGURE 22.3. Clinical features of Klippel–Feil syndrome. This syndrome includes shortening of the neck, a low hairline, and neck stiffness. (*Reprinted with permission from* Staheli LT. *Fundamentals of Pediatric Orthopedics*, 4th ed. Philadelphia: Lippincott Williams & Wilkins, 2008.)

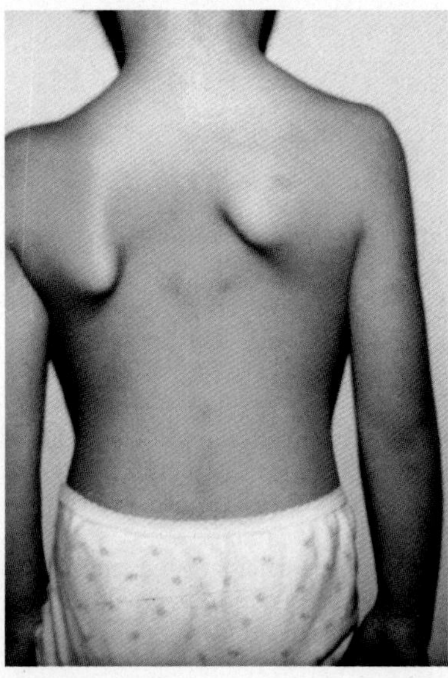

FIGURE 22.4. Sprengel deformity. Note right-sided deformity with elevation of scapula and asymmetry of shoulders and neck when compared with normal left side. (Courtesy of Shriners Hospitals for Children, Houston, Texas.)

- Clinical manifestation: high riding scapula with prominent vertebral border and decreased abduction on affected side (Fig. 22.4).
- Treatment: surgical repair in severe cases to improve shoulder ROM.

Osteogenesis Imperfecta

- Definition: connective tissue disease characterized by recurrent fractures or "brittle bones."
- Histologically: bone mass is decreased and trabeculae are reduced.
- Epidemiology:
  - Incidence 1/20,000 births.
  - Autosomal dominant: 90% of cases are due to gene defect in COL1A1 or COL1 A.
- Clinical manifestations are as follows:
  - Type I/Mild form: distinctly blue sclera at all ages.
  - Variable presentation with few fractures or numerous fractures from birth onward. Fifty percent have premature hearing loss (conductive and sensorineural) as adolescents.
  - Type II/Most severe form: lethal in perinatal period secondary to pulmonary failure. Infants are born either stillborn or IUGR with multiple poorly healed fractures at birth, dark blue-black sclera.
  - Type III/Progressive form: short stature with severe osseous fragility.
  - Type IV/Moderately severe.
- Treatment: Surgical correction of fractures and bisphosphonates.

Osteopetrosis (Osteitis Condensans, Marble Bone Disease, Albers–Schonberg Disease)

- Definition: rare disorder of osteoclastic bone resorption, which results in abnormally dense bones and small bone marrow space. Anemia is a common result.
- Epidemiology: mild autosomal dominant type presents in adulthood, whereas malignant autosomal recessive type presents in infancy.
- Diagnosis: radiographs show increased bone density, transverse shaft bands, and vertical striation of long bones. Also heterotopic calcification of soft tissue may occur.
- Treatment: Allogenic bone marrow transplantation is for the recessive type.

Achondroplasia

- Definition: skeletal dysplasia based on abnormal stature and rhizomelia (disproportion in the length of the upper arms/thighs).
- Epidemiology: most common form of short limb dwarfism and autosomal dominant inheritance with mutation in fibroblast growth factor receptor (FGFR-3).
- Clinical manifestations are as follows:
  - Bowing of extremities and decreased ROM of major joints.
  - Recurrent otitis media and conductive hearing loss.
  - Short fingers and all of equal length.
  - Frontal bossing with risk of foramen magnum stenosis.
  - Lumbar lordosis.
  - Obstructive sleep apnea (Fig. 22.5).
- Diagnosis: radiographs show short thick tubular bones, irregular epiphyseal plates, and cupped ends of bone.
- Treatment: limb lengthening procedures are controversial and growth hormone has no treatment effect.

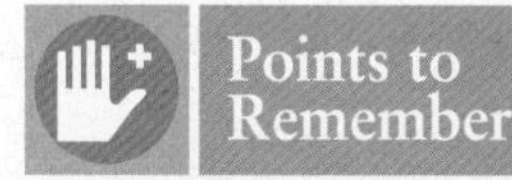

- Two copies of the gene are fatal. If both parents have achondroplasia, there is a 25% chance of fatality with each pregnancy.

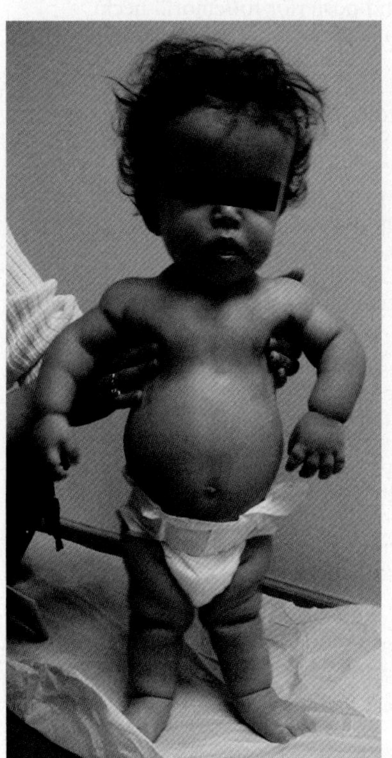

FIGURE 22.5. Achondroplasia. This infant with achondroplasia has tibial bowing, frontal bossing, rhizomelia (the proximal limb segment is shorter than the distal segment), and brachydactyly (short fingers). (Courtesy of Paul S. Matz, MD.)

Morquio Syndrome (Osteochondrodystrophy)

- Definition: mucopolysaccharide storage disorder (MPS IV) causing kyphosis, shortening of spine, short extremities, pectus carinatum, and hypoplastic odontoid (atlantoaxial instability).
- Epidemiology: autosomal recessive.

- Clinical manifestations: children appear normal at birth and then develop skeletal abnormalities between 1 and 4 years as MPS accumulates, resulting in a "duck-waddle" gait.
- Diagnosis: radiographs show flat vertebrae and irregular, malformed epiphyses.

GENERALIZED GROWTH DISTURBANCES

Scoliosis

- Definition: lateral curvature of the spine greater than 10 degrees secondary to rotation of involved vertebrae. Classified by anatomic location: thoracic, lumbar, and rarely cervical. The convexity of the curve is designated right or left position.
- Epidemiology: 80% cases are idiopathic; however, 30% of family members are also affected; therefore, monitor siblings closely.
- Risk factors: females are more likely to need treatment.
- Common associated syndromes: neurofibromatosis, Marfan syndrome, cerebral palsy, muscular dystrophy, poliomyelitis, and myelodysplasia.
- Clinical manifestation: typically asymptomatic; however, if pain occurs, the underlying cause for scoliosis should be sought (e.g., bone or spinal cord malignancy).
- Diagnostic screening examination (Adams forward bend test): patient bends forward 90 degrees with the hands joined midline. An abnormal screen shows asymmetric rib height or paravertebral muscles on one side.
- Diagnosis: clinical examination and AP and lateral standing views of entire spine (Fig. 22.6).
- Treatment: dependant on degree of curvature, skeletal maturity, and risk of progression throughout growth spurt (Table 22.2).

Points to Remember

- Right-sided curvature is most common; left-sided curvature requires a detailed neurological examination.

Points to Remember

- During the adolescent growth, spurt annual curve progression is approximately 5 to 10 degrees per year.

Slipped Capital Femoral Epiphysis

- Definition: displacement of proximal femoral epiphysis due to disruption of growth plate. The femoral head is typically displaced medially and posterior to femoral neck.
- Epidemiology: common in obese African-American males and presents between 10 and 16 years of age.
- Associated syndrome: hypothyroidism.
- Clinical manifestations: vague medial knee pain, groin pain, thigh pain, or limp over protracted period usually without history of trauma. Some patients may present with acute pain and inability to walk.
- Diagnosis: physical examination elicits limitation of internal hip rotation, and AP and frog-lateral radiographs of pelvis show widened epiphyseal plate (Bloomberg's sign) or off-centered Klein's line.
- Treatment: surgical pinning of the slipped femoral head.
- Outcomes: high incidence of degenerative arthritis and possible avascular necrosis of femoral neck if not treated urgently.

Points to Remember

- 30% of individuals will have involvement of contralateral side.

Blount's Disease (Tibia Vara)

- Definition: abnormal stress placed on the medial proximal tibial epiphysis that leads to growth suppression and varus angulation in children greater than 2 years. The various types of tibia vara are outlined in Table 22.3.
- Epidemiology: 70% are bilateral and infantile form is most common. Typically seen in early walkers and obese African-American females.

TABLE 22.2

SCOLIOSIS TREATMENT

Degree of Lateral Curvature	Treatment
<20	Does not require treatment unless the curve progresses during growth spurt
20–40	Bracing considered and monitored closely
40–60	Posterior spinal fusion
>75	Posterior spinal fusion and some degree of pulmonary restriction will result

TABLE 22.3

TYPES OF TIBIA VARA

Type	Age at Presentation (yr)
Infantile	1–3
Late-onset juvenile type	4–10
Late-onset adolescent type	11–14

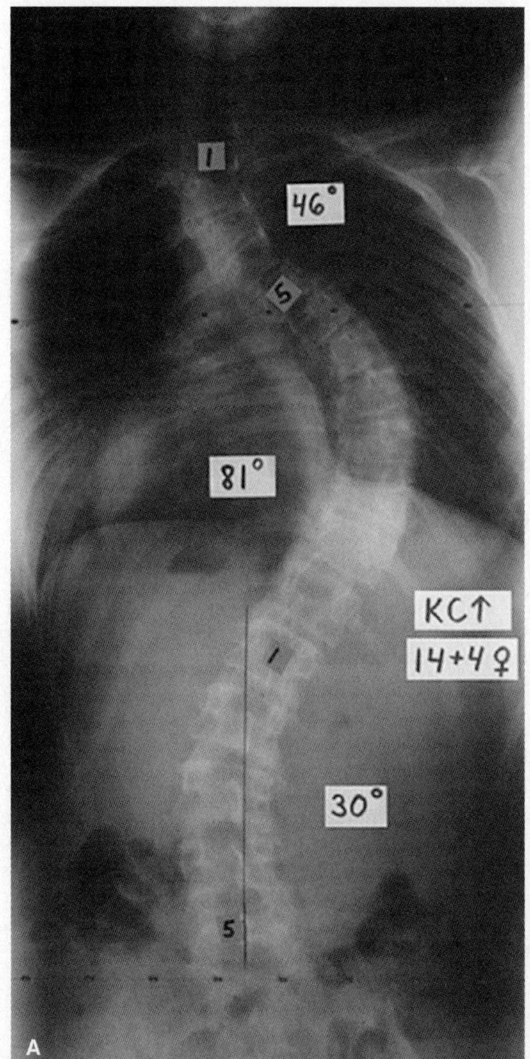

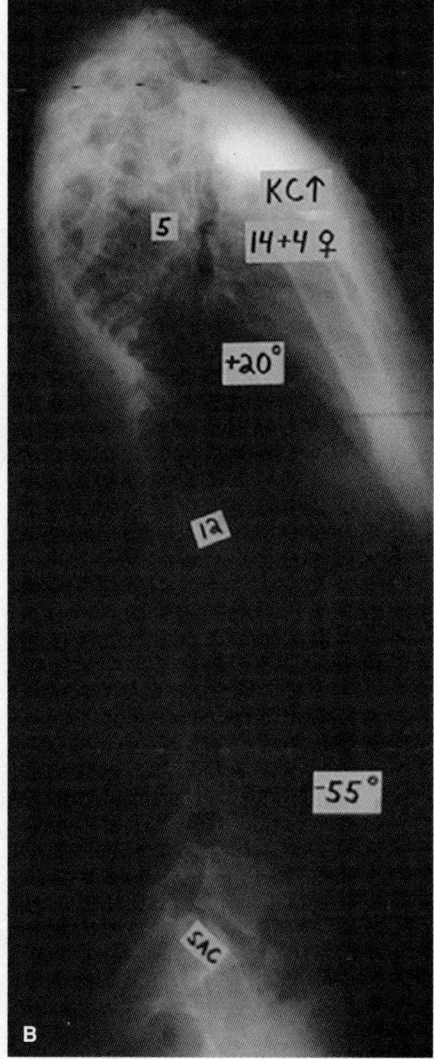

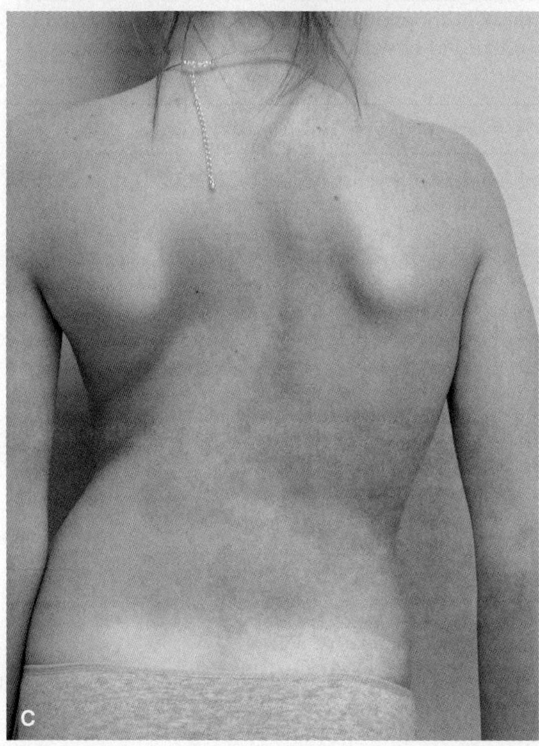

FIGURE 22.6. (**A**) Preoperative upright coronal radiograph demonstrates a large right thoracic curve of 81 degrees with a proximal thoracic curve of 46 degrees above and a lumbar A modifier position. (**B**) The preoperative lateral radiograph demonstrates proximal thoracic kyphosis. Her overall curve classification is 2BN. (**C**) Her preoperative upright clinical photograph demonstrates her significant right thoracic truncal deformity. (*Reprinted with permission from* Frymoyer JW, Wiesel SW, et al. *The Adult and Pediatric Spine*. Philadelphia: Lippincott Williams & Wilkins, 2004.)

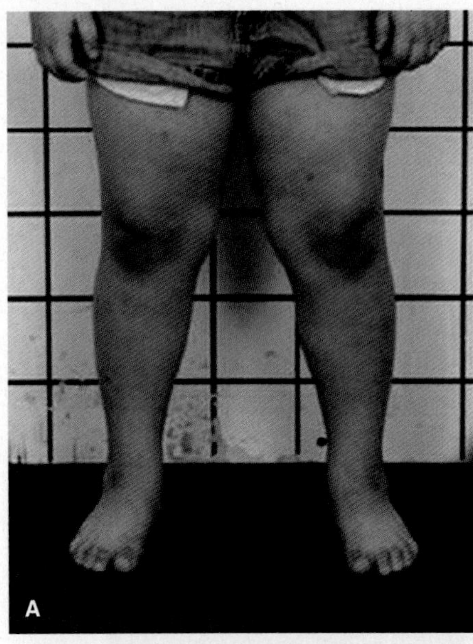

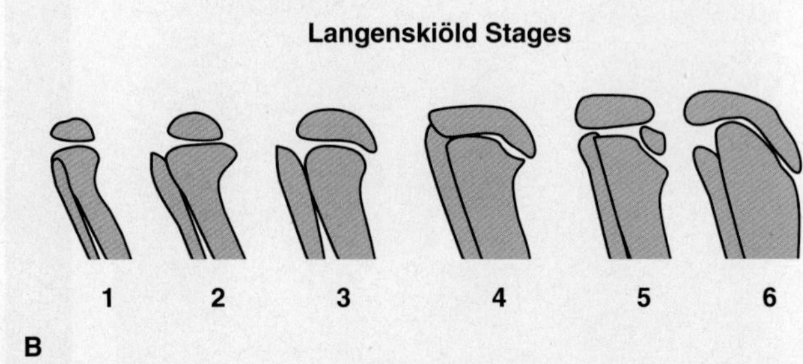

FIGURE 22.7. (A) Blount's disease. Genu varum deformity is seen in this obese male with Blount's disease. (Courtesy of Shriners Hospitals for Children, Houston, Texas.) (B) Langenskiöld classification. This classification is commonly used but sometimes difficult to apply. (*Reprinted with permission from* Staheli LT. *Fundamentals of Pediatric Orthopedics*, 4th ed. Philadelphia: Lippincott Williams & Wilkins, 2008.)

- Clinical manifestations are as follows:
  - Infantile tibia vara presents with bowing and length discrepancy in the lower limbs.
  - Late onset presents with leg shortening may be associated with tenderness over the medial prominence of the proximal tibia.
- Diagnosis: standing AP and lateral radiograph of extremities show varus angulation of the metaphysis, medial sloping of the epiphyses, and irregularity of the growth plates (Fig. 22.7).
- Treatment: varies from observation, bracing to corrective surgery.

Genu Varum (Bowleg)

- Epidemiology: normal from infancy through 2 years of age (Table 24.4) (Fig. 22.8).
- Treatment: typically there is spontaneous resolution. Persistent bowing beyond 2 years, increased bowing, or unilateral bowing requires orthopedic evaluation.

Genu Valgum (Knock-Knee)

- Epidemiology: normal from 2 to 8 years of age (Table 22.4) (Fig. 22.9).

TABLE 22.4

CAUSE OF GENU VARUM AND VALGUM

Causes	Genu Valgum	Genu Varum
Congenital	Fibular hemimelia	
Dysplasia	Osteochondrodysplasias	Osteochondrodysplasias
Developmental	Knock-knee >2 SD	Tibia vara
Trauma	Overgrowth Partial physeal arrest	Partial physeal arrest
Metabolic	Rickets	Rickets
Osteopenic	Osteogenesis imperfecta	
Infection	Growth plate injury	Growth plate injury
Arthritis	Rheumatoid arthritis	

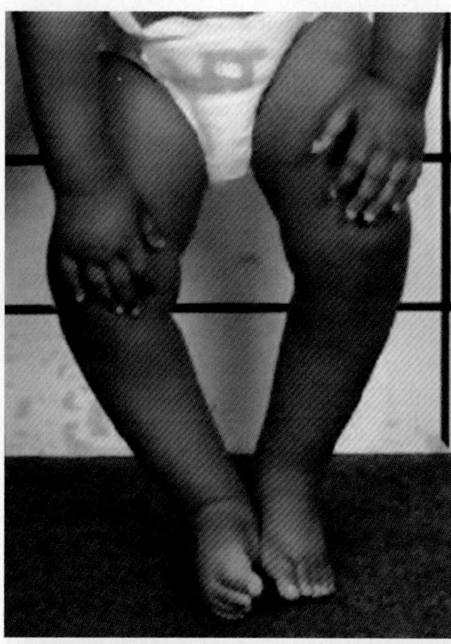

FIGURE 22.8. Infantile tibial bowing. Outward angulation of the tibia bilaterally in an infant. (Courtesy of Shriners Hospitals for Children, Houston, Texas.)

- Treatment: typically no treatment is necessary and there is spontaneous resolution. If angle is greater than 20 degrees, night bracing may be helpful. After 10 years of age if angle is greater than 15 degrees, surgery may be indicated.

Tibial Torsion (Toeing-In)

- Definition: internal rotation of the tibia. There exists 20 degrees of internal rotation at birth and decreases to neutral by 16 months.
- Epidemiology: occurs in males and females equally.
- Clinical manifestation: Noticed by parent when child begins to walk.
- Treatment: this condition improves within the first year of ambulation but will not correct after 4 years of age. Surgical treatment is considered only if there is functional impairment.

Femoral Anteversion (Toeing-In)

- Definition: internal rotation of femur.
- Epidemiology: common in females between 3 and 5 years.

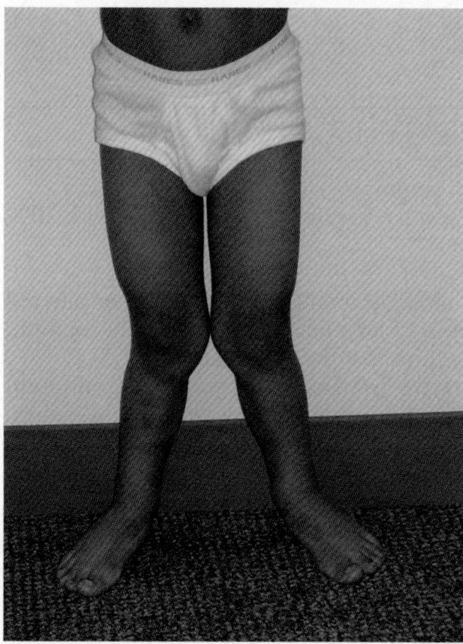

FIGURE 22.9. Genu valgum. A toddler with notable inward angulation of the knees. (Courtesy of Bettina Gyr, MD.)

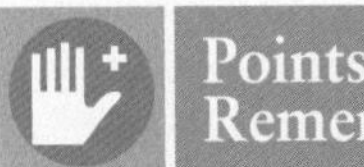

Points to Remember

- Three common causes of toeing-in are metatarsus adductus, femoral anteversion, and tibial torsion.

- Clinical manifestation: child sits in "W" position and stands with "kissing patella's."
- Treatment: corrects spontaneously by 10 years of age. Encourage activities causing external hip rotation: skating and bicycling. Surgical treatment is considered only if there is functional impairment.

Pes Planus (Flat Foot)

- Definition: lack of arch in foot that is normal in infancy and develops within the first 8 years of life.
- Epidemiology: familial inheritance.
- Treatment: orthotic inserts.

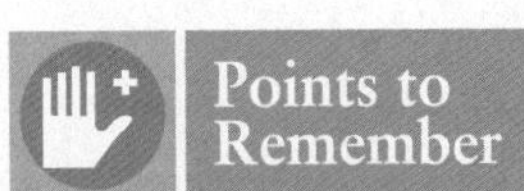

Points to Remember

- All children require detailed neurologic examination and spinal radiographs.

Cavus Foot (High-Arched Foot)

- Associated syndromes: poliomyelitis, Charcot–Marie–Tooth's disease, Friedreich ataxia, and diastematomyelia (splitting of the spinal cord).
- Clinical manifestations: Contracture of toe extensor producing claw toe deformity.
- Treatment: severe symptomatic cases require surgical lengthening of extensor tendon and release of plantar fascia.

OSTEOCHONDROSES

General overview: during normal development, growth plates change from cartilage to bone. Osteochondrosis refers to interruption of the blood supply to epiphysis, followed by localized bony necrosis, and replacement of living bone by "creeping substitution."

Scheuermann's Disease (Juvenile Kyphosis)

- Definition: increased kyphosis in the thoracic or thoracolumbar spine with associated backache and localized changes in the vertebral bodies. In particular, osteochondrosis of the secondary ossification centers occurs in vertebral bodies. The process may be limited to several bodies or may involve the entire dorsal and lumbar spine.
- Epidemiology: affects adolescents between 13 and 16 years with an increased incidence of spondylolysis or spondylolisthesis.
- Risk factors: male gender.
- Associated syndrome: scoliosis.
- Diagnosis: the child is typically seen in the office for poor posture, and Adams Forward bend test is performed from the lateral position of the patient. AP and lateral standing radiographs show wedging of 5 or more in 3 consecutive vertebrae, hyperkyphosis of greater than 40 degrees, and irregular upper and lower vertebral endplates with loss of disk space height.
- NOTE: vertebral plates are poorly formed and develop multiple herniations of the nucleus pulposus known as Schmorl nodes. Schmorl nodes may also be seen in Wilson's disease, sickle cell anemia, and spinal stenosis.
- Treatment: consider bracing and possibly surgical correction if the curve progresses.

Legg–Calve–Perthes Disease (Femoral Head)

- Definition: osteonecrosis of the capital femoral epiphysis.
- Epidemiology: peak age is 4 to 8 years and more often seen in Caucasian males with 20% of cases being bilateral.
- Associated syndrome: sickle cell disease.
- Clinical manifestations: presents with limp, limitation of motion of affected leg, or referred knee pain. Physical examination reveals restriction of hip abduction and internal rotation.
- Diagnosis: AP and frog-leg lateral radiographs can show five stages (Table 22.5).
- Treatment: the goal is to avoid severe degenerative arthritis by supporting the hip until new bone forms. If femur is deep in acetabulum, a normal hip will result. Crutches, physical therapy, bracing and traction are options, and surgery is reserved for severe cases.

Köhler's Disease (Foot Pain)

- Definition: osteonecrosis of the navicular bone.
- Epidemiology: peak incidence in males between 4 and 6 years, and 30% of cases are bilateral.

TABLE 22.5

RADIOGRAPHIC STAGES OF LEGG–CALVE–PERTHES DISEASE

Stage 1	Cessation of growth at the capital femoral epiphysis; smaller femoral head epiphysis; and widening of articular space on affected side
Stage 2	Subchondral fracture; linear radiolucency within the femoral head epiphysis
Stage 3	Resorption of bone
Stage 4	Reossification of new bone
Stage 5	Healed bone

- Clinical manifestation: presents with limp and walks with an increased weight on the lateral side of the foot. Frequently, there is swelling and redness of the soft tissues.
- Diagnosis: lateral radiograph shows narrowing of the navicular AP diameter.
- Treatment: immobilization with short leg weight bearing cast for 6 weeks.

Panner's Disease (Elbow Pain)

- Definition: osteonecrosis of the humerus capitulum.
- Epidemiology: dominant throwing arm in males between 5 and 10 years.
- Clinical manifestations: tenderness on the outside edge of the elbow, and pain generally worsens with activity and eases with rest. Typically, there is inability to completely extend the elbow.
- Diagnosis: radiographs show irregular, flattened capitulum head.
- Treatment: rest from offending activities and long arm splint or cast for severe cases.

Freiberg Disease (Foot Pain)

- Definition: osteonecrosis of metatarsal head.
- Epidemiology: peaks in female adolescents and most commonly involves second metatarsal head.
- Clinical manifestation: presents with vague foot pain, stiffness, and limp exacerbated with activity. Physical examination reveals limited range of motion (ROM), swelling, and tenderness with direct palpation of the MTP joint.
- Diagnosis: radiographs show irregular flattened metatarsal head.
- Treatment: conservative treatment includes activity modification, orthotics, or short-term casting. Surgical treatment is reserved for severe cases to remove loose bodies or to realign the metatarsal head.

Kienböck's Disease (Wrist Pain)

- Definition: osteonecrosis of carpal lunate and disease progression with collapse, fragmentation ultimately leading to arthritis of wrist.
- Epidemiology: peaks in males between 15 and 40 years.
- Clinical manifestation: presents with pain, stiffness, swelling, and diffuse stiffness over the dorsal aspect of the wrist.
- Diagnosis: radiograph of the wrist may reveal any of the following: normal x-ray, sclerosis of lunate, collapse of lunate, or degenerative arthritis of wrist.
- Treatment: splint/casting wrist in neutral position for 3 weeks. Overuse injuries from repetitive microtrauma.

Stress Fractures

- Definition: microfracture in the cortex of the bone resulting from repeated physical stress that exceeds the capability to remodel for support. Stress fractures can occur in any bone of the body (Table 22.6).
- Epidemiology: more common in female adolescents involved in repetitive loading sports: ballet, figure skating, gymnastics, and cheerleading.
- Risk factors: sudden intense training, change in footwear, change in playing surface, and female athlete triad (eating disorder, amenorrhea, and osteoporosis).

TABLE 22.6

COMMON SITES FOR STRESS FRACTURE

Par interarticularis: L4 and L5 (spondylolysis or spondylolisthesis)
Metatarsals: second through fifth
Femur: neck
Tibia
Navicular
Calcaneus

- Clinical manifestations: focal bony pain with a specific maneuver/activity, which gradually worsen.
- Diagnosis: radiographs are typically negative; sclerosis and lucency are apparent only after several months of symptoms. MRI or bone scan may be helpful in difficult cases.
- Treatment: avoidance of all activities that aggravate the injury and evaluate dietary intake of calcium and vitamin. Most heal within 6 weeks and return to play when pain free.
- Complications: development into nonunion fracture. High-risk sites are femoral neck, anterior tibial cortex, navicular, fifth metatarsal, and sesamoids that typically need surgical repair.

Pars Interarticularis Stress Fracture

- Epidemiology: frequently seen in athletes participating in high-level activities that place hyperextension stress on lumbar vertebrae such as gymnastics, football, and lacrosse.
- Clinical manifestations: lumbar back pain that worsens with standing and hyperextension.
- Diagnosis: oblique lumbar view shows a "collar" on scotty dog if spondylolysis or forward translation of vertebral body with spondylolisthesis.
- Treatment: modify activity, occasional brace, strengthen core muscle, and hamstring stretches are recommended. Return to sport when asymptomatic. Spinal fusion is indicated when more than 50% forward slippage in a skeletally immature athlete.

Physeal Stress Fracture

- Definition: widening of the physis as a result of repetitive microtrauma. The most common sites are proximal humeral physis (little league shoulder) and distal radius physis (gymnastics).
- Treatment: rest is required and cast/splint may be helpful to increase patient compliance. Overhead throwing athletes typically require 3 months of complete throwing rest, then gradual return to activity.

Apophysitis

- General overview: apophysis is a prominence that is associated with attachment of muscle-tendon group. It acts as part of the physis responding to large tractions forces of muscle-tendon unit. In the skeletally immature, the apophysis is the weakest site of the tendon-muscle unit and at risk for injury.

Osgood–Schlatter (Tibial Tuberosity Pain)

- Definition: tight quadriceps pulls on the apophysis of the tibial tubercle during rapid growth. This traction induces inflammation of the tibial tubercle.
- Epidemiology: peaks in males between 10 and 15 years.
- Clinical manifestation: pain during stair climbing, running, jumping, and prolonged sitting. Physical examination reveals pain and swelling at the insertion of the patellar tendon into the tibial tubercle.
- Diagnosis: radiographs are typically normal or show small heterotopic ossification anterior to tibial tuberosity (Fig. 22.10).
- Treatment: ice, protective knee pad (Cho–Pat brace), and stretching exercises of quadriceps and hamstrings. Activity modification for 2 to 3 months.

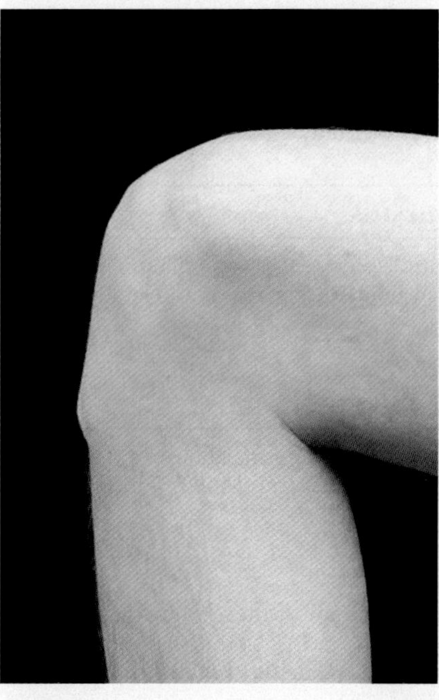

FIGURE 22.10. Osgood–Schlatter disease. Lateral view demonstrating prominence of the tibial tuberosity. (Courtesy of Julie A. Boom, MD.)

Sinding–Larsen–Johansson Disease (Inferior Pole of Patella Pain)

- Definition: traction-induced inflammation at the junction of patellar tendon and distal pole of patella.
- Clinical manifestation: presents with pain during stair climbing, running, jumping, and kneeling. Physical examination reveals pain and swelling at the insertion of patellar tendon into inferior patella.
- Diagnosis: radiographs show elongation of inferior pole of patella.
- Treatment: ice and stretching exercises of quadriceps and hamstrings. Activity modification for 2 to 3 months.

Sever's Disease (Heel Pain)

- Definition: traction-induced inflammation at calcaneal apophysis from Achilles tendon.
- Epidemiology: peak incidence male between 9 and 12 years and typically bilateral.
- Clinical manifestation: presents with diffuse pain and swelling of the heels that worsens with activity and may cause difficulty in ambulating. Physical examination reveals tenderness at posterior aspect of calcaneus.
- Diagnosis: radiographs are not diagnostic.
- Treatment: ice after activity, heel cups, and stretching exercises of Achilles tendon. Short-term activity modification may be necessary in recalcitrant cases.

Medial Elbow Pain (Little League Elbow)

- Definition: traction-induced inflammation at medial epicondyle apophysis. Medial elbow overload can range from apophysitis and avulsion fracture in skeletally immature to rupture of ulnar collateral ligament in skeletally mature.
- Diagnosis: radiographs range from normal to widening of the medial epicondyle.
- NOTE: medial apophysis is the last ossification center in the elbow to close and has the longest exposure to traction forces during throwing.
- Treatment: ice after activity, complete rest from offending activities, stretching and strengthening of shoulder, scapular and core muscles. If the pain is ignored, this can progress to avulsion fracture or UCL rupture.

Osteochondritis Dissecans

- Definition: osteonecrosis of subchondral bone causing osteochondral fragments and loose bodies in joint space.
- Epidemiology: skeletally mature adolescents.

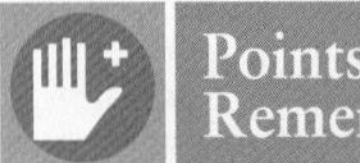

Points to Remember

- Be cautious of diagnosing tendonitis in the skeletally immature who are more at risk for apophysitis, avulsion fractures, and fracture.

- Common sites of occurrence: medial femoral condyle, capitulum, and talus.
- Clinical manifestation: presents with joint pain, effusion, and "locking" sensation of the joint affected.
- Treatment: if skeletally immature, nonsurgical treatment consists of activity modification and immobilization. These lesions take months to heal. If skeletally mature, surgery is required.

Tendonitis and Bursitis

- General overview: tendons and bursa are susceptible to overuse and inflammation from repetitive traction and microtrauma. Typically tendonitis occurs in the skeletally mature adolescent athlete and adults.

Common Pediatric Fractures

- General overview: remodeling of fracture produces almost normal bony appearance in months. As a general rule, the younger the child with a fracture, the more remodeling capability.

Epiphyseal Fractures

- Overview: growth plate is weakest site of bone/ligament unit. Salter–Harris classification was developed to predict the risk of growth arrest (Fig. 22.11).
- Clinical examination: bony pain with an effusion after traumatic event and examination reveals focal tenderness over the physis.
- Treatment: cast immobilization required for Types I and II. Surgical reduction is necessary for Types III, IV, and V.

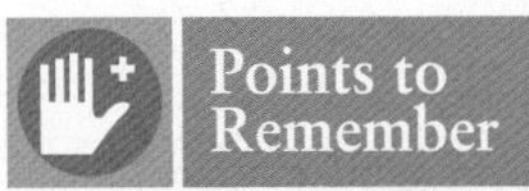

Points to Remember

- Radiographs are not helpful in the diagnosis of Salter-Harris Type I fractures and physical examination is essential. Type V fractures cause nonreversible damage to the growth plate.

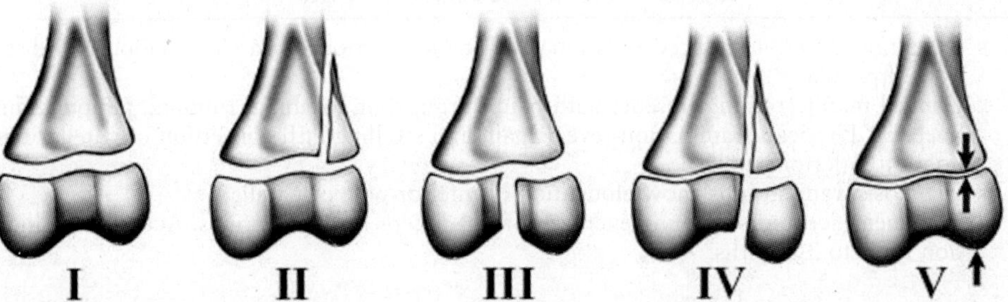

FIGURE 22.11. Salter–Harris classification. (*Reprinted with permission from* Strickland JW, Graham TJ. *Master Techniques in Orthopaedic Surgery: The Hand*, 2nd ed. Philadelphia: Lippincott Williams & Wilkins, 2005.)

Torus Fractures (Fig. 22.12)

- Overview: buckling of cortex due to bone compression.
- Treatment: cast immobilization for 3 to 4 weeks.

Greenstick Fractures (Fig. 22.13)

- Overview: frank cortex disruption on one side and no disruption on the opposite side.
- Treatment: cast immobilization for 4 weeks. Repeat radiograph in 7 to 10 days after initial cast to make certain that the reduction has been maintained in cast.

Clavicle Fracture

- General overview: typically results from traumatic fall on lateral shoulder, fall on outstretched hand, or birth trauma.
- NOTE: Midshaft clavicular fractures are the most common. Distal clavicular fractures require orthopedic evaluation due to high association of ligament injury and nonunion.
- Treatment: neonatal fractures generally heal spontaneously in several weeks without treatment. Midshaft fractures are treated with sling immobilization if compliant. Distal third fractures require sling immobilization and orthopedic consultation.

Supracondylar Fracture of Distal Humerus

- Overview: fractures site above the physis and associated with significant trauma. These fractures have the highest incidence of neurovascular injury due to the close approximation to brachial artery, median nerve, ulnar nerve, and radial nerve.
- Epidemiology: children affected between 2 and 12 years.

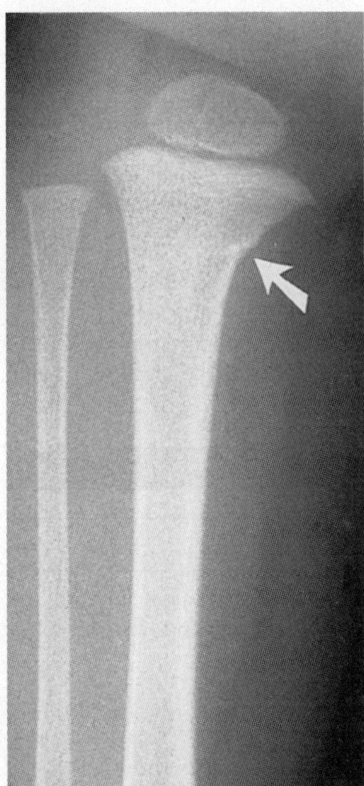

FIGURE 22.12. Torus fracture of the proximal right tibia in a 1-year-old child (**arrow**). (*Reprinted with permission from* Fleisher GR, Ludwig S, Henretig FM, et al. *Textbook of Pediatric Emergency Medicine*, 5th ed. Philadelphia: Lippincott Williams & Wilkins, 2005.)

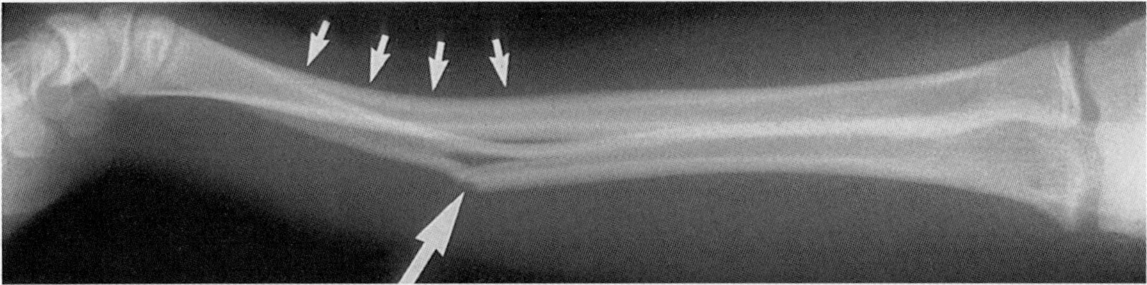

FIGURE 22.13. Greenstick fracture of the ulna (**large arrow**) and a bowing fracture (**small arrows**) of the radius. The extent of bowing can often be fully appreciated only with comparison views of the opposite extremity. (*Reprinted with permission from* Fleisher GR, Ludwig S, Henretig FM, et al. *Textbook of Pediatric Emergency Medicine*, 5th ed. Philadelphia: Lippincott Williams & Wilkins, 2005.)

- Diagnosis: lateral radiograph demonstrates posterior fat pad.
- Treatment: cast immobilization or surgical pinning. Because of concern of nonunion, repeat radiographs are obtained 7 to 10 days after the initial fracture.
- Complications: Volkmann ischemic contracture due to vascular compromise of brachial artery and necrosis of forearm muscles.

Common Pediatric Fractures Secondary to Nonaccidental Trauma

- Metaphyseal fracture (Bucket Handle).
- Spiral fracture of long bones.
- Posterior rib fractures.
- Spinous process fracture.

DISLOCATION/SUBLUXATION

Recurrent Dislocation of Patella

- Epidemiology: common in adolescents with following risk factors: abnormally high patella (patella alta), patellar dysplasia, poorly developed trochlea, or ligamentous laxity.
- Clinical manifestation: severe pain and knee slightly flexed with obvious mass lateral to knee joint if still dislocated. If relocated, large effusion and severe pain are noted on examination.

- Treatment: reduction and immobilization for 4 weeks, then physical therapy. Surgical intervention may be necessary to prevent degenerative arthritis if dislocation/subluxation is recurrent.

Subluxation of Radial Head (Nursemaid Elbow)

- General overview: results from lifting, pulling, or tugging of the child's hand.
- Definition: slippage of radial head under annular ligament.
- Epidemiology: occurs more often in females between 1 and 4 years.
- Clinical manifestations: painful pronated elbow and kept in extension. Physical examination reveals point tenderness over radial head and radiographs are normal.
- Treatment: manipulation of the child's arm so that the annular ligament and radial head return to their normal anatomic positions. Shortly after reduction, the child will begin using arm again.

COMMON SPORTS MEDICINE ISSUES

Preparticipation Physical Examination (PPE)

- General overview: ideally completed 6 weeks prior to the start of preseason training and competition. Goal is to identify disabling conditions, life-threatening conditions, or any predisposition to injury.
- Topics to highlight in history are as follows:
  - Medications, nutritional supplements, and steroid use.
  - Allergies: medicine, food, and environmental.
  - Absence of paired organs—single-organ athletes (eye, kidney, testes).
  - Sickle cell trait—increased risk of rhabdomyolysis and death in extreme training conditions.
  - Cardiac history—important to detect hypertrophic cardiomyopathy, arrhythmia, prolonged QTc, Marfan syndrome, or myocarditis on the basis of history. ECG and ECHO are not required for clearance only if a condition is suspected on the basis of history.
  - Pulmonary history—detect asthma and exercise-induced bronchospasm.
  - Neurologic history: seizure history. Athletes can participate in almost all sports, including contact sports if seizures are well controlled.
  - Female athlete history: screen for female triad—disordered eating, amenorrhea, and osteoporosis.

Concussion

- Definition: trauma-induced neurologic dysfunction that resolves spontaneously. Loss of consciousness and amnesia are not required. Zurich guidelines from 2008 support more recovery time after a young athlete sustains a concussion and no same day return to play. An athlete will miss a minimum of 1 week on the basis of guidelines for gradual return to play in the pediatric athlete.
- Epidemiology: more in female athletes than in male athletes.
- Clinical manifestation: a combination of somatic, emotional, and neurologic symptoms may manifest after a concussion.
- Complications: Second Impact Syndrome is an extremely rare condition in children in which the brain swells rapidly and catastrophically after a second concussion before symptoms from an earlier one have subsided. The gradual return to play guidelines aims specifically at preventing this complication. Return to play guidelines are outlined in Table 22.7.

Points to Remember

- 24 hours are necessary to proceed through each step. If athletes become symptomatic at any step, they revert to the previous step and progress at a slower pace until cleared. The minimum time to return to play is 6 days on the basis of the guidelines.

TABLE 22.7

RETURN TO PLAY GUIDELINES AFTER A SPORTS-RELATED CONCUSSION

Step	Activity
Step 1	No activity and complete rest until asymptomatic. Once postconcussive symptoms resolved, proceed to step 2
Step 2	Light aerobic exercise
Step 3	Sport-specific exercise
Step 4	Noncontact drills
Step 5	Full contact after medical clearance
Step 6	Cleared to return

SAMPLE BOARD REVIEW QUESTIONS

1. A 17-year-old female comes to office after feeling a pop when landing on right knee. There is a large effusion and she is unable to bear weight due to instability. You suspect an ACL tear. Which of the following maneuvers is the most sensitive test to aid in the diagnosis?
   a. Anterior Drawer
   b. Lachman's Test
   c. McMurray's Test
   d. Posterior Drawer
   e. Reverse pivot shift

   Answer: b. Lachman's highest sensitivity and specificity to rule in or out an acute ACL tear. To do this, lay the patient supine. Put the patient's knee in about 20 to 30 degrees flexion and externally rotate the leg. The examiner should place one hand behind the tibia and the other on the patient's thigh. On pulling anteriorly on the tibia, an intact ACL should prevent forward translational movement of the tibia on the femur (firm endpoint). Anterior translation of the tibia associated with a soft or a mushy endpoint indicates a positive test.

2. A 16-year-old female and her mother come to the office for preparticipation physical. She has aspirations of playing basketball in college and has been relatively healthy. Mom is concerned because many of her teammates have torn their ACL and she asks for advice to prevent this injury in her daughter. You recommend which of the following?
   a. Wear turf cleats
   b. Start oral contraception since current research shows a correlation between ovulation and ACL injury
   c. Wear knee braces on both knees
   d. No preventative measures as ACL injury is bad luck due to anatomic differences
   e. Neuromuscular and proprioception training

   Answer: e. Neuromuscular and proprioception training. Research shows that adolescent females are 2 to 10 times more likely than male counterparts to suffer from ACL tears. Studies attribute this increased risk to lack of neuromuscular coordination causing females to land in valgus and extension. Training programs are aimed at training females to land softly, stretching and strengthening the quadriceps/hamstrings, and plyometric drills. Although no ACL injury can be fully prevented, the training programs have shown to decrease the incidence by increasing neuromuscular control and coordination.

3. A 17-year-old male lacrosse player comes to the office with worsening back pain throughout the season. He denies neurologic symptoms. He describes his pain as diffuse lumbar pain worsens after practices and games, which has become more persistent with all shooting maneuvers. Physical examination shows normal strength and reflex testing of both lower extremities. Palpation of spine notes step off of spinous process in L5 region. Straight leg raise test is negative. Hyperextension of back while balancing on one foot reproduces pain in lumbar region. The most likely diagnosis is:
   a. Muscular strain
   b. Spondylolysis
   c. Spondylolisthesis
   d. Disk protrusion
   e. Tumor

   Answer: c. Spondylolisthesis occurs when one vertebral body slips forward in relation with the vertebral body below. In children, it occurs most frequently between L5 and S1. The defect develops at the lamina with the pedicle (pars interarticularis). Diagnosis is made with clinical examination and lateral radiographs show forward slippage of the vertebral body. If only spondylolysis has occurred, the lateral radiograph will be normal and the oblique views with show a defect in pars interarticularis (Scotty dog collar sign). Treatment is observation, stoppage of aggravating activities, physical therapy for hamstring stretching and core strengthening and bracing is optional. Surgical correction is indicated if there is progression and a slip greater 50% with significant growth remaining.

4. A 13-year-old male complains of difficulty fitting in his shoes and rolling his right ankle repeated in gym this spring. He is otherwise healthy and denies pain. Physical examination reveals curled toes and cavus foot deformity of right foot. The test most helpful for diagnosis is:
   a. MRI of cervical spine
   b. MRI of lumbar spine
   c. CT of right foot
   d. AP and lateral radiographs of the right foot

Answer: b. MRI of Lumbar spine—without a history of underlying neuromuscular disorder or known cause of cavus foot deformity, he should undergo diagnostic work-up to rule out unilateral foot deformity. Spinal cord tumor and spinal cord tether both are causes of unilateral cavus deformity and must be ruled out.

5. A 9-year-old male presents with bilateral heel pain notable after soccer practices and games. He is very active on multiple sports teams in one season. He denies night-time pain but occasionally limps after games. Physical examination reveals tenderness at the posterior aspect of the calcaneus bilaterally. There is no obvious swelling. Heel walking in the office reproduces the pain. The next step in management is:
   a. AP and lateral radiographs of both feet
   b. MRI of both feet
   c. Conservative treatment with ice, activity modification, heel lifts, and Achilles stretching
   d. Trial of NSAIDS for 2 weeks
   e. Orthopedic referral for surgical correction

Answer: c. Sever's disease is calcaneal apophysitis that affects active prepubertal children. Pain is typically limited to posterior heel most notable after activity. This is typically a clinical diagnosis. There are no radiographic changes consistent with calcaneal apophysitis. Radiographs are helpful if unilateral or atypical symptoms.

6. A 14-year-old male presents to the office with atraumatic knee effusion. He played in basketball game without incident and awoke the next morning with right-knee swelling. He denies pain and has minimal difficulty in ambulating. Physical examination reveals large knee effusion, no redness or warmth, no direct joint line tenderness, no ligamentous instability. Radiographs did not show evidence of fracture. The next step most helpful for diagnosis is:
   a. MRI of knee to rule out meniscal tear
   b. Oblique x-ray to rule out tibial plateau fracture
   c. Insertion of needle to tap effusion and send for further studies
   d. Watch and wait
   e. Laboratory studies

Answer: c. Insertion of needle to tap effusion and send for further studies is beneficial in this case. There is no history of traumatic injury, and knee examination was normal except for large effusion. Synovial fluid for cell count, differential, culture, and rheumatologic studies are important for accurate diagnosis.

7. A 15-year-old junior varsity football player comes to the sideline after traumatic collision. He seems dazed and slightly ataxic gait noted. Your evaluation shows deficient short-term recall, and he complains of headache, mild nausea, and tinnitus. Repeat examination 15 minutes later reveals full improvement of recall, full neurologic strength throughout, normal gait, no symptoms. The player and coach want him back in the game. As the team physician, your answer for return to play is:
   a. He can return as all symptoms have cleared
   b. He can return since this is his first concussion
   c. He cannot return until second half
   d. He is not cleared to return this game

Answer: d. He is not cleared to return. On the basis of the Zurich guidelines, children under 18 should never return to play the same day. Close monitoring for 24 to 28 hours is required. A gradual return to play is the key in brain recovery, and step-wise guidelines should be strictly enforced in pediatric athlete.

8. A 6-year-old girl presents to the office because she "runs funny." Mom notes her toes turn-in with all running activities. Mom denies functional impairment or daily limitations. Your examination reveals lateral foot curvature bilaterally, internal tibial torsion, and kissing patella's. Gait shows minimal in-toeing with fast walking. Your advice to the parent is:
   a. Orthopedic referral for surgical evaluation
   b. Night-time bracing
   c. Orthopedic referral for bilateral casting
   d. Physical therapy for hip stretching
   e. No treatment necessary

Answer: e. No treatment is necessary. This child has a combination of metatarsus adductus, tibial torsion, and femoral anteversion. Both the metatarsus adductus and tibial torsion are beyond the ages to spontaneously revert. The femoral anteversion may correct in the next few years. Overall, the child has no functional impairments and does not require any treatment.

9. A 12-year-old child suffered a sports-related concussion, and 24 hours after the incident, the child denied all symptoms and examination was normal. The child was eager to play soccer again to prepare for upcoming playoff game. After long discussion, the step-wise guidelines were laid out for the family and child. You called to check-in on her progress and mom notes she will be on step 4 today at practice. Mom says she has been fine except for some headaches in the evenings, inability to concentrate in school, and difficulty sleeping attributed to "nerves" for the big game in 2 days. Your response is:
   a. You are happy with her progress and wish her luck in the big game
   b. Concerned regarding new headaches and refer to neurology for migraine work-up
   c. Advise Tylenol prior to practice to prevent headaches
   d. Advise no game in 2 days and to revert to step 3 throughout the weekend
   e. Order brain MRI to rule out fracture

   Answer: d. This child is symptomatic with activity progression. The goal is to show no postconcussive symptoms while moving through the step-wise guideline. If there are any signs or symptoms, it is best to revert to the prior step for a minimum of 48 hours before progressing forward. The Zurich guidelines state no child should return to sports the same day after diagnosis or with residual symptoms.

10. A 17-year-old African-American male come to the office for preparticipation examination prior to starting college. He will be playing football. His past medical history is notable for exercise induced asthma and uses albuterol inhaler 30 minutes prior to exercise. He had a history of 1 prior concussion 3 years ago and underwent a left ACL repair 4 years ago. He denies supplements. His family members are healthy except for his brother with sickle cell. What are you most concerned about in his history that requires further investigation?
   a. Concussion history
   b. Exercise-induce asthma
   c. Brother with sickle cell
   d. Prior ACL repair
   e. Denial of supplements

   Answer: c. Brother with sickle cell is a red flag. The sickle cell status for this athlete must be identified, and screening test for sickle cell trait is recommended. During intense exertion, the sickle hemoglobin can change the shape and can pose a grave risk for some athletes. In the past 7 years, exertional sickling has killed 9 athletes, ages 12 through 19. Heat, dehydration, altitude, and asthma can increase the risk for and worsen sickling. Confirming sickle cell trait status in all college athletes is now recommended during preparticipation physical examinations. Knowledge of sickle cell trait status can be a gateway to education and simple precautions such as (1) build up slowly in training with paced progressions and longer periods of rest and recovery between repetitions; (2) preseason strength and conditioning programs to enhance the preparedness; (3) cessation of activity with onset of symptoms—muscle "cramping," pain, swelling, weakness, tenderness; and inability to "catch breath," fatigue.

11. A 14-year-old female returns to office for reevaluation of right ankle. She suffered an inversion injury during ballet 6 months prior. She had adequate rest and completed formal physical therapy for ankle strengthening. However, she is unable to fully participate in ballet 6 months later due to persistent swelling, a painful click in ankle, and sensation of locking. You order an MRI of the right ankle to identify:
   a. Osteochondritis dissecans (OCD) lesion of the talus
   b. Ligament rupture
   c. Stress fracture of the calcaneus
   d. Ganglion cyst

   Answer: a. Osteochondritis dissecans is a local abnormality of subchondral bone thought to result from repetitive stress and or trauma. The most common sites are medial femoral condyle, talus, distal humerus, and patella. The goal of treatment is to obtain healing by minimizing shear forces and stimulate new bone formation. Whether treated surgically or nonsurgical, the lesions take months to heal and allow the athlete to return fully to competition.

12. A 13-year-old African-American male presents with left-knee pain. Parents describe insidious onset and deny trauma. The pain has increased over the last 3 weeks and now he walks with a limp. Physical examination reveals a pleasant overweight teenager in no distress. Gait notable for a limp. Knee examination reveals mild tenderness along the patella, no effusion and stable ligaments. He does complain of ipsilateral groin pain with hip examination. You obtain which of the following radiographs?

a. AP and lateral left knee
b. AP, lateral, and sunrise views of left knee
c. AP pelvis and frog-leg views
d. No radiographs are necessary for patellofemoral pain

Answer: c. AP pelvis and frog-leg views are necessary to rule out slipped-capital femoral epiphysis (SCFE). With any joint complaint, it is important to examine the joints above and below. Groin pain and loss of internal hip rotation are concerning in an overweight AA male for hip pathology causing referred knee pain.

13. A 14-year-old male lacrosse player presents to office after feeling a pop over the right hip during a game. After the pop, he was unable to run and had severe pain. He denies trauma and notes approximately 2 months of right-hip pain attributed to hip flexor tendonitis and treated at home. On physical examination, he is unable to bear weight fully on right leg and severe tenderness to palpation over the right ASIS. Resistance testing of the right quadriceps was difficult secondary to pain. AP pelvis radiograph will most likely show:
   a. Avulsion fracture ASIS (anterior superior iliac spine)
   b. No change to the ASIS apophysis
   c. Myositis ossificans
   d. Pelvis fracture
   e. Normal radiograph

   Answer: a. Avulsion fracture of ASIS. History of preceding hip discomfort likely was secondary to apophysitis of ASIS. Continuing to play put the ossification center of ASIS at risk for weakness, further inflammation, and avulsion. The key to this injury is complete rest from all activities, weight bearing as tolerated and crutches if necessary, and completion of physical therapy once pain free. Typically takes 6 to 12 weeks for healing and return to activity.

14. Identify the fracture in Figure 22.14.
   a. Salter Harris I
   b. Salter Harris II
   c. Salter Harris III
   d. Salter Harris IV
   e. Salter Harris V

   Answer: c. Salter Harris III. It is evident the fracture line extends from the physis through the epiphysis only.

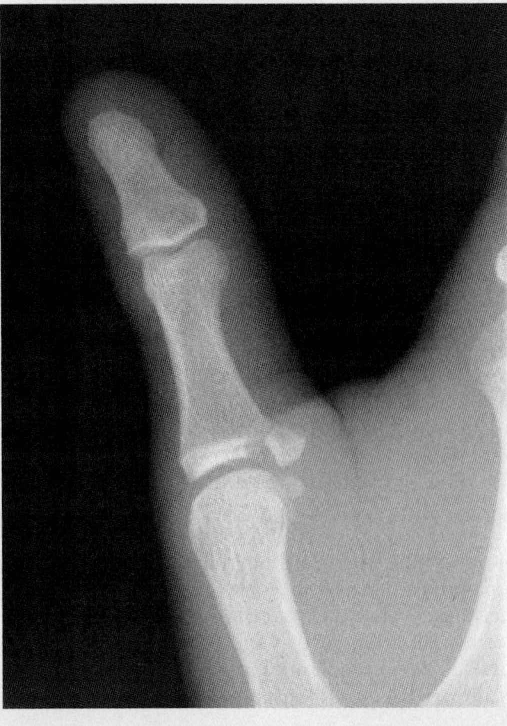

FIGURE 22.14. Salter Harris, Type III. *Reprinted with permission from* Strickland JW, Graham TJ. Master Techniques in Orthopaedic Surgery: The Hand, 2nd ed. Philadelphia: Lippincott Williams & Wilkins, 2005.

15. A 14-year-old male baseball catcher presents to the office with left-ankle swelling and pain. He was involved in a collision during the game and notes ankle swelling developed afterward. He is able to bear weight. Physical examination reveals diffuse lateral left-ankle swelling, mild bruising, and point tenderness along distal fibular physis. Examination of navicular, metatarsals, and ligaments are normal. Radiographs obtained in the office of left ankle were normal and no evidence of fracture. The diagnosis is:

- **a.** Moderate ankle sprain
- **b.** Osteochondritis dissecans lesion of talus
- **c.** High ankle sprain
- **d.** Salter I fracture of distal fibula
- **e.** Muscle strain

Answer: d. Salter I fracture of distal fibula is likely based on clinical examination. Routine radiographs routinely miss Salter I injuries, and it is typically a clinical diagnosis. If a Salter I injury is suspected, conservative treatment in cast, boot, or crutches is appropriate and radiographs can be repeated in 7 to 10 days from injury to determine bony healing.

SUGGESTED READINGS

1. Birrer RB, Griesemer B, Cataletto MB, et al. *Pediatric Sports Medicine for Primary Care*. Philadelphia: Lippincott Williams & Wilkins, 2002.
2. Hay W, Levin M, Sondheimer J, Deterding R, et al. *Current Pediatric Diagnosis and Treatment*, 17th ed. New York: McGraw-Hill, 2006.
3. Metzel J. *Sports Medicine in the Pediatric Office*. Elk Grove Village: American Academy of Pediatrics, 2007.
4. Zitelli B, Davis H, et al. *Atlas of Pediatric Physical Diagnosis*, 5th ed. Philadelphia: Mosby Elsevier, 2007.
5. Griffin L, Greene W. *Essentials of Musculoskeletal Care*, 3rd ed. 2005.

CHAPTER 23 ■ PREVENTIVE PEDIATRICS, BIOSTATISTICS, & ETHICS

MARGARET BREWINSKI

AAP	American Academy of Pediatrics	HDL	High-density lipoprotein
ABER	Auditory brainstem evoked response	HIV	Human immunodeficiency virus
ATV	All terrain vehicle	LDL	Low-density lipoprotein
BMI	Body mass index	LTBI	Latent tuberculosis infection
BP	Blood pressure	MMR	Measles, mumps, and rubella vaccine
CDC	Centers for disease control and prevention	NICU	Neonatal intensive care unit
CMV	Cytomegalovirus	NPV	Negative predictive value
CPSC	Consumer Product Safety Commission	OAE	Otoacoustic emission
CVD	Cardiovascular disease	PPD	Purified protein derivative
DBP	Diastolic blood pressure	PPV	Positive predictive value
DNR	Do not resuscitate	SBP	Systolic blood pressure
DTaP	Diphtheria, tetanus and acellular pertussis vaccine	SCHIP	State Children's Health Insurance Program
ECMO	Extracorporeal membrane oxygenation	SIDS	Sudden infant death syndrome
EDTA	Ethylenediaminetetraacetic acid	TB	Tuberculosis
FN	False negative	TN	True negative
FP	False positive	TP	True positive
		TST	Tuberculin skin test
		UVA	Ultraviolet type A light
		UVB	Ultraviolet type B light

CHAPTER OBJECTIVES

1. Preventive care and anticipatory guidance are two of the most important and fundamental aspects of pediatrics. As children grow and develop, pediatricians have a unique opportunity to help parents establish healthy routines and lay a foundation of healthy lifestyle behaviors for the years to come. In preparation for the Pediatric Board Exam, readers will develop an understanding of key prevention and screening topics in the following areas:
   - Immunization
   - Blood pressure
   - Iron deficiency
   - Lead poisoning
   - Hearing and vision
   - Hypercholesterolemia and hyperlipidemia
   - Tuberculosis
   - Injury prevention
   - Healthy behaviors
   - Overweight and obesity
   - Nutrition
   - Osteoporosis
   - Oral health
2. Additional information important for the boards includes an understanding of biostatistics and epidemiology concepts as well as some basic medical ethics. These topics are straightforward and are easy fodder for board examinations. With just a bit of background knowledge, they can yield high-impact results on examination day. Please remember to see the question sections for additional practice as well. Readers will develop an understanding of key biostatistical, epidemiologic, and ethics topics in the following areas:
   - Study design including randomized control trials, cohort, case-control, cross-sectional, and meta analysis

- Statistical measures
- Ethical considerations for pediatricians

3. To be able to successfully answer the review questions at the end of the chapter.

IMMUNIZATION

The development of vaccines is one of the greatest public health interventions, dramatically reducing morbidity and mortality from a variety of infectious diseases. Currently in the United States, infants, children, and teens are routinely vaccinated against 16 agents. Vaccine schedules are listed in Figures 23.1 to 23.3 and in Table 23.1.

There are several types of vaccines, which are as follows:

1. Live attenuated—organisms have been modified so they cannot cause disease.
2. Killed (inactivated) vaccines—killed bacteria or inactivated viruses.
3. Toxoid vaccines—formalin-inactivated bacterial toxins.
4. Component vaccines—smaller portions (usually proteins or sugars) of the whole bacteria or virus.

General Points

- A previous anaphylactic reaction or a known allergy to a vaccine or vaccine component is a contraindication only to that *specific* vaccine. An adverse or allergic reaction to a vaccine by a sibling or other family member is not a contraindication to vaccination.
- Medically stable premature infants should be vaccinated on the basis of chronological age using the same dose and indications as for full-term infants.
- Children should be vaccinated despite concurrent *mild* illness. Vaccinations should be delayed until patients with *moderate or severe illnesses,* with or without fever, are recovering and no longer acutely ill.
- It is also important for caregivers and household contacts to also be appropriately vaccinated.

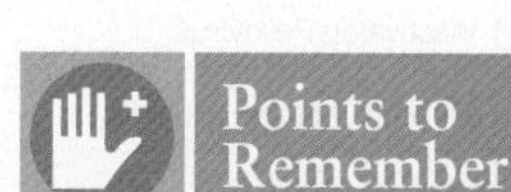

- **Children with mild illness should still receive their vaccines at the scheduled visit. The examination may present a scenario of a child with mild upper respiratory symptoms who comes for a check up and is due for vaccines. In this case, the answer is always to vaccinate the child (if no other contraindications exist) and DO NOT DELAY vaccination due to mild illness.**

Complications to Remember

- Many vaccines can cause mild reactions such as fatigue, vomiting, fever, fussiness and injection site soreness, swelling, or redness.

Recommended Immunization Schedule for Persons Aged 0 Through 6 Years—United States • 2010

For those who fall behind or start late, see the catch-up schedule

Vaccine ▼ Age ▶	Birth	1 month	2 months	4 months	6 months	12 months	15 months	18 months	19–23 months	2–3 years	4–6 years
Hepatitis B	HepB	HepB			HepB						
Rotavirus			RV	RV	RV						
Diphtheria, Tetanus, Pertussis			DTaP	DTaP	DTaP		DTaP				DTaP
Haemophilus influenzae type b			Hib	Hib	Hib	Hib					
Pneumococcal			PCV	PCV	PCV	PCV				PPSV	
Inactivated Poliovirus			IPV	IPV	IPV						IPV
Influenza					Influenza (Yearly)						
Measles, Mumps, Rubella						MMR					MMR
Varicella						Varicella					Varicella
Hepatitis A						HepA (2 doses)				HepA Series	
Meningococcal										MCV	

Range of recommended ages for all children except certain high-risk groups

Range of recommended ages for certain high-risk groups

This schedule includes recommendations in effect as of December 15, 2009. Any dose not administered at the recommended age should be administered at a subsequent visit, when indicated and feasible. The use of a combination vaccine generally is preferred over separate injections of its equivalent component vaccines. Considerations should include provider assessment, patient preference, and the potential for adverse events. Providers should consult the relevant Advisory Committee on Immunization Practices statement for detailed recommendations: **http://www.cdc.gov/vaccines/pubs/acip-list.htm**. Clinically significant adverse events that follow immunization should be reported to the Vaccine Adverse Event Reporting System (VAERS) at **http://www.vaers.hhs.gov** or by telephone, **800-822-7967**.

FIGURE 23.1. CDC vaccine schedule for ages 0 to 6 years. (Source: Department of Health and Human Services, Centers for Disease Control and Prevention.)

Recommended Immunization Schedule for Persons Aged 7 Through 18 Years—United States • 2010
For those who fall behind or start late, see the schedule below and the catch-up schedule

<table>
<tr><th>Vaccine ▼ Age ▶</th><th>7–10 years</th><th>11–12 years</th><th>13–18 years</th></tr>
<tr><td>Tetanus, Diphtheria, Pertussis</td><td></td><td>Tdap</td><td>Tdap</td></tr>
<tr><td>Human Papillomavirus</td><td></td><td>HPV (3 doses)</td><td>HPV series</td></tr>
<tr><td>Meningococcal</td><td>MCV</td><td>MCV</td><td>MCV</td></tr>
<tr><td>Influenza</td><td colspan="3">Influenza (Yearly)</td></tr>
<tr><td>Pneumococcal</td><td colspan="3">PPSV</td></tr>
<tr><td>Hepatitis A</td><td colspan="3">HepA Series</td></tr>
<tr><td>Hepatitis B</td><td colspan="3">Hep B Series</td></tr>
<tr><td>Inactivated Poliovirus</td><td colspan="3">IPV Series</td></tr>
<tr><td>Measles, Mumps, Rubella</td><td colspan="3">MMR Series</td></tr>
<tr><td>Varicella</td><td colspan="3">Varicella Series</td></tr>
</table>

Range of recommended ages for all children except certain high-risk groups

Range of recommended ages for catch-up immunization

Range of recommended ages for certain high-risk groups

This schedule includes recommendations in effect as of December 15, 2009. Any dose not administered at the recommended age should be administered at a subsequent visit, when indicated and feasible. The use of a combination vaccine generally is preferred over separate injections of its equivalent component vaccines. Considerations should include provider assessment, patient preference, and the potential for adverse events. Providers should consult the relevant Advisory Committee on Immunization Practices statement for detailed recommendations: **http://www.cdc.gov/vaccines/pubs/acip-list.htm.** Clinically significant adverse events that follow immunization should be reported to the Vaccine Adverse Event Reporting System (VAERS) at **http://www.vaers.hhs.gov** or by telephone, **800-822-7967.**

FIGURE 23.2. CDC vaccine schedule for ages 7 to 18 years. (Source: Department of Health and Human Services, Centers for Disease Control and Prevention.)

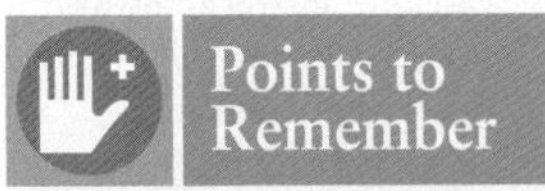

- DTaP side effects are often tested. Know these.

- Additional rare, serious risks associated with specific vaccines include:
  - DTaP: Seizure, inconsolable crying, for 3 hours or more, high fever, and long-term neurologic complications.
  - MMR: Seizure, arthralgia, thrombocytopenia, other neurologic complications.
  - Remember that in the 1990s, a rotavirus vaccine was discontinued due to concerns about a possible association with intussusception. The two rotavirus vaccines currently in use have not been found to pose any increased risk of intussusception. However, since one episode of intussusception predisposes to future episodes, as a precaution, the CDC recommends that children with a history of intussusception should not receive rotavirus vaccine.

SCREENING

Blood Pressure

When to Measure

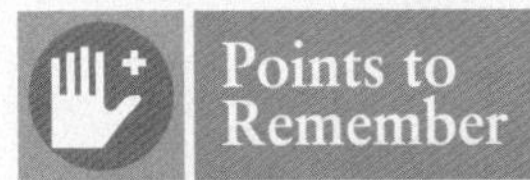

- Regular BP checks should begin at 3 years of age.

All children aged 3 years and above should have their BP checked whenever they are seen in a medical setting, or at least annually.

Children younger than 3 years should have their BP checked under the following circumstances:

- History of prematurity, very low birth weight, or other neonatal complication requiring intensive care.
- Congenital heart disease (repaired or unrepaired).
- Recurrent urinary tract infections, hematuria, or proteinuria.
- Known renal disease or urologic malformations.
- Family history of congenital renal disease.
- Solid-organ transplant.
- Malignancy or bone marrow transplant.
- Treatment with drugs known to raise BP.
- Other systemic illnesses associated with hypertension.
- Evidence of elevated intracranial pressure.

How to Measure

BP should be taken by auscultation with a stethoscope and appropriate size cuff under most circumstances. Automatic BP machines, "oscillometric devices," calculate systolic blood pressure (SBP) and diastolic blood pressure (DBP) from a measurement of mean arterial BP, and results

Catch-up Immunization Schedule for Persons Aged 4 Months Through 18 Years Who Start Late or Who Are More Than 1 Month Behind—United States • 2010

The table below provides catch-up schedules and minimum intervals between doses for children whose vaccinations have been delayed. A vaccine series does not need to be restarted, regardless of the time that has elapsed between doses. Use the section appropriate for the child's age.

Vaccine	Minimum Age for Dose 1	Minimum Interval Between Doses			
		Dose 1 to Dose 2	Dose 2 to Dose 3	Dose 3 to Dose 4	Dose 4 to Dose 5
PERSONS AGED 4 MONTHS THROUGH 6 YEARS					
Hepatitis B	Birth	**4 weeks**	**8 weeks** (and at least 16 weeks after first dose)		
Rotavirus	6 wks	**4 weeks**	**4 weeks**		
Diphtheria, Tetanus, Pertussis	6 wks	**4 weeks**	**4 weeks**	**6 months**	**6 months**
Haemophilus influenzae type b	6 wks	**4 weeks** if first dose administered at younger than age 12 months **8 weeks (as final dose)** if first dose administered at age 12–14 months **No further doses needed** if first dose administered at age 15 months or older	**4 weeks** if current age is younger than 12 months **8 weeks (as final dose)** if current age is 12 months or older and first dose administered at younger than age 12 months and second dose administered at younger than 15 months **No further doses needed** if previous dose administered at age 15 months or older	**8 weeks (as final dose)** This dose only necessary for children aged 12 months through 59 months who received 3 doses before age 12 months	
Pneumococcal	6 wks	**4 weeks** if first dose administered at younger than age 12 months **8 weeks (as final dose for healthy children)** if first dose administered at age 12 months or older or current age 24 through 59 months **No further doses needed** for healthy children if first dose administered at age 24 months or older	**4 weeks** if current age is younger than 12 months **8 weeks** **(as final dose for healthy children)** if current age is 12 months or older **No further doses needed** for healthy children if previous dose administered at age 24 months or older	**8 weeks (as final dose)** This dose only necessary for children aged 12 months through 59 months who received 3 doses before age 12 months or for high-risk children who received 3 doses at any age	
Inactivated Poliovirus	6 wks	**4 weeks**	**4 weeks**	**6 months**	
Measles, Mumps, Rubella	12 mos	**4 weeks**			
Varicella	12 mos	**3 months**			
Hepatitis A	12 mos	**6 months**			
PERSONS AGED 7 THROUGH 18 YEARS					
Tetanus, Diphtheria/ Tetanus, Diphtheria, Pertussis	7 yrs	**4 weeks**	**4 weeks** if first dose administered at younger than age 12 months **6 months** if first dose administered at 12 months or older	**6 months** if first dose administered at younger than age 12 months	
Human Papillomavirus	9 yrs	**Routine dosing intervals are recommended**			
Hepatitis A	12 mos	**6 months**			
Hepatitis B	Birth	**4 weeks**	**8 weeks** (and at least 16 weeks after first dose)		
Inactivated Poliovirus	6 wks	**4 weeks**	**4 weeks**	**6 months**	
Measles, Mumps, Rubella	12 mos	**4 weeks**			
Varicella	12 mos	**3 months** if person is younger than age 13 years **4 weeks** if person is aged 13 years or older			

FIGURE 23.3. CDC catch-up vaccine schedule. (Source: Department of Health and Human Services, Centers for Disease Control and Prevention.)

TABLE 23.1

VACCINE SUMMARY TABLE

Vaccine	Type	Contraindications	Precautions
DTaP Tdap Td	DT—Toxoid P—Component	■ Encephalopathy within 7 days after previous dose ■ Severe life-threatening allergic reaction after prior DTaP	■ Hx of Guillain-Barre ■ Problems within 48 h of prior dose including: collapse, shock, persistent/ inconsolable crying lasting >3 h, fever >40.5 unexplained by another cause ■ Seizures within 3 d of prior dose ■ Underlying progressive neurologic disorder
Hep A	Inactivated	Anaphylaxis to alum or 2-phenoxyethanol	Pregnancy
Hep B	Component	Anaphylaxis to baker's yeast or severe allergic reaction to a prior dose	
Conjugated Hib	Component	Prior allergic reaction to Hib vaccine	
HPV	Component	Severe alleric reaction to HPV vaccine pregnancy	
Influenza (trivalent)	Live attenuated	■ Anaphylaxis to eggs ■ Aspirin or salicylate therapy ■ Pregnancy ■ Hx of Guillain-Barre ■ Hemoglobinopathies, diabetes, or renal dysfunction ■ Chronic pulmonary or cardiovascular system disorder ■ HIV, hematologic, and solid tumors ■ Congenital immunodeficiency, long-term immunosuppressive therapy, including steroids ■ Health care providers for severely immunosuppressed patients	
	Inactivated	Anaphylaxis to eggs	
MMR	Live attenuated	Pregnancy Anaphylaxis to neomycin or gelatin Hematologic and solid tumors, congenital immunodeficiency, long-term immunosuppressive therapy, including steroids, advanced HIV disease untreated, active TB	Anaphylaxis to gelatin Immunoglobulin recently received Thrombocytopenia or hx of TTP
Meningococcal	Component	History of allergic reaction to vaccine or vaccine component	Hx of Guillain-Barre
Pneumococcal	Component	Serious allergic reaction to a previous dose of this vaccine	
Polio (IPV)	Inactivated	Anaphylaxis to neomycin, streptomycin or polymyxin B	Pregnancy
Rotavirus	Live attenuated	Serious allergic reaction to a previous dose of this vaccine	HIV/AIDS or weakened immune system from illness or steriods intussusception
Varicella	Live attenuated	Pregnancy Anaphylaxis to neomycin Untreated, active TB Hematopoietic stem cell transplant	Anaphylaxis to gelatin Advanced HIV disease Immunoglobulin, blood or plasma transfusion recently received
Yellow fever		Anaphylaxis to eggs HIV, hematologic and solid tumors, congenital immunodeficiency, long-term immunosuppressive therapy, including steroids	Pregnancy

Note: A previous anaphylactic reaction to a specific vaccine or its components is a contraindication to further vaccination with this vaccine type.

can vary greatly among different devices. The only situations when oscillometric measurement is preferable are in newborns and young infants in whom auscultation is difficult and in the intensive care setting, where frequent measurements are needed. Aberrant values by oscillometric measurement should be repeated with auscultation.

Definition of Hypertension

In children and adolescents, hypertension is defined as average SBP and/or DBP that is 95th percentile or greater for gender, age, and height on three occasions. Prehypertension is defined as average SBP or DBP levels that are ≥90th percentile but <95th percentile and should be treated with lifestyle changes. Remember that before making a diagnosis of hypertension, the clinician should ensure the proper cuff size is used and document the reading on more than one occasion. For further discussion of hypertension, please refer to the Cardiovascular chapter.

Points to Remember

- The first thing to do if a child has a high BP measurement is to repeat the measurement and rule out sources of error (wrong size cuff, problem with machine, etc.).

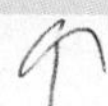

Iron-Deficiency Anemia

Iron deficiency is the most common nutritional deficiency worldwide and the most common hematologic disease of infants and children in the United States. Because of rapid growth and increased physiologic iron need, infants, toddlers, adolescents, and pregnant women are particularly susceptible to iron deficiency.

To screen for iron-deficiency anemia, the AAP recommends a hemoglobin or hematocrit check at least once for all infants between the ages of 9 and 12 months and then again 6 months later in communities or populations with a high prevalence of iron-deficiency anemia. Beyond 2 years of age, universal screening is not recommended, but children should be reevaluated for developing risk factors on a regular basis and screened if necessary. The AAP also recommends screening all adolescents once between ages 11 and 21 years and screening menstruating females annually.

Risk Factors Include

- Children eligible for WIC (women, infants, and children).
- Children of migrant workers.
- Recently arrived refugee or internationally adopted children.
- History of prematurity or low birth weight.
- Infants fed a diet of non-iron-fortified infant formula.
- Infants introduced to cow milk before 1 year of age.
- Breast-fed infants who are receiving inadequate dietary iron after the age of 6 months.
- Children who consume more than 24 oz of cow's milk per day.
- Previous history of iron deficiency.
- Poor or restrictive diet/evidence of low-iron intake.
- Other relevant, predisposing health conditions such as chronic infection/illness, inflammatory disorders, chronic or acute blood loss, or use of medications that interfere with iron absorption.

Points to Remember

- A CBC or HCT to screen for anemia should be checked at the 9- to 12-month well-child visit.

Prevention

For breast-fed infants, complementary foods rich in iron should be introduced around 6 months of age. Infants weaned before 12 months of age should receive iron-fortified infant formula. Bottle-fed infants should only be given formula that is iron fortified. Preterm and low birth weight infants should receive iron supplementation before 6 months of age.

Cow's milk should only be given to children at least 1 year of age and should be limited to no more than 24 oz per day because it:

- is low in iron;
- interferes with iron absorption; and
- can cause gastrointestinal irritation and bleeding in some infants.

Older children and adolescents should include iron-rich foods in their diet.

Points to Remember

- Cow's milk should not be introduced until the child is 1 year of age.

Lead (Fig. 23.4)

Background

Federal regulations requiring the removal of lead from paint, gasoline, and smokestack emissions have resulted in a tremendous decline in childhood lead poisoning over the past several decades. However, many children remain at high risk with about 310,000 children aged 1 to 5 having blood lead levels greater than 10 μg/dL annually. The most common source of lead contamination is ingestion or inhalation of lead-based paint chips or lead-contaminated dust found in old buildings, but lead exposure may also come from contaminated water (usually from pipes in the home), toys, traditional remedies, or being around adults with occupational or recreational exposure (industry, stained glass making).

Screening

As lead levels have declined nationally, screening has trended from a universal to a targeted approach. Screening recommendations remain controversial. At this time, Medicaid eligible children should have a blood lead concentration measured at 1 and 2 years of age. Outside this group, screening should be considered at least once for all children when they are 2 years of age or, ideally, twice, at ages 1 and 2 years. High-risk groups include children in high-risk areas, international adoptees, recent immigrants, those in states or municipalities where screening policies are in place or those with a sibling or close household contact with elevated lead level.

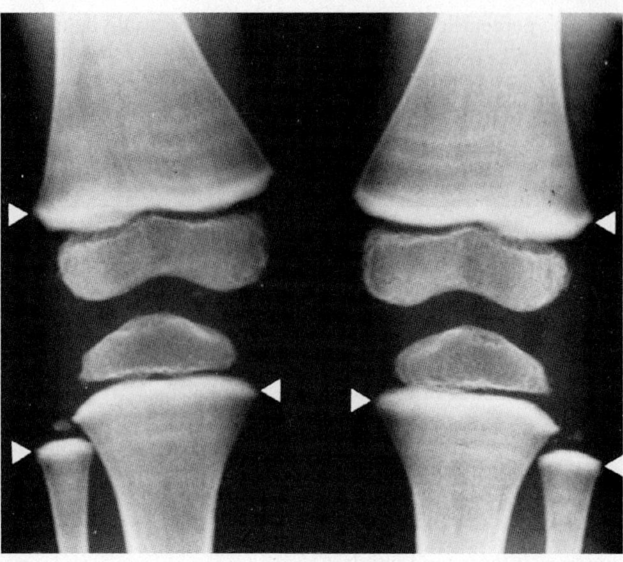

FIGURE 23.4. Lead lines visible at the knee joint on x-ray. (Reprinted with permission from Eisenberg RL. *An Atlas Of Differential Diagnosis.* 4th ed. Philadelphia, PA: Lippincott Williams & Wilkins, 2003.)

Management

Venous samples are preferred. A blood lead concentration greater than 10 μg/dL is considered elevated. However, lead levels less than 10 μg/dL may have effects on behavior and development and should be followed. Key treatment cutoffs to remember are as follows:

- 45 μg/dL chelation therapy with succimer should begin.
- 70 μg/dL, hospitalization for parenteral therapy with EDTA is necessary.

All children with elevated lead levels should have close follow-up. Thorough dietary and environmental histories must be obtained to identify the source of contamination.

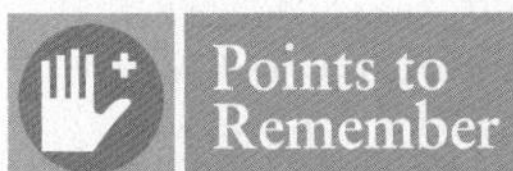

- **Start chelation at 45 μg/dL and hospitalize for parenteral therapy at 70 μg/dL.**

Hearing (Fig. 23.5)

Hearing loss can interfere with multiple aspects of development, including speech, language, and social skills. The earlier intervention and support is provided for a child with hearing loss or impairment, the better the eventual outcome can be.

When to Screen

Newborns: All infants should be screened before 1 month of age, preferably before leaving the hospital nursery. A comprehensive audiological evaluation should be scheduled before 3 months of age for any infant who does not pass the screen. Infants found to have hearing impairment should receive intervention and support services before they are 6-months old.

Children should have their hearing tested again before they enter school, periodically throughout school age, and adolescence, or whenever a concern arises.

Hearing and language development as well as physical inspection of the ear, auditory canal, and tympanic membrane should be performed at each well-child visit.

All infants with a risk factor for hearing loss should undergo thorough audiological assessment at least once by 24 to 30 months of age.

Risk factors for hearing loss in infancy and childhood include:

- Caregiver or physician concern regarding hearing, speech, language, or developmental delay.
- Recurrent or prolonged episodes of otitis media.
- Family history.
- NICU stay longer than 5 days or any of the following regardless of length of stay: ECMO, assisted ventilation, exposure to ototoxic medications (e.g., aminoglycosides) or loop diuretics (e.g., furosemide), and hyperbilirubinemia that requires exchange transfusion.
- Congenital infections—CMV, rubella, and syphilis.
- Craniofacial anomalies.
- Certain syndromes, neurodegenerative disorders, or sensory motor neuropathies (A few key ones: neurofibromatosis, Waardenburg, Alport, Lange–Nielson, Hunter syndrome, Friedreich ataxia, and Charcot–Marie–Tooth syndrome).
- Meningitis.
- Head trauma, especially basal skull/temporal bone fracture that requires hospitalization.
- Chemotherapy.

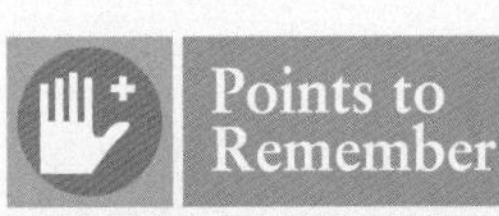

- **If a child is slow to develop language skills, always check for hearing loss as a possible cause.**

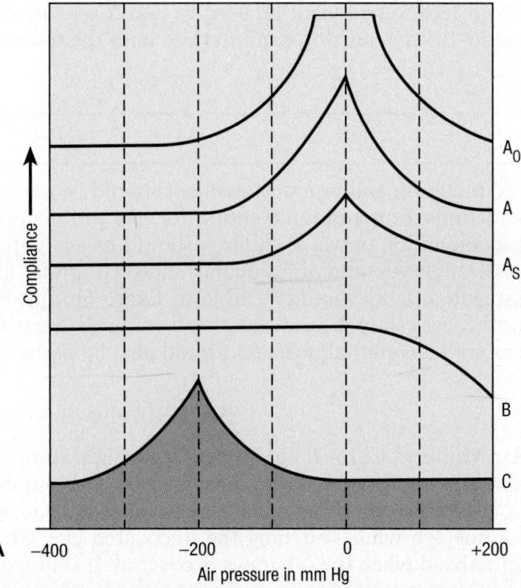

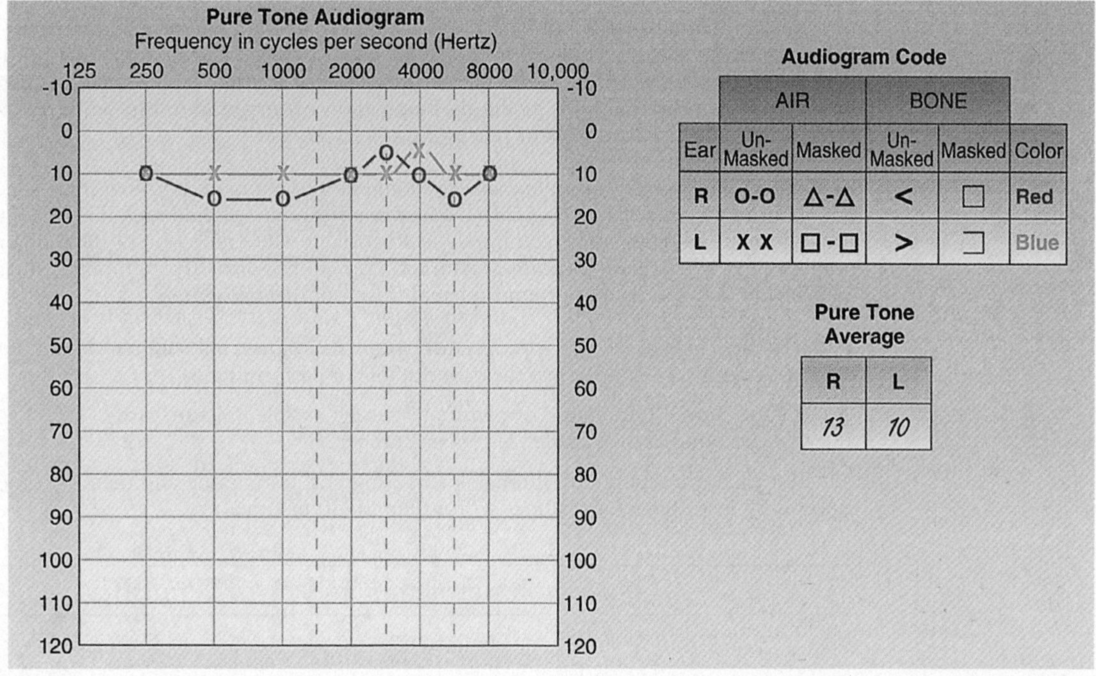

FIGURE 23.5. (**A**) Five tympanograms illustrating various conditions of the middle ear: type A is typical of normal middle ear; type A_s is associated with stiffness of stapes; type A_o is associated with interruptions in the chain of bones or flaccidity of the eardrum membrane; type B suggests fluid in the middle ear; and type C suggests that the pressure within the middle ear is below atmospheric pressure. (*Reprinted with permission from* Stedman's Medical Dictionary. 28th ed. Baltimore, MD: Lippincott Williams & Wilkins, 2005.) (**B**) An audiogram presents a graphic outline of hearing as measured by tones of different pitches ranging from 125 through 8000 cycles per second (cps) or Hertz (Hz). This audiogram shows normal hearing bilaterally. The box on the right indicates the symbols used on an audiogram. (*Reprinted with permission from* Smeltzer SC, Bare BG. *Textbook of Medical-Surgical Nursing*. 9th ed. Philadelphia, PA: Lippincott Williams & Wilkins, 2000.)

Types of Hearing Tests

Otoacoustic emission (OAE) is a screening test that records cochlear response to acoustic stimuli through a microphone and probe assembly placed in the ear canal. This reflects the status of the peripheral auditory system extending only to the cochlear outer hair cells and thus cannot identify neural (eighth nerve or auditory brainstem pathway) dysfunction.

Auditory brainstem evoked response (ABER) delivers acoustic stimuli via an earphone and measures neural activity generated within the cochlea, auditory nerve, and brainstem. This test measures the status of the peripheral auditory system, the eighth nerve, and the brainstem auditory pathway. This is the gold standard hearing test.

Both technologies can be used to detect sensory (cochlear) hearing loss. Temporary outer- or middle-ear dysfunction can interfere with the test and produce a false positive result.

Vision

Eye examination and vision assessment should be performed at every well-child visit to facilitate early identification and intervention for any problems of the visual system. From the first newborn examination onward, children should be evaluated with an ocular history, external assessment of the eyes and lids, ocular motility, pupil and red reflex examination, and vision assessment. Infants should be able to fixate on an object and track objects by 3 months. By 4 months, eyes should be symmetrically aligned. Starting at age 3, age-appropriate visual acuity tests as well as ophthalmoscopy should also be performed.

Brief Review of Visual Tests

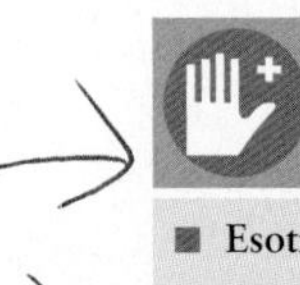

Points to Remember

- Esotropia = uncovered eye moves OUTWARD
- Exotropia = uncovered eye moves INWARD

Ocular Motility. Corneal light reflex: A penlight shone in the child's eyes from about 2 feet away should reflect symmetrically in the center of both pupils.

Cross cover test: The child looks straight ahead with both eyes open, while the examiner covers one eye while watching the uncovered eye. The uncovered eye should remain pointing straight ahead when the other eye is covered. If it moves outward, this is *esotropia* as the uncovered eye corrects by moving outward from its abnormally inward turned position. If it moves inward, this is *exotropia*.

Remember that *strabismus* is any abnormality of ocular alignment. It can occur in children at any age and reflects a problem with eye muscles or some orbital, intraocular, or intracranial process. Do not be fooled by *pseudostrabismus* that is a normal variant most commonly caused by prominent epicanthal folds giving the impression of turned in (esotropia) eyes but does not lead to an abnormal corneal light reflex or cross cover test.

Red Reflex. The red reflex seen in each eye should be a bright reddish-yellow color but can be light gray in brown-eyed patients (Fig. 23.6). Most importantly, it should look the same in both eyes. An abnormal red reflex, most commonly leukocoria, a white reflection of the retina making the pupil appear white, may indicate a cataract, corneal abnormality, retinoblastoma, or retinal detachment and necessitates prompt referral to an ophthalmologist.

Visual Acuity. In general, age-appropriate tests are as follows, but children should be tested with the most cognitively difficult test they are capable of performing.

- Ages 3 to 5: tumbling E or picture tests such as Allen picture cards.
- Ages 6 and above: Snellen letters or numbers.

Test each eye separately, alternately covering and testing one and then the other, at a distance of 10 feet. Refer for readings worse than 20/40 in either eye.

Hypercholesterolemia and Hyperlipidemia

Prevention

All parents of children above 2 years of age should receive healthy diet counseling, including the use of low-fat dairy products. For children between 12 months and 2 years of age for whom overweight or obesity is a concern or who have a family history of obesity, dyslipidemia, or cardiovascular disease, the use of reduced fat milk is appropriate.

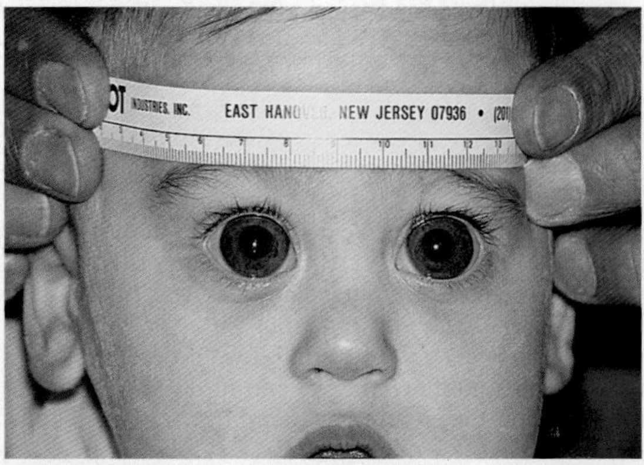

FIGURE 23.6. Corneal clarity is revealed by the red reflex. The ruler on the forehead allows the corneal diameter to be measured without an examination under anesthesia. (*Reprinted with permission from* Tasman W, Jaeger E. *The Wills Eye Hospital Atlas of Clinical Ophthalmology*. 2nd ed. Lippincott Williams & Wilkins, 2001.)

Screening

As of July 2008, the AAP recommends screening children and adolescents with a positive family history of dyslipidemia or early CVD or dyslipidemia (defined as 55 years of age for men and 65 years of age for women). Screening with a fasting lipid profile should take place after 2 years of age but no later than 10 years of age during well-child visits.

- If values are normal, repeat test in 3 to 5 years.
- If family history is unknown or other CVD risk factors are present, such as overweight (BMI ≥85th percentile, <95th percentile), obesity (BMI ≥95th percentile), hypertension (BP ≥95th percentile), cigarette smoking, or diabetes mellitus, children should be screened with a fasting lipid profile annually.

Treatment

1. Nutritional counseling and other lifestyle interventions such as increased physical activity are the primary interventions.
2. For overweight or obese patients and those with high triglycerides or low HDL, weight management is the primary treatment, which includes improvement of diet with nutritional counseling and increased physical activity to produce improved energy balance.
3. For patients aged 8 years and above, medication should be considered if the LDL is:
   - 190 mg/dL.
   - 160 mg/dL with a family history of early heart disease or two additional risk factors.
   - 130 mg/dL if diabetes mellitus is present, medication should be considered.

The initial goal is to lower LDL concentration to less than 160 mg/dL. If additional risk factors are present (strong family history of CVD, obesity, diabetes, and the metabolic syndrome), a target as low as 130 mg/dL or even 110 mg/dL may be necessary.

Tuberculosis

The Tuberculin Skin Test (TST) is the most common method for diagnosing latent TB infection (LTBI) in asymptomatic people. For this test, 5 tuberculin units of purified protein derivative (PPD) are injected intradermally using a 27-gauge needle into the volar aspect of the forearm to create a visible 6- to 10-mm wheal. Universal screening is not recommended as it results in either a low yield of true positives or a large proportion of false positives. Instead, screening should be targeted toward children who are at increased risk for LTBI and tuberculosis disease. Risk assessment for tuberculosis should be performed at first contact with a child and every 6 months thereafter until 2 years of age. After 2 years of age, risk assessment for tuberculosis should be performed annually.

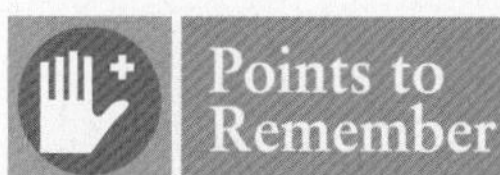

- PPD can be placed concurrently at the time of MMR vaccination.

Risk Factors Include

- Contact with a confirmed or suspected contagious tuberculosis case.
- Radiographic or clinical findings suggesting tuberculosis.
- Travel to or immigration/adoption or substantial contact with persons from countries with endemic infection (Asia, Middle East, Africa, Latin America, former Soviet Union).
- HIV infection.
- Incarcerated adolescents.

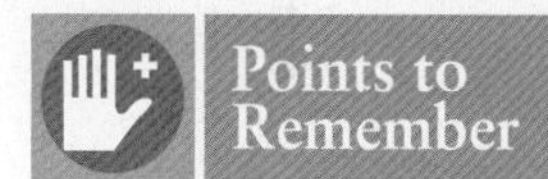

- An initial TST should be performed before initiation of immunosuppressive therapy.

Prevention

Injury Prevention

Review and know the leading causes of death and nonfatal injury for children and adolescents (Figs. 23.7 and 23.8).

Motor vehicle collisions are the leading cause of death among American children aged between 1 and 14 years. Providing proper safety seats and restraints can drastically reduce these deaths. Important guidelines to remember are listed in Table 23.2.

Bicycle Safety. Helmets are a very effective way to prevent the occurrence of up to 88% of serious brain injuries. Helmets absorb some of the impact energy during a crash and dissipate it over a larger area for a slightly longer time. This combined with the protection provided by the skull should help to protect the brain from most severe injuries. Any helmet involved in a crash should be discarded and replaced. All children riding a bike or riding as a passenger on a bike should wear a helmet that meets Consumer Product Safety Commission (CPSC) standards.

Infant cribs should meet the following specifications:

- Slats should be no more than 2 to 3/8 inches apart.
- Lowered crib sides should be at least 9 inches above the mattress support to prevent the infant from falling out. Raised crib sides should be at least 26 inches above the mattress support in its lowest position.

Rank	<1	1–4	5–9	10–14	15–24
1	Congenital Anomalies 5,819	Unintentional Injury 1,610	Unintentional Injury 1,044	Unintentional Injury 1,214	Unintentional Injury 16,229
2	Short Gestation 4,841	Congenital Anomalies 515	Malignant Neoplasms 459	Malignant Neoplasms 448	Homicide 5,717
3	SIDS 2,323	Malignant Neoplasms 377	Congenital Anomalies 182	Homicide 241	Suicide 4,189
4	Maternal Pregnancy Comp. 1,683	Homicide 366	Homicide 149	Suicide 216	Malignant Neoplasms 1,664
5	Unintentional Injury 1,147	Heart Disease 161	Heart Disease 90	Heart Disease 163	Heart Disease 1,076
6	Placenta Cord Membranes 1,140	Influenza & Pneumonia 125	Chronic Low. Respiratory Disease 52	Congenital Anomalies 162	Congenital Anomalies 460
7	Respiratory Distress 825	Septicemia 88	Cerebro vascular 45	Chronic Low. Respiratory Disease 63	Cerebro vascular 210
8	Bacterial Sepsis 807	Perinatal Period 65	Influenza & Pneumonia 40	Cerebro vascular 50	HIV 206
9	Neonatal Hemorrhage 618	Benign Neoplasms 60	Septicemia 40	Septicemia 44	Influenza & Pneumonia 184
10	Circulatory System Disease 543	Cerebro-vascular 54	Benign Neoplasms 38	Benign Neoplasms 38	Complicated Pregnancy 179

FIGURE 23.7. Ten leading causes of death by age group, United States—2006. (Source: National Vital Statistics System, National Center for Health Statistics, CDC.)

- Sides should have a locking, hand-operated latch that will not release unintentionally.
- The mattress should be the same size as the crib so there are no gaps between the mattress and the crib sides.
- Children should not sleep in a crib once they are 35 inches tall.

Safe Sleep to Reduce the Risk of SIDS (Sudden Infant Death Syndrome)

- Infants should ALWAYS be placed on their backs when resting, sleeping, or left alone.
- Supervised tummy time helps to strengthen neck and back muscles but must always be when the baby is awake and supervised.
- The safest place for an infant to sleep is in their own crib or other separate safe sleep surface next to the parent or caregiver's bed.
- No comforters, fluffy blankets, stuffed animals, or other objects should be placed in the crib.
- Research indicates that pacifier use reduces the risk of SIDS.

Walkers

- Parents should be advised not to use baby walkers as they increase the risk of injury and can delay normal muscle control and mental development.

Stairways. Gates should be installed at the top of the stairway as soon as the infant begins crawling and becoming independently mobile.

Rank	<1	1–4	5–9	10–14	15–24
	Age Groups				
1	Unintentional Fall 120,316	Unintentional Fall 828,773	Unintentional Fall 599,540	Unintentional Fall 609,893	Unintentional Struck by/ Against 1,049,015
2	Unintentional Struck by/ Against 32,970	Unintentional Struck by/ Against 370,572	Unintentional Struck by/ Against 399,262	Unintentional Struck by/ Against 580,236	Unintentional Fall 895,255
3	Unintentional Other Bite/ Sting 11,787	Unintentional Other Bite/ Sting 134,641	Unintentional Cut/Pierce 111,914	Unintentional Overexertion 284,190	Unintentional Overexertion 802,676
4	Unintentional Foreign Body 11,508	Unintentional Foreign Body 125,000	Unintentional Pedal Cyclist 95,871	Unintentional Cut/Pierce 136,935	Unintentional MV-Occupant 781,653
5	Unintentional Fire/Burn 10,531	Unintentional Overexertion 83,099	Unintentional Other Bite/ Sting 84,977	Unintentional Pedal Cyclist 114,864	Unintentional Cut/Pierce 464,246
6	Unintentional Other Specified 7,980	Unintentional Cut/Pierce 82,804	Unintentional Overexertion 80,799	Unintentional Unknown/ Unspecified 100,403	Other Assault Struck by/ Against 450,034
7	Unintentional/ Inhalation/ Suffocation 6,297	Unintentional Other Specified 60,323	Unintentional MV-Occupant 60,068	Other Assault Struck by/ Against 81,151	Unintentional Other Specified 214,132
8	Unintentional Unknown/ Unspecified 6,138	Unintentional Fire/Burn 51,651	Unintentional Foreign Body 53,679	Unintentional MV-Occupant 77,504	Unintentional Other Bite/ Sting 188,437
9	Unintentional Overexertion 6,011	Unintentional Unknown/ Unspecified 46,823	Unintentional Other Transport 45,527	Unintentional Other Transport 61,104	Unintentional Unknown/ Unspecified 165,706
10	Unintentional Cut/Pierce 5,863	Unintentional Poisoning 41,737	Unintentional Unknown/ Unspecified 43,323	Unintentional Other Bite/ Sting 58,259	Unintentional Other Transport 148,813

FIGURE 23.8. National estimates of the 10 leading causes of nonfatal injuries treated in hospital emergency departments, United States, 2007. The "Other Assault" category includes all assaults that are not classified as sexual assault. It represents the majority of assaults. (Source: National Electronic Injury Surveillance System—All Injury Program operated by the U. S. Consumer Product Safety Commission.)

TABLE 23.2

PROPER USE OF SAFETY SEATS AND RESTRAINTS FOR INFANTS AND CHILDREN

Age	Guideline
Infants	Rear-facing car safety seat until they are *at least* 1 year of age and weigh 20 pounds. Must be in the car's backseat
Toddlers	Rear-facing or forward-facing car safety seat until child outgrows limits for each position—usually at around 4 years of age and 40 pounds. Must be in the car's backseat
School age	Booster seat until the adult seat belts fit correctly—usually at about 4′ 9″ in height and between 8 and 12 years of age. Must be in the car's backseat
Older children	Children who have outgrown their booster seats should ride in a lap and shoulder belt. May move to the front seat at 13 years of age

Poisonings and Ingestions. Children are at greatest risk for accidental poisoning between the ages of 1 and 3 years when they are more independently mobile, beginning to explore their environment, and prone to putting things in their mouths. Potentially dangerous substances, such as medications, vitamins, household cleansers, and other liquids, should be placed out of a child's reach in a locked cabinet. Parents should be advised to avoid referring to medicine as candy or a treat, and hazardous substances should not be placed in alternate containers, such as drink bottles, which could be confusing to a child. Grandparents, who are likely to take medications, and other caregivers should be informed about these precautions. Parents should be advised about what to do if an ingestion occurs and should have the poison-control phone number readily accessible.

Burn Prevention. Water heater should be set no higher than 120 °F. Working smoke alarm should be installed on every level of the home and be checked monthly. Most home fires are caused by incompletely extinguished cigarettes—another reason for parents not to smoke!

Drowning. Children can drown in less than 2 inches of water. Children should never be left alone around water, including in a bathtub, pails of water, or a swimming pool. Home swimming pools should be entirely enclosed by a fence to separate the pool from the house.

Firearm Safety. According to the AAP, "children in homes where guns are present are in more danger of being shot by themselves, their friends, or family members than of being injured by an intruder." Parents should be advised that the safest thing for their children is not to keep any gun in the home. If parents decide to keep a gun at home, it should be unloaded and stored in a locked place with the ammunition locked separately. Parents should inquire about the possibility of guns in homes or other places their children visit and what safety measures are taken by the owner.

Lawnmower Safety. Ride-on mowers should only be used by teens above 16, and younger children should not be allowed to ride as passengers on the mower. Walk-behind mowers should only be used by children above 12.

Off-Road Vehicles/All Terrain Vehicles (ATVs). Children and adolescents who are not licensed to drive a car should not be allowed to operate off-road vehicles. Injuries frequently occur to passengers, so riding double should be prohibited. Helmets including face shields (designed for motorcycle not bicycle riding), eye protection, and protective, reflective clothing should always be worn. Parents should never permit the use of these vehicles on-road or at night.

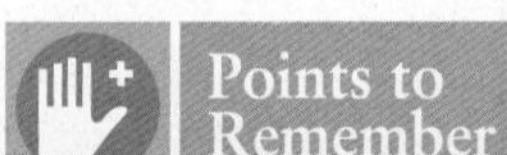

- "Screen time" includes video games, television, movies, and so on and should be limited to no more than 1 to 2 h/d.

Television Viewing. Screen time should be no more than 1 to 2 h/d, and parents should ensure that programs are age and developmentally appropriate. Televisions should not be allowed in children's bedrooms. Children below 2 should be discouraged from watching television in favor of more developmentally enriching activities.

Ultraviolet Radiation and Sun Exposure. The two important types of ultraviolet radiation are UVA and UVB. UVA has a wavelength of 320 to 400 nm and passes easily through the ozone layer, while UVB has a wavelength of 280 to 320 nm and is mostly absorbed by the ozone layer. Though both contribute, UVA is primarily responsible for premature aging of the skin, while the small amount of UVB that gets through the ozone layer causes skin cancer and possibly eye disease such as macular degeneration and cataracts. UVA is strong throughout the day; UVB peaks from 10 AM to 5 PM.

- Avoid outdoor activities or seek shade during the sunniest time of the day (10 AM to 5 PM).
- Shield skin with long sleeves/pants, a hat, and sunscreen of at least SPF 15 with both UVA/UVB protection reapplied regularly.
- Wear sunglasses with 100% UVA/UVB protection.

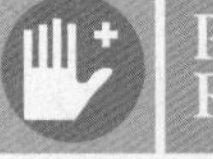
Points to Remember

- If a scenario is presented with a child having recurrent asthma exacerbations, ask about parental tobacco use and counsel as appropriate. Parental smoking is a major trigger of asthma exacerbations in children. For adolescents, be sure to ask if they have experimented with or started smoking.

Substance Use

According to the CDC's 2007 national Youth Risk Behavior Survey that provides data on risk behavior for United States 9th to 12th graders:

- 44% currently use alcohol (at least one drink of alcohol on at least 1 day during the 30 days before the survey).
- 75% have had at least one drink of alcohol ever.
- 25% currently use tobacco.
- 50% have ever tried tobacco products.
- 20% currently use marijuana.
- 38% have tried marijuana at least once.

The AAP recommends pediatricians to include a discussion of substance abuse as a part of routine health care at all well-child visits as part of ongoing anticipatory guidance.

Tobacco. Second-hand smoke: almost 40% of American children are exposed to second-hand smoke, putting them at higher risk for otitis media, SIDS, allergic symptoms, pulmonary problems, including asthma and respiratory infections, and making them more likely to become future smokers themselves. Smoking during pregnancy can lead to miscarriage, prematurity, and low birth weight. Parents should be asked about their own smoking behavior, advised and counseled about quitting, and encouraged to discuss the dangers of smoking and other tobacco use with children and teens.

Overweight and Obesity

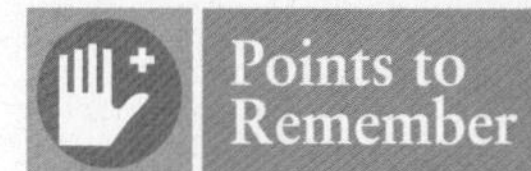

- Pediatric obesity is a hot topic right now and is prime material for boards, so know this section well.

In the United States, we are experiencing an epidemic of pediatric overweight and obesity. On the basis of the most recent CDC National Health and Nutrition Examination Survey from 2003 to 2004, the prevalence of overweight among children aged 2 to 5, 6 to 11, and 12 to 19 is 13.9%, 18.8%, and 17.4%, respectively. Once a child is overweight, it becomes very difficult to change established lifestyle patterns and to successfully return to a healthy weight. In fact, at age 4, children have a 20% risk of carrying extra pounds into adulthood. This risk increases with age as patterns become more ingrained and overweight adolescents have an 80% chance of becoming overweight adults. Overweight children are not only at risk for immediate health effects, such as asthma exacerbations, elevated BP, sleep apnea, gallbladder disease, steatohepatitis, slipped capital femoral epiphysis and other joint disorders, non-insulin dependent diabetes, elevated cholesterol levels, poor self-esteem, and depression, but also for health problems that will continue and progress during their adult years, including early development of atherosclerotic lesions. Aside from the individual health effects, this also represents a tremendous burden on the health care system as pediatric obesity-associated annual hospital costs have increased from $35 million in 1979 to 1981 to $127 million in 1997 to 1999.

Contributing Factors

Childhood overweight is a multifactorial issue. The primary contributing factors include:

- an increase in sedentary behaviors including time spent on the computer, playing video games, and watching TV;
- a decrease in physical activity both at home and in school; and
- an increase in consumption of foods with high caloric density and fat content.

Though some medical conditions such as Prader–Willi syndrome and hypothyroidism can lead to weight gain, they are not sufficient to explain the rise in pediatric overweight on a societal level. Family history also plays a role as overweight parents are more likely to have overweight children. However, this influence is more related to lifestyle and behavior choices rather than a true genetic predisposition. When counseling families about interventions needed to bring a child to an appropriate weight, the difficulty of making major lifestyle changes for the child alone should be explained and all family members should be encouraged to participate.

The mainstays of maintaining a healthy weight include proper nutrition and adequate physical activity. Pediatricians play a major role in educating families and helping to set the foundation for a lifetime of healthy lifestyle choices in their young patients. *BMI should be calculated, graphed against standardized reference charts appropriate for age and gender, and results discussed with the family at each well-child visit starting at age 2.*

Definitions

- *Body mass index* = weight in kg/height in m^2 or = (weight in pounds/height in $inches^2$) × 703.
- *Overweight/obese* = BMI ≥95 percentile.
- *At risk of overweight* = BMI between the 85th and 95th percentile.

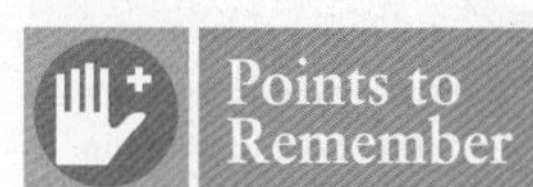

- Know the BMI formula and classifications well!

Physical Activity

While any child may have inadequate physical activity, those at particularly high risk include children who:

- are from a minority population, especially girls, in the preadolescent and adolescent age groups;
- live in poverty;
- have disabilities; or
- reside in apartments or public housing or in neighborhoods where outdoor physical activity is restricted by climate, safety concerns, or lack of recreation facilities.

Recommended Physical Activity. At school: 150 minutes per week for elementary school age (~30 min/d) and 225 minutes per week for middle and high school students (~45 min/d).

Parents should strive to encourage age-appropriate, enjoyable physical activity as a regular part of the family's overall lifestyle. In general, children and adolescents should be physically active for a total of at least 60 minutes per day, inclusive of all school-based and other recreational activities, which does not have to be completed all at once but may be accumulated through multiple, shorter events.

Nutrition

Note: For full discussion of Nutrition, please see Chapter 11.

According to the CDC, the diet of most of the U.S. pediatric population does not meet recommendations set by the Dietary Guidelines for Americans. For children and adolescents 6- to 19-years old, 67% exceed recommended overall fat intake and 72% consumed more saturated fat than recommended. Additionally, 80% of high school students do not eat five or more servings of fruits and vegetables per day. Diet-related anticipatory guidance should be discussed at every well-child visit.

Recommendations. Because of changing nutritional needs for appropriate growth and development, recommendations for daily caloric, protein, and fat intake vary on the basis of age, gender, and physical activity. Knowing the specific guidelines is beyond what will likely be encountered on the board examination. General information to keep in mind is that the AAP recommends:

- balanced caloric intake from a variety of food sources to achieve an appropriate weight;
- a healthful diet in accordance with the U.S. Department of Health and Human Services 2005 Dietary Guidelines for Americans for all children older than 2 years—including low fat dairy products;
- children aged 12 months to 2 years for whom overweight or obesity is a concern or who have a family history of obesity, dyslipidemia, or CVD drink only reduced fat milk;
- limited intake of fruit juice, sugar-sweetened beverages and foods, and salt; and
- increased consumption of fruits, vegetables, and whole grains.

Osteoporosis

To help prevent osteoporosis and maximize optimal bone density development, children and adolescents need sufficient calcium, preferably through dietary sources such as dairy, tofu, calcium-enriched cereals and other grains, legumes and dark, leafy greens. Optimal conditions for bone health, including regular physical activity with a weight-bearing component, are especially important during adolescence when 40% of lifetime bone mass is accumulated. The vast majority of U.S. children and adolescents do not meet recommended calcium intake (Table 23.3).

For healthy, term infants less than 1 year, calcium requirements are adequately met through breast or formula feeding (or breast-feeding plus solid foods from 6 months to 1 year). Deficiency is very rare and additional supplementation is not required. Remember that calcium is more bioavailable from breast milk than from formula.

The following can adversely affect calcium intake or absorption:

- Consumption of soda or non–calcium-enriched juices.
- Poor or overly restrictive diets.
- Caffeine.
- Alcohol.
- Tobacco.
- Kidney disease.

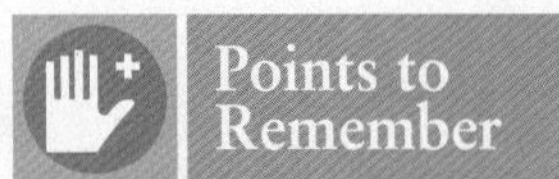

- Breast-feeding infants need a 400 IU dose of Vitamin D supplement each day.

Do not forget vitamin D! Though sun exposure does provide vitamin D, quantifying it is difficult. Therefore, all infants, children, and teens should have a minimum intake of 400 IU of vitamin D per day, given via supplement if dietary intake is not adequate. Because vitamin D content in breast milk is low, breast-fed and partially breast-fed infants should be supplemented with 400 IU per day of vitamin D until the infant is weaned to vitamin D-fortified formula or whole milk.

TABLE 23.3

RECOMMENDED DAILY CALCIUM INTAKE

Age (y)	mg/d of Calcium Needed
1–3	500
4–8	800
9–18	1,300
>18	1,000

Remember that whole milk should not be given until the infant is at least 1 year of age and reduced-fat milk should be used for children over 12 months for whom overweight or obesity is a concern or for those with a family history of obesity, dyslipidemia, or cardiovascular disease.

Oral Health

Poor oral health is an extremely common problem in the pediatric population where more than 40% of children experience tooth decay by the time they start kindergarten. Caries are caused by poor oral hygiene, an acidic oral environment, and overgrowth of oral flora organisms, usually indicated by *Streptococcus mutans* and *Lactobacillus*. Because there is a correlation with maternal dental health and infants can become colonized with these organisms through contact (sharing utensils, kisses, etc), mothers should be educated about the importance of their own dental hygiene.

Prevention recommendations include:

- Never put an infant to sleep with a bottle or allow them to suck on the bottle for periods of time longer than are necessary for feeding.
- Appropriate diet with minimal sugars.
- Twice daily brushing once teeth erupt.
- Once daily flossing once teeth contact each other.
- Routine oral examination beginning at 6 months of age.
- Establishment of a dental home by 1 year of age.

Fluoride. Drinking water: fluoride supplementation of municipal drinking water is a very effective way to reduce dental caries in the community. Additional supplementation is not needed if drinking water fluoride content is at least 0.6 ppm.

If the content is less than 0.6 ppm, the following table should be used to determine supplementation dosage in milligram per day (Table 23.4).

Toothpaste: Nonfluoride toothpaste should be used for young children. Once a child is able to spit instead of swallowing the toothpaste, usually around 2 to 3 years of age, fluoride toothpaste may be used.

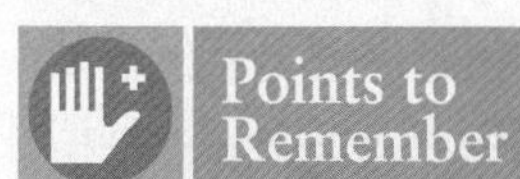
Points to Remember

- Remember this cutoff: a fluoride supplement is needed if water fluoride content is less than 0.6 ppm.

TABLE 23.4

RECOMMENDED DAILY FLUORIDE SUPPLEMENTATION DOSAGE IN MG/D IF WATER FLUORIDE CONCENTRATION IS LESS THAN 0.6 PPM

Age	<0.3 ppm in Drinking Water	0.3–0.6 ppm in Drinking Water
0–6 mo	None	None
6 mo to 3 y	0.25	None
3–6 y	0.5	0.25
6–16 y	1	0.5

STATISTICS AND EPIDEMIOLOGY

Study Designs

Randomized Controlled Trials

The gold standard of experimental studies.

- Description: patients are randomly assigned to one of the two groups—(1) the intervention group that receives the treatment under investigation or (2) the control group that receives either a placebo or the existing standard of care. In a double-blinded study, neither the participant nor the investigator knows to which group a patient belongs.
- Example: two groups of patients are randomly assigned to take either a placebo or a new asthma medicine and are then followed over time to identify differences in outcome.
- Concepts to remember:
  - *Null hypothesis*: the assumption that no difference exists between the two groups being studied.
  - *Type I Error* (also called Alpha error or false positive): determining there *IS* a difference when one *DOES NOT* actually exist. *This results in inappropriately rejecting the null hypothesis.*
  - *Type II Error* (also called Beta error or false negative): determining there *IS NOT* a difference when one *DOES* actually exist. *This results in inappropriately accepting the null hypothesis.*

Points to Remember

- Study design types are frequently tested on board examinations and can mean easy points with mastery of the few pages of concepts described here.

- Advantages:
  1. Minimizes selection bias such as all the patients with difficult to control BP being intentionally put in the treatment group, thus making the new drug look less effective than it actually is.
  2. Minimizes confounding the possibility that by chance all the subjects with a certain risk factor such as smoking will end up in one group or the other.
- Disadvantage: expensive, time-consuming, takes place in a very controlled setting so results may be hard to generalize to people under normal, real-world circumstances.

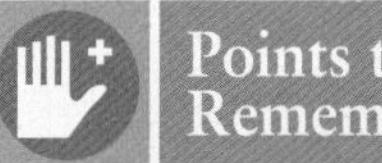

Points to Remember

- Cohort studies start with subjects with the EXPOSURE of interest (i.e., smoking) and then look, either prospectively or retrospectively, for the outcome of interest (i.e., cancer).

Cohort Studies

- Description: patients are selected on the basis of exposures and are then determined to have the outcome under investigation or not. Can be either prospective or retrospective.
- Prospective: children exposed and not exposed to second-hand smoke in the home are followed into adulthood to see what conditions develop.
  1. Advantages: multiple outcomes can be assessed.
  2. Disadvantage: only the exposures defined and followed from the beginning of the study can be assessed, expensive, time-consuming, may lose some subjects to follow-up, and hard to prove causality.
- Retrospective: clinic charts are searched to find all children who were exposed to radiation (x-ray of mother) *in utero,* and their current medical conditions are compared with children who were not exposed.
  1. Advantages: inexpensive as data has already been collected, just needs to be compiled and assessed.
  2. Disadvantage: large potential for bias.

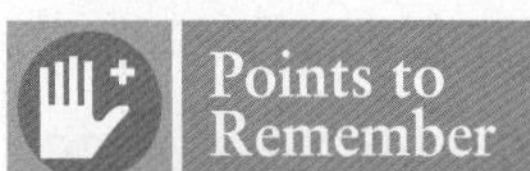

Points to Remember

- Case-control studies start with subjects with and without the OUTCOME of interest (i.e., cancer) and then look to see if the subject has a past history of the exposure (i.e., smoking).

Case-Control Studies

- Description: similar groups of patients currently with and without a condition are assessed for past exposure history.
- Example: groups of children with and without leukemia and similar in other ways (age, gender, race, geographic location, etc.) are compared on the basis of past exposure history.
- Advantages: good for studying rare conditions, are relatively fast and inexpensive to complete, and can consider many different risk factors.
- Disadvantages: can study only one disease outcome, may be difficult to find truly similar case and control groups, and subject to recall bias (participants recalling exposures incorrectly).

Cross-Sectional Studies

- Description: snapshot of the current conditions in a population at a given time.
- Example: telephone survey of all households in a municipal area asking about children in the home with asthma and assessing risk factors.
- Advantages: fast, fairly easy to do, may generate hypotheses for future studies.
- Disadvantages: cannot provide any evidence of causality or temporal relationship.

Meta-Analysis

- Description: combination of the results of different studies examining the same research question.
- Example: the results of several published studies investigating the effectiveness of salt-restricted diets for regulating fluid volume in children with renal disease are combined.
- Advantages: provides overall larger sample size and higher statistical power, may lead to generalization for larger population, and can help identify factors explaining variation.
- Disadvantages: cannot remedy study design flaws or control for factors not controlled for in the original studies (i.e., garbage in, garbage out) and usually only includes previously published studies, meaning some important but unpublished information may be left out, which is particularly concerning since studies not showing any relationship between the variables under investigation are less likely to be published (publication bias).

Statistical Measures

Memorize the following terms:

- **Mean:** sum of values/number of values.
- **Median:** middle number of a series of values when they are arranged in order from lowest to highest. If there is an even number of values in the series, the median is the mean of the two middle numbers.
- **Mode:** value that occurs most frequently in the series.

Case Example

- For the series of numbers 3 4 7 8 8.
- Mean = (3 + 4 + 7 +8 + 8)/5 = 6.
- Median = 7.
- Mode = 8.

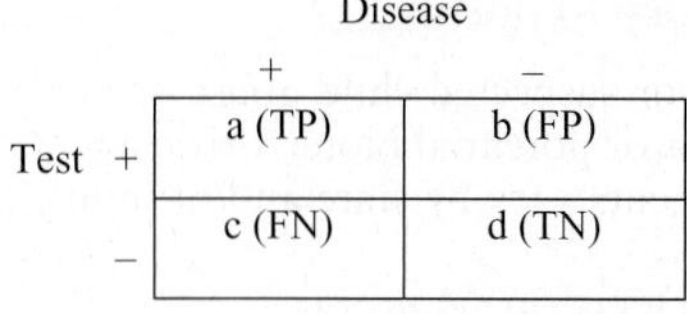

FIGURE 23.9. Chi square.

Prevalence

- *Number of EXISTING cases during a specified time period.*
- Number of people at risk during a specified time period.
  - Example: *American children aged 2 to 18 years with autism in 2003.*
- American children ages 2 to 18 years in 2003.
- Case Example: In a Medicaid insurance population of 15,000 children of school age, 500 were known to have autism in 2003. What is the prevalence of autism in this group?
- Answer: (500/15,000) × 100% = 3.3%.

Incidence

- *Number of NEW cases during a specified time period.*
- Number of people at risk during a specified time period.
  - Example: *American children aged 2 to 18 years with NEW diagnosis of autism in 2003.*
- American children aged 2 to 18 years in 2003.
- Case Example: In a Medicaid insurance population of 15,000 children of school age, 200 were diagnosed with autism in 2003. What is the incidence of autism in this group?
- Answer: (200/15,000) × 100% = 1.3%.

Case-Fatality Rate

- *Number of deaths from a disease in a given time period* × 100.
- Number of cases of the disease in a given time period.
  - Example: *Number of infant deaths from influenza in 2007* × 100.
- Number of infants infected with influenza in 2007.
- Case Example: During an outbreak at a daycare facility, 35 infants were infected with influenza. 3 of the infected infants died. What is the case fatality rate?
- Answer: (3/35) × 100% = 8.6%.

The following terms are descriptors of clinical tests and are calculated using a 2 × 2 (Chi Square) table (Fig. 23.9).

Definitions

Memorize these. They will get you points on the examination.

- **TP** = true positive: those who test positive and actually DO have the disease.
- **TN** = true negative: those who test negative and actually DO NOT have the disease.
- **FP** = false positive: those who test positive and actually DO NOT have the disease.
- **FN** = false negative: those who test negative and actually DO have the disease.
- **Sensitivity** describes the ability of a test to correctly identify persons with the disease and is calculated by a/(a + c) or, in other words, TP/(TP + FN).
- **Specificity** describes the ability of a test to identify persons without a disease and is calculated by d/(b + d) or, in other words, TN/(TN + FP).
- **Positive predictive value** is the probability that a person actually has the disease if the test for the disease is positive and is calculated by a/(a + b) or, in other words, TP/(TP + FP).
- **Negative predictive value** is the probability that a person actually does not have the disease if the test for the disease is negative and is calculated by d/(c + d) or, in other words, TN/(FN + TN).

ETHICS

Confidentiality

The issue of confidentiality is most relevant in caring for adolescents who are by definition going through a time of transition and are more likely to be dealing with high-risk behaviors. Concerns about confidentiality are frequently cited as one reason why adolescents are reluctant to seek care. The AAP makes the following recommendations regarding this issue:

1. The provider should make every effort to encourage the adolescent to involve parents in their care and help the adolescent and parent to adopt healthy communication strategies.
2. Adolescents should have an opportunity for examination and counseling separate from parents.
3. The adolescent must understand under what circumstances the provider will break confidentiality and involve parents (such as a life-threatening emergency) or report information disclosed by the adolescent or found on further testing to authorities (see following sections).

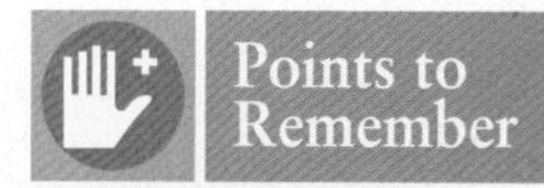

- Reporting of suspected child abuse or neglect is required in all states.

Mandatory Reporting

Federal law requires the reporting of known or suspected child abuse or neglect.

Certain infectious diseases and conditions or potential bioterrorism agents must be reported to authorities; however, specific reportable agents vary by state and/or municipality.

Minors as Decision-Makers

Minors can obtain medical care without parental consent for the following conditions:

- Sexually transmitted diseases.
- Family planning/pregnancy.
- Substance abuse related issues.
- If, by the judgment of the treating physician, there is an immediate/urgent medical need.

NOTE: a minor's ability to undergo an abortion without parental consent varies by state.

Emancipated minors may also obtain medical care without parental consent. The exact legal definition of an emancipated minor varies from state to state but in general applies to adolescents who are:

1. Self-supporting and/or not living at home.
2. Married.
3. Pregnant or already a parent.
4. In the military.
5. Declared to be emancipated by a court.

Points to Remember

- You may be given a scenario of an adolescent who presents for one of these issues and one of the choices will be to call the patient's parent or tell the patient to come back with a parent. Do not fall for these!

Religious and Philosophical Exemptions

Immunizations

For the vast majority of children, the recommended vaccines should be administered to prevent the individual and public health dangers posed by vaccine-preventable diseases. Under normal circumstances where the child is at routine risk for vaccine-preventable diseases, parents have a right to refuse vaccination on religious or philosophical grounds. In this situation, pediatricians should carefully listen to and explore the parent's concerns, make every effort to respond to these concerns given the current knowledge of safety and potential side effects of vaccines and the risks and benefits of choosing to vaccinate or not. If the parent ultimately decides not to vaccinate, the pediatrician should carefully document in the patient's medical record all discussions surrounding the decision not to vaccinate, the counsel provided by the health provider, and consider including a signed refusal waiver. During extenuating circumstance, for example, an outbreak of vaccine-preventable disease, the pediatrician may consider involving state agencies to override the parent's decision on the basis of medical neglect.

Religious exemptions may also come into play when parents refuse treatment for their children's medical conditions. While the U.S. Constitution requires that government not interfere with religious practices or endorse particular religions, the government may intervene when these principles subject a child to possible loss of life or substantial risk of harm.

End of Life Care

End of life care in the pediatric population is emotionally difficult for the patient, the family, and the involved health care providers. The physician's first responsibility is to ensure that the needs of the affected child remain the primary focus and that the child's comfort is maintained to the greatest degree possible at all times. The physician must provide information to the family such as expected outcome, potential risks, benefits, and side effects of treatment options, including, when appropriate, the option of providing only comfort care or withdrawal of care. Physicians should seek to explore the patient and/or family's understanding of the information presented and strive to clarify points of confusion or misunderstanding. For the health care provider, discussions should be guided by the principle of beneficence—meaning the provider has a duty to act in the best interest of the patient.

Until a Do Not Resuscitate (DNR) order has been established for a patient, all attempts at cardiopulmonary resuscitation must be made in the event of patient decompensation.

Organ Transplantation and Donation

The availability of suitable organs for pediatric patients in need is a significant problem. Three percent of people awaiting organ transplantation are children from birth to age 17.

Federal legislation requires that:

- all hospitals participating in Medicare and Medicaid programs refer all potential organ donors to their local organ procurement organization (OPO);

- all families of potential organ donors become aware of their option to donate; and
- all hospitals discuss organ donation with families of deceased patients.

Research Ethics

Because they are a vulnerable population, special issues arise when research is to be conducted involving children and extra scrutiny is necessary to ensure adequate protection of involved children. Some important things to consider are as follows:

- Consent to participate in research is usually being given by proxy from the child's parent or guardian, not directly by the child. It is incumbent upon the researcher to verify that the parent and, when possible, the child have been fully informed of the potential risks and benefits of the research. Ideally, the child's assent should also be obtained.
- Children's cognitive development and social and emotional needs should be considered in the study design and all activities or requirements must be age appropriate.
- The potential for long-term consequences as a result of participation in the study should be considered and explained in the consent process.

General principles of ethical research require that:

- subjects must have all the risks and benefits of participation in the study and any questions arising from the explanation fully explained;
- informed consent must be obtained;
- participation must be voluntary and subjects must be permitted to withdraw from the study at any time; and
- the potential benefits of any study should outweigh the risks.

Institutional ethics committees play three primary roles:

1. consulting on a clinical case when ethical issues arise;
2. creation or revision of institutional policy; and
3. educating health care professionals, patients, and others on ethical issues.

Allocation of Health Care Resources

As of the 2006 U.S. Census, 12% of American children (9.3 million total) were uninsured. Sixty-eight percent of these children were eligible for either Medicaid or the State Children's Health Insurance Program (SCHIP). The main reasons for children being uninsured result from cutbacks in their parent's employer sponsored health plan or being eligible but not properly enrolled in Medicaid or SCHIP.

Eligibility for the two main sources of government sponsored insurance for children are determined on the state level and therefore vary throughout the nation. General guidelines for each program are:

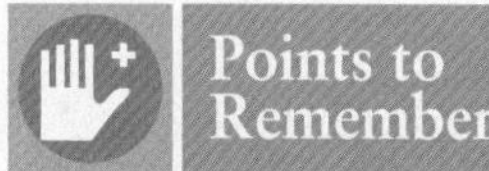

- This is another hot topic given the current debate about health care reform and may show up on the examination. It is a good idea to know the statistics.

Medicaid

- Pregnant women and children under the age of 6 whose family income is at or below 133% of the Federal poverty level (about $28,000 annually for a family of four).
- Children aged 6 to 19 with family income up to 100% of the Federal poverty level (about $21,000 annually for a family of four).

SCHIP

- Children up to age of 19.
- May be part of the state's Medicaid program, completely separate, or a combination of both.
- Generally for children whose parents' income is too high for Medicaid but too low to afford private insurance—usually at or below 200% of the Federal poverty level.

Medical Malpractice

To establish malpractice, four elements must be present:

1. Duty: that the physician–patient relationship exists, usually starting when a physician offers to treat the patient and the patient accepts the physician's care.
2. Breach of duty: the physician has failed to meet the standard of care for his or her specialty and geographic area (e.g., a provider in a rural area cannot be held to the same standard of care as one practicing in a high-level acuity academic setting with more advanced technologies available).

3. Causation: the breach of duty by the physician must be proved to be the cause of the patient's injury or adverse outcome.
4. Damages: the injury or adverse outcome must be assigned a monetary value by the court.

SAMPLE BOARD REVIEW QUESTIONS

1. What is the recommended temperature setting for home water heaters (in degrees Fahrenheit)?
   a. 100
   b. 110
   c. 120
   d. 130

   Answer: c. This is the recommended water heater temperature to prevent accidental scald burns.

2. When providing end of life care for a child, what is the physician's main responsibility?
   a. Helping the child's family prepare for the child's death
   b. Following the instructions given by the family for what degree of care they would like the child to receive
   c. Ensuring the opportunity to donate the child's organs is offered to the family, if medically appropriate
   d. Ensuring that the needs of the child remain the primary focus and that the child's comfort is maintained to the greatest degree possible at all times
   e. Completing all appropriate paperwork and documentation of the child's care

   Answer: d. The physician's primary concern should always be the patient's welfare. While the other options are important and should be addressed as well, the appropriate care of the patient must be the first priority.

3. On the basis of the 2006 U.S. Census, what percentage of American children are uninsured?
   a. 4%
   b. 8%
   c. 12%
   d. 18%
   e. 25%

   Answer: c. The 2006 U.S. Census found that 12% of American children were uninsured.

4. According to the common definition, a patient in which of the following circumstances would likely not be considered an emancipated minor?
   a. Self-supporting and/or not living at home
   b. Employed in a summer job program
   c. Pregnant or already a parent
   d. In the military
   e. Married

   Answer: b. The common definition of emancipated minor includes those adolescents who are self-supporting and/or not living at home, married, pregnant or already a parent, in the military or declared to be emancipated by a court. An adolescent employed in a summer job program may or may not meet one of these criteria, but simply being enrolled in such a program does not confer emancipated minor status.

5. In describing a clinical test, sensitivity is defined as:
   a. The probability that a person actually has the disease if the test for the disease is positive
   b. The ability of a test to identify persons without a disease
   c. The probability that a person actually does not have the disease if the test for the disease is negative
   d. The ability of a test to correctly identify persons with the disease
   e. How well the test distinguishes between two very similar but different variations of a disease

   Answer: d. This is the definition of sensitivity. A helpful way to remember this is that sensitivity rules in and specificity rules out, meaning sensitivity finds those people who do have a disease, whereas specificity helps to exclude those who do not have the disease.

6. What is the correct formula for calculating body mass index (BMI)?
   a. Weight in kg/height in m^2
   b. Weight in pounds/height in m^2

c. Weight in kg/height in inches^2
d. Height in m^2/weight in kg
e. Height in ft^2/weight in pounds

Answer: a. This is the correct formula for calculating BMI. Memorize it and be able to use it. An alternate formula is BMI = (weight in pounds/height in inches^2) × 703. Know both or be able to convert the required elements so you can do the calculation in whichever units are provided.

7. At what age should body mass index (BMI) for children begin being calculated and graphed against standardized reference charts appropriate for age and gender?
a. 1 year
b. 2 years
c. School entry
d. At onset of puberty
e. Whenever the child appears to be overweight

Answer: b. BMI should begin to be calculated and plotted on the appropriate growth chart at the 2-year well-child visit and at each subsequent well-child visit. Children and infants below 2 should still have height/length, weight, and head circumference values measured and plotted on age- and gender-appropriate growth charts at well-child visits, but BMI is not indicated.

8. What is the leading cause of death among American children aged 1 to 14?
a. Infectious diseases
b. Heart disease
c. Motor vehicle collision
d. Cancer
e. Abuse

Answer: c. Unintentional injury is the leading cause of death in this age group, and motor vehicle collision is the major cause of unintentional injury. Cancer, heart disease, and infectious diseases are other causes of death in this age group but not the leading cause.

9. What is considered to be the gold standard hearing test for children?
a. Auditory brainstem evoked response (ABER)
b. Tumbling E test
c. Otoacoustic emission (OAE)
d. Rinne test
e. Red reflex test

Answer: a. The ABER is the gold standard hearing test for children. The OAE and Rinne tests are used to test hearing, but not as the gold standard. The tumbling E test and red reflex tests are ocular tests, not auditory.

10. To screen for iron-deficiency anemia, the AAP recommends a hemoglobin or hematocrit check at what age?
a. 6 months
b. 9 to 12 months
c. 2 years
d. 5 years
e. 10 years

Answer: b. All infants of 9 to 12 months should be screened for iron-deficiency anemia at their well-child visit. Children of other ages should be tested if there is reason for concern, such as poor diet, chronic infection, or a previous history of anemia.

11. What is the correct definition of hypertension for pediatric patients?
a. Average systolic blood pressure and/or diastolic blood pressure that is 90th percentile or greater for gender, age, and height on three occasions.
b. Average systolic blood pressure and/or diastolic blood pressure that is 95th percentile or greater for gender, age, and height on three occasions.
c. Average systolic blood pressure and/or diastolic blood pressure that is 95th percentile or greater for gender, age, and height on at least one occasion.
d. Average systolic blood pressure and/or diastolic blood pressure that is 95th percentile or greater regardless of gender, age, and height on three occasions.
e. Average systolic blood pressure and/or diastolic blood pressure that is 90th percentile or greater for gender, age, and height on one occasion.

Answer: b. This is the correct definition of hypertension for children. The other definitions are either at the wrong percentile, are not repeated on three occasions, or are not considered in light of the patient's gender, age and height. Blood pressure should be measured at all well-child visits beginning at 2 years of age.

12. Which of the following is a contraindication to the DTaP vaccine?
   a. Underlying progressive neurologic disorder
   b. Problems within 48 hours of prior dose including: collapse, shock, persistent/inconsolable crying lasting more than 3 hours, fever above 40.5
   c. Seizures within 3 days of prior dose
   d. Encephalopathy within 7 days after previous dose
   e. Nasal congestion on day due for vaccine administration

Answer: d. This is the only contraindication. Choices a, b, and c are precautions, but not contraindications. Choice e is a mild illness, which is never a contraindication to vaccination.

13. For which of the following vaccines is anaphylaxis to eggs a contraindication for administration?
   a. MMR
   b. HPV
   c. IPV
   d. Influenza
   e. Tdap

Answer: d. Since the process of making influenza vaccine involves the use of eggs, patients with an anaphylactic allergy to eggs should not receive influenza vaccine. The other vaccines listed are not made this way so are not subject to this contraindication.

14. Which of the following vaccines is NOT a live attenuated vaccine?
   a. MMR
   b. Rotavirus
   c. Yellow fever
   d. Varicella

Answer: c. The live attenuated vaccines include influenza, MMR, rotavirus, and varicella.

15. At what blood lead level is hospitalization for parenteral therapy with EDTA necessary?
   a. >10 μg/dL
   b. >20 μg/dL
   c. >50 μg/dL
   d. >60 μg/dL
   e. >70 μg/dL

Answer: d. Start chelation at a blood lead level of 45 μg/dL and hospitalize for parenteral therapy at 70 μg/dL.

SUGGESTED READINGS

AAP Policy Statement. Eye Examination in Infants, Children and Young Adults by Pediatricians. *Pediatrics.* 2003;111:902–907.

AAP Policy Statement. Lead Exposure in Children: Prevention, Detection, and Management. *Pediatrics.* 2005;116:1036–1046.

AAP Recommendations for Preventive Pediatric Health Care. Available online at: http://pediatrics.aappublications.org/cgi/data/120/6/1376/DC1/1.

CDC Guide to Contraindications to Vaccination. September 2003. http://www.cdc.gov/vaccines/pubs/downloads/b_contraindications_guide.pdf.

Daniels, Greer et al. Lipid Screening and Cardiovascular Health in Childhood. *Pediatrics.* 2008;122:198–208.

Medical Research Council Ethics Guide. Medical Research Involving Children. 2004. Available online at: http://www.mrc.ac.uk/Utilities/Documentrecord/index.htm?d=MRC002430.

Section 3 Summaries of Infectious Diseases: Tuberculosis. The Red Book Online. 2006. Available online at: http://aapredbook.aappublications.org/cgi/content/extract/2006/1/3.142.

The Fourth Report on the Diagnosis, Evaluation, and Treatment of High Blood Pressure in Children and Adolescents. *Pediatrics.* 2004;114:555–576.

Wu et al. Screening for Iron Deficiency. *Pediatr Rev.* 2002;23:171–178.

Year 2007 Position Statement: Principles and Guidelines for Early Hearing Detection and Intervention Programs. *Pediatrics.* 2007;120:898–921.

CHAPTER 24 ■ PULMONARY

MEGAN M. TSCHUDY

AAT	Alpha-1-antitrypsin deficiency	GH	Growth hormone
ABC	Airway, breathing, and circulation	HIV	Human immunodeficiency virus
ABG	Arterial blood gas	hMPV	Human metapneumovirus
ABPA	Allergic bronchopulmonary aspergillosis	HSP	Henoch Schonlein purpura
ACE	Angiotensin-converting enzyme	HTN	Hypertension
AIDS	Acquired immune deficiency syndrome	IC	Inspiratory capacity
AOM	Acute otitis media	ICP	Intracranial pressure
ASA	Aspirin	IM	Intramuscular
ASD	Atrial septal defect	IPAP	Inspiratory positive airway pressure
AVM	Arteriovenous malformation	IRT	Immune reactive trypsinogen
BiPAP	Bi-level positive airway pressure	IRV	Inspiratory reserve volume
BOOP	Bronchiolitis obliterans organizing pneumonia	IV	Intravenous
CF	Cystic fibrosis	IVC	Inferior vena cava
CFTR	Cystic fibrosis transmembrane conductance regulator	IVIG	Intravenous Immunoglobulin
		MRI	Magnetic resonance imaging
CHARGE	Coloboma, heart malformation, choanal atresia, retardation of growth and/or development, genital anomalies, and ear anomalies	MRSA	Methicillin-resistant *Staphylococcus aureus*
		NIH	National Institutes of Health
		OSA	Obstructive sleep apnea
		PA	Posterior-anterior
CLE	Congenital lobar emphysema	PCP	Pneumocystis (carinii) jiroveci pneumonia
CMV	Cytomegalovirus	PEEP	Positive end expiratory pressure
CNS	Central nervous system	PFTs	Pulmonary function tests
CP	Cerebral palsy	PO	Oral (per os)
CPAP	Continuous positive airway pressure	RCT	Randomized controlled trial
CRP	C-reactive protein	RSV	Respiratory syncytial virus
CT	Computed tomography	RV	Residual volume
CXR	Chest x-ray	RVH	Right ventricular hypertrophy
EIA	Exercise-induced asthma	TB	Tuberculosis
EKG	Electrocardiogram	TE	Tracheoesophageal
EM	Electron microscopy	TLC	Total lung capacity
ENT	Ear, nose, and throat	TPN	Total parenteral nutrition
EPAP	Expiratory positive airway pressure	URI	Upper respiratory infection
ERV	Expiratory reserve volume	UTI	Urinary tract infection
FDA	Food and drug administration	VATS	Video-assisted thoracoscopic surgery
FEV_1	Forced expiratory volume in 1 second	V_C	Vital capacity
FRC	Functional residual capacity	VP	Ventriculoperitoneal
FTT	Failure to thrive	VSD	Ventricular septal defect
FVC	Forced vital capacity	V_T	Tidal volume
GERD	Gastroesophageal reflux disease	WBC	White blood cell

CHAPTER OBJECTIVES

1. To understand normal lung physiology and diagnostic tests including PFTs and pleural fluid analysis
2. To create a differential diagnosis for common respiratory signs and symptoms including cough, stridor, and wheezing
3. To detail the presentation and management of acute upper airway infections (croup, epiglottitis, and bacterial tracheitis) and lower airway infections (bronchiolitis and pneumonia)
4. To understand the presentation, diagnosis, and acute and chronic management of asthma
5. To detail cystic fibrosis epidemiology, presentation, clinical manifestations, and management
6. To categorize lung disease as restrictive, obstructive, and interstitial and understand the diagnosis, presentation, and management of each group.

INTRODUCTION TO PULMONARY PHYSIOLOGY

Normal Lung Development

By 16 weeks post conception, airways have developed to the point of terminal bronchioles. Alveoli increase in number until 8 years of age, and each alveolus increases in size until it reaches adult size in late adolescence.

Why Do We Breathe?

Two sets of chemoreceptors work to control respiratory drive. Central receptors located in the medulla sense when CO_2 begins to rise and send signals to speed up respirations. Hypercarbia is the main force behind respiratory drive. Peripheral receptors located at the bifurcations of the carotid arteries and arch of aorta normally play a more minor part. These receptors respond to hypoxia and send signals to speed up breathing.

Points to Remember

- *Hypoxic-drive Theory*—People who are chronic CO_2 retainers lose their hypercarbic drive to breathe and rely more on their hypoxemic drive to breathe. Be careful giving oxygen to chronic CO_2 retainers with the concern that they may lose their drive to breathe.

Normal Lung Volumes

Normal lung volumes are shown in Figure 24.1.

History and Physical Examination

A good *history* is a key to determining the presence and etiology of pulmonary disease. Special attention should be paid to the following:

- Classic pulmonary symptoms such as cough, chest pain, shortness of breath, tachypnea, increased work of breathing, hemoptysis, cyanosis, snoring, and exercise intolerance.

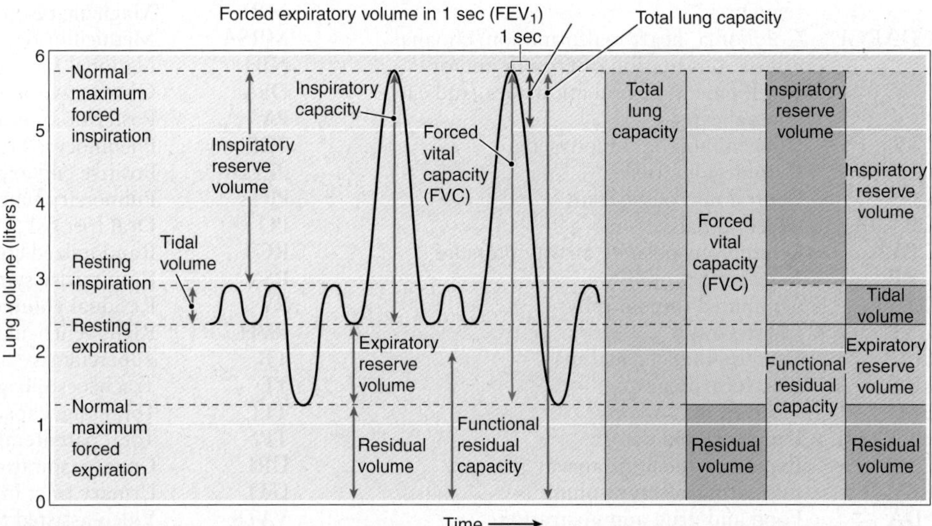

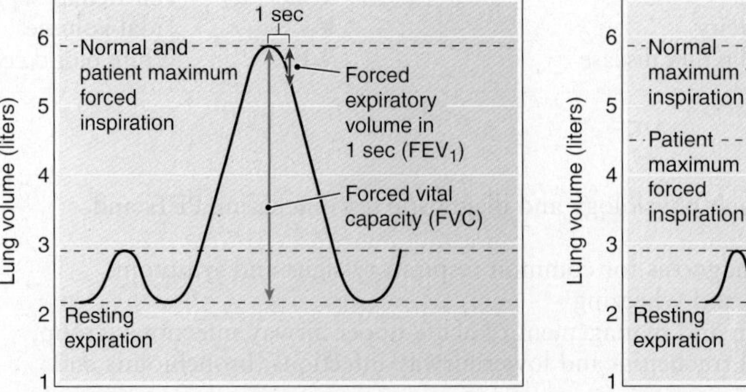

FIGURE 24.1. Spirography. (A) Normal spirogram tracings with lung volumes and capacities. (B) Spirogram in obstructive disease: 1-sec forced expiratory volume (FEV_1) is low; forced vital capacity (FVC) is normal. (C) Spirogram in restrictive disease: both FEV_1 and FVC are low. (*Reprinted with permission from* McConnell TH. *The Nature of Disease Pathology for the Health Professions.* Philadelphia: Lippincott Williams & Wilkins, 2007.)

- Constitutional symptoms such as fever, weight loss, and fatigue.
- Difference between daytime versus night-time symptoms.
- Associations with environmental exposures or changes in the season or weather.
- Chronic diarrhea.
- Failure to thrive.
- Family history.

On *physical examination*, there are also many clues that may point to an etiology.

- Allergic findings (allergic shiners, tearing, or sneezing).
- Clubbing, peripheral edema.
- Cyanosis (central vs. peripheral).
- Chest deformities.
- Abnormal cardiac auscultation or evidence of cor pulmonale.
- Audible stridor, wheeze, labored breathing.
- Organomegaly, generalized lymphadenopathy, ascites.
- Developmental delay, neurologic findings.
- Muscle weakness, tics.
- Failure to thrive, abnormal anthropometric measures.

Points to Remember

- Chronic hypoxemia can lead to pulmonary hypertension and subsequent cor pulmonale because of pulmonary vasoconstriction.
- The kidneys respond to chronic hypoxemia by increasing the production of erythropoietin to raise hemoglobin levels and increase the body's oxygen carrying capacity. Therefore, patients with chronic hypoxemia often have elevated hemoglobin levels.

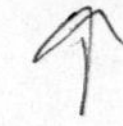

Differential Diagnosis of Common Pulmonary Signs and Symptoms

Stridor

Stridor is created from the turbulence of airflow as is passes through a narrow part of the respiratory tract. It is characterized by a high-pitched, musical breathing sound during inspiration, expiration, or both inspiration and expiration (biphasic). *Inspiratory stridor* is the most common type.

Inspiratory stridor is created by an *extra*thoracic (above the thoracic inlet) obstruction that causes the inward collapse of tissues with inspiration.

Examples

- *Immobile or paralyzed vocal cords* are a common cause of obstruction and stridor during infancy. Etiologies of paralysis include traumatic injury of the recurrent laryngeal nerve, trauma from intubation, or central nervous system bulbar injury such as hydrocephalus. It presents with a high-pitched inspiratory stridor that does NOT change with position, a hoarse or weak cry, and sometimes a weak cough. It is diagnosed via laryngoscopy or bronchoscopy.
- *Laryngomalacia* (poor tone in the structures supporting the larynx) is the *most common cause of inspiratory stridor in the newborn*. During infancy, laryngomalacia presents with variable pitch inspiratory stridor that *worsens when supine* or with feeding and/or agitation. On physical examination, you can see subcostal and suprasternal retractions. Inspiration produces laryngeal narrowing. With expiration, the floppy airway is stented open, resulting in improved symptoms. All of these symptoms improve with age as the cartilage of the larynx becomes more firm. Most infants will outgrow it by 12 to 18 months. If laryngomalacia is severe and causes feeding difficulty or obstructive hypoxia with sleep, surgical supraglottoplasty (trimming of the supraglottis) may be necessary.

Points to Remember

- If a patient experiences persistent stridor after cardiac surgery, think about injury of the left recurrent laryngeal nerve, leading to vocal cord paralysis.

Expiratory stridor is caused by lesions that are *intra*thoracic (below the thoracic inlet).

Examples

- *Tracheomalacia* occurs when weak tracheal rings collapse with expiration. If there is a high obstruction, the stridor can be biphasic. Look for possible TE fistula.
- *Vascular rings* can wrap around the trachea and cause extrinsic compression of the respiratory tract, resulting in expiratory stridor and feeding difficulties. Vascular rings can be diagnosed on a barium esophagram (often first test), bronchoscopy, echocardiogram with Doppler, and/or CT angiogram.

Points to Remember

- Laryngomalacia is the most common cause of stridor in infants and classically worsens with agitation and supine positioning.

Biphasic stridor consists of stridor in both the expiratory and inspiratory phases of respiration.

Example

- *Subglottic stenosis* can be congenital or acquired. Many cases of acquired subglottic stenosis result from prolonged and/or traumatic intubation. Inspiratory stridor more than expiratory stridor. Diagnosis is made by laryngoscopy or bronchoscopy. Severe stenosis may require tracheostomy placement.

Common causes of stridor are shown in Box 24.1.

Points to Remember

- Tracheomalacia usually presents with expiratory or biphasic stridor; in contrast, laryngomalacia presents with inspiratory stridor.

Cough

Cough is a common complaint among infants and children. It can be a normal response intended to assist in clearing airways of mucous and debris as seen with uncomplicated upper respiratory tract infections. Although it is usually benign, coughing can be a symptom of underlying pathology, especially when the cough is chronic. Chronic cough is defined as daily cough for more than 3 weeks and always deserves further evaluation. Conditions associated with chronic cough are listed in Box 24.2.

Box 24.1 Common Causes of Stridor: Inspiratory, Expiratory, and Biphasic

Inspiratory Stridor
- Enlarged tonsils and adenoids
- Pharyngeal/hypopharyngeal masses
- Immobile/paralyzed cords
- Laryngomalacia
- Macroglossia
  - For example, Beckwith–Wiedemann Syndrome, Trisomy 21, congenital hypothyroidism, glycogen storage disease
- Micrognathia
  - For example, Pierre–Robin, Treacher–Collins
- Laryngeal Cyst/Web or Laryngocele (usually presents shortly after birth)
- Infections
  - For example, Laryngotracheitis (croup), Tracheitis, Laryngeal Papilloma, Epiglottitis
- Laryngospasm
  - For example, Hypocalcemia, Reflux, Anesthesia
- Airway Edema
  - For example, Post-extubation, Anaphylaxis

Expiratory Stridor
- Tracheomalacia
- Vascular ring

Biphasic Stridor
- Subglottic stenosis

Points to Remember

- Over-the-counter cough and cold preparations have been shown to be ineffective in children younger than 6 years and can lead to serious adverse side effects, including tachycardia, seizures, change in mental status, and even death. They are not recommended in this age group, and they are not approved by the FDA for use in children younger than 4 years.
- Impaired cough in patients with muscle weakness, CNS dysfunction, cerebral palsy, vocal cord dysfunction, thoracic skeletal deformities, or pain puts the patient at increased risk of pulmonary infections.

Evaluation of chronic cough should be guided by clues in the history and physical examination suggestive of specific pathologies. If no specific clues are present, begin with a chest x-ray, allergy testing, and ENT evaluation. PFTs should be considered in children older than 6 years. If these tests are normal and cough persists, evaluate for gastroesophageal reflux and cystic fibrosis.

Exercise Intolerance

Exercise intolerance is a common complaint in children with underlying lung diseases such as asthma and cystic fibrosis. The differential diagnosis of exercise intolerance, however, should also include nonpulmonary causes such as anemia, muscle weakness, poor conditioning, cardiac disease, depression, and mediastinal masses.

Wheezing

Wheezing refers to the high-pitched musical sound made by air vibrating through narrowed *intra*thoracic airways. Wheezing is classically an expiratory noise but can occur during inspira-

Points to Remember

- *Psychogenic cough*, often referred to as a habit cough, does not result from underlying organic pathology, though it usually begins as a respiratory viral illness is ending. The cough has a harsh or "honking" tone, and patients *do NOT cough during sleep* or when distracted. This is a diagnosis of exclusion and other organic etiologies must be ruled out. Treatment involves reassurance, removal of stressors, and behavior modification.

Box 24.2 Conditions Associated with Chronic Cough

- Asthma
- Recurrent episodes of bronchitis infections (*Chlamydia*, pertussis, *Mycobacterium*)
- Cystic fibrosis
- Primary ciliary dyskinesia
  - Kartagener syndrome
  - Immotile cilia syndrome
- Immunodeficiency
  - Selective IgA deficiency
  - Hypogammaglobulinemia (primary and secondary)
- Anatomic lesions
  - Foreign body
  - Previous esophageal atresia repair
  - Mediastinal tumors
  - Congenital heart disease
- Irritants
  - Milk aspiration (gastroesophageal reflux, tracheoesophageal fistula)
  - Tobacco smoke
  - Pollution
  - Occupational exposure
- Psychogenic cough

(Reprinted with permission from McMillan JA, Feigin RD, DeAngelis C, et al. *Oski's Pediatrics: Principles and Practice*, 4th ed. Philadelphia: Lippincott Williams & Wilkins, 2006.)

TABLE 24.1

DIFFERENTIAL DIAGNOSIS OF WHEEZING

Common Causes	Rare Causes
Aspiration	Aberrant vessels
Direct (e.g., defective swallow, neuromuscular disease)	Alpha$_1$-antitrypsin deficiency
Indirect (gastroesophageal reflux, emesis)	Angioneurotic edema
Asthma (reactive airway disease)	Carcinoid syndrome
Atopic disease	Factitious wheezing
Bronchiectasis	Immotile cilia syndrome (Kartagener syndrome)
Bronchiolitis	Lobar emphysema
Bronchitis	Neoplasm/tumor
Foreign-body aspiration	Psychogenic airway obstruction
Pneumonitis	Pulmonary hemosiderosis (idiopathic, cow's milk allergy, myocarditis associated, Goodpasture disease)
Uncommon Causes	Pulmonary sequestration
Anaphylaxis	Pulmonary vasculitis
Bronchopulmonary dysplasia	Sarcoidosis
Congestive heart failure	Tracheobronchomegaly
Cystic fibrosis	Tracheobronchostenosis
Hypersensitivity pneumonitis	Tracheoesophageal fistula
Allergic bronchopulmonary aspergillosis	Vascular ring/sling
Mediastinal mass/adenopathy	Visceral larva migrans
Pulmonary edema	
Tracheobronchomalacia	
Vocal cord dysfunction/psychogenic airway obstruction	

tion. Asthma is the most common cause of wheezing in children. It is important to remember, however, that "not everything that wheezes is asthma." The differential diagnosis of wheezing is broad and includes inflammatory, infectious, cardiac, and structural conditions that vary by age.

The differential diagnosis for wheezing is shown in Table 24.1.

All children with a first-time episode of wheezing should have a CXR. Further diagnostic testing should be guided by the history and findings on physical examination and may include:

- Trial of bronchodilators to check for reversibility.
- Viral antigen studies and cultures (nasopharyngeal, sputum) to look for infectious cause.
- Imaging
  - Aspiration—modified barium swallow study.
  - Vascular ring/external compression—barium swallow.
  - Infection/mass—CXR.
  - Mass/focal parenchymal defect—CT.
- Sweat test to evaluate for cystic fibrosis.
- Ciliary biopsy to evaluate ciliary function.
- pH probe to evaluate for GERD.
- PFTs to assess fixed airway obstruction (flow volume loop), small airway obstruction, increased airway resistance.
- Airway bronchoscopy +/− bronchoalveolar lavage to evaluate for unusual infectious causes, dynamic airway compression/collapse, mass, and foreign body.

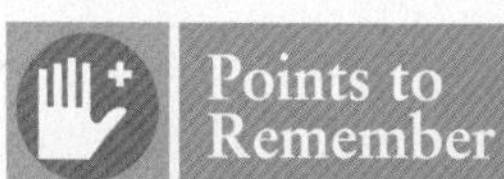

- **Not everything that wheezes is asthma. Always consider other etiologies of wheezing, especially when wheezing is recurrent and/or is not reversed by bronchodilators.**

Pulmonary Diagnostic Tests

Pulse Oximetry

A pulse oximeter works by measuring the differential absorption of light and calculating a ratio of oxyhemoglobin to deoxygenated hemoglobin. It measures oxygen saturation in the blood, and not ventilation.

When using pulse oximeter, make sure that the probe is attached correctly and that the tracing has a good wave form. There are some clinical scenarios, however, where pulse oximetry is inaccurate despite appropriate mechanics, which are as follows:

- *CO poisoning* (elevated carboxyhemoglobin levels cause pulse oximetry to overestimate the level of oxygenated hemoglobin).
- *Methemoglobinemia* (causes pulse oximetry readings to be falsely low, usually in the mid-80s).
- *Impaired perfusion* (may result in decreased correlation; try different parts of the body including fingers, toes, or earlobes).

TABLE 24.2

PFTs IN OBSTRUCTIVE VERSUS RESTRICTIVE PULMONARY DISORDERS

Measure	Obstructive Disorders	Restrictive Disorders
FEV_1/FVC	Decreased	Normal
FEV_1	Decreased	Decreased
FVC	Decreased or Normal	Decreased
TLC	Normal or Increased	Decreased
RV	Normal or Increased	Decreased

Pulmonary Function Tests (PFTs)

Pulmonary function tests (PFTs) are a form of spirometry used to measure lung function. A flow volume loop is generated, which can demonstrate inhaled and exhaled volume and flow. PFTs can be useful in determining whether a pulmonary process is obstructive (asthma, alpha-1-antitrypsin deficiency, etc.) or restrictive (scoliosis, interstitial lung disease, etc.). This is shown in Table 24.2.

Pleural Fluid Analysis

A small number of cells are present in normal pleural fluid. Macrophages make up 75% of these cells.

Pleuritis

Pleuritis is inflammation of the pleura. It begins with an increase in inflammatory cells. Mesothelial cells become more permeable, allowing for more fluid to enter the pleural space than can be reabsorbed, causing a pleural effusion. Complications include effusion with fibrinous loculated pockets or frank pus (empyema).

Clinical Manifestations

- Small effusions may be asymptomatic.
- Chest pain (worse with inspiration).
- Referred shoulder pain and/or upper quadrant abdominal pain.
- Guarding with shallow respirations.
- Increased work of breathing.
- Fever.
- Large effusions can obstruct venous return and lead to decreased cardiac output.

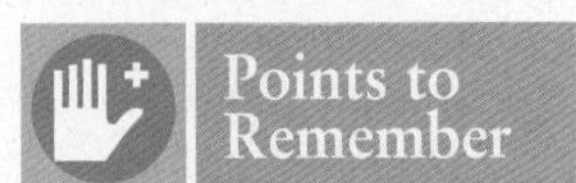

Points to Remember

- CT is a better imaging study than MRI to look at lung parenchyma and interstitial lung disease.

Diagnosis

- Physical examination—pleural friction rub, dullness to percussion, egophony, decreased breath sounds.
- CXR—PA and lateral decubitus views to look for loculation/layering of fluid.
- CT—more precise than CXR; can help distinguish between loculated pus and abscess.
- US—to mark for draining or US-guided thoracentesis.
- Pleural fluid analysis.

Analysis of the pleural fluid can help differentiate exudative versus transudative processes, infectious versus noninfectious etiologies, and provide clues about specific infectious etiologies. This information is shown in Table 24.3.

Points to Remember

- Pleural fluid analysis in rheumatologic disorders such as rheumatoid arthritis and SLE may reveal low glucose.

Pleural Fluid Collections

When developing a differential diagnosis for pleural fluid collections, it is useful to divide them into different fluid types.

- *Empyema* is a thick, purulent fluid combined with cellular debris that clogs normal fluid drainage. It occurs in association with infection.
- *Chylothorax* is caused by a disruption of the thoracic duct, draining chyle into the pleural space.
- *Hemothorax* is blood in the pleural space.
- *Transudate* is caused by systemic factors that change the balance of formation and/or absorption of pleural fluid, for example, heart failure and cirrhosis.
- *Exudate* is caused by local pulmonary factors changing the balance of formation and/or absorption of pleural fluid, for example, bacterial pneumonia, pulmonary embolism, and oncologic process.

Different types of pleural fluid collections and their characteristics are shown in Table 24.4.

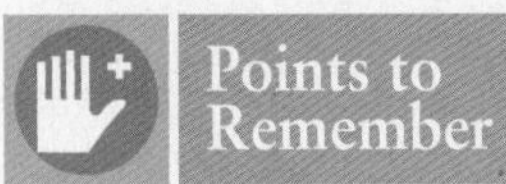

Points to Remember

- Chocolate-colored pleural fluid should make you think of amebiasis.

TABLE 24.3

PLEURAL FLUID ANALYSIS

Fluid Type	Gram Stain/Cell Count	pH	Glucose	Pleural:Serum Ratio
Exudates/ Empyema	PMN predominance	<7.3	<50% serum level	P:S protein ≥0.5 P:S LDH ≥0.6
TB	Lymphocyte predominance		<50% serum level	P:S protein ≥0.5
Chyle	Lymphocyte predominance Triglycerides >110 Protein >3			P:S fat ≥1; P:S protein ≥0.05
Transudate	Low WBC	≥7.3	>50% serum level	P:S protein <0.5 P:S LDH <0.6

TABLE 24.4

PLEURAL FLUID COLLECTIONS

Fluid Collection	Etiology	Presentation/Fluid Make-up	Treatment/Complications
Empyema	*Infections* ■ *Staphylococcus* sp.: most common, especially in young children ■ *Streptococcus* sp.	*Presentation* ■ Often fever *Fluid* ■ Frank Pus	*Treatment* ■ Antibiotics—possibly make pleural fluid sterile ■ Drainage with chest tube ■ May need VATS (video assisted thoracentesis) with decortication *Complications* ■ Bronchopleural fistulas
Chylothorax	*Causes* ■ Thoracic surgery: complication 1% of time ■ Birth injury: thoracic duct leaks with stretch ■ Obstruction of central veins by thrombosis or malignancy	*Presentation* ■ Infants: more often on right side ■ May be bilateral ■ No pain, fever, or signs of infection *Fluid* ■ Chyle appears turbid or white, depending on ingestion of fat ■ Can be clear if fasting or neonate ■ Fat/Triglyceride >110 ■ Lymphocytes ■ Protein >3	*Treatment* ■ Diet low in fat or TPN without intralipids ■ Formula with medium-chain fatty acids ■ If severe can ligate thoracic duct
Hemothorax	*Causes* ■ Trauma ■ Central venous catheter insertion ■ Malignancy metastatic to pleura ■ Pulmonary embolus ■ Coagulopathy ■ Rupture of ductus arteriosus ■ Coarctation or pulmonary ■ AVM ■ Bleeding from aberrant vessels ■ Pleural endometriosis ■ Young female	*Presentation* ■ Often associated with pneumothorax *Fluid* ■ HCT of fluid >50% peripheral HCT *Diagnosis* ■ CXR ■ Confirmed by thoracentesis	*Treatment* ■ Chest tube ■ Hemostasis ■ If bleeding >10 mL/kg/h should have surgical exploration ■ Correct possible coagulopathy
Transudate	*Causes* ■ Cirrhosis ■ Nephrotic syndrome ■ Congestive heart failure (effusion is bilateral) ■ Glomerulonephritis (bilateral or unilateral) ■ Hepatic cirrhosis (right) ■ Malignancies ■ Infectious (viral, *E. coli, Klebsiella pneumoniae, enterococci* or *group A Streptococcus*)	*Presentation* ■ Pleural metastasis or lymphatic obstruction in mediastinum with high back pressure through lymphatics ■ Fever with infectious etiologies *Fluid* ■ Light yellow ■ TG low (<50)	*Treatment* ■ Thoracentesis (remove fluid if symptomatic) ■ Replace fluid removed with IVF ■ May need chest tube ■ Untreated can lead to empyema ■ Damage to the pleura can lead to fibrosis and restrictive lung disease

ACUTE UPPER AIRWAY OBSTRUCTION

Acute upper airway obstruction in children can be a life-threatening emergency. The subglottic region of the larynx is the narrowest point of the pediatric airway and is the most common site of life-threatening upper airway obstruction. Supraglottic obstruction is less common but can be more difficult to manage.

Features of supraglottic versus subglottic acute airway obstruction are as follows:

- *Supraglottic obstruction*—muffled speech, absent cough, tripod position, drooling, and dysphagia.
- *Subglottic obstruction*—hoarse speech, barking cough, and normal swallowing.

Infectious and noninfectious etiologies are as follows:

- Infectious causes of acute upper airway obstruction
  - Croup (acute laryngotracheitis).
  - Epiglottitis.
  - Bacterial tracheitis (acute laryngotracheobronchitis).
- Noninfectious causes of acute upper airway obstruction
  - Foreign body aspiration.
  - Angioedema.

Regardless of the specific etiology, the most important part of management is maintaining the airway. Avoidance of agitation is critical. This includes avoiding painful or stressful procedures such as needlesticks, separation from parents, manipulation by healthcare workers, and radiologic imaging. Ideally, intubation should be done in a controlled setting (i.e., operating room) by expert personnel who are able to do an urgent tracheostomy if needed.

Croup (Laryngotracheitis)

Croup is a common pediatric illness in which a viral infection causes subglottic narrowing at the cricoid cartilage. It is most common in children between 3 months and 4 years of age and usually occurs in the fall and winter months. *Parainfluenza 1* is responsible for 60% of cases. Other etiologies include parainfluenza types 2, 3, and 4, influenza, respiratory syncytial virus (RSV), and adenovirus. Bacterial superinfection can occur but is rare.

Clinical Manifestations

- Nonspecific URI symptoms followed by the development of a *hoarse or "barking" cough.*
- Inspiratory or biphasic stridor.
- Increased work of breathing including retractions, tachypnea, and/or flaring.
- Symptoms usually worsen at night and with agitation.

Diagnosis

- Diagnosis is based on classic clinical findings NOT diagnostic tests.
- Neck film—PA view "steeple sign"—seen in 50% of cases (Fig. 24.2).

Management

- Most children with croup can be managed as outpatients. Indications for hospitalization include hypoxia, stridor at rest, significant respiratory distress, and/or altered mental status.
- Supportive therapy is a mainstay of the treatment. Avoid agitation and provide "cool mist" (humidified O_2 or room air).
- Dexamethasone reduces airway edema and decreases the length and severity of disease. It can be given IV, IM, or PO depending on the level of respiratory distress.
- Nebulized racemic epinephrine is helpful for patients with moderate-to-severe disease. Observe patient for at least 4 hours after giving nebulized epinephrine because of the concern for rebound phenomenon.
- Antibiotics are NOT indicated in cases of uncomplicated croup.

Prognosis

- Croup is a self-limited illness. Most children with mild-to-moderate cases have excellent outcomes. Children with more severe disease require hospitalization and may require intubation and respiratory support.

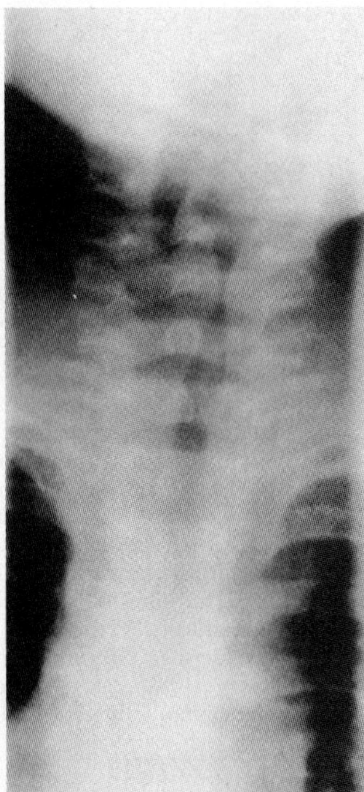

FIGURE 24.2. Steeple Sign. This radiograph shows the characteristic narrowing of the subglottis indicative of acute laryngotracheobronchitis. (*Reprinted with permission from* Cotton RT, Myer CM. *Practical pediatric otolaryngology.* Philadelphia: Lippincott Williams & Wilkins, 1999.)

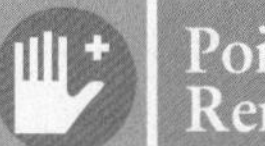

Points to Remember

- *Spasmodic croup* is a variant of acute laryngotracheitis and likely represents a viral infection with an allergic component that causes cough. Children often have no prodrome or minimal coryza. They go to sleep afebrile and without the signs of significant illness, but *awaken* with a barking cough, hoarseness, and stridor. This may happen two to three times per night. Children often respond to mist therapy from a bathroom shower or a vaporizer. Reflux may also be a component.

Epiglottitis

Epiglottitis is a rare life-threatening bacterial infection of the epiglottis. It has an acute onset that can progress to severe respiratory distress within the first 24 hours of illness. The peak age incidence is 2 to 10 years. In the pre-HIB vaccine era, *Haemophilus influenzae* was responsible for the majority of cases of epiglottitis and is still an important cause in children who are unvaccinated. In the post-HIB vaccine era, the most common causes of epiglottitis are *Streptococcus pneumoniae*, *Streptococcus pyogenes*, and *Staphylococcus aureus*.

Clinical Manifestations

- Acute onset of fever, *drooling*, sore throat, dysphagia, and dysphonia.
- Signs of respiratory distress including tachypnea, retractions, and/or inspiratory/biphasic stridor.
- Children usually appear *toxic*.
- Symptoms improve in the "*tripod position*" (leaning forward with chin extended) and worsen when supine.

Points to Remember

- Epiglottitis is rare in the United States, thanks to the Hib vaccine, but is still likely to show up on the boards—watch for an immigrant or child with delayed immunizations.

Diagnosis

- Epiglottitis is a *clinical diagnosis* (do NOT look in their mouth to confirm the diagnosis until airway is secured—once airway is secured, direct visualization may reveal a cherry red epiglottis).
- Lateral neck x-ray reveals "thumbprint sign" (obtain an x-ray only if diagnosis is unclear, patient is nontoxic appearing and can tolerate the procedure safely) (see Fig. 24.3).
- Send CBC and blood culture (bacteremia precedes the development of epiglottitis; thus, in some cases, the pathogen can be identified in a blood culture).

Points to Remember

- Unlike children with croup and bacterial tracheitis, patients with epiglottitis do NOT usually have cough.

Management

- Epiglottitis is a *medical emergency*. Manage ABCs and *be ready to intubate*. Call for back-up quickly. Intubation should be done in a controlled setting and by someone prepared to do an emergent tracheostomy if necessary.
- Avoid agitation. Do not put in an IV or draw blood until airway secured.
- Start antibiotic coverage including a third generation cephalosporin and antistaphylococcal coverage. Consider adding vancomycin to cover MRSA.

Points to Remember

- Because of its rapidly progressive course and potential for complete airway obstruction, epiglottitis always a medical emergency!

Bacterial Tracheitis (Laryngotracheobronchitis)

In otherwise healthy children, bacterial tracheitis represents a serious secondary bacterial infection occurring as a complication of a primary viral croup. It occurs mostly in the fall and winter. It affects patients of all ages and has a peak incidence between 3 months and 4 years of age.

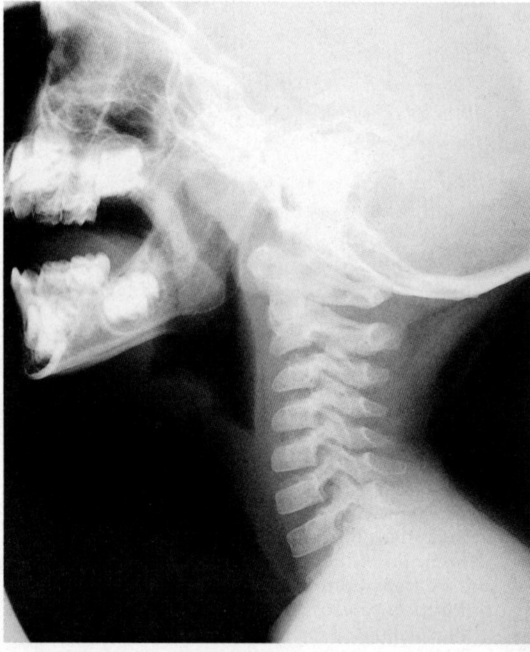

FIGURE 24.3. The patient has epiglottitis. The radiograph demonstrates a swollen epiglottis at the level of the hyoid bone, which is convex on both sides and appears in the shape of a thumbprint. Edema anterior to the epiglottis has obliterated the vallecula, which usually appears as an elongated black shadow. Note the marked swelling of the aryepiglottic folds, projecting inferiorly and posteriorly from the epiglottis, and the arytenoid cartilages at the base of the folds. Because *H. influenzae* type b infection involves all the structures in this area, this disease has alternatively been referred to as "supraglottitis." (*Reprinted with permission from* Fleisher GR, Ludwig S, Baskin MN. *Atlas of Pediatric Emergency Medicine*. Philadelphia: Lippincott Williams & Wilkins, 2004.)

S. aureus is the most common bacterial pathogen. Other etiologies include *Group A streptococcus*, *Streptococcus viridans*, *H. influenzae*, Gram-negative enteric bacteria, and anaerobes. Bacterial tracheitis can also occur as a primary bacterial infection in patients with tracheostomies.

Clinical Manifestations

- Begins as a croup-like illness that acutely worsens with *high fevers*, a *toxic appearance*, and respiratory distress.
- Respiratory symptoms include tachypnea, retractions, prominent *brassy cough*, and stridor. Dysphagia and drooling are NOT prominent symptoms and patients do NOT respond to racemic epinephrine.

Diagnosis

- Bacterial tracheitis is primarily a clinical diagnosis.
- CXR may demonstrate ragged, irregular borders of the trachea.
- Diagnosis can be confirmed via bronchoscopy or at the time of intubation by visualization of inflammation, purulent exudates, and pseudomembranes involving the subglottic area and extending into the trachea. Sputum Gram stain and culture may help identify the specific pathogen. Pneumonia is often associated.

Management

- Manage ABCs and *be ready to intubate*. Can deteriorate rapidly.
- Send CBC and blood culture.
- Start antibiotic coverage including antistaphylococcal coverage. If in an area of highly endemic MRSA, consider treating with vancomycin.
- Typical course is more complicated than croup or epiglottitis—often requires over a week of hospitalization.

Table 24.5 compares characteristics of croup, epiglottis, and bacterial tracheitis.

Foreign Body Aspiration

Foreign body aspiration is a common cause of acute upper airway obstruction in children, especially in toddlers and in children with developmental disabilities. In more than 50% of foreign body aspirations, there is no knowledge of a specific aspiration event. Commonly aspirated foreign bodies include nuts, hotdogs, coins, and seeds.

Clinical Manifestations

- Usually presents as acute onset of respiratory distress, often following a choking or gagging episode.
- Physical examination findings may include tachypnea, retractions, grunting, hypoxia, and/or focally diminished breath sounds and wheezing.
- With delayed diagnosis, children may present with recurrent attacks of coughing and wheezing misdiagnosed as asthma, pneumonia, or bronchiectasis.

TABLE 24.5

DIFFERENTIATION BETWEEN CROUP, EPIGLOTTITIS, AND BACTERIAL TRACHEITIS

	Croup	Epiglottitis	Bacterial Tracheitis
Age	3 mo to 4 y	2–10 y	3 mo to 4 y
Onset	■ URI symptoms first develop	■ Rapid, usually <24 hr	■ Variable
Presentation	■ Inspiratory stridor ■ Hoarse, barking cough	■ Inspiratory stridor ■ High fever ■ Toxic appearing ■ Dysphagia/drooling ■ "Tripod position"	■ Inspiratory stridor ■ Usually high fever ■ Hoarse brassy cough
Etiology	■ Viral	■ Bacterial ■ Prior to Hib vaccine, *Haemophilus influenza* type B most common	■ Viral infection with bacterial superinfection

Diagnosis

- Suspected on the basis of history and physical examination findings.
- CXR may reveal an obvious foreign body, asymmetric obstructive hyperinflation on expiratory views, and/or areas of focal atelectasis. One quarter of patients have normal CXRs.
- If examination and CXR are equivocal, fluoroscopy and/or flexible bronchoscopy can be helpful.

Management

- Initial management includes ABCs.
- Perform Heimlich maneuver in children with asphyxiating foreign bodies. If that fails, proceed quickly to emergent rigid bronchoscopy.
- Children without significant respiratory compromise can undergo urgent rather than emergent removal via rigid bronchoscopy.

Angioedema

Angioedema is an extension of urticaria, which results in deep subcutaneous swelling. It can extend to the face, hands, feet, and genital region. It can be severe enough to result in laryngeal swelling, resulting in airway obstruction. Acute management for angioedema causing upper airway obstruction should include ABCs, epinephrine, and antihistamines.

INFECTIOUS LOWER TRACT DISEASE

Bronchiolitis

Bronchiolitis is an acute viral infection involving the *lower respiratory tract* in which sloughing of epithelial cells, increased mucous secretion, and airway edema cause obstruction of small airways. Bronchiolitis is one of the most common causes of pediatric hospitalization in the United States. It occurs most frequently in the first year of life, and depending on geography, peaks from October to December through March to May. RSV causes 50% to 80% cases. Other pathogens include human metapneumovirus, influenza, adenovirus, rhinovirus, and parainfluenza 1, 2, and 3.

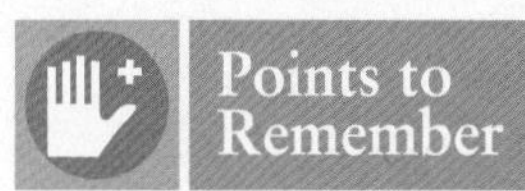

- Risk factors for more severe bronchiolitis include underlying cardiopulmonary disease or immunodeficiency, prematurity, age less than 12 weeks, second-hand smoke exposure, and a family history of asthma.

Clinical Manifestations

- Classic signs and symptoms include fever, rhinitis, cough, tachypnea, flaring, retractions, wheezing, scattered rhonchi/rales, and/or hypoxia.
- *Apnea* can be the primary presentation, especially in younger than *6-weeks old*; young infants can also present with a sepsis-like picture.
- Respiratory distress can lead to poor feeding, resulting in dehydration and lethargy
- Symptoms usually peak at day 5 to 7 of illness.

Diagnosis

- Bronchiolitis is a *clinical* diagnosis defined by a first episode of wheezing at ≤24 months of age plus physical findings of viral infection. Imaging and laboratory studies are not required for diagnosis.
- CXR—often nonspecific; may show air trapping, peribronchial cuffing, atelectasis, patchy consolidation, and/or diffuse interstitial infiltration or it may be normal (Fig. 24.4).

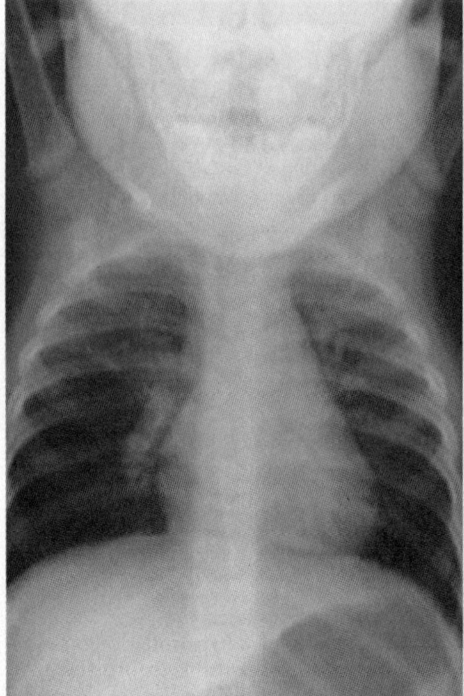
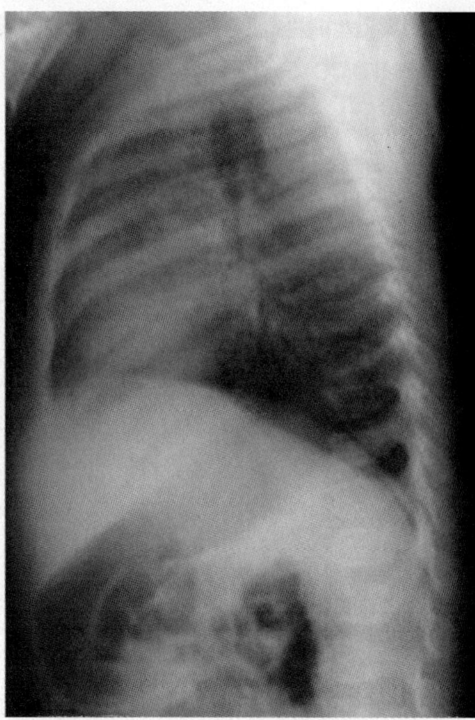

FIGURE 24.4. Chest radiographs of 6-month-old infant with hMPV bronchiolitis, showing hyperinflation and diffuse perihilar infiltrates. (Courtesy of John V. Williams, M.D.; Division of Infectious Diseases, Departments of Pediatrics.)

- ABG—useful in moderate and severe cases to help assess oxygenation and ventilation.
- Viral diagnostics—immunoassay or immunofluorescence and/or viral culture of the nasopharynx can help identify specific viral pathogen (culture is less sensitive but 100% specific).

Management

- Most infants and young children with RSV can be followed as outpatients and do not require specific intervention other than ensuring adequate hydration.
- Criteria for hospitalization include apnea, hypoxemia, moderate respiratory distress, dehydration, inability to sufficiently feed, underlying cardiopulmonary disease or immune deficiency, and unreliable follow-up.
- Supportive care is the mainstay of the treatment and includes supplemental oxygen therapy for $SaO_2 < 90\%$, fluid and nutrition management, and respiratory support if needed.
- Bronchodilators are NOT routinely indicated as RCTs have not shown any benefit. If an individual patient has a beneficial response to a trial of a bronchodilator such as albuterol, therapy can be considered on an individual basis.
- Corticosteroids are NOT routinely indicated and have not been shown to be beneficial.
- Antivirals such as ribavirin have shown inconsistent benefit and are NOT routinely indicated because of questionable efficacy, high cost, and side effects.
- Antibiotics are NOT indicated for uncomplicated bronchiolitis
  - AOM is the most common bacterial infection associated with bronchiolitis, and if present, should be treated with appropriate antimicrobial therapy.
  - UTIs are found in approximately 5% of patients with bronchiolitis, and if present, should be treated with appropriate antimicrobial therapy.
  - Coexisting bacterial pneumonias are very rare and should only be considered in patients with severe prolonged disease.

Prognosis

- Most of the morbidity and mortality associated with bronchiolitis occurs in infants below 12 months of age. Infants with a history of prematurity or underlying cardiopulmonary disease or immunodeficiency are at greater risk for more severe disease.
- Infants and young children with RSV bronchiolitis are at increased risk of developing asthma. It is unclear if this increased risk of asthma is due to the RSV infection itself or rather reflects an underlying predisposition to airway reactivity.
- Reinfection with different viruses or different strains of RSV within the same season is common.

Prevention

Palivizumab (Synagis) is a humanized mouse monoclonal antibody that provides *passive immunity* against RSV and decreases the risk of severe infection. It requires monthly administration during RSV season.

Indications for therapy:

- Chronic lung disease: infants below 24 months who receive medical therapy (supplemental O_2, bronchodilator, diuretic, or chronic corticosteroid therapy) within 6 months of the start of RSV season.
- Hemodynamically significant cyanotic heart disease: infants below 24 months (this does NOT include secundum ASD, small VSD, pulmonary stenosis, uncomplicated aortic stenosis, PDA, or coarctation of the aorta).
- Premature birth (<32 weeks)—infants during RSV season during the first 12 months of life (infants <28 weeks gestation may benefit from prophylaxis during their second RSV season as well).
- Premature (32–35 weeks)—infants below 3 months of age at start of RSV season or born in RSV season AND are at increased risk of exposure because of daycare attendance or a sibling below 5-years old should receive doses until 3-months old (maximum of three monthly doses).

Influenza vaccine—give to all children above 6 months and their caregivers

Avoidance of crowds, tobacco smoke, and daycare in high-risk children

Good Hand Washing. see infectious disease chapter for full discussion.

Pneumonia

In the United States, most cases of pneumonia in children and young adults are due to respiratory viruses and atypical organisms. Depending on the age of the child, approximately 20% to 40% of cases are caused by pyogenic bacteria. Fungal pneumonias are seen almost exclusively in children with underlying immunodeficiency.

- Fever and tachypnea are the most sensitive physical findings in pneumonia, but neither is very specific. Other findings include signs of increased work of breathing (flaring, grunting, retractions) and/or auscultatory findings (crackles, diminished breath sounds).
- Diagnosis is via CXR. WBC and CRP may be elevated.
- Treatment depends on likely specific etiology.

see infectious disease chapter for full discussion.

Points to Remember

- Meconium ileus is present in 15% to 20% of infants with cystic fibrosis and is often the first sign of disease.

Pulmonary Abscess

A pulmonary abscess is caused by an infection and subsequent discrete area of lung necrosis. It can occur at any age and affects the right lung more often than the left. Patients are at increased risk for pulmonary abscess if they have an immunodeficiency, anatomic abnormalities, impaired cough, and/or frequent aspiration.

- Typical organisms that cause pulmonary abscess are *S. aureus*, *S. pneumoniae*, and anaerobic organisms secondary to aspiration.
- Diagnosis is via CXR and/or chest CT.
- Treatment is with long-term antibiotics, ideally tailored to pathogens identified on sputum Gram stain and culture.
- CXR improvement may occur over months.

Points to Remember

- In cystic fibrosis, the systemic immune system is not impaired. Therefore, sepsis and extrasinopulmonary infections are rare in CF patients.

CYSTIC FIBROSIS

Cystic fibrosis (CF) is the most common lethal genetic disease in Caucasians. It is an *autosomal recessive* mutation in the CFTR gene on the long arm of chromosome 7. The *delta F508* mutation *represents 70% of all CFTR mutations*. It results in a 3-base pair deletion that leads to the loss of a single phenylalanine at position 508. Pathologically this mutation leads to changes in epithelial ion transport with overactive sodium pumps and impermeable chloride channels causing thick secretions. The incidence in Caucasians is 1 in 3,000; Hispanics 1 in 10,000; African Americans 1 in 15,000; Asian Americans 1 in 30,000. More than 1,000 different genetic mutations have been identified. Carriers do not show any signs of disease. Estimated carrier rate of CF gene in Caucasians is 1 in 20 to 25. The current life expectancy is middle 30s.

Points to Remember

- Allergic bronchopulmonary aspergillosis (ABPA) can also be seen in 1% to 2% of asthmatics.
- The goal of "pulmonary toilet" is to improve mucous clearance. It includes a combination of chest physical therapy, mucolytics, and bronchodilators.

Clinical Manifestations

- Presentation is usually during infancy or early childhood
  - Infants often present with GI problems including meconium ileus, FTT, steatorrhea, recurrent pulmonary symptoms, and/or lab abnormalities including hypoproteinemia, anemia, and hypokalemic alkalosis.

TABLE 24.6

FEATURES OF CYSTIC FIBROSIS

System	Signs and Symptoms	Treatment	Outcomes/Complications
Sinus/Nasal			
Sinusitis	■ Chronic pansinusitis with abnormal paranasal sinus anatomy	■ Nasal Steroids ■ Nasal saline rinses ■ Antibiotics ■ Surgical intervention	■ Bony erosion of sinuses
Nasal Polyps	■ Nasal polyps (always think about CF in an infant or child with nasal polyps!)	■ Usually benign	■ Occlusion of nasal passages
Pulmonary			
Chronic cough with mucous production and airway obstruction	■ Wheezing, atelectasis and air trapping ■ Obstruction of small airways with thick mucus ■ Inflammation of small and large airways ■ Persistent CXR abnormalities	■ Good pulmonary toilet to improve mucus clearance ■ Chest physical therapy ■ Mucolytics ■ Bronchodilators ■ Some benefit from azithromycin 3 × weekly to reduce inflammation ■ Steroids may be used after weighing the risks/benefits	■ ABPA ■ Pneumothorax—10% ■ Atelectasis ■ Respiratory failure ■ Pulmonary hypertension leading to cor pulmonale ■ Worse prognosis in smokers ■ If severe, may need heart/lung transplant ■ Pulmonary hemorrhage
Infection	Typical pathogens ■ *S. aureus* ■ Nontypeable *H. flu* ■ *Pseudomonas aeruginosa* ■ *Burkholderia cepacia* ■ *Stenotrophomonas maltophilia* ■ Aspergillus fumigatus	■ Broad-spectrum antibiotics including pseudomonas coverage ■ Never eradicate all pathogen, but can control severity	■ Persistent colonization with CF pathogens
Intestinal			
Meconium ileus	■ Abnormal calcifications on prenatal ultrasound ■ Failure to pass meconium ■ Abdominal distention		■ Inspissated meconium in the bowel can serve as a lead point for intussusception
Distal intestinal obstruction syndrome (DIOS)	■ Crampy abdominal pain ■ Emesis	■ May need surgical intervention	■ Microcolon—neonates ■ Perforation—rare
Other GI: rectal prolapse, cholelithiasis, focal biliary cirrhosis, nonspecific steatosis of liver, GERD, intussusception (<1-y-old)			
Pancreas			
Pancreatic insufficiency	■ Fat-soluble vitamin and essential fatty acid deficiencies ■ Malnutrition ■ Growth failure ■ Many never have pancreatic disease	■ Enzyme replacement ■ ADEK (fat-soluble vitamins) ■ High-fat diet ■ Nutrition counseling ■ Salt replacement	■ Hyponatremic dehydration ■ CF-related diabetes
Recurrent pancreatitis Vitamin E deficiency Vitamin K deficiency	■ Autodigestion of pancreas ■ Abnormal bleeding tendency with prolonged PTT	 ■ Replace vitamin E if <5-y old ■ Replace vitamin K as needed	
Hepatobiliary			
Chronic hepatic disease	■ Focal biliary cirrhosis or multilobular cirrhosis		■ Portal hypertension, cirrhosis
Cholecystitis Cholelithiasis	■ Abdominal pain—classically right upper quadrant	■ Intervention as needed	
Cholestasis	■ Emesis		

TABLE 24.6

CONTINUED

System	Signs and Symptoms	Treatment	Outcomes/Complications
Nutritional			
FTT	■ Protein-calorie malnutrition ■ Hypoproteinemia ■ Edema ■ Puberty often delayed	■ Nutritional supplementation, GT feeds, and so on	
Reproductive			
Males	■ Absence of vans deferens → obstructive azoospermia		■ Males infertile
Females	■ Thick cervical mucus		■ Decreased pregnancy rate
Other Tissues			
Hypertrophic pulmonary osteoarthropathy	■ Knee and joint pain	■ x-ray—periosteal thickening of long bones and adjacent joints	

- Children often present with chronic cough, recurrent respiratory and sinus infections, failure to thrive, steatorrhea, and/or rectal prolapse.
- Clinical features of CF are shown in Table 24.6.

Diagnosis

- Sweat chloride iontophoresis (sweat test) = GOLD STANDARD.
  - Interpretation:
    - Normal above 40 mmol/L.
    - Borderline 40 to 59 mmol/L.
    - CF ≥60 mmol/L.
  - Any positive sweat test must be confirmed by a second sweat test or by mutation analysis. False negatives are rare but are more common in infants due to inadequate sample.
- Genetic testing is useful to identify a specific mutation. Many states include CF as part of standard newborn screening
  - Screening is via IRT (immune reactive trypsinogen).
  - False negatives are rare.
  - More than 90% of positives are false positives. If positive, retest in a few weeks and if positive again, perform mutation analysis.
- Fecal fat and stool elastase are helpful but *NOT* diagnostic.

Management

- See Table 24.6.

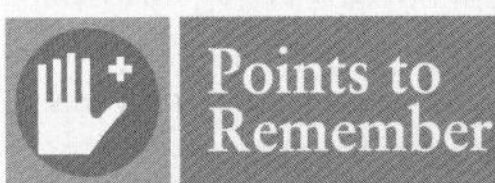

Points to Remember

- The atopic triad: (1) Eczema, (2) Asthma, (3) Allergies.
- Remember that not everything that wheezes is asthma! Always get a CXR in first time wheezers and consider other causes of wheezing such as foreign body aspiration, GERD, bronchiolitis, vascular rings, malignancy, and so on. Never give steroids until a mediastinal mass has been ruled out by CXR since doing so could delay the diagnosis of the specific malignancy.
- "The hygiene hypothesis" suggests that children with frequent respiratory infections or exposure to endotoxin and other bacterial products have lower rates of asthma because early infection modifies the immune system and reduces IgE response to allergens.

OBSTRUCTIVE LUNG DISEASE

Asthma

Asthma is a chronic, *reversible* (either spontaneously or with treatment) inflammatory airway disease. Obstruction of airflow results from edema, airway hyperactivity, bronchial smooth muscle spasm, and excess mucous production. Asthma is a leading cause of morbidity throughout the world and has doubled in prevalence over the past 20 years. The reason for this increase is unclear, but theories include urbanization and increased exposure to pollutants, improved diagnosis, and the hygiene hypothesis. The median age of onset is 4 years. It is more common in boys until puberty and then is more common in girls.

Clinical Manifestations

- Acute exacerbations
  - Patients with acute exacerbations complain of difficulty breathing, chest tightness, and/or cough.
  - Findings on physical examination include diffuse wheezing, diminished breath sounds, prolonged inspiratory:expiratory (I:E) ratio, tachypnea, retractions, flaring, grunting, and/or hypoxia.
  - *Triggers* include viral URI (most common), environmental exposure to irritants, allergen exposure, weather changes (especially exposure to cold dry air), exercise, reflux, and drugs including ASA and B-blockers.

Points to Remember

- In addition to asthma, always remember other etiologies of exercise intolerance including: (1) anemia, (2) muscle weakness, (3) poor conditioning, (4) cardiac disease, and (5) depression/psychological factors.

Points to Remember

- If used correctly, Beta-agonists administered through MDIs with spacer are as effective as nebulizers.
- Tachycardia is a side effect of albuterol. For patients with significant cardiac disease who require beta-agonist therapy, levalbuterol (a selective B1-agonist) can be used as an alternative and is associated with less tachycardia.

Points to Remember

- Theophylline is no longer routinely used for asthma exacerbations because of significant toxicity and multiple drug interactions.

Points to Remember

- GERD can be a significant problem in a child with asthma as irritation from the reflux may cause asthma exacerbations. If a child has worsening asthma symptoms in the setting of reflux, treat the reflux and the asthma may improve.
- Side effects of steroids (dose dependent).

Points to Remember

- In contrast to asthmatics, patients with emphysema respond poorly to bronchodilators.

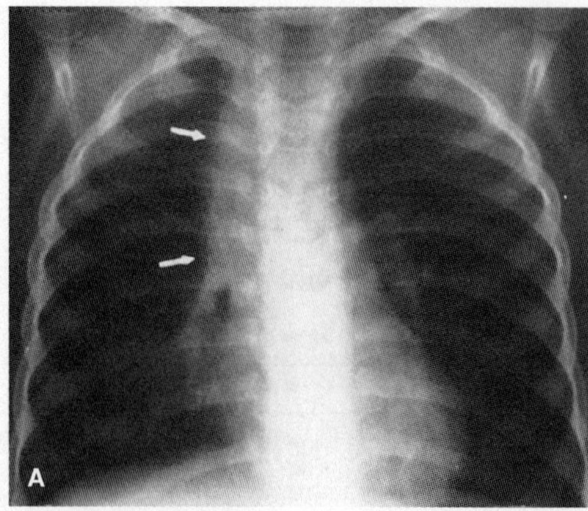

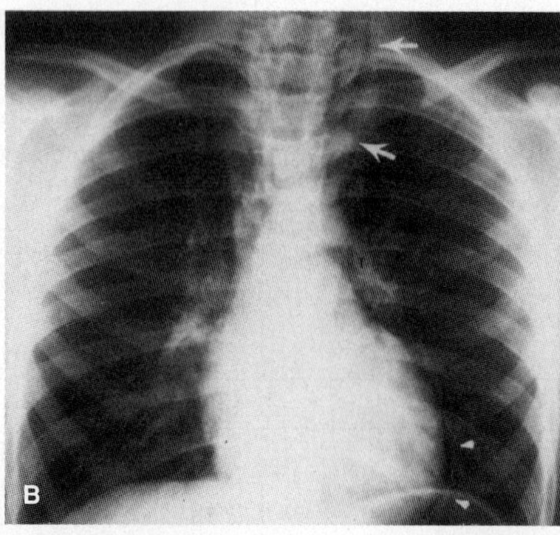

FIGURE 24.5. Pulmonary complications. (**A**) Sublobar atelectasis. Asthmatic child with acute asthma attack. Note area of apparent consolidation in the right paratracheal region (**arrows**). This represents collapse of one portion of the right upper lobe. A subtler finding assisting interpretation is that the minor fissure is slightly elevated. (B) Pneumomediastinum. Asthmatic child with pneumomediastinum with air surrounding the small triangular thymus gland (T), extending as linear sheaths into the neck and superior mediastinum (**upper arrows**) and extending along the lower left cardiac edge (**lower arrows**). (*Reprinted with permission from* Swischuk L. *Emergency Radiology of the Acutely Ill or Injured Child*, 2nd ed. Philadelphia: Lippincott Williams & Wilkins, 1986.)

- Chronic symptoms include cough (worse at night) and exercise intolerance.
- *Exercise-induced asthma* (EIA) is a variant of asthma that is defined as coughing and wheezing within 5 minutes of starting exercising and that improves with rest.

Diagnosis

- Diagnosis is primarily clinical and is partially based on reversibility of symptoms with B-agonist therapy.
- CXR in acute exacerbations demonstrates hyperinflation with increased AP diameter (Fig. 24.5).
- ABG is helpful in patients with severe exacerbations to assess adequacy of oxygenation and ventilation. CO_2 is usually low due to hyperventilation—*a normalizing or increasing CO_2 in an asthmatic with significant respiratory distress is a sign of impending respiratory failure!*
- Allergy testing: 80% children with asthma have positive immediate type allergy skin tests; however, testing is only indicated for patients with allergy symptoms and/or refractory disease.
- PFTs: FEV_1 ≥15% decrease with methacholine challenge and improves with rescue medicine.

Management

Acute Exacerbations

- Give O_2 as needed to keep sats greater than 93% to 95%.
- *Beta-agonists* such as albuterol are the mainstay of the treatment. They can be given as continuous nebulized treatment for severe exacerbations.
- Ipratropium bromide is an anticholinergic bronchodilator useful in the initial management of moderate to severe exacerbations.
- *Corticosteroids* should be given in the initial management of moderate-to-severe exacerbations and should be continued for a total of a 5-day course. Prednisone or prednisolone can be given orally or methylprednisolone can be given IV. Typical PO dose is 2 mg/kg/day (max of 60–80 mg/day).
- Adjunctive therapy for severe exacerbations includes *epinephrine* (given subcutaneously), *magnesium sulfate*, *terbutaline*, and/or heliox.
- *Intubation in asthmatics is problematic* and can result in cardiopulmonary arrest. Reserve intubation for patients with deteriorating mental status and/or imminent pulmonary arrest. Use BiPAP as an alternative whenever possible. If intubation is unavoidable, use ketamine as it has bronchodilator effects that may be beneficial.

Maintenance Therapy and Controller Medications

- Make an asthma action plan! Check and follow daily peak flows.
- Avoid asthma triggers.

TABLE 24.7

CLASSIFICATION OF ASTHMA ACCORDING TO SEVERITY AND RECOMMENDED CONTROLLER MEDICATIONS

	Days with Symptoms	Nights with Symptoms	Preferred Controller Medication	Alternative Controller Medication
Mild intermittent	≤2 per wk	≤2 per mo	No daily medication needed	None
Mild persistent	3–6 per wk	3–4 per mo	Low-dose inhaled corticosteroids	Leukotriene modifiers
Moderate persistent	Daily	≥5 per mo	Low-to-medium-dose inhaled corticosteroids PLUS long acting beta$_2$-agonists	Medium-dose inhaled corticosteroids OR Low-to-medium-dose inhaled corticosteroids PLUS leukotriene modifiers
Severe persistent	Continuous	Frequent	High-dose inhaled corticosteroids PLUS long acting beta$_2$-agonists	Leukotriene modifiers OR oral steroids as needed

- General principles of medication use for chronic asthma management are summarized below in Table 24.7. Please refer to the NIH Asthma Guideline Management Parameters for a more specific stepwise approach to long-term asthma management (http://www.nhlbi.nih.gov/guidelines/asthma/asthsumm.pdf).

Prognosis

- Natural history
  - Sixty percent of children with mild asthma will outgrow their symptoms by adulthood.
  - Only 30% of children with severe asthma will outgrow their symptoms by adulthood.
- Risk factors for persistent asthma include onset of symptoms prior to 3 years of age, eosinophilia, IgE elevation, maternal history of asthma, and allergic rhinitis.
- Risk factors for asthma-related mortality include prior intubation, ≥2 hospitalizations in the last year, ≥3 ED visits in the last year, hospitalization or ED visit in last month requiring steroid treatment, frequent use of albuterol, and history of syncope or hypoxic seizures during asthma attack.

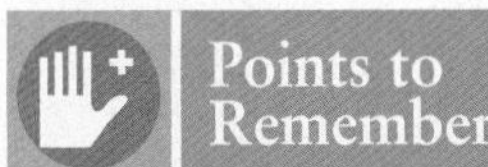

Points to Remember

Side effects of steroids (dose dependent).

- HPA axis suppression (only with prolonged courses; consider taper to minimize suppression; may need stress-dose steroids during acute illness)
- Suppressed immunity (high-dose oral steroids)
- Bone demineralization (long-term oral steroids)
- Impaired growth (low-dose inhaled corticosteroids show no associated with growth delay; medium-to-high-dose inhaled or oral therapy has mild delay in growth for the first year or two of treatment but patients ultimately attain normal height)
- Hyperglycemia (oral steroids)
- Weight gain (long-term oral steroids)
- Oral candidiasis (inhaled steroids)—can be prevented by washing mouth out after each use

Emphysema

Emphysema is a nonreversible enlargement of airspaces distal to the terminal bronchioles along with destruction of alveolar walls. Decreased compliance and elastic lung recoil result. In addition, there is a loss of surface area leading to decreased area for gas exchange. Emphysema is uncommon in children. However, when it is present in children, it is very serious.

Clinical Manifestations

- Lung hyperinflation, wheezing, prolonged expiration, and/or exercise intolerance.
- Often misdiagnosed as refractory asthma.

Diagnosis

- Diagnosis is made by chest CT and lung biopsy, which shows a deficiency of elastic tissue and decreased number of alveoli.
- PFTs with moderate or severe disease will demonstrate a decrease in FEV_1.

Two causes of emphysema that deserve special mention are alpha-1-antitrypsin deficiency and congenital lobar emphysema. These etiologies are included in Table 24.8.

Points to Remember

- Alveoli rapidly increase in number until 8-years old. Therefore, children with severe emphysema in their first years can often dramatically clinically improve as they age.
- Children with severe undertreated asthma can develop emphysematous changes secondary to chronic hyperinflation of lungs that results in loss of elastic recoil.

MISCELLANEOUS OBSTRUCTIVE LUNG DISEASES

Miscellaneous obstructive lung diseases and their characteristics are shown in Table 24.8.

Scimitar Syndrome

Scimitar syndrome is a rare disease of anomalous pulmonary venous return (PAPVR) from all or part of the right lung. It is a well-described constellation of cardiopulmonary anomalies consisting of dextrocardia, situs solitus of the atria and viscera, hypoplasia of the right lung, anomalous

TABLE 24.8

MISCELLANEOUS OBSTRUCTIVE LUNG DISEASES

Disease	Epidemiology/Etiology	Presentation/Diagnosis	Management/Complications
Kartagener Syndrome (Primary ciliary dyskinesia)	■ Prevalence = 1 in 15,000–20,000 (rare) ■ Males = Females ■ AR inheritance is most common ■ Dynein arm defects/mutations cause abnormal ciliary movement → ineffective mucociliary clearance → sinusitis, otitis media, bronchiectasis, and sinopulmonary infections	Presentation ■ Persistent moist cough (starts during infancy) ■ Chronic sinusitis with nasal polyps ■ Situs inversus (50%) ■ Chronic otitis media with hearing loss ■ Bronchitis and bronchiectasis (middle lobe and lingula) ■ Pneumonia ■ Digital clubbing ■ GERD ■ Male and female infertility/ decreased fertility ■ Male—abnormal sperm movement ■ Female—increased ectopic pregnancy ■ Diagnosis ■ CXR shows dextrocardia, hyperinflation, and/or bronchiectasis ■ Evaluation of ciliary motility ■ Ciliary biopsy by nasal/ bronchial brush ■ Ultrastructural examination of cilia from nasal/bronchial brush by electron microscopy = *gold standard*	*Management* ■ Pulmonary toilet to maximize mucous clearance—chest PT, bronchodilators, mucolytics (mesna, acetylcysteine) ■ Antibiotics to treat infections – ■ *H. influenzae* ■ *S. pneumoniae* ■ *S. aureus* ■ *Pseudomonas aeruginosa* ■ Prophylactic antibiotics controversial ■ Sinus surgery ■ Lobectomy—if severe bronchiectasis Outcomes/Complications ■ Early diagnosis and aggressive management is essential ■ PFTs to monitor for decrease in vital capacity, FEV, or TLC ■ 10% have debilitating lung disease
Allergic bronchopulmonary aspergillosis (ABPA)	■ Allergic reaction to aspergillus (noninvasive) ■ Occurs in 11% of patients with CF and in 1%–2% of asthmatics ■ Usually *A. fumigatus*	*Presentation* ■ Prolonged wheeze and cough ■ Productive cough with brownish mucous plugs ■ Low-grade fever ■ NOT responsive to antibiotics *Diagnosis* ■ Peripheral eosinophilia ■ Increased aspergillus IgE Ab ■ Sputum—branching hyphae ■ CXR: recurrent infiltrates ■ Bronchiectasis	*Management* ■ Steroids ≥3 mo ■ Some manage with addition of itraconazole ■ Goal to normalize IgE
Alpha-1-antitrypsin deficiency (AAT)	■ Prevalence is 1 in 3,000–5,000 ■ Caucasian predominance ■ M = F ■ AAT normally acts to protect against damage from proteinase	*Presentation* ■ Children: liver disease predominant (neonatal jaundice, hepatomegaly, ascites) ■ Adults: pulmonary disease predominant (panacinar emphysema) *Diagnosis* ■ Low serum AAT levels	*Management* ■ IV alpha-1-antitrypsin (monthly) ■ If severe need lung transplant *Outcome* ■ Death in childhood rare ■ Death in 40–50s ■ Smokers have much earlier mortality and higher morbidity
Congenital Lobar Emphysema (CLE)	■ Unilobar enlargement due to accumulation of air and/ or fluid ■ Left upper lobe is most commonly affected ■ Can be idiopathic or due to a variety of anatomic defects	*Presentation* ■ Wheezing, SOB, tachypnea, tachycardia, grunting ■ Asymmetry of the chest with hyper-resonance ■ Often presents as severe distress at birth *Diagnosis* ■ Prenatal ultrasound ■ CXR—hyperinflation of one lobe with mediastinal shift and compression of remaining lung ■ CT scan—yield more detailed info	*Management* ■ Distinguish from pneumothorax!! ■ If affected area is small, watchful waiting is appropriate pain management ■ If affected area is large, mechanical ventilation and/or lobectomy may be indicated

systemic arterial blood supply to the right lung, and anomalous pulmonary venous connection of the right lung to the inferior vena cava. The blood returns to the IVC below or just above the diaphragm. The infantile form has high mortality due to a large shunt between the right lung blood supply and the IVC leading to heart failure. In the adult form, the shunt is much smaller and there is a better prognosis.

RESTRICTIVE LUNG DISEASE

Restrictive lung disease is characterized by a decrease in both FVC and TLC. Restrictive lung disease is relatively uncommon in children but can be due to a variety of problems. Causes of restrictive lung disease are shown in Box 24.3.

Interstitial Lung Disease (ILD)

ILD refers to a nonspecific diffuse inflammatory process of the pulmonary interstitium, leading to restrictive lung disease and impaired gas exchange. ILD in children can be idiopathic or due to a known etiology (see Box 24.4).

Clinical Manifestations

- Usually presents with exercise intolerance, dry cough, poor weight gain.
- Duration of symptoms is more than 1 month.
- Physical examination findings include tachypnea, retractions, hypoxemia, wheezing, crackles, failure to thrive, and/or pulmonary hypertension with RVH (loud P2).

Diagnosis

- CXR may show a diffuse reticulonodular interstitial pattern but may also be normal.
- CT scan demonstrates “crazy paving” and “*honeycomb*” appearance.
- PFTs show restrictive pattern.
- Definitive diagnosis is via *lung biopsy*.
- An EKG and echocardiogram should be obtained to evaluate for secondary right heart dysfunction.
- Further evaluation for specific etiologies may include:
  - Blood tests.
  - CBC.
  - Rheumatic disease markers.
  - ACE level (sarcoid).
  - Infectious markers (serology for mycoplasma, etc.).
- UA to look for evidence of glomerulonephritis associated with pulmonary renal syndrome.
- Respiratory samples to evaluate for viral pathogens.
- Bronchoalveolar lavage.

Management

- Supportive care—O_2 as needed.
- Bronchodilators +/− inhaled steroids.
- Immunosuppressive agents.
- Severe cases may need heart/lung transplant.

Box 24.3 Causes of Restrictive Lung Disease

Lung	Pleural Cavity	Chest Wall	Muscle
1. Resection/hypoplasia	1. Pleural thickening	1. Scoliosis	1. Neuromuscular disease
2. Atelectasis	2. Effusion/empyema	2. Splinting due to pain	2. Diaphragmatic paralysis
3. Fibrosis, interstitial lung disease		3. Scleroderma	
4. Pulmonary vascular congestion and increased interstitial fluid secondary to CHF		4. Abdominal visceromegaly/ascites	
5. Tumor			
6. Pneumonia/parenchymal lung diseases			

(Reprinted with permission from McMillan JA, Feigin RD, DeAngelis C, et al. *Oski's Pediatrics: Principles and Practice*, 4th ed. Philadelphia: Lippincott Williams & Wilkins, 2006.)

Box 24.4 Etiologies of Interstitial Lung Disease in Children

- Environment (13%)
  - Hypersensitivity pneumonitis
  - Radiation
- Infection (8%–10%)
  - Bacterial: mycoplasma, chlamydia, legionella
  - Viral: CMV, adenovirus
  - Fungal: PCP, aspergillus, histoplasma
  - Parasitic: visceral larva migrans
  - Can be associated with HIV/AIDS
- Hemorrhagic disorders (5%–8%)
- Aspiration pneumonitis (5%)
- Lymphangiomatosis (4%)
- Sarcoid (2%)
- Neoplasia (Langerhans histiocytosis, etc.)
- Autoimmune
- BOOP
- Drugs (bleomycin, etc.)
- Hemosiderosis
- Idiopathic
- Pulmonary alveolar proteinosis
- Storage/metabolic disorder

Bronchiectasis

Bronchiectasis is the permanent dilatation of the small segments of the respiratory tract (bronchi). It is an irreversible process resulting from damage during inflammation or infection. Common etiologies are cystic fibrosis (CF), chronic aspiration, dysmotile cilia syndromes, and immunodeficiencies.

- Patients present with cough and wheezing. Digital clubbing is often present.
- PFTs demonstrate increased TLC, increased FRC, and decreased VC.
- Ventilation–perfusion mismatch is common.
- Diagnosis should be confirmed via chest CT.
- Treatment includes bronchodilators with postural drainage. Some patients benefit from prophylactic antibiotics.

Hemosiderosis

Hemosiderosis is an abnormal accumulation of hemosiderin in the lungs, leading to diffuse alveolar hemorrhage and bleeding into the lungs. It is NOT hemorrhage from larger arteries. Different forms of hemosiderosis are described in Table 24.9.

Clinical Manifestations

- Recurrent and/or persistent pulmonary symptoms including cough, tachypnea, shortness of breath, increased work of breathing, and hemoptysis.
- Iron-deficiency anemia can lead to pallor and tachycardia.
- Fever may or may not be present (inflammatory response to blood).
- Lung auscultation reveals decreased breath sounds, wheezing, and crackles.
- Transient hepatosplenomegaly (20% cases).
- Long-standing disease may result in clubbing and/or failure to thrive.

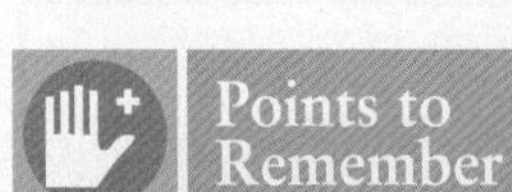

- Do not mistake periodic breathing for apnea. Periodic breathing is when infants take several shallow rapid breaths with 3 or more respiratory pauses less than 20 second interspersed between respirations. It usually occurs during sleep, is not associated with cyanosis or respiratory distress, and is a normal finding in newborns and young infants.

Diagnosis

- CXR demonstrates diffuse, perihilar infiltrates early in the disease process. Later findings include atelectasis, hilar adenopathy, a reticulonodular pattern, and decreased aeration in lower lobes.
- Siderophages (iron laden macrophages) concentrated in gastric fluid, sputum, bronchial washings, or lung biopsy (must use Prussian blue stain to visualize).
- PFTs—establish extent of involvement and show restrictive changes and impaired diffusion; transiently worse after acute bleeding episode.
- Lung biopsy—demonstrates large siderophages in alveolar spaces and interstitium, alveolar epithelial hyperplasia and degeneration, increase in iron content of lung, interstitial fibrosis, and mast cell accumulation.
- Microcytic hypochromic anemia secondary to iron deficiency.

Management

- Treat primary underlying disease.
- Acute episodes of bleeding.
  - Respiratory support—O_2, intubation, PEEP may help with bleeding.

TABLE 24.9

CLASSIFICATIONS OF HEMOSIDEROSIS

Classification	Characteristics
Isolated Pulmonary Involvement	
Idiopathic pulmonary hemosiderosis	■ Usually seen in childhood ■ No gender difference ■ Associated family occurrence ■ Episodic bleeding, worse with viral illness
Cow's milk hypersensitivity = Heiner syndrome	■ ± Elevated WBC and IgE ■ Reattempt to introduce milk every 1–2 y ■ Good prognosis if strict diet restriction
Pulmonary capillary hemangiomatosis	■ Proliferation of capillaries → significant alveolar hemorrhage, hemosiderosis, and pulmonary hypertension
Pulmonary capillaritis	■ Small vessel vasculitis leading to diffuse alveolar hemorrhage
Multisystem Involvement	
Nephritis ■ Goodpasture syndrome	■ Young men ■ Pulmonary hemorrhage may precede renal involvement ■ EM of lung biopsy staining helpful ■ Death from renal failure with 86% 5-y survival rate ■ Poor prognosis—presence of antineutrophil cytoplasm Ab or other Ab
■ Nephritis with immune complexes ■ Nephritis without immune complexes	
Other primary multisystem-associated disease processes: myocarditis, celiac disease, diabetes, collagen-vascular disease, Wegner's granulomatosis, HSP/vasculitides, lymphangioleiomyomatosis, tuberous sclerosis	
Secondary multisystem-associated disease processes: mitral stenosis, congestive heart failure, veno-occlusive disease, clotting disorders, malignancy, immunosuppression, diffuse alveolar injury, insecticides, chemicals (penicillamine, nitrofurantoin, trimellitic anhydride, toxic hydrocarbons, cytotoxic agents)	

  - +/− response to steroids in acute phases; if no response to steroids, use immunosuppressive drugs (Imuran, IVIG).
  - Anemia—transfuse as necessary.
- Lung transplantation—for very severe lung disease.

Complications/Outcomes

- Chronic with remitting relapsing course.
- Repeated exacerbations may lead to chronic pulmonary disease consisting of interstitial fibrosis, pulmonary hypertension, and right-sided heart failure.
- Most deaths are caused by massive intrapulmonary bleeding causing acute respiratory failure or shock.

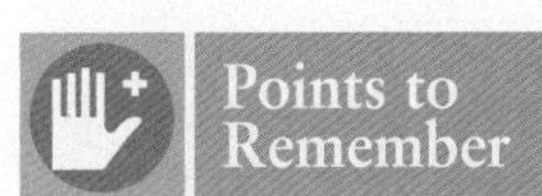

- **In normal individuals, sleep is associated with a decrease in central respiratory drive and upper airway tone, resulting in a mildly increased PCO_2.**

APNEA AND HYPOVENTILATION SYNDROMES

Apnea is defined as a pause in breathing lasting greater than 20 seconds. It can be categorized as either central or obstructive.

- *Central apnea* is apnea secondary to a congenital or acquired decrease in the CNS respiratory drive. Patients with central apnea have normal lungs, airways, and chest walls.
- *Obstructive apnea* is defined as the cessation of airflow at the nose and mouth, despite continued respiratory effort, secondary to upper airway obstruction.

Hypoventilation is defined as inadequate ventilation as measured by an elevated arterial CO_2 tension. Hypoventilation can be due to apnea or inadequate (rather than absent) central ventilatory drive or partial (rather than complete) obstruction.

TABLE 24.10

ETIOLOGIES FOR CENTRAL APNEA

Etiology	Epidemiology	Presentation	Treatment
Arnold–Chiari malformation	■ Central apnea and obstructive aspect if vocal cord paralysis ■ Spina bifida—two-thirds of children with spina bifida display abnormal breathing patterns with sleep	■ Maybe intermittent and appear at any age ■ Morning headache and difficulty swallowing	■ Decrease ICP—VP shunt ■ Ventilator support, +/− tracheostomy
Increased intracranial pressure (ICP)—e.g., Dandy–Walker malformation	■ Central apnea; may have obstructive component if hypotonic	■ Increasing head circumference ■ Papilledema ■ Seizures	■ Decrease ICP—VP shunt ■ Ventilator support, +/− tracheostomy
Congenital central hypoventilation syndrome = Ondine's Curse (*See Neonatology*)	■ Central apnea with normal breathing during wake and hypoventilation with sleep with unknown pathophysiology	■ Presents early in life; symptoms NOT outgrown ■ May be associated with Hirschsprung's disease	■ Ventilatory support at night only or 24 h a day ■ +/− phrenic pacing
Late onset central hypoventilation	■ Morbid obesity due to uncontrollable appetite ■ Central hypoventilation and hypothalamic abnormalities	■ Presents at 1–5 y old ■ Hypothalamic abnormalities ■ GH deficiency ■ Diabetes insipidus ■ Neural tumors with normal cranial MRI	■ Ventilator support, +/− tracheostomy ■ Treat hypothalamic dysfunction
Obesity-hypoventilation syndrome = Pickwickian syndrome	■ Morbid obesity with decreased respiratory drive → hypercapnia and hypoxemia during wake and sleep	Complications ■ Cor pulmonale ■ Restrictive lung disease ■ OSA	■ Reversed by weight loss ■ Some must be supported by mechanical ventilation
Prader–Willi syndrome	■ Chromosome 15 mutation ■ Hypotonia and obesity lead to OSA and restrictive lung disease causing desaturation ■ Abnormal ventilatory control NOT classic central hypoventilation—also associated with obstructive apnea	■ Hypothalamic obesity ■ Mental retardation ■ Hypotonia ■ Hypogonadism ■ Day-time sleepiness common ■ Carotid body dysfunction lead to abnormal ventilator drive	

Other Etiologies: Narcotic overdose, apnea of prematurity (*See Neonatology*).

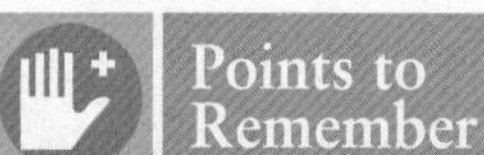

Points to Remember

- CPAP delivers a fixed continuous pressure. BiPAP delivers two levels of pressure: (1) inspiratory positive airway pressure (IPAP) and (2) expiratory positive airway pressure (EPAP), which is a lower pressure to facilitate easier exhalation.
- Recurrent apnea, whether central or obstructive, can lead to cor pulmonale, neurologic impairment (including hyperactivity and poor school performance), and failure to thrive.
- If untreated, long-standing central apnea can result in death from cor pulmonale.

Central Apnea

Congenital Versus Acquired (Table 24.10)

- *Congenital* central apnea can be characterized as neonatal cyanosis without respiratory distress (happy hypoxia). Often these infants exhibit shallow slow breathing not apnea.
- *Acquired* central apnea can present at any age with nonspecific symptoms including lethargy, irritability, poor sleep, and/or headaches, especially in the morning.

Diagnosis

- Diagnosis of hypoventilation requires: (1) assessing gas exchange (blood gas) while awake and sleeping and (2) exclusion of pulmonary and neuromuscular causes of hypoventilation (e.g., diaphragm paralysis).
- Further tests are performed to elicit underlying etiology.

Treatment

- Goal if possible is to treat underlying cause.
- Positive end expiratory pressure (PEEP) via continuous positive pressure (CPAP) or bilevel positive airway pressure (BiPAP) via nasal mask or tracheostomy.
- Diaphragm pacemakers.
- Avoid sedative medications.

Obstructive Apnea and Hypoventilation

Obstructive apnea is defined as occlusion of the upper airway that stops airflow.

Obstructive Sleep Apnea (OSA)

Any pathology that causes obstructive apnea will be likely to cause more problems during sleep than while awake. Obstructive sleep apnea (OSA) results from a combination of abnormal neuromuscular control and anatomic narrowing of the upper airway. During wakefulness, the patient with a narrow airway can compensate by augmenting upper airway muscle tone; thus, OSA does not occur. During sleep, however, there is a decrease in ventilatory drive and in neuromuscular tone that facilitates upper airway collapse. Peak incidence of OSA is between 2- and 6-years old; however, because of the increased rate of obesity, this traditional peak age may be increasing. Incidence is equal in male and females.

Common etiologies of OSA include tonsil and adenoid hypertrophy, obesity, craniofacial anomalies, neuromuscular disorders (e.g., muscular dystrophy), and neurologic disorders involving incoordination of upper airway musculature (Table 24.11).

Presentation

- *Snoring* with labored breathing.
- Episodes of apnea during sleep that resolve with arousal (movement, gasping for air).

Complications

- Chronic hypoxemia can lead to pulmonary HTN and cor pulmonale.
- Failure to thrive secondary to increased work of breathing and decreased growth hormone production.
- Hypertension.
- *Neurobehavioral complications* result from hypoxemia at night and fragmented sleep
  - Hyperactivity, poor school performance, developmental delays.
  - Enuresis.
  - Seizures, asphyxial brain damage, and coma very rare.

Diagnosis

- A history and physical examination consistent with OSA is strongly suggestive of the diagnosis but should be confirmed with *polysomnography*. Polysomnography can determine the severity of OSA.
- Ancillary tests include ABG showing a primary respiratory acidosis with metabolic compensation (acidic pH, elevated HCO_3, elevated pCO_2), CXR or EKG demonstrating right heart failure, and/or CBC with polycythemia.

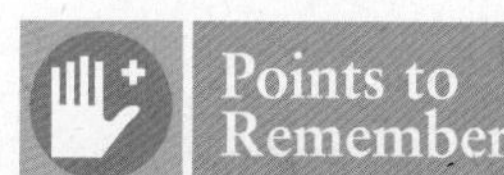

Points to Remember

- **Post-op complications of tonsillectomy and adenoidectomy include bleeding, upper airway edema, pulmonary edema, and respiratory failure.**
- **Snoring without obstruction is NOT an indication for tonsillectomy and adenoidectomy because of risk of post-op complications.**

TABLE 24.11

ETIOLOGIES OF OBSTRUCTIVE APNEA

Etiology	Epidemiology	History	Treatment
Nose			
Allergic rhinitis	■ Common	■ Allergic facies	■ Allergy treatment
Deviated septum	■ Common ■ Ability to move air through only one nostril	■ Trauma to face or nose	■ Surgical correction
Choanal stenosis or choanal atresia		■ Syndromic features ■ CHARGE syndrome	■ Surgical correction
Mouth Macroglossia Hypotonia Poor oral-pharyngeal tone	■ Congenital syndromes—e.g., Trisomy 21, CP, neuromuscular disease	■ Snoring ■ Poor suck or swallow	■ Surgical correction ■ CPAP/BiPAP ■ +/− tracheostomy with respiratory support
Tonsil and Adenoid Hypertrophy	■ Most common cause of obstructive apnea	■ Snoring ■ Apnea ■ Hyperactivity ■ Poor school performance ■ Daytime sleepiness	■ Tonsillectomy +/− adenoidectomy ■ CPAP/BiPAP
Craniofacial Syndromes Treacher–Collins, Pfeiffer	■ Rare syndromes	■ Micrognathia ■ Macroglossia ■ Midface hypoplasia	■ Surgical treatment ■ +/− tracheostomy with ventilatory support

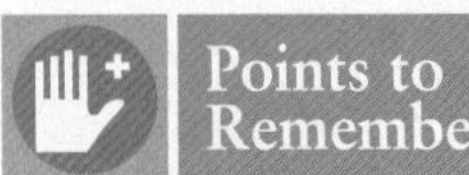

Points to Remember

- Children with OSA are chronic CO_2 retainers and are dependent on hypoxia for their respiratory drive. Do NOT give children with OSA supplemental O_2 without monitoring because it can precipitate respiratory failure.

Treatment

- Surgical corrections are the definitive treatment for most patients with structural abnormalities.
  - Tonsillectomy and adenoidectomy can be curative for patients with tonsil and adenoid hypertrophy.
  - Lip–tongue adhesion for patients with Pierre–Robin sequence and other craniofacial abnormalities.
  - Uvulopharyngoplasty is helpful in patients with cerebral palsy.
- *Weight loss* is a key for obese patients.
- Respiratory support includes nasal *CPAP* or BiPAP to stent open the airways.
- Avoid sedating medications that decrease respiratory drive and airway tone.

SAMPLE BOARD REVIEW QUESTIONS

1. A 6-month-old male with complex congenital heart disease has just undergone open heart surgery requiring cardiac bypass. He was intubated easily for the surgery. The surgery went well and there were no episodes of extended hypoxia. He was extubated within a few hours of returning to the pediatric intensive care unit. After extubation, however, he is noted to have a weak cry and a high-pitched inspiratory sound. His symptoms do not change with position and do not improve with dexamethasone. What is the most likely etiology of his symptoms?
   a. Trauma from traumatic intubation
   b. Bulbar injury secondary to hypoxic event during surgery
   c. Intraoperative injury to the recurrent laryngeal nerve
   d. Laryngomalacia
   e. Congenital subglottic stenosis

   Answer: c. Intraoperative injury to the recurrent laryngeal nerve is a known complication that can occur during open heart surgery. Recurrent laryngeal nerve injury leads to vocal cord paralysis and typically presents as a weak cry and/or stridor in an infant. Although laryngeal edema due to a traumatic intubation is a more common cause of postoperative stridor, there is no history of a traumatic intubation in this patient and stridor due to this etiology would be expected to improve with dexamethasone.

2. A 9-year-old boy presents to your outpatient clinic in September for a school physical. His mother is concerned about a cough that has been present every day for 1 month. When the illness started, he also had a runny nose and his mom thought it was just a normal cold. The runny nose resolved but the cough persisted. He has otherwise been well without fevers or any other systemic or respiratory symptoms. The cough is bothersome to everyone around him but does not seem to distress the child that much. The cough has a honking quality to it, and the only time it goes away is when he is asleep. His past medical history is significant only for seasonal allergies during the early spring season, which improve with antihistamine medication. His mother tells you that she would have brought him in sooner but has been overwhelmed dealing with a recent divorce. What is the best way to initially manage this patient's cough?
   a. Switch to a different oral antihistamine
   b. Educate the patient's mother about psychogenic cough, recommend behavioral strategies, and arrange for follow-up
   c. Start a trial of over-the-counter cough and cold medicine to try to lessen the symptoms of the cough
   d. Perform a pH probe to see if GERD is contributing to cough
   e. Obtain chest CT

   Answer: b. This boy is presenting with a psychogenic cough. Psychogenic cough, also referred to as habit cough, does not result from any underlying organic pathology. Patients are otherwise well and the cough is more bothersome to the people around the patient as compared with the patient. The cough classically has a harsh or honking quality to it. The key to the diagnosis is that patients do not cough during sleep or when distracted. Treatment involves reassurance, removal of stressors, and behavior modification techniques.

3. A 2-year-old girl who recently moved to the United States from Honduras is brought into the ED by her grandmother. She is leaning forward with her chin extended. Her grandmother reports that she has felt warm for the past day, is refusing to eat or drink, and has been drooling a lot. While the nurses are trying to obtain her vital signs, they attempt to lay her down. You note that she appears to be more distressed lying down and resists being in the position. The child is becoming increasingly agitated with inspiratory stridor as the nurses continue their assessment. What is your next immediate step in management?

a. Administer an epinephrine nebulizer treatment
b. Place an IV and administer IV fluids and antibiotics
c. Try to open her mouth and visualize her airway
d. Send nasopharyngeal sample for viral studies
e. Have her grandmother comfort her and avoid further agitation

Answer: e. This patient has epiglottitis. Although epiglottis is rare in the United States secondary to introduction of the HIB vaccine, it is still often tested on the Boards. Watch for a child who is an immigrant, has delayed immunizations, or parents have refused immunization. In the post-HIB vaccine era, the most common causes of epiglottitis in a vaccinated child are *S. pneumoniae*, *S. pyogenes*, and *S. aureus*. Epiglottitis is a clinical diagnosis. Clinical manifestations of epiglottis are fever, drooling, sore throat, dysphagia, and dysphonia. Symptoms worsen when supine and often will improve in the "tripod position" (leaning forward with chin extended). Lateral neck x-rays may reveal a "thumbprint sign." The emergent management of a child is to avoid agitation and be ready to intubate. Further agitation, including IV placement or examination of the oropharynx, should be avoided until the airway is secured. Antibiotics including a third generation cephalosporin and antistaphylococcal should be started immediately after the airway is protected.

4. An 8-month-old male presents to the Emergency Department with inspiratory stridor. His parents noted that he has been constantly sick since he started daycare 2 months ago. He had not been able to attend daycare until he had his 6-month immunizations. This most recent illness began 3 days ago with runny nose and cough. He developed a fever 2 days into the illness that his parent's have been treating acetaminophen. On the day of presentation, his parents became worried because his cough became more hoarse and he was sucking in and using his belly more when he was breathing. Which of the following radiographic findings is most consistent with the most likely diagnosis in this patient?
   a. Chest radiograph with a "steeple sign" (subglottic narrowing)
   b. Lateral neck radiograph with a "thumbprint" sign
   c. Chest radiograph with a focal hyperdensity consistent with an infiltrate
   d. Lateral neck radiograph with widening of the retropharyngeal space
   e. Chest radiograph with asymmetric hyperinflation of lungs between inspiratory and expiratory views

Answer: a. This infant has croup (laryngotracheitis). A classic finding on chest radiograph is a "steeple sign"—subglottic narrowing at the level of the cricoid cartilage. Clinical symptoms include nonspecific URI symptoms followed by a hoarse or barking cough. Children often have increased work of breathing including retractions, tachypnea and/or nasal flaring. Croup is most commonly seen in children aged 3 months to 4 years. Parainfluenza is responsible for the majority of cases. Other viruses can also cause a croup including influenza, respiratory syncytial virus (RSV), and adenovirus. Bacterial superinfection is rare.

5. What is not most important preventive measure for preventing the spread of respiratory syncytial virus (RSV)?
   a. Palivizumab in all children under 6 months during RSV season
   b. Influenza vaccine for caregivers of children under 6 months
   c. Wearing masks around all children who have fever and respiratory symptoms
   d. Good hand washing hygiene
   e. Avoiding crowds, tobacco smoke, and daycare in all children under 6 months

Answer: d. RSV is highly contagious and spread by large droplet. Hand washing is the most effective way to prevent the spread. In the hospital setting, additional measures to prevent nosocomial infections including gowns, gloves, isolation, and cohorting of patients may be employed. However, in the home, clinic, and hospital setting good hand hygiene is the most effective method to prevent the spread of RSV.

6. What is often the primary presentation to an emergency care setting of an infant under 6 weeks with RSV, which is not a common presentation in infants older than 2 months?
   a. Fever
   b. Chest radiograph showing nonspecific air trapping, peribronchial cuffing, and patchy consolidations bilaterally
   c. Apnea
   d. Coexisting urinary tract infection
   e. Improved respiratory status after albuterol nebulizer treatment

Answer: c. Infants less than 6 weeks with RSV are at increased risk of apnea compared to older infants and children, and this is often the primary presentation of such infants to an emergency care setting. Young infants can also present with a sepsis-like picture. Respiratory distress can lead to poor feeding, resulting in dehydration and lethargy. Classic signs and symptoms of RSV in older infants include fever, rhinitis, cough, tachypnea, flaring, retractions, wheezing, and/or hypoxia.

7. A 9-month-old ex full-term Caucasian female presents with severe failure to thrive. She has been followed closely by her pediatrician. Her formula was increased to 22 kcal/oz and then 24 kcal/oz without significant improvement. Her pediatrician also sent stool studies when she found out the patient's mother had switched her formula multiple times because of frequent slimy stools. Stool hemoccult and fecal leukocytes were negative. Bacterial stool cultures and ova and parasite studies were negative. The patient's mother refused metabolic screening when the patient was an infant but seems to be caring for the patient appropriately and allowed the patient to receive all of the recommended immunizations. Which of the following test results is most consistent with the most likely underlying diagnosis in this patient?
   a. Sweat chloride test ≥60 mmol/L
   b. Abdominal x-ray showing air–fluid levels
   c. Bagged urine culture positive for >100,000 colonies of Gram-negative rods
   d. BMP demonstrating hyponatremia from over dilution of formula with mixing
   e. Chest x-ray demonstrating multiple well-defined hyperdensities consistent with pulmonary infiltrates

   Answer: a. This infant has cystic fibrosis (CF). Infants often present with GI problems including failure to thrive, steatorrhea, meconium ileus, or rectal prolapse. Another clue from the question to the diagnosis of CF is that the mother refused newborn metabolic screening. Many states include IRT (immune reactive trypsinogen) to screen for CF on their newborn metabolic screening panels. The gold standard diagnosis for CF is a sweat chloride iontophoresis (sweat test) ≥60 mmol/L. In infants under 6 months, it may be difficult to obtain enough sweat for a valid test result. These infants can be tested by IRT and/or by targeted gene testing.

8. Which of the following is not an extrapulmonary manifestation of cystic fibrosis?
   a. Distal Intestinal Obstruction Syndrome (DIOS)
   b. Thickened cervical mucus in females resulting in decreased fertility
   c. Vitamin B12 deficiency
   d. Increased chance of intussusception if below 1 year
   e. x-rays of long bones and adjacent joints showing periosteal thickening

   Answer: c. Vitamin B12 deficiency is not an extrapulmonary manifestation of CF. Patients with CF have a deficiency of the fat-soluble vitamins A, D, E, and K because of fat malabsorption in the GI tract. Vitamin B12 is not a fat-soluble vitamin.

9. An 8-month-old full-term female is referred to your pulmonary clinic because of wheezing noted by her pediatrician during several well-child visits. Review of the patient's history with her pediatrician and with her mother yield no specific clues as to the etiology of her wheezing. Except for diffuse expiratory wheeze, her physical examination is otherwise normal. Which of the following tests would be helpful in further evaluating the etiology of wheezing in this patient?
   a. Barium swallow
   b. pH probe
   c. Bronchodilator trial
   d. Bronchoscopy with or without bronchoalveolar lavage
   e. All of the above

   Answer: e. Wheezing can be caused by many different etiologies. A thorough history and physical examination will often provide clues as the most likely etiology of wheezing and can help guide your evaluation. When no specific clues are present, however, a more thorough evaluation is often needed. A barium swallow is useful to evaluate for the presence of a vascular ring or external compression of the trachea. A pH probe is useful to evaluate for GERD as underlying etiology contributing to wheezing. A trial of bronchodilators is useful to evaluate for a reactive component. Bronchoscopy with or without bronchoalveolar lavage can be used to evaluate for unusual infectious causes, airway compression or collapse, mass, and foreign body. Although not possible in a child this young, pulmonary functions tests are useful in the evaluation of an older patient with wheezing of unclear etiology to look for fixed airway obstruction, small airway obstruction, and/or increased airway resistance.

10. A 13-year-old African-American female presents to your outpatient clinic for her annual physical. Her mother reports that she has been concerned about her daughter's persistent cough for the last month. The cough is worse at night. The child has a history of asthma with five previous ED visits and one previous hospitalization. She has not been to the ED this winter. She reports using her albuterol on average one time a week because

her chest feels tight. Her previous asthma triggers have been upper respiratory tract infections, tobacco smoke, dust, and mice. Over the past year, her BMI has increased from the 75th percentile to greater than the 95th percentile. On physical examination in your office, she appears to have a normal respiratory effort and her lungs are clear to auscultation bilaterally with good aeration. Of the following, which is the most appropriate management plan for her asthma?

a. Prescribe a 5-day course of oral corticosteroids and arrange for follow-up next week
b. Refer her for skin allergy testing by an allergy specialist
c. Add inhaled corticosteroids to her daily regimen and encourage weight loss
d. Add ipratropium bromide to her rescue regimen of albuterol as needed
e. Start her on a proton pump inhibitor to control any associated GERD

Answer: c. This girl's worsening night-time cough and increased albuterol use are signs that her asthma is currently not well controlled. Adding a daily inhaled corticosteroid would be the first step to improve her asthma control. She should also be encouraged to lose weight as obesity also has an adverse effect on overall asthma severity.

11. Which of the following results of pulmonary function test (PFTS) is consistent with obstructive lung disease?

a. Increased FEV_1/FVC; Increased FEV_1; Increased FVC; Increased TLC; Increased RV
b. Normal FEV_1/FEV; Decreased FEV_1; Decreased FVC; Decreased TLC; Decreased RV
c. Decreased FEV_1/FEV; Decreased FEV_1; Increased FVC; Normal TLC; Normal RV
d. Decreased FEV_1/FEV; Decreased FEV_1; Decreased FVC; Normal TLC; Normal RV

Answer: d. PFTs in obstructive lung disease would show a decreased FEV_1/FEV, decreased FEV_1, decreased FVC, normal TLC, and normal RV. PFTs are a form of spirometry used to measure lung function. They are useful in determining the underlying etiology of a pulmonary process and, in particular, help differentiate between an obstructive versus restrictive process. A restrictive pulmonary processes would be characterized by the results show in B.

12. Which of the following is NOT a cause of obstructive lung disease?

a. Primary Ciliary Dyskinesia
b. Scleroderma
c. Allergic bronchopulmonary aspergillosis (ABPA)
d. Alpha-1-antitrypsin deficiency (AAT)
e. Congenital lobar emphysema (CLE)

Answer: b. All of the processes listed above *except* scleroderma are obstructive pulmonary processes. Scleroderma causes restrictive lung disease.

13. A 17-year-old previously healthy basketball player presents to the emergency department with sudden onset left-sided chest pain that started while he was hanging out with his friends. He says it "hurts worse with breathing." He denies any history of trauma. He says he does not drink alcohol, denies cocaine use, but says that he does smoke some "weed." He has never had pain like this before. On physical examination, he does not appear to be in respiratory distress and his cardiac and pulmonary examinations are normal. EKG and cardiac enzymes are normal. Chest x-ray shows a small (10%) left-sided pneumothorax without any mediastinal shift. What is the best initial management for this patient?

a. Place chest tube immediately
b. Call for surgical consult for consideration of VATS pleural decortications
c. Reassurance and offer referral for drug counseling for marijuana
d. Administer 100% O_2 to see if pneumothorax will resolve spontaneously
e. Needle aspirate chest immediately

Answer: d. The best treatment for a patient who is not in acute distress with a small pneumothorax (without mediastinal shift) is to administer 100% O_2 and observe. This patient has a classic body habitus for a spontaneous pneumothorax—tall and thin male. Often the only clinical symptom of pneumothorax may be chest pain. A small pneumothorax may not be picked up on physical examination. Smoking marijuana has also been linked to spontaneous pneumothorax. If this young man was in acute distress or showed mediastinal shift on chest x-ray, chest needle aspiration would have been the correct answer. Referral for drug counseling for marijuana should be offered to the patient but is not the most critical step in his initial management.

14. Which of the following is a cause of obstructive apnea?
    a. Obstructive sleep apnea (OSA)
    b. Obesity hypoventilation syndrome (Pickwickian Syndrome)
    c. Narcotic overdose
    d. Apnea of prematurity

Answer: a. Obstructive sleep apnea. Apnea is defined as a pause in breathing lasting more than 20 seconds and can be categorized as central versus obstructive. Central apnea is due to lack of CNS respiratory drive, whereas obstructive apnea is due to upper airway obstruction. The most common cause of obstructive apnea in children is OSA. In OSA, there is a decrease in ventilator drive and neuromuscular tone that facilitates upper airway collapse leading to apnea. Obesity is an ever increasingly prevalent risk factor for OSA. Other common etiologies of OSA are tonsil and adenoid hypertrophy, obesity, craniofacial anomalies, neuromuscular disorders (muscular dystrophy), and neurologic disorders involving incoordination of upper airway musculature. All of the other answers listed above are examples of central hypopnea due to insufficient respiratory drive.

15. A 5-year-old obese male presents to your clinic for his 5-year-old well-child check. His mother says that he has been healthy and she does not have any concerns. After further discussions, she says that she has noticed that over the last year he has been snoring a lot more. She has noticed that on a nightly basis she can hear him snoring with the door closed to his room. She says he snores like his "grandfather." She also has noticed that he seems to pause when he is breathing at night. You explain to her that you are concerned that he might have obstructive sleep apnea (OSA). Which of the following statements about OSA is NOT true?
    a. Weight loss is a key in the management of OSA in obese patients
    b. Tonsillectomy and adenoidectomy can be curative to patients who have tonsil and adenoid hypertrophy
    c. Hyperactivity and poor school performance can be complications of OSA
    d. Snoring without obstruction is an indication for tonsillectomy and adenoidectomy
    e. OSA can result in hypertension and cor pulmonale

Answer: d. Snoring without obstruction is not an indication of a tonsillectomy and/or adenoidectomy because of post-op complications. If a sleep study showed obstruction, surgical intervention may be necessary. Post-op complications of tonsillectomy and adenoidectomy include bleeding, upper airway edema, pulmonary edema, and respiratory failure. Surgical corrections are the definitive treatment for most patients with structural abnormalities causing obstruction.

SUGGESTED READINGS

AAP Clinical Practice Guidelines for Diagnosis and Management of Bronchiolitis. American Academy of Pediatrics Subcommittee on Diagnosis and Management of Bronchiolitis Diagnosis and management of bronchiolitis Pediatrics. 2006;118(4):1774–1793. Also available at http://aappolicy.aappublications.org/cgi/reprint/pediatrics;118/4/1774.pdf.

Davis, Pamela. Cystic Fibrosis. Pediatrics in Review. 2001;22(8):257. Also available at http://pedsinreview.aappublications.org/cgi/reprint/22/8/257.

NIH Asthma Guidelines – Guidelines for the Diagnosis and Management of Asthma (EPR-3). Available at http://www.nhlbi.nih.gov/guidelines/asthma.

CHAPTER 25 ■ RENAL AND GENITOURINARY DISORDERS

DANIEL J. SKLANSKY

ACE-I	Angiotensin-converting enzyme inhibitor	Hcg	Human chorionic gonadotropin
ADH	Antidiuretic hormone	HCTZ	Hydrochlorothiazide
ADPKD	Autosomal dominant polycystic kidney disease	HD	Hemodialysis
		HPF	High powdered field
AIN	Acute interstitial nephritis	HTN	Hypertension
Alk phos	Alkaline phosphatase	HUS	Hemolytic uremic syndrome
ARF	Acute renal failure	ICP	Intracranial pressure
ARPKD	Autosomal recessive polycystic kidney disease	IV	Intravenous
		LFT	Liver function test
BM	Basement membrane	LVH	Left ventricular hypertrophy
BMI	Body mass index	MCD	Minimal change disease
BP	Blood pressure	MRI	Magnetic resonance imaging
BUN	Blood urea nitrogen	NICU	Neonatal intensive care unit
Ca	Calcium	NSAID	Nonsteroidal anti-inflammatory drug
Cr	Creatinine		
CRF	Chronic renal failure	OCP	Oral contraceptive pill
CT	Computed tomography	PD	Peritoneal dialysis
DI	Diabetes insipidus	PID	Pelvic inflammatory disease
DM	Diabetes mellitus	PO	Per os (by mouth, orally)
ERSD	End-stage renal disease	RTA	Renal tubular acidosis
FSGS	Focal segmental glomerular sclerosis	SIADH	Syndrome of inappropriate antidiuretic hormone secretion
GBM	Glomerular basement membrane	STD	Sexually transmitted disease
		UA	Urinalysis
GFR	Glomerular filtration rate	US	Ultrasound
GI	Gastrointestinal	UTI	Urinary tract infection
GN	Glomerulonephritis	VCUG	Voiding cystourethrogram
GU	Genitourinary	VUR	Vesicoureteral reflux

CHAPTER OBJECTIVES

1. To understand normal kidney function and related laboratory measures
2. To understand the differential diagnosis and workup of common renal complaints including hematuria and proteinuria
3. To be familiar with the presentation, differential diagnosis, evaluation, and management of common forms of acquired and congenital renal disease in children
4. To be familiar with the workup and treatment of nocturnal and diurnal enuresis.

GENERAL GUIDELINES AND INITIAL EVALUATION

Normal Renal Function

The kidneys regulate water and ion balance and eliminate endogenous and exogenous toxins and other substances from the body. They also secrete hormones, including renin, erythropoietin, and vitamin D.

Urine production relies on two components within the nephron:

1. Glomeruli act as sieves to filter serum, creating ultrafiltrate.

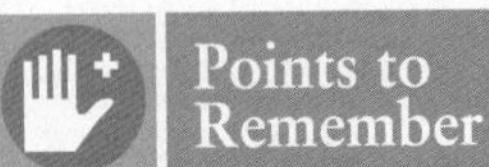

Points to Remember

- In considering pathology for renal diseases, remember that problems with filtration are due to problems with glomeruli, whereas problems with secretion and reabsorption are due to problems with tubules.
- Damaged glomeruli (decreased filtration) and damaged tubules (decreased reabsorption) can result in renal failure with normal urine output.

TABLE 25.1

NORMAL GFR AND SERUM CR LEVELS FOR AGE

Age	GFR (mL/min/1.73 m^2)	Cr (mg/dL)
Neonatal	15–60	Mom's
Infant	Gradual increase	0.2–0.4
Child	120	0.3–0.7
Adolescent	120	0.5–1.0
Adult	120	0.6–1.2

2. Tubules reabsorb and secrete solutes, concentrate the urine, and create and respond to endocrine signals.

Glomerular filtration rate (GFR) represents that amount of ultrafiltrate produced by all of the glomeruli and is measured in units of milliliter per minute. Creatinine clearance is used to estimate GFR because creatinine is not significantly secreted or absorbed in the renal tubules.

GFR and serum Cr vary with age (Table 25.1). GFR is low at birth but gradually increases and reaches adult values by 2 years of age. Serum Cr is lower in infants and children and reaches adult levels during adolescence. Normal Cr values also vary by muscle mass.

Points to Remember

- GFR is best evaluated by the Schwartz formula. No need to memorize it, just know that GFR varies with age and height.
- A high creatinine in the neonatal period reflects the mother's level and does not indicate renal failure in the absence of other findings.

PROTEINURIA

Proteinuria is often found incidentally on a UA obtained for an unrelated reason. It most commonly reflects a benign condition but can also be a sign of serious kidney disease.

Because of low specificity, proteinuria cannot be definitively diagnosed on the basis of urine dipstick results alone, and a urine dipstick showing more than 2+ protein should prompt further testing. The advantages and disadvantages of various methods of testing options for proteinuria are shown in Table 25.2.

Points to Remember

- Urine described as "bubbly" or "frothy" should make you suspicious for proteinuria.

TABLE 25.2

PROTEINURIA TESTING OPTIONS: DIFFERENT ASSAYS HAVE VARYING SENSITIVITY, SPECIFICITY, AND EASE OF USE REGARDING FINDING PROTEIN IN URINE SAMPLES

Test	Advantages	Disadvantages
Urine dipstick	Immediate result	More false positives, not quantitative
Pr:Cr ratio	Only requires one sample	Not as accurate as 24-h collection for protein
24-h urine for protein	Gold standard for severity of protein loss	Very difficult to obtain
Microalbumin/Cr	Good for tracking progression of disease	Not for initial diagnosis

Points to Remember

- Nephrotic range proteinuria is never benign and always warrants further evaluation.

Definitions

- Proteinuria: >0.2 urine spot protein/Cr ratio or >4 mg/m^2/h on 24-hour urine collection.
- Nephrotic range proteinuria: >2.0 urine spot protein/Cr ratio or >40 mg/m^2/h on 24-hour urine collection.

Etiologies of Proteinuria

Benign Causes

- Acute illness, fever, exercise, trauma, and pregnancy can cause transient proteinuria.
- Orthostatic proteinuria is a common cause of proteinuria in teenagers.
  - Proteinuria is present during the day after the patient has been awake and moving.
  - Diagnosis of exclusion based on normal urine protein content on urine collected immediately upon awakening after being recumbent for 12 hours.
  - Not associated with increased risk of long-term kidney problems.

Pathogenic Causes

- Glomerular: nephrotic syndromes, glomerulonephritis, reflux nephropathy, long-standing infections.

- Tubular defects: Fanconi syndrome, reflux nephropathy, metal poisoning, ischemic injury (ATN, etc.).
- Increased protein burden (overwhelms tubular reabsorption): neoplasms, rhabdomyolysis, hemolysis, and so on.

Approach to Proteinuria

1. Complete history focusing on growth, headaches, signs of inflammatory processes such as rash, arthritis, swelling, easy bleeding or bruising, recent illnesses, chronic infections, and family history of kidney disease.
2. Complete physical with special attention given to blood pressure and looking for signs of edema, coagulopathy, and inflammatory processes.
3. Initial laboratories including a repeat UA with microscopy, serum electrolytes, creatinine, albumin, and protein, and urine protein and creatinine; additional laboratories to consider include inflammatory markers, complement levels, and markers of specific diseases.
4. Imaging via a renal US should be obtained for all potentially pathologic proteinuria.
5. Renal biopsy may or may not be indicated depending on suspected diagnosis and response to initial management.

HEMATURIA

Hematuria is defined as more than 5 RBCs/HPF on urine microscopy. It can be further divided into microscopic hematuria and gross hematuria. Microscopic hematuria is often found incidentally on UA or as part of an evaluation for suspected renal disease.

Points to Remember

- Urine dipstick cannot differentiate between hemoglobin, myoglobin, and intact RBCs. Urine microscopy is needed to confirm a diagnosis of hematuria.
- Rifampin and other ingested substances can give the urine a reddish-orangish color that can be mistaken for hematuria—always confirm suspected hematuria with urinalysis!

Definitions

- *Gross hematuria*: visible redness of the urine with more than 5 RBCs/HPF confirmed by urine microscopy.
- *Microscopic Hematuria*: normally colored urine with more than 5 RBCs/HPF on urine microscopy on more than 2 occasions.

Etiologies of Hematuria

Sources of hematuria can be grouped into two major categories according to anatomic origin: (1) post-tubular causes, usually due to extrarenal anatomic trauma, and (2) renal parenchymal disease due to insult to the tubules, glomeruli, or renal interstitial tissue. Findings on UA can help distinguish between these categories (Table 25.3).

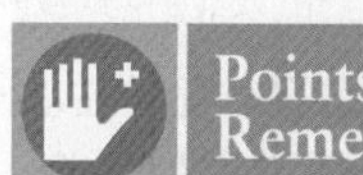

Points to Remember

- Demonstration of proteinuria or RBC casts associated with hematuria virtually always has a glomerular origin.

TABLE 25.3

ETIOLOGIES OF HEMATURIA AND URINE MICROSCOPY FINDINGS ACCORDING TO LOCATION OF DEFECT

	Location of Defect Causing Hematuria	
	Post-Tubular	Renal Parenchymal
Findings on urine microscopy	Normally shaped RBCs	Abnormally shaped RBCs Hemoglobin +/− RBC casts +/− Proteinuria
Diseases	*Structural urinary tract abnormalities:* Hematoma Hydronephrosis Hypercalciuria Renal calculus Renal vein thrombosis Trauma Tumors of kidney or distal collecting system Ureteropelvic junction obstruction Ureterovesicular junction obstruction Vesicoureteral Reflux *Miscellaneous* Cystitis Coagulopathy Infection	Acute tubular necrosis Cystic disease Exercise Familial hematuria Glomerulonephritis Malignant hypertension Papillary necrosis Sickle cell anemia and trait

Points to Remember

- Gross hematuria always warrants further evaluation. If microscopic hematuria is an isolated finding, physical examination is normal, and family/personal history do not reveal any risk factors, it is okay to repeat the UA in 1 month and, if positive, initiate further workup at that time.
- Unless it occurs in the setting of an acute UTI, the combination of proteinuria and hematuria usually bears a poor prognosis.

Approach to Hematuria

1. Complete history focusing on duration and timing of hematuria, trauma, prior surgery, dysuria, urinary frequency or urgency, pain, fever, menstrual history, family history, and medications.
2. Complete physical with special attention given to blood pressure and looking for abdominal masses, abdominal and back pain, urethral abrasions, and genital lesions.
3. Initial laboratories including serum electrolytes and creatinine and urine calcium and creatinine; additional laboratories to consider include an autoimmune panel, complement level, and markers of specific diseases suspected by history or physical.
4. Imaging studies depend on the suspected etiologies but may include plain films, renal ultrasound, abdominal CT, abdominal MRI, and cystoscopy.
5. Renal biopsy may or may not be indicated depending on suspected diagnosis and response to initial management.

ACUTE RENAL FAILURE

Acute renal failure (ARF) is defined as a sudden decrease in renal function as measured by increases in BUN and creatinine. It can occur due to loss of glomerular or tubular function from numerous causes.

Points to Remember

- In female patients with apparent hematuria, always ask about current menstrual status to ensure the blood in the urine is not from contamination.

Etiologies

ARF can be divided in prerenal, renal, and postrenal causes:

1. Prerenal: all types of hypoperfusion, usually secondary to dehydration or distributive shock in children, can cause renal ischemia leading to acute renal failure.
2. Renal:
   a. Glomerular disease: acute glomerulonephritis.
   b. Vascular disease: vasculitis, renal vein thrombosis.
   c. Tubular dysfunction: postischemic, toxic interstitial nephritis.
3. Postrenal: any acute urinary obstruction can cause tubular stasis and elevated tubular pressures leading to ATN.

Points to Remember

- The most common cause of renal failure in neonates is obstruction due to outflow anomalies.

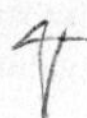

Clinical Manifestations

- Decreased urine output.
- Fluid overload (weight gain, peripheral edema, pulmonary edema).
- Vomiting.
- HTN and sequelae of HTN (headache, papilledema).
- Electrolyte abnormalities (hyperkalemia, acidosis).
- Signs of uremia (pericardial rub).

Treatment

- Correct fluid and electrolyte abnormalities.
- Antihypertensives as needed to control blood pressure.
- Address the underlying etiology.
- May progress to require acute dialysis.

Acute Interstitial Nephritis (AIN)

AIN is an important cause of acute renal failure that deserves special mention. AIN can result from ingestion of many medications and toxins. Presentation may include fever, flank pain, vomiting, and dysuria. Diagnosis is often made by detecting urine eosinophilia and by correlation with recent medication use. The direct mechanisms of damage vary, but the detrimental outcome lies in tubular function, which may return to normal or be permanently altered. Steroids are of questionable benefit. Most patients receive high fluid volumes to dilute and wash through the remaining offending agent.

CHRONIC RENAL FAILURE

Chronic renal failure (CRF) is generally defined as a GFR less than 60 in a non-neonate or other evidence of kidney damage by electrolytes or imaging for more than 3 months. End-stage renal disease (ESRD) is defined by a GFR less than 10% of normal.

Etiologies

- Anything that causes ARF can eventually lead to CRF.
- In infants and young children, CRF is usually secondary to obstructive lesions.
- In older children and adolescents, CRF is usually secondary to glomerular or tubular diseases.

Clinical Manifestations

- Growth failure.
- Nausea and vomiting.
- HTN and its long-term sequelae (e.g., arteriovenous nicking on fundoscopic examination, left ventricular hypertrophy).
- Fluid overload and edema.
- Electrolyte abnormalities.
- Anemia and signs of anemia including tachycardia, murmur, pallor.
- Itching.
- Bone deformities.

Points to Remember

- **Always consider chronic renal failure in a child with growth failure.**

Evaluation

- Evaluate for underlying etiology.
- Monitor laboratories for worsening GFR and electrolyte abnormalities.
- Monitor calcium, phosphorus, and alkaline phosphatase for evidence of bone involvement due to secondary hyperparathyroidism.
- Look for anemia due to decreased production of erythropoietin from diseased kidneys.

Treatment

- Treat underlying etiology if possible.
- Ongoing management of fluids and electrolytes.
- Antihypertensives to control blood pressure.
- Calcium and vitamin D supplementation if there is renal osteodystrophy.
- PRBC transfusions and erythropoietin for severe anemia.
- Patients who progress to ESRD require dialysis and/or renal transplantation.

DIALYSIS

Indications for Dialysis

- Dialysis should be considered in children with acute or chronic renal failure that will result in permanent morbidity if left untreated. In general, patients who become symptomatic from uremia or electrolyte disturbances with signs of mental status change, acidosis, pericardial effusions, and/or EKG changes are candidates for dialysis. It may also be necessary for patients who require fluid removal due to refractory hypertension.
- Dialysis is also indicated to eliminate certain toxins in some accidental or intentional ingestions.

Options for Long-Term Dialysis

Two forms of dialysis—hemodialysis and peritoneal dialysis—are available for patients who require long-term dialysis (Table 25.4).

- Hemodialysis usually requires a stable graft and three weekly trips to a dialysis center, after which the patient is usually fatigued from dramatic fluid shifts and cytokine release associated with the dialysis process.

TABLE 25.4

PERITONEAL DIALYSIS VERSUS HEMODIALYSIS

Factors	Peritoneal Dialysis	Hemodialysis
Fluid shifts	Slow, small volume	Rapid, large volume
Toxin removal	Slow	Rapid
Infection potential	Peritonitis	Graft infection/bacteremia
Convenience	At home overnight	At medical center 3/week
Operative	Initial minor surgery to place catheter	Initial minor surgery to place graft
Growth	PD better than HD	
Functionality	PD patients usually feel better since no acute shifts	

- Peritoneal dialysis can be done in a variety of cycles but consists of indwelling dialysate via a peritoneal catheter. It does not involve large fluid shifts or predispose to fatigue but requires home supplies and daily care.

GLOMERULAR DISEASES

There are numerous renal diseases that manifest with changes in the glomeruli. Although there is some overlap, it is helpful to differentiate between diseases that are mostly nephrotic (primarily protein loss) versus those that are mostly nephritic (primarily inflammatory).

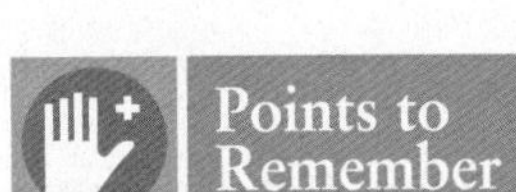

Points to Remember

- Minimal change disease (MCD) is by far the most common cause of nephrotic syndrome in young children.

Nephrotic Syndrome

Nephrotic syndrome is a clinical condition resulting from loss of large amounts of protein in the urine sufficient to cause hypoproteinemia and edema. It is defined by the constellation of *edema*, *massive proteinuria* (>40 mg/m^2/hr), *hypoalbuminemia*, and *hyperlipidemia*. Nephrotic syndrome most often occurs in children less than 10 years and usually has an insidious onset. The most common cause of nephrotic syndrome in children is minimal change disease (MCD).

Clinical Manifestations

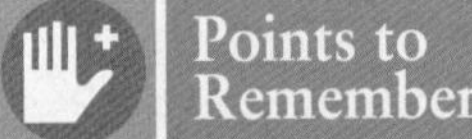

Points to Remember

- In nephrotic syndrome, fluid shifts from the intravascular to the extravascular space as the osmotic load of the intravascular space is depleted due to albumin loss; thus, although they appear edematous and fluid overloaded, patients with nephrotic syndrome are actually intravascularly depleted.

- Physical examination is most notable for edema.
- HTN may or may not be present.
- Laboratory abnormalities include proteinuria, hypoalbuminemia, and hyperlipidemia; hematuria and elevated Cr are uncommon but can occur.
- Secondary risks include:
  - Hypercoagulability from excreting altered ratio of clotting factors.
  - Pulmonary edema and respiratory compromise.
  - Infections (immune compromise from urinary losses of antibodies).

Etiologies

Specific causes of nephrotic syndrome are described in detail in Table 25.5.

General Treatment Strategies

- Control fluid overload with diuretics—but be careful and give albumin as well to prevent further depletion of intravascular volume.
- Control blood pressure with ACE-I as needed.
- Treat any associated infections with appropriate antibiotics.
- Treat underlying etiology.
- NOTE: young children with nephrotic syndrome are presumed to have minimal change disease and should be treated with steroids. If they do not respond to steroid therapy, further evaluation including a renal biopsy is needed.

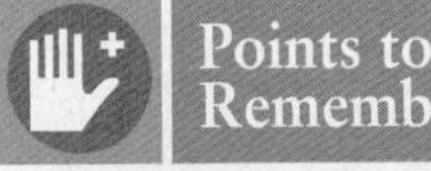

Points to Remember

- Assume that young children with nephrotic syndrome have minimal change disease and treat them with steroids—only obtain a renal biopsy if they do not respond to steroids!

Glomerulonephritis

GN is an inflammatory process characterized by *hematuria* (gross or microscopic), ± proteinuria, *decreased GFR*, and NaCl/H_2O retention usually causing *HTN*. GN is usually caused by immunologic insult via direct humoral autoimmunity to glomerular components or immune complex deposition. It can also result from toxins or cell-mediated immunity.

TABLE 25.5

GLOMERULONEPHROPATHIES

	Who	Mechanism	Symptoms	Diagnosis/Path	Tx	Prognosis
Minimal change (most common!)	Young children	Podocyte loss → protein loss	Rapid onset nephrotic syndrome	Urine maltese crosses Biopsy only if treatment fails	Steroids If steroid refractory, cyclophospamide	Usually resolves Expect relapses
Membranous nephropathy	Older children Autoimmune or infectious cause in about 1/3	Serum IgG complexes → BM damage/ regeneration	Slow onset nephrotic syndrome	Bx → Basement membrane spikes, granular C3, IgG deposits	Steroids likely not effective in changing course	1/3 Remission 1/3 Ongoing proteinuria 1/3 ESRD
Focal segmental glomerular sclerosis (FSGS)	Patients with HIV, hepatitis B, IV drug users, sickle cell disease	Usually a trigger → podocyte loss, sclerosis	Nephrotic syndrome	Biopsy → podocyte loss and sclerosis of glomeruli	Long-term immunosuppression Plasmapheresis	High rate of ESRD in kids
Diabetic nephropathy	Diabetes >5 years	Basement membrane damage from glucose end products	Slow onset nephrotic syndrome	If Bx: thick BM, KW nodules	Control diabetes	Likely ESRD Course depends on DM control

Clinical Manifestations

- Hematuria.
- HTN.
- Laboratory abnormalities may include hematuria, proteinuria, and elevated Cr; depending on the etiology, autoimmune laboratories may also be abnormal.
- May present with acute renal failure.

Etiologies

Specific causes of glomerulonephritis are discussed in detail in Table 25.6.

General Treatment Strategies

- Antihypertensives (ACE-I, etc.).
- Patients with renal failure may progress to require dialysis.
- Most patients require biopsy to establish specific etiology and disease severity.
- Treatment of underlying etiology (many etiologies are treated with immunomodulatory therapy).

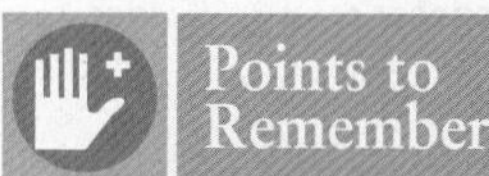

- HUS is most commonly associated with enteric *E. coli* 0157:H7 infections. There is some evidence that treating such infections with antibiotics increases the risk of developing HUS; this is controversial, but it is still best to avoid antibiotics!
- Ninety percent of kids with poststreptococcal GN have low C3 and some will also have low C4. Unlike low complement levels seen in SLE, however, C3 levels in poststreptococcal GN will normalize 1 to 8 weeks after presentation.

CONGENITAL RENAL DISEASES

Unilateral Renal Dysplasia and Agenesis

Unilateral renal dysplasia is the most common multicystic dysplastic kidney disease, sometimes with involution to aplastic kidney (Fig. 25.1). It is often the result of a distal obstruction on the affected side. It can occur as an isolated anomaly or in conjunction with other congenital anomalies. Of note, 40% of patients have contralateral obstruction or VUR.

Clinical Manifestations

- UTIs.
- HTN (due to renin production via damaged kidney).
- Abdominal mass (secondary to obstruction).

Diagnosis

- Renal ultrasound (often discovered on prenatal ultrasound).

Treatment

- Medical management of associated HTN and/or UTIs.
- Nephrectomy is indicated if the child suffers from recurrent UTIs or HTN.

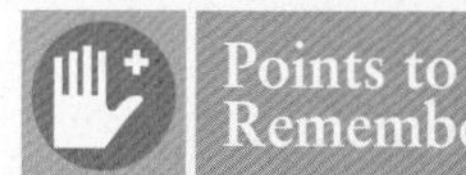

- Be suspicious of renal anomalies in infants with a 2-vessel umbilical cord, abnormal ear morphology, hearing problems, or other major anomalies and consider obtaining a renal ultrasound.

TABLE 25.6

GLOMERULONEPHRITIS

	Who	Mechanism	Symptoms	Diagnosis/Path	Tx	Prognosis
Membrano proliferative GN	Older children	Specific nephritic antibodies→ complement → inflammation	Hematuria, or nephrotic syndrome	Usually low C3, proteinuria. Bx: tram-tracking, C3 deposits	Steroids	Many go on to ESRD
IgA nephropathy	Older children, males > females	IgA deposits cause mesangial inflammation	Nephritic, gross hematuria, often after URI	Normal C3, biopsy: increased mesangial cellularity, IgA immunofluorescence, looks same as HSP	Supportive	Variable, about 20%–40% ESRD
Thin basement membrane	Families, all ages	Type 4 collagen mutation	Benign hematuria	Not necessary if in family, no laboratory changes	None necessary	Normal
Alport syndrome	Usually mid-childhood with family history	Type 4 collagen mutation, usually X-linked	Hematuria, nephritis, hearing loss	Skin or renal biopsy, or family history	None available	ESRD in adulthood
Anti-GBM (Goodpasture if pulmonary involvement)	Older children	IgG to type 4 collagen	Rapid onset of RF, nephritis	Anti-GBM, biopsy: crescents and linear IgG deposits. P and C ANCA common	Immediate plasmapheresis and steroids	Many progress to ESRD
Wegener's	Older children	Poorly understood autoimmune vasculitis	Hematuria, upper/lower respiratory symptoms	C-ANCA, biopsy: crescentic necrosis. Little to no Ig or C3 on biopsy	Steroids, cyclophosphamide	Most respond, half relapse → retreatment
Pauci-immune microscopic polyangiitis	Older children	Autoimmune vasculitis	Similar to Wegener's	P-ANCA (Anti-MPO)	Steroids, cyclophosphamide	Remission, often relapses
Hemolytic uremic syndrome (HUS)	Younger children; exposure to under-cooked meat or animals	*E. coli* 0157:H7 or shiga-like toxin → vasculitis	Bloody diarrhea (but not always!), mental status change, fever, hematuria, hemolytic anemia, thrombocytopenia	Stool toxin, acute creatinine/BUN elevation	Supportive, about 50% need brief dialysis, no antibiotics	Most resolve
Lupus	Girls > boys, African Americans	Immune complex deposition	Hematuria, slower onset	Decreased C3, biopsy: sub-basement membrane deposits	SLE treatment	Depends on control of SLE
Postinfective glomerulonephritis	Boys > girls	Immune complex deposition	Hematuria or full nephritic syndrome weeks after illness; periorbital edema	ASO up, transient low C3, biopsy: BM thickening, crescents	Supportive	Usual full recovery

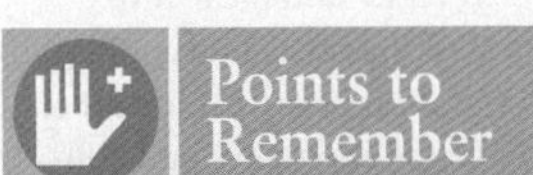

Points to Remember

- **Patients with unilateral renal dysplasia/aplasia have normal function since only one good kidney is needed.**

Prognosis

- Very good if above issues are addressed.

Bilateral Renal Agenesis

Bilateral renal agenesis is associated with several syndromes including Denys–Drash and branchio-oto-renal syndromes and is thought to be a consequence of ureteropelvic occlusion.

Infants with bilateral renal agenesis are stillborn or die from respiratory failure. The condition resulting from renal agenesis is known as *Potter sequence*: lack of urinary output in utero leads to severe oligohydramnios, which causes fatal pulmonary hypoplasia and characteristic flattened facies (Potter facies).

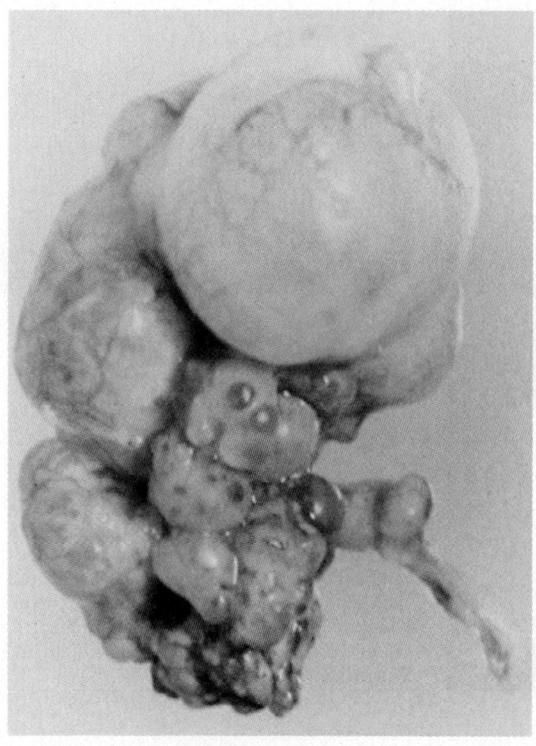

FIGURE 25.1. This multicystic dysplastic kidney is composed of multiple cysts of various sizes. No normal renal parenchyma can be identified. The ureter is cystically dilated at its junction with the renal pelvis and atretic distally. (*Reprinted with permission from* McMillan JA, Feigin RD, DeAngelis C, et al. *Oski's Pediatrics: Principles and Practice*, 4th ed. Philadelphia: Lippincott Williams & Wilkins, 2006.)

Polycystic Kidney Diseases

Autosomal dominant and recessive forms of polycystic kidney disease are distinct entities and have very different clinical manifestations. Table 25.7 shows the features of ADPKD versus ARPKD.

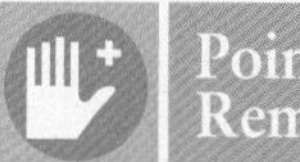

Points to Remember

- ARPKD presents in infancy and quickly progresses to ESRD in 100% of patients. ADPKD presents in adulthood and has a slower and more variable course.
- Do not forget to get head imaging in a patient with ADPKD to evaluate for cerebral aneurysms.

Juvenile Nephronophthisis

Juvenile nephronophthisis (Fig. 25.2) is caused by autosomal recessive mutations involving genes that code for proteins in the cilia of renal epithelial cells. This leads to disintegration of

TABLE 25.7

FEATURES OF AUTOSOMAL DOMINANT AND AUTOSOMAL RECESSIVE POLYCYSTIC KIDNEY DISEASE

	ARPKD	ADPKD
Incidence	1/20,000	1/250
Time of presentation	Early, including perinatally, with oligohydramnios	Usually in adulthood with hematuria, HTN
Presenting symptoms	Infantile abdominal mass, HTN, Potter facies, polyuria, polydipsia	Abdominal mass, family history, UTIs, CRF
Associated findings	Symptomatic hepatic involvement in 50% of infants; can also see cysts in lung and pancreas	Cerebral aneurysms, hepatic cysts
Ultrasound findings	Seen on prenatal US (big, echogenic kidneys with cysts)	US is often normal early in the course of disease
Prognosis	Fast progression to ESRD in 100% of patients	Slow progression to ESRD in middle age or later; ESRD is not 100%—some people do not progress
Treatment	Dialysis, growth hormone, bone growth support, and eventual transplant	BP management, ACE-Is, likely need for transplant

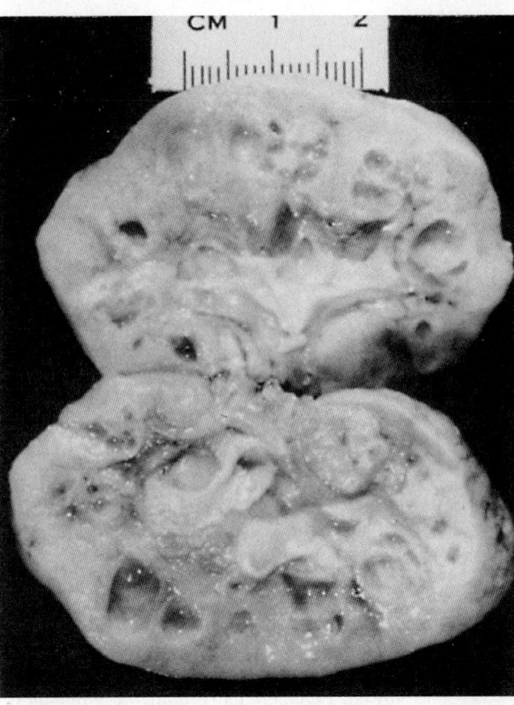

FIGURE 25.2. This kidney from an 11-year-old girl with juvenile nephronophthisis is small and pale. The cortex is somewhat thin, and multiple medullary cysts of various sizes can be seen. (*Reprinted with permission from* McMillan JA, Feigin RD, DeAngelis C, et al. *Oski's Pediatrics: Principles and Practice*, 4th ed. Philadelphia: Lippincott Williams & Wilkins, 2006.)

the tubular basement membrane and an inability to concentrate urine as well as microcystic renal disease. Juvenile nephronophthisis typically presents during childhood or adolescence.

Clinical Manifestations

- Polydipsia and polyuria.
- Anemia (out of proportion to renal disease).
- Associated findings due to ciliary defects may include retinal and midbrain defects.
- Progression to CRF and ESRD.

Differential diagnosis includes diabetes insipidus, *diabetes mellitus*, and other tubular disorders.

Diagnosis

- Renal US may show microcystic medullary disease.
- Renal biopsy reveals disintegration of BM, tubular atrophy, medullary cysts, and interstitial cell infiltration and fibrosis.
- Genetic testing is available but does not identify all mutations.

Treatment

- Supportive treatment focusing on electrolyte and fluid replacement.
- ESRD requires dialysis or renal transplantation.

Prognosis

- Progresses to ESRD but does not recur after renal transplantation.

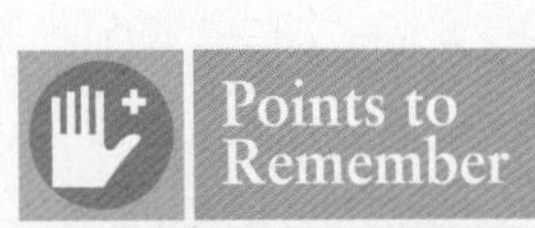

- Cystinosis ≠ Cystinuria. *Cystinuria* results in cystine stone formation due to tubular cystine transporter mutation without direct damage to renal cells. *Cystinosis* results in intracellular cystine accumulation and damage to tubular cells.
- Fanconi syndrome has many etiologies and is characterized by failure to reabsorb electrolytes and nutrients in the proximal tubule of the nephron.

Cystinosis

Cystinosis is an autosomal recessive disease caused by a lysosomal transporter mutation, leading to intracellular cystine accumulation and subsequent Fanconi syndrome from tubular damage. Cystine also accumulates in tissues other than the kidneys, including thyroid, cornea, and pancreas. The most common and most severe form is infantile nephropathic cystinosis, which typically presents around 12 months of age.

Clinical Manifestations

- Chronic renal failure (growth failure, rickets).
- Ocular abnormalities (corneal opacities, visual impairment, photophobia).
- Hypothyroidism.
- Diabetes.
- Infertility.

Diagnosis

- Urinalysis: elevated pH, bicarbonate, glucose, and amino acids due to Fanconi syndrome.
- Slit lamp examination: accumulation of cystine crystals in the cornea.
- Serum cystine levels are normal; urine cystine levels are mildly elevated.
- Confirmation by cystine in leukocytes.

Treatment

- Oral cysteamine (enzyme that cleaves cystine).
- Electrolyte and vitamin D replacement.
- Growth hormone can be used for short stature.
- Renal transplantation.

Prognosis

- Progresses to ESRD but does not recur in transplanted kidney; cystine continues to accumulate in other tissues and causes associated morbidity and mortality.

Congenital Nephrotic Syndrome

Congenital nephrotic syndrome is defined as nephrotic syndrome occurring in the first 3 months of life. Congenital nephrotic syndrome is usually Finnish-type, which is an autosomal recessive condition in which a nephrin mutation leads to loss of foot processes with subsequent proteinuria and injury to the nephrons.

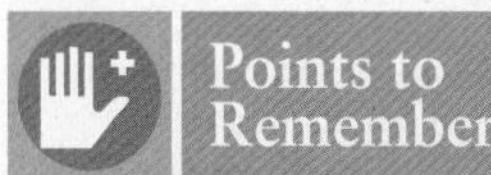

- **Half of patients with congenital nephrotic syndrome have clinical evidence of nephrotic syndrome at birth. The remaining half develop nephrotic syndrome within the first 3 months of life.**

Clinical Manifestations

- Nephrotic syndrome (edema, infections, hypothyroidism, thromboembolic disease).
- Small for gestational age.
- Prematurity.
- Failure to thrive.
- ESRD develops by age 3 to 8 years.

Differential diagnosis includes minimal change disease, FSGS, Denys–Drash syndrome, and diffuse mesangial sclerosis.

Diagnosis

- Laboratory abnormalities include those of nephrotic syndrome (hypoalbuminemia, hyperlipidemia).
- Elevated alpha-fetoprotein and/or polyhydramnios.
- Ultrasound may show polycystic appearance.
- Genetic testing is available for nephrin mutations.

Treatment

- Supportive treatment of complications including fluid and electrolyte management, T4 replacement for hypothyroidism, and ACE-Is for hypertension.
- Definitive treatment is bilateral nephrectomy, dialysis, and eventual transplantation.

Prognosis

- Rapid progression to ESRD.
- Twenty-five percent transplant failure in Finnish-type due to rejection of wild-type nephrin protein in new kidney.

Familial Nephritis (Alport Syndrome)

Alport syndrome is an inherited type of glomerulonephritis caused by mutations of collagen IV. Eighty-five percent of cases are X-linked dominant, but some mutations are autosomal recessive and autosomal dominant.

Clinical Manifestations

- Usually presents with hematuria, proteinuria, and HTN.
- High-frequency hearing loss (progressive; usually becomes clinically evident during late childhood or early adolescence).
- Ocular changes (up to 30% of patients).

Diagnosis

- Skin and renal biopsies for collagen IV fibers.
- Audiology revealing sensorineural hearing loss.
- Ophthalmologic examination demonstrating perimacular spots or lenticonus anterior.

Treatment

- Supportive therapy including fluid and electrolyte management and antihypertensives.

Prognosis

- Men with all forms of Alport syndrome develop progressive HTN; ESRD develops in most by age 30; progressive hearing loss eventually affects all frequencies.
- Women with X-linked Alport syndrome are usually asymptomatic and often have benign hematuria. Some may develop renal impairment late in life.
- Women with autosomal dominant and autosomal recessive Alport's usually progress to ESRD in early adulthood, much like men.

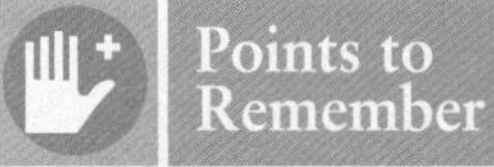

Points to Remember

- Many of the medications commonly used in the NICU are nephrotoxic, including vancomycin, aminoglycosides, furosemide, thiazides, and acyclovir.
- Nephrogenic diabetes insipidus (DI) causes excessive urine losses of water due to an inability of the distal tubules to respond to ADH. Children with DI generally present with polydipsia and will continue to produce a high urine output even if fluid restricted. They must be allowed free access to fluids to allow their thirst drive to regulate their volume status.

ACQUIRED RENAL DISEASES

Toxin-Induced Renal Injury

Acute renal failure can be caused by endogenous and exogenous nephrotoxins and can take the form of AIN, progressive tubular injury, nephrogenic DI, or crystal formation. Examples of endogenous nephrotoxins include hemoglobin, myoglobin, and uric acid. Examples of nephrotoxic medications are shown in Table 25.8. Toxin-induced renal injury is often reversible with prompt removal of the offending agent.

Nephrolithiasis

Nephrolithiasis is much less common in children than in adults and often presents nonspecifically—thus, a high index of suspicion is needed to make the diagnosis in children.

The most common cause of nephrolithiasis in children is idiopathic or familial hypercalciuria. Other risk factors include chronic UTIs, stone-forming medications, high rates of cell turnover with purine loss, and metabolic disorders leading to hyperexcretion of amino acids and salts.

Types and etiologies of nephrolithiasis in children are shown in Table 25.9.

Points to Remember

- The most common cause of nephrolithiasis in children is idiopathic or familial hypercalciuria.

Clinical Manifestations

- Nonspecific abdominal pain (no peritoneal signs).
- Vomiting.
- Hematuria.
- Flank pain (not positional).
- May copresent with a UTI (dysuria, urinary frequency, urinary urgency).

Differential diagnosis includes appendicitis, ovarian torsion, pancreatitis, biliary obstruction, pyelonephritis, and bowel obstruction.

Diagnosis

- UA may reveal hematuria.
- Imaging—abdominal x-ray first, then US or CT if x-ray is negative.

TABLE 25.8

NEPHROTOXIC MEDICATIONS AND TYPE OF RENAL INJURY

AIN	Tubular Injury	Nephrogenic DI	Crystals
Sulfonamides	Radio contrast	Lithium	Sulfonamides
Beta-lactams	Aminoglycosides	Demeclocycline[a]	Acyclovir
NSAIDS			Methotrexate
Amphotericin B			
Vancomycin			

[a]Used to treat SIADH.

TABLE 25.9

TYPES AND ETIOLOGIES OF RENAL CALCULI

Calcium[a]	Struvite	Uric Acid	Xanthine	Cystine
Hypercalciuria Hyperoxaluria	Proteus UTI	Tumor lysis Gout Lesch–Nyhan	Allopurinol Xanthinuria	Cystinosis

[a]Most common.

- Evaluation should also include:
  - BUN/Cr to evaluate renal function.
  - Serum calcium to look for hypercalcemia.
  - 24-hour urine collection for calcium, electrolytes, and pH (hypercalciuria is defined as calcium excretion >3 mg/kg/d).
  - Straining the urine to obtain stones for analysis.

Points to Remember

- **Calcium stones are the most common type of renal calculi and are usually easily visible on x-ray. Not all other types of stones are visible on x-ray, and diagnosis is via US or CT.**

Treatment

- Hydration with 1.5 to 2 × maintenance IV fluids.
- Pain management.
- Urine should be strained for stones to use for analysis and to document stone passage.
- Surgical removal or lithotripsy for large stones (usually >7 mm) unable to pass.
- Treatment of underlying etiology is as follows:
  - Normocalcemic hypercalciuria: thiazide diuretics (increase tubular calcium reabsorption), mild reduction in dietary calcium, low Na/high K diet.
  - Hypercalcemic hypercalciuria: reduce serum calcium based on etiology of hypercalcemia.
  - Antibiotics for associated UTIs.
  - Removal of medication causing stones.

Renal Tubular Acidosis (RTA)

Renal tubular acidosis is a biochemical syndrome characterized by a persistent *hyperchloremic (non-anion gap) metabolic acidosis* caused by abnormalities in the renal regulation of bicarbonate concentration. RTA syndromes have a wide variety of pathogenic mechanisms and causes and are usually identified as part of the evaluation of a child with failure to thrive or unexplained acidosis. Children with RTAs may also have histories of repeated episodes of dehydration and anorexia.

RTAs can be categorized as Type I, II, or IV on the basis of their specific etiology. Table 25.10 provides a discussion of the different types of RTAs, their diagnosis, and treatment.

Points to Remember

- **Type II RTA is common in premature infants in the perinatal period. It is also seen in Fanconi syndrome.**

TABLE 25.10

CHARACTERISTICS OF TYPE I, II, AND IV RTA

Type	I (Distal)	II (Proximal)	IV (Hyperkalemic)
Etiology	↑H+ secretion → $NaHCO_3$ loss	↓ Bicarbonate reabsorption	Pseudo- or true hypoaldosteronism
Laboratories			
Urine pH	>5.5	<5.5	<5.5
Urine citrate	↓	↑	↑
Plasma K	Normal or ↓	Normal or ↓	↑
Treatment	Bicarbonate	Aggressive bicarbonate, possible thiazide	Bicarbonate, mineralocorticoid

ENURESIS

Enuresis refers to the involuntary discharge of urine beyond the age of expected continence. Most cases are idiopathic, and only 10% of children with enuresis have an underlying disease process causing their enuresis. Pathologic enuresis can result from processes causing increased

TABLE 25.11

DIFFERENTIAL DIAGNOSIS OF ENURESIS

Diagnostic Categories of Differential Diagnosis	Examples
Increased urinary output	Diabetes mellitus, diabetes insipidus, sickle cell disease, excessive water intake
Increased bladder irritability	Urinary tract infection, constipation, pregnancy, bladder spasm
Structural problems	Ectopic ureter, epispadias (females), partial urethral valves, and thickened bladder wall (males)
Abnormal sphincter control	Spinal cord abnormalities, sphincter weakness, neurogenic bladder

Reprinted with permission from McMillan JA, Feigin RD, DeAngelis C, et al. *Oski's Pediatrics: Principles and Practice*, 4th ed. Philadelphia: Lippincott Williams & Wilkins, 2006.

urine output, increased bladder irritability, structural problems, and abnormal sphincter control and are shown in Table 25.11.

Approach to Enuresis

1. Complete history focusing on prior continence history, timing of incontinence, family history, fluid and caffeine intake, bed time routine, polyuria, polydipsia, history of UTIs, prior urologic procedures.
2. Complete physical examination focusing on GU, spine, and abdominal portions looking for external anomalies indicative of abnormal internal GU structures, signs of spina bifida that could lead to a neurogenic bladder, and for abdominal mass that could indicate obstructive uropathy.
3. Laboratories to consider include urinalysis, urine culture, serum electrolytes, and hemoglobin.
4. Imaging studies to consider include renal US, spine MRI, and urodynamics.

Patterns of Enuresis

Enuresis can be separated into nocturnal enuresis (night-time wetting) versus diurnal enuresis (daytime wetting) and primary versus secondary enuresis.

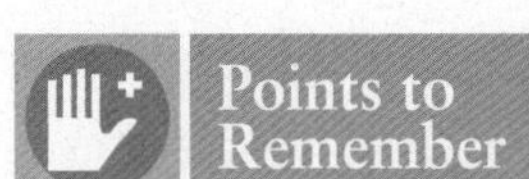
Points to Remember

- Fifty percent of children with one parent with a history of bed-wetting will also wet the bed.

Primary Nocturnal Enuresis

- Defined as night-time incontinence after 6 years of age with no preceding period of dryness or less than 6 months dryness at a time.
- Rarely pathologic and often familial.
- Usually resolves spontaneously with time (10%–15% of school-age children have nocturnal enuresis compared to <1% of adolescents).
- *Alarm systems* are by far the most effective treatment; motivational therapies, bladder exercises, fluid restriction, and caffeine elimination are all moderately effective; DDAVP can be used for sleepovers but should not be used on a long-term basis.

Secondary Nocturnal Enuresis

- Defined as night-time incontinence after a dry period of at least 6 months.
- Causes include UTI, DI, DM, neurological disease, tethered cord, new caffeine intake, and new excessive fluid intake before bed.
- Psychological changes or stressors may also be involved with regression.
- Consider US for obstructive process and MRI for concerns about spinal etiology.
- Treat any associated infectious, endocrine, and neurologic conditions.
- Otherwise, may attempt alarm if no signs of organic disease or psychological red flags.

Primary Diurnal Enuresis

- Defined by lack of consistent daytime continence by the age of 4.
- Often due to urge or stress incontinence in girls and by constipation in both genders.
- Consider congenital anatomic urologic or neurologic lesions: ectopic ureter, postobstructive leaking, spinal cord lesion, neurogenic bladder, congenital DI.
- Diagnosis: UA, serum electrolytes, imaging for anatomic disorder as above.

- For stress/urge incontinence, do bladder exercises to gradually increase bladder capacity
  - Anticholinergics are helpful for bladder spasms.

Secondary Diurnal Enuresis

- Defined by daytime wetting after continent for a 6-month period.
- Etiologies include constipation, tethered cord, DI, DM, new obstruction, UTI, and busy little girl syndrome.
- Busy little girl syndrome is when a child is so involved in activity that he or she does not interrupt activity to get to bathroom in time; more common in girls than boys; treatment is via behavioral modification and voiding schedule.
- Treatment of other etiologies of secondary diurnal enuresis involve correction of underlying abnormality.

Points to Remember

- **Dysuria may be caused by stones, very concentrated urine, trauma, stricture, abuse, urinary tract infections, STDs, or vulvovaginitis. Start with a history, careful examination, and UA.**

HYPERTENSION

Proper blood pressure measurement is essential and is outlined in Box 25.1 and Figure 25.3. Because normal blood pressure varies with height, age, and sex, elevated blood pressure in children is defined relative to age-based norms, which as follows:

- Normal blood pressure: BP below 90% for age/height/sex.
- High normal or borderline blood pressure elevation: BP 90% to 95% for age/height/sex
- High blood pressure: BP above 95% for age/height/sex.
- ***Hypertension: BP above 95% on at least three separate occasions.***

Hypertensive urgency is defined as BP greater than 99th percentile, often with headache or vomiting, but no signs of end organ damage.

Hypertensive emergency is defined as BP greater than 99th percentile with end organ effects such as encephalopathy, seizure, and/or renal dysfunction.

Hypertension can be classified as primary or secondary.

Points to Remember

- **"White coat HTN" or "situational HTN" is when a patient has a transiently elevated blood pressure because of the stress/anxiety of having his or her blood pressure taken.**

Box 25.1 Proper Blood Pressure Measurement

At rest for 3–5 mins
Right arm at heart level resting on solid surface
Width of cuff bladder about 40% of mid-humoral circumference
Length of cuff bladder 80%–100% of mid-humoral circumference
Inflate to 20 mm Hg above point at which radial pulse is gone
Deflate at 2–3 mm/sec
First Korotkoff sound = systolic, disappearance of last sound = diastolic

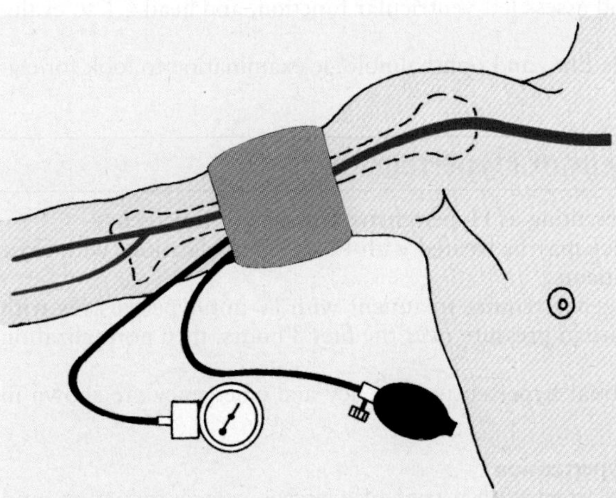

FIGURE 25.3. Proper alignment of arm, length, and width of blood pressure cuff. (*Reprinted with permission from* Springhouse. Lippincott's Visual Encyclopedia of Clinical Skills. Philadelphia: Wolters Kluwer Health, 2009.)

Primary HTN (Essential HTN)

- Defined as HTN without a specific underlying medical cause.
- More likely in older children, especially those who are obese and/or have a family history of essential HTN.
- Usually asymptomatic.

Secondary HTN

- Defined as HTN due to a specific underlying etiology.
- More likely in younger children.
- Because of numerous possible etiologies (Box 25.2).
- More likely to be symptomatic from the HTN itself and/or from the underlying etiology.

Points to Remember

- There is an association between primary HTN and metabolic syndrome.

Box 25.2 Etiologies of Secondary HTN

Renal: parenchymal or tubular damage, obstruction
Endocrine: Cushing syndrome, hyperthyroidism hyperparathyroidism, congenital adrenal hyperplasia
Nephron: glomerulonephritis, congenital renal diseases
Alcohol
Lots of food: obesity
Meds: corticosteroids, oral contraceptives, NSAIDs, decongestants, drugs of abuse, licorice
ICP increase leading to Cushing's triad
Sleep apnea
Tumor: aldosteronoma, pheochromocytoma, neuroblastoma, neurofibromatosis
Renal artery stenosis or vein thrombosis
Coarctation of the aorta
Preeclampsia

Points to Remember

- In general, the younger the patient, the higher the blood pressure, and with less family history of HTN, secondary forms of hypertension are more likely.
- Preeclampsia is important to consider in adolescent females with acute hypertension—do not forget to check an Hcg!

Approach to Hypertension

1. Complete history with special attention to past medical history, family history of autoimmune or kidney disorders, medication use, recent infections, and the presence of headaches, fatigue, vomiting, hematuria, frothy urine, visual changes, neurologic abnormalities.
2. Complete physical examination with special attention looking for papilledema, fundoscopic arteriovenous nicking, increased cardiac impulse, murmurs, renal bruits, mental status changes, and/or edema.
3. Laboratories to consider include electrolytes, BUN, Cr, fasting lipid panel, LFTs, autoimmune studies, and urine hcg.
4. Imaging to consider includes renal US to look for renal abnormalities, echocardiogram to evaluate structure of heart and assess left ventricular function, and head CT to evaluate for intracranial pathology.
5. Other studies to consider include EKG and ophthalmologic examination to look for evidence of end organ dysfunction.

Points to Remember

- Cushing's triad consists of hypertension, bradycardia, and an abnormal breathing pattern. It is a medical and/or surgical emergency as it indicates elevated ICP.

Treatment of Hypertension

Acute Management of Hypertension Presenting as Hypertensive Urgency or Emergency

- Patients with hypertensive urgency may be treated with IV or PO medications with close follow-up as inpatients or outpatients.
- Patients with hypertensive emergency require treatment with IV antihypertensives with the goal of less than 25% decrease in pressure over the first 8 hours, then normalization in the next 1 to 2 days.
- Classes of medications used to treat hypertensive urgency and emergency are shown in Table 25.12.

Points to Remember

- When treating a hypertensive emergency, avoid decreasing the BP too quickly because cerebral vessels adapt to high pressure, and a sudden drop in BP can cause cerebral hypoperfusion and consequent ischemic brain injury.

Long-Term Management of Chronic Hypertension

- For patients with primary HTN, start with a trial of exercise, calorie reduction, and sodium restriction before treating with medications.

TABLE 25.12

COMMON MEDICATIONS USED TO TREAT HYPERTENSIVE URGENCY AND EMERGENCY

Drug	Mechanism	Concerns
Hydralazine	Direct vasodilator	Lupus-like syndrome
Nifedipine	Ca^{2+} channel blocker	Rapid drop in BP
Nitroprusside	NO pathway dilator	Cyanide toxicity
Assorted β-Blockers (-lol)	β-adrenergic blockade	Bradycardia

Data from National High Blood Pressure Education Program Working Group on High Blood Pressure in Children and Adolescents, The fourth report on the diagnosis, evaluation, and treatment of high blood pressure in children and adolescents. *Pediatrics.* 2004;114(2 Suppl 4th Report):555–576, with permission.

TABLE 25.13

PHARMACOLOGIC TREATMENT OPTIONS FOR CHRONIC HTN

Class	Usage	Concerns/Contraindications
Diuretics: HCTZ, furosemide	Best long-term safety in adults	Excessive urination, electrolyte change
β-Blockers (-lol)	May be best with LVH, concomitant anxiety	Fatigue, bradycardia, asthma
ACE-Inhibitors (-pril)	Males, diabetics	Teratogenic
Ca^{2+} channel blockers (-ipine)	Q-day dosing	Mild including rash, edema
Clonidine	7 d patch → ↑ compliance	Fatigue, depression

Points to Remember

- **Obstructive uropathies are the most common cause of renal dysplasia in the neonate.**

- Pharmacologic treatment is indicated for patients with refractory primary HTN and patients with secondary HTN. Classes of commonly used medications are shown in Table 25.13.
- Treatment of secondary HTN also involves correction of underlying etiology.

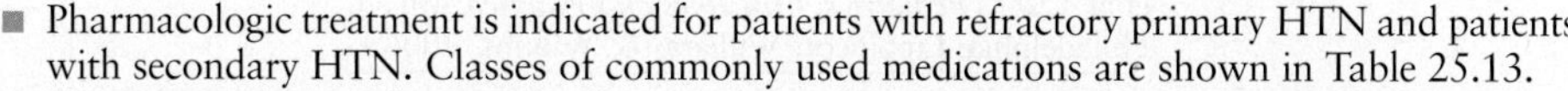

GENITOURINARY SYSTEM

Obstructions of the Urinary Tract

Obstructions of the urinary tract are relatively common in infants and young children and can exist in several different forms (Figs. 25.4–25.7). Obstructive uropathies usually cause some degree of hydronephrosis (static fluid in the collecting system) and can ultimately lead to permanent renal damage and failure.

General signs and symptoms associated with obstructive uropathies include abdominal pain, abdominal masses, growth failure, urinary tract infections, irritability, and poor urine output.

Specific obstructive uropathies are discussed in Table 25.14.

Points to Remember

- **Hydronephrosis is static fluid in the collecting system and can be bilateral or unilateral. It is usually the result of vesicoureteral reflux (VUR) or obstructed flow of urine.**

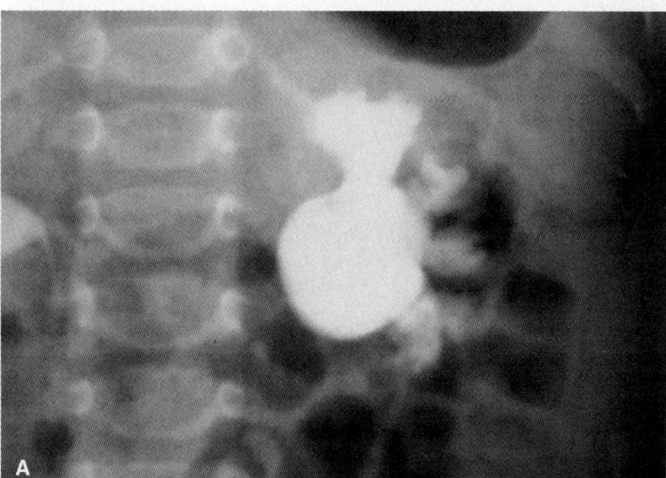

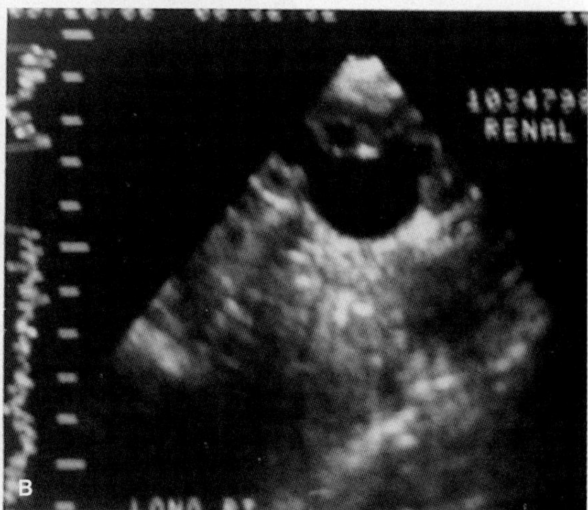

FIGURE 25.4. Ureteropelvic junction obstruction demonstrated by (A) intravenous pyelography and (B) renal ultrasound. (*Reprinted with permission from* McMillan JA, Feigin RD, DeAngelis C, et al. *Oski's Pediatrics: Principles and Practice*, 4th ed. Philadelphia: Lippincott Williams & Wilkins, 2006.)

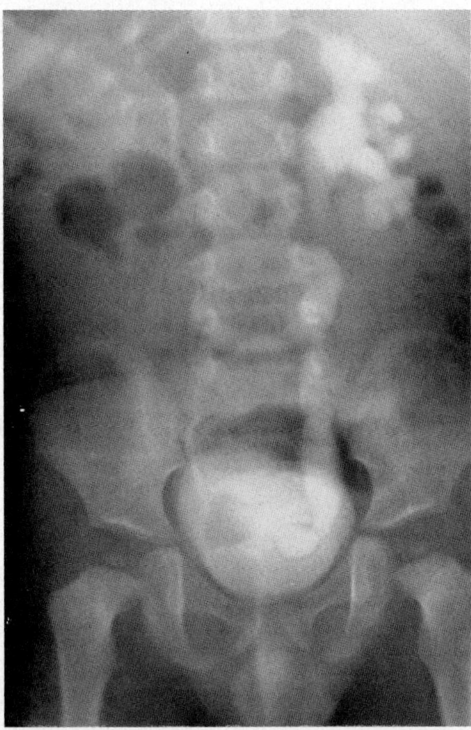

FIGURE 25.5. A simple ureterocele is shown in this intravenous pyelogram. Note the ureteral dilation and swelling of the distal ureter. (*Reprinted with permission from* McMillan JA, Feigin RD, DeAngelis C, et al. *Oski's Pediatrics: Principles and Practice*, 4th ed. Philadelphia: Lippincott Williams & Wilkins, 2006.)

Vesicoureteral Reflux

Vesicoureteral reflux is the leakage of urine proximally from vesicourethral valves with retrograde flow. It is thought to be due to a shortened submucosal portion of the ureter, leading to a perpendicular insertion of the ureter into the bladder and a short valve. VUR is graded I through V on the basis of severity (Fig. 25.8).

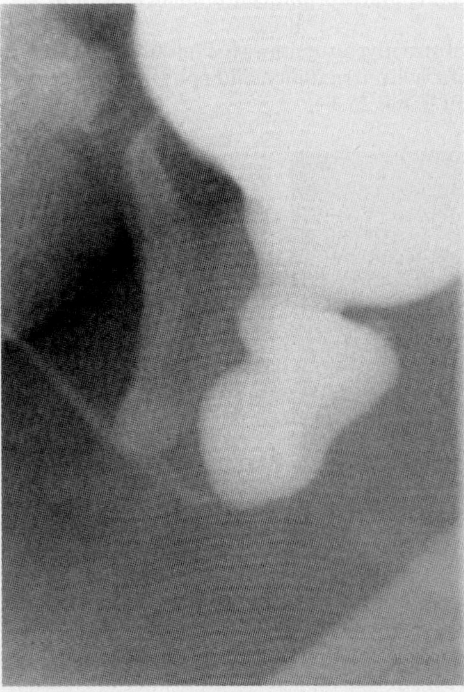

FIGURE 25.6. A newborn boy with typical radiographic findings of posterior urethral valves. (*Reprinted with permission from* Gonzales ET, Jr. Genitourinary disorders in the neonate. In: Whitaker RH, Woodard JR, eds. *Paediatric Urology*. London: Butterworth, 1985.)

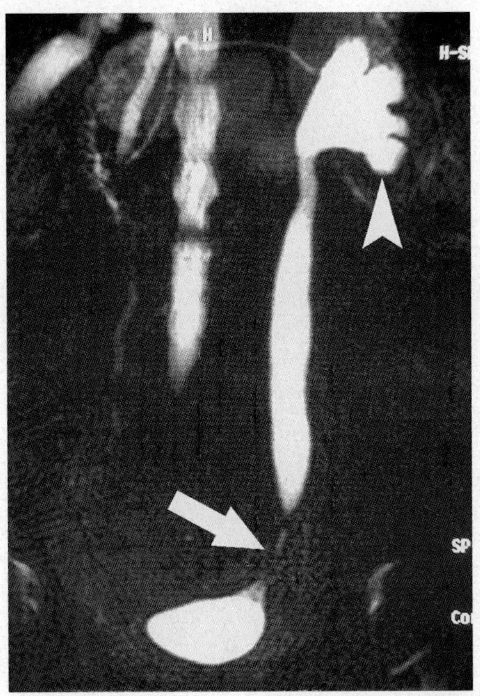

FIGURE 25.7. Benign ureteral stricture. Coronal thick-slab static MR urogram image demonstrates smoothly tapered stricture (**arrow**) of distal ureter related to prior stone disease and instrumentation. Stricture has resulted in hydronephrosis (**arrowhead**). (*Reprinted with permission from* Leyendecker JR, Brown JJ. *Practical Guide to Abdominal and Pelvic MRI*. Philadelphia: Lippincott Williams & Wilkins, 2004.)

Clinical Manifestations

- Usually presents with UTI or pyelonephritis; can also present with reflux nephropathy and renal failure.
- Physical examination findings may include abdominal mass, hypertension, and growth failure.

Diagnosis

- Renal US may demonstrate hydronephrosis.
- VCUG is the gold standard for diagnosis of VUR.

TABLE 25.14

OBSTRUCTIVE UROPATHIES IN INFANTS AND CHILDREN

	Definition	Clinical Manifestations	Diagnosis	Treatment	Prognosis
Hydronephrosis	Static fluid in collecting system	May be incidental finding or due to workup for obstruction or UTI	Ultrasound	Depends on etiology	Depends on etiology
Ureteropelvic junction (UPJ) obstruction	Collection of urine distal to UPJ, often due to fibrosis	Obstructive symptoms (sometimes seen on prenatal US)	Ultrasound and VCUG	Surgical relief of obstruction	Good if treated early
Ureterocele	Cystic dilatation of ureter within bladder	Obstructive symptoms or prenatal US	VCUG best. *Cobra head* on x-ray	None if not obstructive. Else, transurethral incision	Excellent
Posterior urethral valve	*Only in boys*, obstructive leaflets in prostatic urethra	Bilateral hydronephrosis on prenatal US, poor urine output, obstructive symptoms	VCUG	Surgical valvectomy, likely ureterostomies while bladder recovers from high pressures	Variable, but many go to ESRD even if treated. Cr >1.0 at presentation → poor prognosis
Duplicated collecting system	Duplication of any part of collecting system	Often on US for UTI. With obstruction if other anatomic problems	US or VCUG	Resection if urinary stasis or severe VUR. High incidence in siblings	Usually very good

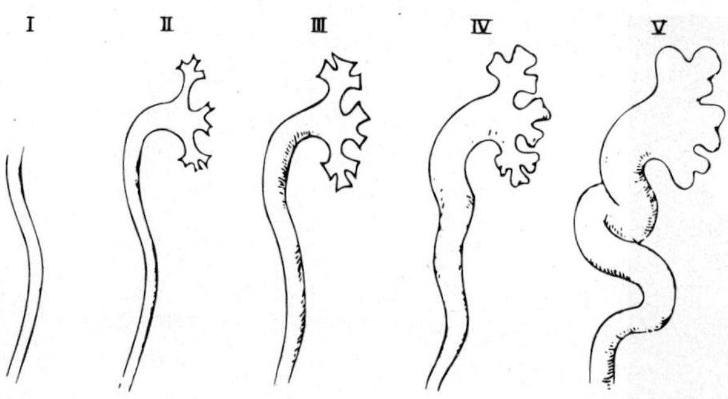

FIGURE 25.8. Classification of vesicoureteral reflux. (*Reprinted with permission from* Report of the International Reflux Study Committee. Medical versus surgical treatment of primary vesicoureteral reflux. *Pediatrics.* 1981;67:392–400.)

- Nuclear scan is useful to assess the degree of scarring in severe cases

Treatment

Table 25.15 outlines the basic principles of management of VUR according to grade.

- Depending on the severity and associated complications, prophylactic antibiotics may be indicated to prevent UTIs associated with VUR (this is controversial but is still the standard of care).
- Operative management is indicated in severe cases. Table 25.16 discusses surgical options for managing VUR.

Prognosis

- Depending on severity, most cases of VUR resolve spontaneously.
- Prognosis is excellent with early detection and appropriate follow-up.
- Untreated, VUR associated with recurrent UTIs and reflux nephropathy can lead to chronic scarring and renal failure.

Points to Remember

- **Hypospadias plus undescended testicles should suggest female pseudohermaphroditism.**

TABLE 25.15

INDICATIONS FOR PROPHYLACTIC ANTIBIOTICS AND OPERATIVE TREATMENT IN VUR

Type	Antibiotic Prophylaxis	Spontaneous Resolution	Surgical Treatment Needed
I–II	Debated	75%	If repeat UTIs on antibiotics, scarring, persistent very long term
III–IV	Yes	25% for grade 4	If persistent
V	Yes	<25%	On presentation if scarring, or if persistent

TABLE 25.16

SURGICAL OPTIONS FOR MANAGEMENT OF SEVERE VUR

Method	Inpatient Post op	Effectiveness	Invasiveness
Reimplantation	Yes	99%	Open operation
Deflux	No	85%	Transurethral

[a]Deflux is an agent injected into valve sites transurethrally to increase valve bulk.

CONGENITAL GU ANOMALIES

Chordee

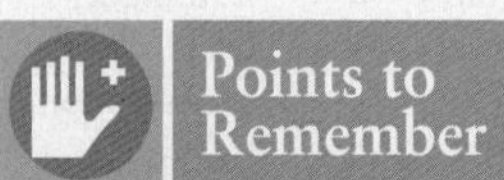
Points to Remember

- **Chordee is a common associated lesion with many congenital male urogenital abnormalities.**

Chordee is the downward curvature of erect penis due to paucity or scarring of tissue on ventral surface of penis (Fig. 25.9). It can occur as an isolated deformity but is often associated with hypospadias or other anomalies.

Presentation

- Seen with erection in infant.

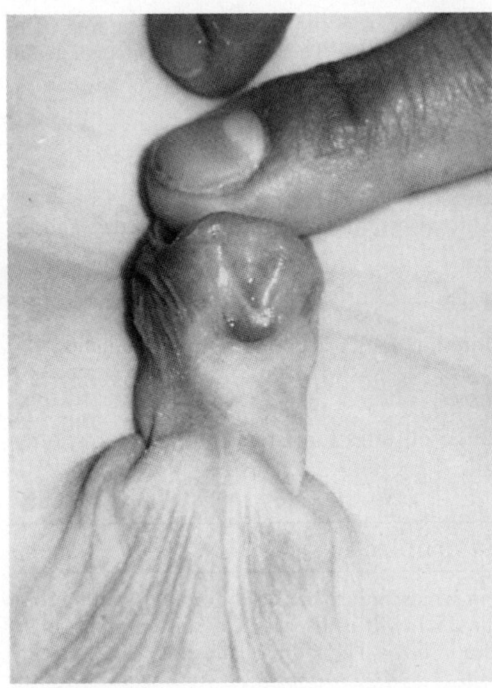

FIGURE 25.9. Severe chordee and deficiency of the ventral penile skin is seen. (*Reprinted with permission from* McMillan JA, Feigin RD, DeAngelis C, et al. *Oski's Pediatrics: Principles and Practice*, 4th ed. Philadelphia: Lippincott Williams & Wilkins, 2006.)

Treatment

- Lysis of ventral adhesions for minor repairs, tissue graft for severe cases.

Prognosis

- Good.

Hypospadias

Hypospadias occurs when the urethral plate fails to close, resulting in an abnormally placed urinary meatus on the ventral side of the penis rather than at the tip of the penis (Fig. 25.10).

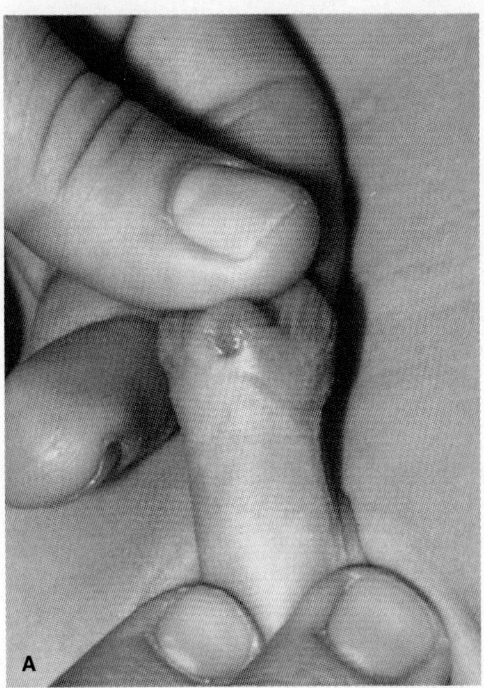

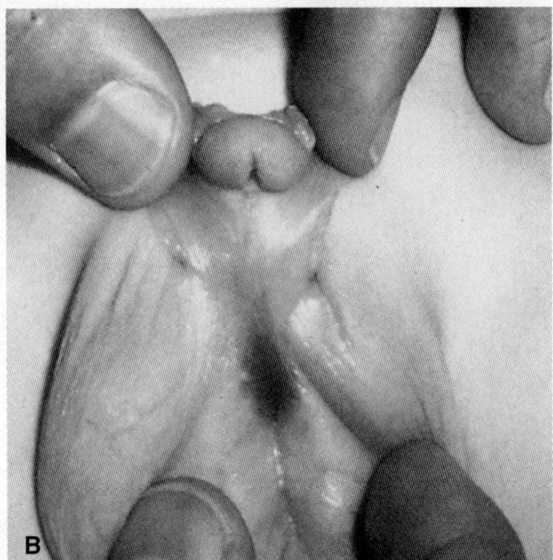

FIGURE 25.10. Two cases of hypospadias with varying degrees of involvement. (**A**) A distal meatus without evidence of concomitant chordee. (**B**) A perineal hypospadias with severe chordee. (*Reprinted with permission from* McMillan JA, Feigin RD, DeAngelis C, et al. *Oski's Pediatrics: Principles and Practice*, 4th ed. Philadelphia: Lippincott Williams & Wilkins, 2006.)

Hypospadias is the most common penile anomaly and can occur as an isolated finding or in association with chordee, bifid scrotum, and other anomalies. There is a high concordance in siblings.

Presentation

- Urination from ventral portion of penis.
- If very distal defect, may be covered by foreskin.
- Full GU examination should be performed to assess for viable foreskin for repair and for associated anomalies.

Treatment

- Surgical reconstruction of urethra using foreskin and correction of other anomalies.

Prognosis

- Good cosmetic outcome, but high complication rates for fistulas and strictures, often requiring further minor operations.

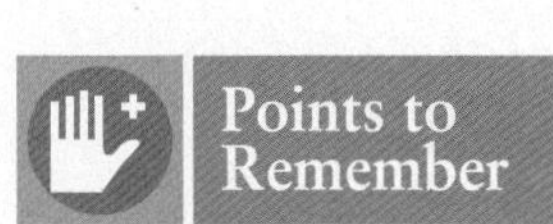

- **Do not circumcise a male who may need genital repair, especially with hypospadias.**

Bladder Exstrophy

Bladder exstrophy is a rare congenital anomaly in which failure of the abdominal wall to close properly results in protrusion of the bladder (Fig. 25.11). It is also associated with abnormalities of the pelvic bone, bifid genitalia, and chordee in boys. The kidneys and ureters are usually normal as are other organ systems.

Presentation

- May or may not be identified on prenatal U/S.
- Defect is obvious at birth with exposed, open bladder fused to midline lower abdominal wall.

Treatment

- Initial management in the delivery room includes covering the lesion with a translucent sterile dressing.
- Definitive management with complex multistaged operations including bladder closure with externalized bladder neck, repairing genitals, and eventual connection of bladder neck to repaired urethra.

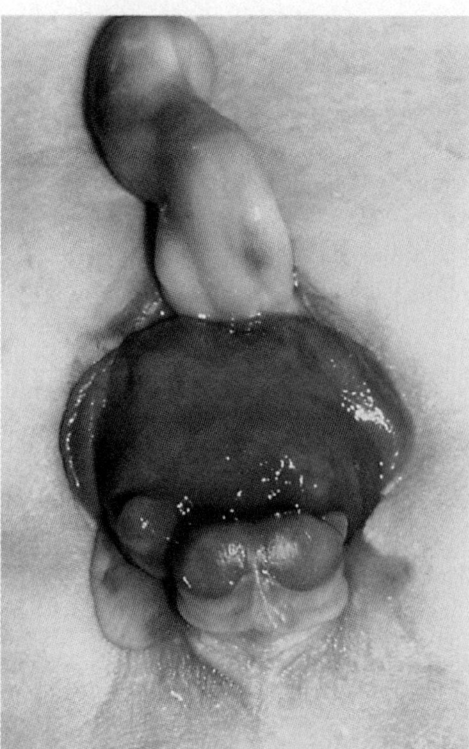

FIGURE 25.11. A typical example of classical bladder exstrophy. (*Reprinted with permission from* Gonzales ET, Jr. Genitourinary disorders in the neonate. In: Whitaker RH, Woodard JR, eds. *Paediatric Urology*. London: Butterworth, 1985.)

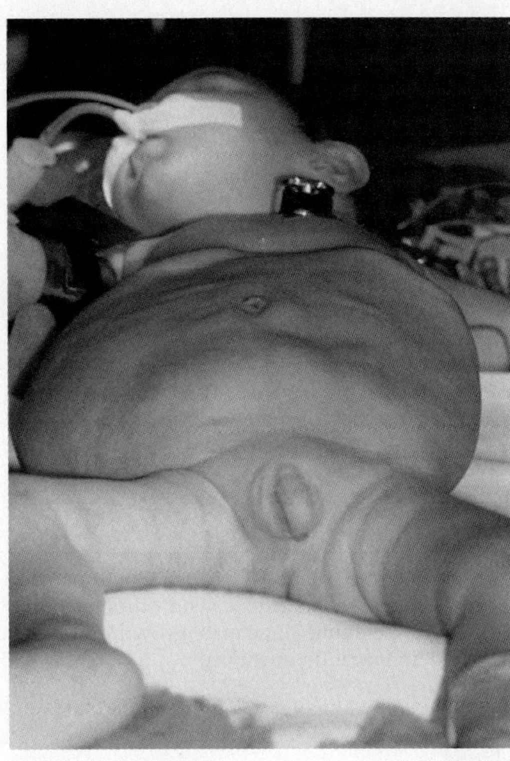

FIGURE 25.12. Typical appearance of a child with Prune–Belly syndrome. (*Reprinted with permission from* Gonzales ET, Jr. Genitourinary disorders in the neonate. In: Whitaker RH, Woodard JR, eds. *Paediatric Urology*. London: Butterworth, 1985.)

- Iliac osteotomies are often required to make room for the bladder.

Prognosis

- Improved surgical techniques allow many but not all patients to achieve urinary continence and acceptable sexual function.

Prune–Belly Syndrome (Eagle–Barrett)

Prune–Belly syndrome occurs only in boys and involves a rare absence of abdominal musculature with abdominal testes and dilated but unobstructed urinary collecting system (Fig. 25.12). A wide spectrum of disease exists, from subtle-to-severe GU anomalies, with possible urethral atresia, dysmorphic kidneys, and patent urachus.

Presentation

- GU anomalies are often identified on prenatal US, and lack of abdominal muscular is usually obvious at birth, but subtle cases may present later with renal failure.
- US will confirm GU anomalies.

Treatment

- Early surgery is not recommended unless there is urethral involvement.
- It is, however, advised to have orchiopexy within 1 year.
- Patients will likely require ureteral implantation due to valve incompetence and reflux leading to UTIs and may require abdominoplasty later in life.

Prognosis

- Patients frequently have infertility and may progress to renal failure if they have severe anomalies or delayed repair.
- Abdominal weakness can limit activity and affect physical appearance.

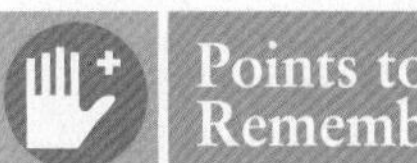

Points to Remember

- **Retractile testis can easily be mistaken for cryptorchidism—be sure to do a careful examination in a warm room with warm hands and confirm your findings with ultrasound if necessary.**

Cryptorchidism

Cryptorchidism is the failure of one or both of the testes to descend, resulting in inguinal or abdominal testes. It is relatively common, occurring in 4% of newborns and 30% of premature infants.

Presentation

- Careful palpation on physical examination reveals an empty scrotal sac, possibly with palpation of the testis in the inguinal canal.
- Confirmation via US.

Treatment

- Because many cases will resolve spontaneously within the first year of life, orchiopexy is usually deferred until approximately 12 months of age.

Prognosis

- Outcomes are excellent with early treatment.
- Delayed treatment can result in infertility, especially if bilateral.
- Of note, testes with a history of maldescent have a tenfold increased risk of testicular cancer, and although orchiopexy does not decrease the risk of malignancy, it does increase the likelihood that a malignancy will be detected and treated earlier.

Micropenis

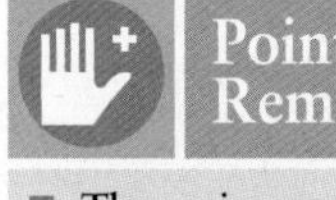
Points to Remember

- The penis may appear small in obese males but actually be normal in size.

Micropenis is defined as a stretched penis less than 2.5 cm in a term newborn or less than the age-appropriate norm in an older child. Micropenis is often seen in genetic syndromes including Prader–Willi syndrome or with endocrine abnormalities including inadequate growth hormone, abnormalities in testosterone pathway hormones, and androgen insensitivity.

Presentation

- Usually at birth, sometimes during childhood.

Treatment

- Testosterone or growth hormone therapy depending on etiology.
- Usually there is no surgical intervention in childhood.
- Likely need counseling later in life.

Prognosis

Points to Remember

- If you see a child with hypoglycemia and micropenis, think about growth hormone deficiency.

- Variable depending on condition.
- Some eventually achieve normal penile length.

Phimosis

Phimosis is defined as scarring or narrowing of the prepuce that prevents its retraction.

Presentation

- Normal in infants, but can persist into later childhood or occur as result of trauma or infection.

Treatment

- Do not attempt blunt retraction.
- Consider circumcision if scarring or very narrowed in boys over 3 years.

Prognosis

- Excellent with time for infants.
- Circumcision may be required for older boys.

Paraphimosis

Paraphimosis is defined as the incarceration and ischemia of the glans after insult or flipped retraction of the prepuce (Fig. 25.13).

Presentation

- Severe pain.
- Edema.

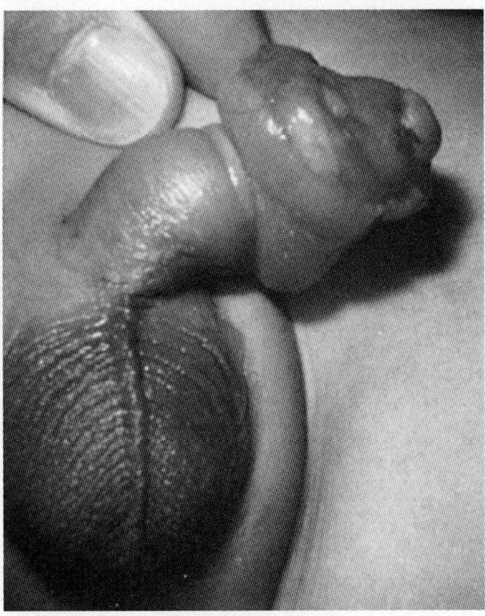

FIGURE 25.13. Paraphimosis. A foreskin that is left in a retracted position leads to venous congestion and edema of the foreskin. (*Reprinted with permission from* Fleisher GR, Ludwig S, Henretig FM, et al. *Textbook of Pediatric Emergency Medicine*, 5th ed. Philadelphia: Lippincott Williams & Wilkins, 2005.)

Treatment

- If identified early, reduction of prepuce back over the glans may be sufficient.
- If prepuce very edematous or not mobile, may require incision and/or circumcision.

Prognosis

- Can lead to necrosis if not treated.
- Excellent with early intervention.

Ambiguous Genitalia

Ambiguous genitalia are often seen with in utero overproduction of androgen in XX infants, androgen insensitivity, or underproduction in XY infants (Fig. 25.14). The most common cause of ambiguous genitalia is congenital adrenal hyperplasia in female infants (male infants with CAH have normal external male genitalia).

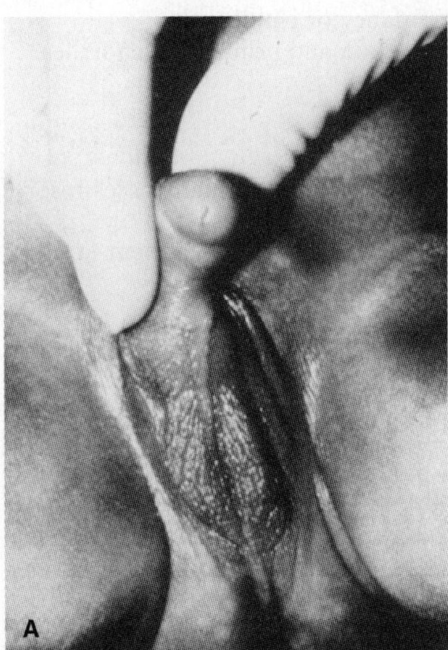

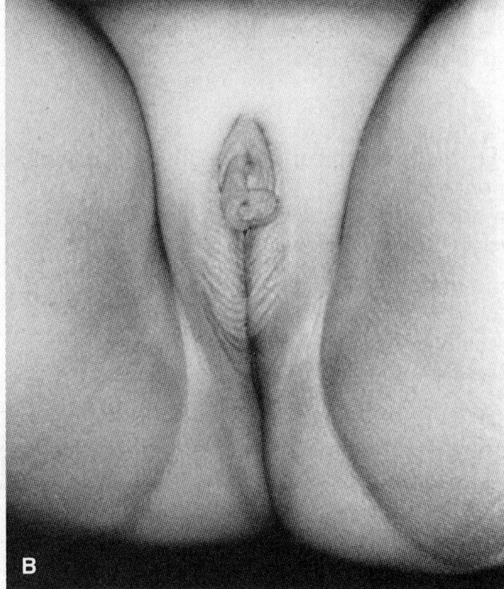

FIGURE 25.14. (**A**) Infant with 46,XX congenital adrenal hyperplasia. The degree of virilization of this infant resulted in an initial male gender assignment. Note the well-formed phallus, scrotum with rugae, and mild hypospadias. No gonads were palpable. (**B**) Infant with early testicular regression syndrome. Severe undervirilization of genitalia in a 46,XY infant with early testicular loss. (*Reprinted with permission from* McMillan JA, Feigin RD, DeAngelis C, et al. *Oski's Pediatrics: Principles and Practice*, 4th ed. Philadelphia: Lippincott Williams & Wilkins, 2006.)

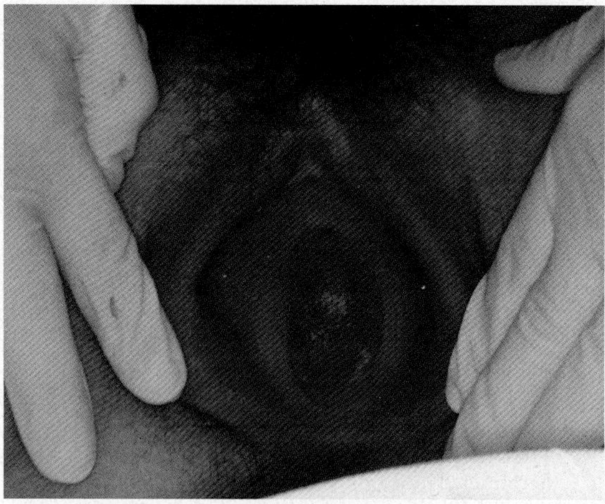

FIGURE 25.15. Imperforate hymen. (*Reprinted with permission from* Fleisher GR, Ludwig S, Baskin MN. *Atlas of Pediatric Emergency Medicine*. Philadelphia: Lippincott Williams & Wilkins, 2004.)

Presentation

- At birth.

Treatment

- Depends on underlying physiology and likely gender identity as predicted by hormonal exposure in utero.
- Gender reassignment approached with extreme caution.
- Very controversial.

Prognosis

- Variable depending on underlying etiology, physical appearance, surgical outcome, and ability to correlate physical appearance and function with eventual gender identity.

Imperforate Hymen

Imperforate hymen is a relative common finding in which the hymen completely obstructs vaginal flow (Fig. 25.15). It is usually an idiopathic congenital abnormality but can be secondary to inflammation and subsequent scaring as a result of sexual abuse.

Presentation

- Can be detected on careful physical examination in infancy or childhood.
- Undiagnosed adolescents may present with abdominal pain and primary amenorrhea.
- Confirmation via US.

Treatment

- May defer treatment in neonate or young child until adolescence as many cases resolve spontaneously.
- In adolescents with hematocolpos, OCPs can be tried as an initial treatment strategy before proceeding to surgical lysis and evacuation.

Prognosis

- Usually good, likely retained fertility.
- Risk for endometriosis in adolescents with retrograde menstrual flow.

MALE ACQUIRED GU ABNORMALITIES

Testicular Torsion

Absence of the posterior attachment to scrotum (*Bell-clapper deformity* [Fig. 25.16]) predisposes testes to torsion.

Presentation

- Severe acute testicular or abdominal pain.
- Vomiting.

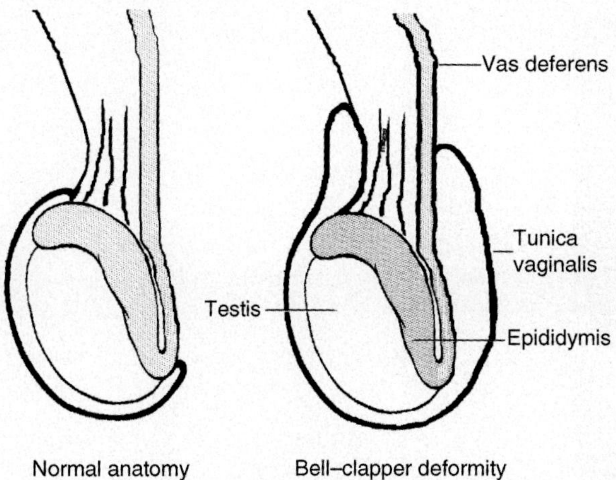

FIGURE 25.16. Bell-clapper deformity associated with testicular torsion. (*Reprinted with permission from* Siroky MB, Oates RD, Babayan RK. *Handbook of Urology: Diagnosis & Therapy*, 3rd ed. Lippincott Williams & Wilkins, 2004.)

- Loss of cremasteric reflex.
- High-riding testicle.
- Improvement of testicular pain with outward rotation of testicle.

Differential diagnosis includes testicular trauma, infection, torsion of the appendix testis, distal kidney stones, and appendicitis.

Diagnosis

- Gold standard is Doppler ultrasound.

Treatment

- Testicular torsion is a *surgical emergency*.
- Manual reduction can be attempted and is sometimes successful.
- Even if manually reduced, however, surgical intervention for evaluation and orchiopexy is required.
- Must also explore and likely repair other side since anatomic predisposition often bilateral.

Prognosis

- Good if addressed within hours.
- Delay in treatment with prolonged ischemia can result in testicular necrosis.

Testicular Appendiceal Torsion

Testicular appendiceal torsion is the torsion of one of several small testicular appendages.

Presentation

- Similar to that of testicular torsion except there is a normal cremasteric reflex and normal testicular position.
- Classic physical examination finding is the *blue dot sign* (from engorged hypoxic appendage (Fig. 25.17)).

Diagnosis

- US is needed to confirm the diagnosis and rule out testicular torsion.

Treatment

- NSAIDs.

Prognosis

- Pain usually resolves within 2 weeks.
- No long-term sequelae.

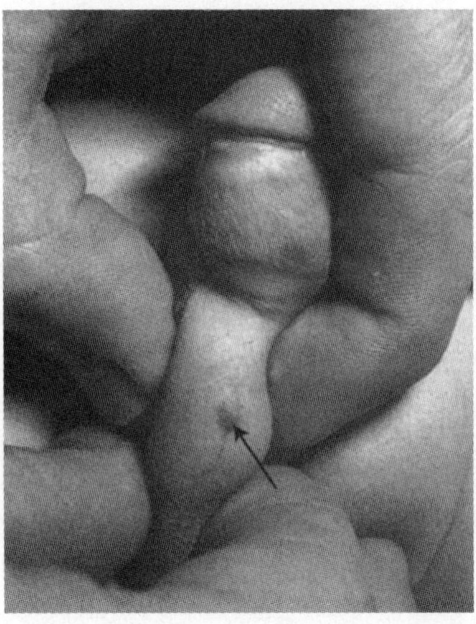

FIGURE 25.17. Blue dot sign for testicular appendiceal torsion. (*Reprinted with permission from* Graham SD, Keane TE. *Glenn's Urologic Surgery*, 7th ed. Philadelphia, Lippincott Williams & Wilkins, 2009.)

Pediatric Male Genitourinary Infections

Infection may occur in the seminal, urinary, or shared tracts and present with urinary pain, scrotal pain or swelling, or discharge. Table 25.17 summarizes the symptoms and methods of diagnosis and treatment of common male GU infections.

TABLE 25.17

PEDIATRIC MALE GU INFECTIONS

Infection	Sx	Dx	Tx
Epididymitis	Testicular pain, redness, and warmth. +/− Fever May present like testicular torsion in young males	UA: pyuria, bacteriuria, ↑ urinary WBCs make torsion unlikely US to r/o torsion. Usually caused by STDs in older kids, *E. coli* in prepubertal	Antibiotics, bed rest. US in prepubertal male for anomalies
Orchitis	Severe pain, fever, and swelling. Nausea, vomiting, abdominal pain common	Think mumps in postpubertal males, most commonly unilateral	Same
Urethritis	Pain with urination, discharge	Culture, PCR for gonorrhea and chlamydia in sexually active boys. Possibly viral. Consider trauma	Likely antibiotics

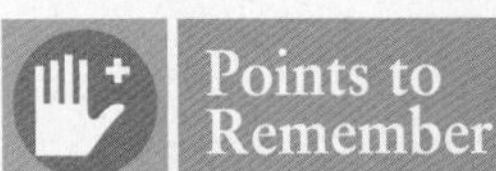

Points to Remember

- **Priapism is a serious condition involving persistent penile erection that may result in permanent damage from vascular stasis and ischemic injury. It is often associated with sickle cell disease, leukemia, spinal cord lesions, and phosphodiesterase inhibiting medications. Treatment involves systemic or local medical therapy with beta-agonists or alpha-blockers and may require surgical intervention to relieve pressure.**

Pediatric Scrotal and Testicular Masses

Intrascrotal masses in boys may be painful or painless, present at any age, and may be benign or serious in nature. Table 25.18 outlines symptoms and treatment in the most common masses.

FEMALE ACQUIRED ABNORMALITIES

Labial Adhesions

Labial adhesions can be congenital but more often result from inflammation.

Clinical Manifestations

- Usually asymptomatic.
- Usually noted on routine examination or because of parental concern.

Treatment

- Usually none since most are asymptomatic and resolve by adolescence.

TABLE 25.18

SCROTAL/TESTICULAR MASSES IN CHILDREN

Condition	Illuminates?	Examination	Etiology/Therapy/Prognosis
Hydrocele (Fig. 25.18)	Yes	Soft or firm, smooth	Patent processus vaginalis. Usually resolves by 1 year. If not, risk of hernia → operatively close processus. Good outcome
Spermatocele	Yes	Firm, attached to posterior testis	From epididymis, usually asymptomatic. No treatment unless pain due to size
Varicocele	No	*"Bag of worms,"* valsalva worsens *Usually left*	Because of left testicular vein or internal spermatic vein valves. Usually not noticeable until standing. Ligation of veins if pain or testicular change. Good outcome
Neoplasm	No	Hard, irregular, new	Various cancers, requires imaging, exploration, oncologic management
Hernia	No	May reduce, peristalsis	Requires operative repair, urgent if incarcerated

- Medical management with estrogen cream or surgical lysis are options for persistent or symptomatic adhesions.

Prognosis

- Excellent.

Ovarian Torsion

Ovarian torsion may often occur in children with normal anatomy, but there is an *increased risk with ovarian masses* or other adnexal abnormalities.

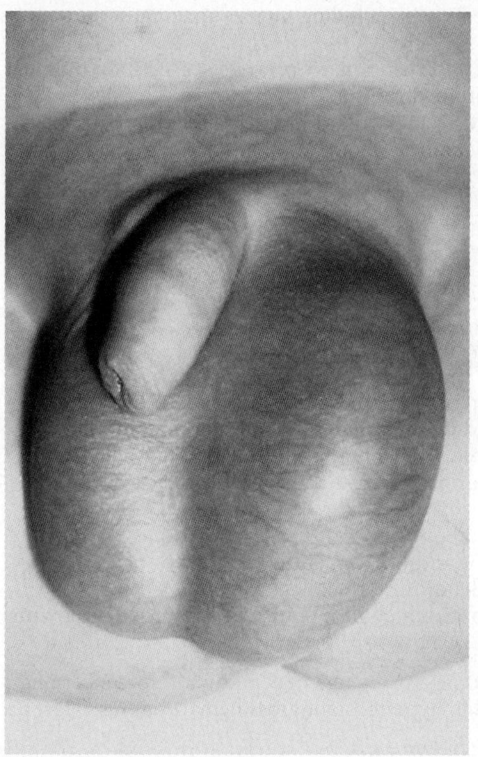

FIGURE 25.18. A large, tense hydrocele. (*Reprinted with permission from* McMillan JA, Feigin RD, DeAngelis C, et al. *Oski's Pediatrics: Principles and Practice*, 4th ed. Philadelphia: Lippincott Williams & Wilkins, 2006.)

Clinical Manifestations

- Acute onset of severe unilateral lower abdominal pain (can be colicky), vomiting.
- Adnexal mass may be palpable on pelvic examination.

Differential diagnosis includes appendicitis, nephrolithiasis, pyelonephritis, PID, ruptured ovarian cyst, and ectopic pregnancy.

Diagnosis

- US with Doppler to evaluate for ovarian edema and to assess blood flow.

Treatment

- Emergent operative detorsion.

Prognosis

- Excellent with early treatment.
- Delay leads to necrosis of ovary.

Ovarian Cyst

Ovarian cysts are very common, especially in adolescents. Most cysts are functional cysts (from follicle or corpus luteum), but benign and malignant neoplasms are occasionally seen.

Presentation

- With imaging for another reason, or with pain upon rupture.
- Follicular cyst rupture may coincide with ovulatory pain (mittelschmerz).

Differential diagnosis includes ovarian torsion, appendicitis, nephrolithiasis, PID, ectopic pregnancy, pancreatitis, neoplasms, endometriosis, and UTI.

Diagnosis

- Usually able to diagnose type of cyst with US.
- But may require CT or MRI to better assess tissue type.
- Chronicity of bleeding in the case of hemorrhagic cysts.

Treatment

- Simple, nonhemorrhagic cysts less than 10 cm in size—no therapy other than pain control.
- Complex cysts may prompt workup for neoplasm including further imaging, serum oncologic markers, and possible biopsy.
- Hemorrhagic cysts may require surgical intervention to prevent scarring or ongoing blood loss into the peritoneal or retroperitoneal cavities.
- OCPs help reduce the incidence of future cysts but do not affect the course of a preexisting cyst.

Prognosis

- Simple cysts usually do not impact health.
- Expect complete cyst resolution in 1 to 2 months.

SAMPLE BOARD REVIEW QUESTIONS

1. A 5-year-old male with an unremarkable past medical history presents to clinic with a 5-day history of increasing facial edema and frothy urine. His vital signs are normal, and his examination is otherwise unremarkable. You obtain studies showing high serum triglycerides, hypoalbuminemia, and high urine protein. The next step should be:
   a. Treat with oral glucocorticoids
   b. Obtain renal ultrasound
   c. Obtain ESR, CRP, ANA, ANCA, C3, and C4 to identify etiology of process
   d. Arrange for renal biopsy to obtain definitive tissue diagnosis
   e. Arrange follow-up visit in 1 week to watch clinical course before proceeding with further workup or treatment

   Answer: a. This child has nephrotic syndrome. At the age of 5 and with no concerning features on history or physical like headache, hypertension, gross hematuria, rash, fever, or joint pain, the diagnosis is most likely minimal change disease. The most appropriate course of action is to treat empirically with oral glucocorticoids and proceed with further workup or treatment only in the case of treatment failure.

2. A full-term girl by last menstrual period born to a mother with no prenatal care is born via spontaneous vaginal delivery. It is noticed that there is very little amniotic fluid. The infant is apneic and has a flattened face. Despite aggressive interventions including intubation and mechanical ventilation, she expires due to respiratory failure. What is the most likely primary cause of her condition?
   a. Congenital diaphragmatic hernia
   b. Bilateral renal agenesis
   c. Placental abruption
   d. Congenitally acquired infection
   e. Maternal drug use

   Answer: b. This neonate has Potter sequence secondary to oligohydramnios, resulting in flattened face and pulmonary hypoplasia. Bilateral renal agenesis is the only answer that explains the lack of amniotic fluid necessary to cause this cascade of symptoms.

3. A 5-year-old girl is brought to your clinic by her parents for anticipatory guidance about kidney disease that runs in the family. Her paternal grandmother requires dialysis and her father has been on medication for his kidneys for several years due to increasing blood pressure and findings on ultrasound. Further family history reveals that the girl's paternal aunt died suddenly last year, but the family refused an autopsy. What is the most likely potential cause of sudden death in this patient if she has the kidney disease that runs in her family?
   a. Arrhythmia from electrolyte disturbance
   b. Obstructive hypertrophic cardiomyopathy
   c. Overwhelming sepsis
   d. Pulmonary embolism
   e. Ruptured cerebral aneurysm

   Answer: e. This child most likely has autosomal dominant polycystic kidney disease. It is a relatively common disorder, with an incidence of approximately 1/250 people. It is associated with cerebral aneurysms in about 10% of patients, which tend to run in families and is possibly the cause of death of the girl's aunt.

4. You are taking care of an 18-year-old male admitted for initiation of dialysis due to end-stage renal disease. His past medical history is significant for gradually worsening renal function, hematuria, and sensorineural hearing loss. His parents are both well, with no known health problems, but his maternal uncle had a similar course and required renal transplantation at age 20. The patients' mother likely has:
   a. Hearing loss
   b. Asymptomatic microscopic hematuria
   c. A decreased glomerular filtration rate
   d. Cystic changes on renal ultrasound
   e. Joint hyperextensibility

   Answer: b. This family exhibits inheritance and symptoms characteristic of X-linked Alport's disease. Although autosomal forms exist, X-linked disease is the most common form and explains why the patient's mother is asymptomatic. Alport's disease is a defect in type 4 collagen that affects basement membranes. Most female carriers do not have any of the above signs or symptoms of disease but often have asymptomatic hematuria.

5. Concerned parents bring in their 8-year-old son for evaluation of marked polydipsia and polyuria over the past several weeks. His serum electrolytes are normal, including normal serum glucose. Urinalysis is negative for glucose, protein, and hemoglobin but does reveal a very low specific gravity. When admitted and not allowed to drink, he continues to produce copious amounts of dilute urine and loses weight. The most likely medication associated with this condition is:
   a. Methylphenidate
   b. Sertraline
   c. Levetiracetam
   d. Lithium
   e. Risperidone

   Answer: d. This child has diabetes insipidus (DI) as evidenced by his laboratory finding and the lack of hyperglycemia or psychogenic polydipsia. DI can be central due to lack of antidiuretic hormone (ADH) production or nephrogenic due to poor renal collecting system response to ADH. On the basis of the history alone, this child could have central or nephrogenic DI, but the medication notorious for causing nephrogenic DI is lithium.

6. You have admitted a 7-year-old boy for acute hypertension, headache, decreased renal function, hematuria, and proteinuria. His glomerular filtration rate at presentation is concerning but eventually recovers to baseline health without any management other than observation and careful fluid and electrolyte management. Serum studies are significant for low C3 and C4 and high antistreptolysin O titers. On the basis of his clinical picture, you make a likely diagnosis and reassure his parents. What finding would be most concerning for an alternative diagnosis at a clinic visit 3 months after hospitalization?
   a. Borderline hypertension
   b. Decreased C3 and C4
   c. Microscopic hematuria
   d. Microscopic proteinuria
   e. Normal energy

   Answer: b. This child had an episode of acute glomerulonephritis (GN). In his age group, as a male, and with a high ASO, his symptoms are most likely to be due to postinfectious GN from streptococcal infection. Hypertension is a feature in many but not all patients with this condition. Microscopic proteinuria and hematuria are expected up to a year after diagnosis. Borderline hypertension is nonspecific and could have existed prior to diagnosis. Normal energy is not concerning. Persistently low serum complement indicates ongoing immune complex deposition in the glomeruli, suspicious for IgA nephropathy, or other vasculitis.

7. A 15-year-old male comes to clinic for a routine visit after a lapse in medical care for several years. His blood pressure is greater than the 95th percentile for age and height. He does not complain of any symptoms of hypertension. His BMI is 38. The next step in the workup of his hypertension should be:
   a. Obtain at least two more blood pressure measurements over the next several weeks
   b. Obtain electrolytes and urinalysis
   c. Obtain hemoglobin A1 C and fasting glucose
   d. Obtain renal ultrasound and echocardiogram
   e. Obtain fasting lipid panel

   Answer: a. To make a diagnosis of hypertension in this child, he needs to have 3 separate measurements that are over the 95th percentile. All of the other options are likely to be necessary in his workup eventually given that he likely has essential hypertension and possible metabolic syndrome.

8. You are taking care of a 12-day-old male who was born at 28 weeks gestational age and is being managed in the neonatal intensive care unit. He is not on any medications and is receiving a combination of enteral feeds and parenteral nutrition. Despite excellent respiratory status and an unremarkable clinical course, his serum pH is persistently low at 7.25 to 7.30. Which of the following is correct about the most likely disease in this child?
   a. Will result in a urine pH above 7
   b. Will result in decreased urine citrate
   c. Will result in hyperkalemia
   d. Will improve with time
   e. Will require mineralocorticoid supplementation

   Answer: d. Type 2 renal tubular acidosis (RTA) is very common in premature neonates and is characterized by the dumping of bicarbonate from the proximal tubules. The distal nephrons function better and are still able to acidify urine to some extent; thus, urine is usually acidic, unlike the more severe distal defect in type 1 RTA. Type 2 RTA associated with prematurity usually resolves with time. It can be treated with bicarbonate supplementation. Type 4 RTA may respond to mineralocorticoid supplementation.

9. Concerned parents bring in their 8-year-old boy with a chief complaint of ongoing bedwetting. They state that he has never been consistently dry and that this problem is now getting embarrassing for him and inconvenient for them. His father also wet the bed during childhood, with spontaneous resolution at age 12. The boy is otherwise well, has no significant past medical history, is growing normally, does not have any difficulty with daytime continence, and has no urinary symptoms. His vital signs and examination are normal. You tell his parents that the intervention most likely to succeed in helping him achieve night-time continence is:
   a. Eliminate caffeine from his diet
   b. Prohibit fluids prior to bed time

c. Insist that he urinates immediately before going to bed
d. Prescribe a bed-wetting alarm
e. Have him see a psychologist to work through likely underlying issues

Answer: d. This child has a classic case of primary nocturnal enuresis defined by nighttime incontinence after 6 years of age with no preceding period of dryness or less than 6 months dryness at a time. The positive family history is typical. There are no red flags for other diagnoses in this case. Bed-wetting alarm is by far the most effective intervention for this child. Options A, B, and C may also be helpful but are not nearly as effective. There is nothing in the history that indicates the child needs to see a psychologist.

10. Parents ask you about the prognosis of their 9-month-old girl recently diagnosed with cystinosis. They have heard that children with her syndrome require special interventions regarding kidney health and ask you what to expect:
a. Kidney transplant is likely to be necessary but is temporizing since cystine will reaccumulate in the new kidney
b. She should be started on vitamin D
c. Kidney problems will likely occur much later in life and they should focus on other organs now
d. Hey kidneys will not be affected by the disease
e. Her kidney damage will result in high serum cystine that will damage her other organs

Answer: b. Cystinosis affects multiple organ systems including the kidneys with symptomatic Fanconi syndrome with electrolyte disturbances and progression to ESRD in childhood. The disease does not recur in transplanted kidneys because the defect involves intracellular storage of cystine, not elevated blood levels. Like most children with kidney dysfunction, she should be treated with vitamin D to increase calcium absorption and to prevent renal osteodystrophy from calcium wasting with secondary hyperparathyroidism.

11. Parents bring their 2-week-old son in for a routine visit. He has been feeding, growing, and sleeping well, but they have noticed some clear fluid coming out of his umbilicus. On examination, you are able to detect an open tract in his umbilicus and notice that his abdomen is abnormally soft, even when he is crying. He also seems to have easily palpable bilateral flank masses and you cannot palpate his testes. What is the most likely diagnosis?
a. Posterior urethral valve
b. Multicystic dysplastic kidneys
c. Congenital nephrotic syndrome
d. Prune–Belly syndrome
e. Throckmorton syndrome

Answer: d. The above description is classic for Prune–Belly syndrome with poor abdominal musculature, hydronephrosis from severe vesicoureteral reflux or partial obstruction, patent urachus, and intra-abdominal testes. Posterior urethral valve and multicystic dysplastic kidneys are not associated with patent urachus, undescended testes, or abdominal wall changes. Congenital nephrotic syndrome would not present with any of the above symptoms.

12. An 8-year-old male presents to the emergency department with a chief complaint of vomiting and sudden onset extreme unilateral scrotal/testicular pain. Which of the following is true about the possible diagnosis that would require the most urgent action to prevent serious morbidity?
a. He will have an exaggerated cremasteric reflex
b. The scrotum may be transilluminated with a light
c. The diagnostic study of choice is scrotal/testicular ultrasound
d. Observing the "blue dot" portends a worse outcome
e. The painful side will have a low-riding testicle

Answer: c. The most urgently important diagnosis to make in this child is testicular torsion since it must be corrected quickly to avoid testicular necrosis. The diagnostic test of choice is a scrotal ultrasound looking at blood flow to the testis. The testis may be able to be manually reduced with external rotation in the "open book" maneuver, but this is often unsuccessful and emergent surgical correction is likely to be required. Even if manual reduction is successful, surgery is needed to secure the testis and explore the contralateral scrotum for a similar defect in anchoring. The cremasteric reflex is often absent in patients with testicular torsion, and the torsed testis is usually high riding. The blue dot sign would be reassuring since it is a sign of a torsed testicular appendage rather than testicular torsion.

13. When examining a 14-year-old boy, you notice a unilateral scrotal mass. The patient says he notices it the most in the shower and thinks he noticed it within the last year. He does not have any abnormal urethral discharge, dysuria, or systemic symptoms. It is mildly uncomfortable with palpation but is not significantly painful and is otherwise asymptomatic. It does not transilluminate, becomes much smaller when supine, and feels wormy. You suspect that the source of the mass is:

a. Dilated veins in the scrotum
b. A collection of sperm in the epididymis
c. Malignant cells spilling out of the testicular capsule
d. Defect in the processus vaginalis leading to accumulation of fluid in the scrotum
e. Bowel that is herniated into the scrotum

Answer: a. This child has a classic case of varicocele, consisting of dilated tortuous veins in the scrotum. The condition is thought to be due to defective valves or increased pressure on the left testicular vein. The other choices describe spermatocele (B), malignancy (C), hydrocele (D), and hernia (E).

14. A 16-year-old girl is admitted to your service for observation because of abdominal pain. She reports that she has had this type of pain on numerous other occasions over the past year, that the pain lasts for a few days, and that it is getting worse every time. She has never had a fever with these symptoms. She denies any sexual activity and has not yet reached menarche. On examination, she has a diffusely tender, distended abdomen, and has Tanner 5 sexual features. She is afebrile and has a normal white blood cell count and C-reactive protein. Pancreatic and hepatic inflammatory markers are also normal. One serious complication from her most likely diagnosis is:

a. Premature ovarian failure
b. Ovarian torsion
c. Endometriosis
d. Anemia
e. Pelvic inflammatory disease

Answer: c. The keys to this question are that this girl has no sign of infection, has worsening periodic abdominal pain, exhibits Tanner 5 sexual maturity, and has not yet menstruated. Her diagnosis is most likely hematocolpos secondary to an imperforate hymen. Backup of blood flow in the GU tract with increased pressure may result in retrograde flow through the fallopian tubes, resulting in abdominal endometriosis. She is not likely to be more anemic than if she had been having her periods and losing blood normally. She denies sexual activity and is afebrile, making PID less likely. There is also nothing to suggest ovarian torsion or ovarian failure.

15. A 15-year-old girl presents to the emergency department due to acute onset left-sided abdominal pain without fever or vomiting. Routine laboratories including CBC and UA are unremarkable, and she does not have clinical signs of appendicitis on physical examination. Aside from tenderness to palpation on the left side of her abdomen, she does not have any other physical findings. She has Tanner 4 secondary sexual development and reached menarche 2 years ago. She denies sexual activity and has not had any vaginal symptoms. Her periods are regular and her last period started 2 weeks ago. Pelvic and transvaginal ultrasound do not show any abnormalities. After thorough workup, her pain improves significantly without medication or other intervention. What is true about her most likely diagnosis?

a. She requires urgent operative intervention to save her ovary from becoming necrotic
b. Her symptoms are most likely to risky sexual behavior
c. She will also likely develop acne, acanthosis nigricans, and hirsutism
d. This pain is likely to recur but is not harmful to internal organs or fertility
e. The diagnosis would have been made on CT

Answer: d. This patient presents with classic mittelschmerz, or pain associated with ovulation, which is indeed likely to recur at some point. The quick spontaneous resolution, unilateral nature, timing, negative sexual history, and normal ultrasound all point to this diagnosis. There are no indications that she has ovarian torsion or polycystic ovarian syndrome. A ruptured ovarian cyst could cause unilateral pain but does not usually resolve so quickly and ultrasound usually shows cysts, follicles, or free fluid on ultrasound.

SUGGESTED READINGS

Chan J, Williams D, Roth K. Kidney Failure in Infants and Children. *Pediatr Rev.* 2002;23;47.
Roth K, Amaker B, Chan J. Nephrotic Syndrome: pathogenesis and management. *Pediatr Rev.* 2002;23;237.
McMillan J, et al. Diseases of the genitourinary system. *Oski's Pediatrics*, 4th ed. 2006:1818–1914.

INDEX

Note: Pages followed by f and t indicate figure and table, respectively.